# CLINICAL GENOMICS

*Practical Applications in*
*Adult Patient Care*

# CLINICAL GENOMICS

*Practical Applications in Adult Patient Care*

*Editors*

**Michael F. Murray MD**
Director of Clinical Genomics
Genomic Medicine Institute
Geisinger Health System
Danville, PA

**Mark W. Babyatsky MD**
Adjunct Professor
Department of Medicine
Columbia University Medical Center
New York, NY

**Monica A. Giovanni MS, CGC**
Director of Clinical Genomic Strategy
Genomic Medicine Institute
Geisinger Health System
Danville, PA

*Associate Editors*

**Fowzan S. Alkuraya MD**
Professor of Human Genetics
Department of Genetics
King Faisal Specialist Hospital and Research Center
Riyadh, Saudi Arabia

**Douglas R. Stewart MD**
Investigator, Clinical Genetics Branch
Division of Cancer Epidemiology and Genetics
National Cancer Institute
Rockville, MD

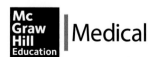

New York  Chicago  San Francisco  Athens  London  Madrid
Mexico City  Milan  New Delhi  Singapore  Sydney  Toronto

ISBN 978-0-07-162244-8
MHID 0-07-162244-6

This book was set in Times LT Std by Cenveo® Publisher Services.
The editors were James Shanahan and Regina Y. Brown.
The production supervisor was Catherine H. Saggese.
Production management was provided by Sapna Rastogi, Cenveo Publisher Services.
RR Donnelley was printer and binder.

This book is printed on acid-free paper.

Catalog-in Publication Data is on file for this title at the Library of Congress.

*To the many patients and those who care for them worldwide whose participation in genetic and genomic research have allowed this knowledge to accumulate.*

# CONTENTS

# CONTRIBUTORS

**Noura S. Abul-Husn, MD, PhD**
Resident, Internal Medicine-Medical Genetics
Departments of Medicine and Genetics and Genomic Medicine
Mount Sinai School of Medicine
New York, NY

**Tariq Ahmad, MD**
Cardiology Fellow
Department of Medicine
Duke University School of Medicine
Durham, NC

**Haya Al-Saud, MSc**
Department of Genomics of Common Diseases
School Of Public Health, Imperial College London
London, UK

**Fowzan S. Alkuraya, MD**
Professor of Human Genetics
Department of Genetics
King Faisal Specialist Hospital and Research Center
Riyadh, Saudi Arabia

**Abdulrahman Alsultan, MD, FAAP**
Assistant Professor
Department of Pediatrics, King Khalid University Hospital and
   College of Medicine
King Saud University
Riyadh, Saudi Arabia

**Raymond M. Anchan, MD, PhD**
Assistant Professor
Dept of Obstetrics, Gynecology and Reproductive Biology
Brigham and Women's Hospital and Harvard Medical School
Boston, MA

**Justin P. Annes, MD, PhD**
Assistant Professor
Division of Endocrinology
Stanford University Medical Center
Stanford, CA

**Mohammed T. Ansari, MBBS, MMedSc, MPhil.**
Associate Investigator
Clinical Epidemiology Program,
Ottawa Hospital Research Institute
Ottawa, Canada

**Ines Armando, PhD**
Associate Professor
Division of Nephrology, Department of Medicine
University of Maryland School of Medicine
Baltimore, MD

**Matthew J. Armstrong, MBChB, BSc, MRCP**
Wellcome Trust Clinical Research Fellow, Honorary SpR in
   Hepatology
Centre of Liver Research
University of Birmingham
Birmingham, UK

**Mark W. Babyatsky, MD**
Adjunct Professor
Department of Medicine
Columbia University Medical Center
New York, NY

**Alice Bailey, BA**
Clinic Coordinator
The "22q and You" Center
The Children's Hospital of Philadelphia
Philadelphia, PA

**Ravikumar Balasubramanian, MD, PhD, MRCP**
Instructor in Medicine
Harvard Reproductive Endocrine Sciences Center
Massachusetts General Hospital and Harvard Medical School
Boston, MA

**Manisha Balwani, MD, MS**
Assistant Professor
Genetics and Genomic Medicine
Mount Sinai School of Medicine
New York, NY

**Adi Bar-Lev, MD**
Fellow
Department of Medicine
Brigham and Women's Hospital
Boston, MA

**Carl Barnes, MD**
Associate Professor
Department of Medicine
Veterans Hospital
Denver, CO

**Merrill D. Benson, MD**
Professor Pathology and Laboratory Medicine, Medicine and
   Medical and Molecular Genetics
Department of Pathology & Laboratory Medicine
Indiana University School of Medicine
Indianapolis, IN

**Mitchel S. Berger, MD, FACS, FAANS**
Kathleen M. Plant Distinguished Professor, Chairman,
   Department of Neurological Surgery,
   Director, Brain Tumor Surgery Program and
   Director, Neurosurgical Research Centers,
   Brain Tumor Research Center
Department of Neurological Surgery
University of California San Francisco
San Francisco, CA

**Kailash P. Bhatia, MD, DM, FRCP**
Professor
Institute of Neurology
University College London
London, UK

**Frederick R. Bieber, MD**
Associate Professor
Department of Pathology
Brigham and Women's Hospital
Boston, MA

**Joann Bodurtha, MD, MPH**
Professor of Pediatrics and Oncology
McKusick-Nathans Institute of Genetic Medicine
Johns Hopkins University
Baltimore, MD

**Carolyn Bondy, MD**
Scientist Emeritus
Program in Developmental Endocrinology and Genetics
NICHD, NIH
Clinical Center,
Bethesda, MD

**Philip M. Boone, PhD**
MD/PhD Student
Department of Molecular and Human Genetics
Baylor College of Medicine
Houston, TX

**Ronald A. Booth, PhD**
Assistant Professor
Department of Pathology and Laboratory Medicine
The Ottawa Hospital
Ottawa, Canada

**Erwin Bottinger, MD**
Professor
Department of Medicine
Mount Sinai School of Medicine
New York, NY

**Riley Bove, MD**
Instructor in Neurology
Department of Neurology
Brigham and Women's Hospital
Boston, MA

**Esteban Braggio, PhD**
Assistant Professor
Department of Medicine
Mayo Clinic Scottsdale
Scottsdale, AZ

**Rebecca Breslow, MD**
Instructor
Division of Rheumatology, Immunology and Allergy, Department of Medicine
Brigham and Women's Hospital and Harvard Medical School
Boston, MA

**Scott E. Brodie, MD, PhD**
Professor
Department of Ophthalmology
Mount Sinai School of Medicine
New York, NY

**Lawrence C. Brody, PhD**
Senior Investigator and Chief, Genome Technology Branch
National Human Genome Research Institute
National Institutes of Health
Bethesda, MD

**David G. Brooks, MD, PhD**
Medical Head
Translational Development
Tesaro, Inc.
Waltham, MA

**Matthew Brown, MBBS, MD, FRACP, FAA**
Director, University of Queensland Diamantina Institute
Human Genetics Group
University of Queensland
Brisbane, Queensland, Australia

**Sara J. Brown, MRCP**
Wellcome Trust Intermediate Clinical Fellow,
Clinical Senior Lecturer & Hon Consultant Dermatologist,
   Division of Molecular Medicine
University of Dundee
Dundee, UK

**Ramon Brugada, MD, PhD, FACC, FESC**
Director Cardiovascular Genetics Center, Dean School Of
   Medicine
Cardiovascular Genetics Center, Department Of Medicine
School Of Medicine, University Of Girona-Idibgi
Girona, Spain

**Merlin G. Butler, MD, PhD**
Director, Division of Research
Professor of Psychiatry, Behavioral Sciences and Pediatrics,
   Department of Psychiatry & Behavioral Sciences and Pediatrics
Kansas University Medical Center
Kansas City, KS

**Rodrigo Calado, MD, PhD**
Assistant Professor
Department of Medicine
Center for Cell-Based Therapy
Sao Paulo, Brazil

**Susanna Campion, PhD**
Senior Research Scientist
Malaria Programme
Welcome Trust Sanger Institute (WTSI)
Hinxton, Cambridge, United Kingdom

**Oscar Campuzano Larrea, BSc, PhD**
Post-Doc Investigator
Cardiovascular Genetics Center, Department Of Medicine
School Of Medicine, University Of Girona-Idibgi
Girona, Spain

**Antonio Cao, MD**
Professor
Institute of Neurogenetics and Neuropharmacology
Consiglio Nazionale delle Ricerche
Cagliari, Italy

**Juan C. Cardet, MD**
Clinical Research Fellow in Medicine
Division of Rheumatology, Immunology and Allergy,
Department of Medicine
Brigham and Women's Hospital
Boston, MA

**David J. Carey, PhD**
Associate Chief Research Officer
The Sigfried and Janet Weis Center for Research
Geisinger Health System
Danville, PA

**Varun Chawla, MD, MPH**
Nephrologist
Chabot Nephrology Medical Group
Fremont, CA

**Sruti Chandrasekaran, MBBS**
Fellow
Department of Medicine
University of Maryland School of Medicine
Baltimore, MD

**Charissa Y. Chang, MD**
Assistant Professor
Department of Medicine
Mount Sinai School of Medicine
New York, NY

**Benjamin K. Chen, MD, PhD**
Associate Professor
Department of Medicine
Mount Sinai School of Medicine
New York, NY

**Daniel C. Chung, MD**
Clinical Chief, Gastrointestinal Unit
Director, GI Cancer Genetics Program
Department of Medicine
Massachusetts General Hospital
Boston, MA

**Janice Y. Chyou, MD**
Cardiology Fellow
Department of Medicine
New York University Langone Medical Center
New York, NY

**Lee C. Claridge, BM, BS (Hons), MRCP (UK)**
Consultant Hepatologist
Liver Unit
St James's University Hospital
Leeds, UK

**Deirdre Cocks Eschler, MD**
Fellow
Department of Medicine
Mount Sinai School of Medicine
New York, NY

**Elizabeth A. Comen, MD**
Attending Physician
Department of Medicine
Memorial Sloan-Kettering Cancer Center
New York, NY

**Christopher D. T. Corbett, MBBS, MRCP**
Hepatology Registrar
Liver Unit
Queen Elizabeth Hospital
Birmingham, UK

**Ingrid Cristian, MD**
Assistant Professor of Pediatrics
Department of Pediatrics
Nemours Children's Hospital
Orlando, FL

**Carlo M. Croce, MD**
Professor and Chair
Department of Molecular Virology, Immunology, and Medical
    Genetics
Ohio State University
Columbus, OH

**William F. Crowley, Jr., MD**
Daniel K. Podolsky Professor of Translational Medicine, Director,
    Harvard Reproductive Endocrine Sciences Center
Department of Medicine
Massachusetts General Hospital
Boston, MA

**Benjamin S. Daniel, MBBS**
Associate Faculty
Department of Dermatology
St George Hospital, University of New South Wales
Sydney, Australia

**Philip L. De Jager, MD, PhD**
Associate Professor of Neurology
Department of Neurology
Brigham and Women's Hospital
Boston, MA

**Yun Deng, MD**
Postdoctoral Research Fellow
Department of Medicine
David Geffen School of Medicine, University of California,
Los Angeles
Los Angeles, CA

**Joshua C. Denny, MD, MS**
Associate Professor
Departments of Biomedical Informatics and Medicine
Vanderbilt University
Nashville, TN

**Robert J. Desnick, MD**
Dean and Chairman Emeritus
Genetics and Genomic Sciences
Mount Sinai School of Medicine
New York, NY

**Kristine Dickinson**
Genetics Assistant The "22q and You" Center
The Children's Hospital of Philadelphia
Philadelphia, PA

**Harold C. Dietz, MD**
Victor A. McKusick Professor of Genetics and Medicine
McKusick-Nathans Institute of Genetic Medicine
Johns Hopkins University
Baltimore, MD

**Jill S. Dolinsky, RN, MS, CGC**
Genetic Counselor
Clinical Genetics
Ambry Genetics
Aliso Viejo, CA

**Fatima Donia Mili, MD, PhD**
Senior Service Fellow
Division of Blood Disorders
The Centers for Disease Control and Prevention
Atlanta, GA

**Rajkumar Dorajoo, PhD**
Department of Genomics of Common Diseases
School Of Public Health, Imperial College London
London, UK

**Henry L. Dorkin, MD**
Associate Professor
Department of Pediatrics
Boston Children's Hospital
Boston, MA

**Stephanie Dukhovny, MD**
Clinical Fellow
Department of Obstetrics, Gynecology, and Reproductive Biology
Brigham and Women's Hospital
Boston, MA

**Lisa Edelmann, PhD**
Associate Professor
Genetics and Genomic Medicine
Mount Sinai School of Medicine
New York, NY

**Stacey Eggert, PhD**
Genetics Fellow
Departments of Obstetrics, Gynecology and Reproductive Biology and Pathology
Brigham and Women's Hospital
Boston, MA

**Francesca M. Elli**
Endocrinology Unit, Department of Medical Sciences
Università degli Studi di Milano
Milan, Italy

**Charis Eng, MD, PhD, FACP**
Hardis/ACS Professor and Chair
Genomic Medicine Institute
Cleveland Clinic
Cleveland, OH

**W. Andrew Faucett, MS, CGC**
Director of Policy and Education
Office of the Chief Scientific Officer
Geisinger Health System
Danville, PA

**Faisal Fecto, MD, PhD**
Postdoctoral Fellow
Department of Neurology and Clinical Neurosciences
Northwestern University Feinberg School of Medicine
Chicago, IL

**W. Gregory Feero, MD, PhD**
Faculty
Maine-Dartmouth Family Medicine Residency
Augusta, ME

**James M. Fernandez, MD, PhD**
Staff Physician
Department of Allergy & Immunology
Cleveland Clinic Foundation
Cleveland, OH USA

**John K. Fink, MD**
Professor
Department of Neurology
University of Michigan; and Geriatric Research, Education, and Clinical Center, Ann Arbor Veterans Affairs Medical Center
Ann Arbor, MI, USA

**Edward A. Fisher, MD, PhD, MPH**
Leon H. Charney Professor of Cardiovascular Medicine
Departments of Medicine, Pediatrics and Cell Biology
New York University Langone Medical Center
New York, NY

**Rebecca C. Fitzgerald, PhD**
Professor and MRC Programme Leader
MRC Cancer Cell Unit
Hutchinson/MRC Research Centre
University of Cambridge
Cambridge, United Kingdom

**Rafael Fonseca, MD**
Co-director, Hematologic Malignancies Program, Deputy Director, Mayo Clinic Cancer Center
Department of Medicine
Mayo Clinic Scottsdale
Scottsdale, AZ

**David N. Franz, MD**
Director, Tuberous Sclerosis Clinic
Department of Pediatrics
Cincinnati Children's Hospital Medical Center
Cincinnati, OH

**Scott Friedman, MD**
Professor
Department of Medicine
Mount Sinai School of Medicine
New York, NY

**Christopher A. Friedrich, MD, PhD**
Associate Professor
Division of Medical Genetics
University of Mississippi Medical Center
Jackson, MS

**Charlotte Frise, MA, MRCP**
Specialist Registrar
Obstetric & General Medicine
Oxford University Hospitals NHS Trust
Oxford, UK

**Phillippe Froguel, MD, PhD**
Professor of Genomic Medicine, Head of the Department of
    Genomics of Common Diseases
Department of Genomics of Common Diseases
School Of Public Health, Imperial College
London, UK

**Terry Fry, MD**
Head, Blood and Marrow Transplant Section
Pediatric Oncology Branch
National Cancer Institute
Bethesda, MD

**Michele Gabree, MS, CGC**
Genetic Counselor
Center for Cancer Risk Assessment
Massachusetts General Hospital
Boston, MA

**Manish Gala, MD**
Clinical and Research Fellow in Gastroenterology
Department of Medicine
Massachusetts General Hospital
Boston, MA

**Renzo Galanello, MD**
Professor
Department of Public Health and Clinical and Molecular
    Medicine
University of Cagliari
Cagliari, Italy

**Judy E. Garber, MD, MPH**
Professor of Medicine
Center for Cancer Genetics and Prevention
Dana Farber Cancer Institute
Boston, MA

**Bruce D. Gelb, MD**
Professor
Pediatrics, and Genetics and Genomic Sciences
Mount Sinai School of Medicine
New York, NY

**Behzad Gerami-Naini, PhD**
Assistant Professor
Department of Oral and Maxillofacial Pathology, Oral Medicine
    and Craniofacial Pain
Tufts University, School of Dental Medicine
Boston, MA

**Neera Ghaziuddin, MD, MRCP**
Associate Professor of Psychiatry
Department of Psychiatry
University of Michigan
Ann Arbor, MI

**Monica A. Giovanni, MS, CGC**
Director of Clinical Genomic Strategy
Genomic Medicine Institute
Geisinger Health System
Danville, PA

**Mark Goodarzi, MD, PhD**
Associate Professor of Medicine
Division Director, Division of Endocrinology, Diabetes and
    Metabolism
Cedars-Sinai Medical Center
Los Angeles, CA

**Omri Gottesman, MD**
Assistant Professor
Department of Medicine
Mount Sinai School of Medicine
New York, NY

**Evgenia Gourgari, MD**
Pediatric Endocrinology Fellow
Section on Endocrinology and Genetics, Program on
    Developmental Endocrinology & Genetics (PDEGEN)
National Institutes of Health
Bethesda, MD

**Sylvie Grandemange, PhD**
Engineer
Laboratoire de génétique des maladies rares et auto-
    inflammatoires
Montpellier, France

**Robert C. Green, MD, MPH**
Associate Professor of Medicine
Division of Genetics, Department of Medicine
Brigham and Women's Hospital and Harvard Medical School
Boston, MA

**Mark H. Greene, MD**
Chief, Clinical Genetics Branch
Division of Cancer Epidemiology and Genetics
National Cancer Institute
Rockville, MD

**Elizabeth G. Grubbs, MD**
Assistant Professor
Department of Surgical Oncology
University of Texas M.D. Anderson Cancer Center
Houston, TX

**Dong-Chuan Guo, PhD**
Assistant Professor
Department of Internal Medicine
The University of Texas Medical School at Houston
Houston, TX

**Richard J. H. Smith, MD**
Professor
Department of Otolaryngology-Head and Neck Surgery
University of Iowa
Iowa City, IA

**Karen Hanson, MS, MBA**
Medical Science Liaison
Sequenom, Inc.
San Diego, CA

**John Hardy, PhD**
Professor
Reta Lila Weston Institute
University College London
London, United Kingdom

**Chellamani Harini, MD**
Instructor in Neurology
Division of Epilepsy and Clinical Neurophysiology
Boston Children's Hospital
Boston, MA

**Heather L. Harrell, MD, JD**
Research Associate
Institute for Bioethics, Health Policy, and Law
University of Louisville School of Medicine
Louisville, KY

**David J. Harris, MD**
Lecturer on Pediatrics
Division of Genetics and Metabolism
Boston Children's Hospital
Boston, MA

**Vijay Hegde, MD**
Postdoctoral Fellow
Department of Pathology
Brigham and Women's Hospital
Boston, MA

**Robert A. Hegele, MD**
Distinguished University Professor
Department of Medicine and Robarts Research Institute
University of Western Ontario
London, ON, Canada

**Rebecca S. Heist, MD, MPH**
Assistant Professor
MGH Cancer Center
Massachusetts General Hospital, Harvard Medical School
Boston, MA

**J. Fielding Hejtmancik, MD, PhD**
Senior Investigator
Ophthalmic Genetic and Visual Function Branch, National Eye
    Institute
National Institutes of Health
Bethesda, MD

**Amy L. Hernandez, MS, CGC**
Director of Genetic Counseling
Laboratory for Molecular Medicine
Partners Center for Personalized Genetic Medicine
Boston, MA

**Ray E. Hershberger, MD**
Professor of Medicine and Director, Division of Human Genetics
Department of Internal Medicine
Wexner Medical Center at The Ohio State University
Columbus, OH

**Michael Heuser, MD**
Attending Physician
Department of Hematology, Hemostasis, Oncology, and Stem Cell
    Transplantation
Hannover Medical School
Hannover, Germany

**Michael S. Hildebrand, PhD**
Fellow
Department of Otolaryngology-Head and Neck Surgery
University of Iowa
Iowa City, IA

**Grant Hill-Cawthorne, MA, MB, Bchir, MRCP**
PhD Student
Pathogen Genomics Laboratory, Biological and Environmental
    Sciences and Engineering
King Abdullah University of Science and Technology
Thuwal, Mekkah, Kingdom of Saudi Arabia

**Irene Hinterseher, MD, PhD**
Senior Physician
Fachärztin für Chirurgie und Gefäßchirurgie
Charité Universitätsmedizin Berlin
Berlin, Germany

**Kurt Hirschhorn, MD, PhD**
Medicine Chairman of Pediatrics Emeritus; Professor
Pediatrics and Genetics and Genomic Sciences
Mount Sinai School of Medicine
New York, NY

**Carolyn Y. Ho, MD**
Medical Director, Cardiovascular Genetics Center
Department of Medicine
Brigham and Women's Hospital
Boston, MA

**Erin P. Hoffman, MS, CGC**
Genetic Counselor
Department of Medicine
Brigham and Women's Hospital
Boston, MA

**Mark Hoffman, PhD**
Associate Professor of Pediatrics and Biomedical and Health
    Informatics
School of Computing and Engineering
University of Missouri-Kansas City
Kansas City, MO

**Ronald Hoffman, MD**
Professor
Department of Medicine
Mount Sinai School of Medicine
New York, NY

**W. Craig Hooper, PhD**
Division of Blood Disorders
The Centers for Disease Control and Prevention
Atlanta, GA

**Julie E. Hoover-Fong, MD, PhD**
Assistant Professor
Department of Pediatrics
Mount Sinai School of Medicine
New York, NY

**Mimi I. Hu, MD**
Assistant Professor
Dept. of Endocrine Neoplasia & Hormonal Disorders
University of Texas M.D. Anderson Cancer Center
Houston, TX

**Jennifer Huang, MD**
Instructor
Dermatology Program
Boston Children's Hospital
Boston, MA

**Peter Hulick, MD, MMSc**
Head, Division of Medical Genetics
Department of Medicine
NorthShore University HealthSystem
Evanston, IL

**Rachel J. Hundley, PhD**
Assistant Professor of Pediatrics
Developmental Medicine
Monroe Carell Jr. Children's Hospital at Vanderbilt
Nashville, TN

**Shirish Huprikar, MD**
Professor
Department of Medicine
Mount Sinai School of Medicine
New York, NY

**Michael Iannuzzi, MD, MBA**
Edward C. Reifenstein Professor and Chair
Department of Medicine
SUNY Upstate Medical University
Syracuse, NY

**Maria V. Irazabal, MD**
Research Fellow
Translational Polycystic Kidney Disease Center
Mayo Clinic
Rochester, MN

**David J. Irwin, MD**
Fellow
Departments of Neurology, Pathology, and Laboratory Medicine
Perelman School of Medicine at the University of Pennsylvania
Philadelphia, PA

**Seema Jamal, MS, CGC**
Genetic Counselor
Department of Pediatrics, Division of Genetic Medicine
University of Washington
Seattle, WA, USA

**Saumya S. Jamuar, MBBS, MRCPCH**
Fellow
Division of Genetics and Metabolism
Boston Children's Hospital
Boston, MA

**Nicholas E. Johnson, MD**
Experimental Therapeutics Fellow
Department of Neurology
The University of Rochester
Rochester, NY

**Lynn B. Jorde, PhD**
H.A. and Edna Benning Presidential Professor and Chair
Department of Human Genetics
University of Utah School of Medicine
Salt Lake City, UT

**Pedro A. Jose, MD, PhD**
Professor
Department of Medicine
University of Maryland School of Medicine
Baltimore, MD

**Tisha R. Joy, MD**
Assistant Professor
Department of Medicine
University of Western Ontario
London, ON, Canada

**Joseph Kannry, MD**
Associate Professor Director, EMR Clinical Transformation
   Group
Department of Medicine
Icahn School of Medicine at Mount Sinai
New York, NY

**Sunil Kapur, MD**
Cardiology Fellow
Department of Medicine
Brigham and Women's Hospital
Boston, MA

**Amel Karaa, MD**
Instructor
Departments of Genetics and Neurology
Massachusetts General Hospital
Boston, MA

**Brian D. Kent, MB**
Respiratory and Sleep Physician
Department of Respiratory Medicine
Guy's and St. Thomas' Hospitals
London, United Kingdom

**Aline Ketefian, MD**
Fellow
Division of Reproductive Endocrinology and Infertility
Cedars-Sinai Medical Center
Los Angeles, CA

**Ahmed Khattab, MD**
Fellow
Department of Pediatrics
Mount Sinai School of Medicine
New York, NY

**Brian Kirmse, MD**
Assistant Professor
Department of Genetics and Metabolism
Children's National Medical Center
Washington, DC

**Daniel Kiss, MD**
Medical Resident
Department of Internal Medicine
Hospital of the University of Pennsylvania
Philadelphia, PA

**Christian A. Koch, MD, PhD**
Professor of Medicine
Department of Medicine/Endocrinology
University of Mississippi Medical Center
Jackson, MS

**Isabella Kone-Paut, MD**
Professor of Pediatrics
Service de pédiatrie générale et rhumatologie pédiatrique
APHP, CHU de Bicêtre, Université de Paris Sud
Le Kremlin-Bicêtre, France

**Christian Kratz, MD**
Professor and Department Head
Pediatric Hematology and Oncology
Hannover Medical School
Hannover, Germany

**Marcin Krawczyk, Dr. med.**
Department of Internal Medicine II
Saarland University Medical Center
Homburg, Germany

**Darcy A. Krueger, MD, PhD**
Assistant Professor
Department of Pediatrics
Cincinnati Children's Hospital Medical Center
Cincinnati, OH

**S. Helena Kuivaniemi, MD, PhD**
Staff Scientist
The Sigfried and Janet Weis Center for Research
Geisinger Health System
Danville, PA

**Jody L. Kujovich, MD**
Assistant Professor of Pediatrics and Medicine, Director,
    Women's Hemostasis and Thrombosis Clinic
The Hemophilia Center
Oregon Health and Science University
Portland, OR

**Hiroki Kurahashi, MD, PhD**
Professor
Division of Molecular Genetics
ICMS, Fujita Health University
Toyoake, Aichi, Japan

**Fuat Kurbanov, PhD**
Post-Doctoral Fellow
Department of Medicine, Infectious Diseases
Johns Hopkins University
Baltimore, MD

**Andre Kushniruk, PhD**
Professor
School of Health Information Science
University of Victoria
Victoria, BC

**Neal K. Lakdawala, MD**
Instructor
Department of Medicine
Harvard Medical School and Brigham and Women's Hospital
Boston, MA

**Frank Lammert, Dr. med.**
Professor
Department of Internal Medicine II
Saarland University Medical Center
Homburg, Germany

**Blair R. Leavitt, MDCM, FRCPC**
Professor
The Centre for Molecular Medicine and Therapeutics Child and
    Family Research Institute
Child and Family Research Institute, BC Children's Hospital,
    University of British Columbia
Vancouver, BC

**Charles Lee, PhD**
Director
Institute for Genomic Medicine
The Jackson Laboratory
Farmington, CT

**Dru F. Leistritz, MS, CGC**
Genetic Counselor
Department of Pathology
University of Washington
Seattle, WA

**Oksana Lekarev, DO**
Assistant Professor
Department of Pediatrics
Weill Cornell Medical College
New York, NY

**Caryn Lerman, PhD**
Professor of Psychology in Psychiatry
Department of Psychiatry
University of Pennsylvania
Philadelphia, PA

**Harvey L. Levy, MD**
Senior Physician in Medicine and Genetics
Division of Genetics and Metabolism
Boston Children's Hospital
Boston, MA

Howard Levy, MD, PhD
Assistant Professor
Division of General Internal Medicine & McKusick-Nathans
    Institute of Genetic Medicine
Johns Hopkins University
Baltimore, MD

Ming D. Li, PhD
Jean and Ronald Butcher Professor
Head, Section of Neurobiology
Vice Chair for Research, Department of Psychiatry and NB
    Sciences
University of Virginia
Charlottesville, VA

Noralane Lindor, MD
Professor
Medical Genetics
Mayo Clinic
Scottsdale, AZ

W. Marston Linehan, MD
Chief
Urologic Oncology Branch
National Cancer Institute
Bethesda, MD

Nicola Longo, MD, PhD
Professor and Chief
Medical Genetics/Pediatrics
University of Utah
Salt Lake City, UT

Helen C. Looker, MD
Clinical Senior Research Fellow
Division of Population Health Sciences
University of Dundee School of Medicine
Dundee, UK

James E. Loyd, MD
Professor of Medicine
Department of Medicine
Vanderbilt University Medical Center
Nashville, TN

James R. Lupski, MD, PhD, D.Sc. (Hons)
Cullen Professor and Vice Chairman Genetics
Department of Molecular and Human Genetics
Baylor College of Medicine
Houston, TX

Tom H. M. Ottenhoff, MD, PhD
Professor
Department of Infectious Diseases
Leiden University Medical Center
Leiden, Netherlands

Lucy MacKillop, MA, FRCP
Consultant Obstetric Physician
Maternal high-risk maternity service
Oxford University Hospitals NHS Trust
Oxford, UK

Kenneth D. Macneal, BS, MBA
University of Denver
Denver, CO

Calum A. Macrae, MD, PhD
Associate Professor
Department of Medicine
Brigham and Women's Hospital
Boston, MA

Simon Mallal, MBBS
Professor of Medicine
Center for Translational Immunology & Infectious Diseases
    Vanderbilt University, Nashville TN
Director, Institute for Immunology and Infectious Diseases,
    Murdoch University, Murdoch, Western Australia

Leslie Manace-Brenman, MD
Assistant Professor
Department of Medicine
University of California, San Francisco
San Francisco, CA

Giovanna Mantovani, MD, PhD
Endocrinology Unit, Department of Medical Sciences
Università degli Studi di Milano
Milan, Italy

Deborah Marsden, MBBS
Assistant Clinical Professor of Pediatrics
Division of Genetics and Metabolism
Boston Children's Hospital
Boston, MA

George M. Martin, MD
Professor
Department of Pathology
University of Washington
Seattle, WA

John O. Mascarenhas, MD
Assistant Professor
Department of Medicine
Mount Sinai School of Medicine
New York, NY

James Mastrianni, MD, PhD
Director, Center for Comprehensive Care and Research on
    Memory Disorders
Department of Neurology
University of Chicago
Chicago, IL

Donna M. McDonald-McGinn, MS, CGC
Associate Director, Clinical Genetics
Program Director, The "22q and You" Center
The Children's Hospital of Philadelphia
Philadelphia, PA

Kimberly R. McDonald, MD
House Officer
Department of Pediatrics
University of Mississippi Medical Center
Jackson, MS

**Peter J. McGuire, MS, MD**
Genetic Disease Research Branch
National Human Genome Research Institute
National Institutes of Health
Bethesda, MD

**Melvin McInnis, MD, FRCP**
Professor of Psychiatry
Department of Psychiatry
University of Michigan
Ann Arbor, MI

**W. H. Irwin McLean, FRSE FMedSci**
Professor of Human Genetics
Dermatology and Genetic Medicine, Division of Molecular
    Medicine
University of Dundee
Dundee, UK

**Walter T. McNicholas, MB BCh BAO, MD, FRCPC, MRCPI,
    FRCPC**
Director, Pulmonary and Sleep Disorders Unit,
Newman Professor
Pulmonary and Sleep Disorders Unit
St. Vincent's University Hospital
Dublin, Ireland

**Robert R. McWilliams, MD**
Associate Professor of Oncology
Division of Medical Oncology
Mayo Clinic
Rochester, MN

**Lakshmi Mehta, MD**
Associate Professor
Genetics and Genomic Medicine
Mount Sinai School of Medicine
New York, NY

**Eugen Melcescu, MD**
Post-Doctoral Fellow
Department of Medicine/Endocrinology
University of Mississippi Medical Center
Jackson, MS

**Francesca Menconi**
Department of Medicine
Mount Sinai School of Medicine
New York, NY

**Federica Mescla, MD**
Negri Bergamo Laboratories and the Daccò Centre
Mario Negri Institute for Pharmacological Research
Milan, IT

**Dianna M. Milewicz, MD, PhD**
President George H. W. Bush Chair of Cardiovascular Medicine,
    Director, Division of Medical Genetics
Director MD/PhD Program
Department of Internal Medicine
The University of Texas Health Science Center at Houston
Houston, TX

**Jeffrey M. Milunsky, MD**
Co-Director
Center for Human Genetics
Cambridge, MA

**Beau Mitchell, MD**
Clinical Assistant Professor
Department of Pediatrics
Weill Cornell Medical College
New York, NY

**Braxton D. Mitchell, PhD**
Professor
Department of Medicine
University of Maryland School of Medicine
Baltimore, MD

**Matthew Morris, PhD**
Assistant Professor
Department of Family and Community Medicine
Meharry Medical College
Nashville, TN

**Cynthia Morton, PhD**
William Lambert Richardson Professor of Obstetrics, Gynecology
    and Reproductive Biology and Professor of Pathology, Harvard
    Medical School, and Director of Cytogenetics, Brigham and
    Women's Hospital
Departments of Obstetrics, Gynecology and Reproductive Biology
    and Pathology
Brigham and Women's Hospital and Harvard Medical School
Boston, MA

**Richard T. Moxley III, MD**
Director, Neuromuscular Disease Center
Helen Aresty Fine & Irving Fine Professor of Neurology
Director, Neuromuscular Disease Center
Department of Neurology, The University of Rochester
Rochester, NY

**Maureen Murphy-Ryan, MD**
Psychiatry Fellow
Department of Psychiatry
Washington University School of Medicine
St. Louis, MO

**Michael F. Murray, MD**
Director of Clinical Genomics
Genomic Medicine Institute
Geisinger Health System
Danville, PA

**Dedee F. Murrell, MA, BMBCh, FAAD, MD, FACD**
Professor and Head of Dermatology
Department of Medicine
St George Hospital, University of New South Wales
Sydney, Australia

**Yusuke Nakamura, MD, PhD**
Professor
Knapp Center for Biomedical Discovery
The University of Chicago
Chicago, IL

**Serge P. Nana-Sinkam, MD**
Associate Professor
Department of Medicine
Ohio State University
Columbus, OH

**Goutham Narla, MD, PhD**
Assistant Professor
Department of Medicine
Case Western Reserve University
Cleveland, OH

**Ramzi H. Nasir, MD, MPH**
Attending Physician in Developmental Behavioral Pediatrics
Division of Developmental Medicine
Boston Children's Hospital
Boston, MA

**Shyamala C. Navada, MD**
Assistant Professor
Department of Medicine
Mount Sinai School of Medicine
New York, NY

**Eric J. Nestler, MD, PhD**
Professor and Chair
Department of Neurosciences
Mount Sinai School of Medicine
New York, NY

**Maria I. New, MD**
Professor
Departments of Pediatrics and Genetics and Genomic Medicine
Mount Sinai School of Medicine
New York, NY

**Anna Newlin, MS, CGC**
Genetic Counselor
Center for Medical Genetics
NorthShore University HealthSystem
Evanston, IL

**Vipan Nikore, MD**
Staff Physician
Medicine Institute
Cleveland Clinic
Cleveland, OH

**Haruki Nishizawa, MD, PhD**
Associate professor
Department of Obstetrics and Gynecology
Fujita Health University School of Medicine
Toyoake, Aichi, Japan

**Maina Noris, MD**
Laboratory Chief
Immunology and Genetic of Rare Diseases and Organ
   Transplantation
Mario Negri Institute for Pharmacological Research
Milan, IT

**Fabio P. Nunes, MD**
Associate Medical Advisor
Eli Lilly and Company
Indianapolis, Indiana

**Darren D. O'Rielly, PhD**
Senior Clinical Scientist
Faculty of Medicine
Memorial University of Newfoundland
St. John's, Newfoundland, Canada

**Kenneth Offit, MD, MPH**
Chief, Clinical Genetics Service
Department of Medicine
Memorial Sloan-Kettering Cancer Center
New York, NY

**Alexander R. Opotowsky, MD, MPH**
Assistant Professor
Department of Pediatrics
Boston Children's Hospital and Brigham and Women's Hospital
Boston, MA

**Raffaella Origa, MD**
Researcher
Department of Public Health and Clinical and Molecular
   Medicine
University of Cagliari
Cagliari, Italy

**Junko Oshima, MD, PhD**
Research Professor
Department of Pathology
University of Washington
Seattle, WA

**Gretchen Oswald, MS, CGC**
Genetic Counselor
McKusick-Nathans Institute of Genetic Medicine
Johns Hopkins University
Baltimore, MD

**Michael Paconowski, PharmD, MPH**
Associate Director for Genomics and Targeted Therapy
Office of Clinical Pharmacology
U.S. Food and Drug Administration
Silver Spring, MD

**Arnab Pain, PhD**
Associate Professor, Pathogen Genomics
Computational Bioscience Research Center, Chemical Life
   Sciences and Engineering Division
King Abdullah University of Science and Technology
Thuwal, Mekkah, Kingdom of Saudi Arabia

**Faith J. Pangilinan, PhD**
Staff Scientist
National Human Genome Research Institute
National Institutes of Health
Bethesda, MD

**Melissa A. Parisi, MD**
Chief, Intellectual and Disabilities Branch
Eunice Kennedy Shriver National Institute of Child Health &
   Human Development (NICHD)
National Institutes of Health
Bethesda, MD

**Alan A. Parsa, MD**
Fellow
Department of Medicine
Cedars-Sinai Medical Center
Los Angeles, CA

**Marzia Pasquali, PhD**
Professor
Pathology Department
University of Utah
Salt Lake City, UT

**Thomas J. Payne, PhD**
Professor
Department of Otolaryngology and Communicative Sciences
University of Mississippi Medical Center
Jackson, MS

**Anthony A. Philippakis, MD, PhD**
Fellow
Department of Medicine
Brigham and Women's Hospital
Boston, MA

**Elizabeth J. Phillips, MD**
Professor of Medicine
Director of Personalized Immunology, Vanderbilt University,
   Nashville TN
Institute of Immunology & Infectious Diseases, Murdoch
   University
Murdoch, Australia

**Scott R. Plotkin, MD**
Associate Professor
Pappas Center for Neuro-Oncology
Massachusetts General Hospital
Boston, MA

**Annapurna Poduri, MD, MPH**
Assistant Professor of Neurology
Division of Epilepsy and Clinical Neurophysiology
Boston Children's Hospital
Boston, MA

**Martin Pollak, MD**
Professor of Medicine
Division of Nephrology, Department of Medicine
Beth Israel Deaconess Medical Center
Boston, MA

**Reed E. Pyeritz, MD, PhD**
Vice Chair for Academic Affairs;
   Director, Center for the Integration of Genetic Healthcare
   Technologies;
   Professor of Medicine,
   Senior Fellow, Center for Bioethics;
   Senior Fellow, Leonard Davis Institute of Health Economics
Department of Medicine
Perelman School of Medicine at the University of Pennsylvania
Philadelphia, PA

**John M. Quillin, PhD, MPH, MS, CGC**
Assistant Professor
Department of Human and Molecular Genetics
Virginia Commonwealth University
Richmond, VA

**Daniel J. Rader, MD**
Cooper-McLure Professor of Medicine and Pharmacology
Chief, Division of Translational Medicine and
   Human Genetics Associate Director, Institute for
   Translational Medicine and Therapeutics
Perelman School of Medicine at the University of Pennsylvania
Philadelphia, PA

**Proton Rahman, MD**
Professor of Medicine
Faculty of Medicine
Memorial University of Newfoundland
St. John's, Newfoundland

**Huma Q. Rana, MD**
Instructor
Department of Medicine
Dana Farber Cancer Institute
Boston, MA

**Uma Rao, MD**
Professor of Psychiatry and Behavioral Sciences; Director, Center
   for Molecular and Behavioral Neuroscience; Endowed Chair in
   Brain and Behavior Research
Center for Molecular and Behavioral Neuroscience
Meharry Medical College
Nashville, TN

**Ellen S. Regalado, MS, CGC**
Genetic Counselor/Instructor
Department of Internal Medicine
The University of Texas Medical School at Houston
Houston, TX

**Heidi Rehm, PhD**
Assistant Professor of Pathology
Director, Laboratory for Molecular Medicine
Brigham and Women's Hospital and Harvard Medical School
Boston, MA

**Giuseppe Remuzzi, MD**
Professor
Negri Bergamo Laboratories and the Daccò Centre
Mario Negri Institute for Pharmacological Research
Milan, IT

**Marcos I. Restrepo, MD, MSc, FCCP**
Investigator, Assistant Professor
Department of Medicine
University of Texas Health Science Center at San Antonio
San Antonio, TX

**Matthew RG Taylor, MD, PhD**
Director, Adult Medical Genetics Program
Department of Medicine
University of Colorado Denver
Denver, CO

Paul M. Ridker, MD
Eugene Braunwald Professor of Medicine
Department of Medicine
Brigham and Women's Hospital
Boston, MA

Nahir Rivera, PharmD
Pharmacist
Department of Pharmacy Practice
University of Puerto Rico – Medical Sciences Campus
San Juan, Puerto Rico

Eve A. Roberts, MD, MA, FRCPC
Adjunct Professor of Paediatrics, Medicine and Pharmacology
University of Toronto
Toronto, ON

Philip Robinson, MB ChB, FRACP
Rheumatologist & PhD Student
Human Genetics Group
University of Queensland Diamantina Institute
Brisbane, Queensland, Australia

Hobart L. Rogers, PharmD, PhD
Lieutenant Commander, U.S. Public Health Service
Office of Clinical Pharmacology
U.S. Food and Drug Administration
Silver Spring, MD

Henry Rosenberg, MD
Director of Medical Education
Department of Medical Education and Clinical Research
Saint Barnabas Medical Center
Livingston, NJ

Mark A. Rothstein, JD
Herbert F. Boehl Chair of Law and Medicine
Director, Institute for Bioethics, Health Policy, and Law
University of Louisville School of Medicine
Louisville, KY

Gualberto Ruano, MD, PhD
Director
Genetic Research Center
Hartford Hospital
Hartford, CT

Henrik Rueffert, MD
Department of Anesthesiology and Intensive Care Medicine
HELIOS Kliniken
Borna, Germany

Ornella J. Rullo, MD
Clinical Instructor
Division of Pediatric Rheumatology
Mattel Children's Hospital, University of California, Los Angeles
Los Angeles, CA

Silke Ryan, MD, PhD
Consultant in Respiratory and Sleep Medicine
Pulmonary and Sleep Disorders Unit
St. Vincent's University Hospital and Conway Institute, University
    College Dublin
Dublin, Ireland

Arturo Saavedra, MD, PhD, MBA
Assistant Professor in Dermatology, Medicine and
    Dermatopathology
Department of Dermatology
Brigham and Women's Hospital and Harvard Medical School
Boston, MA

Marc S. Sabatine, MD
Chairman of TIMI Study Group
Department of Medicine
Brigham and Women's Hospital
Boston, MA

Sadia Saeed, MSc
Department of Genomics of Common Diseases
School Of Public Health, Imperial College London
London, UK

Solomon Sager, MD
Cardiology Fellow
Division of Cardiology
University of Miami Miller School of Medicine and Jackson
    Memorial Hospital
Miami, FL

Birendra P. Sah, MD
Assistant Professor
Department of Pulmonary/Critical Care
SUNY Upstate Medical University
Syracuse, NY

Melissa Savage, MS, CGC
Manager
Medical Education and Clinical Affairs
Natera
San Carlos, CA

John A. Sayer, MB ChB, PhD
Senior Clinical Lecturer in Nephrology
Institute of Genetic Medicine
Newcastle University
Newcastle upon Tyne, Tyne and Wear, United Kingdom

Gretchen Schneider, MS, CGC
Professor of the Practice
Genetic Counseling Program
Brandeis University
Waltham, MA

Susanne A. Schneider, MD, PhD
Consultant Neurologist
Department of Neurology
Christian Albrechts University of Kiel
Kiel, Germany

Elizabeth K. Schorry, MD
Associate Professor
Department of Pediatrics
Cincinnati Children's Hospital Medical Center
Cincinnati, OH

**Matthew Schu, MS. Ed, MS**
Division of Biomedical Genetics,
Department of Medicine
Boston University School of Medicine
Boston, MA

**David A. Schwartz, MD**
Professor and Chair
Department of Medicine
University of Colorado School of Medicine
Aurora, CO

**Arthur Z. Schwartzbard, MD**
Assistant Professor
Department of Medicine
New York University Langone Medical Center
New York, NY

**Marvin I. Schwarz, MD**
Professor of Medicine
Department of Medicine
University of Colorado School of Medicine
Denver, CO

**Stuart A. Scott, PhD**
Assistant Professor
Genetics and Genomic Sciences
Mount Sinai School of Medicine
New York, NY

**Christine E. Seidman, MD**
Thomas W. Smith Professor of Medicine, Director, Cardiovascular
    Genetics Center
Department of Medicine
Brigham and Women's Hospital
Boston, MA

**Richard L. Seip, PhD**
Senior Scientist
Department of Cardiology
Hartford Hospital
Hartford, CT

**Lecia V. Sequist, MD, MPH**
Associate Professor
MGH Cancer Center
Massachusetts General Hospital, Harvard Medical School
Boston, MA

**Jessica C. Shand, MD**
Clinical Fellow
Pediatric Oncology Branch
National Cancer Institute
Bethesda, MD

**Nicholas B. Shannon, PhD (Cantab), BSc (Ebol)**
Research Associate
Cambridge Research Institute
Cambridge, United Kingdom

**A. Eliot Shearer, MD**
Clinical Research Fellow
Department of Otolaryngology – Head and Neck Surgery
University of Iowa
Iowa City, IA

**Alan Shiels, PhD**
Professor
Department of Ophthalmology and Visual Sciences
Washington University School of Medicine
St. Louis, MO

**Dolores Shoback, MD**
Professor of Medicine
Department of Medicine
University of California San Francisco
San Francisco, CA

**Brian Shuch, MD**
Research Fellow
Urologic Oncology Branch
National Cancer Institute
Bethesda, MD

**Teepu Siddique, MD**
Professor and Director, Neuromuscular Medicine/Neurogenetics
    Division
Department of Neurology and Clinical Neurosciences
Northwestern University Feinberg School of Medicine
Chicago, IL

**Lewis R. Silverman, MD**
Associate Professor
Department of Medicine
Mount Sinai School of Medicine
New York, NY

**Katherine Sims, MD**
Director Mitochondrial Clinic
Neurology Department, Massachusetts General Hospital
Professor of Neurology, Harvard Medical School
Boston, MA

**Pamela Sklar, MD, PhD**
Professor
Departments of Psychiatry, Neurosciences, and Genetics and
    Genomic Medicine
Mount Sinai School of Medicine
New York, NY

**Thomas J. Smith, MD**
Professor of Oncology
Sidney Kimmel Comprehensive Cancer Center
Johns Hopkins University
Baltimore, MD

**Jung Sook Ha, MD, PhD**
Associate Professor
Department of Laboratory Medicine
Keimyung University School of Medicine
Daegu, South Korea

**Elizabeth A. Sparks, APNG**
McKusick-Nathans Institute of Genetic Medicine
Johns Hopkins University
Baltimore, MD

**Martin H. Steinberg, MD**
Professor of Medicine
Department of Medicine
Boston University Medical Center
Boston, MA

**Douglas R. Stewart, MD**
Investigator, Clinical Genetics Branch
Division of Cancer Epidemiology and Genetics
National Cancer Institute
Rockville, MD

**James K. Stoller, MD, MS**
Chairman, Education Institute Cleveland Clinic; Jean Wall
    Bennett Professor of Medicine, Cleveland Clinic Lerner
    College of Medicine; Samson Global Leadership Academy
    Endowed Chair
Educational Institute
Cleveland Clinic
Cleveland, OH

**Constantine A. Stratakis, MD, DMSci**
Scientific Director, Senior Investigator
Eunice Kennedy Shriver National Institute of Child Health &
    Human Development (NICHD)
National Institutes of Health
Bethesda, MD

**Aaron Sturrock, MRCP**
Department of Medical Genetics
University of British Columbia
Vancouver, BC

**Prasanth Surumpudi, MD**
Fellow
Division of Endocrinology/Metabolism
David Geffen School of Medicine, University of California,
Los Angeles
Los Angeles, CA

**Talia H. Swartz, MD**
Assistant Professor
Department of Medicine
Mount Sinai School of Medicine
New York, NY

**Ronald Swerdloff, MD**
Professor of Medicine
Chief, Division of Endocrinology/Metabolism
David Geffen School of Medicine, University of California,
    Los Angeles
Los Angeles, CA

**Eva Szarek, PhD, MProjMg**
Fellow
Eunice Kennedy Shriver National Institute of Child Health &
    Human Development (NICHD)
National Institutes of Health
Bethesda, MD

**Wen-Hann Tan, BMBS**
Attending Physician in Genetics
Division of Genetics
Boston Children's Hospital
Boston, MA

**Polakit Teekakirikul, MD**
Clinical Fellow in Medicine
Department of Medicine
Mount Auburn Hospital and Harvard Medical School
Cambridge, MA

**Kathryn Teng, MD**
Director, Center for Personalized Health
Medicine Institute
Cleveland Clinic
Cleveland, OH

**Josephy V. Thakuria, MD, MMSc**
Attending Physician
Division of Medical Genetics
Massachusetts General Hospital
Boston, MA

**Chloe L. Thio, MD**
Associate Professor
Department of Medicine, Infectious Diseases
Johns Hopkins University
Baltimore, MD

**Felicitas Thol, MD**
Attending Physician
Department of Hematology, Hemostasis, Oncology, and Stem Cell
    Transplantation
Hannover Medical School
Hannover, Germany

**Paul D. Thompson, MD**
Director, Cardiology and Cardiovascular Research
Department of Cardiology
Hartford Hospital
Hartford, CT

**Peter Tishler, MD**
Associate Professor
Division of Medical Genetics
Brigham and Women's Hospital and Harvard Medical School
Boston, MA

**Yaron Tomer, MD**
Professor
Department of Medicine
Mount Sinai School of Medicine
New York, NY

**Vicente Torres, MD, PhD**
Director
Translational Polycystic Kidney Disease Center
Mayo Clinic
Rochester, MN

Isabelle Touitou, MD, PhD
Professor of Genetics
Laboratoire de génétique des maladies rares et auto-
    inflammatoires
CHRU de Montpellier, France; INSERM U844, Montpellier,
    France; Université Montpellier 1, UM1
Montpellier, France

Gerard C. Tromp, PhD
Staff Scientist
The Sigfried and Janet Weis Center for Research
Geisinger Health System
Danville, PA

Betty P. Tsao, PhD
Professor
Department of Medicine
University of California, Los Angeles
Los Angeles, CA

Hensin Tsao, MD, PhD
Associate Professor
Dermatology Department
Harvard Medical School
Boston, MA

Ahmet Z. Uluer, DO, MS
Director, Adult Cystic Fibrosis Program
Department of Medicine
Brigham and Women's Hospital and Boston Children's Hospital
    Cystic Fibrosis Center
Boston, MA

Ryan Ungaro, MD
Fellow
Department of Medicine
Mount Sinai School of Medicine
New York, NY

Esther van de Vosse, PhD
Assistant Professor
Department of Infectious Diseases
Leiden University Medical Center
Leiden, Netherlands

Vivianna Van M. Deerlin, MD, PhD
Associate Professor
Department of Pathology and Laboratory Medicine
Perelman School of Medicine at the University of Pennsylvania
Philadelphia, PA

Oriol S. Vidal, MD, PhD
Staff Pulmonologist
Servei de Pneumologia
Hospital de la Canta Creu i Sant Pau
Barcelona, Spain

Steven G. Waguespack, MD
Associate Professor and Deputy Department Chair
Dept. of Endocrine Neoplasia & Hormonal Disorders
University of Texas M.D. Anderson Cancer Center
Houston, TX

Mona Walimbe, MD
Clinical Fellow
Department of Medicine
University of California San Francisco
San Francisco, CA

Shawn S. Wallery, MD
Neuromuscular Medicine Fellow
Department of Neurology and Clinical Neurosciences
Northwestern University Feinberg School of Medicine
Chicago, IL

Christopher E. Walsh, MD, PhD
Associate Professor
Department of Medicine
Mount Sinai School of Medicine
New York, NY

Kyle M. Walsh, PhD
Assistant Professor
Division of Neuroepidemiology
University of California San Francisco
San Francisco, CA

Ethylin Wang Jabs, MD
Professor
Genetics and Genomic Sciences
Mount Sinai School of Medicine
New York, NY

Ronald Wapner, MD
Professor
Department of Obstetrics and Gynecology
Columbia University Medical Center
New York, NY

Melissa Wasserstein, MD
Associate Professor
Genetics and Genomic Sciences
Mount Sinai School of Medicine
New York, NY

Grant W. Waterer, MBBS, PhD
Professor of Medicine
School of Medicine and Pharmacology Royal Perth Hospital Unit
University of Western Australia
Perth, Australia

Bryn D. Webb, MD
Instructor
Pediatrics, Genetics and Genomic Sciences
Mount Sinai School of Medicine
New York, NY

James Weisfeld-Adams, MD
Instructor
Genetics and Genomic Sciences
Mount Sinai School of Medicine
New York, NY

Constance Weismann, MD
Assistant Professor
Pediatrics
Yale University School of Medicine
New Haven, CT

**Scott Weiss, MD, MS**
Professor of Medicine
Department of Medicine
Harvard Medical School
Boston, MA

**Shelly Weiss, MS, CGC**
Regional Medical Specialist
Preventive Care
Myriad Genetics
Salt Lake City, UT

**Duane R. Wesemann, MD, PhD**
Associate Professor of Medicine
Division of Rheumatology, Immunology and Allergy,
Department of Medicine
Brigham and Women's Hospital and Harvard Medical School
Boston, MA

**David C. Whitcomb, MD, PhD**
Giant Eagle Professor of Cancer Genetics
Professor of Medicine, Cell Biology & Physiology, and Human
   Genetics
Chief Division of Gastroenterology, Hepatology and Nutrition
Department of Medicine
University of Pittsburgh Medical Center
Pittsburgh, PA

**Janey L. Wiggs, MD, PhD**
Associate Professor of Ophthalmology
Harvard Medical School
Massachusetts Eye and Ear Infirmary
Boston, MA

**Louise Wilkins-Haug, MD, PhD**
Associate Professor
Department of Obstetrics, Gynecology, and Reproductive
Biology
Brigham and Women's Hospital
Boston, MA

**Marc S. Williams, MD**
Director
Genomic Medicine Institute
Geisinger Health System
Danville, PA

**Wojciech Wisniewski, MD, PhD**
Assistant Professor
Department of Molecular and Human Genetics
Baylor College of Medicine
Houston, TX

**Margaret R. Wrensch, MPH, PhD**
Stanley D. Lewis and Virginia S. Lewis Endowed Chair in Brain
   Tumor Research
Department of Neurological Surgery
University of California San Francisco
San Francisco, CA

**Katie Wusik, MS, CGC**
Genetic Counselor
Department of Pediatrics
Cincinnati Children's Hospital Medical Center
Cincinnati, OH

**Paraskevi Xekouki, MD, DMedSci**
Fellow
Eunice Kennedy Shriver National Institute of Child Health &
   Human Development (NICHD)
National Institutes of Health
Bethesda, MD

**Amy Yang, MD**
Assistant Professor
Genetics and Genomic Medicine
Mount Sinai School of Medicine
New York, NY

**Mabel Yau, MD**
Instructor
Department of Pediatrics
Mount Sinai School of Medicine
New York, NY

**Elaine H. Zackai, MD**
Director
Clinical Genetics
Children's Hospital of Philadelphia
Philadelphia, PA

**Ulrich M. Zanger, PhD**
Deputy Head and Section Head
Molecular and Cell Biology
Dr. Margarete Fischer-Bosch Institute of Clinical Pharmacology
Stuttgart, Germany

**Hitoshi Zembutsu, MD, PhD**
Assistant Professor
Laboratory of Molecular Medicine
The Institute of Medical Science, The University of Tokyo
Tokyo, Japan

# FOREWORD

At medical and scientific conferences in the last few years, the iPad has been the most popular raffle prize donated by conference sponsors. At the most recent genomic medicine conference I attended, the raffle prize was a free personal genome sequence, delivered to the winner on an iPad! As the cost of sequencing is dropping faster than the cost for computing power and storage, the genome sequence will soon cost less than the iPad that's used to deliver it.

There are many other indicators of the mind-boggling pace of technology advances and plummeting price for genome sequencing. Recently, the National Institutes of Health (NIH) has requested grant applications for pilot studies to determine the potential role of whole genome sequencing during newborn screening, when virtually every baby born in the United States has a small blood sample taken by a heel stick. Having a complete genomic profile from birth would obviate the need for any future blood or DNA sampling in order to obtain genetic testing information; one would only access the data from a patient's electronic health record, personal health vault, or their smart phone.

Besides the stunning technical advances, application of large-scale sequencing has led to unexpected and game-changing biological and medical insights. At the top of my list for these changes has been the realization in oncology that a tumor's genomic profile of mutations is more important in determining the appropriate choice of chemotherapeutic agent than the organ in which a tumor originates (eg, breast or lung), necessitating a complete revamping of cancer taxonomy for diagnosis and treatment and promising much improved survival rates.

Another potentially widespread application for rapid sequencing is identification of infectious agents involved in hospital outbreaks, where it is now possible to determine exactly when, where, and by whom the infection was introduced to the hospital. Such molecular microbiology by genome sequencing may soon be done as a routine screening procedure prior to hospital or emergency department admission on all patients.

Increasingly, genome sequencing has been used to identify the etiology of diseases in children with complex, undiagnosed conditions. In the most famous of these cases, Nick Volcker, a young boy in Wisconsin with a severe Crohn-like disease was not only diagnosed by sequencing as having a mutation in a gene on the X chromosome, but knowledge of the specific gene causing his clinical symptoms led to the correct treatment and a complete cure. The story of using DNA sequencing to save the life of a gravely ill child was documented in a series of articles in the Milwaukee Journal Sentinel that was awarded a Pulitzer Prize.

In 2012, Stephen Kingsmore's group in Kansas City pushed the envelope of genome sequencing to show that sequencing and genome interpretation could be performed in less than 50 hours in babies in the neonatal intensive care unit (NICU), arriving at accurate medical diagnoses and appropriate treatments far faster than the sequential testing procedures for individual disorders usually followed in this setting. This demonstration of "stat sequencing" has made the potential clinical relevance of genome sequencing a reality for many previous skeptics.

But how do physicians and healthcare providers make sense of the vast amount of new genomic data and its potential clinical implications? Although we still don't know what much of our genome does, there are many clinical situations where sufficient evidence now exists for the use of genomic information to optimize patient care and treatment. Therefore, it is timely to see a comprehensive textbook and practical guide to the use of this information across a broad spectrum of adult diseases—from individual differences in drug response, cardiac and cancer risks, to Alzheimer and other neurological and psychiatric disorders. I applaud both the timing and the effort of the editors and the authors of this volume, as well as the American College of Physicians for their role in supporting this effort.

The organization and style make this a very practical handbook for internists, primary care physicians, and other healthcare providers, with concise presentations of key information needed for diagnosis, management, and treatment across approximately 200 different clinical conditions.

Physicians today are increasingly dealing with patients who have surfed the Web to obtain information potentially relevant to their health. In the next few years, patients will increasingly individualize this research based on knowledge of their unique genomic profile and expect their physicians and healthcare system to act as "Genome Health Navigators" to provide precise and optimum health and wellness guidance.

David H. Ledbetter, PhD
*Executive Vice President &*
*Chief Scientific Officer*
*Geisinger Health System*
*Danville, PA*

# ACKNOWLEDGMENT

The editors wish to acknowledge the support of Ms. Jamie Valerius, Dr. Richard Maas and Dr. David Ledbetter without whom this project would not have succeeded.

# 1 Clinical Genomics–an Introduction

Monica A. Giovanni, Mark W. Babyatsky, and Michael F. Murray

The use of genomic sequence data in a clinical setting is truly a new phenomenon in this 21st century. In the year 1999, no human ever had their genome sequenced; by 2009 there were seven individuals who had their genome sequenced [ref Wade NYT], and it has been predicted by some that the millionth person will have their genome sequenced in calendar year 2014. Although it is not clear if or when the remarkable uptake of this technology might level off, it is clear that this technology will increasingly affect the way medicine is practiced. All healthcare practitioners will be increasingly asked to put this data into an appropriate clinical context, and this book is designed to assist you in this effort.

Genomics has the potential to improve our approach to care in almost every aspect of medicine from cancer to infectious diseases. This book is organized according to the standard medical and surgical subspecialties of clinical care and, in addition, has dedicated sections to areas that are not classic clinical subspecialties in adult care such as metabolomics and pharmacogenomics. The pharmacogenomics section describes the use of genetic sequence information to guide the choice and dosage of therapeutic agents. We expect that the knowledge base for all of the book's sections will continue to grow.

We are moving into an increasingly DNA-first world of clinical medicine, where the DNA sequence data will be available for decision making prior to the patient's visit to your office or hospital. In this DNA-first world, we will all need point-of-care decision support and we hope in these early years of genomic medicine that you find this book to be useful in your decision support needs. In addition to the detailed information in this book, several online resources including annotated genomic glossaries are available and listed in the supplementary materials.

Importantly, enthusiasm about genomic medicine should not lead to an abandonment of the classic tools of clinical medicine that are needed to inform care. First and foremost among these tools are the history and physical examination. The importance of environmental influences on health must not be overlooked [ref Willett]. While this text gives great attention to the "nature" side of the nature versus nurture equation, there are many other sources of important information on the role of environment in all diseases including that which is considered as "genetic" [ref Harrisons].

## The Evolving Role for Family Health History

Family health history has been used in clinical medicine for generations as a proxy for genetic information in efforts to predict disease risk in patients. In contrast to its previous application, in the era of DNA-first genomic medicine, family health history will increasingly be used to add context to the DNA sequence data.

Since every patient will be revealed to have rare genetic changes, so rare that they may only exist within their immediate family, the health history of others in the family who share these changes will be necessary in order to gain insight into how these changes will affect health. It will only be through knowing how these changes played out for the patient's immediate relatives that we will be able to interpret some sequence variations in the patient who is being seen. It is because of this "interpretative need" that we will ultimately require detailed family health histories that are annotated with DNA sequence variant information.

At the current time, patients can be engaged in the gathering of detailed family health history to maximize the time of busy providers. The US Surgeon General's My Family Health Portrait (available at https://familyhistory.hhs.gov) provides a web-based tool that allows patients to enter data regarding their own personal medical history as well as that of relatives. This data can be analyzed as a pedigree image or in a table format providing valuable information to care providers. In this interim time, before we arrive at "genomically annotated" family health history tools, we can use such currently available tools to guide disease risk interpretation via classical methodologies.

## Ethical, Legal, and Social Implications

The application of genomics in clinical medicine presents ethical challenges for clinicians. The risk of genetic discrimination remains a prominent concern around the use of genetics in healthcare. Despite all efforts surrounding privacy, it is recognized that health information cannot be considered entirely private. A step forward in assuaging concern and protecting the public was achieved in 2008 when the US congress passed the Genetic Information Nondiscrimination Act (GINA) into federal law. GINA serves to protect individuals from discrimination on the basis of genetic information with respect to employability and health insurability. Genetic information is defined as information about genetic testing performed on individuals and their relatives as well as information about family health history. Importantly, the protection afforded by GINA does not protect individuals from discrimination in life, disability, and long-term care insurance.

There are also ethical considerations in the application of genetic technology that affect the relationship between the patient and the healthcare provider. Genetic testing, in any form, is viewed as distinct from other laboratory tests used routinely in medicine. Obtaining truly informed consent is vital to ensure that patient and provider expectations are in line. Due to the nature of genetic testing, it is possible to discover misattributed paternity or incest. Also, the heritable nature of genetic findings requires that patients be counseled on the duty to share their genetic status with at-risk relatives.

Recently, more focus has been placed on research into ethical, legal, and social implication (ELSI) issues; most published studies stem from scientists engaged in genomic and clinical research, the legal profession, and bioethicists. Fortunately, social scientists and population researchers are increasingly engaged in conducting and guiding research efforts. Engaging both scientific and nonscientific stakeholders in these important initiatives are important for the future of both genomics or systems biology research as well as the promise of personalized medicine to unlock the clinical potential of the great strides already made. ELSI issues are increasingly debated in the "public square" of the press and various community organizations; engagement with the public will help in the navigation of public acceptance of these efforts.

## Genetic and Genomic Testing

DNA-based diagnostic testing has evolved significantly over the last 50 years. While new technologies yield great promise and have delivered diagnostic successes, there remains a role for older technologies to answer some diagnostic questions.

*Karyotyping*, also called chromosome analysis, was developed in the mid 1950s as a method to visualize human chromosomes under a light microscope. Karyotype analysis is still a very useful diagnostic test to investigate for aneuploidy such as Down syndrome (trisomy 21), Turner syndrome (45, X), or Klinefelter syndrome (47, XXY) or to identify chromosomal rearrangements such as translocations, inversions, or large-scale deletions or duplications. *Fluorescence in situ hybridization (FISH)*, often performed in conjunction with karyotype analysis, uses sequence-specific probes to fluoresce chromosomal regions to investigate targeted regions such as the breakpoint cluster region-Abelson murine leukemia (BCR-ABL) fusion created by the reciprocal translocation of chromosomes 9 and 22 creating the Philadelphia chromosome associated with chronic myelogenous leukemia (CML).

*Genotyping* is a simple and inexpensive method for determining an individual's genetic makeup at a single genetic locus. Genotyping is the tool of choice in conditions in which there are few genetic variations that account for the vast majority of disease; an example is sickle cell anemia in which one mutation in the *HBB* gene, Glu6Val, causes the formation of sickle-shaped red blood cells. While this variant could be identified using advanced technologies, they are not necessary to make the molecular diagnosis. Genotyping is also used for carrier screening for cystic fibrosis, Tay-Sachs disease, and many other conditions in which there are a relatively small number of known variations causing disease. This method allows for a cost-effective approach for population-based screening programs.

*Sanger sequencing*, first developed in 1977, is still held as the gold standard for the determination of gene sequence. Sanger sequencing produces a long contiguous DNA sequence read that can be used to determine the full sequence of a gene of interest. This method is preferred when the condition in question is caused by variation at any point within a known gene. When a clinician suspects hereditary breast and ovarian cancer based on personal and family history, full gene sequencing of *BRCA1* and *BRCA2* is the appropriate diagnostic test to determine if there is a variation at any location within the two gene sequences.

Deletion and duplication testing is necessary in those conditions in which deletion or duplication of multiple nucleotides,

exons, or even genes is the mechanism of disease. Small-scale deletions and duplications of nucleotides or exons can be detected by *multiplex ligation-dependent probe amplification (MLPA)*, which is commonly used in the diagnostic workup for Duchenne muscular dystrophy in which multiexon deletions are a common cause of disease. Large-scale deletions or duplications of multiple genes can be detected by *array-based comparative genomic hybridization (aCGH)*; aCGH, also known as chromosomal microarray, can detect variations in copy number at a resolution of 5000 to 10,000 nucleotide bases (5-10 kb) depending on the testing platform. It is the diagnostic test of choice in evaluation of individuals with developmental delay and autism in which large-scale genomic deletions and duplications are reported.

*Next-generation sequencing* methods utilize high-throughput, massively parallel cycles to generate short sequence fragments that can be compiled to provide the sequence of multiple genes. This technology is employed in multigene panels which test for conditions with genetic heterogeneity such as hypertrophic cardiomyopathy or hearing loss. Next-generation sequencing approaches are also used in whole genome and whole exome sequence generation. Using this technology requires repetitive sequencing of DNA fragments in order to generate enough read depth to confidently make a base call at each locus. Multiscale biology technologies promise to afford simultaneous determination of DNA, ribonucleic acid (RNA), and protein pathways.

**BIBLIOGRAPHY:**

**Family History**

1. Centers for Disease Control and Prevention. Awareness of Family Health History as a Risk Factor for Disease—United States, 2004. *MMWR Morb Mortal Wkly Rep.* 2004;53(44):1044-1047.

2. Guttmacher AE, Collins FS, Carmona RH. The family history—more important than ever. *N Engl J Med.* 2004;351(22):2333-2336.

3. Pyeritz RE. The family history: the first genetic test, and still useful after all those years? *Genet Med.* 2012;14(1):3-9.

4. U.S. Preventive Services Task Force. Genetic risk assessment and BRCA mutation testing for breast and ovarian cancer susceptibility: recommendation statement. *Ann Intern Med.* 2005;143(5):355-361.

**ELSI**

1. Clayton EW. Ethical, legal, and social implications of genomic medicine. *N Engl J Med.* 2003;349(6):562-569.

2. McLean N, Delatycki MB, Macciocca I, Duncan RE. Ethical dilemmas associated with genetic testing: which are most commonly seen and how are they managed? *Genet Med.* 2012: [Epub ahead of print].

3. Offit K. Personalized medicine: new genomics, old lessons. *Hum Genet.* 2011;130(1):3-14.

4. Soden SE, Farrow EG, Saunders CJ, Lantos JD. Genomic medicine: evolving science, evolving ethics. *Per Med.* 2012;9(5):523-528.

**Genetic and Genomic Testing**

1. Dave BJ, Sanger WG. Role of cytogenetics and molecular cytogenetics in the diagnosis of genetic imbalances. *Semin Pediatr Neurol.* 2007;14(1):2-6.

2. Lee C, Iafrate AJ, Brothman AR. Copy number variations and clinical cytogenetic diagnosis of constitutional disorders. *Nat Genet.* 2007;39(suppl 7):S48-S54.

3. Shendure J, Ji H. Next-generation DNA sequencing. *Nat Biotechnol.* 2008;26(10):1135-1145.

4. Wade N. Cost of decoding a genome is lowered. NYT 2009; August 10.

# 2 Primary Care and Genomics

Vipan Nikore and Kathryn Teng

## Introduction

The primary care physician's (PCP's) decision framework and toolkit have evolved over the past two centuries. Diagnosis in the 19th century was driven by a patient's history and physical examination. External cues interpreted by the physician's senses served as input—the data was what the clinician could hear from the patient's story, visualize, touch, smell, or even taste as was the case with tasting urine to diagnose diabetes.

The 20th century marked the addition of advanced diagnostic modalities such as laboratory testing, tissue analysis, and imaging that allowed physicians to interpret the body's internal cues invisible to the naked eye. At times, this new medical technology led to the extinction of various parts of the history and physical examination, but more often it served as adjunct information.

The 21st century will be remembered as a time when genomic information became a key driver of clinical decisions. Although genomic information is also an internal cue invisible to the naked eye, it differs from traditional laboratory values and imaging. Genomic information is a permanent fingerprint that provides clues to historic and future states and insight into the pathophysiology of why the body reached a particular state, whereas laboratory values and imaging are snapshots of a patient's state at a moment in time. Our hope is that use of genomic information might improve our ability to screen for disease, make accurate diagnoses, and allow for more appropriate therapies.

In this era of genomic-informed medicine, we will learn about new categories of diseases and mechanisms of disease that we did not previously know existed. Through genome sequencing technology, we can pool large populations of patients with similar symptoms and find genetic patterns, enabling us to discover novel disease-causing alleles and providing explanations for previously unexplained conditions. The genomic revolution promises to improve quality of care for patients and decrease cost for the healthcare system by driving more appropriate utilization of resources and decreasing adverse drug events. Adverse drug events and medication errors result in 700,000 emergency department visits, 120,000 hospitalizations, and $3.5 billion in medical costs. Even a modest decrease in adverse events would result in substantial savings.

The remainder of this chapter will help clinicians understand how we might apply genomic information in our clinical practices.

## The Basics—Speaking the Language

Before we can discuss the clinical applications of genomics, let us review a few basic terms and concepts:

- An organism's complete set of DNA is called its *genome*. Virtually every single cell in the body contains a complete copy of the approximately 3 billion DNA base pairs that make up the human genome.
- With its four-letter language, DNA contains the information needed to build the entire human body. A *gene* traditionally refers to the unit of DNA that carries the instructions for making a specific protein or set of proteins. Each of the estimated 20,000 protein coding genes in the human genome codes for an average of three proteins.
- Located on 23 pairs of chromosomes packed into the nucleus of a human cell, genes direct the production of proteins with the assistance of enzymes and messenger molecules. Specifically, an enzyme copies the information in a gene's DNA into a molecule called *messenger ribonucleic acid RNA (mRNA)*. The mRNA travels out of the nucleus and into the cell's cytoplasm, where the mRNA is read by a tiny molecular machine called a ribosome, and the information is used to link together small molecules called amino acids in the right order to form a specific protein.
- Remarkably, over the human genome is more than 99% conserved, meaning that individuals differ in less than 1% of their genetic code.
- *Genetics* is the study of a particular gene.
- *Genomics* is the study of the function and interactions of the DNA in a genome. Genomics has a broader and more ambitious reach than genetics. Although more than 1800 single gene disorders have been identified, the study of genomics continues to hold great promise because new study techniques allow for the investigation of common multifactorial disorders caused by the interaction of genes and environment. Some of these interactions might confer a protective or pathologic role in the expression of these diseases.
- *Single-nucleotide polymorphism (SNP)* is a variation of a single base pair on the DNA molecule. Scientists are studying how SNPs (pronounced as "snips"), in the human genome correlate with disease, drug response, and other phenotypes.
- *Genome-wide association studies (GWAS)* are one type of research used in genomics to associate specific genetic variations with particular diseases. The method involves scanning the genomes from many different people and looking for genetic markers that can be used to predict the presence of a disease. Once such genetic markers are identified, they can be used to understand how genes contribute to the disease and develop better prevention and treatment strategies.
- *Personalized medicine* is the tailoring of medical treatment to the individual characteristics of each patient. In order to do this, we classify individuals into subpopulations that differ in their susceptibility to a particular disease or their response to a specific treatment. Preventative or therapeutic interventions can then be concentrated on those who will benefit, sparing expense and side effects for those who will not.
- *Pharmacogenetics* is the study of a person's genetic makeup affecting the body's response to drugs.

### How Will Advances in Genomics Affect the PCP's Daily Practice, and What Can We Do to Be Prepared?

In the following section, we will list and demonstrate several concepts which PCPs will need to incorporate into clinical practice. To illustrate a typical PCP encounter, we will use fictional patient Jane Doe, a 38-year-old woman who presents to Dr. Smith's office for a preventive care visit.

☞**FAMILY HEALTH HISTORY REMAINS ESSENTIAL:** During medical training, many physicians hear "it's all about the history." As medicine advances into a new world influenced by genomics, a thorough family health history remains the cornerstone of an appropriate diagnosis and evaluation. Family health history continues to provide clinical utility as a proxy for genetic, environmental, and behavioral risk to health. It is critical to inform risk stratification, allowing for judicious use of screening and opening the door to early and even prophylactic treatment.

Despite its clear clinical utility, there is ample evidence that family health history is underutilized across the healthcare community, with most practitioners asking infrequently and inconsistently about their patients' family health history. On average, PCPs spend less than 3 minutes collecting family health history. Given that one of the largest barriers to the collection of family health history is time, here are some existing solutions to this challenge:

- Electronic family health history collection tools: A very useful example is the US Surgeon General tool, found at https://familyhistory.hhs.gov/
- Use of ancillary staff to collect and obtain family health history information either by phone in advance or while the patient is waiting.
- Office-based family health history questionnaires, which can be e-mailed or taken home. This approach requires careful thought on how to integrate the information gathered into the patient's medical record.

During Ms. Doe's preventive care visit, Dr. Smith obtains a complete family health history. He notes that her paternal aunt had breast cancer in her 40s. He also notes that she is of Ashkenazi Jewish ancestry.

☞**LEARNING GENETICS—A LIFELONG RESPONSIBILITY:** The application of genomics is spreading from rare disorders to common conditions and patients are beginning to approach PCPs with questions about personalized medicine. Unfortunately, the primary care workforce has felt inadequate delivering genetic services and yet they must remain up to date with advances in genomics in order to recognize diseases with either a genetic etiology or implication for therapy. GWAS are rapidly discovering new genetic markers to predict disease on a weekly basis. The challenge is how to keep up with the rapid rate of genomic discoveries across the disease spectrum. Several online resources will help the PCP remain up to date. Point-of-care resources available through electronic health record systems or personal electronic applications will gain further development soon as well.

Dr. Smith knows that deleterious mutations of the breast cancer genes *BRCA1* and *BRCA2* are common in the Ashkenazi Jewish population and are strongly associated with early-onset breast cancer. This concerns him and he decides to pursue a more aggressive investigation into Ms. Doe's health.

☞**GENETIC TESTING IS EVOLVING:** As a result of genomic discoveries, increasing numbers of clinical guidelines suggest incorporating genetic tests into the standard of care. PCPs have been slow to adopt genetic testing, but we foresee a time when genetic or genomic testing will be routine. The decision about whether to order a genetic test is similar to the decision making for other tests. As with other tests, we should continue to consider clinical validity, pretest probability, sensitivity, specificity, cost, and clinical utility when deciding if testing is appropriate.

Clinically, there are several situations when genetic testing is indicated.

- *Prenatal diagnosis* includes invasive (eg, amniocentesis, chorionic villus sampling [CVS]) and noninvasive (eg, maternal serum screen, ultrasound, alpha-fetoprotein [AFP]) testing and can be performed to assess risk and/or diagnose abnormalities in a pregnancy. Risk factors such as maternal age, ethnicity, and family history should be considered.
- *Population-based screening* of an entire population. The most common application is newborn screening (eg, phenylketonuria).
- Diagnostic testing based on a *positive family history* can be ordered for those with a family history suggestive of hereditary disease as well as for those with a family member with previous positive genetic test. Genetic counselors, allied health professionals specializing in family history assessment and genetic testing, can assist PCPs with assessment and ordering.
- *Diagnostic testing* should be ordered if symptoms or other information suggest hereditary disease (ie, alpha-1-antitrypsin for a young person with symptoms or pulmonary function tests suggesting emphysema).
- *Pharmacogenetic testing* should be ordered if a patient is to be prescribed a drug with a known or recommended pharmacogenetic indication.

As more genetic tests become available and costs decrease, it will be important for PCPs to have available references and access to genetic specialists to understand when testing is warranted and how it might be helpful.

Because of her strong family history, Dr. Smith refers Ms. Doe for genetic counseling. The genetic specialist collects and confirms her family history and recommends ordering testing for BRCA mutations. This test returns positive result for a BRCA1 mutation.

☞**PREVENTION AND PREDICTION OF DISEASE—A PERSONALIZED AND EMPOWERED APPROACH:** Personalized medicine is the shift from the "one size fits all" approach to health maintenance to more dynamic screening. The use of family health history and genetic testing can sometimes enhance our ability to tailor screening recommendations to specific subpopulations based on demographics or patient risk factors. One example commonly encountered in primary care practice is the recommendation for early colonoscopy screening for those with a first-degree relative with colon cancer.

Interestingly, just the discussion of family health history can improve outcomes with at-risk patients. Individuals with a family history of disease are not only more knowledgeable about risk factors for that disease, but discussing their increased familial risk has been shown to motivate these patients to greater compliance with disease screening and higher rates of adherence to medical recommendations.

As part of her visit, Jane Doe and Dr. Smith discuss preventive health actions for her. Based on American Cancer Society guidelines, an annual screening mammogram is recommended for women at average risk of breast cancer starting at age 40. Based on her positive gene test, however, Dr. Smith follows the NCCN management guidelines, including mammogram and breast magnetic resonance imaging (MRI), as well as referral for discussion of risk-reducing treatment options.

☞**THERAPIES FOR PATIENTS WILL BE MORE INDIVIDUALIZED:** Our current practice of treating patients is based on population studies. Present-day recommendations are based on research subjects who may or may not be representative of the patient in front of us. The goal of personalized medicine is to move to an individualized approach to treatment. There are already examples of cancer therapeutics that are being targeted to the individual characteristics of the tumor or the metabolic profile of the patient.

Approximately 70 drugs currently list pharmacogenetic indicators. Clinical practice guidelines, recommendations, and statements on pharmacogenetic testing exist for many commonly prescribed drugs, such as codeine, statins, selective serotonin reuptake inhibitors, and warfarin. It will be important for PCPs to consider such information when prescribing these types of drugs. This is an area of great opportunity for us to develop the systems and tools to integrate pharmacogenetic information into clinical practice.

Jane Doe's mammogram shows an area of concerning calcifications. This area is biopsied and read by the pathologist as an invasive ductal carcinoma. After discussion of bilateral mastectomy given her positive *BRCA* test results, Jane opts for lumpectomy with lymph node resection. Tumor margins are clear, as are lymph nodes, giving a favorable prognosis. Her tumor is sent for several tests, including Oncotype Dx test which predicts risk for recurrent cancer. Her tests return several weeks later showing an Oncotype Dx score that places her at high risk for recurrent cancer. Based on these results, she is advised to undergo chemotherapy, a pathway she would not have been advised to take without the Oncotype Dx test score.

While on chemotherapy, Jane Doe develops leg swelling and is found to have a blood clot in her leg. She is admitted to her local hospital and started on intravenous heparin with plans to transition her to an oral blood thinner, warfarin, to treat this blood clot. Jane had enrolled in a research study 5 years ago as a control subject, during which she underwent some pharmacogenetic testing and was informed that she was a poor metabolizer of warfarin. She shares this information with Dr. Smith, who orders clinical CYP2C9 and VKORC1 pharmacogenetic testing and confirms that Ms. Doe indeed is a poor metabolizer of warfarin. Based on this information, he elects to start her on a smaller dose of warfarin than normal. She reaches her target warfarin level earlier than expected and returns home.

☞**A GENETICS SPECIALIST WILL BE A MEMBER OF THE CARE TEAM:** Given our expanding knowledge of the contribution of genetics and genomics to disease risk and treatment, referrals to genetics specialists will be in greater demand. Medical geneticists and genetic counselors serve as important members of the healthcare team who facilitate the appropriate use of genetics and genomics in clinical practice. The American Board of Medical Genetics is one of the 24 medical specialty boards that exist, but there is a shortage of medical geneticists. Improved access to genetics specialists and novel models to provide this access will be important to provide optimal care to patients. Given the shortage of genetics specialists in the workforce, it is essential that the PCP be empowered and educated to detect and diagnose the more common genetic diseases.

Several months after her surgery, Jane Doe presents for a follow-up visit. She expresses concern about her family members and their risk for breast cancer. Because of Ms. Doe's *BRCA1* mutation-positive status, Ms. Doe's sister, age 42, seeks a referral to a genetics specialist. When she finds out that she has also inherited the family's *BRCA1* gene mutation, she elects to undergo prophylactic salpingo-oophorectomy.

☞**GENETIC KNOWLEDGE WILL RESULT IN CHANGES IN DOCUMENTATION:** With the increased use of genetics and genomics to inform clinical care, it is likely that our traditional "SOAP note" documentation will change as well. Rather than our usual classification of patients, it is quite likely that we will classify them by genetic risk groups, and not just by traditional race or ethnicity.

Jane Doe's SOAP note may now read "Ms. Doe is a 38-year-old *BRCA1* positive, homozygous CYP2C9*3 and VKORC1-1639 polymorphism positive woman who presents for follow-up visit."

☞**THE GENETICS OF MULTIFACTORIAL DISEASE WILL CONTINUE TO BE EXPLORED:** Most diseases seen in adult primary care practice are felt to have multifactorial etiology with genetic and environmental factors both playing a part in causing disease. Some examples of multifactorial diseases include diabetes, obesity, coronary artery disease and stroke, and many cancers. The role of genetics in these multifactorial diseases continues to be investigated. In some cases, as with diabetes, we know that having a single first-degree relative with diabetes confers a higher risk for developing diabetes than age, body mass index, waist circumference, physical activity, diet, and hypertension. In addition, the cumulative prevalence of diabetes is 3.5 times higher in individuals with one first-degree relative with diabetes as compared to those without a family history. Many scientists continue to search for genetic markers, which either track with or cause disease, and together with family history may help better predict risk for developing a given disease.

☞**PERSONAL GENOMIC TESTING IS A REALITY OF CURRENT DAY MEDICINE:** Personal genomic companies have arisen in recent years, offering genomic risk profiles to patients based on SNP profiling. While these genomic profiles have been slow to gain acceptance among medical professionals due to their very limited clinical utility, there is a growing interest in personal genomics by the patient community. We anticipate that it will be a matter of time before we are asked to incorporate the results of personal genomic testing into clinical care and at the very least, help our patients to interpret their risk profiles. While existing literature indicates that patients do not experience increase in anxiety when learning about their risk for disease through personal genomic testing, there continues to be confusion and misperceptions about the risk conferred by SNP testing. Additional focus on education will be needed for both clinicians and patients to successfully navigate SNP profiling.

☞**ETHICAL, LEGAL, AND SOCIETAL IMPLICATIONS NEED TO BE CONSIDERED:** The incorporation of genetic risk into regular patient care has several implications and considerations:

- *Reimbursement for genetic-informed care*: PCPs will need better reimbursement for counseling and preventive care, and further efforts will be needed to enable the coverage of appropriate genetic testing and pharmacogenetic testing.
- *Privacy and confidentiality*: With the passing of the Genetic Information Nondiscrimination Act (GINA) in 2008, great strides were taken to protect individuals from discrimination based on genetic information. GINA prohibits discrimination in health coverage and employment based on genetic information but does not yet protect for life or disability insurance. We will need to continue to advocate for these protections.
- *Sharing of health information*: The move toward electronic health records should facilitate the sharing of patient information among healthcare practitioners and institutions, including the use of existing genetic information. We will need to create innovative ways to share genetic information with healthcare

providers and family members so as to improve health outcomes without compromising individual privacy.

- *Patient expectations and demand*: As people learn about the power of genomics, patient demand for genetic-informed care will likely to increase. With the continued rise in healthcare spending in the United States, we will all have to take responsibility so that those who might benefit most from interventions have equal access and that we spend our resources judiciously.

These are just some of the social and ethical questions that may arise in clinical practice. As we are the advocates for our patients and consumers of health care, we will need to help shape these conversations and solutions.

## Conclusion

In 1876, Alexander Graham Bell made history's first telephone call in Brantford, Ontario. Fifty years later the telephone found its way into mainstream use. In 1903, the Wright Brothers piloted the first airplane in Kitty Hawk, North Carolina. Fifty years later commercial aviation began to sprout. In 1953, Watson and Crick deduced the structure of DNA in a laboratory in Cambridge, England. Fifty years later we sequenced the entire human genome and are now on the verge of an explosion in practical day-to-day applications of DNA.

The promise of personalized medicine will only be fully realized if PCPs embrace new approaches to assessment. PCPs are often the first point of contact in the healthcare system for patients, and therefore genomic literacy of PCPs is required to transition genetic and genomic knowledge from the laboratory bench to patient's bedside.

The genomic revolution has made it an exciting time to be involved in medicine. Adding genomics to our decision analysis adds complexity, but if we as clinicians understand it, it grants us an opportunity to provide more precise diagnoses and improved treatments for our patients.

**BIBLIOGRAPHY:**

1. Committee on Identifying and Preventing Medication Errors, Aspden P, Wolcott J, Bootman JL, Cronenwett LR, eds. *Preventing Medication Errors: Quality Chasm Series*. Washington, DC: The National Academies Press; 2007.

2. Feero WG, Guttmacher AE, Collins FS. Genomic medicine—an updated primer. *N Engl J Med*. 2010;362:2001-2011.

3. O'Connor TP, Crystal RG. Genetic medicines: treatment strategies for hereditary disorders, *Nat Rev Genet*. 2006;7:261-276.

4. Definition from The National Human Genome Research Institute Glossary. http://www.genome.gov/glossary/, Accessed October, 2011.

5. Rich EC, Burke W, Heaton CJ, et al. Reconsidering the family history in primary care. *J Gen Intern Med*. 2004;19:273-280.

6. Green R. Summary of workgroup meeting on use of family history information in pediatric primary care and public health. *Pediatrics*. 2007;120:S87-S100.

7. Yang Q, Liu T, Valdez R, Moonesinghe R, Khoury MJ. Improvements in ability to detect undiagnosed diabetes by using information on family history among adults in the United States. *Am J Epidemiol*. 2010;171:1079-1089.

8. Acheson LS, Wiesner GL, Zyzanski SJ, Goodwin MA, Stange KC. Family history-taking in community family practice: implications for genetic screening. *Genet Med*. 2000;2:180-185.

9. Scheuner MT, Sieverding P, Shekelle PG. Delivery of genomic medicine for common chronic adult diseases: a systematic review. *JAMA*. 2008;299:1320-1334.

10. The National Human Genome Research Institute. http://www.genome.gov; National Center for Biotechnology Information. http://www.ncbi.nlm.nih.gov, Accessed October, 2011.

11. Zimmern RL, Kroese M. The evaluation of genetic tests. *J Public Health (Oxf)*. 2007;29:246-250.

12. Burke W, Laberge AM, Press N. Debating clinical utility. *Public Health Genomics*. 2010;13:215-223.

13. Chung WK. Implementation of genetics to personalize medicine. *Gend Med*. 2007;4:248-265.

14. Baptiste-Roberts K, Gary TL, Beckles GL, et al. Family history of diabetes, awareness of risk factors, and health behaviors among African Americans. *Am J Public Health*. 2007;97:907-912.

15. Qureshi N, Kai J. Informing patients of familial diabetes mellitus risk: how do they respond? A cross-sectional survey. *BMC Health Serv Res*. 2008;8:37.

16. Frueh FW, Amur S, Mummaneni P, et al. Pharmacogenomic biomarker information in drug labels approved by the United States food and drug administration: prevalence of related drug use. *Pharmacotherapy*. 2008;28:992-998.

17. Scott SA. Personalizing medicine with clinical pharmacogenetics. *Genet Med*. 2011;13:987-995.

18. Cooksey JA, Forte G, Benkendorf J, Blitzer MG. The state of the medical geneticist workforce: findings of the 2003 survey of American Board of Medical Genetics certified geneticists. *Genet Med*. 2005;7:439-443.

19. Cooksey JA, Forte G, Flanagan PA, Benkendorf J, Blitzer MG. The medical genetics workforce: an analysis of clinical geneticist subgroups. *Genet Med*. 2006;8:603-614.

20. ABMG Number of Certified Genetic Specialists 2011. http://www.abmg.org/pdf/SpecalistsByState.pdf, Accessed May, 2013.

21. Schwarz PE, Li J, Lindstrom J, Tuomilehto J. Tools for predicting the risk of type 2 diabetes in daily practice. *Horm Metab Res*. 2009;41:86-97.

22. Lindstrom J, Tuomilehto J. The diabetes risk score: a practical tool to predict type 2 diabetes risk. *Diabetes Care*. 2003;26:725-731.

23. Valdez R. Detecting undiagnosed type 2 diabetes: family history as a risk factor and screening tool. *J Diabetes Sci Technol*. 2009;3:722-726.

24. Bloss CS, Schork NJ, Topol EJ. Effect of direct-to-consumer genomewide profiling to assess disease risk. *N Engl J Med*. 2011;364:524-534.

25. Gollust SE, Gordon ES, Zayac C, et al. Motivations and perceptions of early adopters of personalized genomics: perspectives from research participants. *Public Health Genomics*. 2012;15:22-30.

# 3 Pharmacogenomic Information in Drug Labeling

Hobart L. Rogers and Michael Pacanowski

## KEY POINTS

- *Drug summary:*
  - Pharmacogenomic information is contained in the labeling of many drugs; the type of data available determine whether the results of a test are clinically actionable or useful.
  - Pharmacogenomic tests can be used to select patients for therapy based on their ability to identify responders, predict adverse events, or guide drug dosing.
- Most pharmacogenomic labeling has focused on drugs that
  - Have a narrow therapeutic index
  - Exhibit highly variable pharmacokinetics or responses
  - Are used to treat morbid or mortal conditions
  - Have serious toxicities
- Several examples exist where knowledge of a patient's genotype can significantly influence the benefit-risk profile of a drug product and aid therapeutic decision making. Some examples of this include
  - Warfarin—*CYP2C9* and *VKORC1* genotypes predict stable warfarin doses and risk for severe bleeding.
  - Clopidogrel—*CYP2C19* genotype identifies individuals with low active metabolite exposure and diminished responses who may benefit from drugs not metabolized by *CYP2C19*.
  - Abacavir—*HLA-B*5701* genotype identifies patients at risk for severe hypersensitivity reactions that should not receive the drug.
  - For a comprehensive list of all drugs with pharmacogenomic information appearing in their labels see http://www.fda.gov/Drugs/ScienceResearch/ResearchAreas/Pharmacogenetics/ucm083378.htm.

In the last decade, new tools and methods to explore the human genome have tremendously accelerated discovery of genetic markers for disease susceptibility, prognosis, and drug response. Hence, many clinicians are now faced with staying abreast of the enormous amount of genomic information being generated. Numerous resources are available to keep prescribers informed of important information related to drugs, including the FDA-approved drug label. With greater ability to characterize the genetic underpinnings of drug exposure (ie, pharmacokinetics) and response, whether intended effects or toxicities, drug labels will increasingly incorporate pharmacogenomic information and serve as a key resource for genetic biomarker information. In this chapter, we highlight some of the considerations that go into labeling drugs with pharmacogenomic biomarker information, as well as some translational challenges borne out in recent years.

## General Labeling Considerations

Prescription drug labeling is intended to provide a summary of the essential scientific information needed for the safe and effective use of a drug, so that clinicians are able to make informed prescribing decisions. The CFR§ Sec. 201.56 states that labels meet the following requirements: (1) The label must contain a summary of the essential scientific information needed for the safe and effective use of the drug. (2) The label must be informative and accurate and must be updated when new information becomes available. (3) The label must be based where possible on data derived from human experience and no claims may be made if there is inadequate evidence of safety or lack of efficacy.

Currently, pharmacogenomic information appears in the labeling of dozens of drugs, covering nearly all therapeutic areas (Fig. 3-1; a comprehensive listing of these labels can be found on the FDA website). To date, most pharmacogenomic labeling has focused on drugs that (1) have a narrow therapeutic index, (2) exhibit highly variable pharmacokinetics or responses, (3) are used to treat morbid or mortal conditions, or (4) have serious toxicities. Drugs with these characteristics tend to be the most difficult to use in the absence of clinical monitoring tools, and are thus amenable to genetic testing as a means of assessing an individual's probability of benefit or risk.

Clinical testing for patient selection or dose adjustment is not necessary for most drugs although numerous examples of clinically relevant pharmacogenomic interactions do exist. As shown in Fig. 3-1, most pharmacogenomic labeling is related to genetic defects in drug metabolism that affect drug concentrations (eg, because of CYP2D6 polymorphisms). Generally, doses are to be reduced in patients that cannot metabolize a particular drug, but genotyping does not always need to be performed prospectively.

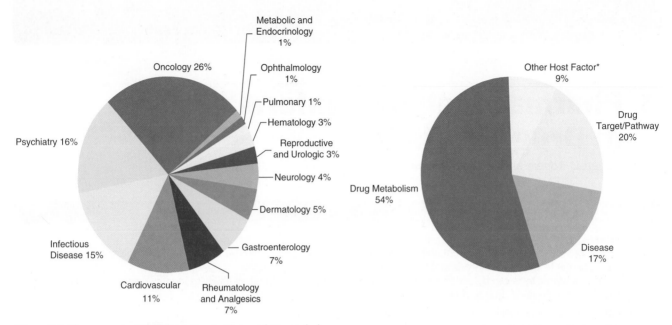

***Figure 3-1*** Pharmacogenomic Information in Approved Drug Labels.
The figure illustrates the therapeutic areas and nature of pharmacogenomic information in the labels of 74 unique molecules. *Other host factors include errors of inborn metabolism (eg, glucose-6-phosphate dehydrogenase [G6PD deficiency]) and immunologic factors (eg, human leukocyte antigen [HLA] type).

For instance, tetrabenazine is a drug that exhibits very high concentrations in CYP2D6 poor metabolizers at a certain dose threshold. Therefore, genotyping is recommended if that dose is reached to determine whether the dose should be increased further, so as to avoid toxicities. In the case of prodrugs, on the other hand, inability to activate the drug because of genetic polymorphisms may result in loss of efficacy, as discussed in the clopidogrel example later in this chapter.

Many examples exist where the genetic information is used to characterize the drug target in order to select patients for treatment, particularly for oncology drugs. A classic example is trastuzumab which is indicated for breast cancer patients whose tumors express HER2 since clinical trials for this drug were conducted only in patients whose tumors expressed this marker. More recently, KRAS mutations were found in postmarketing trials to significantly influence the outcome of antiepidermal growth factor receptor (anti-EGFR) therapy in metastatic colorectal cancer patients, which resulted in revisions to the panitumumab and cetuximab labels. Additionally, genetic factors that are major predictors of response to standards of care or disease prognosis are also captured in labeling, such as *IL28B* genotype for peg-interferon and the direct-acting antiviral drugs, which are used to treat chronic hepatitis C. This information may not be used to select patients per se, but may be used to determine the most appropriate treatment strategy.

Pharmacogenomic information may appear in a variety of forms within the drug label, depending on the implications of the biomarker on appropriate use of the medication. The quantity and quality of pharmacogenomic information depend in part on the strength of the relationship between the biomarker and the outcome of interest, the predictive utility of the biomarker, the severity of

the outcome, availability of alternative therapies or feasibility of dose adjustment, and numerous other contextual factors. For example, genetic information may be described in the Clinical Pharmacology section for informational purposes if the drug is metabolized by an enzyme that is known to have genetic variations, but might only be critical to dosage and administration if it is necessary to modify the dosing regimen to prevent toxicities. Understanding the relevance and clinical utility of pharmacogenomic information is not only important for all healthcare practitioners, but also helps to provide targeted therapy to decrease side effects while increasing efficacy. In the following sections, we would review three scenarios where genetic factors were found to be important markers of response, but varied with respect to labeling recommendations and uptake in clinical practice.

## Warfarin—A Lesson in Pharmacogenomic Influence on Pharmacokinetics and Dynamics

Warfarin is the most cited drug for drug-related mortality and widely recognized as a drug with a narrow therapeutic index due to increased bleeding risk from its anticoagulation effect. Approximately 25% of patients experience bleeding within the first 6 months of initiating therapy. Consequently, warfarin requires continuous pharmacodynamic monitoring (ie, international normalized ratio [INR] testing) with dose adjustments to achieve the targeted response; the usual, stable doses of warfarin that patients receive can range anywhere between 1 and 10 mg daily. Clinicians have been accounting for a number of demographic factors (age, height, body weight, and interacting drugs) to control for the large variability in response to warfarin. Despite accounting for these factors, responses remain variable, leading to adverse effects and poor patient outcomes. Thus, warfarin represents a good candidate for pharmacogenetic testing because it is highly effective but has significant safety issues and remarkably wide variability in response.

Within the last decade, genetic variants in the key enzyme that metabolizes warfarin, cytochrome P450 2C9 (CYP2C9), and the target of warfarin, vitamin K oxide reductase (VKORC1), were found to be the major determinants of warfarin dose requirements. Specifically, patients who have CYP2C9 gene variants metabolize warfarin at a much slower rate, which results in higher warfarin concentrations. Moreover, patients who have a variant in the VKORC1 gene may be sensitive or resistant to warfarin. Together these two genetic factors account for approximately 40% of the variability in warfarin dose requirements. Thus, accounting for the genetic status of both of these factors can help clinicians to predict the stable dose of warfarin.

The relationship between warfarin dose and CYP2C9 and VKORC1 genotype has been unequivocally established in over 4000 patients. In the Medco-Mayo Warfarin Effectiveness Study (MM-WES), 896 patients randomly assigned to a pharmacogenetic strategy had significantly decreased hospitalizations (28%) for bleeding or thromboembolism compared to a matched historical control group of 2688 patients. However, conflicting data have been presented regarding the utility of a prospectively genotyping patients and making treatment decisions. A number of studies are currently underway to further examine the clinical utility of genetic testing to modify warfarin dosing (www.clinicaltrials.gov).

In January 2010, the label for warfarin was revised to provide specific dosing recommendations based on CYP2C9 and VKORC1 genotype information (Table 3-1). The current label takes into account both the patient's VKORC1 and CYP2C9 status to recommend a dosing range tailored to an individual's genetics.

The current clinical conundrum with warfarin is that most patients are not aware of their VKORC1 or CYP2C9 status at the initiation of therapy. If this information is available the prescriber may be inclined to target doses in the table above. At the present time, because genomic information is not typically known, most of this targeted dosing is performed after the initial administration of warfarin. However, in the future the widespread use of genotyping and quick assay turn-around time will allow "real-time" decision making a common part of warfarin dosing. In the case of warfarin, pharmacogenomics allows us to predict doses, identify those patients that should be more vigilantly monitored, as well as identify patients who might be better served by an alternative therapy such as dabigatran.

## Clopidogrel—an Example of Variable Response

Clopidogrel is an antiplatelet prodrug that irreversibly inhibits adenosine diphosphate (ADP)-induced activation of platelets. Clopidogrel is currently approved for prevention of cardiovascular (CV) events in patients with acute coronary syndromes, recent myocardial infarction (MI), recent stroke, or established peripheral artery disease. Clopidogrel is among the most commonly used drugs with over 25 million prescriptions in 2010. However, responses to clopidogrel are highly variable, with approximately one in three individuals not exhibiting an antiplatelet response. Patients with diminished responses, therefore, may be at higher risk for CV events. Since clopidogrel is used to prevent life-threatening events and antiplatelet responses are not routinely monitored in clinical practice, genotyping strategies could be used to improve treatment outcomes.

As a prodrug, clopidogrel must be converted to its active form by the cytochrome P450 (CYP) enzyme system, one of which is CYP2C19. Polymorphisms in the gene encoding CYP2C19 result in a nonfunctional protein. Therefore, patients who have a nonfunctional allele on both chromosomes, referred to as CYP2C19 poor metabolizers, would be expected to produce less active metabolite and have diminished effectiveness. Pharmacokinetic studies have shown that individuals with one or two dysfunctional CYP2C19 alleles (intermediate and poor metabolizers, respectively) do indeed have lower clopidogrel active metabolite concentrations compared to extensive metabolizers (EMs). These findings have been substantiated by numerous antiplatelet response studies that consistently show diminished antiplatelet response in intermediate and poor metabolizers. Moreover, the majority of clinical outcome studies have also shown that patients who were CYP2C19 poor metabolizers had higher rates of CV events such as death, MI, stroke, urgent revascularization, and stent thrombosis.

Based on the accumulation of a substantial amount of data from pharmacokinetic, pharmacodynamic, and outcome studies the Food and Drug Administration (FDA) updated the label of clopidogrel with the following Boxed Warning:

WARNING: Diminished effectiveness in poor metabolizers: The effectiveness of Plavix is dependent on its activation to an active metabolite by the CYP system, principally CYP2C19. Plavix at recommended doses forms less of that metabolite and has a smaller effect on platelet function in patients who are CYP2C19 poor metabolizers. Poor metabolizers with acute coronary syndrome or undergoing percutaneous coronary

**Table 3-1 Range of Expected Therapeutic Warfarin Doses Based on CYP2C9 and VKORC1 Genotypes**

| | VKORC1 | | | CYP2C9 | | |
|---|---|---|---|---|---|---|
| | *1/*1 | *1/*2 | *1/*3 | *2/*2 | *2/*3 | *3/*3 |
| GG | 5-7 mg | 5-7 mg | 3-4 mg | 3-4 mg | 3-4 mg | 0.5-2 mg |
| AG | 5-7 mg | 3-4 mg | 3-4 mg | 3-4 mg | 0.5-2 mg | 0.5-2 mg |
| AA | 3-4 mg | 3-4 mg | 0.5-2 mg | 0.5-2 mg | 0.5-2 mg | 0.5-2 mg |

intervention treated with Plavix at recommended doses exhibit higher CV event rates than do patients with normal CYP2C19 function. Tests are available to identify a patient's *CYP2C19* genotype; these tests can be used as an aid in determining therapeutic strategy. Consider alternative treatment or treatment strategies in patients identified as CYP2C19 poor metabolizers.

This labeling change advises prescribers to consider alternative treatments for patients who are known to be CYP2C19 poor metabolizers (about 2%-3% of the white and black populations, up to 20% of Southeast Asian populations), such as other drugs that are not subject to activation by CYP2C19 like prasugrel or ticagrelor.

As with warfarin, genetic testing prior to clopidogrel treatment has been limited in clinical practice. In a survey of the American College of Cardiology, CYP2C19 genetic testing was ordered for 6% of patients starting clopidogrel and 4% of patients already taking the medication. Also like warfarin, prospective studies to evaluate genotyping strategies are under way to establish the utility of genotyping to guide antiplatelet drug choices or dosing for intermediate or poor metabolizers.

## Abacavir—a Lesson in Safety Pharmacogenomics

Abacavir is an efficacious HIV-1 protease inhibitor, but 5% to 8% of patients develop a serious immunologically mediated hypersensitivity reaction that consists of fever, rash, gastrointestinal (GI), and respiratory symptoms that become more severe with prolong dosing. This serious adverse reaction limited its use in therapy. Moreover, the symptoms of this hypersensitivity are nonspecific and can be difficult to distinguish from infection and other inflammatory diseases.

Two studies were published that found a significant association within the major histocompatibility complex (MHC) region, specifically the HLA-B*5701 variant, and abacavir-induced hypersensitivity. The frequency of the *HLA-B*5701 allele in European populations is approximately 6%, and the odds of developing hypersensitivity among carriers versus noncarriers is approximately ninefold higher. Following this original signal for association, three historical control studies found that prospectively implementing HLA-B*5701 genotyping reduced the incidence of abacavir hypersensitivity from 7% to 10% to less than 0.7%. Thus, HLA-B*5701 was found to be unequivocally associated with hypersensitivity reactions, and prospective screening, based on observational studies, appeared to be effective at reducing the incidence of this potentially severe adverse drug reaction.

In order to definitively establish the clinical utility of *a priori* HLA-B*5701 screening, a large, randomized, double-blind, prospective clinical trial was conducted in 19 different countries to test the effectiveness of prospective HLA-B*5701 screening in preventing the hypersensitivity reaction to abacavir. *HLA-B*5701 allele was present in 5.6% of the prospectively tested patients, and these patients were excluded from treatment. In the control arm, in which patients were not screened for HLA-B*5701, 7.8% developed hypersensitivity (2.7% immunologically confirmed), while in the experimental arm, HLA-B*5701 screening reduced the incidence

of hypersensitivity to 3.4% (eliminating immunologically confirmed hypersensitivity).

Based on the results of this large, randomized trial, the FDA provided the following Boxed Warning for abacavir:

WARNING: Risk of hypersensitivity reactions, lactic acidosis, and severe hepatomegaly: Patients who carry the *HLA-B*5701 allele are at high risk for experiencing a hypersensitivity reaction to abacavir. Prior to initiating therapy with abacavir, screening for the *HLA-B*5701 allele is recommended; this approach has been found to decrease the risk of hypersensitivity reaction. Screening is also recommended prior to reinitiation of abacavir in patients of unknown HLA-B*5701 status who have previously tolerated abacavir. HLA-B*5701-negative patients may develop a suspected hypersensitivity reaction to abacavir; however, this occurs significantly less frequently than in HLA-B*5701-positive patients.

In addition to being described in the FDA-approved label, prospective testing for HLA-B*5701 is recommended before initiating treatment with abacavir according to the HIV treatment guidelines. This genetic test has very good performance characteristics (eg, positive and negative predictive value), giving prescribers confidence in the results of the test. In the small subset of patients who are carriers of the *HLA-B*5701 allele, another protease inhibitor should be chosen. Abacavir provides a good example of how pharmacogenetic testing can drive clinical decision making and positively influence patient outcomes. The development of the HLA-test for abacavir is an exceptional example where a prospective trial unequivocally established the utility of genotyping to avoid adverse outcomes.

## Future Directions

Advances in technology have driven innovation in the field of pharmacogenomics at an incredible rate. The cost of genotyping is continuing to decrease dramatically. As a result, numerous clinically relevant genetic associations are being discovered. Several examples exist where the discovery of genetic biomarkers for drug response have translated to clinical tests that select patients for treatment. The most notable have been in the area of oncology, such as KRAS testing for cetuximab and panitumumab and HER2 testing for trastuzumab. Genetic testing is becoming more common in other therapeutic areas, such as infectious diseases with the advent of drug response or toxicity biomarkers such as HLA-B*5701 for abacavir and IL28B genotyping for peg-interferon or ribavirin. However, a general lag in implementing the pharmacogenomic discoveries in the clinic currently exists, largely because of the perceived need for large, clinical utility trials, despite the challenges of conducting such trials. Additionally, drug developers and regulators are facing new challenges such as ensuring the identification of the proper subset of genetic responders along with the additional codevelopment of diagnostic devices that would identify the genetic subpopulations most likely to benefit from treatment. With more prospective use of biomarkers in premarketing clinical trials, pharmacogenomic information in drug labels will be more and more prevalent, as will the number of drugs with companion diagnostics.

## Supplementary Hyperlinks

**Genomics: Table of Pharmacogenomic Biomarkers in Drug Labels**

http://www.fda.gov/Drugs/ScienceResearch/ResearchAreas/Pharmacogenetics/ucm083378.htm

### BIBLIOGRAPHY:

1. Budnitz DS, Pollock DA, Weidenbach KN, Mendelsohn AB, Schroeder TJ, Annest JL. National surveillance of emergency department visits for outpatient adverse drug events. *JAMA.* 2006;296:1858-1866.

2. Beyth RJ, Quinn L, Landefeld CS. A multicomponent intervention to prevent major bleeding complications in older patients receiving warfarin. A randomized, controlled trial. *Ann Intern Med.* 2000;133:687-695.

3. Manolopoulos VG, Ragia G, Tavridou A. Pharmacogenetics of coumarinic oral anticoagulants. *Pharmacogenomics.* 2010;11:493-496.

4. International Warfarin Pharmacogenetics Consortium, Klein TE, Altman RB, et al. Estimation of the warfarin dose with clinical and pharmacogenetic data. *N Engl J Med.* 2009;360:753-764.

5. Epstein RS, Moyer TP, Aubert RE, et al. Warfarin genotyping reduces hospitalization rates results from the MM-WES (medco-mayo warfarin effectiveness study). *J Am Coll Cardiol.* 2010;55:2804-2812.

6. Drugs.com. Top 200 Pharmaceutical Drugs. http://www.drugs.com/top200.html. Accessed November 8, 2011.

7. Gurbel PA, Bliden KP, Hiatt BL, O'Connor CM. Clopidogrel for coronary stenting: response variability, drug resistance, and the effect of pretreatment platelet reactivity. *Circulation.* 2003; 107:2908-2913.

8. Giusti B, Gori AM, Marcucci R, Saracini C, Vestrini A, Abbate R. Determinants to optimize response to clopidogrel in acute coronary syndrome. *Pharmgenomics Pers Med.* 2010;3:33-50.

9. Mega JL, Close SL, Wiviott SD, et al. Cytochrome p-450 polymorphisms and response to clopidogrel. *N Engl J Med.* 2009;360:354-362.

10. Varenhorst C, James S, Erlinge D, et al. Genetic variation of CYP2C19 affects both pharmacokinetic and pharmacodynamic responses to clopidogrel but not prasugrel in aspirin-treated patients with coronary artery disease. *Eur Heart J.* 2009;30:1744-1752.

11. Brandt JT, Close SL, Iturria SJ, et al. Common polymorphisms of CYP2C19 and CYP2C9 affect the pharmacokinetic and pharmacodynamic response to clopidogrel but not prasugrel. *J Thromb Haemost.* 2007;5:2429-2436.

12. Mega JL, Simon T, Collet JP, et al. Reduced-function CYP2C19 genotype and risk of adverse clinical outcomes among patients treated with clopidogrel predominantly for PCI: a meta-analysis. *JAMA.* 2010;304:1821-1830.

13. Lewin J. New frontiers in personalized medicine. *New Frontiers in Personalized Medicine: Cardiovascular Research and Clinical Care*; January 6, 2011; Washington, DC.

14. Mallal S, Nolan D, Witt C, et al. Association between presence of HLA-B*5701, HLA-DR7, and HLA-DQ3 and hypersensitivity to HIV-1 reverse-transcriptase inhibitor abacavir. *Lancet.* 2002;359:727-732.

15. Hetherington S, Hughes AR, Mosteller M, et al. Genetic variations in HLA-B region and hypersensitivity reactions to abacavir. *Lancet.* 2002;359:1121-1122.

16. Hughes DA, Vilar FJ, Ward CC, Alfirevic A, Park BK, Pirmohamed M. Cost-effectiveness analysis of HLA B*5701 genotyping in preventing abacavir hypersensitivity. *Pharmacogenetics.* 2004;14:335-342.

17. Zucman D, Truchis P, Majerholc C, Stegman S, Caillat-Zucman S. Prospective screening for human leukocyte antigen-B*5701 avoids abacavir hypersensitivity reaction in the ethnically mixed French HIV population. *J Acquir Immune Defic Syndr.* 2007;45:1-3.

18. Martin AM, Nolan D, Gaudieri S, et al. Predisposition to abacavir hypersensitivity conferred by HLA-B*5701 and a haplotypic Hsp70-hom variant. *Proc Natl Acad Sci USA.* 2004; 101:4180-4185.

19. Rauch A, Nolan D, Martin A, McKinnon E, Almeida C, Mallal S. Prospective genetic screening decreases the incidence of abacavir hypersensitivity reactions in the western Australian HIV cohort study. *Clin Infect Dis.* 2006;43:99-102.

20. Mallal S, Phillips E, Carosi G, et al. HLA-B*5701 screening for hypersensitivity to abacavir. *N Engl J Med.* 2008;358:568-579.

# 4 Common Cytochrome P450 Polymorphisms and Pharmacogenetics

Ulrich M. Zanger

## KEY POINTS

- *Disease summary:*
  - In this chapter, relatively common (>1% frequency) and ethically diverse genetic polymorphisms of drug-metabolizing cytochrome P450s (CYPs) will be reviewed. In general, these variants
  - Affect pharmacokinetics and response to drugs which are substrates of these enzymes
  - Are not usually associated with drug-independent clinical phenotypes
  - Have pharmacokinetic phenotypes categorized as poor, intermediate, normal (extensive), and ultrarapid metabolizer (UM)
  - Have clinical phenotypes which depend on the particular pharmacologic situation (drug, prodrug, therapeutic index, etc)
- *Differential diagnosis:*
  - Intoxication, drug-drug interaction, allergy
- *Monogenic forms:*
  - CYP polymorphisms are monogenically inherited as autosomal recessive (poor or intermediate metabolizers) or dominant (UMs) traits.
- *Twin studies:*
  - The few mono- or dizygotic twin studies available indicate a large contribution of genetic factors to drug oxidation phenotype: heritability of antipyrine 4-hydroxylation rate, which is mainly catalyzed by CYP3A4, was estimated at 0.88 and that of the caffeine metabolic ratio, a marker of CYP1A2, at 0.72.
- *Environmental factors:*
  - Drug-drug interactions (inhibition, induction), food constituents, circadian rhythm
- *Genome-wide associations:*
  - GWAS revealed associations between CYP2C9 genotype and final dose of warfarin, an anticoagulant metabolized by the enzyme. Further, single-nucleotide polymorphisms (SNPs) in the regulatory region of the *CYP1A* locus were associated with habitual coffee consumption; this association is likely based on the major role of CYP1A2 as the rate-limiting enzyme for metabolism of caffeine.

## Common Characteristics of Cytochrome P450 Polymorphisms

The influence of heritable genetic polymorphisms in genes encoding drug-metabolizing CYPs on drug pharmacokinetics and drug response is well documented. Clinically relevant polymorphisms exist in CYPs 2B6, 2C9, 2C19, 2D6, and 3A4/5 (see later). In each of these genes, several individual SNPs are found in coding and/or noncoding gene regions, which influence either gene expression or enzymatic activity (Table 4-1). The *CYP2D6* gene is also known for its numerous large-scale structural variants including a variety of gene copy number variants (CNV). Variants that lead to lower or higher expression of the enzyme are expected to decrease or increase the clearance of all enzyme substrates in a similar manner, respectively, whereas nonsynonymous coding SNPs may lead to substrate-dependent effects.

Different terms are in use for the associated pharmacokinetic phenotypes. In the case of CYP2D6 and CYP2C19, poor metabolizer (PM) refers to homozygous or compound heterozygous carriers of alleles with a complete lack of function (null allele). An efficient (or extensive) metabolizer (EM) refers to the normal phenotype, usually representing the most common phenotype mode in the population. Intermediate metabolizers (IMs) harbor either one normal or one functionally deficient allele, thus resulting in impaired drug oxidation capacity. Lastly, the UM originates

from three or more functional *CYP2D6* alleles or from a functionally more active *CYP2C19* allele. When referring to other CYPs, these terms are not appropriate because the lack of common null alleles and the functional overlap with enzymes of similar substrate selectivity preclude the occurrence of more than two distinct phenotypic modes. In these cases, the terms slow metabolizer and rapid (normal) metabolizer are more appropriate. The CYP-specific drug oxidation phenotype can be determined in vivo by using selective model substrates (Table 4-1).

The individual polymorphisms within one gene are often linked to each other, giving rise to complex haplotype patterns and overlapping genotype-phenotype correlations. The wild type or reference haplotype was usually defined as the first historically described gene variant and therefore does not necessarily represent the most frequent allele. Individual allele frequencies may thus vary between << 1% and greater than 50%. Allele frequencies of SNPs and CNVs typically vary greatly between different ethnicities.

The consequences of polymorphic drug metabolism for drug therapy need to be considered within their pharmacologic context. Loss-of-function variants will lead to reduced clearance and increased plasma concentrations of the drug itself, while gain-of-function variants will lead to increased clearance and lower plasma drug concentrations. If the drug itself is pharmacologically active and the metabolite is inactive, this should result in higher and lower drug effect and potentially drug-related toxicity due to overdosing. In the case of a prodrug, the opposite consequences are

*Table 4-1  Pharmacogenetic Polymorphisms of Cytochrome P450s*

| Gene | Associated Medications[a] | Variant[b] | Frequency[c] | Effect |
|------|---------------------------|------------|--------------|--------|
| CYP2B6 | Artemether, artemisinin, *bupropion*, cyclophosphamide, diazepam, efavirenz, ketamine, meperidine, methadone, nevirapine, propofol, selegiline, sertraline | CYP2B6*4<br>c.785A>G(rs2279343) | 0.00 AA, Af<br>0.04 Ca<br>0.07 As | K262R<br>↑ expression & activity |
| | | CYP2B6*6<br>c.516G>T (rs3745274)<br>c.785A>G(rs2279343) | 0.33-0.5 AA, Af<br>0.15-0.20 As<br>0.24-0.27 Ca | Q172H, K262R<br>↓ expression & activity (most substrates) |
| | | CYP2B6*18<br>c.983T>C (rs28399499) | 0.04-0.12 AA, Af<br>0.00 As, Ca, Hs | I328T ↓↓ expression & activity (null allele) |
| | | CYP2B6*22<br>-82T>C (rs34223104) | 0.00-0.025 AA, Af, As<br>0.024 Ca, Hs | ↑ expression & activity<br>↑ inducibility (in hepatocytes) |
| CYP2C9 | Candesartan, celecoxib, *diclofenac*, flurbiprofen, glimepiride, glipizide, glyburide, ibuprofen, indomethacin, irbesartan, meloxicam, naproxen, piroxicam, rosuvastatin, *tolbutamide*, S-warfarin, zaltoprofen | CYP2C9*2<br>c.430C>T (rs1799853) | 0.00-0.02 AA, Af<br>0.00-0.02 As, Pc<br>0.10-0.17 Ca<br>0.065 Hs | R144C<br>↓ activity (substrate-dependent) |
| | | CYP2C9*3<br>c.1075A>C (rs1057910) | 0.00-0.01 Af, AA<br>0.02-0.06 As<br>0.06 Ca | I359L<br>↓↓ activity (substrate-dependent) |
| CYP2C19 | Amitriptyline, citalopram, clomipramine, clobazam, clopidogrel, diazepam, lansoprazole, *S-mepheny-toin*, nelfinavir, omeprazole, pantoprazole, proguanil, venlafaxine, voriconazole | CYP2C19*2<br>c.681G > A (rs4244285) | 0.10-0.17 AA, Af<br>0.22-0.32 As, Pc<br>0.06-15 Ca<br>0.15 Hs | Splicing defect<br>Null allele |
| | | CYP2C19*3<br>c.636G>A (rs4986893) | 0.00-0.01 Af, Ca, Hs<br>0.03-0.07 As, Pc | W212X<br>Null allele |
| | | CYP2C19*17<br>-806C>T (rs12248560) | 0.15-0.27 AA, Af<br>0.00-0.02 As<br>0.21-0.25 Ca | Promoter variant<br>↑ expression & activity |
| CYP2D6 | Amitriptyline, aripiprazole, atomoxetine, carvedilol, chlorpromazine, clomiphene, clomipramine, codeine, *debrisoquine*, *dextromethorphan*, dihydrocodeine, donepezil, galantamine, haloperidol, imipramine, mexiletine, metoprolol, mianserin, mirtazapine, nortriptyline, ondansetron, paroxetine, perhexiline, *propafenone*, risperidone, tamoxifen, thioridazine, timolol, tramadol, tropisetron, venlafaxine, zuclopenthixol | CYP2D6*4<br>1846G>A (rs3892097) | 0.15-0.25 Ca<br>0.01-0.10 AA, Af, As, Hs | Splicing defect<br>Null allele |
| | | CYP2D6*5 | 0.03-0.06 all ethnicities | Gene deletion<br>Null allele |
| | | CYP2D6*10<br>100C>T (rs1065852) | 0.08-0.12 AA, Af<br>0.40-0.70 As | P34S<br>↓ expression & activity |
| | | CYP2D6*17<br>1023C>T (rs28371706)<br>2850C>T (rs16947) | 0.14-0.24 Af<br>0.00 As, Ca | T107I, R296C<br>↓ expression & activity |
| | | CYP2D6*41<br>2988G>A (rs28371725) | 0.09 Ca<br>0.01-0.06 Af, As, Pc, Hs | Splicing defect<br>↓ expression & activity |
| | | CYP2D6*Nxn | 0.01-0.09 Ca<br>up to 0.30 Af, Ar | Increased gene copy number<br>↑ expression & activity |

*(Continued)*

*Table 4-1* **Pharmacogenetic Polymorphisms of Cytochrome P450s (Continued)**

| Gene | Associated Medications[a] | Variant[b] | Frequency[c] | Effect |
|------|---------------------------|------------|--------------|--------|
| CYP3A4 | Antipyrine, atorvastatin, carbamazepine, cisapride, cyclosporine, erythromycin, felodipine, ifosfamide, *midazolam*, nifedipine, paracetamol, quetiapine, quinidine, ritonavir, simvastatin, tacrolimus, *testosterone*, tramadol, verapamil, vincristine, zolpidem | CYP3A4*22 15389 C>T (rs35599367) | 0.043 AA 0.043 As 0.025-0.08 Ca | Intron 6 ↓ expression & activity |
| CYP3A5 | (All CYP3A4 substrates) Saquinavir, tacrolimus, verapamil | CYP3A5*3 6986A>G rs776746 | 0.37 AA 0.12-0.35 Af 0.66-0.75 As, Hs 0.88-0.97 Ca | Splicing defect ↓ expression & activity |

[a]Substrates shown are primarily metabolized by the respective CYP. Highly selective probe substrates are italicized.

[b]Key mutations only shown; allele nomenclature refers to the CYP Allele Nomenclature website.

[c]AA, African American; Af, African; Ar, Arabian; As, Asian; Ca, Caucasian; Hs, Hispanic; Pc, Polynesian.

to be expected. An example for the latter is the increased formation of morphine from codeine by CYP2D6 ultrarapid metabolizers. Less clear consequences may arise if both the drug and the metabolites are pharmacologically active. An analysis of adverse drug reaction studies published between 1995 and 2000 identified 27 drugs frequently cited in connection with an adverse drug reaction. Remarkably, 59% of these 27 drugs are metabolized by at least one polymorphic enzyme, compared to only 7% of randomly selected top-selling drugs, emphasizing the clinical significance of pharmacokinetic polymorphisms.

## CYP2B6 Enzyme Characteristics and Clinical Pharmacogenetics

*CYP2B6* is the only functional gene of the *CYP2B* subfamily located on chromosome 19. In humans, CYP2B6 is a minor hepatic P450 contributing approximately 2% to 4% to the total hepatic P450 pool, but exhibits large interindividual variability of expression. This variability is in part explained by the fact that human and rodent *CYP2B* genes are strongly inducible by phenobarbital and other xenobiotics which act as ligands to the constitutive androstane receptor (CAR) (NR1I3) and the pregnane X receptor (PXR) (NR1I2). On ligand binding these orphan nuclear receptors dimerize with the retinoid X receptor (RXR) to bind to DNA response elements in various CYP gene promoters including CYP2B6. Ligands of these receptors include rifampicin, barbiturates, cyclophosphamide, statins, and others.

The CYP2B6 enzyme metabolizes many diverse chemicals including not only clinically used drugs but also pesticides and other environmental chemicals. Therapeutically important drugs metabolized mainly by CYP2B6 include the prodrug cyclophosphamide, which is activated by 4-hydroxylation, the non-nucleoside reverse transcriptase inhibitor efavirenz, the atypical antidepressant and smoking cessation agent bupropion, the antimalarial artemisinin, the anesthetics propofol and ketamine, and others (Table 4-1). CYP2B6 can also be reversibly or irreversibly inhibited by a variety of agents, including clopidogrel, thiotepa, ticlopidine, or voriconazole, which can lead to drug-drug interactions.

The *CYP2B6* gene is extensively polymorphic with numerous variants in the coding and noncoding regions of the gene. The most common variant *CYP2B6*6* harbors two amino acid changes (Gln172His and Lys262Arg) and occurs with a frequency of 15% and 60% in different populations (Table 4-1). The c.516G>T [Gln172His] polymorphism was identified as the major causal variant for decreased expression due to incorrect splicing of the CYP2B6 pre-mRNA, which results in a shorter mRNA that lacks exons 4 to 6. Another important functionally deficient allele is *CYP2B6*18* (c.983C>T [I328T]), which occurs predominantly in African subjects with allele frequencies of 3% to 8%. *CYP2B6*22* is associated with increased activity due to a TATA-box polymorphism that rearranges the promoter occupancy and also results in synergistically enhanced CYP2B6 inducibility in human primary hepatocytes. Additional alleles with low or absent function occur at low frequency in different populations (see CYP Allele website, listed later).

The major clinical role of *CYP2B6* polymorphism is in HIV therapy, as CYP2B6 is the major enzyme responsible for 8-hydroxylation of efavirenz. This drug is a component of common highly active antiretroviral therapy regimes. Patients with subtherapeutic plasma concentrations can develop resistance and treatment failure, whereas those with elevated plasma levels are at increased risk of central nervous system (CNS) side effects, which can lead to treatment discontinuation in a fraction of patients. Homozygosity for the 516T variant is associated with severalfold higher median efavirenz levels compared to carriers of only one or no T allele as shown in numerous clinical studies. In one prospective study, the dose of efavirenz could be successfully reduced and CNS-related side effects decreased, demonstrating the feasibility of genotype-based dose adjustment. In addition to efavirenz, *CYP2B6* genotype likely also affects plasma levels of nevirapine, cyclophosphamide, bupropion, and methadone.

## CYP2C9 Enzyme Characteristics and Clinical Pharmacogenetics

CYP2C9 belongs to the *CYP2C* gene subfamily, which also harbors CYP2C8 and CYP2C19 as functional but less abundant proteins. CYP2C9 is one of the major drug-metabolizing CYPs in human liver. It accepts weak acidic substances as substrates, including the anticoagulant warfarin, the anticonvulsants phenytoin and valproic acid, the angiotensin receptor blockers candesartan and losartan, oral antidiabetics like glyburide and tolbutamide, and most nonsteroidal anti-inflammatory drugs (NSAIDs). Commonly used substrates for CYP2C9 phenotyping are diclofenac and tolbutamide (Table 4-1). CYP2C9 inhibition has been observed by amiodarone, fluconazole, sulfaphenazole, voriconazole, and, notoriously, tienilic acid (irreversible inhibition leading to LKM2 autoantibodies). Inhibition can be clinically important, for example in the case of warfarin treatment.

Two variant alleles of CYP2C9 have clinical relevance (Table 4-1): CYP2C9*2 [R144C] and CYP2C9*3 [I359L] occur with low frequency in African and Asian populations, but at higher frequency in Caucasians and Hispanics (Table 4-1). Expressed mutant CYP2C9.2 and CYP2C9.3 proteins have reduced intrinsic clearance, although the degree of activity reduction appears to depend on the particular substrate. The widely used marker substrate diclofenac is not a sensitive substrate to detect the *2/*3 activity difference. Compared to the *2 allele, the *3 allele is more severely affected and can be reduced 70% to 90% for some substrates. In vivo, this results in clearance reductions of more than 70% in *3/*3 homozygotes and in about half of the clearance for heterozygotes. Other more rare alleles with decreased function are also known.

Numerous studies have demonstrated the clinical significance of the CYP2C9*2 and *3 polymorphisms for most drug substrates mentioned in Table 4-1. Due to their common occurrence in Caucasians, there are about 1% to 2% of homozygous (*2/*2, *3/*3) and hemizygous (*2/*3) carriers that are at risk of adverse effects such as hypoglycemia following treatment with hypoglycemic drugs, gastrointestinal bleeding from NSAIDs, and serious bleeding from warfarin treatment. The anticoagulant warfarin is the best-studied clinical application of CYP2C9 pharmacogenetics. Variants in CYP2C9 but also in the vitamin K epoxide reductase complex subunit 1 (VKORC1) affect warfarin dosing and response, reported by several retrospective and prospective studies. The influence of CYP2C9 polymorphisms on the metabolism of first- and second-generation sulfonylurea hypoglycemic drugs has also been well established. In contrast, only limited data is available for the role of CYP2C9 polymorphism in the NSAID-related risk for gastrointestinal bleeding.

## CYP2C19 Enzyme Characteristics and Clinical Pharmacogenetics

Compared to CYP2C8 and CYP2C9, CYP2C19 is less abundant in liver. However, the CYP2C19 polymorphism (also known as the mephenytoin polymorphism) has marked impact on the metabolism of numerous drugs (Table 4-1), including the proton pump inhibitors omeprazole and pantoprazole, the antiplatelet agent clopidogrel, and several antidepressants. CYP2C19 can be transcriptionally induced via nuclear receptors CAR and PXR. Inhibition of CYP2C19 occurs by some substrates like clopidogrel and omeprazole, as well as by fluvoxamine, ticlopidine, and voriconazole.

The two most important null alleles are CYP2C19*2, which occurs almost exclusively in Caucasians, and CYP2C19*3, which occurs primarily in Asians (Table 4-1). The causal mutation of the *2 allele is located in exon 5 and affects the consensus splice site, whereas that of *3 in exon 4 creates a premature stop codon. A further clinically relevant variant is the promoter variant -806C>T (*17) which is associated with increased activity in some studies. Further rare null alleles and variants with unknown phenotypic penetrance are also known.

The clinical significance of CYP2C19 has been extensively documented. For example, the CYP2C19 polymorphism clearly affects Helicobacter pylori eradication success by triple therapy in patients with ulcers. As CYP2C19 metabolizes proton pump inhibitors, the increase in intragastric pH and treatment outcome depend on CYP2C19 genotype, with PM subjects showing significantly higher eradication rates compared to EMs. Since proton pump inhibitors are also used in the treatment of nonulcer dyspepsia, reflux esophagitis, gastroesophageal reflux disease (GERD), the Zollinger-Ellison syndrome, and prevention and treatment of NSAID-associated damage, healing rates of these symptoms are also influenced by CYP2C19 genotype.

CYP2C19 is a genetic determinant of the efficacy of the platelet aggregation inhibiting thienopyridine, clopidogrel. Numerous clinical studies have confirmed that CYP2C19 PMs have a significantly lower anticoagulation effect from clopidogrel, which is associated with an increased risk of major adverse cardiovascular events. Pharmacokinetic effects associated with CYP2C19 genotype are also known for several antidepressants, benzodiazepines, the antifungal agent voriconazole, and the antimalarial drug proguanil, although an influence of CYP2C19 genotype on clinical pharmacodynamic outcome for most of these drugs remains so far controversial. Several clinical studies also confirmed a clinical impact of the gain-of-function allele CYP2C19*17, for example, for omeprazole, clopidogrel, escitalopram, and tamoxifen. However, not all studies have identified a significant effect of CYP2C19*17.

## CYP2D6 Enzyme Characteristics and Clinical Pharmacogenetics

CYP2D6 is the only protein-coding gene of the CYP2D locus on chromosome 22q13, which also harbors two pseudogenes, CYP2D7 and CYP2D8P. CYP2D6 is considered to be essentially a noninducible gene not significantly influenced by smoking, alcohol consumption, or gender. Hepatic CYP2D6 protein content varies dramatically from person to person. CYP2D6 is also expressed in several extrahepatic tissues, most notably in the gastrointestinal tract and in different areas of the human brain. In fetal liver, CYP2D6 is virtually undetectable but expression surges within hours after birth.

CYP2D6 metabolizes a large number of drugs from different therapeutic classes including antiarrhythmics (eg, propafenone, mexiletine, flecainide), tricyclic and second-generation antidepressants (eg, amitriptyline, paroxetine, venlafaxine), antipsychotics (aripiprazole, risperidone), beta-blockers (bufuralol, metoprolol), as well as anticancer drugs (tamoxifen), opioid analgesics (codeine, tramadol), and many others (Table 4-1). Test drugs that can be used to determine the CYP2D6 drug oxidation phenotype are debrisoquine, dextromethorphan, metoprolol, or sparteine. CYP2D6 inhibition occurs by numerous compounds that bind to the enzyme with high affinity, for example, quinidine, fluoxetine, haloperidol, and paroxetine. Some of these inhibitors are potent enough to change the apparent phenotype of the patient, a phenomenon known as phenocopying.

*CYP2D6* polymorphisms comprise a wide spectrum of genetic variants, ranging from null alleles to severalfold gene amplification. The CYP2D6 PM phenotype occurs in 5% to 10% of Caucasian populations but at much lower incidence in other races (Table 4-1). The most frequent null allele is *CYP2D6\*4*, which harbors a consensus splice site mutation (1846G>A) that leads to absence of detectable protein in the liver and accounts for 70% to 90% of all PMs. The *CYP2D6* gene deletion allele *\*5* is present at a frequency of approximately 3% to 6% in most populations. Several null alleles of lower frequency are also known. Heterozygous carriers of one defective and one normal allele of *CYP2D6* tend to have a lower median enzyme activity. The IM phenotype is caused by the presence of one partially defective allele (in Caucasians *\*41*, in Asians *\*10*, and in Africans *\*17*), in combination with another partially active or null allele such as *\*4*. Structural variations at the *CYP2D* locus include variants with deleted, duplicated, or otherwise recombined genes. *CYP2D6* gene duplications occur with different functional and nonfunctional alleles, which is important for phenotype prediction. The overall frequency of the gene duplications in Caucasians is between 1% and 5% whereas in some Arabian, Eastern African, and Pacific populations it can reach 10% and even up to 50% and more. Studies documenting the clinical importance of *CYP2D6* polymorphisms in adverse drug reactions involving agents that are either inactivated or activated by the enzyme include investigations on metoprolol, propafenone and other antiarrhythmics, amitriptyline and other antidepressants, antipsychotics, codeine and other opioids, tamoxifen, and the chemically related infertility drug clomiphene.

## CYP3A4/5 Enzyme Characteristics and Clinical Pharmacogenetics

The human CYP3 family consists of the only subfamily, CYP3A, which comprises the four CYPs 3A4, 3A5, 3A7, and 3A43. CYP3A4 is one of the most abundant CYPs in human liver and intestine, whereas CYPs 3A5, 3A7, and 3A43 are generally minor forms; CYP3A7 is more abundantly expressed in fetal liver than in adult liver. *CYP3A* genes, in particular *CYP3A4*, are highly inducible via ligands of the nuclear xenosensors PXR and CAR, including barbiturates, rifampicin, and statins. Additional ligand-dependent transcriptional regulators of CYP3A4 include the bile acid receptor FXR, the glucocorticoid receptor, the oxysterol receptor LXR, and the vitamin D receptor. CYP3A4 and CYP3A5 have largely overlapping substrate specificity and together account for the metabolism of approximately 30% to 40% of all clinically used drugs (Table 4-1). Typical substrates are immunosuppressants like cyclosporin A and tacrolimus, macrolide antibiotics like erythromycin, anticancer drugs including taxol, cyclophosphamide, ifosfamide, tamoxifen, benzodiazepines, the HMG-CoA reductase inhibitors simvastatin and atorvastatin, antidepressants, opioids, and many more.

CYP3A4 drug oxidation phenotype is strongly variable but unimodally distributed. Although there is evidence for substantial heritability, most of the currently known *CYP3A4* polymorphisms are either rare or lack phenotypic effect. An exception is the recently discovered CYP3A4\*22 (Table 4-1), a promising intron 6 variant showing association with decreased expression in liver and hepatocytes and in vivo pharmacokinetic and pharmacodynamic phenotypes, including statins, tacrolimus, and cyclosporine.

In contrast to CYP3A4, expression of CYP3A5 in liver is polymorphic as only a fraction of about 5% to 10% of Caucasians, but 60% or more of Africans or African Americans express this isoform due to a common mutation in intron 3 that leads to aberrant splicing and a truncated protein, and occurs in all ethnic groups at various frequency (Table 4-1). Despite the pronounced polymorphic expression of CYP3A5, there is a lack of penetrance to pharmacokinetics and pharmacodynamics, mainly due to the overlap in substrate selectivity among the CYP3A enzymes. Associations with *CYP3A5* genotype were reported in particular for the immunosuppressant tacrolimus, the antihypertensive verapamil, and the HIV protease inhibitor saquinavir.

***Genetic Testing:*** The presence of the pseudogenes, structural variants, and numerous SNPs at the *CYP* loci requires particular caution in the design of genotyping assays. Coamplification of pseudogenes, unexpected recombination events, and failure to account for important variants (eg, due to ethnic variation) can lead to erroneous interpretation of genotype. The most comprehensive commercially available platform for *CYP2D6* and *CYP2C19* genotyping is the AmpliChip CYP450 (Roche). This microarray has probes to identify 33 *CYP2D6* alleles, including most confirmed variants responsible for absent or impaired enzyme activity and seven gene duplications, as well as two *CYP2C19* variant alleles.

Genetic testing is not routinely available. The clinical utility of testing depends on drug, CYP, and clinical situation and is currently being debated and assessed in numerous clinical trials.

***Future Directions:*** The CYPs and polymorphisms selected for this chapter represent the best-studied and clinically most relevant examples. Future directions on these and other polymorphic *CYP* genes should include basic as well as clinical aspects. Among the basic aspects, it will be interesting to see how many rare mutations exist among these genes, and its contribution to the total variability. Current progress in the 1000 Genomes project and by targeted resequencing suggests that the number of unknown rare polymorphisms and private mutations could indeed make a major contribution to interindividual variability. This would be of particular relevance for those CYPs that are so far considered as essentially nonpolymorphic. However, the task is a difficult one, because available in vitro test systems are time consuming and unreliable; in vivo testing on the other hand is impractical due to the low SNP frequencies, and prediction of mutation effects even more difficult, especially for intronic and promoter variants. Furthermore, polymorphisms in trans-acting genes, for example, genes that influence monooxygenase activity (eg, NADPH: CYP reductase, cytochrome b5) or in the numerous regulatory genes involved in transcriptional, post-transcriptional, and post-translational regulation have so far not been systematically investigated. These directions may ultimately reveal the true genetic contribution to variable CYP-dependent drug metabolism phenotype. Future clinical directions should focus on the proper evaluation of clinical outcomes and ultimately the clinical utility as well as practicality of CYP genotyping. A pharmacogenetic test is considered clinically useful when it can be shown to improve drug therapy in terms of efficacy or safety, whereas practicality requires development of a suitable infrastructure, including testing facility, instructed personnel, and incorporation into the general healthcare system. Important is that *CYP* genotyping alone cannot be the answer. For each drug, the relevant genes have to be defined and tested, along with other factors (sex, age, health and nutritional condition, and many more), in order to exploit the full potential of pharmacogenetics for drug therapy. Systems biology approaches, in particular physiology-based pharmacokinetic and pharmacodynamic modeling of the complex interplay between the many levels and facets of drug-organism interactions should also be expected to make major contributions in the future toward implementing pharmacogenetic testing in personalized medicine.

## BIBLIOGRAPHY:

1. Meyer UA. Pharmacogenetics—five decades of therapeutic lessons from genetic diversity. *Nat Rev Genet.* 2004;5(9):669-676.

2. Eichelbaum M, Ingelman-Sundberg M, Evans WE. Pharmacogenomics and individualized drug therapy. *Annu Rev Med.* 2006;57:119-137.

3. Zanger UM, Turpeinen M, Klein K, Schwab M. Functional pharmacogenetics/genomics of human cytochromes P450 involved in drug biotransformation. *Anal Bioanal Chem.* 2008;392(6): 1093-1108.

4. Phillips KA, Veenstra DL, Oren E, Lee JK, Sadee W. Potential role of pharmacogenomics in reducing adverse drug reactions: a systematic review. *JAMA.* 2001;286(18):2270-2279.

5. Zanger UM, Klein K, Saussele T, Blievernicht J, Hofmann MH, Schwab M. Polymorphic CYP2B6: molecular mechanisms and emerging clinical significance. *Pharmacogenomics.* 2007;8(7):743-759.

6. Telenti A, Zanger UM. Pharmacogenetics of anti-HIV drugs. *Annu Rev Pharmacol Toxicol.* 2008;48:227-256.

7. Rosemary J, Adithan C. The pharmacogenetics of CYP2C9 and CYP2C19: ethnic variation and clinical significance. *Curr Clin Pharmacol.* 2007;2(1):93-109.

8. Jonas DE, McLeod HL. Genetic and clinical factors relating to warfarin dosing. *Trends Pharmacol Sci.* 2009;30(7):375-386.

9. Klotz U. Clinical impact of CYP2C19 polymorphism on the action of proton pump inhibitors: a review of a special problem. *Int J Clin Pharmacol Ther.* 2006;44(7):297-302.

10. Zanger UM, Raimundo S, Eichelbaum M. Cytochrome P450 2D6: overview and update on pharmacology, genetics, biochemistry. *Naunyn Schmiedebergs Arch Pharmacol.* 2004;369(1):23-37.

11. Schaeffeler E, Schwab M, Eichelbaum M, Zanger UM. CYP2D6 genotyping strategy based on gene copy number determination by TaqMan real-time PCR. *Hum Mutat.* 2003;22(6):476-485.

12. Sadee W, Wang D, Papp AC, et al. Pharmacogenomics of the RNA world: structural RNA polymorphisms in drug therapy. *Clin Pharmacol Ther.* 2011;89(3):355-365.

## WEBSITES:

1. The Human Cytochrome P450 (CYP) Allele Nomenclature Database http://www.cypalleles.ki.se/

2. PharmGKB: Pharmacogenomics Knowledge Base http://www.pharmgkb.org/

3. Substrates, inhibitors, inducers of P450 isozymes at the Indiana University School of Medicine Division of Clinical Pharmacology http://medicine.iupui.edu/clinpharm/ddis/

4. Cytochrome P450 Homepage. A comprehensive cytochrome P450 website http://drnelson.uthsc.edu/CytochromeP450.html

5. Cytochrome P450 nomenclature (HUGO Gene Nomenclature Committee) http://www.genenames.org/genefamilies/CYP

## Supplementary Information

### OMIM REFERENCES:

[1] Cytochrome P450, Subfamily IIB, Polypeptide 6; CYP2B6 (OMIM# 123930)

[2] Poor Metabolism of Efavirenz; CYP2B6 (OMIM# 614546)

[3] Cytochrome P450, Subfamily IIC, Polypeptide 9; CYP2C9 (OMIM# 601130)

[4] Coumarin Resistance; CYP2C9 (OMIM# 122700)

[5] Cytochrome P450, Subfamily IIC, Polypeptide 19; CYP2C19 (OMIM# 124020)

[6] Poor Drug Metabolism, CYP2C19-Related (OMIM# 609535)

[7] Cytochrome P450, Subfamily IID, Polypeptide 6; CYP2D6 (OMIM# 124030)

[8] Poor/Ultrarapid Drug Metabolism, CYP2D6-Related (OMIM# 608902)

[9] Cytochrome P450, Subfamily IIIA, Polypeptide 4; CYP3A4 (OMIM# 124010)

[10] Cytochrome P450, Subfamily IIIA, Polypeptide 5; CYP3A5 (OMIM# 605325)

### Alternative Names:

- The *CYP* genes and enzymes mentioned here are named according to the internationally valid cytochrome P450 gene nomenclature rules. Previously used alternative names are no longer in use (for a compilation of alternative names and historically used symbols see website 5).

*Key Words:* Cytochrome P450, drug metabolism, pharmacogenetics, pharmacogenomics, phase I enzyme, polymorphism, xenobiotic

# 5 Thiopurine Methyltransferase Pharmacogenetics

Ronald A. Booth and Mohammed T. Ansari

## KEY POINTS

- *Clinical utility of thiopurine methyltransferase analysis:*
  - Various guidelines recommend pre-thiopurine therapy thiopurine methyltransferase (TPMT) assessment in managing chronic inflammatory conditions.
  - There is insufficient evidence base to recommend pretherapy TPMT assessment.
  - Decreased or absent TPMT activity is associated with increased risk of myelotoxicity and leukopenia in patients treated with thiopurine medications (azathioprine [AZA] or 6-mercaptopurine [6-MP]).
  - Decreased or absent TPMT activity is not associated with hepatitis or pancreatitis in patients treated with thiopurine medications (AZA or 6-MP).
  - Reduced or absent TPMT activity does not place patients at risk of disease.
- *Medication(s) affected:*
  - Thiopurine drugs AZA and 6-MP. Limited effects on 6-thioguanine (6-TG), as TPMT is not the major metabolic enzyme.
- *Drug-related adverse events:*
  - Thiopurine treatment may be associated with anemia, myelotoxicity and leukopenia, hepatitis, and pancreatitis.
- *TPMT deficiency:*
  - The presence of mutant TPMT alleles or decreased TPMT enzymatic activity increases the risk of thiopurine treatment-related myelotoxicity and leukopenia.
- *Non-TPMT–associated myelosuppression:*
  - Normal TPMT testing does not rule out all the risk of myelotoxicity for patients on thiopurine medications.
- *Analytic methods:*
  - Genotyping—most common mutant alleles (*TPMT*2, *TPMT*3A, *TPMT*3B, and *TPMT*3C) are routinely available through reference laboratories.
  - Enzymatic analysis—less commonly available, but is the preferred method as it will also detect rare mutations not identified by genetic screening. Recent blood transfusions (within 90 days) can produce incorrect results.

## Thiopurine Drugs and Metabolic Pathway

*Biochemistry:* AZA, 6-MP, and 6-TG are thiopurine-based pro-drugs that have no intrinsic biologic activity, and require extensive metabolism for activity (Fig. 5-1). After oral administration of AZA or 6-MP, between 27% and 83% is available as biologically active metabolites. AZA is often used clinically, as it is more stable and soluble than 6-MP. AZA doses are higher because the molecular weight of 6-MP is 55% of that of AZA.

In the gut, approximately 90% of AZA is converted to 6-MP, a thiopurine analogue of the purine base hypoxanthine, by cleavage of the imidazolyl moiety which is thought to be catalyzed through the action of glutathione transferase. 6-MP is then enzymatically converted to its active metabolite, deoxy-6-thioguanosine 5' triphosphate (6-tGN), through successive enzymatic conversions by hypoxanthine-guanine phosphoribosyl transferase (HGPRT) and inosine monophosphate dehydrogenase (IMPDH). Inactivation of 6-MP (and hence AZA) occurs primarily through S-methylation by thiopurine S-methyltransferase (TPMT), and to a minor degree by catabolism, to thiouric acid by xanthine oxidase (XO). 6-TG is converted to its active metabolite (6-tGN) in a single step involving HGPRT, while inactivation occurs through two pathways. The major metabolic pathway involves guanine deaminase (GD) and aldehyde oxidase (AO) to form inactive 6-thiouric acid. Metabolism by TPMT, to form inactive 6-methyl-TG, is a minor contributor to

drug inactivation. TPMT also plays a minor role in directly methylating and inactivating 6-tGN.

Incorporation of 6-tGN into DNA triggers cell-cycle arrest and apoptosis through the mismatch repair pathway. Until recently, this was considered the primary mechanism of action. However, recent evidence has suggested other mechanisms of immunosuppression not directly related to 6-tGN incorporation into DNA. Metabolism by TPMT of 6-thiomercaptopurine (6-tIMP), an intermediate metabolite, to produce 6-methyl–tIMP has been shown to inhibit de novo purine synthesis in lymphocytes, which likely contributes to the immunosuppressive effects of thiopurines. Furthermore, accumulation of 6-tGN in lymphocytes has been demonstrated to decrease the expression of TRAIL, TNFRS7, and α-4 integrin, effectively decreasing inflammation. Thiopurine drugs have also been shown to induce apoptosis in T cells through modulation of Rac1 activation on CD28 costimulation. Rac1 is a GTPase upstream of MEK, NF-κB, and bcl-xL. On binding of 6-thio-GTP with Rac1, activation of its downstream mediators is blocked, inducing apoptosis.

*Toxicity:* TPMT represents the predominant inactivation pathway of thiopurines in hematopoietic cells. Thiopurine-based drugs have been associated with various toxic adverse events, including myelosuppression, hepatotoxicity, pancreatitis, and flu-like symptoms, among others. One of the most serious dose-dependent reactions is myelosuppression, which is believed to be caused by increased 6-tGN levels (the active metabolite), either due to overdosing or a

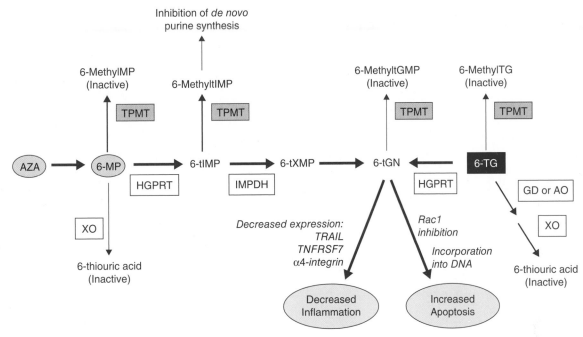

***Figure 5-1*** Metabolic Pathways of Thiopurine Drugs.
Reproduced with permission from Agency for Healthcare Research and Quality. Assessment of Thiopurine Methyltransferase Activity in Patients Prescribed Azathioprine or Other Thiopurine-Based Drugs. Evidence Report No 196, Published December 2010.

decreased rate of thiopurine metabolism due to impaired activity of the TPMT enzyme.

## TPMT Polymorphisms

The TPMT gene is located on chromosome 6 at 6p22.3. It is approximately 27 kb in size and contains nine exons. A nonfunctional TPMT pseudogene has also been identified on chromosome 18 at 18q21.1. TPMT is widely expressed in many tissues, but TPMT expression in lymphocytes, red blood cells, and bone marrow is most relevant clinically for immunosuppression by thiopurine drugs. To date, at least 30 variant (or mutant) alleles of TPMT have been identified, the majority of which have been associated with lower TPMT enzymatic activity or protein expression (Table 5-1).

Several studies have highlighted the importance of thiopurine drug metabolism by TPMT, as decreased activity of TPMT may place patients at higher risk of developing drug-related toxicity. The four most common alleles (*TPMT*\*2, *TPMT*\*3A, *TPMT*\*3B, and *TPMT*\*3C) seen in Caucasians, Asians, and Africans account for approximately 80% to 95% (dependent on ethnicity) of individuals with lower TPMT activity. When comparing genotype to phenotype (enzymatic activity), homozygous mutant individuals have very low or absent enzymatic activity while those heterozygous for a mutant allele demonstrate intermediate enzymatic activity between those of noncarrier and homozygous individuals. The frequency of the common alleles within each ethnic group varies, as does the overall number of individuals with lower TPMT activity. Heterozygous individuals with intermediate enzymatic activity comprise 5% to 15% of patients, while approximately 0.3% are homozygous, with very low or absent enzymatic activity. Individuals with intermediate or low or absent TPMT activity are otherwise healthy, but in theory more prone to thiopurine-related adverse events. Notwithstanding, up to 70% of patients

with thiopurine-related adverse events have normal TPMT activity; other factors such as viral infections, concomitant drug therapy, and other disturbances in the thiopurine metabolic pathway are likely to play a role.

## Utility and Dosing Strategies of Thiopurine Therapy

***Clinical Utility of Thiopurine Drugs:*** Thiopurines (AZA, 6-MP, and 6-TG) make up a class of immunosuppressive and chemotherapeutic drugs that is used effectively in the treatment of chronic autoimmune inflammatory conditions, hematologic malignancies, and prevention of organ transplant rejection. The clinical response to thiopurines varies according to the nature of disease, dose, and individual patient metabolism of the drugs.

AZA and 6-MP are currently widely used as steroid-sparing agents in chronic autoimmune inflammatory conditions, including pemphigoid, inflammatory bowel disease, and rheumatoid arthritis, among others. AZA and 6-MP are effective in inducing remission in 50% to 60% of inflammatory bowel disease patients, and permit steroid reduction or withdrawal in up to two-thirds of patients. Clinical response rates using AZA to treat nonbullous inflammatory dermatoses can be as high as 75%. However, use of AZA or 6-MP in other chronic inflammatory disorders including lupus and rheumatoid arthritis has been variable, and they are often not the primary drugs of choice. When used among organ transplant patients, although AZA has been associated with a 5-year renal graft survival ranging from 70% to 92%, use of AZA and 6-MP in transplantation has declined somewhat in favor of other immunosuppressive drugs. Both 6-MP and 6-TG have been used effectively in treatment of childhood acute lymphoblastic leukemia, with remission rates (5-year relapse-free survival) of approximately 80% using 6-MP.

Table 5-1 **TPMT Genetic Polymorphisms**

| Allele | Nucleotide | Amino Acid Substitution | Enzyme Activity | Allele Frequencies, % | | |
|---|---|---|---|---|---|---|
| | | | | White | African | Asian |
| TPMT*1 | WT | | Wild-type | | | |
| TPMT*2 | 277G→C | 80Alanine→proline | Low | 0-0.7 | 0-0.4 | 0 |
| TPMT*3A | 460G→A<br>719A→G | 154Alanine→threonine<br>240Tyrosine→cysteine | Low | 2.24-8.6 | 0-0.8 | 0-0.3 |
| TPMT*3B | 460G→A | 154Alanine→threonine | Significant decrease on in vitro assay | 0-0.13 | 0 | 0 |
| TPMT*3C | 719A→G | 240Tyrosine→cysteine | Decrease on in vitro assay | 0.1-0.8 | 2.4-10.1 | 0.6-4.75 |
| TPMT*3D | 460G→A<br>719A→G<br>292G→T | 154Alanine→threonine<br>240Tyrosine→cysteine<br>98Glutamic acid→stop | Intermediate | <0.1 | | |
| TPMT*4 | _1G→A (intron 9) | Splicing defect | Low | 0.002 | | |
| TPMT*5 | 146T→C | 49Leucine→serine | Decrease on in vitro assay | 0.0018[a] | | |
| TPMT*6 | 539A→T | 180Tyrosine→phenylalanine | Low | | | 0.2 |
| TPMT*7 | 681T→G | 227Histidine→glutamine | Intermediate | 0.3 | | |
| TPMT*8 | 644G→A | 95Arginine→histidine | Intermediate | | 0.2 | |
| TPMT*9 | 356A→C | 119Lysine→threonine | Intermediate or normal | 0.2 | | |
| TPMT*10 | 430G→C | 144Glycine→arginine | Decrease on in vitro assay | 1 patient (1 in 41 screened) | | |
| TPMT*11 | 395G→A | 132Cysteine→tyrosine | Low | 1 patient | | |
| TPMT*12 | 374C→T | 125Serine→leucine | Decrease on in vitro assay | 1 patient[a] | | |
| TPMT*13 | 83A→T | 28Glutamic acid→valine | Decrease on in vitro assay | 1 patient[a] | | |
| TPMT*14 | 1A→G | 1Methionine→valine | Low | 1 patient | | |
| TPMT*15 | 1G→A (intron 7) | Splicing defect | Low | 1 patient | | |
| TPMT*16 | 488G→A | 163Arginine→histidine | Intermediate | 0.1 | <0.1 | |
| TPMT*17 | 124C→G | 42Glutamine→glutamic acid | Intermediate | 0.1 | | |
| TPMT*18 | 211G→A | 71Glycine→arginine | Intermediate | 0.1 | | |
| TPMT*19 | 365A→C | 122Lysine→threonine | Normal | <0.1 | | |
| TPMT*20 | 712A→G | 277Lysine→glutamic acid | Intermediate | <0.1 | | |
| TPMT*20[b] | 106G→A | 36Glycine→serine | Significant decrease on in vitro assay | | 0.003 | |

20

| | | | | |
|---|---|---|---|---|
| TPMT*21 | 205C→G | 69Leucine→valine | Intermediate | <0.1 |
| TPMT*22 | 488G→C | 163Arginine→proline | Intermediate | <0.1 |
| TPMT*23 | 500C→G | 167Alanine→glycine | Low | 1 patient (but none in 200 screened) |
| TPMT*24 | 537G→T | 179Glutamine→histidine | Intermediate | <0.1 |
| TPMT*25 | 634T→C | 212Cysteine→arginine | Intermediate | <0.1 |
| TPMT*26 | 117T→C | 208Phenylalanine→leucine | Intermediate | 1 patient |
| TPMT*27 | 19T→G | 107Tyrosine→aspartic acid | Intermediate | 1 patient (but none in 220 screened) |

[a]Ethnicity not determined.

[b]Originally called TPMT*20, but another paper by the same group refers to this allele as TPMT*24.

TPMT, thiopurine S-methyltransferase.

Adapted from Annals of Internal Medicine.

Since myelosuppression in organ transplant and cancer patients pose several potential confounders (namely, concomitant myelosuppressive treatment and the short-term complications induced by procedures or disease), the following discussion on the clinical utility of TPMT analysis is restricted to populations with chronic autoimmune diseases.

## Clinical Utility of TPMT Analysis

Currently, there is no evidence that the presence of one or more mutant TPMT alleles causes disease or places one at increased risk for a disease. However, the presence of a mutant allele has been suggested to increase the risk of thiopurine-related drug toxicity, particularly when using AZA or 6-MP (6-TG is not metabolized to as great an extent by TPMT). Therefore, a fraction of patients prescribed thiopurines are at greater risk of developing drug-related toxicity. Until the availability of TPMT analysis, all patients were prescribed a standard starting dose of either AZA or 6-MP. The current starting dose for AZA ranges from 1 to 2.5 mg/kg/d and 0.75 to 1.25 mg/kg/d for 6-MP.

***Assessment of TPMT Status Prior to Treatment:*** Various clinical guidelines suggest measuring TPMT enzymatic activity or screening for TPMT alleles associated with reduced enzymatic activity before starting patients with chronic autoimmune diseases on thiopurine drugs. However, measuring TPMT activity may not by itself lead to reduced adverse events during thiopurine therapy since regular monitoring and continued dosage adjustments are also routinely undertaken, and other factors and concomitant therapies may also influence outcomes. Determinations of complete blood counts, including platelet counts are recommended weekly during the first month, twice monthly for the second and third months of treatment, then monthly or more frequently if dosage alterations or other therapy changes are necessary.

Indeed, a recent systematic review of the literature investigating the assessment of TPMT activity in patients prescribed thiopurines, we found very limited evidence to recommend pretreatment TPMT assessment. To date the utility of TPMT pretesting has been investigated in a single randomized trial. Newman et al. randomized 333 patients (with just one patient homozygous for TPMT mutation) with chronic inflammatory conditions into either a group that had prior TPMT genotyping or one without pretesting to investigate the utility of pretreatment TPMT analysis. Over a 4-month period, no significant differences between starting doses administered with or without prior knowledge of TPMT genotype were observed in both the noncarriers and heterozygous carrier patients. However, in the genotyped treatment arm, heterozygotes received significantly lower doses of TPMT when compared with noncarriers. Most patients in both groups were given starting doses lower than 2 mg/kg/d including those with predisclosed noncarrier genotype. About 7% of those in whom noncarrier genotype was predisclosed received AZA doses greater than or equal to 2 mg/kg/d, as compared to 8.4% of those in whom noncarrier genotype was found out after the fact. Furthermore, there was no significant difference between the two groups in terms of mean AZA prescribed dose at the end of the study period. As the trial was terminated early because of recruitment problems, it was underpowered to detect clinical events and drug dosing. No significant differences were noted in the outcomes of mortality, serious adverse events, neutropenia, and pancreatitis; whereas significantly higher odds were observed for hepatitis in the group randomly assigned to receive TPMT genotyping before therapy (odds ratio, 2.54 [95% CI, 1.08-5.97]).

In conclusion, the utility of pretesting for TPMT status before initiating thiopurine treatment remains equivocal. Insufficient evidence demonstrated that this strategy was effective to reduce harm or was superior to the established clinical standard of hematologic monitoring.

***Thiopurine Toxicity Associated With TPMT Status:*** We have previously confirmed earlier reports that reduced TPMT enzymatic activity or the presence of a TPMT variant allele is associated with an increased risk of myelotoxicity (enzymatic activity only) and leukopenia in chronic inflammatory disease patients. We found that compared with noncarriers, heterozygous and homozygous genotypes were both associated with higher risk of leukopenia (odds ratios, 4.29 [95% CI, 2.67-6.89] and 20.84 [95.4% CI, 3.42-126.89], respectively). Compared to patients with intermediate and normal TPMT enzymatic activities, those with low TPMT activities had odds of 14.53 (95% CI, 2.78, 76.01) and 19.12 (95% CI, 4.56, 80.24) for myelotoxicity and 2.74 (95% CI, 1.54, 4.86) and 2.56 (95% CI, 1.41, 4.67) for leukopenia, respectively. There was no significant association of reduced TPMT activity (or presence of mutant allele) with anemia, hepatitis, or pancreatitis.

## Molecular Genetics and Molecular Mechanism

***Analytic Methods:*** *Genetic analysis* is routinely available through reference laboratories. The majority of laboratories screen for the three to four most common mutant alleles which account for 80% to 95% of deficient patients. The most commonly identified mutant alleles are *TPMT*2, *TPMT*3A, *TPMT*3B, and *TPMT*3C. See Table 5-1 for a list of mutations identified to date. Analytic methods include restriction fragment length polymorphism (RFLP), denaturing high-performance liquid chromatography (HPLC), and direct sequencing. Although genetic analysis is readily available, it has the potential to misclassify patients with reduced TPMT activity as normal, since most laboratories only screen for the high prevalence alleles. Indeed, meta-analysis of 19 studies that genotyped all ethnicity-specific mutations with a known prevalence greater than 1% yielded a pooled sensitivity of 79.90% (CI, 74.81%-84.55%) for identification of a carrier genotype (heterozygous or homozygous) in patients with subnormal enzymatic activity (intermediate or low).

*Enzymatic analysis* is the preferred method of TPMT assessment. Although it is technically more complicated, it should detect any patients with reduced TPMT activity regardless of the mutant allele present. Since TPMT activity is based in red blood cells, one major limitation of enzymatic analysis is with patients that have undergone recent blood transfusions. It is suggested that TPMT testing should not be done within 2 to 3 months of any blood transfusions. In patients with recent history of blood transfusion, TPMT genotyping may instead be determined. It has been suggested that sulfasalazine use may affect TPMT analysis. One in vitro study showed concentration-dependent inhibition of TPMT from 11% to 55%, in the presence of 80 to 640 mol/L sulfasalazine.

TPMT enzymatic activity is normally determined by measuring the formation of 6-methylmercaptopurine (6-MMP) from 6-MP, with S-adenosyl-L-methionine (SAM) as the methyl donor. This was originally described by Weinshilboum et al., who used radiolabeled SAM. More recently, 6-MMP has also been measured using HPLC or mass spectrometry.

**Influence of drugs in vivo TPMT activity:** Our systematic review also included a review of the effects of a number of drugs on TPMT activity, including 5-aminosalicylate, sulfasalazine, mesalazine, AZA, mesalamine, ac-5-aminosalicylate, syringic acid, prednisone, prednisolone, 6-methylprednisolone, cyclophosphamide, methotrexate, trimethoprim-sulfamethoxazole, SKF 525-A, 3,4-dimethoxy-5-hydroxybenzoic acid, trimethoprim, vincristine, dexamethasone, L-asparaginase. Studies showing potential clinical significant effects were conducted in vitro, and therefore their in vivo influence on TPMT activity remains unknown. Two studies reported significant inhibition. 3,4-dimethoxy-5-hydroxybenzoic acid decreased TPMT activity by 97% in vitro. One in vitro study showed concentration-dependent inhibition of TPMT from 11% to 55%, in the presence of 80 to 640 mol/L sulfasalazine. One study reported 147% to 148% stimulation of TPMT activity in vitro by methotrexate and trimethoprim. However in a clinical diagnostic laboratory in many cases the red cells are rinsed prior to assay, which should remove extracellular inhibitory compounds. Six in vivo studies demonstrated no clinically relevant interactions. While the coadministration of interfering drugs will likely not affect the in vitro measurement of TPMT, these drugs may alter the in vivo activity of TPMT and hence the true in vivo TPMT may not be reflected by the measured TPMT activity. Care should be taken when prescribing AZA and 6-MP in combination with other drugs that may inhibit TPMT activity, although we did not find any evidence demonstrating clinically significant sequelae.

**Future Directions:** There is insufficient evidence of examining the effectiveness of TPMT pretreatment enzymatic or genetic testing to minimize thiopurine-related toxicity in patients with chronic autoimmune diseases. As a priority, well-powered, good quality, randomized controlled studies need to be conducted, in diverse and representative patient populations, to compare the effectiveness of TPMT genotyping and phenotyping with one another, and with no TPMT testing. These studies should be large enough to include a sizable number of patients homozygous for the variant alleles and should be pragmatic in conduct, mimicking routine clinical practice.

## BIBLIOGRAPHY:

1. Sahasranaman S, Howard D, Roy S. Clinical pharmacology and pharmacogenetics of thiopurines. *Eur J Clin Pharmacol.* 2008; 64:753-767.

2. Seki T, Tanaka T, Nakamura Y. Genomic structure and multiple single-nucleotide polymorphisms (SNPs) of the thiopurine S-methyltransferase (TPMT) gene. *J Hum Genet.* 2000;45:299-302.

3. Escousse A, Guedon F, Mounie J, et al. 6-Mercaptopurine pharmacokinetics after use of azathioprine in renal transplant recipients with intermediate or high thiopurine methyl transferase activity phenotype. *J Pharm Pharmacol.* 1998;50(11):1261-1266.

4. Gisbert JP, Gomollon F. Thiopurine-induced myelotoxicity in patients with inflammatory bowel disease: a review. *Am J Gastroenterol.* 2008;103:1783-1800.

5. Colombel JF, Ferrari N, Debuysere H, et al. Genotypic analysis of thiopurine S-methyltransferase in patients with Crohn's disease and severe myelosuppression during azathioprine therapy. *Gastroenterology.* 2000;118:1025-1030.

6. Menter A, Korman NJ, Elmets CA, et al. Guidelines of care for the management and treatment of psoriasis with traditional systemic agents. Guidelines of care for the management of psoriasis and psoriatic arthritis. *J Am Acad Dermatol.* 2009;61(3):451-485.

7. Lichtenstein GR, Abreu MT, Cohen R, Tremaine W. American Gastroenterological Association Institute medical position statement on corticosteroids, immunomodulators, and infliximab in inflammatory bowel disease. *Gastroenterology.* 2006;130: 935-939.

8. U.S. Food and Drug Administration—Center for Drug Evaluation and Research. Overview: Imuran [website]. http://www.accessdata.fda.gov/drugsatfda_docs/label/2011/016324s034s035lbl.pdf. Accessed Mar 8, 2011.

9. Booth RA, Ansari MT, Loit E, et al. Assessment of thiopurine S-methyltransferase activity in patients prescribed thiopurines: a systematic review. *Ann Intern Med.* 2011;154:814-823.

10. Newman WG, Payne K, Tricker K, et al. A pragmatic randomized controlled trial of thiopurine methyltransferase genotyping prior to azathioprine treatment: the TARGET study. *Pharmacogenomics.* 2011;12(6):815-826.

11. Loit E, Tricco AC, Tsouros S, Sears M, Ansari MT, Booth RA. Pre-analytic and analytic sources of variations in thiopurine methyltransferase activity measurement in patients prescribed thiopurine-based drugs: A systematic review. *Clin Biochem.* Jul 2011;44(10-11):751-757.

## Supplementary Information

### OMIM REFERENCE:

[1] Thiopurine S-Methyltransferase (TPMT); (#187680)

**Key Words:** Pharmacogenomics, thiopurine. thiopurine S-methyltransferase, TPMT, azathioprine, 6-mercaptopurine

# 6 Pharmacogenetics of Warfarin

Stuart A. Scott and Robert J. Desnick

## KEY POINTS

- *Drug summary:*
  - Warfarin (Coumadin) is a commonly prescribed vitamin K antagonist for the prevention of thromboembolism. However, the drug has a very narrow therapeutic index and a large interindividual variability in response, in part due to inherited genetic variability within genes involved in warfarin pharmacokinetics and pharmacodynamics.
  - Clinical indications for anticoagulation therapy include atrial fibrillation, mechanical heart valves, deep venous thrombosis, and dilated cardiomyopathies.
  - Interindividual and interethnic variability in therapeutic warfarin dose requirements is responsible for frequent adverse drug reactions and underutilization due to its toxicity.
  - Several factors affect warfarin dosage, including age, body weight, concomitant medications, and DNA sequence variants in cytochrome P450 2C9 (*CYP2C9*) and vitamin K epoxide reductase subunit 1 (*VKORC1*).
  - Common variant *CYP2C9* and *VKORC1* alleles are associated with impaired warfarin metabolism and sensitivity to warfarin, respectively, both resulting in lower therapeutic dose requirements.
  - Individuals with impaired warfarin metabolism and/or increased sensitivity require decreased dosage to avoid their international normalized ratio (INR) increasing beyond the target range (typically 2-3). Increased INR values can be associated with morbidity and mortality due to major bleeding episodes.
  - Although many variant *CYP2C9* and *VKORC1* alleles are found in several major racial and ethnic groups, some are specific to various subpopulations.
  - Pharmacogenetic dosing algorithms including both clinical and genetic variables have been developed that predict the therapeutic warfarin dose.
  - Clinical testing for variant *CYP2C9* and *VKORC1* alleles is available and generalized FDA-approved dosing recommendations are now noted on the warfarin package insert.
- *Monogenic forms:*
  - Rare heterozygous coding region *VKORC1* mutations cause warfarin resistance (OMIM #122700). These mutations make *VKORC1* less susceptible to warfarin inhibition, and generally result in doses in excess of 80 mg/wk to maintain appropriate anticoagulation. Homozygosity for these rare mutations results in combined deficiency of vitamin K-dependent clotting factors type 2 (OMIM #607473), which is responsive to oral administration of vitamin K.
- *Family history or heritability:*
  - The genetic determinants of warfarin dose variability are inherited germline variants, not acquired mutations.
- *Environmental factors:*
  - Age, diet, gender, body size, comorbidities, and concomitant medications are other factors that influence warfarin dosing.
- *Genome-wide associations:*
  - To date, three genome-wide association studies (GWAS) primarily using Caucasian patients have confirmed previous *CYP2C9* and *VKORC1* candidate gene studies, and have identified a small role for cytochrome P450 4F2 (*CYP4F2*) in warfarin dose variability.
- *Pharmacogenomics:*
  - *CYP2C9*, *VKORC1*, and *CYP4F2* have been estimated to account for approximately 10%, 25%, and 2.5% of the variability in warfarin dosing among individuals. Although the variant alleles of these genes may be less common in certain racial or ethnic groups, their effect on warfarin dose variability remains constant.

## Clinical Characteristics, Management, and Treatment

Warfarin is the most commonly used oral anticoagulant worldwide. Indications for warfarin therapy include the treatment and prevention of venous and arterial thromboembolism, including deep venous thrombosis, pulmonary embolus, atrial fibrillation, and mechanical heart valves. Treatment is often prolonged and the use of anticoagulants is steadily increasing with an aging population. For example, in the United States, approximately 2 million new patients start warfarin therapy every year. Despite a long history of clinical use, warfarin treatment remains very challenging due to its narrow therapeutic index and large interindividual variability in patient response.

***Narrow Therapeutic Index:*** Although warfarin is highly efficacious at the appropriate level of anticoagulation, it is less effective when anticoagulation levels are too low, and there is a significant risk of major bleeding complications when levels are too high. The rates of major bleeding in practice are approximately 7% to 8% per year; however, even minor bleeding can lead to withdrawal of therapy and repeat clinic and/or emergency room visits. The best predictors of bleeding complications are the INR and the variability in anticoagulation control. The risk of over-anticoagulation, and therefore of bleeding risk, is highest during the dose-titration period of warfarin use. Thus, genotype-guided warfarin dosing could reduce the risk of major bleeding and discontinuation of an efficacious therapy. In contrast, the effectiveness of warfarin is substantially reduced by insufficient levels of anticoagulation.

Specifically, the risk of thromboembolism increases dramatically as the INR falls below 2. In addition to these serious clinical concerns, patients who have out-of-range INR values must be reassessed, often requiring dosage changes, generating additional clinic visits, blood tests, and costs.

***Interindividual Dosing Variability:*** Although the average maintenance warfarin dose is 4 to 6 mg/d, there is a very wide range of doses required to achieve the same INR among individuals, varying by as much as 20-fold. Despite this, warfarin initiation remains largely empirical, with the majority of patients started on 5 mg/d during the initiation phase of treatment. Daily doses subsequently are titrated by INR until stable therapeutic warfarin doses are determined, which typically requires time (weeks), regular INR testing, frequent dose changes, and patient compliance. Even with careful follow-up, over- and under-anticoagulation are common during the initiation phase, reflected in high monthly bleeding rates during the first weeks of treatment. Reductions in the time that patients are over- or under-anticoagulated have been associated with reductions in bleeding, thromboembolism, and healthcare costs. Given INR values continue to fluctuate even after therapeutic INRs are attained on stable warfarin doses, patients typically require intermittent INR testing throughout their treatment.

***Pharmacogenetics:*** The response to warfarin is multifactorial. Patient, clinical, and environmental factors that influence warfarin dose requirements include adherence, age, gender, body size, treatment indication, diabetes mellitus, liver disease, malignancy, comedications, alcohol, and diet, among others. Importantly, recent evidence has indicated that a significant proportion of the variation in warfarin dose requirements can be attributed to common pharmacogenetic variation among genes involved in warfarin pharmacokinetics and pharmacodynamics, most notably *CYP2C9* and *VKORC1*, respectively. Together, common single-nucleotide polymorphisms (SNPs) within *CYP2C9* and *VKORC1* account for approximately 35% of warfarin dosing variability and notable variants are listed in Table 6-1. The identification of variant *CYP2C9* and *VKORC1* alleles in association with warfarin dosing prompted the FDA-approved warfarin product insert revision noting the availability of clinical genetic testing with dosing recommendations, and the recent inclusion of *CYP2C9* and *VKORC1* genotypes into pharmacogenetic-based dosing algorithms.

## Screening and Counseling

***Screening:*** Genotyping of *CYP2C9* and *VKORC1* variants is commercially available and should be performed prior to initiation of warfarin treatment or when treating a patient with a highly variable and unstable INR.

***Counseling:*** The *CYP2C9*, *VKORC1*, and *CYP4F2* pharmacogenetic variants, located at chromosome 10q23.33, 16p11.2, and 19p13.12, respectively, are inherited as autosomal codominant traits. They are not acquired mutations. Although specific alleles may have differing effects on enzymatic activity (eg, *CYP2C9* variants), they are fully penetrant. There are numerous *CYP2C9* variants with different frequencies in various ethnic and racial groups; however, *2* (p.R144C) and *3* (p.I359L) are the most commonly tested. For current information on variant *CYP2C9* alleles, refer to the Home Page of the Human Cytochrome P450 (CYP) Allele Nomenclature Committee: http://www.cypalleles.ki.se/cyp2c9.htm.

Like other CYP450 enzymes, CYP2C9 participates in the metabolism of several clinically important drugs and xenobiotics. In addition to warfarin, CYP2C9 also metabolizes tolbutamide, phenytoin, losartan, and anti-inflammatory drugs such as ibuprofen. Thus, carriers of variant *CYP2C9* alleles may also have altered metabolism of other clinically important medications. For additional pharmacogenetic information on CYP2C9, refer to the Pharmacogenomics Knowledge Base: http://www.pharmgkb.org.

Since 2006, the warfarin label has included a black box indicating that warfarin treatment can cause major or fatal bleeding, which is more likely to occur during the starting period and with a higher dose. Patients should be informed that genotyping provides improved warfarin dosing; however, all available clinical data should be taken into consideration with genetic testing results. For example, several drugs have been shown to be either inducers or inhibitors of CYP2C9, which can also influence warfarin dosing. It is estimated that the currently identified clinical and genetic variables together account for approximately 45% to 55% of the variation in warfarin dosing. To facilitate the clinical implementation of pharmacogenetic algorithm-guided warfarin dosing, the Clinical Pharmacogenetics Implementation Consortium (CPIC) has recently published a practice guideline for *CYP2C9* and *VKORC1* genotype-directed warfarin therapy.

## Molecular Genetics and Molecular Mechanism

Numerous studies have investigated the genetic contribution to interindividual variability in warfarin dosing, interrogating polymorphisms in candidate genes that encode metabolizing enzymes, the warfarin target in the vitamin K cycle, the gene responsible for vitamin K-dependent protein γ-carboxylation, and polymorphisms within the coagulation factors themselves, among others. Although a number of genes have been identified with moderate statistical influence on warfarin dosage, two genes, *CYP2C9* and *VKORC1*, have reproducibly been found to account for approximately 10% and 25% of the variability in warfarin dose, respectively. The principal genes involved in the pharmacokinetic and pharmacodynamic pathways of warfarin are illustrated in Fig. 6-1.

Although warfarin is a racemic mixture of R- and S-warfarin enantiomers, the more active isomer is S-warfarin. CYP2C9 is responsible for the majority of hepatic S-warfarin metabolism by converting the drug to the inactive 6-hydroxy and 7-hydroxy metabolites which are excreted in the urine. Like other CYP450 enzymes, the *CYP2C9* gene is highly polymorphic with over 35 reported variant alleles (http://www.cypalleles.ki.se/cyp2c9.htm). *CYP2C9*1* represents the reference sequence and wild-type allele. The most commonly studied variants are *2* (p.R144C) and *3* (p.I359L), which have allele frequencies of approximately 15% and 6% in Caucasians, respectively, but are less common in other racial and ethnic groups. In vitro studies have shown that *2* and *3* are functionally defective, exhibiting only approximately 70% and 5% of wild-type activity toward S-warfarin, respectively. Consequently, carriers of these alleles have impaired in vivo warfarin metabolism and, therefore, require lower maintenance doses of the drug. Several studies have confirmed the association between *CYP2C9* genotype and graded reductions in

*Table 6-1 Pharmacogenetic Considerations in Warfarin Dosing*

| Gene (Chromosome Location) | Associated Variant [effect on protein; dbSNP number] | Goal of Testing | Frequency of Risk Allele | Putative Functional Significance | Associated Phenotype |
|---|---|---|---|---|---|
| *CYP2C9* (10q23.33) | *2: c.430C>T [p.R144C; rs1799853]<br>*3: c.1075A>C [p.I359L; rs1057910]<br>*4: c. 1076T>C [p. I359T; rs56165452]<br>*5: c.1080C>G [p.D360E; rs28371686]<br>*6: c.818delA [p.K273fs; rs9332131]<br>*8: c.449G>A [p.R150H; rs7900194]<br>*11: c.1003C>T [p.R335W; rs28371685]<br>*13: c.269T>C [p.L90P; rs72558187] | Safety | Varies with ethnicity (see Scott et al., 2010) | Reduced activity | Deficient warfarin metabolism (lower therapeutic dose) |
| *VKORC1* (16p11.2) | *Warfarin sensitivity tag-SNPs:*<br>c.-1639G>A (rs9923231)<br>c.174-136C>T (1173C>T) (rs9934438)<br>c.283+124G>C (1542G>C) (rs8050894)<br>c.283+837C>T (2255C>T) (rs2359612)<br>Also known as "haplotype group A." | Safety | Varies with ethnicity (see Scott et al., 2010) | Reduced expression | Warfarin sensitivity (lower therapeutic dose) |
| *VKORC1* (16p11.2) | *Coding region mutations:*<br>c.85G>T [p.V29L; rs28940302]<br>c.106G>T [p.D36Y; rs61742245]<br>c.121G>T [p.A41S]<br>c.134T>C [p.V45A; rs28940303]<br>c.172A>G [p.R58G; rs28940304]<br>c.196G>A [p.V66M; rs72547529]<br>c.383T>G [p.L128R; rs28940305] | Safety | - p.D36Y: 1 in 12 Ashkenazi Jewish<br>- p.V66M: 1 in 100 African Americans<br>- Others: rare | Pharmaco-dynamic inhibition | Warfarin resistance (significantly increased therapeutic dose) |
| *CYP4F2* (19p13.12) | *3: c.1297G > A [p.V433M; rs2108622] | Safety | Varies with ethnicity (see Scott et al., 2010) | Reduced enzyme levels | Reduced vitamin $K_1$ metabolism (slightly increased therapeutic dose) |

warfarin dosage and these alleles are considered strong risk factors for over-anticoagulation and bleeding events when patients are initiated with standard doses (5 mg/d). In other ethnic groups such as African Americans and Asians, *2 and *3 are rare (~1%-3% allele frequencies); however, other *CYP2C9* variants are also observed. Although fewer studies have reported on the in vivo and/or in vitro association between the other *CYP2C9* alleles and warfarin dose, the available data indicate that *4 (p. I359T), *5 (p.D360E), *6 (p.K273fs), *8 (p.R150H), *11 (p.R335W), and *13 (p.L90P) have decreased enzymatic activity which results in impaired warfarin metabolism and reduced therapeutic doses (Table 6-1).

Warfarin acts as a vitamin K antagonist by inhibiting the regeneration of reduced vitamin K, an essential cofactor for the clotting cascade. The target enzyme for warfarin is VKORC1, which catalyzes the rate-limiting step in the vitamin K cycle. The identification of the *VKORC1* gene in 2004 prompted several investigations on the role of its genetic variability in oral anticoagulant drug response. Although very rare, homozygous *VKORC1* coding region mutations cause multiple coagulation factor deficiency type 2, whereas heterozygous mutations cause warfarin resistance (Table 6-1). Of note, not all patients requiring very high maintenance doses of warfarin carry *VKORC1* mutations. Other factors, such as noncompliance and excessive vitamin K intake, can contribute to a warfarin

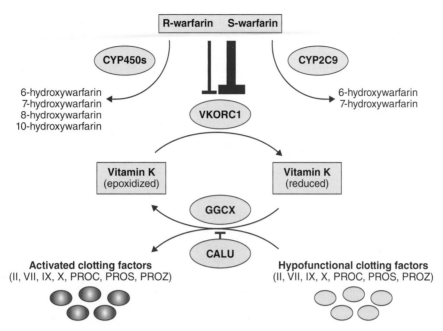

***Figure 6-1*** Warfarin Pharmacokinetics and Pharmacodynamics.

resistance phenotype independent of *VKORC1* status. The most common coding region mutation that is associated with elevated warfarin doses is the *VKORC1* p.D36Y variant found in approximately 1 in 12 individuals of Ashkenazi Jewish decent.

In contrast, common SNPs in regulatory regions of *VKORC1* correlate strongly with warfarin dose response across the normal dose range. Although several *VKORC1* polymorphisms in high linkage disequilibrium have been investigated in relation to warfarin (Table 6-1), two are widely studied and are the most common *VKORC1* alleles incorporated in clinical genotyping assays: c.-1639G>A and c.174-136C>T (1173C>T). Both of these intronic SNPs tag the same haplotype group, previously referred to as "haplotype A," and have reproducibly been shown to significantly correlate with warfarin dosage due to reduced hepatic *VKORC1* expression among individuals with the variant haplotypes. Specifically, carriers of the c.-1639A or c.174-136T alleles have lower therapeutic warfarin doses than individuals with c.-1639G or c.174-136C, and genotyping either of these alleles is estimated to account for approximately 25% of warfarin dosing variability. Like *CYP2C9*, the frequency of these variant *VKORC1* alleles vary between racial and ethnic groups, with allele frequencies of approximately 10%, 45%, and 70%, found among African American, Caucasian, and Asian individuals, respectively. Importantly, the effects of *VKORC1* c.-1639G>A or c.174-136C>T are additive with *CYP2C9* as similar *VKORC1*-mediated warfarin dosage effects are observed in patients with wild-type *CYP2C9* as those with variant *CYP2C9* genotypes.

In addition to *CYP2C9* and *VKORC1*, several studies have investigated other candidate genes to identify additional variants that influence warfarin dosing. Although some statistical associations have been observed in *GGCX*, *APOE*, *CALU*, and other genes in the warfarin pathway, all have had only a small impact on dosing variability and few have been independently reproduced. Three GWAS using primarily Caucasian patient cohorts have been reported, which confirmed the primary roles for both *CYP2C9* and *VKORC1* in warfarin dosing, and also identified a smaller role for *CYP4F2*. CYP4F2 has since been shown to be a vitamin $K_1$

oxidase, whereby the identified nonsynonymous SNP associated with warfarin dosing, c.1297G>A (p.V433M; rs2108622), results in reduced capacity to metabolize vitamin $K_1$. Thus, patients carrying this allele are predisposed to elevated hepatic levels of vitamin $K_1$, necessitating a higher warfarin dose for a therapeutic anticoagulant response. Although p.V433M (*CYP4F2*3*) was only responsible for approximately 1% to 2.5% of the remaining variation in warfarin dose, patients homozygous for this allele required 1 to 2.5 mg/d more warfarin to achieve stable anticoagulation than wildtype homozygotes, indicating that this variant may have clinical utility. Like *CYP2C9* and *VKORC1*, the frequency of *CYP4F2*3* varies between ethnic groups and is uncommon in the African-American population.

***Genetic Testing:*** Clinical genetic testing for variant *CYP2C9* and *VKORC1* alleles is available in selected laboratories and several different genotyping platforms exist, some of which are FDA approved. The majority of platforms interrogate *CYP2C9*2* (p. R144C) and *3* (p.I359L), and *VKORC1* c.-1639G>A (or c.174-136C>T); however, some offer more expanded allele coverage, which may be more suitable for non-Caucasian patients. In addition, some clinical laboratories may also include subpopulation-specific alleles (eg, p.D36Y for the Ashkenazi Jewish population) and/or the *CYP4F2*3* (p.V433M) variant.

Using genotype information to guide warfarin dose initiation has the potential to improve dosing accuracy, reduce the time to attain a stable dose, and may lead to improved outcomes in warfarin-treated patients, such as decreased hemorrhagic or thrombotic events associated with supra- or subtherapeutic anticoagulation, respectively. Several dosing algorithms have been developed that incorporate demographic, clinical, and genetic variables (including variant *CYP2C9* and *VKORC1* alleles), and some are freely available online (http://www.warfarindosing.org/). Consequently, some clinical diagnostic laboratories use these algorithms and provide a recommended warfarin dose based on genotype and provided clinical information; other laboratories will interpret the genetic results by suggesting higher or lower doses than usual. Additionally, some laboratories will refrain from any formal warfarin

*Table 6-2* **Range of Expected Therapeutic Warfarin Doses Based on CYP2C9 and VKORC1 Genotypes**[a]

| VKORC1 (c.-1639G>A) | CYP2C9 | | | | | |
|---|---|---|---|---|---|---|
| | *1/*1 | *1/*2 | *1/*3 | *2/*2 | *2/*3 | *3/*3 |
| G/G | 5-7 mg | 5-7 mg | 3-4 mg | 3-4 mg | 3-4 mg | 0.5-2 mg |
| G/A | 5-7 mg | 3-4 mg | 3-4 mg | 3-4 mg | 0.5-2 mg | 0.5-2 mg |
| A/A | 3-4 mg | 3-4 mg | 0.5-2 mg | 0.5-2 mg | 0.5-2 mg | 0.5-2 mg |

[a]Adapted from the warfarin product insert: http://www.accessdata.fda.gov/drugsatfda_docs/label/2010/009218s108lbl.pdf. Accessed May 23, 2013.

dosing recommendations and interpret the *CYP2C9* and *VKORC1* genotype results by indicating their impact on warfarin metabolism and warfarin sensitivity, respectively. For example, patients with a *CYP2C9*1/*3* and *VKORC1* c.-1639G/A genotype would carry one variant allele from each gene and thus have both impaired warfarin metabolism and increased sensitivity to warfarin, likely necessitating a reduced therapeutic warfarin dose to achieve stable anticoagulation.

In early 2010, to facilitate physician interpretation of clinical *CYP2C9* and *VKORC1* genotyping, the FDA updated the Dosage and Administration section of the warfarin label to include a table containing stable maintenance doses observed in large patient cohorts with different combinations of *CYP2C9* and *VKORC1* variants (Table 6-2). The label recommends healthcare providers to consider these ranges in choosing the initial dose. Moreover, the label also states that patients with variant *CYP2C9* genotypes may require a prolonged time (>2-4 weeks) to achieve an optimal INR effect for a given dosage regimen.

Of note, these FDA-approved dosing recommendations are based on the three common genetic variants in *CYP2C9* and *VKORC1*. Less frequent *VKORC1* coding region mutations (eg, p.D36Y, p.V66M) are dominant and typically would result in much higher warfarin doses, regardless of the *CYP2C9* and/or *VKORC1* c.-1639G>A variants. In addition, the recommended dose ranges do not include the *CYP2C9* alleles that are prevalent in non-Caucasian populations. For example, the African-American and Hispanic populations also have variant *5, *6, *8, and *11 alleles, which also are associated with impaired warfarin metabolism and lower therapeutic dose requirements.

**Future Directions:** The genetic determinants of interindividual warfarin dosing variability have been intensively studied in order to identify DNA variants that influence dosage and, therefore, enable more accurate dose selection during the initiation of treatment. Although several candidate genes have been interrogated, common variants in *CYP2C9* and *VKORC1* have reproducibly been shown to be important in warfarin dosing. Randomized clinical trials currently are underway that will establish if using pharmacogenetic-based dosing algorithms to determine the initial dose of warfarin results in improved anticoagulation control and safer dosing. However, the majority of pharmacogenetic-based dosing algorithms have been designed based on studies using Caucasian individuals. As such, future directions in the warfarin pharmacogenetics field will undoubtedly identify racial- and ethnic-specific genetic variants that are unique or more prevalent among certain subpopulations. For example, recent studies identified the *VKORC1* p.D36Y allele that results in higher warfarin doses in the Ashkenazi

Jewish population (1 in 12 individuals), and the variant *CYP2C9*8* (p.R150H) and *CALU* (rs339097) alleles that are prevalent among African-American individuals. Furthermore, as rapid clinical genotyping for genes involved in warfarin dosing becomes more commonplace and standard of care, future studies will also determine the cost-effectiveness of such testing. However, of utmost importance to the warfarin pharmacogenetics field is adequate and appropriate physician education of clinical warfarin genetic testing and how to properly interpret these laboratory results for optimal and personalized patient care.

**BIBLIOGRAPHY:**

1. Caldwell MD, Awad T, Johnson JA, et al. CYP4F2 genetic variant alters required warfarin dose. *Blood.* 2008;111:4106-4112.

2. Cooper GM, Johnson JA, Langaee TY, et al. A genome-wide scan for common genetic variants with a large influence on warfarin maintenance dose. *Blood.* 2008;112:1022-1027.

3. Gage BF, Eby C, Johnson JA, et al. Use of pharmacogenetic and clinical factors to predict the therapeutic dose of warfarin. *Clin Pharmacol Ther.* 2008;84:326-331.

4. Flockhard DA, O'Kane D, Williams MS, et al. Pharmacogenetic testing of CYP2C9 and VKORC1 alleles for warfarin. *Genet Med.* 2008;10:139-150.

5. International Warfarin Pharmacogenetics Consortium. Estimation of the warfarin dose with clinical and pharmacogenetic data. *N Engl J Med.* 2009;360:753-764.

6. Limdi NA, Veenstra DL. Warfarin pharmacogenetics. *Pharmacotherapy.* 2008;28:1084-1097.

7. Lubitz SA, Scott SA, Rothlauf EB, et al. Comparative performance of gene-based warfarin dosing algorithms in a multiethnic population. *J Thromb Haemost.* 2010;8:1018-1026.

8. Schelleman H, Limdi NA, Kimmel SE. Ethnic differences in warfarin maintenance dose requirement and its relationship with genetics. *Pharmacogenomics.* 2008;9:1331-1346.

9. Scott SA, Khasawneh R, Peter I, et al. Combined CYP2C9, VKORC1, and CYP4F2 frequencies among racial and ethnic groups. *Pharmacogenomics.* 2010;11:781-791.

10. Takeuchi F, McGinnis R, Bourgeois S, et al. A genome-wide association study confirms VKORC1, CYP2C9, and CYP4F2 as principal genetic determinants of warfarin dose. *PLoS Genet.* 2009;5:e1000433.

11. Wadelius M, Pirmohamed M. Pharmacogenetics of warfarin: current status and future challenges. *Pharmacogenomics J.* 2007;7:99-111.

12. Wu AH, Wang P, Smith A, et al. Dosing algorithm for warfarin using CYP2C9 and VKORC1 genotyping from a multi-ethnic population: comparison with other equations. *Pharmacogenomics.* 2008;9:169-178.

13. Johnson JA, Gong L, Whirl-Carrillo M, et al. Clinical Pharmacogenetics Implementation Consortium Guidelines for CYP2C9 and VKORC1 genotypes and warfarin dosing. *Clin Pharmacol Ther.* 2011;90:625-629.

14. Scott SA, Edelmann L, Kornreich R, et al. Warfarin pharmacogenetics: CYP2C9 and VKORC1 genotypes predict different sensitivity and resistance frequencies in the Ashkenazi and Sephardi Jewish populations. *Am J Hum Genet.* 2008;82:495-500.

## Supplementary Information

### OMIM References:

[1] Coumarin Resistance (#122700)

[2] Combined Deficiency of Vitamin K-Dependent Clotting Factors Type 2 (#607473)

[3] Cytochrome P450 2A6 (#122720)

[4] Cytochrome P450 2C9 (#601130)

[5] Cytochrome P450 4F2 (#604426)

[6] Vitamin K Epoxide Reductase Complex, Subunit 1; VKORC1 (#604426)

### Alternative Names:

- Warfarin Sensitivity
- Warfarin Resistance
- Coumarin Resistance
- Warfarin Poor Metabolizer

*Key Words:* Warfarin, coumarin, sensitivity, resistance, cytochrome P450 2C9 (CYP2C9), vitamin K epoxide reductase subunit 1 (VKORC1), cytochrome P450 4F2 (CYP4F2)

# 7 Clopidogrel Pharmacogenomics

Janice Y. Chyou and Marc S. Sabatine

## KEY POINTS

- *Drug summary:*
  - Clopidogrel blocks the P2Y$_{12}$ adenosine diphosphate (ADP) receptor on the surface of platelets and thus inhibits platelet activation.
  - Despite established clinical efficacy, an inadequate response to clopidogrel has been observed in up to 30% of compliant patients. Such variability has been labeled as "clopidogrel nonresponsiveness," "clopidogrel hyporesponsiveness," and "clopidogrel resistance."
- *Pharmacogenomics:*
  - Clopidogrel is a prodrug that is subject to extensive CYP450 metabolism.
  - The genes encoding the relevant metabolizing enzymes have known functional polymorphisms.
  - In particular, the *CYP2C19*2* polymorphism is a loss-of-function variant that has been associated with lower levels of the active clopidogrel metabolite, diminished inhibition of ADP-induced platelet aggregation, and an increased risk of death and ischemic events in the setting of clopidogrel therapy and percutaneous coronary intervention.

## Clopidogrel Therapy

**Indications of Clopidogrel Use:** As part of dual antiplatelet therapy (aspirin + ADP receptor blocker) for acute coronary syndrome (ACS), percutaneous coronary intervention (PCI), antithrombotic therapy for primary stroke prevention in atrial fibrillation patients who are indicated for but are not candidates for warfarin therapy.

As monotherapy for secondary prevention of stroke as an alternate to Aggrenox (dipyridamole + aspirin) and for management of mixed atherothrombosis (defined as recent ischemic stroke, recent myocardial infarction (MI), or symptomatic peripheral arterial disease).

**Clopidogrel Pharmacology:** Clopidogrel is an oral thienopyridine ingested as a prodrug and undergoes extensive metabolism (Fig. 7-1). Absorption of the prodrug can be influenced by the xenobiotic efflux pump P-gp (encoded by *ABCB1*). If the prodrug is absorbed, approximately 85% is inactivated via hydrolysis by esterases into a carboxylic acid metabolite. The remaining 15% requires biotransformation by the hepatic cytochrome 450 system into an active thiol metabolite. The active metabolite, formed within several hours, irreversibly binds the P2Y$_{12}$ ADP receptor on the surface of platelets, leading to inhibition of ADP-dependent platelet activation and aggregation. Full antiplatelet effects occur within 4 to 6 hours and lasts for the lifetime of the platelet. Up to 30% of patients have a marginal degree of platelet inhibition in response to a standard 300 mg loading dose of clopidogrel.

## Clopidogrel Pharmacogenomics

Polymorphism of genes involved in clopidogrel absorption, metabolism, and binding of active metabolites have been explored (see Fig. 7-1 for pathway; see Table 7-1 for notable genetic polymorphisms). However, association between polymorphism of *CYP2C19* and clopidogrel response have been most consistently replicated and that *CYP2C19* polymorphism was the only significant polymorphism noted in a genome-wide association studies (GWAS) investigating genetic influence of clopidogrel response.

**CYP2C19 (boldfaced in Table 7-1):** *Reduced function variants:* Reduced-function variants in *CYP2C19* have been associated with lower levels of the active clopidogrel metabolite, diminished inhibition of ADP-induced platelet aggregation, and an increased risk of death and ischemic events in the setting of clopidogrel therapy and PCI.

In particular, the *2 variant (rs4244285) creates an aberrant splice site, leading to synthesis of a truncated, nonfunctional CYP2C19 protein. The *CYP2C19*2* genotype accounts for about 12% of the variation in clopidogrel response, when considering age, body mass index (BMI), and lipid levels, about 22% of variation in clopidogrel response can be explained. Less common reduced-function alleles include the nonfunctional *3 allele and the reduced-function *4, *5, *6, *7, and *8 alleles.

Enhanced function variant: The *CYP2C19*17* allelic variant has been linked to increased transcriptional activity of the CYP2C19 enzyme, leading to extensive clopidogrel metabolism. As such, the *CYP2C19*17* allelic variant has been associated with greater inhibition of ADP-induced platelet aggregation and an increased risk of bleeding; however, stent thrombosis in the setting of clopidogrel therapy does not seem to be affected.

## Management and Treatment

The Food and Drug Administration (FDA) added a black box warning to the Plavix label, noting diminished effectiveness in poor metabolizers, defined as having two loss-of-function alleles. The black box warning states, "Consider alternative treatment of treatment strategies in patients identified as CYP2C19 poor metabolizers."

However, limited evidence are available to guide potential therapeutic modifications for individuals with *CYP2C19*2* allele. Potential therapeutic modifications include escalation of clopidogrel dosage or switching to a different P2Y$_{12}$ ADP receptor blocker not subject to the same pharmacogenetic interactions:

- *Escalation of clopidogrel dosage*: Higher clopidogrel loading and maintenance dose (up to 1200 mg loading and 150 mg daily as maintenance) may improve platelet inhibition in carriers of

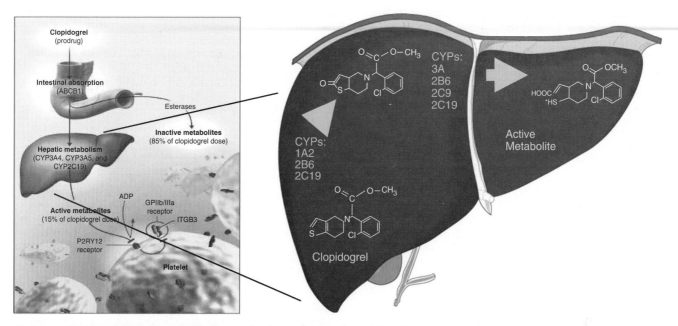

*Figure 7-1* Clopidogrel Absorption, Metabolism, and Action Pathway. Adapted from Simon T, Verstuyft C, Mary-Krause M, et al. Genetic determinants of response to clopidogrel and cardiovascular events. *N Engl J Med*. 2009;360:363-375.

reduced function *CYP2C19* alleles. The safety of long-term therapy with such high doses is unclear. Higher-dose clopidogrel during the first week post-PCI was studied (in all-comers, regardless of genotype) by the CURRENT-OASIS7 trial and reported at the 2009 European Congress of Cardiology. A loading dose of 600 mg with post-PCI maintenance dose of 150 mg for the first week followed by 75 mg daily thereafter was noted to reduce in-stent thrombosis and cardiovascular (CV) events compared to a loading dose of 300 mg followed by maintenance dose of 75 mg daily. The high-dose arm was associated with a modest increase in CURRENT-defined major bleeds but with no increase in TIMI major bleeds, intracranial hemorrhage, fatal bleeds, or coronary artery bypass graft (CABG)-related bleeds.

- *Prasugrel* is a third-generation thienopyridine P2Y$_{12}$ ADP receptor blocker. In PCI for ACS, compared to clopidogrel, prasugrel was found to have superior efficacy in reduction of the composite of CV death, MI, or stroke, including stent thrombosis; however, prasugrel was associated with increased risk of bleeding. Prasugrel was approved for use in PCI for ACS by the FDA in July 2009. Of note, responses to prasugrel, as measured by active drug metabolism levels, platelet aggregation inhibition, or clinical CV event rates, were not affected by *CYP2C19* polymorphism.
- *Ticagrelor*, an oral active reversible direct antagonist of platelet ADP P2Y$_{12}$, is a potential antiplatelet alternative to clopidogrel under FDA review. The PLATO trial found ticagrelor (loading dose of 180 mg with 90 mg twice-daily maintenance dose) to be superior to clopidogrel (loading dose of 300-600 mg with 75 mg daily maintenance dose) in reduction of vascular death, MI, or stroke, but with an increase in the rate of nonprocedure-related bleeding, in ACS.
- Neither of these third-generation agents has been studied in elective PCI.
- Other novel antiplatelet agents are actively being studied in clinical trials.

***Genetic Testing:*** (Fig. 7-2) Pharmacogenetic testing is not part of the current standard of care of clopidogrel therapy and there is a lack of consensus for whether individuals should be tested. The predictive value of pharmacogenetic testing for clopidogrel is still being defined.

Commercial testing kits for clopidogrel pharmacogenetics are being developed but have not been widely tested or standardized and reimbursement policy by insurance companies is unknown.

Feasibility and utility of clopidogrel pharmacogenetic testing may be compromised by cost and delay in return but the cost may be offset by the availability of clopidogrel in generic form in the near future.

Platelet function testing is currently used more widely than genetic testing. However, there remains controversy regarding the utility of platelet function testing, which remains a variable and imperfect surrogate for the risk of clinical events.

The observations of racial variability in *CYP2C19* polymorphism in addition to platelet function assays may help identify patients for testing.

Prospective clinical trials are needed to further evaluate if testing indeed improves outcome, if pharmacogenetic testing is superior to platelet function testing, and if testing of all-comers versus only the high-risk population is most feasible. These questions will need to be answered before pharmacogenetic testing of *CYP2C19* polymorphism can be recommended as part of standard of care for clopidogrel therapy.

***Future Directions:*** Future directions include research on novel antiplatelet agents, determination of optimal antiplatelet agent, and dosing in patients with reduced function of *CYP2C19* alleles, efficacy and safety of high clopidogrel loading dose in patients with or without *CYP2C19* reduced function allele, development of a standardized algorithm for approaching patients indicated for clopidogrel therapy, as well as elucidation of the role of genetic screening and counseling in clopidogrel therapy.

**Table 7-1 Key Susceptibility Variants Studied**

| Candidate Gene (Chromosome Location) | Encodes for | Variant Studied [effect on protein] | Frequency of Risk Allele | Associated Disease Phenotype and Relative Risk |
|---|---|---|---|---|
| *ABCB1* (7q21.1) | P-glycoprotein drug-efflux transporter, involved in intestinal absorption of clopidogrel | C3435T (rs1045642) | | • *Biochemical*: lower levels of the active metabolite<br>• *Clinical*: higher rate of cardiovascular events |
| *CYP3A4* (7q22.1) | Eponymous protein involved in clopidogrel metabolism | IVS10+12G>A | | • Association unclear: some reported association with reduced GPIIb/IIIa activation and enhanced clopidogrel response, while others showed no significant association with ADP-induced platelet aggregation |
| *CYP3A5* (7q22.1) | | *3 (rs776746, G6986A) [nonfunctional] | | • Association unclear: some showed an association with increased atherothrombotic events while others noted no significant association with antiplatelet effect or clinical outcome in setting of clopidogrel therapy |
| **CYP2C19 (10q24.1-q24.3)** | **Eponymous protein essential in the two-step CYP450 hepatic metabolism of clopidogrel prodrug** | **\*2 (rs4244285, G681A) [aberrant splice site; nonfunctional]** | • **15%-30% of whites**<br>• **40% of blacks, 55% of East Asians** | • ***Biochemical*: relative reduction of 25% in platelet inhibition and 32.4% in plasma exposure to the active metabolite**<br>• ***Clinical*: 1.5 to 2.4 times increased risks of cardiovascular events and 3 times increased risk of stent thrombosis** |
| | | **\*17 (rs12248560, C806T) [enhanced-function allele]** | • **22% of European, 0%-2% Asian, 28% Sub-Saharan African by HapMap** | • ***Biochemical*: enhanced inhibition of ADP-induced platelet aggregation**<br>• ***Clinical*: increased risk of bleeding, but without significant influence on stent thrombosis**<br>• **Both biochemical and clinical phenotypic effects exaggerated in subjects homozygous for \*17 allele** |
| *P2RY12* (3q24-q25) | Receptor for active clopidogrel metabolite | T744C | | • No significant change in clopidogrel response |

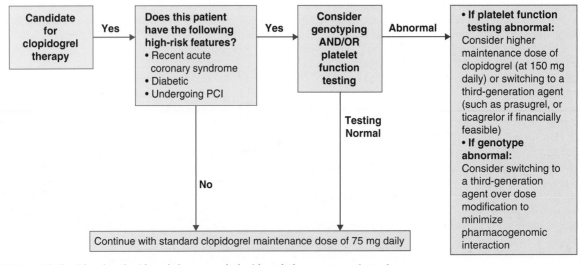

*Figure 7-2* Potential Algorithm for Clopidogrel Therapy and Clopidogrel Pharmacogenetic Testing.

**BIBLIOGRAPHY:**

1. Yusuf S, Zhao F, Mehta SR, et al. Effects of clopidogrel in addition to aspirin in patients with acute coronary syndromes without ST-segment elevation. *N Engl J Med*. 2001;345:494-502.

2. Sabatine MS, Cannon CP, Gibson CM, et al. Addition of clopido-grel to aspirin and fibrinolytic therapy for myocardial infarction with ST-segment elevation. *N Engl J Med*. 2005;352:1179-1189.

3. Chen ZM, Jiang LX, Chen YP, et al. Addition of clopidogrel to aspirin in 45,852 patients with acute myocardial infarction: ran-domised placebo-controlled trial. *Lancet*. 2005;366:1607-1621.

4. Sabatine MS, Cannon CP, Gibson CM, et al. Effect of clopidogrel pretreatment before percutaneous coronary intervention in patients with ST-elevation myocardial infarction treated with fibrinolytics: the PCI-CLARITY study. *JAMA*. 2005;294:1224-1232.

5. Mehta SR, Yusuf S, Peters RJ, et al. Effects of pretreatment with clopidogrel and aspirin followed by long-term therapy in patients undergoing percutaneous coronary intervention: the PCI-CURE study. *Lancet*. 2001;358:527-533.

6. Steinhubl SR, Berger PB, Mann JT 3rd, et al. Early and sus-tained dual oral antiplatelet therapy following percutaneous coronary intervention: a randomized controlled trial. *JAMA*. 2002;288:2411-2420.

7. ACTIVE Investigators, Pogue J, Hart RG, et al. Effect of clopido-grel added to aspirin in patients with atrial fibrillation. *N Engl J Med*. 2009;360:2066-2078.

8. Sacco RL, Yusuf S, Cotton D, et al. Aspirin and extended-release dipyridamole versus clopidogrel for recurrent stroke. *N Engl J Med*. 2008;359:1238-1251.

9. CAPRIE Steering Committee. A randomised, blinded, trial of clopidogrel versus aspirin in patients at risk of ischaemic events (CAPRIE). *Lancet*. 1996;348:1329-1339.

10. Taubert D, Kastrati A, Harlfinger S, et al. Pharmacokinetics of clopidogrel after administration of a high loading dose. *Thromb Haemost*. 2004;92:311-316.

11. Kandzari DE, Berger PB, Kastrati A, et al. Influence of treatment duration with a 600-mg dose of clopidogrel before percutaneous coronary revascularization. *J Am Coll Cardiol*. 2004;44:2133-2136.

12. Gurbel PA, Bliden KP, Hiatt BL, et al. Clopidogrel for coro-nary stenting: response variability, drug resistance, and the effect of pretreatment platelet reactivity. *Circulation*. 2003;107: 2908-2913.

13. Simon T, Verstuyft C, Mary-Krause M, et al. Genetic determinants of response to clopidogrel and cardiovascular events. *N Engl J Med*. 2009;360:363-375.

14. Shuldiner AR, O'Connell JR, Bliden KP, et al. Association of cytochrome P450 2C19 genotype with the antiplatelet effect and clinical efficacy of clopidogrel therapy. *JAMA*. 2009;302: 849-857.

15. Mega JL, Close SL, Wiviott SD, et al. Cytochrome P-450 poly-morphisms and response to clopidogrel. *N Engl J Med*. 2009; 360:354-362.

16. Collet JP, Hulot JS, Pena A, et al. Cytochrome P450 2C19 poly-morphism in young patients treated with clopidogrel after myocar-dial infarction: a cohort study. *Lancet*. 2009;373:309-317.

17. Sibbing D, Koch W, Gebhard D, et al. Cytochrome 2C19*17 allelic variant, platelet aggregation, bleeding events, and stent thrombo-sis in clopidogrel-treated patients with coronary stent placement. *Circulation*. 2010;121:512-518.

18. Giusti B, Gori AM, Marcucci R, et al. Relation of cytochrome P450 2C19 loss-of-function polymorphism to occurrence of drug-eluting coronary stent thrombosis. *Am J Cardiol*. 2009;103:806-811.

19. de Morais SM, Blaisdell J, Nakamura K, Meyer UA, Goldstein JA. The major genetic defect responsible for the polymorphism of S-mephenytoin metabolism in humans. *J Biol Chem*. 1994;269: 15419-15422.

20. Taubert D, von Beckerath N, Grimberg G, et al. Impact of P-glycoprotein on clopidogrel absorption. *Clin Pharmacol Ther*. 2006;80:486-501.

21. Simon T, Mary-Krause M, Quteineh L, et al. Genetic determinants of response to clopidogrel and cardiovascular events. *N Engl J Med*. 2009;360:363-375.

22. Angiolillo DJ, Fernandez-Ortiz A, Bernardo E, et al. Contribution of gene sequence variations of the hepatic cytochrome P450 3A4 enzyme to variability in individual responsiveness to clopidogrel. *Arterioscler Thromb Vasc Biol*. 2006;26:1895-1900.

23. Giusti B, Gori AM, Marcucci R, et al. Cytochrome P450 2C19 loss-of-function polymorphism, but not CYP3A4 IVS10 + 12G/A and P2Y12 T744C polymorphisms, is associated with response variability to dual antiplatelet treatment in high-risk vascular patients. *Pharmacogenet Genomics*. 2007;17:1057-1064.

24. Suh JW, Koo BK, Zhang SY, et al. Increased risk of atherothrom-botic events associated with cytochrome P450 3A5 polymorphism in patients taking clopidogrel. *CMAJ*. 2006;174:1715-1722.

25. Brandt JT, Close SL, Iturria SJ, et al. Common polymorphisms of CYP2C19 and CYP2C9 affect the pharmacokinetic and pharma-codynamic response to clopidogrel but not prasugrel. *J Thromb Haemost*. 2007;5:2429-2436.

26. Smith SM, Judge HM, Peters G, et al. Common sequence vari-ations in the P2Y12 and CYP3A5 genes do not explain the vari-ability in the inhibitory effects of clopidogrel therapy. *Platelets*. 2006;17:250-258.

27. Mega JL, Close SL, Wiviott SD, et al. Cytochrome P-450 poly-morphisms and response to clopidogrel. *N Engl J Med*. 2009; 360:354-362.

28. Desta Z, Zhao X, Shin JG, Flockhart DA. Clinical significance of the cytochrome P450 2C19 genetic polymorphism. *Clin Pharma-cokinet*. 2002;41:913-958.

29. Shuldiner AR, O'Connell JR, Bliden KP, et al. Association of cytochrome P450 2C19 genotype with the antiplatelet effect and clinical efficacy of clopidogrel therapy. *JAMA*. 2009;302:849-857.

30. Cuisset T, Frere C, Quilici J, et al. Role of the T744C polymor-phism of the P2Y12 gene on platelet response to a 600-mg loading dose of clopidogrel in 597 patients with non-ST-segment elevation acute coronary syndrome. *Thromb Res*. 2007;120:893-899.

31. Angiolillo DJ, Fernandez-Ortiz A, Bernardo E, et al. Lack of association between the P2Y12 receptor gene polymorphism and platelet response to clopidogrel in patients with coronary artery disease. *Thomb Res*. 2005;116:491-497.

32. Plavix (clopidogrel bisulfate) tablets—Prescribing Informa-tion. http://products.sanofi-aventis.us/PLAVIX/PLAVIX.html, Accessed March 3, 2010.

33. Gladding P, Webster M, Zeng I, et al. The pharmacogenetics and pharmacodynamics of clopidogrel response: an analysis from the PRINC (Plavix Response in Coronary Intervention) trial. *JACC Cardiovasc Interv*. 2008;1:620-627.

34. Mehta SR, Bassand JP, Chrolavicius S, et al. Design and ratio-nale of CURRENT-OASIS 7: a randomized, 2 x 2 factorial trial evaluating optimal dosing strategies for clopidogrel and aspirin in patients with ST and non-ST-elevation acute coronary syndromes managed with an early invasive strategy. *Am Heart J*. 2008;156: 1080-1088.

35. Niitsu Y, Jakubowski JA, Sugidachi A, Asai F. Pharmacology of CS-747 (prasugre, LY640315), a novel, potent antiplatelet agent with in vivo P2Y12 receptor antagonist activity. *Semin Thromb Hemost*. 2005;31:184-194.

36. Wiviott SD, Braunwald E, McCabe CH, et al. Prasugrel versus clopidogrel in patients with acute coronary syndromes. *N Engl J Med*. 2007;357:2001-2015.

37. Mega JL, Close SL, Wiviott SD, et al. Cytochrome P450 genetic polymorphisms and the response to prasugrel: relationship to pharmacokinetic, pharmacodynamic, and clinical outcomes. *Circulation*. 2009;119:2553-2560.

38. Wallentin L, Becker RC, Budaj A, et al. Ticagrelor versus clopidogrel in patients with acute coronary syndromes. *N Engl J Med.* 2009;361:1045-1057.

39. Holmes DR Jr, Dehmer GJ, Kaul S. ACCF/AHA clopidogrel clinical alert: approaches to the FDA "boxed warning." A report of the American College of Cardiology Foundation Task Force on Clinical Expert Consensus Documents and the American Heart Association. *Circulation.* 2010;56:321-341.

40. Breet NJ, van Werkum JW, Bouman HJ, et al. Comparison of platelet function tests in predicting clinical outcome in patients undergoing coronary stent implantation. *JAMA.* 2010;303:754-762.

## Supplementary Information

**OMIM References:**

[1] Drug Metabolism, Poor, CYP2C19-Related; CYP2C19 (#609535)

[2] Cytochrome P450, Subfamily IIC, Polypeptide 19; CYP2C19 (#124020)

**dbSNP References:**

[1] rs4244285 *[Homo sapiens]*

[2] rs776746 *[Homo sapiens]*

[3] rs12248560 *[Homo sapiens]*

**Alternative Names:**

- Plavix
- Clopidogrel Resistance

***Key Words:*** Clopidogrel, Plavix, pharmacogenomics, stent, in-stent thrombosis, stent thrombosis, antiplatelet resistance

# 8 Tamoxifen Pharmacogenetics

Hitoshi Zembutsu and Yusuke Nakamura

## KEY POINTS

- *Drug summary:*
  - Tamoxifen is widely used antiestrogen therapy for pre- and postmenopausal women with metastatic breast cancer, for prevention of recurrence as adjuvant therapy, and for women with a high risk of developing breast cancer as chemoprevention.
  - Five years of adjuvant tamoxifen safely reduces 15-year risks of breast cancer recurrence.
  - The most frequent adverse events by tamoxifen treatment is hot flash (>60%).
- *Pharmacogenomics:*
  - Endoxifen is an active metabolite of tamoxifen, and has the higher affinity to estrogen receptors (ERs) and greater potency in suppressing estrogen-dependent breast cancer cell proliferation than tamoxifen.
  - CYP2D6 plays an important role in biotransformation of tamoxifen into its active metabolites including endoxifen.
  - There is a large interindividual variability in the metabolism of drugs that can be explained largely by *CYP2D6* genetic polymorphisms affecting the enzymatic activity and expression level.
  - Women with reduced CYP2D6 enzymatic activity display low endoxifen concentrations and are expected to have poor response to tamoxifen therapy.

## Indication, Efficacy, and Side Effects of Tamoxifen

**Indication for Tamoxifen:** Tamoxifen is an antagonist of the ER in breast tissue via its active metabolite, hydroxytamoxifen or endoxifen. Tamoxifen has been proven to be effective in the adjuvant treatment and metastatic tumor of breast cancer. Tamoxifen is indicated for the treatment of patients with

- Pre- and postmenopausal breast cancer
- ER-positive breast cancer

**Efficacy of Tamoxifen:** Adjuvant tamoxifen therapy is a major endocrine treatment option, especially for women who have ovarian estrogenic activity that cannot be regulated by aromatase inhibitors. Five-year adjuvant tamoxifen treatment effectively reduces recurrence of ER-positive tumors. Tamoxifen is also approved for the chemoprevention of breast cancer for women with high risk of developing the disease.

**Side Effects of Tamoxifen:** Side effects caused by tamoxifen are relatively mild compared to chemotherapy, but are rarely severe enough to require discontinuation of treatment. The adverse event observed most commonly in patients treated with tamoxifen is hot flashes. Table 8-1 shows the frequency of adverse events of tamoxifen in the NSABP B-14 study which is randomized to 5-years tamoxifen or placebo following primary surgery.

## Screening and Counseling

**Screening:** Although expression level of ER or the number of cancer cells expressing ER in breast cancer tissue are usually evaluated before initiation of tamoxifen treatment, genetic screening is not yet clinically available for selection of patients who should be treated with tamoxifen in adjuvant setting or to metastatic tumor. However, for chemopreventive use of tamoxifen, the high risk for breast cancer can be assessed by a family history consistent with

high risk, or *BRCA1* or *BRCA2* mutation. It has been estimated that women could benefit from tamoxifen as chemoprevention medication for breast cancer. However, even in the most favorable of situations, this medication is not acceptable to many women, because the efficacy of tamoxifen in preventing breast cancer is limited to ER-positive tumors.

**Counseling:** Women who are at high risk for breast cancer are confronted with multiple decisions regarding breast cancer risk management including tamoxifen treatment as preventive medication. According to the National Comprehensive Cancer Network, women who have no pre-existing breast cancer, but are considered to be at high risk for breast cancer (a family history consistent with high risk, or *BRCA* mutation) and to have low risk of adverse events, may have indication of treatment by tamoxifen to reduce the risk of breast cancer. However, this medication increases the risk of endometrial cancer, thromboembolic events, and vasomotor adverse events. Discussion of risks and benefits of preventive tamoxifen therapy by doctors and the other health providers is important to patient's decision making.

## Management and Treatment

Tamoxifen is more beneficial for women whose breast cancer cells express ERs. A tissue sample obtained from breast biopsy or surgical resection is usually used to determine whether cancer cells are ER-positive or negative. ER can be measured by enzyme immunoassay (EIA) or immunohistochemistry (IHC) assay. The progesterone receptor (PgR), which is transcriptionally upregulated as a downstream effect of activated ER, can also be measured by EIA and IHC. However, according to the recommendation of the St. Gallen International Conference, IHC is recently thought to be more useful than EIA in the assessment of hormone receptor status for breast cancer patients.

**Pharmacogenetic Applications:** Tamoxifen is metabolized to more active or inactive metabolites by the enzymes including cytochrome P450s (CYPs), sulfotransferases (SULTs), and

*Table 8-1* **Side Effects of Tamoxifen**

| Side Effect | Events in Patients With 20 mg of TAM (%) |
|---|---|
| Hot flashes | 64 |
| Fluid retention | 32 |
| Vaginal discharge | 30 |
| Nausea | 26 |
| Irregular menses | 25 |
| Weight loss (5% or more) | 23 |
| Skin changes | 19 |
| Increased SGOT | 5 |

UDP-glucuronosyltransferases (UGTs). Recent data support that genetic polymorphisms in these drug-metabolizing enzymes contribute to individual differences in plasma concentrations of active metabolites of tamoxifen and clinical outcome after tamoxifen therapy. Among them, the genetic polymorphism of *CYP2D6* is most extensively investigated. It was recently reported that drug transporters are involved in the transport of active tamoxifen metabolites and pharmacogenetic evaluation of transporter genes suggests that they are involved in the variable clinical outcome observed in patients treated with tamoxifen.

## Molecular Mechanisms

Tamoxifen is known to be metabolized in liver and gut wall in humans to several primary and secondary metabolites that exhibit a range of pharmacologic activity. Hence, the differences in systemic exposure of the active metabolites should influence the variable responses of tamoxifen in patients with breast cancer. Tamoxifen can be considered as a prodrug. The parental drug itself has weak affinity to ER but is biotransformed into active

and inactive metabolites. CYP450 enzymes including CYP2B6, CYP2C9, CYP2C19, CYP2D6, and CYP3A are involved in the process to increase the affinity to ER (Fig. 8-1). Endoxifen, which is a metabolite of tamoxifen, is formed predominantly by the CYP2D6-mediated oxidation of N-desmethyl tamoxifen; N-desmethyl tamoxifen, the most abundant tamoxifen metabolite, is generated from tamoxifen by N-desmethylation with CYP3A (Fig. 8-1). Endoxifen has a potency which is equivalent to the potency of 4-hydroxytamoxifen in vitro, and it reaches greater than sixfold higher plasma concentrations than 4-OH tamoxifen in patients receiving tamoxifen. The hydroxylated metabolites undergo conjugation by phase II enzymes such as SULTs and/or uridine diphosphate–UGTs (Fig. 8-1).

***Genetic Variants That Contribute to Tamoxifen Efficacy:*** Recently, many studies have reported the clinical relevance of *CYP2D6* genotypes on outcomes for breast cancer patients treated with tamoxifen. There is a large interindividual and ethnic variability in the metabolism of drugs by CYP2D6 that can be explained largely by genetic polymorphisms affecting the enzyme activity and expression level. Some of these alleles are associated with reduced enzymatic activity (eg, *CYP2D6*\*10, \*17, \*41) or with no enzymatic activity (eg, \*3, \*4, \*5, \*6). The typical CYP2D6 phenotype is usually classified into three groups: poor metabolizers (PMs), intermediate metabolizers (IMs), and extensive metabolizers (EMs). Endoxifen, which is an active form of tamoxifen metabolized by CYP2D6, is a potent antiestrogen metabolite in breast cancer cells that functions through targeting ER-alpha for degradation by the proteasome, blocking ER-alpha transcriptional activity, and inhibiting estrogen-induced breast cancer cell proliferation. It has been hypothesized that women with a reduced CYP2D6 enzyme activity and low endoxifen concentration might have poorer treatment outcomes. In 2009, Schroth et al. published the largest retrospective analysis of 1325 German and North American patients with an early-stage breast cancer treated with adjuvant tamoxifen. With a median follow-up of 6.3 years, the authors observed that women with reduced CYP2D6 activity had a significantly higher incidence of recurrence (HR, 1.4; 95% CI, 1.04-1.9) than those with EMs. However,

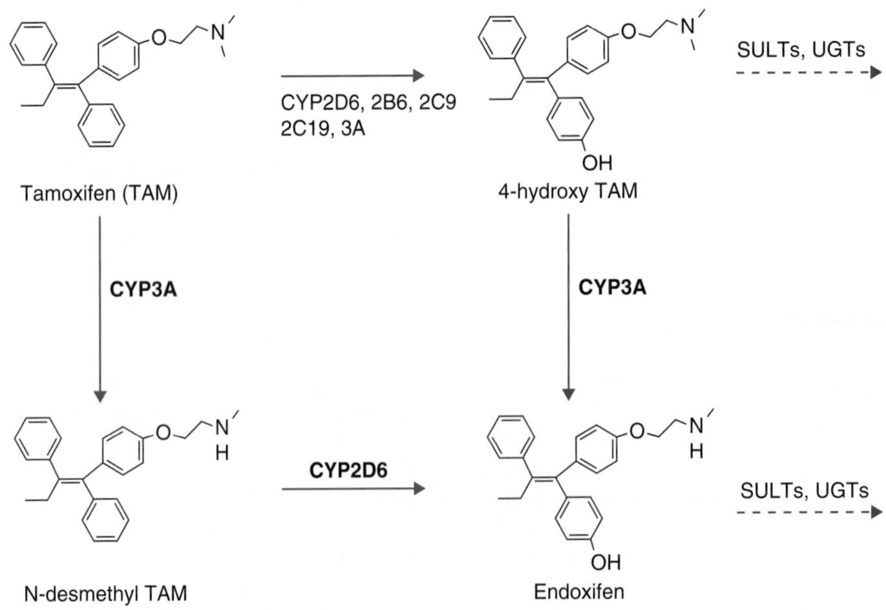

*Figure 8-1* Schematic Representation of the Metabolism of Tamoxifen by the Cytochrome P450 (CYP) System.

several smaller studies have reported discordant results. Most of the *CYP2D6*-tamoxifen studies have been retrospective and lack uniformity in genotyping methods, clinical background of patients, and tamoxifen dose. Because the result of *CYP2D6*-tamoxifen study is still controversial, *CYP2D6* genotype test is not yet applied for routine clinical use. However, some experts agree that *CYP2D6* test may be useful for personalized tamoxifen therapy after robust confirmatory data would be available from adequately powered prospective trials.

***Future Direction:*** There have been some discrepant reports questioning the association between *CYP2D6* genotype and clinical outcome after tamoxifen treatment. One of the reasons for these controversial results among the studies might reflect considerable heterogeneities in tamoxifen treatment regimen, coverage of genetic polymorphisms of *CYP2D6*, and most importantly selection of study participants. The studies involving patients receiving combination of tamoxifen and other therapies tend to show no positive association between *CYP2D6* genotypes and the recurrence rate or disease-free survival after tamoxifen therapy. In contrast, studies in which the participants were restricted only to patients with tamoxifen monotherapy have revealed positive associations. These lines of evidence indicate that the employment of patients receiving combination therapy with tamoxifen and other drugs might be inappropriate to evaluate the association of *CYP2D6* genotype with tamoxifen response.

Personalized tamoxifen therapy could improve the treatment efficacy in patients with breast cancer. *CYP2D6* genotype test may be more practical than plasma tamoxifen or endoxifen monitoring because CYP2D6 metabolizer status of a patient can be identified easily and rapidly before starting tamoxifen therapy. Recent *CYP2D6*-tamoxifen studies suggest that genotype-guided tamoxifen administration may be beneficial for breast cancer patients in terms of optimizing the treatment of breast cancer. The findings of large, well-designed clinical trials may support such a change in clinical practice.

## Bibliography:

1. Davies C, Godwin J, Gray R, et al. Relevance of breast cancer hormone receptors and other factors to the efficacy of adjuvant tamoxifen: patient-level meta-analysis of randomised trials. *Lancet.* 2011;378:771-784.

2. Visvanathan K, Chlebowski RT, Hurley P, et al. American society of clinical oncology clinical practice guideline update on the use of pharmacologic interventions including tamoxifen, raloxifene, and aromatase inhibition for breast cancer risk reduction. *J Clin Oncol.* 2009;27:3235-3258.

3. Zembutsu H, Sasa M, Kiyotani K, Mushiroda T, Nakamura Y. Should CYP2D6 inhibitors be administered in conjunction with tamoxifen? *Expert Rev.* 2011;11:185-193.

4. Kurosumi M. Significance of immunohistochemical assessment of steroid hormone receptor status for breast cancer patients. *Breast Cancer.* 2003;10:97-104.

5. Kiyotani K, Mushiroda T, Imamura CK, et al. Significant effect of polymorphisms in CYP2D6 and ABCC2 on clinical outcomes of adjuvant tamoxifen therapy for breast cancer patients. *J Clin Oncol.* 2009;28:1287-1293.

6. Stearns V, Johnson MD, Rae JM, et al. Active tamoxifen metabolite plasma concentrations after coadministration of tamoxifen and the selective serotonin reuptake inhibitor paroxetine. *J Natl Cancer Inst.* 2003;95:1758-1764.

7. Desta Z, Ward BA, Soukhova NV, Flockhart DA. Comprehensive evaluation of tamoxifen sequential biotransformation by the human cytochrome P450 system in vitro: prominent roles for CYP3A and CYP2D6. *J Pharmacol Exp Ther.* 2004;310:1062-1075.

8. Sistonen J, Sajantila A, Lao O, Corander J, Barbujani G, Fuselli S. CYP2D6 worldwide genetic variation shows high frequency of altered activity variants and no continental structure. *Pharmacogenet Genomics.* 2007;17:93-101.

9. Sideras K, Ingle JN, Ames MM, et al. Coprescription of tamoxifen and medications that inhibit CYP2D6. *J Clin Oncol.* 2010;28:2768-2776.

10. Lim HS, Ju Lee H, Seok Lee K, Sook Lee E, Jang IJ, Ro J. Clinical implications of CYP2D6 genotypes predictive of tamoxifen pharmacokinetics in metastatic breast cancer. *J Clin Oncol.* 2007;25:3837-3845.

11. Schroth W, Goetz MP, Hamann U, et al. Association between CYP2D6 polymorphisms and outcomes among women with early stage breast cancer treated with tamoxifen. *JAMA.* 2009;302:1429-1436.

12. Hoskins JM, Carey LA, McLeod HL. CYP2D6 and tamoxifen: DNA matters in breast cancer. *Nat Rev Cancer.* 2009;9:576-586.

13. Ramon y Cajal T, Altes A, Pare L, et al. Impact of CYP2D6 polymorphisms in tamoxifen adjuvant breast cancer treatment. *Breast Cancer Res Treat.* 2009;119:33-38.

14. Kiyotani K, Mushiroda T, Hosono N, et al. Lessons for pharmacogenomics studies: association study between CYP2D6 genotype and tamoxifen response. *Pharmacogenet.* 2010;9:565-568.

---

## Supplementary Information

**OMIM Reference:**

[1] Cytochrome P450, Subfamily IID, Polypeptide 6; CYP2D6 (#124030)

**Alternative Names:**
- Personalized Tamoxifen Therapy
- Made-to-Order Medicine for Tamoxifen Therapy
- Tamoxifen Pharmacogenomics

***Key Words:*** Tamoxifen, endoxifen, breast cancer, CYP2D6, genotype, pharmacogenomics, personalized therapy, clinical outcome, disease-free survival

# 9 Statin-Induced Neuromyopathy

Richard L. Seip, Nahir Rivera, Gualberto Ruano, and Paul D. Thompson

## KEY POINTS

- *Disease summary:*
  - Statins may cause a series of musculoskeletal and neuromuscular disturbances and diseases, including rhabdomyolysis and mild serum creatine kinase (CK) elevations. Genetic factors have been associated with an increased risk of statin-induced myopathy.
  - Statins or 3-hydroxy-3-methylglutaryl coenzyme A reductase inhibitors are widely prescribed because of their cardiovascular benefits. Statins are well tolerated by most patients at low starting dosages but can produce statin-induced neuromyopathy and their usage is ultimately limited by toxicity.
  - The American College of Cardiology (ACC)/American Heart Association (AHA)/National Heart, Lung, and Blood Institute (NHLBI) definitions and terminology are widely used in the literature and therefore used here. They have defined four syndromes:
    - Statin myopathy (any muscle complaints related to statins)
    - Myalgia (muscle complaints without serum CK elevation)
    - Myositis (muscle complaints with CK elevation >10 ULN [upper limit of normal])
    - Rhabdomyolysis (CK activity >10-fold ULN with an elevated creatinine level consistent with brown urine and urinary myoglobin)
  - Muscle complaints encompass aches, cramps, pain, tenderness, weakness, fatigue, and heaviness and are broadly categorized as neuromuscular side effects (NMSEs).
  - NMSE occur in approximately 10% of patients during high-dose therapy, affecting compliance to therapy. NMSEs vary in extent among drugs and from patient to patient.
  - Increased serum CK activity provides the predominant means for assessing the degree of muscle injury, with elevation of CK activity to greater than 10-fold ULN suggested as indicating severe statin-induced neuromyopathy. Elevation of CK to greater than fourfold ULN with statin therapy may warrant testing for underlying metabolic muscle disease. However, serum CK activity correlates poorly with the more common and less severe NMSE, can be normal in patients with NMSE, and is not an effective clinical marker for common NMSE.
- *Differential diagnosis:*
  - Muscle pain can be caused by bursitis, myofascial pain, muscle strain, osteoarthritis, radiculopathy, and tendonitis. Other etiologies for muscle complaints or an increased CK level are increased physical activity, trauma, falls, accidents, seizure, shaking chills, hypothyroidism, viral infections, carbon monoxide poisoning, polymyositis, dermatomyositis, alcohol abuse, and drug abuse (cocaine, amphetamines, heroin, or phencyclidine [PCP]).
- *Monogenic forms:*
  - No single gene cause of NMSE is known to exist.
- *Family history:*
  - One-third of the patients with myopathy have family members who also experienced symptoms associated with lipid-lowering drugs. The presence of family history almost doubles the risk of the adverse reaction.
- *Twin studies:*
  - None available.
- *Environmental factors:*
  - Physical exercise, addition of a new drug, or paradoxically, rest, or assuming the lying position may trigger symptoms. The disparate nature of these factors suggests more than one pathophysiology.
- *Genome-wide associations:*
  - To date there exist two published genome wide studies of statin response. Severe statin myopathy has been strongly associated with the *SLCO1B1* *5 variant.
- *Pharmacogenomics:*
  - Statin efficacy (low-density lipoprotein-cholesterol [LDL-C] lowering, prevention of major adverse cardiovascular events) and the safety factors of NMSE and myositis strongly influence patient drug selection. Emerging studies are focused on predicting the balance of statin efficacy (LDL-C lowering, prevention of major adverse cardiovascular events) versus Safety.

## Diagnostic Criteria and Clinical Characteristics

***Diagnostic Criteria for Statin-Induced Myopathy:*** Diagnostic evaluation should include (see Fig. 9-1)

- Assessment of family history to evaluate for predisposition to myopathy.
- Physical examination focusing on tenderness to palpation and findings consistent with other causes of myopathy.
- A CK level should be drawn and patients with elevated CK levels should be asked about recent strenuous exercise, significant alcohol, grapefruit or pomegranate juice ingestion, and the use of red yeast rice supplements or of medications that might interact with the statins. Also, a workup for other possible causes of myopathy should be initiated.
- If the patient complains of brown urine or if CK levels are markedly elevated (>10 × ULN), renal function and urine myoglobin should be evaluated.
- A muscle biopsy should be considered if the patient's symptoms and/or the CK elevation persist after withdrawal of the lipid-lowering drug.

***Clinical Characteristics:*** The clinical characteristics for statin-induced NMSE depend on the patient, ranging from myalgia, lassitude, and fatigue to frank proximal muscle weakness. Patients may experience an aching or cramping sensation in their muscles, nocturnal leg cramps, and tendon pain. Sensations may be widespread and increase with exercise, though paradoxically, some patients report sensations upon rest or lying down. Symptoms develop within 4 weeks to 4 years after initiation of statin therapy, and more often in response to high dose. The addition of a new drug can trigger myopathy.

The most frequent NMSE reported in 832 patients suffering statin-associated myopathy were heaviness, stiffness, and cramps in 57.9% of patients, and stiffness and cramps in 13.1% of patients. Most patients reported diffuse pain, but complaints focused on a given location, mostly in the lower limbs. Other symptoms were muscle weakness during physical activity and tendonitis, the latter reported by 24.4% of the patients. Most patients do not present with elevated CK activity.

Statins are used on a long-term basis and it is important to know which drugs may interact with them. Various medications may interact with statins, increasing serum concentrations and the risk of myopathy, rhabdomyolysis, and acute renal failure. Table 9-1 describes drug interactions and their prevention.

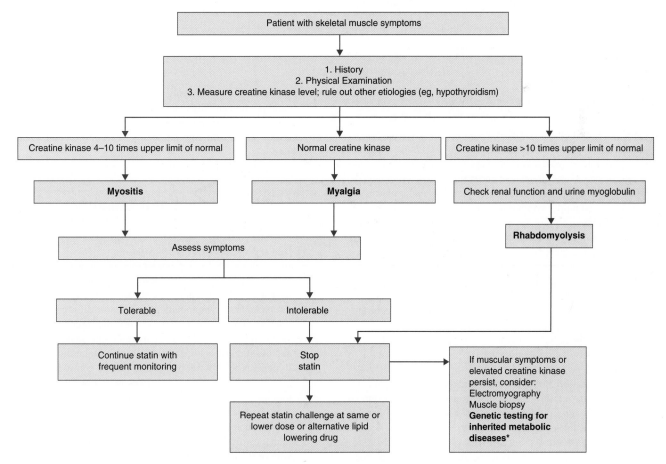

***Figure 9-1*** Algorithm for Diagnosis and Treatment of Statin-induced Myopathy.
Modified from Sathasivam S, Lecky B, 2008.
*Genetic tests listed in Table 9-2 correspond to inherited muscle diseases that have been found to be more prevalent in patients with statin myopathies (see references 7, 36)

*Table 9-1 Pharmacokinetic Considerations in Statin Induced Neuromyopathy (SINM)*

| Gene | Protein Function | Associated Medications | Polymorphisms | Frequency | Outcome |
|------|------------------|------------------------|---------------|-----------|---------|
| CYP2D6 | Cytochrome CYP450 metabolizing enzyme | Fluvastatin Atorvastatin, simvastatin | *3, *4, and *5 produce null activity | *3 and *5: 0.02 in European Caucasians *4: 0.1-0.2 in North Americans | *3, *5: higher incidence of fluvastatin intolerability in homozygotes *4: atorvastatin and simvastatin-induced myopathy |
| CYP3A5 | Cytochrome CYP450 metabolizing enzyme | Lovastatin, pravastatin, simvastatin, atorvastatin | *3 and *5 produce decreased activity | *3: Caucasian ~0.05 African >0.60 Asian 0.2-0.3 *5: not available | *3: homozygotes greater risk for muscle damage *5: elevated plasma concentration of simvastatin |
| SLCO1B1 (OATP1B1) | Organic anion transporting polypeptide C which transports statins into hepatocytes | Simvastatin, pravastatin, atorvastatin, rosuvastatin, pitavastatin | *5 is associated with compromised hepatic uptake of the drug | 0.15-0.28 | Mild myopathy, serum CK ↑ Drug clearance ↓; plasma statin levels ↑ |
| ABCB1 | Intestinal P-glyco-protein efflux transporter | Atorvastatin, simvastatin | Various | Varied | Elevated plasma statin levels |

## Screening and Counseling

**Screening:** Measurement of CK is a widely used screening diagnostic test for suspected muscle disease since it has relative predominance in skeletal muscle and is not falsely elevated by hemolysis. However, it may cause diagnostic uncertainty. Most symptomatic patients do not have elevated CK levels and an elevated level can be found in a patient mildly symptomatic or asymptomatic with respect to NMSE. Obtaining a pretreatment, baseline CK level is relatively inexpensive. It should be considered in patients who are at high risk of experiencing muscle toxicity, such as the elderly or when combining statin with an agent known to increase myotoxicity, or in patients suspected of carrying an inherited muscle disease (see Table 9-3). When measuring CK levels during statin therapy, clinicians should recognize that marked, clinically important CK elevations are rare and are usually related to physical exertion or other causes.

Currently genetic testing before or during the course of statin therapy is not part of clinical guidelines or physician practice.

**Counseling:**

☞**INHERITANCE, PENETRANCE:** One-third of the patients with myopathy have family members who also experienced symptoms associated with lipid-lowering drugs. The presence of family history almost doubles the risk of the adverse reaction.

☞**GENOTYPE-PHENOTYPE CORRELATION:** The *rs4149056* variant in the *SLCO1B1* gene is associated with increased risk of elevated CK (>3- to >10-fold ULN) in response to simvastatin 80 mg/d. *SLCO1B1* encodes the organic anion transporter 1B1 protein, which is responsible for hepatic uptake and, indirectly, clearance of most statins. The C allele produces deficient transport. Individuals carrying two copies of the risk-allele (CC genotype) had an 18% chance of developing myopathy over 5 years. For those carrying only one or no copy of the C allele, the chances of developing myopathy were 2.8% and 0.4%, respectively.

## Management and Treatment

**Management:**

☞**DISCONTINUATION OF THERAPY:**

- In patients who develop intolerable muscle symptoms with or without a CK elevation and in whom other etiologies have been ruled out, the statin should be discontinued. Once the patient is asymptomatic, the same or different statin at a lower dose can be restarted to test the reproducibility of symptoms. Recurrence of symptoms with multiple statins and doses requires initiation of other lipid-altering therapy.
- In patients who develop tolerable muscle complaints or are asymptomatic with CK four times the ULN, statin therapy may be continued at the same or reduced doses and symptoms may be used to guide, stop, or continue therapy.
- Statin therapy should be stopped in patients who develop rhabdomyolysis (CK >10,000 IU/L or CK >10 times the ULN with or without an elevation in serum creatinine or requiring intravenous (IV) hydration therapy). IV hydration therapy in a hospital setting should be instituted if indicated for patients experiencing rhabdomyolysis. Once recovered, the risk versus benefit of statin therapy should be carefully reconsidered.

☞COENZYME Q10: Coenzyme Q10 ($CoQ_{10}$) is a mitochondrial respiratory chain component with redox function. It has been postulated that $CoQ_{10}$ (ubiquinone) deficiency contributes to statin-induced myopathy. It is not clear if supplementation with $CoQ_{10}$ relieves the discomfort. Two randomized trials have shown differing results. In one, 32 statin-treated patients who received $CoQ_{10}$ (100 mg/d) showed significant improvement in myopathic pain (no change in CK elevation) compared to controls receiving vitamin E (400 IU/d). In contrast, another study of 44 patients found no differences in myalgia scores or in statin tolerance. A randomized double-blind trial is in progress to test the hypothesis that $CoQ_{10}$ supplementation reduces the intensity of NMSE during statin treatment in 135 patients with documented statin myalgia (ClinicalTrials.gov Identifier: NCT01140308).

☞PHARMACOGENETICS: Some gene variants affect LDL-C lowering (eg, *APOE*, *HMGCR*), and others modulate statins' capacity to prevent major adverse coronary event (MACE) (*CLMN*, *KIF6*, *LDLR*, *CETP*, *ADAMTS1*, *F5*, and *F7*). These are reviewed elsewhere. Single-nucleotide polymorphisms (SNPs) associated with or contributing to genetic predisposition for statin myopathy have been identified (Table 9-1), of which only *SLCO1B1* has been confirmed. Emerging studies are focused on predicting the balance of statin efficacy (LDL-C lowering, prevention of major adverse cardiovascular events) versus safety.

## Molecular Genetics and Molecular Mechanism

Recent studies suggest that some patients who develop statin-induced myopathy may have inherited defects in skeletal muscle genes. Clinicians should always consider the possibility of previous unknown skeletal myopathies in patients presenting with statin-induced muscle symptoms.

*Genetic Testing:* Genetic testing for determining predisposition to NMSE prior to the initiation of statin therapy is not clinically validated. However, recent studies found the *SLCO1B1* *5 allele (*rs4149056* T>C) to be associated with an increased risk of elevated CK (>3 × to >10 × ULN) in patients taking high-dose simvastatin.

The prevalences of carrier status for McArdle disease and carnitine palmitoyltransferase deficiency are 20-fold and 11-fold higher in patients with severe statin myopathy (Table 9-2). Testing for inherited muscle metabolic diseases in patients with statin myopathy is ongoing and DNA samples may be sent to Dr. Georgirene Vladutiu, Robert Guthrie Biochemical & Molecular Genetics Laboratory, Kaleida Health Laboratories (www.rgbmgl.org).

*Table 9-2 Inherited Muscle Disease Associated Susceptibility Variants*

| Gene (Disease) | Protein Function | Mutations | Frequency | Outcome |
|---|---|---|---|---|
| *CPT2* (carnitine palmitoyl-transferase deficiency) | Carnitine palmitoyl-transferase allows acyl CoA into the mitochondrial matrix for β-oxidation of fatty acids, an energy source for sustained skeletal muscle exercise | Most common: p.S113L p.Q413fs p.P50H | Mutant allele frequencies in newborn screening: • S113L: 0.00037 • Q413fs: 0.0025 • P50H: <0.0025 | Rhabdomyolysis in heterozygotes and homozygotes |
| *PYGM* (McArdle disease) | Muscle glycogen phosphorylase catalyzes conversion of glycogen to glucose | Most common: p.R50X (others not listed here) | Heterozygosity for mutations: • Statin myopathy: 0.123 • General population: 0.006 | Rhabdomyolysis in heterozygotes |
| *AMPD1* (myoadenylate deaminase [MADA] deficiency) | Converts adenosine 5 monophosphate to inosine monophosphate, an important regulator of ATP levels in skeletal muscle | Most common: p.Q12X and p.P48L (others not listed here) | Homozygosity for mutant allele: • Severe statin myopathy: 0.065 • General population: 0.02 | Rhabdomyolysis in homozygotes only |
| Mitochondrial DNA mutations (mitochondrial myopathy, encephalopathy, lactic acidosis, and stroke-like episodes [MELAS]) | Enzymes that participate in the oxidative phosphorylation pathway | Most common: A3243G, T3271C, A3260G | A3243G is most common General population: 0.0024-0.000014 | Mutations produce symptoms in muscle and neurological tissues, provoked by statin therapy |

*Table 9-3  Statin-Drug Interactions*

| Object Drugs | Precipitant Drugs | Comments | Management |
|---|---|---|---|
| 1. Lovastatin<br>2. Simvastatin | 1. Clarithromycin<br>2. Erythromycin<br>3. Fluconazole<br>4. Itraconazole<br>5. Ketoconazole<br>6. Posaconazole<br>7. Troleandomycin<br>8. Voriconazole | Lovastatin and sim-vastatin undergo extensive first-pass metabolism by CYP3A4; antimicrobials that inhibit CYP3A4 increase the risk of myopathy, rhabdomyolysis, and acute renal failure. | **Use only if benefit outweighs risk**<br>Alternative:<br>1. *Statin*—**Pravastatin** is not metabolized by CYP450 isoenzymes. **Fluvastatin** and **rosuvastatin** are metabolized by CYP2C9 and may be affected by fluconazole and voriconazole. **Atorvastatin** undergoes less first-pass metabolism by CYP3A4; the extent to which CYP3A4 inhibitors increase the risk of atorvastatin-induced myopathy is not clear, but some cases have been reported.<br>2. *Azole antifungals*—Fluconazole appears to be a weaker inhibitor of CYP3A4 than itraconazole or ketoconazole. In larger doses it may inhibit CYP3A4 and should be used cautiously with lovastatin or simvastatin. Single doses of fluconazole would be unlikely to increase the risk of statin toxicity. **Terbinafine** does not appear to inhibit CYP3A4.<br>3. *Macrolides*—**Azithromycin** and **dirithromycin** do not appear to inhibit CYP3A4 and would not be expected to interact with lovastatin or simvastatin. *Circumvent/minimize*: Consider stopping lovastatin or simvastatin during short-term azole antifungal use.<br>*Monitor*: If antimicrobials that inhibit CYP3A4 are used with lovastatin or simvastatin, the patient should be alert for muscle pain or weakness (myopathy) and myoglobinuria (dark urine). |
| 1. Lovastatin<br>2. Simvastatin | 1. Diltiazem<br>2. Verapamil | Lovastatin and sim-vastatin undergo extensive first-pass metabolism by CYP3A4; calcium channel blockers that inhibit CYP3A4 increase the statin serum concentrations, increasing the risk of myopathy, rhabdomyolysis, and acute renal failure. | **Assess risk and take action if necessary**<br>Alternative:<br>1. *Statin*—**Pravastatin** is not metabolized by CYP450 isoenzymes, while **fluvastatin** and **rosuvastatin** are metabolized by CYP2C9—thus, they are not affected by CYP3A4 inhibition. **Atorvastatin** undergoes less first-pass metabolism by CYP3A4; the extent to which CYP3A4 inhibitors increase the risk of atorvastatin-induced myopathy is not clear, but some cases have been reported.<br>2. *Calcium channel blockers*—Calcium channel blockers other than diltiazem and verapamil are unlikely to inhibit the metabolism of statins.<br>*Monitor*: If either diltiazem or verapamil is used with lovastatin or simvastatin, the patient should be alert for evidence of myopathy (muscle pain or weakness) and myoglobinuria (dark urine). Myopathy is usually associated with increased serum CK concentrations. |

*(Continued)*

Table 9-3 **Statin-Drug Interactions (Continued)**

| Object Drugs | Precipitant Drugs | Comments | Management |
|---|---|---|---|
| 1. Lovastatin<br>2. Simvastatin<br>3. Atorvastatin | 1. Fenofibrate<br>2. Gemfibrozil | Combined use of statins and fibrates may increase the risk of myopathy, which may lead to rhabdomyolysis and acute renal failure. The risk of myopathy with combined use of statins and fenofibrate may be less than with gemfibrozil. | **Assess risk and take action if necessary**<br>Alternative:<br>1. *Statin*—Although definitive incidence data are not available, the risk of myopathy during concurrent **pravastatin** or **fluvastatin** with gemfibrozil or fenofibrate appears to be minimal.<br>*Monitor*: The manufacturers of simvastatin and rosuvastatin suggest that when these drugs are combined with gemfibrozil, the daily dose should not exceed 10 mg (Merck & Co., 2004 2908 /id; Astra-Zeneca, 2010 3187 /id). For lovastatin, daily doses should not exceed 20 mg when given with a fibrate. If any statin is used with gemfibrozil or another fibrate, the patient should be monitored for evidence of myopathy (muscle pain or weakness) and myoglobinuria (dark urine). Myopathy is usually associated with increased serum CK concentrations. |
| 1. Lovastatin<br>2. Simvastatin<br>3. Atorvastatin | 1. Amiodarone<br>2. Amprenavir<br>3. Atazanavir<br>4. Conivaptan<br>5. Cyclosporine<br>6. Darunavir<br>7. Delavirdine<br>8. Fluvoxamine<br>9. Grapefruit<br>10. Indinavir<br>11. Nefazodone<br>12. Nelfinavir<br>13. Quinupristin<br>14. Ritonavir<br>15. Saquinavir<br>16. Telithromycin | Lovastatin and simvastatin undergo extensive first-pass metabolism by CYP3A4; inhibitors of CYP3A4 increase the risk of myopathy, in some cases leading to rhabdomyolysis, and acute renal failure. | **Use only if benefit outweighs risk**<br>Alternative:<br>1. *Statin*—**Pravastatin** is not metabolized by CYP450 isoenzymes. **Fluvastatin** and **rosuvastatin** are metabolized by CYP2C9 and will not be affected by CYP3A4 inhibitors. **Atorvastatin** undergoes less first-pass metabolism by CYP3A4; the extent to which CYP3A4 inhibitors increase the risk of atorvastatin-induced myopathy is not clear, but some cases have been reported.<br>2. *Antidepressants*—**Sertraline, citalopram, venlafaxine**, and **paroxetine** appear less likely to inhibit CYP3A4 than fluvoxamine. **Fluoxetine** appears to be a weak inhibitor of CYP3A4.<br>*Circumvent/minimize*: If CYP3A4 inhibitors will be used short term, consider stopping lovastatin or simvastatin while the CYP3A4 inhibitor is being given. Grapefruit juice consumption should be limited to one glass or one whole grapefruit per day.<br>*Monitor*: Patients receiving lovastatin or simvastatin and a CYP3A4 enzyme inhibitor should be alert for evidence of muscle pain or weakness (myopathy) and myoglobinuria (dark urine). |

**Future Directions:** Genetic markers for the statin response phenotypes for safety (NMSE, CK elevation) and efficacy (LDL-C lowering, prevention of MACE) appear largely phenotype specific suggesting separate pathophysiology pathways. Continuing research is focused on construction of a physiogenomic-based safety or efficacy model that consolidates the NMSE and CK elevation, and LDL cholesterol reduction components. In the future, the existence of genotypes may help clinicians prescribe statins so as to minimize side effects and maximize efficacy.

**BIBLIOGRAPHY:**

1. Golomb BA, Criqui MH, White H, Dimsdale JE. Conceptual foundations of the UCSD Statin Study: a randomized controlled trial assessing the impact of statins on cognition, behavior, and biochemistry. *Arch Intern Med*. 2004;164:153-162.

2. Thompson PD, Clarkson P, Karas RH. Statin-associated myopathy. *JAMA*. 2003;289:1681-1690.

3. Pasternak RC, Smith SC Jr., Bairey-Merz CN, Grundy SM, Cleeman JI, Lenfant C. ACC/AHA/NHLBI clinical advisory on the use and safety of statins. *Stroke*. 2002;33:2337-2341.

4. Bruckert E, Hayem G, Dejager S, Yau C, Begaud B. Mild to moderate muscular symptoms with high-dosage statin therapy in hyperlipidemic patients—the PRIMO study. *Cardiovasc Drugs Ther.* 2005;19:403-414.

5. McKenney JM, Davidson MH, Jacobson TA, Guyton JR. Final conclusions and recommendations of the National Lipid Association Statin Safety Assessment Task Force. *Am J Cardiol.* 2006;97: C89-C94.

6. Vladutiu GD, Simmons Z, Isackson PJ, et al. Genetic risk factors associated with lipid-lowering drug-induced myopathies. *Muscle Nerve.* 2006;34:153-162.

7. Vladutiu GD. Genetic predisposition to statin myopathy. *Curr Opin Rheumatol.* 2008;20:648-655.

8. Phillips PS, Haas RH, Bannykh S, et al. Statin-associated myopathy with normal creatine kinase levels. *Ann Intern Med.* 2002;137:581-585.

9. Vladutiu GD. Genetic predisposition to statin myopathy. *Curr Opin Rheumatol.* 2008;20:648-655.

10. Sathasivam S, Lecky B. Statin induced myopathy. *BMJ.* 2008; 337:a2286.

11. Franc S, Dejager S, Bruckert E, Chauvenet M, Giral P, Turpin G. A comprehensive description of muscle symptoms associated with lipid-lowering drugs. *Cardiovasc Drugs Ther.* 2003; 17:459-465.

12. Link E, Parish S, Armitage, J, et al. SLCO1B1 variants and statin-induced myopathy—a genomewide study. *N Engl J Med.* 2008;359:789-799.

13. Barber MJ, Mangravite LM, Hyde CL, et al. Genome-wide association of lipid-lowering response to statins in combined study populations. *PLoS ONE.* 2010;5:e9763.

14. Voora D, Shah SH, Spasojevic I, et al. The SLCO1B1*5 genetic variant is associated with statin-induced side effects. *J Am Coll Cardiol.* 2009;54:1609-1616.

15. Ruaño G, Windemuth A, Seip RL, Wu AHB, Thompson PD. Physiogenomics of statin safety and efficacy. *J Lipidol.* 2007;1:444.

16. Seehusen DA, Asplund CA, Johnson DR, Horde KA. Primary evaluation and management of statin therapy complications. *South Med J.* 2006;99:250-256.

17. Sorokin AV, Duncan B, Panetta R, Thompson PD. Rhabdomyolysis associated with pomegranate juice consumption. *Am J Cardiol.* 2006;98:705-706.

18. Baer AN, Wortmann RL. Myotoxicity associated with lipid-lowering drugs. *Curr Opin Rheumatol.* 2007;19:67-73.

19. Al-Sulaiman AA, Al-Khamis FA. Statin-induced myopathy: a clinical perspective. *Bahrain Medical Bulletin.* 2009;31:1-5.

20. Oshiro C, Mangravite L, Klein T, Altman R. PharmGKB very important pharmacogene: SLCO1B1. *Pharmacogenet Genomics.* 2010;20:211-216.

21. Marcoff L, Thompson PD. The role of coenzyme Q10 in statin-associated myopathy: a systematic review. *J Am Coll Cardiol.* 2007;49:2231-2237.

22. Young JM, Florkowski CM, Molyneux SL, et al. Effect of coenzyme Q(10) supplementation on simvastatin-induced myalgia. *Am J Cardiol.* 2007;100:1400-1403.

23. Mangravite LM, Wilke RA, Zhang J, Krauss RM. Pharmacogenomics of statin response. *Curr Opin Mol Ther.* 2008;10:555-561.

24. Seip RL, Duconge J, Ruaño G. Genotype guided statin therapy. In: Wu AHB, Yeo J, eds. *Pharmacogenomic Testing in Current Clinical Practice: Implementation in the Clinical Laboratory.* Humana Press; 2010.

25. Sachse C, Brockmoller J, Bauer S, Roots I. Cytochrome P450 2D6 variants in a Caucasian population: allele frequencies and phenotypic consequences. *Am J Hum Genet.* 1997;60:284-295.

26. Payami H, Lee N, Zareparsi S, et al. Parkinson's disease, CYP2D6 polymorphism, and age. *Neurology.* 2001;56:1363-1370.

27. The International HapMap Consortium. A haplotype map of the human genome. *Nature.* 2005;437:1299-1320.

28. Keskitalo JE, Kurkinen KJ, Neuvoneni PJ, Niemi M. ABCB1 haplotypes differentially affect the pharmacokinetics of the acid and lactone forms of simvastatin and atorvastatin. *Clin Pharmacol Ther.* 2008;84:457-461.

29. Vladutiu GD. Personal communication. Robert Guthrie Biochemical & Molecular Genetics Laboratory, Kaleida Health Laboratories. 7-28-2010.

30. Morisaki T, Gross M, Morisaki H, Pongratz D, Zollner N, Holmes EW. Molecular basis of AMP deaminase deficiency in skeletal muscle. *Proc Natl Acad Sci USA.* 1992;89:6457-6461.

31. Manwaring N, Jones MM, Wang JJ, et al. Population prevalence of the MELAS A3243G mutation. *Mitochondrion.* 2007;7: 230-233.

32. Chinnery PF, Johnson MA, Wardell TM, et al. The epidemiology of pathogenic mitochondrial DNA mutations. *Ann Neurol.* 2000;48:188-193.

33. Ruaño G, Thompson PD, Windemuth A, et al. Physiogenomic analysis links serum creatine kinase activities during statin therapy to vascular smooth muscle homeostasis. *Pharmacogenomics.* 2005;6:865-872.

34. Ruaño G, Thompson PD, Windemuth A, et al. Physiogenomic association of statin-related myalgia to serotonin receptors. *Muscle Nerve.* 2007;36:329-335.

35. Oh J, Ban MR, Miskie BA, Pollex RL, Hegele RA. Genetic determinants of statin intolerance. *Lipids Health Dis.* 2007;6:7.

36. Ghatak A, Faheem O, Thompson PD. The genetics of statin-induced myopathy. *Atherosclerosis.* 2009.

37. Hansten PD, Horn JR. *The Top 100 Drug Interactions: A Guide to Patient Management, Year 2008.* Freeland, WA: H & H Publications; 2008.

38. Merck & Co. I. Zocor Label. November 2004. Whitehouse Station, NJ, Merck & Co, Inc. 2004.

39. Astra-Zeneca. Crestor Label. 2010. Wilmington, DE, AstraZeneca Pharmaceuticals LP. 2010.

40. Merke Sharpe & Dohme. Mevacor (Lovastatin) Label. 2010. Morgantown, WV, Mylan Pharmaceuticals, Inc. 2010.

## Supplementary Information

**OMIM Reference:**

[1] Solute Carrier Organic Anion Transporter Family, Member 1B1; SLCO1B1 (#604843)

**Alternative Names:**
- OAT1B1
- Organic Ion Transporter 1B1

*Key Words:* HMG-CoA reductase inhibitor, myalgia, myositis, creatine kinase

# 10 Abacavir Pharmacogenomics

Elizabeth J. Phillips and Simon Mallal

## KEY POINTS

- *Disease summary:*
  - Abacavir is a nucleoside reverse transcriptase inhibitor used in combination therapy for the treatment of the human immunodeficiency virus type 1 (HIV-1) that has been associated with a hypersensitivity reaction in approximately 8% of those starting the drug.
  - Abacavir hypersensitivity reaction is characterized by greater than or equal to two progressive symptoms typically starting from the second week of therapy (median 9 days) with fever, malaise, nausea, vomiting, diarrhea, and later mild-to-moderate skin rash (present in 70% of patients).
  - Symptoms of abacavir hypersensitivity resolve rapidly with 24 to 72 hours after drug discontinuation.
  - A previous clinical history compatible with abacavir hypersensitivity is a contraindication to future rechallenge as severe morbidity and even mortality characterized by hypotension and shock has been described.

- *Differential diagnosis:*
  - The symptoms and signs associated with abacavir hypersensitivity are nonspecific and may be confused with other diseases occurring in HIV-positive patients such as infections, immune restoration disease, and hypersensitivity reactions associated with other drugs (eg, nevirapine, amprenavir or fosamprenavir, trimethoprim-sulfamethoxazole etc).

- *Family history:*
  - A description of the disease in a father and daughter, and predilection for white race, were early clues to the genetic basis.

- *Environmental factors:*
  - A higher prevalence of true immunologically mediated abacavir hypersensitivity syndrome is seen in white race which is related to the high prevalence of HLA-B*5701 in this group. There are no other demographic or environmental factors known to predispose to abacavir hypersensitivity.

- *False-positive clinical diagnosis and skin patch testing:*
  - The apparent low sensitivity of HLA-B*5701 for clinically diagnosed abacavir hypersensitivity was related to high false-positive clinical diagnosis which caused a differential misclassification error in the original studies. Randomized double-blinded HIV treatment studies involving abacavir consistently showed 2% to 7% diagnosed abacavir hypersensitivity in the arm not receiving abacavir.
  - Early barriers to the widespread implementation of HLA-B*5701 as a screening test included the doubt shed on the sensitivity of HLA-B*5701 for abacavir hypersensitivity and the generalizability of the test to nonwhite ethnic groups.
  - Early studies on a abacavir skin patch test showed a high proportion of patients meeting stringent clinical criteria for abacavir hypersensitivity were patch test positive and later on that 100% of patch test-positive patients with a clinical history compatible with abacavir hypersensitivity carried HLA-B*5701. This suggested that patch testing would be useful in a research context to increase the specificity of the diagnosis of abacavir hypersensitivity.

- *Pharmacogenomics and evidence leading to translation of HLA-B*5701 testing into clinical practice:*
  - In 2002, two independent groups published on the association between the major histocompatibility class I allele, HLA-B*5701 and abacavir hypersensitivity reactions.
  - Subsequent case control studies suggested an apparent low sensitivity for HLA-B*5701 in blacks and other nonwhite races but this was found to be related to the low prevalence of HLA-B*5701 in blacks and the high false-positive clinical diagnosis of abacavir hypersensitivity.
  - Observational studies have been important to establish the utility of HLA-B*5701 in real clinical practice, showing significant reduction in both true and false-positive diagnosis of abacavir hypersensitivity.
  - Two seminal studies published in 2008 confirmed the 100% negative predictive value of HLA-B*5701 for true immunologically abacavir hypersensitivity generalizable across ethnicity:
    - PREDICT-1 study: This was a randomized double-blinded controlled study in HIV treatment-naïve patients enrolling 1956 (84% Caucasian) subjects from 265 centers across Europe and Australia. The design was to randomize patients to (1) exclusion from abacavir based on positive HLA-B*5701 versus (2) no real-time HLA-B*5701 screening and clinical monitoring and thereby ascertain the clinical utility of HLA-B*5701 screening to prevent abacavir hypersensitivity. The coprimary endpoints of clinical diagnosis of abacavir hypersensitivity and clinical diagnosis + patch test positivity were utilized. There were no cases of patch test-positive abacavir hypersensitivity in the screened arm confirming 100% negative predictive value of HLA-B*5701 for immunologically confirmed abacavir hypersensitivity.
    - SHAPE study: The PREDICT-1 study enrolled predominantly Caucasian Europeans and did not answer the question of the generalizability of the 100% negative predictive value of HLA-B*5701 to black race. The SHAPE study was a case control study that retrospectively identified black and white patients meeting clinical criteria for abacavir hypersensitivity versus control patients who had tolerated abacavir for at least 3 months and applied HLA-B*5701 and abacavir skin patch testing. All whites and blacks with positive skin patch test results carried HLA-B*5701 suggesting 100% negative predictive value of HLA-B*5701 for abacavir hypersensitivity across white and black race.

## Laboratory and Clinical Implementation

Feasible, cost-effective, and quality assured laboratory testing has been key to the success of routine implementation of HLA-B*5701 screening for abacavir screening in the developed world. Polymerase chain reaction (PCR)-based techniques allow for batching of samples and are sensitive, specific, and significantly less costly than sequence-based human leukocyte antigen (HLA) typing. In addition, the development of a monoclonal antibody recognizing the HLA-B17 serotype (which includes all HLA-B57 and HLA-B58 subtypes) promises that flow cytometry-based methods may be cost-effective and offer the best turn-around-time in the routine HIV clinic.

## Screening and Counseling

The availability and evidence for HLA-B*5701 screening to predict and prevent abacavir hypersensitivity was critical to a change of treatment guidelines that moved abacavir to a first-line agent in combination with other drugs for the treatment of HIV. All current national and international treatment guidelines currently recommend that abacavir be used only in HLA-B*5701-negative individuals.

The burden of morbidity and mortality associated with abacavir hypersensitivity syndrome is related to rechallenge following the initial exposure which represents immunologically priming associated with a period of systemic exposure. This means that the safest approach is to prevent genetically predisposed individuals from first exposure to abacavir. The prevalence of HLA-B*5701 carriage differs across ethnicity being highest in Northern European Caucasians (6%-8%) and lowest among Asians and sub-Saharan Africans (<1%). Despite this, due to population admixture, the clinical difficulty in phenotyping individuals according to race and the high rate of false-positive diagnosis of abacavir

hypersensitivity screening for HLA-B*5701 is likely to be cost-effective across different racial groups. The implications for HLA-B*5701 screening across black and white patients is shown in Fig. 10-1.

## Future Directions

A strong body of clinical and basic science currently supports that HLA-B*5701 is necessary but not sufficient for the development of abacavir hypersensitivity. This makes HLA-B*5701 a robust and ideal screening test for the prediction and prevention of abacavir hypersensitivity. Since 2008, HLA-B*5701 screening has been widespread in the developed world and there have been no HLA-B*5701 negative clinical and immunologically confirmed cases of abacavir hypersensitivity. However, this does not completely rule out the possible association between a, as yet undiscovered, rare class I allele and abacavir hypersensitivity. For this reason, patients who develop clinical symptoms and signs of abacavir hypersensitivity despite negative HLA-B*5701 screening should be carefully studied with skin patch and ex vivo studies. In addition, since the positive predictive value derived from the PREDICT-1 study was 55%, 45% of those excluded from abacavir on the basis of positive HLA-B*5701 status would have tolerated abacavir. Some preliminary work looking for factors to explain this tolerance has suggested that the basis may lie outside of the major histocompatibility complex (MHC).

In keeping with the specificity of HLA-B*57:01 for abacavir hypersensitivity, abacavir specific CD8+ T cell responses can be consistently demonstrated after 10-14 day culture in abacavir naïve HLA-B*57:01 positive healthy blood donors but not donors with other HLA types. Furthermore two independent groups have resolved the crystal structure of abacavir-HLA-B*57:01-peptide and confirmed that abacavir binds within the antigen-blinding cleft of HLA-B*57:01 and form contacts with its hydrophobic F pocket. This interaction changes the chemistry and shape of the antigen binding cleft which leads to a change of the repertoire of peptides

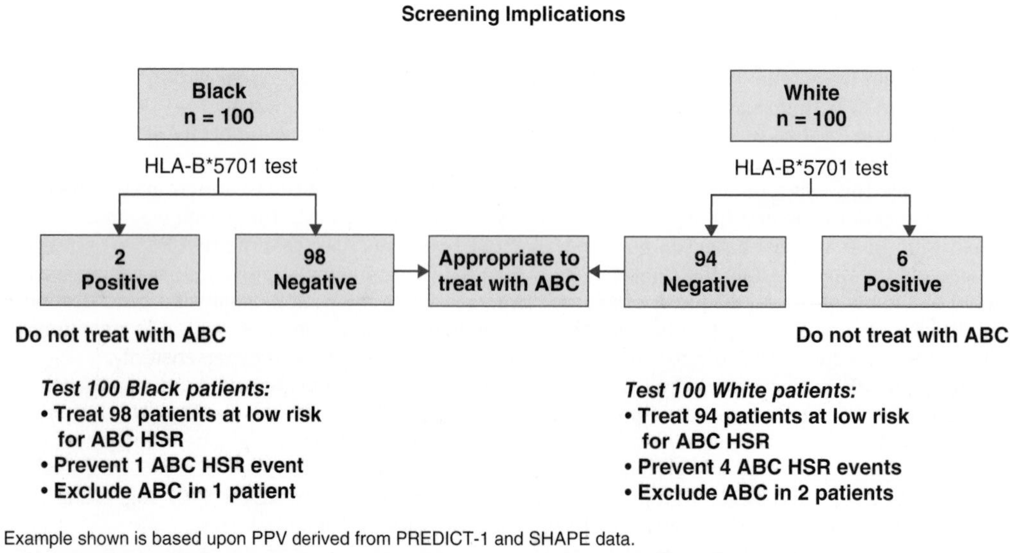

**Screening Implications**

*Example shown is based upon PPV derived from PREDICT-1 and SHAPE data.*

***Figure 10-1*** Flow Diagram Demonstrates the Predicted Percentages of Those Testing Positive for HLA B*5701 in Two Different Cohorts. Adapted from Phillips E, Mallal S. Abacavir hypersensitivity in Uptodate, added October 2008.

presented to CD8+ T cells and may induce alloreactivity similar to that seen with solid organ transplant rejection.

## BIBLIOGRAPHY:

1. Hetherington S. Hypersensitivity reactions during therapy with the nucleoside reverse transcriptase inhibitor abacavir. *Clin Ther.* 2001;23:1603-1614.

2. Shapiro M, Ward KM, Stern JJ. A near-fatal hypersensitivity reaction to abacavir: case report and literature review. *AIDS Read.* 2001;11:222-226.

3. Phillips E, Mallal S. Drug hypersensitivity in HIV. *Curr Opin Allergy Clin Immunol.* 2007;7:324-330.

4. Peyrieere H, Guillemin V, Lothe A, et al. Reasons for early abacavir discontinuation in HIV-infected patients. *Ann Pharmacother.* 2003;37:1392-1397.

5. Phillips E, Sullivan JR, Knowles SR, et al. Utility of patch testing in patients with hypersensitivity syndromes associated with abacavir. *AIDS.* 2002;16:2223-2225.

6. Phillips E, Wong GA, Kaul R, et al. Clinical and immunogenetic correlates of abacavir hypersensitivity. *AIDS.* 2005;19:979-981.

7. Mallal S, Nolan D, Witt C, et al. Association between presence of HLA-B*5701, HLA-DR7 and HLA-DQ3 and hypersensitivity to HIV-1 reverse transcriptase inhibitor abacavir. *Lancet.* 2002; 359:727-732.

8. Hetherington S, Hughes AR, Mosteller M, et al. Genetic variations in HLA-B region and hypersensitivity reactions to abacavir. *Lancet.* 2002;359:1121-1122.

9. Hughes AR, Mosteller N, Bansal AT, et al. Association of genetic variation in HLA-B region with hypersensitivity in some, but not all, populations. *Pharmacogenomics.* 2004;5:203-211.

10. Rauch A, Nolan D, Martin A, et al. Prospective genetic screening decreases the incidence of abacavir hypersensitivity reactions in the Western Australian HIV cohort study. *Clin Infect Dis.* 2006;43:99-102.

11. Mallal S, Phillips E, Carosi G, et al. HLA-B*5701 screening for hypersensitivity to abacavir. *N Eng J Med.* 2008;358:568-579.

12. Saag M, Balu R, Phillips E, et al. High sensitivity of human leukocyte antigen-B*5701 as a marker for immunogenetically confirmed abacavir hypersensitivity in White and Black patients. *Clin Infect Dis.* 2008;46:1111-1118.

13. Hammond E, Almeida CA, Mamotte C, et al. External quality assessment of HLA-B*5701 reporting: an International multicentre survey. *Antivir Ther.* 2007;12:1027-1032.

14. Martin AM, Nolan D, Mallal S. HLA-B*5701 typing by sequence-specific amplification: validation and comparison with sequence-based typing. *Tissue Antigens.* 2005;65:571-574.

15. Hammond E, Mamotte C, Noland D, et al. HLA-B*5701 typing: evaluation of an allele-specific polymerase chain melting assay. *Tissue Antigens.* 2007;70:58-61.

16. Martin AM, Krueger R, Almeida CA, et al. A sensitive and rapid alternative to HLA typing as a genetic screening test for abacavir hypersensitivity syndrome. *Pharmacogenet Genomics.* 2006;16:353-357.

17. Department of Health and Human Services Panel on Antiretroviral Guidelines for Adults and Adolescents. Guidelines for the use of antiretroviral agents in HIV-1 infected adults and adolescents: November 3, 2008 [online]. http://aidsinfo.nih.gov/contentfiles/AdultandAdolscentGL.pdf. Accessed September 16, 2009.

18. Hammer SM, Eron Jr. JJ, Reiss P. et al. Antiretroviral treatment of adult HIV infection: 2008 recommendations of the International AIDS Society-USA panel. *JAMA.* 2008;300:555-570.

19. Chessman D, Kostenko L, Lethborg T, et al. Human leukocyte antigen class-I restricted activation of CD8+ T cells provide the immunogenetic basis of a systemic drug hypersensitivity. *Immunity.* 2008;28:822-832.

20. Phillips E, Nolan D, Thorborn D, et al. Genetic factors predicting abacavir hypersensitivity and tolerance in HLA-B*5701 positive individuals. *Eur J Dermatol.* 2008;18:247.

21. Illing PT, Vivian JP, Dudek NL et al. Immune self-reactivity triggered by drug-modified HLA-peptide repertoire. *Nature.* 2012; 28:554-558.

22. Ostrov DA, Grant BJ, Pompeu YA et al. Drug hypersensitivity caused by alteration of the MHC-presented self-peptide repertoire. *Proc Natl Acad Sci.* 2012;109:9959-9964.

23. Norcross MA, Luo S, Lu L et al Abacavir induces loading of novel self-peptides into HLA-B*57: 01: an autoimmune model for HLA-associated drug hypersensitivity. *AIDS.* 2012;26:F21-9.

## Supplementary Information

*Key Words:* Abacavir, HIV, hypersensitivity

# 11 Coronary Artery Disease

Tariq Ahmad and Paul M. Ridker

## KEY POINTS

- *Disease summary:*
  - Coronary artery disease (CAD) is a multifactorial disorder that results from interplay between genetic and environmental factors.
  - CAD is the most common cause of death worldwide.
  - CAD is a progressive disease process that generally begins in childhood and manifests clinically in mid-to-late adulthood. It results from the accumulation of atherosclerotic changes within the walls of coronary arteries. The distribution of lipid and connective tissue, and the degree of inflammation in the atherosclerotic lesions determine whether they are stable or at risk of rupture, and subsequent thrombosis, causing acute coronary syndromes (ACSs).
  - Hypertension, hypercholesterolemia, smoking, and diabetes are major risk factors for CAD. However, they do not account for up to 15% to 20% of patients with myocardial infarction (MI); such patients often have a family history of CAD, pointing to an integral role of genetics in the development of this disease.
  - Commonly used CAD risk prediction models such as the Framingham risk score take into account known risk factors such as age, plasma lipid levels, blood pressure, tobacco use, and type 2 diabetes. Newer models such as the Reynolds risk score additionally include family history as an independent risk factor but the exact mechanisms by which risk of CAD is inherited remain unclear.
- *Hereditary basis:*
  - Monogenic causes of lipid disorders exist. The more commonly encountered premature CAD is highly heritable and common variation in several genes has been shown to be associated with increased risk.
- *Environmental factors:*
  - Age, tobacco, sedentary lifestyle, high-fat or -salt diet, hypertension
- *Monogenic forms:*
  - Familial hypercholesterolemia (FH), familial defective apolipoprotein B or ApoB (FDB), autosomal dominant hypercholesterolemia, autosomal recessive hypercholesterolemia (ARH), sitosterolemia, primary hypoalphalipoproteinemia
- *Genome-wide associations:*
  - More than a dozen genetic loci related to CAD have been found. Currently, testing for any of them has not been clinically validated for risk prediction or to guide treatment (Table 11-1).
- *Pharmacogenomics:*
  - The Food and Drug Administration (FDA) has approved *CYP2C19* genotype testing to determine if patients may be poor metabolizers of clopidogrel, an agent commonly used to prevent rethrombosis among CAD patients (Table 11-2). Pharmacogenomic data has demonstrated increased risk of statin-related myopathy based on variation in the *SLCO1B1* gene.
- *Differential diagnosis:*
  - Thromboangiitis obliterans, Kawasaki disease, pericarditis, myocarditis, coronary artery anomaly, coronary artery vasospasm, cardiomyopathy, esophageal disorders

## Diagnostic Criteria and Clinical Characteristics

The manifestations of CAD are quite broad, ranging from asymptomatic to ACSs and sudden cardiac death. Equally broad and intricate are the diagnostic criteria and clinical characteristics used for risk stratification and choice of treatment. Here we provide a brief overview of the characteristics and testing of patients with stable disease and those with ACS. It must be noted that majority of patients with CAD are asymptomatic and physicians rely on ever improving methods of risk stratification to guide their management. Diagnostic evaluation of suspected CAD begins with a clinical assessment.

***Clinical Characteristics:***

**Chronic CAD**

- Dyspnea on exertion; substantial chest pain (angina) from cardiac stressors with radiation to the neck, jaw, shoulders, arm, or abdomen; palpitations, syncope or presyncope, and fatigue

*Table 11-1  CAD- or MI-Associated Susceptibility Variants*

| Candidate Gene(s), Chromosome Location | Associated Variant | Relative Risk (95% CI) | Risk Allele, Frequency | Putative Functional Significance |
|---|---|---|---|---|
| CELSR2-PSRC1-SORT1, 1p13.3 | rs599839 | 1.24 (1.12-1.38) | A, 77% | LDL metabolism |
| MIA3, 1q41 | rs17465637 | 1.14 (1.09-1.19) | C, 72% | Cellular proliferation |
| PCSK9, 1p32.3 | rs11206510 | 1.15 (1.10-1.21) | T, 81% | LDL metabolism |
| WDR12, 2q33.1 | rs6725887 | 1.17 (1.11-1.23) | C, 14% | Unknown |
| MRAS, 3q22.3 | rs9818870 | 1.15 (1.11-1.19) | T, 15% | Intracellular signaling, cellular proliferation |
| PHACTR1, 6p24.1 | rs12526453 | 1.12 (1.08-1.17) | C, 65% | Unknown |
| MTHFD1L, 6q25.1 | rs6922269 | 1.23 (1.13-1.35) | A, 30% | Homocysteine metabolism |
| LPA, 6q26-6q27 | rs3798220 | 1.47 (1.35-1.60) | C, 2% | Lp(a) metabolism |
| LPA, 6q26-6q27 | rs10455872 | 1.68 (1.43-1.98) | G, 7% | Lp(a) metabolism |
| CDKN2A/2B, 9p21.3 | rs1333049 | 1.29 (1.25-1.34) | C, 56% | Unknown, cellular proliferation suggested |
| CXCL12, 10q11.21 | rs1746048 | 1.17 (1.11-1.24) | C, 84% | Inflammation, chemokines |
| HNF1A, 12q24 | rs2259816 | 1.08 (1.05-1.11) | T, 37% | Inflammation, metabolic syndrome, lipids |
| SH2B3, 12q24 | rs3184504 | 1.13 (1.08-1.18) | T, 40% | Inflammation |
| LDLR, 19p13.2 | rs1122608 | 1.15 (1.10-1.20) | G, 75% | LDL metabolism |
| SLC5A3-MRPS6-KCNE2, 21q22.11 | rs9982601 | 1.20 (1.14-1.27) | T, 13% | Lp(a) levels |

## ACSs

- Angina that is new in onset, progressive, or at rest. Relieved by nitroglycerin or rest.
- Vagal symptoms such as diaphoresis and nausea; shortness of breath, dizziness; sense of impending doom.
- New S4 on physical examination, mitral regurgitation murmur, paradoxical S2, increased jugular venous pressure (JVP), lung crackles.

## Diagnostic Testing for CAD:

**Screening of Asymptomatic Middle-Aged Individuals**

- Fasting lipid profile: Total cholesterol, high-density lipoprotein-cholesterol (HDL-C), low-density lipoprotein-cholesterol (LDL-C), and triglyceride levels
- Inflammatory markers (high-sensitivity C-reactive protein [hs-CRP])
- Ankle-brachial index (ABI)
- Blood pressure

*Table 11-2  Pharmacogenetic Considerations in the Treatment of CAD*

| Gene | Associated Medications | Goal of Testing | Variants | Function | Effect |
|---|---|---|---|---|---|
| SLCO1B1 | Statins | Prediction of statin-related myopathy | rs4149056 CC—high risk TT—low risk | SLCO1B1 encodes the organic anion-transporting polypeptide OATP1B1, which mediates the hepatic uptake of various drugs, including most statins and statin acids | 4.5 × risk of myopathy per risk allele Homozygotes—17 × greater risk |
| CYP2C19 | Clopidogrel | Identification of clopidogrel nonresponders | *1A, *2A, *3, *4, *5A, *6, *7, *8, *9, *10, *12, *13, *14, *17 | CYP2C19, a member of the cytochrome P450 mixed-function oxidase system, is involved in the metabolism of several important classes of drugs, including clopidogrel | Based on genetic variation of these alleles, individuals are classified as poor, intermediate, and extensive metabolizers |

**Evaluation of Suspected or Chronic CAD**

- Electrocardiogram (ECG) and ECG stress testing
- Rest or stress transthoracic echocardiography (TTE)
- Nuclear imaging studies (treadmill nuclear stress test, a dipyridamole [Persantine] or adenosine nuclear stress test, and a dobutamine nuclear stress test)
- Electron beam computed tomography (CT) scanning
- Percutaneous coronary angiography

**Evaluation of ACS**

- ECG
- Measurement of biomarkers of myocardial necrosis (serum troponin I or T, creatinine kinase myocardial band [CK-MB])
- TTE
- Nuclear imaging studies
- Percutaneous coronary angiography

## Screening and Counseling

**Screening:** Screening for suspected familial forms of CAD should begin by consideration of Mendelian lipid disorders, the best established genetic risk factors for CAD. These involve key genes in lipid metabolism pathways and should be screened for via a careful family history, lipid profile, and physical examination for presence of associated findings such as xanthomas. They include autosomal dominant hypercholesterolemia due to mutations in the *LDLR*, *PCSK9*, and *APOB* genes, autosomal recessive hypercholesterolemia due to mutations in the *ARH* gene, and sitosterolemia due to mutations in the *ABCG5* and *ABCG8* genes. These disorders are reviewed elsewhere in the book. Linkage studies for MI or CAD have also identified several loci and genes, including *MEF2A*, *LRP6*, *ALOX5AP*, and *LTA4H*. These findings have not been reliably replicated and their role as candidate genes in familial CAD remains unclear.

The majority of patients with a family history of CAD would not be expected to have rare mutations within these genes. Instead, they would likely have a combination of risk variants at several loci that collectively increase their risk of CAD. Single-nucleotide polymorphisms (SNPs) uncovered by several genome-wide association studies (GWAS) for CAD are presented in Table 11-1.

While the GWAS approach has led to finding several validated genetic associations, their clinical application is limited and testing of these variants to inform risk is currently not recommended. SNPs associated with CAD consistently show small-to-modest relative risks (1-1.3), and only explain a small proportion of the variance in risk (1%-5%). Genetic scores incorporating these loci have not been shown to more informative than conventional risk factors. A recent study showed that, after adjustment for traditional CAD risk factors, a risk score comprised of 101 SNPs associated with CAD or intermediate phenotypes such as hypertension, diabetes, and lipid levels, did not improve risk prediction beyond traditional risk factors. Despite this, a number of companies offer direct-to-consumer testing for CAD and patients may ask their physicians to interpret the results of such testing. Currently, there is no proven clinical utility to using this information for risk prediction or for making treatment decisions. Therefore, established risk prediction algorithms such as the Framingham risk score (http://hp2010.nhlbihin.net/atpiii/CALCULATOR.asp?usertype=prof) or the Reynolds risk score

(http://www.reynoldsriskscore.org) that take into account a patient's family history should be used to assess risk.

**Counseling:** Genetic counseling related to Mendelian lipid disorders are discussed elsewhere. Patients with a family history of CAD should be counseled about their increased risk (~two times that of people without a family history), even after controlling for traditional risk factors. For example, the Framingham Offspring Study found that individuals with at least one parent with a history of premature CAD (<55 years in men, <65 in women) had up to twice the risk as someone without a family history, even after controlling or established risk factors. Therefore, these patients and their families would benefit from early screening of lipids and risk stratification, which can be done using online calculators of risk that take into account family history, such as the Reynolds risk score (see earlier). Currently, the use of genetics for risk prediction or for making treatment decisions in these patients has not been shown to be of benefit and is not recommended.

## Treatments and Pharmacogenetics

**Management:** The management of CAD is complicated and nuanced beyond the scope of this chapter. Here we review the medications commonly used to manage patients with CAD, along with any pharmacogenetic considerations. While several genetic markers have been found to predict the individual response to many medications used in CAD, and testing for some is commercially available, the use of genomics to guide management is currently only recommended for the use of clopidogrel.

**HMG-CoA Reductase Inhibitors (Statins):** Statins are a mainstay of preventive cardiology and numerous studies have shown them to cause dramatic reductions in incidence and recurrence of CAD. They lower cholesterol by inhibiting HMG-CoA reductase, the rate-limiting enzyme in cholesterol synthesis. Current guidelines for treatment goals related to statin use depend on estimations of CAD risk. Numerous studies have suggested that common genetic polymorphisms might modify the response to statin therapy. These include polymorphisms in the *HMGCR*, *APOE*, *PCSK9*, *LDLR*, and *APOB* genes. However, these findings have either been inconsistent, or lack the confirmation of well-designed randomized controlled trials that show testing to improve outcomes. Interestingly, variation within the *KIF6* gene has been associated with both increased risk of CAD and greater response to statin therapy, and while commercial laboratories offer testing, validation in large prospective studies has failed to confirm this association. Several studies have also shown that the risk of developing side effects of statin use are related to reduced-function SNPs in the *SLCOB1* gene.

**Aspirin:** Acetylsalicylic acid, or aspirin, is the most widely used medication in the world for prevention of cardiovascular disease. In doses ranging from 75 to 300 mg/d, aspirin has been shown effective in primary prevention in adults at increased risk for CAD and those who have survived ACS. Aspirin's mechanism of action is via irreversible inhibition of platelet cyclo-oxygenase 1 (COX1), which reduces thromboxane generation and inhibits platelet-mediated thrombus formation. Studies have found evidence for several genetic polymorphisms (*COX1*, *COX2*, *GPIIIa*, *GP1a*, *GPVI*, *GNB3*, *P2Y1R*, and *P2Y12R*) influencing aspirin response but these results are inconclusive. This is inconsistent with the strong heritability demonstrated for aspirin phenotypes and may be due to the lack of adequately sized studies that test a comprehensive list of genetic variants. A few data demonstrate that pharmacogenetic considerations in aspirin intake influence clinical outcomes; one report suggested that carriers of a variant in the *LPA* gene had increased cardiovascular risk, and appeared to benefit more from aspirin than noncarriers.

**Beta-Adrenergic Blockers:** Beta-blockers are prescribed to millions of Americans for hypertension, angina, recovery after MI, and heart failure. These medications reduce myocardial oxygen demand by inhibiting the effects of adrenergic activation on the cardiovascular system, thus leading to less angina, infarction, and protection from arrhythmias. Genetic variation in at least two different genes has reproducibly shown to modify treatment effect. These include polymorphisms in genes that regulate beta-adrenergic signaling (*ADRB1, ADRB2*). Pending results of trials that show differential outcomes based on consideration of these variants, testing is not recommended.

**Calcium Channel Blockers:** Calcium channel blockers are coronary vasodilators that produce reductions in myocardial oxygen demand via negative ionotropy and reductions in arterial pressure. They have not been shown to improve life expectancy in CAD, and are used for treatment of angina and hypertension. Despite extensive use of these medications, very few studies have looked at interactions between genetic variants and treatment effects. Recently, two studies showed that polymorphisms in the *CACNA1C* gene which encodes the alpha-1c subunit of L-type calcium channel were associated with treatment response. However, these data and others are preliminary and require replication.

**ACE Inhibitors/Angiotensin Receptor Blockers:** Angiotensin-converting enzyme inhibitors (ACEIs) or angiotensin receptor blockers (ARBs) are widely used for hypertension and heart failure. They are also used to reduce the progression of diabetic nephropathy and in chronic heart failure, where their benefits lie beyond an antihypertensive effect. Several pharmacogenetic studies have looked at whether SNPs can predict individual differences in ACEI response. Polymorphisms in the *AGT, AGTR1,* and *ACE* genes have been implicated but the findings have been inconsistent and warrant further investigations. The pharmacogenetic actions of ARBs with several polymorphisms have been investigated but suffer from lack of replication and disparate results across different drugs within the same class.

**Adenosine Diphosphate Receptor Blockers:** The standard of care for treatment of patients who have experienced ACSs and percutaneous coronary intentions with stenting is dual antiplatelet therapy with aspirin and the thienopyridine inhibitors of the platelet adenosine diphosphate (ADP) receptors. Some patients (2%-14% of the US population), due to genetic variation in the cytochrome P450 gene, *CYP2C19,* have diminished pharmacokinetic and pharmacodynamic responses to clopidogrel and an increased rate of death from CAD. Therefore, the FDA has issued a black box warning alerting patients and healthcare professionals that the drug can be less effective in people who cannot metabolize the drug to convert it to its active form. They suggest alternative dosing of clopidogrel or consideration of other antiplatelet medications for these patients. Commercial testing is available to assess *CYP2C19* genotype to determine if a patient is a poor metabolizer, and point-of-care assays are under development. The effect of prasugrel, a third-generation thienopyridine that is a more potent platelet inhibitor than clopidogrel does not appear to be modified by *CYP* genetic variants.

## Molecular Genetics and Molecular Mechanism

The GWA methodology, as applied to finding genetic determinants of CAD, has yielded many genetic variants in diverse loci that relate to both clinical outcomes and intermediate phenotypes. These variants confirm what we have known about the molecular biology of atherosclerosis and provide us with a list of candidate genes that are shedding new light on the mechanism of disease.

GWAS on intermediate phenotypes of CAD such as plasma lipid concentrations, blood pressure, diabetes, obesity, and inflammatory markers such as CRP have pinpointed established regulators of known pathways, many in genes that cause Mendelian disorders, and others such as *HMGCR* that are already drug targets. These studies have also identified numerous loci that are clarifying the complexity behind perturbations in regularly measured clinical parameters. Findings from such efforts are updating our understanding of clinical phenotypes long observed to be related to CAD and are yielding targets for the next generation of effective medications. For example, the identification of, *PCSK9,* a novel gene involved in lipid metabolism has led to ongoing efforts to develop PCSK9 inhibitors.

Many of the SNPs associated with CAD are within pathways that modify plasma lipid levels and a few exist in regions of the genome not clearly linked to known risk factors. One of these regions, the 9p21 locus, is considered to be one of the major discoveries of GWAS for CAD. Risk variants at the 9p21 locus are not associated with traditional or novel risk factors for CAD and do not reside within any protein coding genes. SNPs at this locus have been associated with other vascular phenotypes, such as peripheral artery disease and abdominal aneurysm, raising the possibility that the mechanism involves a vascular abnormality. At the time of writing this chapter, however, a definite answer remains elusive.

**Future Directions:** The use of GWAS has provided the field of Cardiovascular Genetics with an abundance of genetic candidates that will likely uncover novel mechanisms for CAD. Deep sequencing and functional analyses of the candidate loci are ongoing with the goal of pinpointing causal variants. Additionally, causal variants that have not been found via this approach are expected to be identified by the next-generation sequencing technology.

The clinical application of these findings has been hampered by the fact that these loci only explain a small proportion of the interindividual variability in risk of CAD. Efforts are ongoing to pinpoint this unexplained variance by searching for rare variants, elucidating gene and environment interactions, characterizing between-population heterogeneity, and applying more comprehensive sequencing methods. As more disease-associated variants are uncovered and more sophisticated genetics risk scores are constructed, their value in risk prediction would be based on their ability to add prognostic value beyond what is afforded by asking patients about their family history. The clopidogrel example shows us that use of genetic variants for personalized treatment has already proved useful and, in the future, may allow us to more accurately predict both therapeutic response and safety of medications prior to prescribing them.

**BIBLIOGRAPHY:**

1. Robin NH, Tabereaux PB, Benza R, Korf BR. Genetic testing in cardiovascular disease. *J Am Coll Cardiol.* 2007;50:727-737.
2. Musunuru K, Kathiresan S. Genetics of coronary artery disease. *Annu Rev Genomics Hum Genet.* 2009.

3. Paynter NP, Chasman DI, Pare G, Buring JE, Cook NR, Miletich JP, Ridker PM. Association between a literature-based genetic risk score and cardiovascular events in women. *JAMA*.303:631-637.

4. Berger JS, Jordan CO, Lloyd-Jones D, Blumenthal RS. Screening for cardiovascular risk in asymptomatic patients. *J Am Coll Cardiol 2010;*.55:1169-1177.

5. Lloyd-Jones DM, Nam BH, D'Agostino RB Sr., et al. Parental cardiovascular disease as a risk factor for cardiovascular disease in middle-aged adults: a prospective study of parents and offspring. *JAMA*. 2004;291:2204-2211.

6. Mangravite LM, Wilke RA, Zhang J, Krauss RM. Pharmacogenomics of statin response. *Curr Opin Mol Ther*. 2008;10:555-561.

7. Chasman DI, Posada D, Subrahmanyan L, Cook NR, Stanton VP Jr., Ridker PM. Pharmacogenetic study of statin therapy and cholesterol reduction. *JAMA*. 2004;291:2821-2827.

8. Iakoubova OA, Sabatine MS, Rowland CM, et al. Polymorphism in KIF6 gene and benefit from statins after acute coronary syndromes: results from the PROVE IT-TIMI 22 study. *J Am Coll Cardiol*. 2008;51:449-455.

9. Ridker PM, MacFadyen JG, Glynn RJ, Chasman DI. Kinesin-like protein 6 (KIF6) polymorphism and the efficacy of rosuvastatin in primary prevention. *Circ Cardiovasc Genet*. 2011;4:312-317.

10. Vladutiu GD, Isackson PJ. SLCO1B1 variants and statin-induced myopathy. *N Engl J Med*. 2009;360:304.

11. Goodman T, Ferro A, Sharma P. Pharmacogenetics of aspirin resistance: a comprehensive systematic review. *Br J Clin Pharmacol*. 2008;66:222-232.

12. Feher G, Feher A, Pusch G, Lupkovics G, Szapary L, Papp E. The genetics of antiplatelet drug resistance. *Clin Genet*. 2009;75:1-18.

13. Ahmad T, Voora D, Becker RC. The pharmacogenetics of antiplatelet agents: towards personalized therapy? *Nat Rev Cardiol*. 2011;8(10):560-571.

14. Arnett DK, Claas SA. Pharmacogenetics of antihypertensive treatment: detailing disciplinary dissonance. *Pharmacogenomics*. 2009;10:1295-1307.

15. Steinhubl SR. Genotyping, clopidogrel metabolism, and the search for the therapeutic window of thienopyridines. *Circulation*. 2010; 121:481-483.

16. Horton JD, Cohen JC, Hobbs HH. PCSK9: a convertase that coordinates LDL catabolism. *J Lipid Res*. 2009;50(suppl):S172-S177.

## Supplementary Information

**Alternative Names:**
- Cardiovascular Disease (CVD)
- Coronary Heart Disease (CHD)

# 12 Metabolic Syndrome

Tisha R. Joy and Robert A. Hegele

## KEY POINTS

- *Disease summary:*
  - Metabolic syndrome (MetS) is a complex genetic disorder, involving the interaction of multiple genetic loci with environmental factors.
  - MetS consists of three of the five following criteria: increased waist circumference (Table 12-1); triglyceride (TG) level greater than or equal to 150 mg/dL (1.7 mmol/L) *or* drug treatment for elevated TG; high-density lipoprotein-cholesterol (HDL-C) less than 40 mg/dL (1 mmol/L) in males or less than 50 mg/dL (1.3 mmol/L) in females *or* drug treatment for reduced HDL-C level; systolic blood pressure (SBP) greater than or equal to 130 mm Hg and/or diastolic blood pressure (DBP) greater than or equal to 85 mm Hg *or* antihypertensive drug treatment in a patient with a history of elevated blood pressure (BP); fasting glucose greater than or equal to 100 mg/dL (5.6 mmol/L) *or* drug treatment for elevated glucose.
  - Individuals with MetS have a twofold increased risk for cardiovascular disease (CVD) and fivefold increased risk for type 2 diabetes (DM2) compared to individuals without MetS.
- *Differential diagnosis:*
  - MetS is polygenic in nature and may be often evident in individuals with coexistent DM2, HIV lipodystrophy, or polycystic ovary syndrome. Rare monogenic forms of lipodystrophy such as familial partial lipodystrophy (FPLD), congenital generalized lipodystrophy (CGL), and acquired partial lipodystrophy (APL) are often considered extreme forms of MetS.
- *Monogenic forms:*
  - Extreme forms of MetS may be evident in monogenic forms of lipodystrophy such as FPLD, CGL, and APL.
- *Family history:*
  - There may be a family history of one or more of the components of MetS. In the genetic lipodystrophies with MetS phenotype, FPLD is inherited in an autosomal dominant fashion, while CGL is inherited as an autosomal recessive trait.
- *Environmental factors:*
  - The components of MetS may be exacerbated by environmental factors. For example, hypertension can be aggravated by excessive salt. Dietary components such as intake of saturated fat or simple carbohydrates can influence the onset and severity of dysglycemia and dyslipidemia. Overall, obesity is a significant moderator of all components of MetS.
- *Genome-wide association studies:*
  - Many associations have been reported for common MetS, especially its individual components. There is no evidence at present for any added diagnostic, prognostic, or therapeutic value of genetic evaluation for common single-nucleotide polymorphism (SNP) genotypes or risk allele scores for the component quantitative traits in common MetS presentation.
- *Pharmacogenomics:*
  - There is no demonstration yet of a potential role for pharmacogenetic evaluation in common MetS. FPLD2 (due to mutant *LMNA*) appears to be more responsive to therapy with thiazolidinediones than is FPLD3 (due to mutant *PPARG*).

## Diagnostic Criteria and Clinical Characteristics

***Diagnostic Criteria for Metabolic Syndrome:*** Although several different definitions for MetS have been proposed, six different organizations have recently issued a joint statement in an attempt to harmonize the definition of MetS. According to their report, three of the following five criteria are required to make a diagnosis of MetS:

- Elevated waist circumference based on population- and country-specific definitions. Although consensus regarding worldwide waist circumference criteria is still pending, the joint statement recommends using International Diabetes Federation (IDF) thresholds for non-Europeans and IDF or American Health Association/National Heart, Lung, and Blood Institute (AHA/NHLBI) thresholds for those of European origin (Table 12-1).
- TG level greater than or equal to 150 mg/dL (1.7 mmol/L) *or* drug treatment for elevated TGs

- HDL-C less than 40 mg/dL (1 mmol/L) in males or less than 50 mg/dL (1.3 mmol/L) in females *or* drug treatment for reduced HDL-C level
- SBP greater than or equal to 130 mm Hg and/or DBP greater than or equal to 85 mm Hg *or* antihypertensive drug treatment in a patient with a history of elevated BP
- Fasting glucose greater than or equal to 100 mg/dL (5.6 mmol/L) *or* drug treatment for elevated glucose

***Clinical Characteristics:***

- MetS represents a clustering of risk factors for the development of CVD and DM2.
- These risk factors include central adiposity, hypertension, hypertriglyceridemia, hypoalphalipoproteinemia, and dysglycemia.
- Insulin resistance is often present, and may be clinically manifest as acanthosis nigricans.
- Atherogenic dyslipidemia characterized by elevated serum TG, apolipoprotein B (ApoB), small low-density lipoprotein (LDL) particles, and reduced HDL-C level is often demonstrated in these patients.

*Table 12-1 Waist Circumference Thresholds for Definition of Abdominal Obesity in MetS[1]*

| Population | Waist Circumference Cutoffs (cm) | |
| --- | --- | --- |
| | Males | Females |
| Caucasian | ≥102 | ≥88 |
| Asian | ≥90 | ≥80 |
| Middle East, Mediterranean, Sub-Saharan Africa | ≥94 | ≥80 |
| Ethnic Central and South American | ≥90 | ≥80 |

- Individuals with MetS have a twofold increased risk for CVD and fivefold increased risk for DM2 compared to individuals without MetS.
- Most individuals with MetS will also demonstrate increased hepatic and visceral adiposity.
- Polycystic ovaries and hirsutism may be evident in women.

### Differential Diagnosis:

- In most individuals, MetS is polygenic in nature and is often evident in individuals with coexistent DM2, HIV lipodystrophy, or polycystic ovary syndrome.
- Less commonly, the cause of MetS can be monogenic in the form of certain lipodystrophies such as FPLD, CGL, and APL.
- The genetic basis has been revealed in two subtypes of FPLD, CGL, and some patients with APL (see later).
- These monogenic forms of lipodystrophy are often considered extreme forms of MetS.
- 10% of individuals with severe forms of MetS have demonstrated mutations in the *LMNA* gene.
- FPLD is the most common genetic lipodystrophy, commences at puberty, and is characterized by gradual and progressive loss of subcutaneous fat from the extremities and variable subcutaneous fat loss in the trunk.
- Compared to individuals with FPLD2, those with FPLD3 have less extensive adipose tissue loss clinically but more severe metabolic complications.
- CGL is typically evident in infancy due to the muscular phenotype of affected individuals, who demonstrate significant generalized loss of subcutaneous fat.
- APL typically develops in adulthood and is often accompanied by other autoimmune conditions.
- Hirsutism and polycystic ovaries commonly occur in FPLD.
- Increased visceral, hepatic, and intramyocellular fat as well as acanthosis nigricans are often present in CGL and FPLD.

## Screening and Counseling

Common MetS is very heavily influenced by nongenetic factors, such as poor diet and inactivity. For the majority of patients in whom there is not a suspicion of a rare syndromic form of MetS, such as an inherited lipodystrophy syndrome, there is no specific benefit to screening family members for a molecular genetic diagnosis.

For FPLD, molecular diagnosis can help and can provide a means for diagnosis of affected family members presymptomatically. However, no presymptomatic intervention other than diet and exercise seems effective in delaying onset or reducing the severity of the metabolic disturbances. Medical advice for carriers of such rare mutations would include lifestyle advice and appropriate pharmacologic intervention when specific clinical and biochemical features arise.

## Management and Treatment

Regardless of whether the MetS is polygenic or monogenic in nature, the overall goal for management is to reduce the risk for future CVD as well as DM2.

Management of MetS focuses on management of each of the individual components of MetS—central adiposity, hypertension, dyslipidemia, and dysglycemia.

### Lifestyle Intervention:

- First-line intervention to improve all parameters of MetS with the following goals:
  - Weight loss of 7% to 10% of baseline weight during the first year of therapy, followed by further weight loss to achieve an ideal body mass index (BMI) of less than 25 kg/m$^2$.
  - Regular moderate-intensity aerobic activity of at least 30 minutes (preferably 60 minutes) 5 d/wk (preferable daily).
  - Dietary modification consisting of total fat and saturated fat intake of 25% to 35% and less than 7% of total calories, respectively; total cholesterol intake less than 200 mg/d; and decreased trans fat intake.
- Smoking cessation is also recommended to reduce future CVD risk.

### Hypertension:

- If BP is greater than or equal to 120/80 mm Hg, initiate or maintain lifestyle intervention as above but also focus on alcohol moderation (<2 standard alcoholic drinks per day in men and <1 drink per day in women), sodium restriction (<2.4 g sodium/d), and adoption of Dietary Approaches to Stop Hypertension [DASH] diet with increased consumption of fresh fruits, vegetables, and low-fat dairy products.
- If BP is greater than or equal to 140/90 mm Hg (or ≥130/80 mm Hg with coexistent DM), add BP medication according to nation-specific guidelines to achieve target BP.

### Dyslipidemia:

- Nation-specific guidelines should be followed.
- Lifestyle modification as discussed earlier is key first step.
- See Table 12-2 for management guidelines for dyslipidemia based on risk stratification according to National Cholesterol Education Program Adult Treatment Panel (NCEP ATP III) guidelines:
  - Primary goal is achievement of target low-density lipoprotein-cholesterol (LDL-C).
  - Secondary target is achievement of non–HDL-C level appropriate for risk category if TG is greater than or equal to 200 mg/dL.
  - Tertiary goal is to improve HDL-C levels to the extent possible with either intensification of lifestyle therapy or standard pharmacologic therapies (niacin or fibrates) in males with HDL-C less than 40 mg/dL or females with HDL-C less than 50 mg/dL.

*Table 12-2 Recommended Therapeutic Targets for Dyslipidemia in Individuals With MetS*

| | Very High-risk Patients | High-risk Patients | Moderately High Risk | Moderate Risk | Low Risk |
|---|---|---|---|---|---|
| 10-year CHD risk (calculated by the Framingham risk score) | >20% but likely to have major event during next few years | >20% | 10%-20% and ≥2 major risk factors[a] | <10% and ≥2 major risk factors[a] | <10% and 0-1 major risk factors[a] |
| LDL-C target (mg/dL) | <70 | <100 | <130 (<100 optional) | <130 | <160 |
| Non–HDL-C target (mg/dL) | <100 | <130 | <160 (<130 optional) | <160 | <190 |

[a]Risk factors include cigarette smoking, hypertension (BP ≥140/90 mm Hg or on antihypertensive medication), low HDL-C (<40 mg/dL), family history of premature CHD (first-degree male or female relative <55 or <65 years, respectively).

CHD, coronary heart disease; HDL-C, high-density lipoprotein-cholesterol; LDL-C, low-density lipoprotein-cholesterol.

***Dysglycemia:***
- In those individuals with impaired fasting glucose or impaired glucose tolerance, lifestyle management seems more effective than pharmacologic therapy in delaying the progression toward DM2.
- Once diagnosed with DM2, the initial steps would be lifestyle management with or without pharmacologic management to achieve a glycosylated hemoglobin (HbA$_{1c}$) according to nation-specific guidelines.

***Pharmacogenetics:***
- There is no demonstration yet of a potential role for pharmacogenetic evaluation in common MetS.
- FPLD2 (due to mutant *LMNA*) appears to be more responsive to therapy with thiazolidinediones (TZDs) than is FPLD3 (due to mutant *PPARG*).

# Molecular Genetics and Molecular Mechanisms

***Common MetS:***
- SNP genotypes that have been found from genome-wide association studies (GWAS) to be determinants of the individual components, such as TG, HDL-C, BP, waist circumference, and glucose, contribute to the clinical construct called *MetS*, which is defined by the individual components.

***Monogenic MetS:***
- The molecular genetic basis of some of the inherited lipodystrophies—which can be seen as extreme monogenic forms of MetS—has been defined.

***Partial Lipodystrophies:***
- FPLD2 results from heterozygous mutations in *LMNA* encoding nuclear lamin A/C (MIM 150330).
- FPLD3 (MIM 604367) results from heterozygous mutations in the *PPARG* gene encoding peroxisome proliferator-activated receptor gamma.
- Other genes that cause variant FPLD include *CAV1*, encoding caveolin-1.
- APL is sometimes associated with rare heterozygous mutations in *LMNB2*, encoding nuclear lamin B2.

- The mechanism causing FPLD2 and other laminopathies due to mutations within or near the lamin DNA-binding domain could be altered interactions of transcription factors or other DNA-binding molecules with the nuclear lamina.
- The clinical and biochemical disturbances in FPLD3 subjects are out of proportion to the extent of lipodystrophy compared with FPLD2 subjects, suggesting that the *PPARG* mutations might have additional effects on metabolism.

***Generalized Lipodystrophies:***
- Berardinelli-Seip congenital lipodystrophy (BSCL) type 1 is caused by mutations in the *AGPAT2* gene, which encodes 1-acylglycerol-3-phosphate *O*-acyltransferase 2.
- BSCL2 (MIM 606158) is caused by mutations in seipin, a 398-amino acid integral membrane protein localized to the endoplasmic reticulum.

Thus, rare monogenic lipodystrophies occur as the result of mutations in genes encoding two nuclear envelope structural components (*LMNA* and *LMNB2*), a nuclear hormone receptor (*PPARG*), an integral endoplasmic reticulum membrane protein (*seipin*) and a lipid biosynthetic enzyme (*AGPAT2*). There are no obvious unifying mechanistic links or pathways that account for lipodystrophy phenotype and associated MetS profile that result in this wide range of causative gene products.

***Genetic Testing:*** DNA sequencing of *LMNA* and related genes causing rare monogenic lipodystrophy and insulin resistance syndromes is available at some commercial laboratories and in a few research laboratories. The value of knowing the precise mutation underlying a lipodystrophy phenotype in a particular patient, beyond establishing a molecular diagnosis, is not clear.

There is also no evidence at present for any added diagnostic, prognostic, or therapeutic value of genetic evaluation for common SNP genotypes or risk allele scores for the component quantitative traits in common MetS presentation.

***Future Directions:*** Translation of the diagnostic and therapeutic value for genotyping common variants in common MetS needs to be solved. Further molecular heterogeneity is likely to be discovered among lipodystrophy patients who lack a molecular diagnosis. An unresolved question is whether the metabolic disturbances in lipodystrophies develop secondarily to adipose tissue repartitioning or result from a direct effect of the individual mutant gene product. Combining next-generation genomic and comprehensive phenomic perspectives will improve understanding of common MetS and perhaps HIV-associated lipodystrophy.

## BIBLIOGRAPHY:

1. Alberti KG, Eckel RH, Grundy SM, et al. Harmonizing the metabolic syndrome: a joint interim statement of the International Diabetes Federation Task Force on Epidemiology and Prevention; National Heart, Lung, and Blood Institute; American Heart Association; World Heart Federation; International Atherosclerosis Society; and international association for the Study of Obesity. *Circulation*. 2009;120:1640-1645.

2. Alberti KG, Zimmet P, Shaw J. The metabolic syndrome—a new worldwide definition. *Lancet*. 2005;366:1059-1062.

3. Grundy SM, Cleeman JI, Daniels SR, et al. Diagnosis and management of the metabolic syndrome: an American Heart Association/National Heart, Lung, and Blood Institute Scientific Statement. *Circulation*. 2005;112:2735-2752.

4. Decaudain A, Vantyghem MC, Guerci B, et al. New metabolic phenotypes in laminopathies: LMNA mutations in patients with severe metabolic syndrome. *J Clin Endocrinol Metab*. 2007;92:4835-4844.

5. Hegele RA, Joy TR, Al-Attar SA, Rutt BK. Thematic review series: Adipocyte Biology. Lipodystrophies: windows on adipose biology and metabolism. *J Lipid Res*. 2007;48:1433-1444.

6. Chobanian AV, Bakris GL, Black HR, et al. The Seventh Report of the Joint National Committee on Prevention, Detection, Evaluation, and Treatment of High Blood Pressure: the JNC 7 report. *JAMA*. 2003;289:2560-2572.

7. Campbell NR, Khan NA, Hill MD, et al. 2009 Canadian Hypertension Education Program recommendations: the scientific summary—an annual update. *Can J Cardiol*. 2009;25:271-277.

8. Executive Summary of The Third Report of The National Cholesterol Education Program (NCEP) Expert Panel on Detection, Evaluation, And Treatment of High Blood Cholesterol in Adults (Adult Treatment Panel III). *JAMA*. 2001;285:2486-2497.

9. Genest J, McPherson R, Frohlich J, et al. 2009 Canadian Cardiovascular Society/Canadian guidelines for the diagnosis and treatment of dyslipidemia and prevention of cardiovascular disease in the adult—2009 recommendations. *Can J Cardiol*. 2009;25:567-579.

10. Knowler WC, Barrett-Connor E, Fowler SE, et al. Reduction in the incidence of type 2 diabetes with lifestyle intervention or metformin. *N Engl J Med*. 2002;346:393-403.

11. Chiasson JL, Josse RG, Gomis R, Hanefeld M, Karasik A, Laakso M. Acarbose for prevention of type 2 diabetes mellitus: the STOP-NIDDM randomised trial. *Lancet*. 2002;359:2072-2077.

12. Canadian Diabetes Association 2008 Clinical Practice Guidelines for the Prevention and Management of Diabetes in Canada. *Can J Diabetes*. 2008;32:S1-S201. http://www.diabetes.ca/files/cpg2008/cpg-.pdf. Accessed December, 2009.

13. Standards of medical care in diabetes—2009. *Diabetes Care*. 2009;32(suppl 1):S13-S61.

14. Joy T, Hegele RA. Genetics of metabolic syndrome: is there a role for phenomics? *Curr Atheroscler Rep*. 2008;10:201-208.

15. Grundy SM, Cleeman JI, Merz CN, et al. Implications of recent clinical trials for the National Cholesterol Education Program Adult Treatment Panel III guidelines. *Circulation*. 2004;110:227-239.

# 13 Dyslipidemia

Daniel Kiss and Daniel J. Rader

## KEY POINTS

- *Disease summary:*
  - Hyperlipidemia describes the phenotype of elevated blood lipids, predisposing a patient to atherosclerotic vascular disease. The overall heritability of blood lipids is often due to the interaction of a variety of alleles.
  - Classic Mendelian monogenic lipoprotein disorders, while rare, have provided profound insight into lipoprotein metabolism and atherosclerotic vascular disease.
  - Originally characterized by Fredrickson and Levy by the type of lipoprotein that accumulated in the circulation, the modern approach to classic Mendelian monogenic disorders emphasizes the molecular basis of the disease and the defect in cholesterol metabolism.
  - Within the population, blood lipid variation is typically the consequence of variation at multiple loci, in addition to significant effect from the environment.
- *Hereditary basis:*
  - Monogenic forms of lipoprotein disorders will be emphasized here, however for the majority of patients with lipid disorders, no one causative allele or mutation can be identified.
    - Genome-wide-association studies (GWAS) have identified a large number of novel loci associated with plasma lipid traits. This application of genomic medicine has uncovered numerous potential targets for therapy, as well as provided insight into the complex interplay of multiple alleles which gives rise to hyperlipidemia in most patients encountered in clinic.
    - In the population, the degree of variation in the major plasma lipid traits attributable to genetic variance is estimated to be approximately 50%. The Framingham Heart Study showed that heritability for single time point measurements of low-density lipoprotein-cholesterol (LDL-C), high-density lipoprotein-cholesterol (HDL-C), and triglycerides (TGs) is 0.59, 0.52, and 0.48, respectively.
- *Differential diagnosis:*
  - The vast majority of cases of hyperlipidemia are discovered on routine screening and are infrequently due to a monogenic lipoprotein disorder. However, the presence of markedly elevated lipids or lipoproteins, xanthomas, accelerated atherosclerosis, or other clinical manifestations of hyperlipoproteinemia are suggestive of a monogenic disorder. It is important to screen for secondary causes such as nephrotic syndrome, obstructive liver disease, and hypothyroidism before making a diagnosis of a monogenic disorder and before initiating therapy.

## Genetic Differential Diagnosis

***Diagnostic Criteria and Clinical Characteristics of Disorders of Elevated LDL-C and Normal TGs:***

- Elevated LDL-C (generally >200 mg/dL)
- TGs normal (generally <200 mg/dL)

Often accompanied by one or more of the following:

- Tendinous xanthomas
- Premature corneal arcus
- Accelerated symptomatic cardiovascular disease (CVD)
- Family history of substantially elevated cholesterol and/or premature CVD

☞**CLINICAL CHARACTERISTICS:** These patients may present for the first time with premature symptomatic atherosclerotic cardiovascular disease. Alternatively, they may be discovered to have markedly elevated cholesterol on routine screening, which is now recommended for all adults. They typically report a family history of hypercholesterolemia and/or early cardiovascular disease. The exceptions to this are the recessive disorders sitosterolemia and autosomal recessive hypercholesterolemia (ARH). On physical examination, patients may have tendon xanthomas at the Achilles tendons or dorsum of the hands, feet, or knees. Patients that are homozygous for familial hypercholesterolemia often develop CVD in childhood.

***Diagnostic Criteria and Clinical Characteristics of Disorders of Decreased HDL:***

- Very low density lipoprotein (VLDL), less than 10th percentile and generally less than 20 mg/dL

Sometimes accompanied by one or more of the following:

- Planar xanthomas
- Enlarged tonsils, hepatosplenomegaly
- Corneal arcus
- Progressive renal disease
- Premature atherosclerotic CVD

☞**CLINICAL CHARACTERISTICS:** These disorders have a great degree of clinical variability based on the underlying gene defect. Deficiency of ApoA-I is associated with planar xanthomas and corneal opacities, as well as premature CVD. However, structural mutations in ApoA-I, for example those heterozygous for Arg173Cys (ApoA-I Milano), have no increased risk of CVD despite their low HDL. Some structural mutations in ApoA-I form amyloid deposits and cause amyloidosis. Tangier disease presents with profoundly low HDL (<5 mg/dL), hepatosplenomegaly, and pathognomonic enlarged orange tonsils secondary to deposition of cholesterol in the reticuloendothelial (RE) system. Lecithin-cholesterol acyltransferase (LCAT) deficiency is characterized by low HDL-C (<10 mg/dL), corneal opacification, and hypertriglyceridemia. The homozygous form of LCAT deficiency also suffers

*Table 13-1* **Mendelian Disorders Causing Elevated LDL-C Levels and Normal TGs**

| Syndrome | Gene Symbol | Pathogenesis |
|---|---|---|
| Familial hypercholesterolemia | LDLR | Loss of function mutation in the LDL receptor (LDLR), reducing clearance of LDL |
| Familial defective apolipoprotein B-100 | APOB | Mutation in the region of ApoB-100 that binds the LDLR, hindering clearance of LDL |
| Autosomal dominant hypercholesterolemia | PCSK9 | Gain of function mutation in proprotein convertase subtilisin/kexin type 9, which causes degradation of the LDLR, thus reducing LDL clearance |
| Autosomal recessive hypercholesterolemia | LDLRAP1 | Loss of function mutation causing decreased receptor-mediated endocytosis of the LDLR, reducing LDL clearance |
| Sitosterolemia | ABCG5 and ABCG8 | Markedly increased absorption and decreased excretion of plant sterols and cholesterol, down regulating the LDLR and reducing LDL clearance |

*Table 13-2* **Mendelian Disorders Causing Low Levels of HDL-C**

| Syndrome | Gene Symbol | Pathogenesis |
|---|---|---|
| ApoA-I deficiency | APOA | ApoA-I gene deletion or mutations preventing synthesis of the ApoA-I protein results in the virtual absence of HDL from the plasma, effectively impairing reverse cholesterol transport and leading to premature atherosclerotic CVD. |
| ApoA-I structural mutations | APOA | Results in the synthesis of structurally abnormal ApoA-I, resulting in rapid catabolism and reduced plasma levels of HDL-C. Generally no increased risk of atherosclerotic CVD. Some structural mutations in ApoA-I form amyloid deposits and cause amyloidosis. |
| Tangier disease | ABCA1 | Lack of ABCA1, a key transporter of cholesterol efflux from cells to free ApoA-I, reduces the assembly of mature HDL by the liver and intestine and results in rapid catabolism of ApoA-I, with extremely low levels of HDL-C. Cells of the reticuloendothelial (RE) system have impaired cholesterol efflux and accumulated cholesterol, resulting in large tonsils and spleen. Relationship to CVD remains uncertain. |
| LCAT deficiency | LCAT | Impaired cholesterol esterification in HDL, resulting in inability to generate mature HDL and rapid catabolism of ApoA-I. All patients develop corneal opacification due to unesterified cholesterol. Some patients develop progressive renal disease. |

*Table 13-3* **Mendelian Disorders Causing Elevated TGs**

| Syndrome | Gene Symbol | Pathogenesis |
|---|---|---|
| Familial chylomicronemia syndrome (type I hyperlipoproteinemia) | LPL and APOC-II | Deficiency in the lipolytic enzyme LPL or its required cofactor ApoC-II causes impaired lipolysis of chylomicron and VLDL TGs and greatly elevated fasting TGs, sometime resulting in pancreatitis. |
| GPIHBP1 deficiency | GPIHBPI | Loss of endothelial attachment for LPL leads to reduced lipolysis and hyperchylomicronemia. |
| ApoA-V deficiency | APOA5 | Lack of ApoA-V, which helps to promote LPL-mediated lipolysis of chylomicron TGs leads to elevated TGs. |
| Familial dysbetalipoproteinemia (type III hyperlipoproteinemia) | APOE | Impaired ability for ApoE-2 and other much rare variants of ApoE to effectively bind lipoprotein receptors, resulting in delayed clearance of chylomicron and VLDL remnants. |

from hemolytic anemia and progressive renal failure. Other than ApoA-I deficiency, these other Mendelian forms of extreme low HDL are not generally associated with premature atherosclerotic CVD.

### Diagnostic Criteria and Clinical Characteristics of Disorders of Increased TGs:

- Fasting TGs greater than 500 mg/dL and often greater than 1000 mg/dL for the first three and fasting TGs greater than 250 mg/dL for the last.

Many patients may have one or more of the following:

- Eruptive xanthomas
- History of pancreatitis
- Other characteristics of the metabolic syndrome
- Premature CVD

☞CLINICAL CHARACTERISTICS: In these disorders, hypertriglyceridemia is due to excess chylomicrons and/or VLDL. In familial chylomicronemia syndrome, patients often present in childhood with severe abdominal pain secondary to pancreatitis. Physical examination may reveal lipemia retinalis or eruptive xanthomas; however these patients are not at increased risk of cardiovascular disease. Serum TGs are often over 1000 mg/dL. In GPIHBP1 deficiency and ApoA-V deficiency, significantly elevated TGs are common, although chylomicronemia is rare. Familial hypertriglyceridemia is suggested by the presence of elevated TGs (>500 mg/dL) in the absence of significantly elevated total cholesterol (<250 mg/dL). These patients have a propensity for pancreatitis. Familial dysbetalipoproteinemia often will present with premature coronary disease, with physical examination revealing distinctive xanthomas: tuberoeruptive and palmar. Laboratory findings of familial dysbetalipoproteinemia reveal elevated cholesterol and TGs, with normal HDL-C. These patients are at increased risk for atherosclerotic CVD.

## Screening and Counseling

**Screening:** As in many conditions in medicine, an accurate history and physical examination is paramount in the diagnostic evaluation of a patient with hyperlipidemia. Patients with elevated LDL-C may display CVD at an early age, as well as have evidence of xanthomas and corneal arcus. Patients with familial chylomicronemia may have bouts of pancreatitis beginning in childhood; a high index of suspicion is essential to uncovering the diagnosis. With regards to laboratory findings, the current recommendation is that every patient of age 20 years should be screened with a fasting lipid panel measuring TGs, HDL, and total cholesterol. From these data, LDL is calculated. Importantly, if the fasting TG level is greater than 400 mg/dL then the conventional formula for calculating LDL-C is inaccurate. Further evaluation or treatment is determined by the specific lipid disorder. In pediatric populations, the American Academy of Pediatrics endorses screening children with a family history of early CVD, however consensus as to screening guidelines have not yet been universally adopted.

Once hyperlipidemia is identified, the next step is to rule out secondary causes of elevated lipids. Standard workup for elevated LDL-C includes a thyroid-stimulating hormone (TSH), fasting glucose, basic metabolic panel for assessment of renal function, and liver function tests to rule out cholestatic liver disease. Patients with HDL less than 10th percentile should be questioned about use of anabolic steroids and any other drug use. Rarely, occult malignancies can cause marked reduction in HDL. Patients with TG greater than 500 mg/dL should be carefully questioned about alcohol use, diet, and physical activity and nephrotic syndrome should be excluded. In parallel with ruling out secondary causes of hyperlipidemia, an extensive family history and possible evaluation of family members' lipid profile should be obtained.

If the patient has LDL-C greater than the 95th percentile and secondary causes have been excluded, a genetic cause is likely. The presence of xanthomas and an autosomal dominant pattern of inheritance is consistent with familial hypercholesterolemia, familial dysbetalipoproteinemia, or autosomal dominant hypercholesterolemia. There is no benefit to further diagnostic testing as treatment is identical. If the history reveals an autosomal recessive pattern of inheritance, sitosterolemia and autosomal recessive hypercholesterolemia should be suspected. In particular, sitosterolemia should be ruled out in this setting by measuring plasma levels of phytosterols, sitosterol, and campesterol. This diagnosis has implications for therapy.

If the patient has HDL less than 20 mg/dL and no secondary causes, it is likely due to a genetic etiology. Plasma ApoA-I levels should be obtained. An HDL and ApoA-I less than 5 mg/dL is strongly suggestive of Tangier disease, especially if there is evidence of hepatosplenomegaly or enlarged tonsils. Severe corneal opacification is very suggestive of LCAT deficiency, and this can be confirmed in specialized laboratories with an LCAT activity assay.

If the patient has TGs greater than 1000 mg/dL, the patient most likely has chylomicronemia. Often, there is a genetic component to chylomicronemia, although this condition is heavily influenced by environmental factors. A postheparin lipolytic assay can be performed in specialized laboratories. If TGs are in the range of 250 to 750 mg/dL and if the cholesterol is elevated to a similar degree, then type III hyperlipoproteinemia should be considered. The disorder can be diagnosed by beta quantification to determine the ratio of VLDL-C to TGs or by genotyping to detect homozygosity of the *APOE2* allele.

**Counseling:** Counseling for these patients is appropriate depending on the particular Mendelian monogenic disorder. In the case of familial hyperlipidemia, the penetrance of the disorder approaches 90%. In these patients, advanced CVD may manifest in childhood, prompting early lipid-lowering therapy. However, many of these conditions have a variable penetrance, which can be greatly affected by diet, exercise, and lifestyle factors. Additionally, while these disorders are recognized by a particular phenotype, such as elevated LDL without hypertriglyceridemia, numerous mutations in a particular gene may be responsible, further confounding genetic counseling. Genes where a particular mutation is responsible for a genotype are outlined in Table 13-4, as are inheritance patterns. It is important to remember that in the majority of patients, hyperlipidemia is polygenic, and that one particular mutation or inheritance pattern may not be apparent.

## Management and Treatment

**Diet and Lifestyle Modification:** While many patients with hyperlipidemia will need pharmacotherapy, diet and lifestyle modification play an enormous and often underappreciated role

Table 13-4 Molecular Genetic Testing

| Gene | Loci | Testing Modality | Mutation Type | Inheritance Pattern |
|------|------|------------------|---------------|---------------------|
| LDLR | 19p13.2 | Skin biopsy measuring fibroblast LDLR function or sequencing of the LDLR gene | Caused by >1000 mutations in LDLR gene | Homozygotes for this condition display a more severe phenotype; heterozygotes display a codominant phenotype |
| APOB | 2p24.1 | Can be detected directly by genetic assay (not recommended, as it does not affect management) | Mutations in the LDLR-biding domain of ApoB-100, in particular a substitution of glutamine for arginine at position 3500 | Autosomal dominant |
| PCSK9 | 1p32.3 | Measurement of PCSK9 in plasma or sequencing of the PCSK9 gene | Missense and nonsense mutations in PCSK9 | Autosomal dominant |
| LDLRAP1 | 1p36.11 | Can test fibroblasts and lymphocytes for LDLR function or sequencing of the LDLRAP gene | Mutations in LDLR adaptor protein | Autosomal recessive |
| ABCG5 ABCG8 | 2p21 | Gas chromatography demonstrates increased sitosterol in plasma | Defect in either gene will cause dysfunction of heterodimer protein product | Autosomal recessive |
| APOA1 | 11q23.3 | Measurement of ApoA-I in plasma; sequencing of the APOA gene | Missense and nonsense mutations in APOA1, heterozygotes for Arg173Cys account for ApoA-1 Milano | Varies depending on mutation |
| ABCA1 | 9q31.1 | Skin biopsy measuring fibroblast ABCA1 function | Loss of function mutations in both alleles | Autosomal codominant |
| LCAT | 16q22.1 | Measurement of plasma LCAT activity in specialized laboratory; sequencing of LCAT gene | Loss of function mutation in both alleles | Autosomal recessive, although heterozygotes sometimes have modestly reduced HDL-C levels |
| LPL APOC | 8p21.3 19q13.32 | Assay of TG lipolytic activity in postheparin plasma, confirmed with molecular sequencing | Loss of function mutation in either gene | Autosomal recessive |
| APOE | 19q13.32 | Lipoprotein ultracentrifugation with assessment of the VLDL-C to TG ratio; genotyping of the APOE2 allele | Substitution of a cysteine for an arginine at position 158 | Most commonly seen in individuals with homozygosity for ApoE-2/E2 |
| GPIHBP1 | 8q24.3 | Sequencing of GPIHBP1 gene | Loss of function mutation in both alleles | Autosomal recessive |
| APOA5 | 11q23.3 | Sequencing of APOA5 gene | Loss of function mutation in both alleles | Autosomal codominant |

in disease management. Specific recommendations vary depending on the predominant lipid derangement. Patients with elevated LDL-C often benefit from reduction of dietary fat and cholesterol; frequently prescribed is the "Step I diet," recommended by the American Heart Association. Restriction in dietary fat and carbohydrates is appropriate for patients with very elevated TGs. Additionally, all patients benefit from weight loss, cardiovascular exercise, and smoking cessation. Sitosterolemia and hypertriglyceridemia are disorders that are responsive to dietary intervention. All patients with hypercholesterolemia benefit from consultation with an experienced dietician.

***HMG-CoA Reductase Inhibitors (Statins):*** Statins are the cornerstone of lipid-lowering pharmacotherapy and work by inhibiting a key enzyme in cholesterol synthesis. Statins are the most potent class of lipid-lowering pharmacotherapies. The magnitude of LDL reduction varies widely among individuals. Once a patient begins statin therapy, the response to increasing therapy is more modest; doubling the dose will decrease plasma LDL-C by 6%. Statins also have a modest effect on TGs and HDL. Numerous studies have validated the efficacy of statins, and current recommendations from the National Cholesterol Education Panel/Adult Treatment Panel III (NCEP III/ATP) for patients with coronary heart disease or an equivalent establish a target LDL of at least less than 100 mg/dL and in very high-risk patients an optional goal of less than 70 mg/dL. Statins are well tolerated, with the most common side effects being myalgias and a slight increase in transaminases.

***Bile Acid Sequestrants:*** These medications function to decrease cholesterol adsorption in the distal ileum by binding to bile acids in the gut lumen. In order to maintain the bile acid pool, the liver diverts cholesterol to the biliary system from the circulation. This functions to lower serum LDL-C levels. Care must be used for patients who have concurrent hypertriglyceridemia, as these medications may increase serum TGs. The most common side effects are bloating and constipation. Bile acid sequestrants are often used as an adjunct to statin therapy or with ezetimibe in patients who are statin-intolerant.

***Cholesterol Absorption Inhibitors:*** The only medication in this class with Food and Drug Administration (FDA) approval is ezetimibe. Ezetimibe functions by inhibiting NPC1L1, a protein that has a role in cholesterol intestinal absorption. The mean serum reduction of LDL-C is 18% with this medication, with negligible effects on TGs and HDL. Ezetimibe is used as monotherapy only in statin-intolerant patients. While often an adjunct in statin therapy, mortality benefit in these patients is controversial.

***Fibrates:*** This class of medication functions as agonists of PPARα, which stimulates lipoprotein lipase (LPL) activity. The primary role of these medications is to decrease pancreatitis by lowering TG levels, particularly in patients with TG levels greater than 500 mg/dL. They are generally well tolerated; the most common side effect is dyspepsia. Care must be used when prescribed with statins, as these medications can increase the risk of myopathy. These medications are considered first line for management of hypertriglyceridemia.

***Fish Oils (Omega-3 Fatty Acids):*** Fish oil tablets consist of highly concentrated N-3 polyunsaturated fatty acids (n-3 PUFA) are often used to lower fasting TG levels. These medications may result in a mild increase in LDL-C and are useful in combination with other lipid-lowering therapy. Fish oils are exceedingly safe and well tolerated. While fish oils have been associated with a mild

prolongation of bleeding time, this has not been associated with a clinically significant risk of hemorrhage.

***Niacin:*** This B-complex vitamin reduces the flux of nonesterified fatty acids to the liver, which is thought to decrease production of VLDL. Niacin has primarily been used to increase HDL levels, with a modest effect on LDL and TGs. Recently, the AIM-HIGH study found no benefit to the addition of niacin to statin therapy in patients with hyperlipidemia. However, more studies need to be done before the role of niacin in hyperlipidemia is determined. The most common side effect of niacin is cutaneous flushing, which can be minimized by coadministration of aspirin.

***New therapies for severe hypercholesterolemia:*** Two new classes of lipid-lowering drugs act by reducing VLDL and apoB production and are approved for homozygous FH. Lomitapide is a small molecule inhibitor of the microsomal triglyceride transfer protein (MTP) and reduces VLDL production by inhibiting the loading of lipids onto newly synthesized apoB. Mipomersen is an antisense oligonucleotide directed against the apoB mRNA that is administered subcutaneously and reduces VLDL production by reducing apoB synthesis. Both drugs effectively reduce LDL-C in patients with hoFH and severe hypercholesterolemia. Due to their mechanism, both also increase hepatic fat and variably increase transaminases. In addition, lomitapide can cause GI side effects and mipomersen can cause skin reactions and flu-like reactions. These medicines can only be prescribed by registered and qualified physicians.

***LDL Apheresis:*** This treatment modality consists of passing a patient's plasma through a column that selectively removes LDL-C, and returning the delipidated blood to the patient. This is considered the last line of therapy for patients with extremely elevated LDL-C who are intolerant of lipid-lowering medications or who are unable to achieve adequate reduction in serum LDL-C. Patients with CVD on maximal lipid-lowering therapy and an LDL greater than 200 mg/dL are candidates for this therapy, as are patients with LDL greater than 300 mg/dL and no CVD. This treatment is only available at specialized lipid centers and consists of every-other-week sessions.

## Molecular Genetics and Molecular Mechanism

Specific genes and loci are detailed in Table 13-4, as are inheritance patterns and mutation type.

***Genetic Testing:*** The role of genetic testing depends on the type of Mendelian monogenic disorder suspected. For example, in autosomal dominant causes of elevated LDL-C without hypertriglyceridemia, there is no utility to further diagnostic workup as management is the same for familial hypercholesterolemia, familial dysbetalipoproteinemia or autosomal dominant hypercholesterolemia. However, determining the underlying pathophysiology may alter therapy. Different testing modalities for specific monogenic disorders are outlined in Table 13-4.

**BIBLIOGRAPHY:**

1. Teslovich T, Musunuru K, Smith A, et al. Biological, clinical and population relevance of 95 loci for blood lipids. *Nature.* August 2010;466(7307):707-713.

2. Calandra S, Tarugi P, Speedy HE, Dean AF, Bertolini S, Shoulders CC. Mechanisms and genetic determinants regulating sterol adsorption, circulating LDL levels and sterol elimination: implications for classification and disease risk. *J Lipid Research*. Nov 2011;52(11):1885-1926.

3. Naoumova R, Thompson G, Soutar A. Current management of severe homozygous hypercholesterolemias. *Curr Opin Lipidol*. Aug 2004;15(4):413-422.

4. Tibolia G, Norata G, Artali R, Meneghetti F, Catapano. Proprotein convertase subtilisin/kexin type 9 (PCSK9): from structure-function relation to therapeutic options. *Nutr Metab Cardiovasc Dis*. Nov 2011;21(11):835-843.

5. Fitzgerald M, Mujawar Z, Tamehiro N. ABC transporters, atherosclerosis, and inflammation. *Atherosclerosis*. 2010;211(2):361-370.

6. Calabresi L, Franceschini G. Lecithin: cholesterol acyltransferase, high-density lipoproteins, and atheroprotection in humans. *Trends Cardiovasc Med*. July 2010;20(2):50-53.

7. Smelt A, de Beer F. Apolipoprotein E and familial dysbetalipoproteinemia: clinical, biochemical, and genetic aspects. *Semin Vasc Med*. Nov 2004;4(3):249-257.

8. Young S, Davies B, Voss C, Gin P, et al. GPIHBP1, an endothelial cell transporter for lipoprotein lipase. *J Lipid Research*. 2011;52:1869-1884.

9. Schaefer E, Santos R, Asztalos. Marked HDL deficiency and premature coronary heart disease. *Curr Opin Lipidol*. 2010;21:289-297.

10. Cleeman J. Executive Summary of the Third Report of the National Cholesterol Education Program Expert Panel on Detection, Evaluation and Treatment of High Blood Cholesterol in Adults. *JAMA*. 2001;285(19):2486-2497.

## Supplementary Information

### OMIM REFERENCES:

[1] Familial Hypercholesterolemia; LDLR (#606945)

[2] Familial Defective Apolipoprotein B-100; APOB (#107730)

[3] Autosomal Dominant Hypercholesterolemia; PCSK9 (#607786)

[4] Autosomal Recessive Hypercholesterolemia; LDLRAP1 (#605747)

[5] Sitosterolemia; ABCG5/ABCG8 (#605459/605460)

[6] ApoA-I Deficiency; APOA (#107680)

[7] ApoA-I Structural Mutations; APOA (#107680)

[8] Tangier Disease; ABCA1 (#600046)

[9] LCAT Deficiency; LCAT(#606967)

[10] Familial Chylomicronemia Syndrome; LPL/APOC-II (#609708)

[11] GPIHBP1 Deficiency; GPIHBPI (#612757)

[12] ApoA-V Deficiency; APOA5 (#606368)

[13] Familial Dysbetalipoproteinemia; APOE (#107741)

*Key Words:* Familial hypercholesterolemia, familial defective apolipoprotein B-100, autosomal dominant hypercholesterolemia, autosomal recessive hypercholesterolemia, sitosterolemia, ApoA-I deficiency, ApoA-I structural mutations, Tangier disease, LCAT deficiency, familial chylomicronemia syndrome, GPIHBP1, ApoA-V deficiency, familial dysbetalipoproteinemia, genome-wide association studies

# 14 Hypertriglyceridemia

Tisha R. Joy and Robert A. Hegele

## KEY POINTS

- *Disease summary:*
  - Common hypertriglyceridemia can be considered a polygenic disorder, involving the interaction of often multiple genetic loci, many yet to be identified, and environmental factors.
  - Hypertriglyceridemia can be divided into primary versus secondary causes.
  - Although clinical manifestations of hypertriglyceridemia are often rare, those with primary hypertriglyceridemia may have eruptive xanthoma, tuberous xanthoma, palmar xanthoma, or lipemia retinalis.
  - Both primary and secondary hypertriglyceridemia can present with pancreatitis, particularly if triglyceride (TG) levels exceed 1000 mg/dL.

- *Differential diagnosis:*
  - For primary hypertriglyceridemia, the differential includes lipoprotein lipase (LPL) deficiency, apolipoprotein (Apo) C-II, familial hypertriglyceridemia, familial combined hyperlipidemia while the most common secondary causes of hypertriglyceridemia are obesity, excess alcohol consumption, diabetes (poorly controlled), hypothyroidism, and medications such as thiazides, antipsychotic medications, antiretroviral medications.

- *Monogenic forms:*
  - A few individuals with plasma TG levels greater than 95th percentile have rare monogenic disorders resulting from homozygous loss-of-function mutations, including in the *LPL* and Apo genes *APOC2* and *APOA5*.

- *Family history:*
  - A family history of severe hypertriglyceridemia, recurrent pancreatitis in affected members, or of cutaneous manifestations increase the likelihood of primary hypertriglyceridemia.

- *Environmental factors:*
  - Several environmental factors such as obesity, diabetes, hypothyroidism, pregnancy, alcohol intake, and certain medications can exacerbate hypertriglyceridemia in those with a genetic predisposition to hypertriglyceridemia.

- *Genome-wide association studies:*
  - For children with suspected LPL deficiency, sequencing of candidate genes is now the most expeditious method to make a diagnosis. Genome-wide association studies (GWAS) have shown that for common hypertriglyceridemia, common small-to-moderate effect variants and rare large-effect mutations are both determinant of triglyceride levels, but there is no allelic risk score yet established. Thus, genetic screening for common, less severe hypertriglyceridemia in adults is not presently recommended.

- *Pharmacogenomics:*
  - There is no evidence yet that genotypes for common single-nucleotide polymorphism (SNP) variants from GWAS determine pharmacogenetic response of hypertriglyceridemia to interventions.

## Diagnostic Criteria for Hypertriglyceridemia

According to the National Cholesterol Education Program Adult Treatment Panel III (NCEP ATP III), the severity of hypertriglyceridemia can be classified as follows:

- Normal — Less than 150 mg/dL (<1.7 mmol/L)
- Borderline high — 150 to 199 mg/dL (1.7-2.25 mmol/L)
- High — 200 to 499 mg/dL (2.26-5.63 mmol/L)
- Very high — Greater than or equal to 500 mg/dL (≥5.64 mmol/L)

**Clinical Characteristics:** Although most patients with hypertriglyceridemia have no clinical manifestations, those with primary causes of hypertriglyceridemia (see later) or severe elevations in plasma TG levels may have characteristic clinical findings. Several variations of xanthoma may be evident in primary hypertriglyceridemia. Eruptive xanthomas are small (2-5 mm in diameter) raised yellow lesions that occur most typically on the trunk, buttocks, or extremities while tuberous xanthomas are larger (<3 cm in diameter), reddish or orange, shiny, nontender, mobile nodules present on extensor surfaces. The former is most often encountered where there is marked elevation in chylomicrons, such as in familial hyperchylomicronemia (type I hyperlipidemia) or mixed (type V) hyperlipidemia, while the latter is often seen in type III hyperlipidemia (or familial dysbetalipoproteinemia). The presence of yellowish deposits within palmar creases (palmar xanthomas) is pathognomonic for type III hyperlipidemia. Individuals with types I or V hyperlipidemia may also exhibit hepatosplenomegaly, recurrent epigastric pain with predisposition to pancreatitis, focal neurologic symptoms such as irritability, as well as lipemia retinalis. Lipemia retinalis refers to a milky appearance of the retinal vessels, often when TG levels exceed 3100 mg/dL (~35 mmol/L). Pancreatitis can occur in individuals with primary or secondary hypertriglyceridemia, and the risk for pancreatitis is greatly increased once TG levels are greater than 1000 mg/dL (>11.3 mmol/L).

**Differential Diagnosis:** Hypertriglyceridemia can be classified into primary and secondary causes (Table 14-1).

*Table 14-1  Primary and Secondary Causes of Hypertriglyceridemia*

| Primary | Secondary |
|---|---|
| Familial hyperchylomicronemia (type I) <br>• Clinical manifestations such as cutaneous eruptive xanthoma, lipemia retinalis, failure to thrive, recurrent epigastric pain, hepatosplenomegaly, pancreatitis, focal neurologic symptoms evident since childhood <br>• Significant elevations in triglyceride levels (>1000 mg/dL or >11 mmol/L) <br>• Prevalence 1 in 10 <br>• AR; due to deficiency of lipoprotein lipase (LPL) or its cofactor, apolipoprotein C-II (ApoC-II) <br>Familial dysbetalipoproteinemia (type III) <br>• Characterized by elevations in IDL resulting in equimolar elevation in plasma total cholesterol and triglyceride levels <br>• Clinical manifestations include tuberous and palmar xanthoma <br>• Elevations in atherogenic IDL results in increased risk for CVD <br>• Prevalence 1 to 2 in 20,000 <br>• Homozygous for ApoE-2 <br>Familial hypertriglyceridemia (type IV) <br>• Moderate elevations in triglycerides (265-890 mg/dL or 3-10 mmol/L) often accompanied by ↓ HDL-C levels <br>• Isolated elevation in VLDL, not chylomicrons <br>• Associated with increased risk of CVD, obesity, DM2, hypertension, hyperuricemia, insulin resistance <br>• Prevalence 5% to 10%; polygenic most likely <br>Primary mixed hyperlipidemia (type V) <br>• Similar clinical manifestations as type I but develops in adulthood <br>• Frequently exacerbated by secondary factors <br>• Less severe functional deficiency or likelihood of gene mutations in *LPL* or *APOC2* <br>• Population prevalence 1 in 10 | Type 2 diabetes—particularly poor glycemic control <br>Obesity, metabolic syndrome <br>Alcohol <br>High-fat or high-carbohydrate intake <br>Minimal physical activity <br>Hypothyroidism <br>Lipodystrophies—genetic or acquired <br>Renal disease—uremia or glomerulonephritis in particular <br>Pregnancy <br>Autoimmune disorders such as SLE <br>Medications, including <br>• Estrogen <br>• Tamoxifen <br>• Glucocorticoids <br>• Antihypertensives—thiazide diuretics, nonselective beta-blockers <br>• Bile acid-binding resins <br>• Cyclophosphamide <br>• Antiretroviral medications (protease inhibitors) <br>• Antipsychotic medications, particularly second-generation antipsychotics such as clozapine and olanzapine |

AD, autosomal dominant; AR, autosomal recessive; CVD, cardiovascular disease; DM2, type 2 diabetes; HDL, high-density lipoprotein; HDL-C, high-density lipoprotein-cholesterol; IDL, intermediate-density lipoprotein; SLE, systemic lupus erythematosus; VLDL, very low density lipoprotein.

## Screening and Counseling

For children with suspected LPL deficiency, sequencing of candidate genes is now the most expeditious method to make a diagnosis, supplanting biochemical assessment of LPL activity in plasma collected after a bolus injection of heparin intravenously. But besides establishing the diagnosis, knowing the nature of the mutation does not yet appear to have any bearing on medical advice or interventions for these rare patients. If a molecular diagnosis is made, family members can be screened: heterozygotes typically have a much less severe TG phenotype or can even have normal TGs. Genetic screening for common, less severe hypertriglyceridemia in adults is not presently recommended.

## Management and Treatment

The management of hypertriglyceridemia can be considered as two domains—nonpharmacologic and pharmacologic intervention.

The specific therapeutic intervention depends on the initial severity classification of hypertriglyceridemia according to NCEP ATP III guidelines. These guidelines primarily focus on achieving LDL-C targets and secondarily focus on achieving non–HDL-C targets. The non–HDL-C value refers to LDL + VLDL cholesterol calculated as total cholesterol—HDL-C. The target for non–HDL-C in individuals with high serum TGs is 30 mg/dL higher than their respective LDL-C target within the appropriate risk category (Table 14-2).

*Nonpharmacologic Intervention:*
• Identify and rectify secondary causes of hypertriglyceridemia if possible (listed in Table 14-1).
• Initiate nonpharmacologic intervention in all individuals with hypertriglyceridemia.
• Weight loss and increased aerobic physical activity can result in mild-to-moderate decreases in TG levels.
• Recommend low fat (<10%-15%) and low simple carbohydrate diet.
• In individuals with type I hyperlipidemia, the mainstay of treatment is a very low-fat diet (<10%-15% of total calories from fat); medium chain fatty acids can be used as an alternate source

*Table 14-2 Non–HDL-C Goals in Individuals With Hypertriglyceridemia*

| | Very High-risk Patients | High-risk Patients | Moderately High Risk | Moderate Risk | Low risk |
|---|---|---|---|---|---|
| **10-year risk for CHD** | >20% but likely to have major event during next few years | >20% | 10%-20% and ≥2 major risk factors[a] | <10% and ≥2 major risk factors[a] | < 10% AND 0 to 1 major risk factors[a] |
| **LDL-C target (mg/dL)** | <70 | <100 | <130 (<100 optional) | <130 | <160 |
| **Non–HDL-C target (mg/dL)** | <100 | <130 | <160 (<130 optional) | <160 | <190 |

[a]Major risk factors include cigarette smoking, hypertension (BP ≥140/90 mm Hg or on antihypertensive medication), low HDL-C (<40 mg/dL), family history of premature CHD (first-degree male or female relative <55 or <65 years, respectively).

CHD, coronary heart disease; HDL-C, high-density lipoprotein-cholesterol; LDL-C, low-density lipoprotein-cholesterol.

of fats. Importantly, fat-soluble vitamin essential fatty acid supplementation may be required.

- Omega-3 fatty acids may reduce TGs by approximately 40%.
- Reduction in alcohol consumption, abstinence from alcohol, particularly if triglyceride levels are greater than 2000 mg/dL (>22.5 mmol/L).

***Pharmacologic Intervention:***

- Pharmacologic interventions should be utilized according to nation-specific recommendations.
- For example, according to NCEP ATP III guidelines, pharmacologic intervention is typically reserved for those individuals with high to very high TG elevations (Table 14-3).

***Pharmacogenetics:***

- For patients with proven homozygous LPL deficiency, treatment with currently available medications is suboptimal; furthermore, there is no obvious correlation between mutation type and the response to treatment.
- For adult patients with severe hypertriglyceridemia, about 10% are heterozygous for a rare loss-of-function mutation in *LPL* or *APOC2* or *APOA5* genes. These individuals are less responsive to treatment with fibrates than are patients with the same biochemical phenotype, but are not carriers of such mutations.

- There is no evidence yet that genotypes for common SNP variants from GWAS determine pharmacogenetic response of hypertriglyceridemia to interventions.

## Molecular Genetics and Molecular Mechanisms

***Rare Monogenic Severe Hypertriglyceridemia:*** A few individuals with plasma TG levels greater than 95th percentile have rare monogenic disorders resulting from homozygous loss-of-function mutations, including in the *LPL* and Apo genes, *APOC2* and *APOA5*.

***Polygenic Severe Hypertriglyceridemia:*** According to the "common-disease-common-variant" model, genetic predisposition is comprised of multiple, common genetic variants, each with small-to-modest effects on TG levels in combination with modifier genes or environmental factors. Alternatively, the "heterogeneity" model maintains that genetic contribution to complex traits is comprised of numerous rare genetic variants. In reality, a blend of these models—in which a mosaic of many variants, frequent and rare, with effect size ranging from small to large—seems to explain the genetic basis of hypertriglyceridemia.

*Table 14-3 Recommended Interventions for Individuals With Hypertriglyceridemia Based on NCEP ATP III Guidelines*

| Triglyceride Elevation | Triglyceride Level | Goal | Intervention |
|---|---|---|---|
| Borderline high | 150 to 199 mg/dL (1.7-2.25 mmol/L) | Achieve LDL-C target | • Weight reduction, increased physical activity |
| High | 200 to 499 mg/dL (2.26-5.63 mmol/L) | Achieve LDL-C target Achieve secondary target of non–HDL-C | • Weight reduction, increased physical activity<br>• Pharmacologic therapy in high-risk individuals to achieve non–HDL-C goal by<br> • Intensifying LDL-C–lowering therapy<br> • Using nicotinic acid or fibrate |
| Very high | ≥500 mg/dL (≥5.64 mmol/L) | Initial goal is to achieve TG <500 mg/dL to avoid pancreatitis Once TG <500 mg/dL, focus on LDL-C target | • Weight reduction, increased physical activity<br>• Very low-fat diet (≤15% of caloric intake)<br>• Fibrate or nicotinic acid |

Near the median population TG level, recent GWAS identified approximately eight common associated SNPs with small effect sizes (1%-2% per gene). When these common SNPs were studied in patients with TG levels greater than 1000 mg/dL, virtually all of them showed moderate associations and cumulatively contributed to approximately 30% of disease susceptibility. Combining markers increased hypertriglyceridemia risk: those with six risk alleles had an almost monogenic odds ratio (OR) of 25. In addition, rare heterozygous loss-of-function mutations were strongly associated with type 5 hyperlipidemia (OR ~50), albeit in only approximately 10% of patients. Thus, common small-to-moderate effect variants and rare large-effect mutations are both determinants of hypertriglyceridemia.

***Genetic Testing:*** For children with suspected LPL deficiency, sequencing of candidate genes is now the most expeditious method to make a diagnosis. At this time, it is not obvious that knowing the molecular diagnosis has any role in altering medical advice or interventions for these patients. There is no evidence that genetic testing for common, less severe hypertriglyceridemia in adults is currently warranted or would alter treatment advice or clinical prognostication.

***Future Directions:*** Progress in understanding the genes determining hypertriglyceridemia has rapidly accelerated thanks to high-throughput automated DNA sequencing and genotyping, which complement traditional approaches such as candidate gene association studies, linkage studies, and the use of animal models. Phenomic analysis (deep phenotyping), systems biology, and network approaches may help further integrate experimental data. Newly identified genes represent potential new drug targets, so it is critical to define the metabolic roles of the gene products. The value of somatic LPL gene therapy in patients with monogenic LPL deficiency is currently being evaluated.

Future GWAS should focus on samples covering a wide range of geographic ancestries and should also be performed in patients with hypertriglyceridemia. Next-generation sequencing of the whole genome will provide an agnostic approach to identify additional causative genes in hypertriglyceridemic patients. Accounting for the genetic determinants of such intimately associated metabolic states as obesity and diabetes will be essential. Also, because drugs and diet play a key role in the management of hypertriglyceridemia, pharmacogenetic and nutrigenetic studies should be undertaken.

The definition of new pathways and targets will inform new drug design and eventually lead to evidence-based changes in practice. However, predicting the precise evolution and consequences of dyslipidemia in any single individual might remain elusive, because of the confounding influence of the environment, nonlinear interactions between genes and environment, and stochastic effects in these networks of pathways.

## BIBLIOGRAPHY:

1. Executive Summary of The Third Report of The National Cholesterol Education Program (NCEP) Expert Panel on Detection, Evaluation, And Treatment of High Blood Cholesterol In Adults (Adult Treatment Panel III). *JAMA*. 2001;285:2486-2497.

2. Yuan G, Al-Shali KZ, Hegele RA. Hypertriglyceridemia: its etiology, effects and treatment. *CMAJ*. 2007;176:1113-1120.

3. Rouis M, Dugi KA, Previato L, et al. Therapeutic response to medium-chain triglycerides and omega-3 fatty acids in a patient with the familial chylomicronemia syndrome. *Arterioscler Thromb Vasc Biol*. 1997;17:1400-1406.

4. Press M, Hartop PJ, Prottey C. Correction of essential fatty-acid deficiency in man by the cutaneous application of sunflower-seed oil. *Lancet*. 1974;1:597-598.

5. Goldberg RB, Sabharwal AK. Fish oil in the treatment of dyslipidemia. *Curr Opin Endocrinol Diabetes Obes*. 2008;15:167-174.

6. Brunzell JD. Clinical practice. Hypertriglyceridemia. *N Eng J Med*. 2007;357:1009-1017.

7. Genest J, McPherson R, Frohlich J, et al. 2009 Canadian Cardiovascular Society/Canadian guidelines for the diagnosis and treatment of dyslipidemia and prevention of cardiovascular disease in the adult—2009 recommendations. *Can J Cardiol*. 2009;25:567-579.

8. Wang J, Cao H, Ban MR, et al. Resequencing genomic DNA of patients with severe hypertriglyceridemia (MIM 144650). *Arterioscler Thromb Vasc Biol*. 2007;27:2450-2455.

9. Hegele RA. Plasma lipoproteins: genetic influences and clinical implications. *Nat Rev Genet*. 2009;10:109-121.

10. Stroes ES, Nierman MC, Meulenberg JJ, et al. Intramuscular administration of AAV1-lipoprotein lipase S447X lowers triglycerides in lipoprotein lipase-deficient patients. *Arterioscler Thromb Vasc Biol*. 2008;28:2303-2304.

11. Grundy SM, Cleeman JI, Merz CN, et al. Implications of recent clinical trials for the National Cholesterol Education Program Adult Treatment Panel III guidelines. *Circulation*. 2004;110:227-239.

# 15 Familial Hypercholesterolemia

Edward A. Fisher and Arthur Z. Schwartzbard

## KEY POINTS

- *Disease summary:*
  - Familial hypercholesterolemia (FH) is an autosomal dominant, monogenic disorder of lipoprotein metabolism characterized by strikingly elevated low-density lipoprotein-cholesterol (LDL-C), the presence of xanthomas, and premature atherosclerosis.
  - FH is most often caused by a defect in the gene that encodes for the apolipoprotein B or E (ApoB or E) (LDL) receptor (LDLR). Over 1000 different mutations of this receptor have been identified since it was first discovered by Goldstein and Brown in the late 1970s.
  - Impairment in, or in severe cases, a complete absence of function of, LDLR results in reduced clearance of LDL particles from the circulation into many cell types. Because over 60% of total body LDLR is in the liver, decreased clearance of LDL particles by this organ has a particularly potent effect on plasma LDL-C levels. Hypercholesterolemia is present from birth. LDL particles begin to be retained in arterial sites early on in life and their uptake by macrophages turn them into foam cells, the fundamental building block of an atherosclerotic plaque.
  - The FH homozygote frequency is estimated to be 1:1,000,000 worldwide compared with the heterozygote frequency of 1:500.

- *Differential diagnosis:*
  - The differential diagnosis includes sitosterolemia, cerebrotendinous xanthomatosis, familial combined hyperlipidemia, polygenic hypercholesterolemia, familial defective ApoB-100, autosomal recessive hypercholesterolemia (ARH), and cholesterol 7 alpha-hydroxylase deficiency based on either clinical presentation (usually xanthoma) or laboratory testing (elevated LDL-C), or family history of elevated LDL or premature coronary artery disease (CAD).

- *Monogenic forms:*
  - Most often caused by a mutation of one or both copies of the gene that encodes for the LDLR, located on chromosome 19p13.

- *Family history:*
  - The prevalence of heterozygous FH is drastically higher in first-degree relatives of patients with the disorder estimated at one in two. Having a known case of FH in the family lowers the LDL cutoff needed to confirm the diagnosis (Table 15-1).

- *Environmental factors:*
  - For patients with homozygous FH, risk is related to an extremely high level of LDL-C that is relatively insensitive to modifications by lifestyle factors. In contrast, for heterozygous FH, the phenotypic expression of the disease is related not only to the severity of the LDLR defect, but also to traditional dietary, genetic, behavioral, and cultural factors. For example, Hill et al. studied a large cohort of heterozygous FH patients and found that men who smoked or had low HDL levels had the greatest risk for developing CAD. This was in contrast to women in whom CAD was most associated with elevated triglycerides or the presence of hypertension.

- *Genome-wide associations:*
  - Not surprisingly, the LDLR comes up in genome-wide association studies (GWAS) as associated with both LDL-C levels and risk of myocardial infarction. There are also a number of other genes that are significant in determining LDL-C levels that are not related to the LDLR, such as ApoB, proprotein convertase subtilisin/kexin type 9 (PCSK9), and sortillin. An important lesson from the GWAS on lipids, the largest incorporating up to 100,000 individuals of European descent, is that the same genes that cause Mendelian disorders also harbor common variants that result in small but significant changes in lipid levels. Much of the remaining inheritability may ultimately be attributable to these novel variants.

- *Pharmacogenomics:*
  - Many believe that the response to treatment is likely a function of the particular mutation causing FH but few studies have been conducted to answer this question rigorously.

## Diagnostic Criteria and Clinical Characteristics

**Diagnostic Criteria for FH:** Conventionally, the diagnosis of FH has been based on elevated total cholesterol levels in subjects belonging to families with high frequencies of premature CAD. Tendon xanthomas are thought to be nearly pathognomonic of FH, but are insensitive as a diagnostic marker.

Three sets of diagnostic criteria utilizing population-based algorithms have been used extensively for clinical diagnosis: the Simon Broome Register Group in United Kingdom, the Make Early Diagnosis to Prevent Early Death program in United States, and the Dutch Lipid Clinic Network (Table 15-1 and Fig. 15-1).

Laboratory data should show an elevated total cholesterol level, a plasma LDL-C level above the age- and gender-related 95th percentile for the local population, a normal triglyceride level, and often a slightly low serum HDL-C. Secondary causes of

**Table 15-1** *LDL-C Cut Points for Diagnosis of Heterozygous FH: Degree of Relationship to an Affected Relative*

| Age (Years) | LDL-C Cut Point (MG/DL) | | | |
|---|---|---|---|---|
| | First-Degree Relative | Second-Degree Relative | Third-Degree Relative | General Population |
| < 20 | 155 | 165 | 170 | 200 |
| 20–29 | 170 | 180 | 185 | 220 |
| 30–39 | 190 | 200 | 210 | 240 |
| ≥ 40 | 205 | 215 | 225 | 260 |

Reproduced with permission from Williams RR, Hunt SC, Schumacher MC, et al. Diagnosing heterozygous familial hypercholesterolemia using new practical criteria validated by molecular genetics *Am J Cardiol*. 1993; 72:171-176.

hyperlipidemia such as thyroid disease and kidney disease should be excluded. Once there is high clinical suspicion, genetic testing for an LDL-receptor mutation known to cause FH is the only way to make an unequivocal diagnosis. After a mutation has been identified for a specific pedigree, genetic mapping can be used to identify individuals with FH. The large assortment of mutations known to cause FH makes screening the general population impractical.

*Clinical Characteristics:* The characteristic findings on physical examination are excessive cholesterol deposits which are either visible or palpable. The Achilles tendon is the most common site of xanthoma formation (tendon deposits), followed by the dorsum of the foot, extensor tendons of the hand, and the tibial tuberosity. Deposits in the eyelid (xanthelasma) or cornea (arcus cornealis) are common but not specific for FH.

**Homozygous FH** patients express few, if any functional LDLRs as a result of mutations to both alleles and have plasma LDL levels that can reach greater than 1000 mg/dL. Tendon xanthomas, cutaneous xanthoma (yellow-orange lesions on the skin), and CAD are regularly seen before the age of 25, and in some, as early as 4 years of age. Approximately 50% will also develop a characteristic supravalvular aortic stenosis due to atherosclerotic involvement of the aortic root.

**Heterozygous FH** patients have plasma LDL-C levels two- to fivefold higher than normal and without treatment, clinically significant CAD usually occurs at the mean age of 45 to 48 years in men and 55 to 58 in women. The prevalence of xanthoma increases with age, eventually occurring in 70% of heterozygous patients.

(1) TC >6.7 mmol/L if under 16 years old or
TC >7.5 mmol/L if over 16 years old or
LDL-C 4.9 mmol/L if over 16 years old
(2) Xanthomata in first or second-degree relative
(3) Family history of myocardial infarction under age 60 in first-degree relative or family history of myocardial infarction under age 50 in a second-degree relative
(4) Family history of TC >7.5 mmol/L in a first-or second-degree relative

**Figure 15-1** The Four Criteria Used by the Simon Broome Registry in the United Kingdom. "Definite" FH is met if both 1 and 2 are present. "Possible" FH is met if both 1 and 3, or 1 and 4 are present.

## Screening and Counseling

*Screening:* The wide array of mutations and phenotypic variability seen in FH, as well as mutations in other genes, such as ApoB and *PCSK9*, which can cause clinical and laboratory presentations similar to FH, in conjugation with the lack of sophisticated diagnostic and public health resources, has made it difficult to develop a cost-effective, genetic screening program for the general population, or even those with premature CAD.

Patients deemed to have definite, possible, or probable FH based on the population-based algorithms described earlier should have family screening performed at a center with expertise in lipid risk management. Screening for this disease can begin as early as age 2 to 3 years if suspicion is high.

Cascade testing (screening relatives of FH probands) can be performed with the same clinically based criteria as described earlier. However, some data suggests that up to 25% of family members could be incorrectly classified on the basis of cholesterol testing alone.

The Dutch have the most experience with cascade testing using genetic testing. From data collected, this method would likely identify 60% to 80% of patients with definite FH, but much fewer when the diagnosis is only probable or possible. The main drawbacks are that many mutations in the LDLR may still be unknown, there are likely genes responsible for phenocopies of FH which are yet to be identified, and current techniques are relatively insensitive at screening the whole *LDLR* gene.

*Counseling:* Although FH is monogenic and penetrance is almost complete, the phenotypic expression, in terms of onset of severity of atherosclerotic disease, varies considerably even among individuals who share the same genetic defect. As mentioned earlier, for heterozygotes in particular, the phenotype depends not only on the level of dysfunction of the LDLR, but also genetic, metabolic, and environmental factors.

The psychologic effects of being labeled with FH must be considered prior to screening. Significant anxiety can come with the diagnosis of FH—both for patient and family. Screening has the potential to lead to family conflict as some will prefer to be tested while others will refuse. This may be particularly difficult when children are diagnosed and expected to drastically alter their lifestyles and when counseled regarding the status of potential progeny.

## Management and Treatment

High levels of LDL-C have been consistently shown to be associated with CAD risk. The chance of a man with heterozygous FH suffering a myocardial infarction is 5% before age 30, 50% by age 50, and 85% by age 60. Corresponding values for women are less than 1% before age 30, 15% by age 50, and 50% by age 60. Therefore, without treatment to reduce LDL-C concentrations, many of these patients will develop progressive and obstructive atherosclerotic cardiovascular disease and impaired endothelial function at a time in their lives when they are expected to be active members of society. There are no guidelines for the degree of LDL lowering specific to this population, but most agree they should fit in the most aggressive lipid-lowering category. Since this often requires an LDL-C reduction of greater than 50%, a multimodality approach using both dietary modification and drug therapy is often used. There is an absence of large, randomized drug trials in the FH population. Therefore, while many of the lipid-lowering drugs have not been proven to decrease mortality or cardiovascular events, it is reasonable to use a multidrug regimen to bring the LDL-C as low as possible, barring any serious adverse side effects.

**Diet**: Diet alone is not adequate for the treatment of patients with FH, but should still be the cornerstone of any management program. By reducing the amount of saturated fat consumed, reducing dietary cholesterol, eating more food with plant stanol and sterol esters, and including foods rich in fiber that can bind bile acids, both LDL production and removal rates can be favorably affected. For example, estimates suggest that a diet consisting of whole grains, legumes, fruits, vegetables, nuts, fish, fat-free dietary products, and no more than 100 mg/d of cholesterol, 20% of calories from fat, and 6% from saturated fatty acids reduced plasma LDL-C levels by 18% to 21% in heterozygous FH adults and children. Dietary cholesterol and fat restriction is not recommended before the age of 2 years because it can negatively affect neural development and growth. Regular visit with a nutritionist who is experienced in lipid management is encouraged.

*Pharmacotherapy:*

- **Statins:** Since their introduction in 1987, hydroxymethylglutaryl coenzyme A reductase inhibitors (statins) have proven in multiple large double-blind placebo controlled trials that they are the most effective drug at lowering circulating LDL-C levels and reducing the risk of CAD. By inhibiting the rate-limiting step in cholesterol synthesis, where HMG-CoA is converted to mevalonate, statins decrease the hepatic cholesterol pool which in turn stimulates the production of LDL receptors. Even in the homozygous FH population, a group without any functional LDL-R's, both atorvastatin and simvastatin have been shown to lower LDL-C levels by decreasing hepatic production and secretion of lipoproteins. The ASAP trial demonstrated the benefit of more aggressive lipid lowering in FH using atorvastatin 80 mg/d for a period of 2 years (51% LDL-C reduction and a decrease in intima-media thickness [IMT] of 0.031 mm) compared with 40 mg/d (41% LDL-C reduction and a decrease in IMT of 0.036 mm). At present, high-dose atorvastatin, rosuvastatin, or simvastatin should be the initial regimen since they are the most potent statins as monotherapy. Multiple randomized, placebo-controlled studies have shown that starting statin therapy even at a young age is safe and efficacious and should be considered in those with FH in whom the life-time risk of CAD is even higher based on additional risk factors (male sex, a family history of premature CAD, markedly elevated LDL-C, low HDL-C, cigarette smoking, and elevated lipoprotein [a]). In a randomized, double-blind, placebo-controlled trial, Wiegman et al. showed that 2 years of pravastatin therapy induced significant regression of carotid atherosclerosis (based on carotid IMTs) in children (aged 8-18 years old) with FH, with no adverse effects on growth, sexual maturation, hormone levels, or liver or muscle tissue.

- **Ezetimibe** can be used when a multidrug regimen is needed. It blocks the Niemann-Pick C1-like 1 (NPC1L1) cholesterol transporter on enterocytes, thereby reducing the absorption of dietary and biliary cholesterol (by >50%) by preventing its transport into enterocytes. In the general population, multiple randomized double-blind, placebo-controlled trials have been performed and consistently show ezetimibe at a dose of 10 mg daily reduces LDL-C by approximately 17% as monotherapy and by an additional 14% when added to a baseline regimen

of simvastatin. In the double-blind, 24-month ENHANCE trial, 720 patients with heterozygous FH were randomized to receive 80 mg of daily simvastatin plus placebo or plus 10 mg of ezetimibe. The primary endpoint was the change in carotid IMT. Despite the large additional reduction in LDL-C with ezetimibe (56% vs 39%), there was no statistically significant difference in carotid IMT or in the small number of cardiovascular events. Of note, approximately 80% of patients in both treatment groups had previously been on statins and the carotid IMT in both groups was near normal at the start of the trial (potentially masking the beneficial effect of ezetimibe). In contrast, The SHARP (study of Heart and Renal Protection) trial was able to provide clinical evidence of the beneficial effects of ezetimibe in combination with simvastatin among patients with chronic kidney disease. About 9438 patients with no prior history of CAD were randomized to receive ezetimibe 10 mg daily with simvastatin 20 mg versus placebo versus simvastatin 20 mg daily as monotherapy. After 4.9 years, patients randomized to the ezetimibe or simvastatin combination arm experienced a 17% reduction in major atherosclerotic events (*p* .0022) and a 15.3% reduction in major vascular events (*p* 0.0012) compared with the placebo group.

- **Bile acid sequestrants** (cholestyramine, colesevelam, colestipol) lower cholesterol by binding bile acids in the intestine and are used most often when a multidrug regimen is needed, or if a patient is younger than 10 years of age. They can reduce LDL-C by 10% to 30% when used as monotherapy, and work well in combination with statins. Welchol (colesevelam) has also been shown to lower hemoglobin $A_{1C}$ in diabetic patients when added to a baseline hypoglycemic regimen. Their use is often limited by noncompliance secondary to gastrointestinal side effects.

- **Nicotinic acid** is the best drug for raising HDL-C. It also has some (10%-15%) LDL-C lowering effect. Niacin is a useful component of multidrug regimens in adults with FH. Its mechanism of action is not clearly defined, but it may involve several actions including partial inhibition of release of free fatty acids from adipose tissue, and increased lipoprotein lipase activity. Its use is often limited by side effects, of which the most bothersome is flushing.

- **LDL apheresis**, a procedure similar to hemodialysis, requires extracorporeal circulation of the patient's blood through filters that can selectively absorb LDL, thereby markedly lowering LDL-C and lipoprotein (a) levels. Since the only data to suggest its use is from clinical experience, and its use is expensive and impractical (biweekly), it should be started only after maximal drug therapy has failed to achieve target LDL levels. FDA-approved indications for LDL apheresis and criteria for Medicare reimbursement include those with homozygous FH and those with heterozygous FH who have failed a 6-month trial of diet and maximally tolerated combination drug therapy (at least two separate classes) who still have an LDL-C of more than 200 mg/dL in those with CAD and more than 300 mg/dL in those without documented CAD.

*Children:* The optimal age at which to safely start treatment of children with heterozygous FH is unknown. It is currently recommended by the American Academy of Pediatrics to initiate cholesterol-lowering therapy in children with considerable elevations in LDL (>190 mg/dL without other risk factors, >160 mg/dL in children with two or more risk factors) or a family history of early atherosclerotic disease. The current scientific statement from the American Heart Association recommends initial treatment in children with statins at age 10 years or more for males and after onset of the menses in females, taking into account the level of LDL-C, the presence of xanthoma, and family history. As mentioned earlier, early start of statins has been shown to reduce IMT progression in FH adolescents (a surrogate endpoint for cardiovascular risk), although longer-term data in children is still needed. It is recommended that homozygous FH children receive early initiation of combined therapy including LDL apheresis, high-dose statins, and a cholesterol absorption inhibitor.

*Pharmacogenetics:* As of 2005, there were 12 studies conducted in FH patients which tried to estimate the effect of the LDL-R genotype on statin therapy efficacy. Seven of these showed LDL reduction by various statins is genotype-dependent. The remaining did not detect any relationship. There is some pharmacogenetic evidence, however, that responses to statins in the general population are influenced by variations in the 3'-UTR (untranslated region) of the *LDLR* gene and in the genetic region regulating HMG-CoA reductase. In addition, the combined presence of both of these haplotypes (seen in greater prevalence in the African-American population) is associated with a further reduction in the lipid-lowering response to statin treatment. Pharmacogenomic research on existing drugs is still needed to determine the effectiveness and safety of genotype-tailored dosages and individualized therapy.

## Molecular Genetics and Molecular Mechanism

While mutations in the *LDLR* gene account for the majority of identified mutations that cause FH, there are mutations in other genes that contribute to the disease phenotype (described below). Some of these (such as familial defective ApoB) can result in phenocopies of heterozygous FH.

The *LDLR* gene is located on the short arm of chromosome 19 and consists of 18 exons that span 45 kilobases (kb). The gene encodes an 860 amino acid, transmembrane polypeptide which has five functional domains. Mutations in each domain have been shown to impair LDLR function. The N-terminus, for example, contains the LDL-binding domain that recognizes ApoB-100; ApoB-100 is the protein portion of LDL and the major ligand for the LDLR. Overall, over 1000 mutations have been described to affect the LDLR, ranging from single-nucleotide substitutions to major deletions. If a novel mutation is identified, in vitro testing may be performed to determine if it is phenotypically relevant (although this can often be determined clinically). The clinically significant mutations are generally divided into five subgroups based on their phenotypic effects on receptor function—complete loss of function without protein synthesis, failed protein transport to the cell membrane, LDL-binding defect, failure to internalize LDL once bound, and failure to recycle the receptor back to the cell surface once internalized. In general, receptor-negative alleles (those without any protein synthesis) are associated with a more elevated LDL-C and CAD risk than are receptor-defective alleles. The majority of mutations identified to date involve exon 4 which codes for a repeat required for both LDL binding via ApoB-100 and very low density lipoprotein (VLDL) binding via ApoE.

In the mid 1980s, Innerarity and colleagues showed that the FH phenotype could also be caused by mutations in the ApoB-100 gene. The 29-exon ApoB-100 gene is located on chromosome 2, spans 43 kb, and is responsible for the 4536 amino acid protein component of LDL which serves as the sole ligand for the LDLR. There are only five hypercholesterolemic mutations of ApoB-100 known to cause this phenotype. The most common mutation, a substitution of glutamine for arginine at position 3500 of the protein, results in an LDL particle with a mutant ApoB-100 and a reduced affinity for the LDLR. The LDL particles containing mutant ApoB-100 then accumulates in the circulation, causing an often less severe phenotype than the classic FH described earlier. This autosomal dominant disorder, deemed familial defective ApoB-100 is estimated to account for 2% to 6% of patients with a clinical diagnosis of FH.

In 1973, Khachadurian and Uthman described a Lebanese family in which all four offspring had the clinical features of homozygous FH (severe hypercholesterolemia and huge tendon xanthomas) and yet both parents had normal plasma cholesterol levels. This rare, genetic defect was named ARH. Mutations in LDLR adaptor protein 1 (*LDLRAP1*; also known as *ARH*), located on chromosome 1, prevent normal internalization of the LDLR from the cell surface to endosomes and therefore accumulation of the receptor on the cell surface. Ultimately, this leads to failure of clearance of LDL from plasma and the clinical phenotype of ARH. The majority of patients described are Italian, specifically of Sardinian origin. Compared with classic FH, the clinical phenotype is similar, but more variable, generally less severe, and more responsive to lipid-lowering therapy.

The most recently identified gene to cause the FH phenotype is also inherited in an autosomal dominant fashion and was first described in French families in the 1990s. Mutations in this gene (located on chromosome 1), which encodes a protease named proprotein convertase subtilisin/kexin type 9 (PCSK9), is estimated to account for 2% of patients with FH in Northern Europe. Normally, this enzyme is involved in degrading the LDLR protein in the lysosome of the cell and preventing it from recycling. One of the eight hypercholesterolemic missense mutations identified as a gain-of-function mutation is Asp374Tyr and it is associated with severe elevations in LDL-C.

There are variations in other genes that may have minimal effects on phenotype in the normal population, but pronounced effects in the FH patients. These include mutations in the lipoprotein lipase (LPL) gene, ApoE gene, cholesteryl ester transfer protein gene, and microsomal triglyceride transfer protein gene. There are ongoing studies to better elucidate their role in this disease. The genomes of over 100,000 individuals of European ancestry were screened for common variants associated with plasma lipids in a GWAS published in 2010. Fifty-nine novel loci were identified that showed genome-wide significant associations, 22 of which were specific for LDL-C.

*Genetic Testing:* The general opinion at present seems to be that genetic analysis should be limited to founder populations in which only a few LDLR mutations account for most cases of FH (such as in France, Canada, and Lebanon), and several countries have programs in place at national levels. If a specific mutation as been identified in a proband, screening the rest of the pedigree becomes more straightforward and feasible to diagnose on the molecular level desired.

*Future Directions:* DNA testing for specific mutations could identify groups of patients within this cohort with higher or lower risk than average for CAD so that lipid-lowering treatment could be adjusted.

☞**INVESTIGATIONAL DRUG THERAPIES:** Many patients with FH may need LDL-C lowering beyond that achievable with combinations of currently available medications, even those who are able to lower LDL-C by 70% with a multiple-drug regimen.

Administration of an antisense oligonucleotide to human ApoB (mipomersen) that interferes with the synthesis of ApoB-100 mRNA is in advanced development and has shown striking results in Phase III studies both as monotherapy and in combination with statins. Data from a 26-week study of 124 patients with heterozygous FH (on maximally tolerated doses of statin) receiving mipomersen, a once-weekly subcutaneous injection, versus placebo showed a 28% reduction in LDL cholesterol in the study group, compared with a 5% reduction in the placebo group. About 90% of patients experienced injection-site reactions. Further studies evaluating the impact of increased hepatic fat accumulation, a finding shown on magnetic resonance imaging (MRI) after use of mipomersen, over a longer period of time are needed.

Microsomal triglyceride transfer protein inhibitors (MTP-Is) can drastically reduce LDL-C and ApoB levels by blocking the assembly of VLDLs in the liver. Initially, concerns of drug-related side effects, most importantly hepatic fat accumulation and elevated liver function tests (LFTs), overshadowed the drugs potent LDL-C lowering potential. However, promising data from the first 10 patients from a Phase III study of patients with homozygous FH being treated with an MTP-I called lomitapide (AEGR-733/BMS-201038) was presented in 2009. At 6 months, the mean LDL-C level reduction observed as compared to baseline was 44% (range + 19%-93%) on top of traditional background therapy. Despite a minimal-modest increase in hepatic fat accumulation noted on MRI, only three subjects experienced transitory LFT elevations that required dose reduction; however, no subjects discontinued due to elevated LFTs. Long-term follow-up data for the 29 patients recruited is expected in 2011.

Changes in the *PCSK9* gene help to regulate LDLR protein levels and function. Cohen et al. first identified loss-of-function mutations in *PCSK9* in humans that lowered plasma LDL-C in the Dallas Heart Study. In a later observational study, moderate lifelong reduction in the plasma level of LDL-C was associated with a substantial reduction in the incidence of coronary events (88% reduction in black subjects with a 28% reduction in LDL and 47% reduction in white subjects with a 15% reduction in LDL), even in populations with a high prevalence of non–lipid-related cardiovascular risk factors. Animal models using antisense oligonucleotides targeted at PCSK9 have demonstrated increased levels of LDLR and resulting reductions in LDL-C and this has become an attractive new target for LDL-lowering therapy. Phase I trials have been completed using REGN727 and showed LDL reductions of 60% in healthy volunteers after subcutaneous dosing every 2 weeks. Other clinical trials are underway.

**BIBLIOGRAPHY:**

1. Soutar A. Familial hypercholesterolemia: mutations in the gene for the low-density-lipoprotein receptor. *Mol Med Today.* 1995;1: 90-97.

2. Tabas I, Williams KJ, Borén J. Subendothelial lipoprotein retention as the initiating process in atherosclerosis: update and therapeutic implications. *Circulation.* 2007;116(16):1832-1844.

3. Ose L. Familial hypercholesterolemia from childhood to adults. *Cardiovasc Drugs Ther.* 2002;16:289-293.

4. Williams RR, Hunt SC, Schumacher MC, et al. Diagnosing heterozygous familial hypercholesterolemia using new practical criteria validated by molecular genetics. *Am J Cardiol.* 1993;72:171-176.

5. Hill JS, Hayden MR, Frohlich J, Pritchard PH. Genetic and environmental factors affecting the incidence of coronary artery disease in heterozygous familial hypercholesterolemia. *Aterioscler Thromb.* 1991;11(2):290-297.

6. Pirruccello J, Kathiresan S. Genetics of lipid disorders. *Curr Opin Cardiol.* 2010;25:238-242.

7. Musunuru K, Kathiresan S. Genetics of coronary artery disease. *Annu Rev Genomics Hum Genet.* 2010;11:91-108.

8. Van Aalst-Cohen E, Jansen A, Jongh S, de Sauvage Nolting P, Kastelein J. Clinical, diagnostic, and therapeutic aspects of familial hypercholesterolemia. *Semin Vasc Med.* 2004;4:31-41.

9. Van Aalst-Cohen E, Jansen A, Jongh S, de Sauvage Nolting P, Kastelein J. Clinical, diagnostic, and therapeutic aspects of familial hypercholesterolemia. *Semin Vasc Med.* 2004;4:31-41.

10. Marks D, Thorogood M, Neil A, Humphries S. A review of the diagnosis, natural history, and treatment of familial hypercholesterolemia. *Atherosclerosis.* 2003;168:1-14.

11. Ose L. An update on familial hypercholesterolemia. *Ann Med.* 1999;31(suppl 1):13-18.

12. Nussbaum RL, McInnes RR, Willard HF. *Thompson and Thompson: Genetics in Medicine.* Philadelphia, PA: Saunders; 2004.

13. Leren TP, Finborud Th, Manshaus TE, et al. Diagnosis of familial hypercholesterolemia in general practice using clinical diagnostic criteria or genetic testing as part of cascade genetic screening. *Community Genet.* 2008;11:26-35.

14. Bhatnagar D. Diagnosis and screening for familial hypercholesterolemia: finding the patients, finding the genes. *Ann Clin Biochem.* 2006;43:441-456.

15. Connor We, Connor SL. Importance of diet in the treatment of familial hypercholesterolemia. *Am J Cardiol.* 1993;72: D42- D53.

16. Marais AD, Naoumova RP, Firth JC, Penny C Neuwirth CK, Thomspson GR. Decreased production of low density lipoprotein by atorvastatin after apheresis in homozygous familial hypercholesterolemia. *J Lipid Res.* 1997;38:2071-2078.

17. Raal FJ, Pilcher GJ, Illingworth Dr., et al. Expanded-dose simvastatin is effective in homozygous familial hypercholesterolemia. *Atherosclerosis.* 1997;135:249-256.

18. Smilde TJ, van Wissen S, Wollersheim H, Trip MD, Kastelein JJ, Stalenhoef AF. Effect of aggressive versus conventional lipid lowering on atherosclerosis progression in familial hypercholesterolemia (ASAP): a prospective, randomized, double-blind trial. *Lancet.* 2001;357:577-581.

19. Wiegman A, Rodenburg J, de Jongh S, et al. Family history and cardiovascular risk in familial hypercholesterolemia: data in more than 1000 children. *Circulation.* 2003;107:1473-1478.

20. Wiegman A, Hutten B, de Groot E, et al. Efficacy and safety of statin therapy in children with familial hypercholesterolemia. *JAMA.* 2004;292(3):331-337.

21. Yatskar L, Fisher E, Schwartzbard A. Ezetimibe: rationale and role in the management of hypercholesterolemia. *Clin Cardiol.* 2006;29:52-55.

22. Dujovne CA, Ettinger MP, McNeer JF, et al. Efficacy and safety of a potent new selective cholesterol absorption inhibitor, ezetimibe, in patients with primary hypercholesterolemia. *Am J Cardiol.* 2002;90(10):1092-1097.

23. Knopp RH, Gitter H, Truitt T, et al. Effects of ezetimibe, a new cholesterol absorption inhibitor, on plasma lipids in patients with primary hypercholesterolemia. *Eur Heart J.* 2003;24(8): 729-741.

24. Davidson MH, McGarry T, Bettis R, et al. Ezetimibe coadministered with simvastatin in patients with primary hypercholesterolemia. *J Am Coll Cardiol.* 2002;40(12):2125-2134.

25. Kastelein JJ, Akdim F, Stroes ES, et al. Simvastatin with or without ezetimibe in familial hypercholesterolemia. *N Engl J Med.* 2008;358(14):1431-1443.

26. The SHARP collaborative group. Study of heart and renal protections (SHARP): randomized trial to assess the effects of lowering low-density lipoprotein cholesterol among 9,438 patients with chronic kidney disease. *Am Heart J*. 2010;160(5):785-794.

27. Hopkins P. Familial hypercholesterolemia—improving treatment and meeting guidelines. *Int J Cardiol*. 2003;89:3-23.

28. Moriarty P. LDL-apheresis therapy. *Curr Treat Options Cardiovasc Med*. 2006;8:282-288.

29. Kavey RE, Allada V, Daniels SR, et al. Cardiovascular risk reduction in high-risk pediatric patients: a scientific statement from the AHA expert panel on population and prevention science; the councils on cardiovascular disease in the young, epidemiology and prevention, nutrition, physical activity and metabolism, high blood pressure research, cardiovascular nursing, and the kidney in heart disease; and the interdisciplinary working group on quality of care outcomes research. *Circulation*. 2006;114:2710-2738.

30. Despoina M, Dedoussis G. Familial hypercholesterolemia and response to statin therapy according to LDLR genetic background. *Clin Chem Lab Med*. 2005;43(8):793-801.

31. Mangravite L, Medina M, Cui J, et al. Combined influence of LDLR and HMGCR sequence variation on lipid-lowering response to simvastatin. *Aterioscler Thomb Vasc Biol*. 2010;30:1485-1492.

32. Hopkins P. Familial hypercholesterolemia—improving treatment meeting guidelines. *Int J Cardiol*. 2003;89:13-23.

33. Bhatnagar D. Diagnosis and screening for familial hypercholesterolemia: finding the patients, finding the genes. *Ann Clin Biochem*. 2006;43:441-456.

34. Austin M, Hutter C, Zimmern R, Humphries S. Genetic causes of monogenic heterozygous hypercholesterolemia: a HuGE prevalence review. *Am J Epidemiol*. 2004;160:407-420.

35. Cohen J, Kimmel M, Polanski A, Hobbs H. Molecular mechanisms of autosomal recessive hypercholesterolemia. *Curr Opin Lipidol*. 2003;14:121-127.

36. Soutar A, Naomova R, Traub L. Genetics, clinical phenotype, and molecular cell biology of autosomal recessive hypercholesterolemia. *Art Thromb Vasc Biol*. 2003;23:1963-1970.

37. Teslovich TM, Musunuru K, Smith A, et al. Biological, clinical and population relevance of 95 loci for blood lipids. *Nature*. 2010;466:707-713.

38. Stein EA. Other therapies for reducing LDL cholesterol: medications in development. *Endocrinol Metab Clin North Am*. 2009;38:99-119.

39. Goldberg AC. Novel therapies and new targets of treatment for familial hypercholesterolemia. *J Clin Lipidol*. 2010;4:350-356.

40. Cuchel M, Meagher E, Marais A, et al. A phase III study of microsomal triglyceride transfer protein inhibitor lomitapide (AEGR-733) in patients with homozygous familial hypercholesterolemia: interim results of 6 months. *Circulation*. 2009;120:S441.

41. Cohen J, Pertsemlidis A, Kotowski IK, et al. Low LDL cholesterol in individuals of African descent resulting from frequent nonsense mutations in PCSK9. *Nat Genet*. 2005;27:161-165.

42. Cohen JC, Boerwinkle E, Mosley T, Hobbs H. Sequence variations in PCSK9, low LDL, and protection against coronary heart disease. *N Eng J Med*. 2006;354:1264-1272.

43. Regeneron Pharmaceuticals. Press release. http://files.shareholder.com/downloads/REGN/0x0x387214/534aaeb6-5e66-4e8f-86a9-0f9cac20d72f/REGN%20Investor%20Day%20Early%20Clinical%20Development1.pdf. Accessed July 15, 2010.

# 16 Hypertension

Ines Armando and Pedro A. Jose

## KEY POINTS

- *Disease summary:*
  - Hypertension is a disease than can be caused by mutations in single genes (monogenic hypertension), nonidentifiable causes (essential hypertension) or secondary to other diseases (secondary hypertension).
  - **Essential (primary) and secondary hypertension:** It accounts for 95% of all cases of hypertension, and is traditionally defined as high blood pressure for which an obvious secondary cause cannot be determined. However, several gene variants are claimed to cause essential hypertension. In the remaining 5% of the cases, the cause of hypertension is secondary to conditions such as primary hyperaldosteronism, excess glucocorticoids, pheochromocytoma, or renal disease.
  - **Monogenic hypertension:** Most monogenic forms of hypertension have renal origins. The consequence of a defective gene in each of these forms of hypertension is abnormally increased sodium transport in the distal nephron causing an expansion of the circulating plasma volume and increase in cardiac output (Table 16-1). All hereditary forms of hypertension lead to a suppression of the renin-angiotensin system due to plasma volume expansion.
  - The estimated prevalence of hypertension (in the United States derived from the NHANES 2005-2008) in adults 20 years or older is 33.5% (28.5% ≥18 years) which is approximately 76 million US adults and nearly equal between men (34.1%) and women (32.7%). The prevalence of hypertension varies by age, gender, and race or ethnicity and is also affected by behavior such as the intake of dietary sodium and potassium, weight, waist to hip ratio, alcohol consumption, and physical activity. The prevalence of essential hypertension is highest in non-Hispanic Blacks (43%-46%) and lowest in Asian Americans (30%). Among Americans 65 years and older, more women than men have hypertension.
  - Blood pressure is regulated by a complex group of interacting genes and essential hypertension is a polygenic disease. About half of the blood pressure variability is thought to be genetically determined but the variation of blood pressure is the result of an interaction among genes and environmental factors.
  - Early fetal environment may be linked to long-term health and lifespan consequences in the adult, including essential hypertension. Low birth weight babies have higher blood pressures, even after correction for various modifiers such as sex, cigarette smoking, and weight.
  - Hypertension is strongly associated with major cardiovascular risks such as premature cardiovascular disease, congestive heart failure, left ventricular hypertrophy, stroke, chronic kidney disease, and end-stage renal disease. In 2008, high blood pressure was responsible for about one in six deaths of US adults and was the single largest risk factor for cardiovascular mortality, accounting for about 45% of all cardiovascular deaths.
- *Differential diagnosis:*
  - The correct measurement of blood pressure, including the use of an appropriately sized cuff and sphygmomanometer that is properly calibrated and validated is critical.
- *Family history:*
  - Blood pressure heritability estimated from family studies is about 20%. The predictive strength of family history as a risk factor is doubled with one hypertensive first-degree relative and increases nearly fourfold with two such relatives.
- *Twin studies:*
  - Twin studies showed blood pressure heritability of about 60%. Genome-wide scans for blood pressure in extremely discordant and concordant sib pairs for blood pressure have revealed loci in several genes that are linked to hypertension but the specific gene variants have not been identified.
- *Environmental factors:*
  - The most important environmental factors in the development of hypertension at the population level are obesity, high sodium chloride intake, low potassium intake, physical inactivity, heavy alcohol consumption, and psychosocial stress.
- *Genome-wide associations:*
  - Genetic studies of essential hypertension have used two approaches: family-based linkage studies and the study of the association of candidate genes in a population-based design. Several chromosomal loci have been linked to hypertension. Common genetic variants associated with blood pressure and hypertension identified through genome-wide association studies (GWAS) in adult populations only account for about 1% to 2% of the variance of blood pressure (Table 16-2). Genome-wide mapping studies have linked loci in several chromosomes to essential hypertension, but these studies have not yet led to the identification of specific gene variants that may be causal. Linkage studies have been successful in the identification of rare and highly penetrant alleles but lack the power to detect alleles conferring moderate risks that may be the case in essential hypertension. Even if a disease risk locus is identified by linkage, the power of linkage disequilibrium to detect an association with a specific variant may be limited if multiple variants at each locus confer disease susceptibility. However, although their individual associations may not reach significance, the combination of variants may explain a substantial proportion of blood pressure variance.

**Table 16-1** *Monogenic Forms of Hypertension*

| Gene | Mutation | Inheritance | Syndrome |
|---|---|---|---|
| ENaC (*SCNN1B and SCNN1G*) | C terminal of β and γ subunits (constitutive activation) | Autosomal dominant | Liddle syndrome |
| 11β-hydroxysteroid dehydrogenase type 2 (*HSD11B2, 11βHSD2*) | Loss of function | Autosomal recessive | Apparent mineralocorticoid excess |
| *CYPB1* and *CYPB2* | Fusion of the two genes | Autosomal dominant | Glucocorticoid-remediable aldosteronism |
| *WNK1* and *WNK4* | *WNK1* gain of function/*WNK4* loss of function | Autosomal dominant | Pseudohyperaldosteronism type II (Gordon syndrome) |
| *KLHL3* | Loss of function | Dominant or recessive | Increased activity of sodium chloride cotransporter |
| *CUL3* | *KLHL3* loss of function | Dominant | |
| Mineralocorticoid receptor (*NR3C2*) | S810L-activating mutation of the mineralocorticoid receptor | Unknown | Hypertension exacerbated by pregnancy |
| 11β-hydroxylase; 17α-hydroxylase, (*CYP11B1;CYP17*) | *CYP11B1* exons 6-8*CYP17* random mutations | Unknown | Mineralocorticoid excess |

## Diagnostic Criteria and Clinical Characteristics

***Diagnostic Criteria of Hypertension:*** In adults aged 18 years and older normal blood pressure is defined as systolic blood pressure less than 120 mm Hg and diastolic blood pressure less than 80 mm Hg measured, at least twice, in the sitting position with feet on the floor, after at least a 5-minute rest. Hypertension is defined as systolic blood pressure equal to or greater than 140 mm Hg or diastolic blood pressure equal to or greater than 90 mm Hg. Systolic blood pressure from 140 to 159 mm Hg or diastolic blood pressure 90 to 99 mm Hg is considered stage 1 hypertension. Systolic blood pressure equal to or greater than 160 mm Hg or diastolic blood pressure equal to or greater than 100 mm Hg is considered stage 2 hypertension. Systolic blood pressure from 120 to 139 mm Hg or diastolic blood pressure from 80 to 89 mm Hg systolic is prehypertension.

Subjects with hypertension have blood pressure greater than 135/85 mm Hg when awake and more than 120/75 mm Hg when asleep. Hypertension that is not observed in the clinic or doctor's office is called masked hypertension while hypertension observed only in the clinic or doctor's office is called white coat hypertension.

In children and adolescents, hypertension is defined as repeatedly (≥3) measured systolic or diastolic blood pressure (fifth Korotkoff sound) at or greater than the 95th percentile adjusted for age, height, and sex. Systolic or diastolic blood pressures from the 95th percentile to 5 mm Hg about the 99th percentile is stage 1 hypertension while blood pressures greater than 5 mm Hg above the 99th percentile is stage 2 hypertension. Prehypertension in children is defined as systolic or diastolic blood pressure equal to or greater than the 90th percentile but less than the 95th percentile, adjusted for height, weight, and sex.

***Clinical Characteristics:*** There are no signs or symptoms in uncomplicated hypertension.

## Screening and Counseling

***Screening:*** Blood pressure measurement in parents and relatives may give a clue as to the genetic pattern of hypertension.

***Counseling:*** Lifestyle modification, similar to those used in the Dietary Approaches to Stop Hypertension (DASH), appropriate weight and waist to hip ratio, limitation of dietary sodium chloride intake, moderate alcohol intake of no more than two drinks per day and increased physical activity are recommended. Additionally, smoking cessation is also recommended to improve cardiovascular health. The benefits of these interventions include lowering of blood pressure, enhancement of antihypertensive efficacy, and reduction of cardiovascular risks.

## Management and Treatment

The primary goal of antihypertensive therapy is to reduce cardiovascular and renal morbidity and mortality using the least intrusive means possible. The Joint National committee on Prevention, Detection, Evaluation, and Treatment of High Blood Pressure (JNC 7) and US national guidelines recommend systolic blood pressure below 140 mm Hg and diastolic blood pressure below 90 mm Hg in all hypertensive patients. However, there may be a J-shaped curve, in which blood pressure below a critical level (which remains to be determined) may be associated with increased cardiovascular risk.

In patients with hypertension and diabetes or chronic kidney disease, the recommended blood pressure goal is less than 130/80 mm Hg.

The JNC 7 recommends that low-dose thiazide-type diuretics should be used as initial therapy for most patients with hypertension either alone in stage 1 hypertension, or in combination with other agents such as angiotensin-converting enzyme (ACE) inhibitors,

*Table 16-2 Disease-Associated Susceptibility Variants*

| Candidate Gene | Chromosome Location | Associated Variant (Odds Ratio) | Associated Disease Phenotype |
|---|---|---|---|
| **Sympathetic nervous system** | | | |
| $\alpha_{1A}$ adrenergic receptor (*ADRA1A*) | 8p21-p11.2 | 347 Arg 2547G | |
| $\alpha_{2B}$ adrenergic receptor (*ADRA2B*) | 2p13-q13 | In/del 216C>A | |
| $\alpha_{2A}$ adrenergic receptor (*ADRA2A*) | 10q24-q26 | In/del 216C>A | |
| $\beta_2$ adrenergic receptor (*ADRB2*) | 5q31-q32 | C79G (1.38) A46G A16G +491C/T | Severe hypertension |
| Tyrosine hydroxylase (*TH*) | 11p15.5 | C-824T rs2070762 | |
| Phenylethanolamine N-methyltransferase (*PNMT*) | 17q21 | G-353A G367A/G161A haplotype | |
| Solute carrier family 6, member 2, (norepinephrine transporter) (*SLC6A2*) | 16q12.2 | Promoter 3 A→G | |
| **Renin-angiotensin–aldosterone system** | | | |
| Angiotensinogen (*AGT*) | 1q42-q43 | G-217A (1.37); G-152A; A-20C; A-793G (1.88) G6A; T31A; T68C; M235T (rs699) T174M (1.74) | Salt sensitivity |
| Angiotensin-converting enzyme (*ACE*) | 17q23 | In/del C8342T A12292G A15990G | |
| Angiotensin II type 1 receptor (*AGTR1*) | 3q21-q25 | A1166C (rs5186) CA-repeat, A44221G rs4524238 | Salt sensitivity |
| Renin (*REN*) | 1q32 | *Hind*III RFLP *Mbo*I RFLP *Bgl*I RFLP 1205C>T 10607G>A Exon 9 G1051A C-4021T In/del | |
| Aldosterone synthase (*CYP11B2*) | 8q21 | T-344C (rs79996) A6547G rs3802230 (532G>T) | |
| Mineralocorticoid receptor nuclear receptor subfamily 3, group C, member 2 (*NR3C2*) | 4q31.1-31.2 | rs11737660 rs6810951 rs10519963 c.-2G>C (rs2070951) rs5522 | |
| 11β-hydroxysteroid dehydrogenase type 2 (*HSD11B2, 11βHSD2*) | 16q22 | G534A G-209A | Salt sensitivity |
| **Vasoactive peptides/substances** | | | |
| Apelin (*APLN*) | Xq25 | rs3761581 (A/C) T-1860C (via haplotypes) | |
| Apelin receptor (*APLNR*) | 11q12 | rs7119375 (G/A) | |
| Bradykinin receptor β₂ (*BDKRB2*) | 14q32.1-q32.2 | C181T | |

*Table 16-2  Disease-Associated Susceptibility Variants (Continued)*

| Candidate Gene | Chromosome Location | Associated Variant (Odds Ratio) | Associated Disease Phenotype |
|---|---|---|---|
| Endothelin 1 (*EDN1*) | 6p24-p23 | K198N | |
| Endothelin 2 (*EDN2*) | 1p34 | A985G | |
| Endothelin receptor type A (*EDNRA*) | 4q31.22 | 5′ UTR G→A<br>Exon 8 C→T | |
| Atrial natriuretic peptide receptor, type A (*NPRA*) | 1q21-q22 | In/del 15,129 (3′ UTR)<br>CT dinucleotide repeat polymorphism within the 5′-flanking region | |
| Atrial natriuretic peptide precursor A (*NPPA*) | 1p36.21 | rs5063 | Development of hypertension |
| Prostacyclin synthase, prostaglandin I2 synthase (*CYP8A1*) | 20q13.11 | G1662A | |
| Nitric oxide synthase 3 (*NOS3*) | 7q36 | G10T, intron 23<br>G894T (rs1799983)<br>T-786C (rs2070744)<br>rs3918226 promoter region (1.9) | Salt sensitivity |
| **Oxidative stress and inflammation** | | | |
| Catalase (*CAT*) | 11p13 | CATH2 haplotype (three variants in the promoter and 5′-UTR) | |
| CC-chemokine receptor 2 (*CCR2*) | 3p21 | V64I | |
| CC-chemokine receptor 5 (*CCR5*) | 3p21 | CCR5Δ32 | |
| Heme oxygenase-1 (*HMOX-1*) | 22q12 | T-413A<br>rs9607267 | |
| Transforming growth factor $\beta_1$ (*TGF β1*) | 2p22-p21 | +869T/C (2.50) | |
| Tumor necrosis factor $\alpha$ (*TNFA*) | 6p21.3 | C-850T | |
| TNF receptor 2 (*TNFRSF1B*) | 1p36.22 | CA repeat in intron 4 (CA16) | |
| E selectin (*SELE*) | 9q34.2 | C602A<br>T1559C | |
| **Channels, transporters, sodium homeostasis** | | | |
| Chloride channel, kidney A (*CLCNKB*) | 8q23 | rs1010069<br>rs1805152<br>rs848307<br>rs1739843 | Salt sensitivity<br>Salt sensitivity<br>Salt sensitivity<br>Salt sensitivity |
| Chloride channel, kidney B (*CLCNKB*) | 1p36 | T481S | |
| ENaC $\alpha$ subunit (*SCNN1A*) | 12p13.3 | A2139G | |
| ENaC $\beta$ subunit (*SCNN1B*) | 16p13-p12 | G589S<br>intronic i12-17CT substitution<br>GT dinucleotide short tandem repeat | |
| ENaC $\gamma$ subunit1 (*SCNN1G*) | 16p13-p12 | G-173A | |
| Sodium bicarbonate exchanger (*SLC4A5*) | 2p13 | hcv1137534 | |
| Serum- and glucocorticoid-regulated kinase (*SGK1*) | 6q23 | Intron 6 TT/CT<br>rs2758151<br>rs9402751 | <br>Salt sensitivity<br>Salt sensitivity |
| Neural precursor cell expressed developmentally downregulated 4-like (*NEDD4L*) | 18q21 | 296921-296923delTTG, rs2288774<br>rs2288775<br>rs3865418<br>rs4149601 | <br>Salt sensitivity<br>Salt sensitivity |

*(Continued)*

*Table 16-2 Disease-Associated Susceptibility Variants (Continued)*

| Candidate Gene | Chromosome Location | Associated Variant (Odds Ratio) | Associated Disease Phenotype |
|---|---|---|---|
| Protein kinase, lysine-deficient 4 (*WNK4*) | 17q21-q22 | G1662A<br>G/A intron 10, bp 1156666<br>Exon 8 G1155942T<br>Exon 8 A589S C1163527T | |
| Protein kinase, lysine-deficient 1 (*WNK1*) | 12p13.3 | rs11885<br>rs11554421<br>rs34880640 | |
| Vasopressin receptor 1A (*AVPR1A*) | 12q14-q15 | D12S398 | |
| Uromodulin (*UMOD*) | 16p12.3 | rs13333226 | |
| ATPase, Ca++ transporting (*ATP2B1*) | 12q21.3 | rs2070759 (1.17)<br>rs11105378 (1.31) | |
| Ste20-related proline-alanine–rich kinase (*STK39*) | 2q24.3 | rs6749447<br>rs3754777 | |
| **Dopaminergic system** | | | |
| Dopamine D1 receptor (*DRD1*) | 5q35.2 | A-48G<br>G-94A (rs 5326) | |
| Dopamine D2 receptor (*DRD2*) | 11q23 | Taq1 | |
| G protein-dependent receptor kinase 4 (*GRK4*) | 4p16.3 | R65L (rs296036)<br>A142V (rs1024323)<br>A486V (rs1801058) | Salt sensitivity |
| **Cellular structure (cytoskeleton, gap junctions)** | | | |
| Connexin 40 (*GJA5*) | 1q21.1 | -44AA/+71GG (1.87/2.10) | |
| α-adducin (*ADD1*) | 4p16.3 | G460W<br>rs4961<br>rs17833172 | Salt sensitivity<br>Salt sensitivity |
| β-adducin (*ADD2*) | 2p14-p13 | C1797T<br>rs3755351 | |
| **Lipid metabolism** | | | |
| 20-HETE synthase (*CYP4A11*) | 1p33 | T8590C<br>rs1558139 | |
| Lipoprotein lipase (*LPL*) | 8p22 | IVS4-214C→T | |
| **Glucose metabolism** | | | |
| Glucagon receptor (*GCGR*) | 17q25 | G40S | |
| Glycogen synthase 1 (*GYS1*) | 19q13.3 | *Xba*I RFLP | |
| Insulin receptor (*INSR*) | 19p13.2 | R1 (*Rsa*I) RFLP<br>Insertion polymorphism<br>CA repeat (intron 9)<br>GAG-1040-GAA (SSCP)<br>*Nsi*I RFLP (exon 8) | |
| **GPCR signaling** | | | |
| Guanine nucleotide binding protein, subunit 3 (*GNB3*) | 12p13 β3 | C825T (rs5443)<br>rs1129649 | Salt sensitivity |
| Regulator of G-protein signaling 2 (*RGS2*) | 1q31 | In/del<br>1891-1892 TC In/del (1.69)<br>rs34717272 | |
| **Other** | | | |
| 5,10-methylenetetrahydrofolate reductase (*MTHFR*) | 1p36.3 | rs1801133<br>C677T | Development of hypertension |

In/del : insertion/deletion. Variants are termed as in the original reference.

angiotensin receptor blockers (ARBs), calcium channel blockers (CCBs) or beta-blockers in stage 2 hypertension. However, the use of thiazide-type diuretics, because of toxic effects, in the treatment of essential hypertension has been questioned.

*Pharmacogenetics/Pharmacogenomics:* Genotyping for certain gene variants may aid in the diagnosis of salt sensitivity (Table 16-2). Genetic screening may be an effective mechanism to identify salt-sensitive normotensive and hypertensive subjects. As an example, genotyping for *GRK4* variants has a 70% predictive value for hypertension in Ghanaians and 94% predictive accuracy for salt sensitivity in Japanese. Pharmacogenomics of essential hypertension is in its early stages. Patients with adducin (*ADD1*) G460T may respond better to ouabain antagonists. Patients with *NEDD4L* rs4149601 G allele may be more responsive to beta-adrenergic blocker or diuretic monotherapy. In South African black patients with mild-to-moderate hypertension, carriers of *GRK4* R65 and *GRK4* R65L or *GRK4* A142 and *GRK4* A142V may have a good response to low-sodium diet.

## Molecular Genetics and Molecular Mechanism

Refer also to Table 16-2.

*Renal Mechanisms:* Many studies on the pathogenesis of essential hypertension have focused on the kidney because of its importance in the long-term regulation of blood pressure. Essential hypertension is associated with increased sodium transport in the renal proximal tubule and medullary thick ascending limb, although increased distal tubular transport has also been reported. In contrast, monogenic hypertension is caused by increased sodium transport mainly in the distal nephron. Essential hypertension has been attributed to increased extracellular fluid volume, caused by a failure of the kidneys to eliminate sodium chloride and water at normal blood pressure levels. Sodium in the interstitial fluid affects the expression of the hypertensive phenotype. The impaired renal sodium handling in essential hypertension may be the result of abnormal regulation of natriuretic and antinatriuretic pathways. Variants in genes expressing proteins that increase renal sodium transport or vascular smooth muscle cells reactivity, as well as genes expressing proteins that normally decrease renal sodium transport have been found to be associated with essential hypertension.

*Nonrenal Mechanisms: Secondary Role of the Kidney:* A primary role of neuroendocrine and cardiac mechanisms in the pathogenesis of hypertension with a secondary role played by vasoconstrictor and vasodilatory agents from the endothelial cells has also been documented. Hormones regulate blood pressure both by renal and nonrenal mechanisms. The sympathetic nervous system is important in the pathogenesis of essential hypertension and may regulate blood pressure by extrarenal mechanisms. Humans with essential hypertension have increased sympathetic nervous activity outside the kidney.

*Genes Associated With Antinatriuretic or Vasoconstrictor Pathways:*

☞SYMPATHETIC NERVOUS SYSTEM: Increased sympathetic activity has been demonstrated in salt-sensitive hypertension. Common variants of the tyrosine hydroxylase gene, the enzyme catalyzing the rate-limiting step in the synthesis of catecholamines, are associated with hypertension. Several polymorphisms of adrenergic receptors, as well as the enzyme catalyzing the synthesis of epinephrine and the norepinephrine transporter that mediates norepinephrine reuptake in nerve terminals, are also associated with essential hypertension.

☞RENIN-ANGIOTENSIN–ALDOSTERONE SYSTEM (RAAS): The renin-angiotensin–aldosterone (RAAS) is the most important regulator of renal sodium transport and the major system involved in the increase in renal sodium transport, especially under conditions of sodium deficit. Several polymorphisms of angiotensinogen, angiotensin-converting enzyme, renin, and angiotensin AT1 receptor, as well as aldosterone synthase, the mineralocorticoid receptor, and 11β-hydroxysteroid dehydrogenase, the enzyme that inactivates 11-hydroxysteroid in the kidney and protects the mineralocorticoid receptor from occupation by glucocorticoids, have been reported to be associated with hypertension.

☞ENDOTHELIN: Endothelins have multiple effects; they mediate vasoconstriction in vascular muscle cells, vasodilation via the endothelial cells, and decrease or increase sodium transport in a nephron segment endothelin-receptor dependent manner. Polymorphisms in two of the endothelin isopeptides and the endothelin receptor A are associated with high blood pressure.

☞REACTIVE OXYGEN SPECIES AND INFLAMMATION: Some polymorphisms in genes regulating inflammation and the production of reactive oxygen species (ROS) are also associated with essential hypertension. In nonphagocytic cells, ROS regulate vascular tone and cell growth; inflammation may be an important mechanism that contributes to the maintenance of high blood pressure initiated by other primary processes.

☞RENAL SODIUM TRANSPORTERS AND CHANNELS: The activity of renal channels and transporters is a common final pathway in the regulation of renal transport of sodium and other ions. Common variants in the amiloride-sensitive epithelial sodium channel (ENaC) and in ENaC regulators *NEDD4L, WNK1, WNK4, SGK1*, as well as the renal chloride channel (*CLCNK*), are associated with hypertension and salt sensitivity. Polymorphisms in the *STK39* gene, which encodes a serine/threonine kinase that interacts with WNK kinases and cation-chloride cotransporters, are associated with the susceptibility to high blood pressure.

*Genes Associated With Natriuretic or Vasodilator Pathways:*

☞VASOACTIVE PEPTIDES OR SUBSTANCES: ADRENOMEDULLIN (ADM): ADM and ADM2 or intermedin are widely distributed in the body, including blood vessels and the kidney. ADM and ADM2 or intermedin can reduce blood pressure and increase sodium excretion, in part through an increase in renal NO activity. *ADM* 1984G is associated with lower sodium excretion but also lower systolic blood pressure.

Apelin decreases blood pressure by stimulating NO release and induces a diuresis by decreasing vasopressin secretion. Variants in the gene encoding for apelin and the apelin receptor are also associated with hypertension. Several polymorphisms of endothelial NO synthase (*eNOS*) have been associated with essential hypertension. A meta-analysis of 53 studies showed that the effect of *eNOS* G894T SNP may be dependent on total cholesterol status.

☞ATRIAL NATRIURETIC PEPTIDE: Common genetic variants at the natriuretic peptide precursor A (*NPPA*) and the atrial natriuretic peptide receptor contribute to interindividual variations in blood pressure and hypertension.

☞DOPAMINERGIC SYSTEM: Dopamine produced in the kidney (mainly by proximal tubules) acts in an autocrine/paracrine manner to regulate renal ion transport. The inhibition of renal transport of sodium and other ions occurs in multiple segments of the nephron, including the proximal and distal convoluted tubule, thick ascending limb of Henle, and cortical collecting duct. The ability of dopamine to increase sodium excretion is impaired in humans with essential hypertension, which has been related to polymorphisms in the promoter region of the D1-like receptor (D1R) gene (*DRD1*) G-94A (rs5326). The inhibitory effect of dopamine and D1R agonists on sodium transport is impaired in hypertension. The decreased function of D1R in hypertension may be related to a state of constitutive desensitization due to the presence of activating variants of *GRK4*, including *GRK4 R65L, A142V,* and *A486V.* Several studies in different ethnic groups have shown that *GRK4* gene variants are associated with essential hypertension. Salt-sensitive hypertensive Japanese patients carrying at least three *GRK4* gene variants have an impaired natriuretic response to a dopaminergic drug, and salt-sensitive hypertension can be correctly predicted in 94% of the cases.

☞Eicosanoids: The loss-of-function 20-hydroxyeicosatetraenoic acid (HETE) synthase (*CYP4A11*) 8590C allele is associated with hypertension and, in normotensive individuals, with higher blood pressure regardless of salt intake. Among hypertensive individuals, the C allele is associated with salt sensitivity. 20-HETE increases blood pressure by vasoconstriction but can also decrease blood pressure by decreasing renal sodium transport, especially at the proximal tubule and thick ascending limb of Henle.

*Genes That Do Not Normally Decrease Renal Sodium Transport:* Adducin: Adducins are cytoskeletal proteins that regulate the membrane organization of spectrin-actin. The inhibition of Na$^+$K$^+$-ATPase activity is mediated, in part, by internalization of its subunits involving the actin-microtubule cytoskeleton.

Human carriers of *ADD1 460W, WNK1 GG, and NEDD4L* GG need a greater increase in systolic blood pressure to excrete the same amount of sodium relative to the carriers of *ADD1G460, WNK1 AA, and NEDD4L* AA. *ADD1460WW, ACE* DD, and *CYP11B2* 344CC may also contribute to the risk of salt-sensitive hypertension.

*Genetic Testing:* The utility of genetic testing for essential hypertension is not yet fully realized. The interaction among different genes, behavior, and environment needs to be considered before widespread testing is undertaken.

*Future Directions:* Multiple criteria have been promulgated to identify genetic variants associated with complex traits (such as salt sensitivity and hypertension). These include linkage and association methods and circumstantial evidence (eg, comparison of wild-type and variant biochemistry and physiology). Animal investigations are useful, however, gene overexpression and deletion studies in mice have not always taken into account the salt sensitivity of the strain of mice in which the genetic manipulation is undertaken. For example, the C57BL/6 strain of mice from Jackson Laboratories have an impaired ability to excrete a sodium load, which results in an increase in blood pressure when salt intake is increased. Other strains (eg, SJL mice) are salt-resistant. Many genes have been proposed to be causal of hypertension but many of these variants, including those identified by GWAS, have not been shown to produce hypertension in mice, except for those in the promoter region of *AGT* and coding region of *GRK4.* Finally, somatic mutations in the kidney, in addition to germline mutations, may underlie the pathogenesis of essential hypertension.

## Bibliography:

1. Lenfant C, Chobanian AV, Jones DW, Roccella EJ, Joint National Committee on the Prevention, Detection, Evaluation, and Treatment of High Blood Pressure. The Seventh Report of the Joint National Committee on Prevention, Detection, Evaluation, and Treatment of High Blood Pressure (JNC 7): resetting the hypertension sails. *Hypertension.* 2003;41(6):1178-1179. (http://www.nhlbi.nih.gov/guidelines/hypertension/jnc7full.pdf, Accessed July, 2013.)

2. Roger VL, Go AS, Lloyd-Jones DM, et al. Heart disease and stroke statistics—2012 update: a report from the American Heart Association. *Circulation.* 2012;125(1):e2-e220.

3. Boyden LM, Choi M, Choate KA, et al. Mutations in kelch-like 3 and cullin 3 cause hypertension and electrolyte abnormalities. *Nature.* 2012;482(7383):98-102.

4. Harrap SB. Blood pressure genetics: time to focus. *J Am Soc Hypertens.* 2009;3(4):231-237.

5. Taal HR, Verwoert GC, Demirkan A, et al. Genome-wide profiling of blood pressure in adults and children. *Hypertension.* 2012;59(2):241-247.

6. Sanada H, Jones JE, Jose PA. Genetics of salt-sensitive hypertension. *Curr Hypertens Rep.* 2011;13(1):55-66.

7. Johnson JA. Pharmacogenomics of antihypertensive drugs: past, present and future. *Pharmacogenomics.* 2010;11(4):487-491.

8. Lanzani C, Citterio L, Glorioso N, et al. Adducin- and ouabain-related gene variants predict the antihypertensive activity of rostafuroxin, part 2: clinical studies. *Sci Transl Med.* 2010;2(59):59ra87.

9. Lupton SJ, Chiu CL, Lind JM. A hypertension gene: are we there yet? *Twin Res Hum Genet.* Aug 2011;14(4):295-304.

10. Moore JH, Williams SM. New strategies for identifying gene-gene interactions in hypertension. *Ann Med.* 2002;34:88-95.

11. Glazier AM, Nadeau JH, Aitman TJ. Finding genes that underlie complex traits. *Science.* 2002;298:2345-2349.

12. Jain S, Tillinger A, Mopidevi B, et al. Transgenic mice with -6A haplotype of the human angiotensinogen gene have increased blood pressure compared with -6G haplotype. *J Biol Chem.* 2010;285:41172-41186.

## Supplementary Information

**OMIM References:**

[1] Hypertension Essential; (#145500)

[2] Liddle Syndrome; (#177200)

**Alternative Names, Symbols:**
- EHT

*Key Words:* High blood pressure, cardiovascular disease, kidney, sodium transport

# 17 Stroke and Cerebrovascular Disease

Tisha R. Joy and Robert A. Hegele

## KEY POINTS

- *Disease summary:*
  - Stroke is an umbrella term for the rapid loss of neurologic function in a particular vascular territory, with symptoms lasting greater than 24 hours.
  - The causes of stroke are broadly defined as either ischemic or hemorrhagic.
  - Clinical manifestations depend on the vascular territory affected, with the middle cerebral artery (MCA) being most commonly affected.
  - Management of stroke involves identifying the onset and duration of symptoms, assessing and maintaining normal vital signs, evaluating whether the patient with acute stroke is a candidate for thrombolysis, and longer-term risk factor management.

- *Differential diagnosis for stroke:*
  - Several phenomena may present similar to stroke, including transient ischemic attacks ([TIAs], which manifest as neurologic deficits lasting <24 hours), migraines, Todd paresis, head trauma, brain tumors, and metabolic and/or toxic insults (such as hypoglycemia, hypothyroidism, renal or liver failure, certain drug intoxications).

- *Monogenic forms:*
  - Monogenic forms of stroke include (1) syndromes that feature ischemic or hemorrhagic stroke as the primary or key component, or (2) multisystem syndromes or conditions that contain stroke as a secondary component.

- *Family history:*
  - A family history of early cardiovascular disease increases the likelihood for the development of ischemic stroke. A family history of cerebral aneurysms may be relevant for hemorrhagic stroke risk.

- *Environmental factors:*
  - For ischemic stroke, the classical determinants of atherosclerosis, such as smoking, poor diet, obesity, hyperlipidemia, and hypertension can increase the risk for stroke, as can the use of certain medications, such as hormone replacement therapy.

- *Genome-wide association studies (GWAS):*
  - GWAS findings of stroke as a clinical end point are relatively inconsistent, while GWAS of risk factors and intermediate traits, such as plasma lipids and hypertension, show much more consistency across studies.

- *Pharmacogenomics:*
  - Preventive therapies for embolic stroke, specifically Coumadin (warfarin), show replicable associations with interindividual genomic variation. Also, interindividual differences in the susceptibility to serious side effects from statins, used widely in stroke prevention, appear to have a genetic basis.

## Diagnostic Criteria and Clinical Characteristics

**Diagnostic Criteria:** Stroke is defined as the rapid loss of neurologic function in a particular vascular territory caused by either ischemia or hemorrhage, with symptoms lasting greater than 24 hours. Ischemic strokes can be subdivided according to cause: thrombotic or embolic. Meanwhile, hemorrhagic strokes are subdivided according to location of bleeding: parenchymal (intracerebral hemorrhage [ICH]) or subarachnoid hemorrhage (SAH) (Fig. 17-1). The diagnosis of stroke depends on accurate history and physical examination, and confirmed by appropriate neuroimaging.

**Clinical Characteristics:** The exact clinical characteristics of a stroke depend on the vascular territory affected, with the MCA most often affected. See Fig. 17-2 for types of vessels affected and their respective clinical characteristics.

**Differential Diagnosis:** Several phenomena may present similar to stroke, including TIAs, migraines, Todd paresis, head trauma, brain tumors, and metabolic and/or toxic insults (such as hypoglycemia, hypothyroidism, renal or liver failure, certain drug intoxications). Of these, TIAs are most often difficult to distinguish from strokes,

since the only difference between the two phenomena is duration of symptoms. Neurologic deficits secondary to TIAs resolve within 24 hours. Unfortunately, due to the need for early intervention with thrombolytic therapy in patients with ischemic strokes, time is often not enough to determine whether a patient's symptoms are due to stroke or TIA.

## Screening and Counseling

**Monogenic forms:** Once a firm molecular diagnosis has been made for a rare monogenic form of stroke or for the broader multisystem disorder that includes stroke as a component, family members can be tested in a cascade manner for the specific mutation.

**Hemorrhagic stroke:** Most forms of inherited cerebral aneurysmal disease have no molecular basis determined. When a strong familial tendency is suspected, relatives of a proband with cerebral aneurysms can be screened not with molecular techniques, but instead with noninvasive imaging technologies for clinically silent aneurysms, which if detected, can be pre-emptively treated surgically.

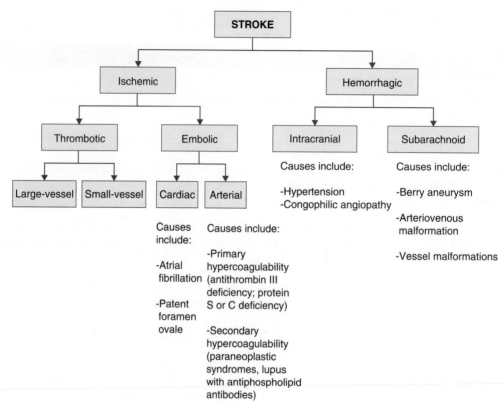

***Figure 17-1*** Clinical Approach to Strokes.

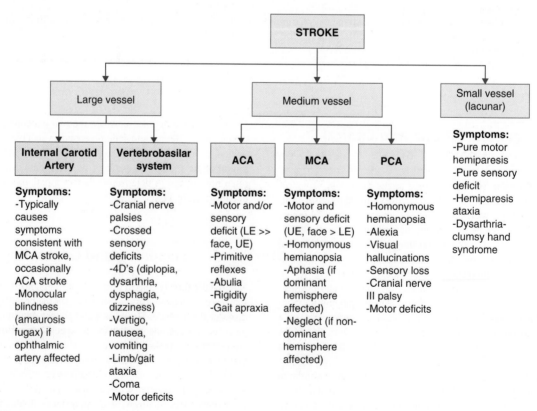

***Figure 17-2*** Clinical Characteristics of Stroke Dependent on Vascular Territory Affected.
ACA, anterior cerebral artery; LE, lower extremity; MCA, middle cerebral artery; PCA, posterior cerebral artery; UE, upper extremity.

**Common complex ischemic stroke:** Family members of a patient who has suffered a common, later-onset ischemic stroke, should themselves be screened for the presence of modifiable risk factors, such as hypertension, dyslipidemia, or diabetes. Appropriate lifestyle interventions—diet, weight loss, and exercise—together with appropriate drug treatments can be instituted following clinical guidelines for the prevention of cardiovascular and cerebrovascular disease.

## Management and Treatment

Timing is essential to the management of patients with stroke. Immediate management of patients presenting with symptoms suggestive of a stroke includes assessment of airway, breathing, and circulation (ABC), ensuring euglycemia and euvolemia, and evaluating underlying reversible or life-threatening causes. Determining the exact onset of symptoms is critical to determining whether the patient is a candidate to thrombolytic therapy.

### Acute Management:

☞NONPHARMACOLOGIC INTERVENTION:

- Assess ABCs, check blood sugar to ensure not hypoglycemic.
- Obtain accurate history, including exact onset of symptoms and potential causes for presentation.
- Perform thorough physical examination to rule out immediate life-threatening of presenting symptoms (hypoglycemia, hemorrhage).
- Neurologic examination with the aid of the National Institutes of Health Stroke Scale (NIHSS).
- Routine investigations including complete blood count, electrolytes, creatinine, international normalized ratio (INR), activated partial thromboplastin time, oxygen saturation, markers of cardiac ischemia, and electrocardiogram.
- Noncontrast brain computed tomography (CT) or brain magnetic resonance imaging (MRI) to assess for hemorrhage and rule out causes other than ischemic stroke. (Imaging of the brain must be performed prior to stroke-specific therapy, particularly thrombolysis.)
- Ancillary tests such as toxicology screen, liver enzymes, blood alcohol level, beta-hCG (in women of reproductive potential), arterial blood gases (if hypoxia suspected), chest x-ray (if lung disease suspected), lumbar puncture (if subarachnoid hemorrhage suspected and no blood demonstrated on CT), and electroencephalogram (if seizures suspected), depending on clinical situation.
- Maintain euvolemia and adequate oxygenation, if hypoxic.
- Maintain euglycemia and avoid extremes in blood pressure.
- Maintain normal body temperature; use antipyretics as needed.
- Cardiac monitoring.
- Dysphagia precautions as necessary.

☞PHARMACOLOGIC INTERVENTION:

- Evaluate if patient is candidate for thrombolysis with intravenous (IV) recombinant tissue plasminogen activator (rtPA) based on inclusion and exclusion criteria in Table 17-1.
- Intravenous thrombolysis is ideally administered within the first 3 hours of symptom onset.
- A more select group of patients may be considered eligible for thrombolysis within 4.5 hours of onset of symptoms. The eligibility criteria for treatment in the 3- to 4.5-hour window are similar to those for patients treated earlier, with the following additional exclusion criteria:

- Age greater than 80 years
- Use of oral anticoagulants regardless of INR
- Severe stroke with baseline NIHSS score greater than 25
- History of diabetes and prior ischemic stroke
- Intra-arterial thrombolysis is an option in patients who are evaluated within 6 hours of symptoms but who are ineligible to receive IV rtPA because of recent surgery or other procedures.

### Subacute and Long-Term Management:

☞NONPHARMACOLOGIC INTERVENTION:

- Close monitoring in specialized stroke centers during the acute and subacute period for signs of neurologic deterioration secondary to edema, hemorrhage post-thrombolysis, or extension of the infarct.
- Maintain euvolemia and adequate oxygenation, if hypoxic.
- Maintain euglycemia and avoid extremes in blood pressure.
- Maintain normal body temperature; use antipyretics as needed.
- Dysphagia precautions as necessary with assessment by speech language pathology prior to reinitiation of oral intake.
- Depending on clinical manifestations, involvement of the following ancillary healthcare members is required:
  - Occupational therapy
  - Physiotherapy
- Investigate for and institute appropriate therapy for other risk factors such as
  - Hyperlipidemia
  - Hypertension
  - Carotid stenosis
  - Aneurysm or arteriovenous malformation
- Thus, other possible investigations may include
  - Carotid Doppler ultrasound
  - Echocardiogram with bubble study
  - MRI/MR angiography (MRA)
- If persistently severe deficits, transfer to rehabilitation center once acute management and risk factor control has been undertaken within the specialized stroke care units.

☞PHARMACOLOGIC INTERVENTION:

- Aspirin 325 mg daily within 24 to 48 hours after stroke onset
- Anticoagulation with Coumadin in patients with atrial fibrillation or certain hypercoagulability syndromes
- Treatment of hyperlipidemia, hypertension, and other concomitant medical conditions
- Deep vein thrombosis prophylaxis using subcutaneous anticoagulants in immobilized patients

☞PHARMACOGENETICS:

- Individuals who are at the extremes of responsiveness to Coumadin (warfarin) differ according to single-nucleotide polymorphism (SNP) genotypes of the genes encoding enzyme cytochrome P450 2C9 (*CYP2C9*, namely *2 and *3 polymorphisms) and vitamin K epoxide reductase complex subunit 1 (*VKORC1*, namely 1639G>A and 3730G>A). There is emerging evidence that this genotyping can reduce morbidity.
- Individuals homozygous for the rare allele of the rs4363657 SNP located within the *SLCO1B1* gene encoding organic anion-transporting polypeptide OATP1B1 have approximately 20-fold increased risk of severe statin-related myopathy, although this genetic testing is not yet approved for routine use.

*Table 17-1 Inclusion and Exclusion Criteria For Patients With Ischemic Stroke Potentially Able To Receive rtPA*

| Inclusion | Exclusion |
|---|---|
| • Diagnosis of ischemic stroke causing measurable neurologic deficit<br>• Onset of symptoms < 3 hours before beginning treatment<br>• Aged ≥ 18 years | • Significant head trauma or prior stroke in prior 3 months<br>• Symptoms suggestive of subarachnoid hemorrhage<br>• History of prior intracranial hemorrhage<br>• Arterial puncture at non-compressible site in previous 7 days<br>• Intracranial neoplasm, arteriovenous malformation, or aneurysm<br>• Recent intracranial or intraspinal surgery<br>• Elevated blood pressure (systolic > 185 mmHg or diastolic > 110 mmHg)<br>• Active internal bleeding<br>• Acute bleeding diathesis, including but not limited to<br>  • Platelet count < 100,000/mm³<br>  • Heparin received within 48 hours, resulting in abnormally elevated aPTT greater than the upper limit of normal<br>  • Current use of anticoagulant with INR > 1.7 or PT > 15 seconds<br>  • Current use of direct thrombin inhibitors or direct factor Xa inhibitors with elevated sensitive laboratory tests (such as aPTT, INR, platelet count, and ECT; TT; or appropriate factor Xa activity assay)<br>• Blood glucose concentration < 50 mg/dL (2.7 mmol/L)<br>• CT demonstrates multilobar infarction (hypodensity >1/3 cerebral hemisphere)<br><br>*Relative exclusion criteria*[a]<br>• Only minor or rapidly improving stroke symptoms (clearing spontaneously)<br>• Pregnancy<br>• Seizure at onset with postictal residual neurological impairments<br>• Major surgery or serious trauma within previous 14 days<br>• Recent gastrointestinal or urinary tract hemorrhage (within previous 21 days)<br>• Recent acute myocardial infarction (within previous 3 months) |

[a]Patients may receive fibrinolytic therapy despite one or more relative exclusions provided that there has been careful consideration and weighting of the risk to benefit.

aPTT, activated partial thromboplastin time; CT, computed tomography; ECT, ecarin clotting time; INR, international normalized ratio; rtPA, recombinant tissue plasminogen activator; TT, thrombin time.

## Molecular Genetics and Molecular Mechanisms

• A stroke is the clinical culmination of many complex processes and interacting pathways, none of which is individually a necessary or sufficient cause.
• The pathways are broadly suggested by the clinical subtypes: hemorrhagic versus ischemic.
• Divergent pathophysiologies include cardiac arrhythmias, disordered coagulation, defective arterial wall structure and function, and altered metabolic, inflammatory, and immune mechanisms, each of which in turn has a genetic component.
• Intermediate phenotypes, also referred to as biomarkers, subphenotypes, endophenotypes, subclinical traits or disease attributes, including imaging phenotypes of stroke, such as carotid intima media thickness are targeted measures of disease progression that may be more directly related to a specific disease etiology.
• Monogenic forms of stroke include
  • Syndromes or conditions which feature ischemic or hemorrhagic stroke as the primary or key component, such as cerebral autosomal dominant arteriopathy with subcortical infarcts and leucoencephalopathy (CADASIL) due to mutations in

*NOTCH3*, Moyamoya disease (bilateral intracranial carotid artery occlusion associated with telangiectatic vessels in the region of the basal ganglia) or the syndrome of mitochondrial myopathy, encephalopathy, lactic acidosis, and stroke-like episodes (MELAS) due to mutations in the mitochondrial genome.
• Multisystem syndromes or conditions which contain stroke as a secondary component, such as Fabry disease (alpha-galactosidase deficiency), sickle cell disease, homocystinuria, and certain connective tissue disorders, such as Ehlers-Danlos syndrome, which causes dissection of the carotid or vertebral arteries.
• Monogenic disorders that affect key pathogenic pathways in ischemic stroke, such as monogenic cardiac dysrhythmias (eg, atrial fibrillation), cardiomyopathies (eg, dilated cardiomyopathy), coagulopathies (eg, antithrombin III deficiency), dyslipidemias (familial combined hyperlipidemia), and vasculopathies (eg, Kawasaki disease).
• Complex genetic susceptibility uncovered by recent GWAS have somewhat inconsistent findings (Table 17-2) compared to GWAS performed in other complex traits. If replicated and validated, several loci identified by GWAS represent new pathways and potential molecular targets.

*Table 17-2* **Stroke-Associated Susceptibility Variants From GWAS**

| Candidate Gene (Chromosome Location) | Associated Variant (effect on protein) | Relative Risk | Frequency of Risk Allele | Putative Functional Significance | Associated Disease Phenotype | First Author of Reference |
|---|---|---|---|---|---|---|
| PRKCH (14q22) | rs2230500 1425A/G V374I | OR 1.66 (1.44-2.09) $p = 9.84$ E-6 | A: 0.018 JPT HapMap A: 0.227 cases A: 0.188 controls (Cerebral infarct) | None assessed | Ischemic stroke | Kubo |
| AGTRL1 (11q12) | rs9943582 -154C/T[a] (C allele risk allele) | OR 1.30 (1.14-1.47) $p = 6.6$ E-5 | C: 0.631 JPT HapMap | None assessed | Ischemic stroke | Hata |
| PITX2 (4q25) | rs2200733 C/T | OR 1.26 (1.17-1.35) $p = 2.18$ E-10 All groups including replication | T: 0.132 All groups (CEU) | None assessed | Ischemic stroke | Gretarsdottir |
| ZFHX3 (16q22) | rs7193343 71586660C/T | OR 1.11 (1.04-1.17) $p = 5.4$ E-4 (all groups) | T: 0.150 CEU HapMap | None assessed | Ischemic stroke | Gudbjartsson |
| NINJ2 (12p13) | rs11833579 | HR 1.41 (1.27-1.56) $p = 2.3$ E-10 | A:0.23 cases A:0.225 CEU HapMap | None assessed | Ischemic stroke | Ikram |
| CELSR1 (22q13) | rs6007897 C/T[a] T2268A | OR 1.85 (1.29-2.61) $p = 6.0$ E-4 | C: 0.023 JPT HapMap | None assessed | Ischemic stroke | Yamada |

[a]All single-nucleotide polymorphism (SNP) nomenclature is oriented relative to the forward nucleotide strand.

## Genetic Testing:

- Prediction of Coumadin response by genotyping of *VKORC1* and *CYP2D9* has recently been suggested by the United States Food and Drug Administration (FDA), with some caveats. No other genetic testing has yet been recommended as part of screening for susceptibility to common stroke.
- Screening for specific monogenic forms as part of cascade family testing or to clarify diagnosis at the molecular level might be considered as more information on monogenic stroke phenotypes and genotypes accumulates.
- For common stroke, there is no evidence yet that including allele scores from GWAS genotypes will enhance current prediction algorithms, such as the Framingham stroke score.

## Future Directions:

- Future genomic analysis of stroke will need to evaluate individuals from multiple ethnicities.
- Phenomics entails both the collection of a wide breadth of fine resolution phenotypes and the careful analysis of phenotype data to extract the most information possible. Due to the large degree of clinical heterogeneity in stroke patients, phenomics may particularly benefit the genomic analysis of stroke.
- Hierarchical cluster analysis may be used to identify subgroups of patients with a more homogeneous disease pathophysiology. Phenotypic classification of study participants is of utmost importance, and efforts continue to improve the classification of stroke patients.

- Next-generation sequencing technologies promise to interrogate the genome at the resolution of a single base pair. Deep resequencing, in which a candidate region is sequenced in samples of cases and controls, has successfully identified genes that appear to contain an excess, or accumulation, of rare sequence changes in a range of phenotypes. Technologic progression from deep resequencing to whole genome sequencing will present challenges for data storage, analysis, and interpretation.

**BIBLIOGRAPHY:**

1. Lee JK, Bae CJ. Neurology. In: Stoller JK, Michota FA Jr., Mandell BF, eds. *The Cleveland Clinic Foundation Intensive Review of Internal Medicine.* 5th ed. Philadelphia, PA: Wolters Kluwer/ Lippincott Williams & Wilkins; 2009.

2. Jauch EC, Saver JL, Adams HP Jr, et al. Guidelines for the early management of adults with ischemic stroke: a guideline for healthcare professionals from the American Heart Association/ American Stroke Association. *Stroke.* 2013;44(3):870-947.

3. Del Zoppo GJ, Saver JL, Jauch EC, et al. Expansion of the time window for treatment of acute ischemic stroke with intravenous tissue plasminogen activator: a science advisory from the American Heart Association/American Stroke Association. *Stroke.* 2009;40(8):2945-2948.

4. Dichgans M. Genetics of ischemic stroke. *Lancet Neurol.* 2007;6(2): 149-161.

5. Kubo M, Hata J, Ninomiya T, et al. A nonsynonymous SNP in PRKCH (protein kinase C eta) increases the risk of cerebral infarction. *Nature Genet.* 2007;39(2):212-217.

6. Hata J, Matsuda K, Ninomiya T, et al. Functional SNP in an Sp1-binding site of AGTRL1 gene is associated with susceptibility to brain infarction. *Hum Mol Genet*. 2007;16(6):630-639.

7. Gretarsdottir S, Thorleifsson G, Manolescu A, et al. Risk variants for atrial fibrillation on chromosome 4q25 associate with ischemic stroke. *Ann Neurol*. 2008;64(4):402-409.

8. Gudbjartsson DF, Holm H, Gretarsdottir S, et al. A sequence variant in ZFHX3 on 16q22 associates with atrial fibrillation and ischemic stroke. *Nat Genet*. 2009;41(8):876-878.

9. Ikram MA, Seshadri S, Bis JC, et al. Genomewide association studies of stroke. *N Eng J Med*. 2009;360(17):1718-1728.

10. Yamada Y, Fuku N, Tanaka M, et al. Identification of CELSR1 as a susceptibility gene for ischemic stroke in Japanese individuals by a genome-wide association study. *Atherosclerosis*. 2009;207(1):144-149.

# 18 Thrombophilia

Jody L. Kujovich

## KEY POINTS

- *Disease summary:*
  - The term thrombophilia refers to an inherited or acquired predisposition to thromboembolism.
  - Inherited thrombophilias include deficiencies of the three natural anticoagulant proteins antithrombin (AT), protein C (PC), and protein S (PS), and specific mutations in the genes for factor V (factor V Leiden) and prothrombin (prothrombin 20210G>A).
  - Inherited thrombophilias increase the risk for a first venous thromboembolism (VTE) 2- to 20-fold but are not major risk factors for arterial thromboembolism.
  - Although the risks vary, inherited thrombophilias are not strongly predictive of recurrent VTE after an initial episode.
  - The clinical expression of an inherited thrombophilia reflects a complex interplay between genetic and acquired risk factors.

- *Hereditary basis:*
  - Deficiencies of the three natural anticoagulant proteins AT, PC, and PS are typically inherited as autosomal dominant traits. However, rare homozygous or compound heterozygous patients have been reported and they have a much more severe phenotype.
  - Mutations in the factor V Leiden and prothrombin 20210G>A predispose to thrombophilia both in the heterozygous and homozygous states but the latter tends to confer higher risk (see later).

- *Differential diagnosis:*
  - The differential diagnosis of VTE includes multiple inherited and acquired thrombophilic disorders.
  - Because these disorders are clinically indistinguishable, laboratory testing is required for diagnosis in each case.
  - Acquired thrombophilias include antiphospholipid antibodies, high levels of several clotting factors (factors VIII, IX, XI), myeloproliferative disorders and paroxysmal nocturnal hemoglobinuria (PNH).
  - Homozygosity and compound heterozygosity for two common polymorphisms in the 5,10-methylenetetrahydofolate reductase (MTHFR) gene (C677T, A1298C) predispose to mild hyperhomocysteinemia. MTHFR polymorphisms do not increase the risk for VTE independent of homocysteine levels and genetic testing is not recommended.

## Diagnostic Criteria and Clinical Characteristics

***Diagnostic Criteria:*** At least one of the following (Fig. 18-1)

- Identification of factor V Leiden or prothrombin 20210G>A mutation
- Abnormal activated PC (APC) resistance assay confirmed by a genetic test for factor V Leiden
- Low AT activity
- Low PC activity
- Low free PS antigen (and/or PS activity)

The diagnosis of AT, PC, or PS deficiency also requires

- Exclusion of acquired causes of a deficiency
- Repeat testing on a separate sample to confirm a low protein level
- Demonstration of a deficiency in family members in difficult cases

Thrombophilia testing should include tests for inherited and acquired disorders (Table 18-1):

- APC resistance or DNA assay for factor V Leiden
- DNA assay for prothrombin 20210G>A
- AT activity
- PC activity
- Free PS antigen
- Immunoassays for anticardiolipin and beta-2-glycoprotein-1 antibodies
- Multiple coagulation tests for a lupus inhibitor.

Measurement of homocysteine is discouraged since lowering levels with vitamin supplements does not reduce thrombotic risk. Clotting factor levels (eg, factor VIII, factor IX) are not routinely included since the cutoff values for identifying high-risk individuals are not well defined.

The APC resistance assay is a partial thromboplastin time (PTT)-based screening test with almost 100% sensitivity and specificity for the factor V Leiden mutation. The DNA test is required to confirm a positive screening assay, and to distinguish heterozygotes and homozygotes. Molecular genetic tests for factor V Leiden and prothrombin 20210G>A are not affected by acute thrombosis, illness, or antithrombotic agents.

Functional assays of AT and PC activity detect both quantitative and qualitative defects. The PS activity assay is less reliable but is useful to confirm the diagnosis and detect rare qualitative defects Anticoagulant protein levels may be temporarily reduced by acute thrombosis, disseminated intravascular coagulation (DIC), surgery, liver disease, and nephrotic syndrome. Testing is optimally performed several months after an acute VTE episode when the patient is not on anticoagulation. Therapeutic dose heparin can reduce AT levels by up to 30%. Proteins C and S levels are lowered by vitamin K deficiency and warfarin therapy. PS levels fall during pregnancy, estrogen contraception, and acute or chronic inflammation. Testing should be delayed for at least 2 to 3 weeks after stopping warfarin, and several months after delivery or discontinuation of estrogen.

***Clinical Characteristics:*** The primary clinical manifestation of inherited thrombophilia is VTE (deep venous thrombosis [DVT] and pulmonary embolism). DVT usually involves the legs but also occurs in upper extremities. Less commonly, thrombosis develops in unusual locations such as cerebral, hepatic, portal and renal veins.

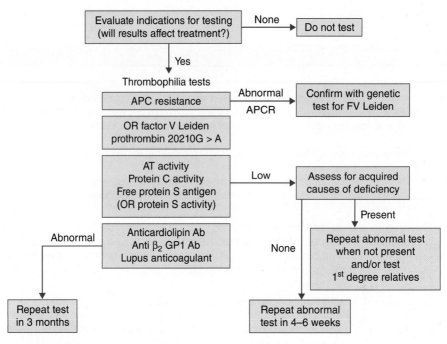

**Figure 18-1** Algorithm for diagnostic testing for thrombophilia.

Inherited thrombophilia may increase the risk of pregnancy loss and possibly other obstetric complications such as pre-eclampsia, fetal growth restriction, and placental abruption. Despite a modest increase in relative risk, the absolute risk of fetal loss is low and most thrombophilic women have normal pregnancies.

Inherited thrombophilias are not major risk factors for arterial thrombosis. The contribution of a single thrombophilic mutation to these complex diseases is likely to be small. Arterial thromboembolism may occur paradoxically through a patent foramen ovale in the heart of individuals with venous thrombosis.

☞**VTE RISK:** Inherited thrombophilias increase the relative risk for a first episode of VTE (Table 18-2). AT deficiency is the most clinically severe disorder, conferring a 10- to 20-fold increase in relative risk. PC and PS deficiency are associated with 5- to

10-fold increase in thrombotic risk. The relative risk for VTE is increased four to sevenfold and two to fourfold in factor V Leiden and prothrombin 20210G>A heterozygotes, respectively.

Approximately 30% of individuals with an incident VTE will develop recurrent thrombosis within the subsequent 8 years. The risk of recurrence depends on the type of initial event (spontaneous vs provoked by a transient risk factor) and other clinical factors. Heterozygosity for either factor V Leiden or prothrombin 20210G>A has at most a mild effect (odds ratio [OR] ~1.5) on recurrence after treatment of a first VTE. Deficiencies of AT, PC, or PS increase the risk of recurrence, particularly in members of thrombosis-prone families. Factor V Leiden and prothrombin 20210G>A homozygotes or double heterozygotes have a higher risk of recurrent VTE than those with a single heterozygous mutation.

**Table 18-1 *Genetic Differential Diagnosis***

| Diagnosis | Gene Symbol | Test Method | Mutation | Factors Affecting Testing |
|---|---|---|---|---|
| Factor V Leiden | F5 | Targeted mutation analysis | 1691G>A | Reliable during acute VTE, DIC, liver disease, warfarin, heparin |
| Prothrombin 20210G>A | F2 | Targeted mutation analysis | 20210G>A c.*97G>A | Reliable during acute VTE, DIC, liver disease, warfarin, heparin |
| Antithrombin deficiency | SERPINC1 | Antithrombin activity | >200 reported[a] | ↓ by acute VTE, heparin, DIC, liver disease |
| Protein C deficiency | PROC | Protein C activity | >160 reported[a] | ↓ by Vit K def., warfarin, acute VTE, DIC, liver disease |
| Protein S deficiency | PROS1 | Free protein S antigen (or protein S activity) | 300 reported[a] | ↓ by Vit K def., warfarin, acute VTE, DIC, liver disease, estrogen, pregnancy, inflammation |

[a]A list of laboratories offering sequence analysis of entire coding region is available at Gene Tests.

DIC, disseminated intravascular coagulation; VTE, venous thromboembolism; Vit, vitamin; def., deficiency.

Table 18-2 *Inherited Thrombophilia: Estimated Prevalence and Risk of VTE*[a]

| Thrombophilia | Prevalence: General Population (%) | Prevalence: Patients with VTE (%) | Relative Risk VTE (OR) | Annual Incidence VTE (%/year) |
|---|---|---|---|---|
| Antithrombin deficiency | 0.02-0.17 | 0.5-1 | 10-20 | 1.77 |
| Protein C deficiency | 0.14-0.50 | 3 | 7 | 1.52 |
| Protein S deficiency | 0.16-0.21 | 2 | 5-10 | 0.4-1.5 |
| FV Leiden[b] (heterozygous) | 5 | 15-20 | 4-7 | 0.49 |
| FV Leiden[b] (homozygous) | 0.065-0.2 | 0.01 | 18-80 | 1.30 |
| Prothrombin 20210 G>A[b] (heterozygous) | 2-3 | 6 | 2-4 | 0.34 |
| Prothrombin 20210 G>A[b] (homozygous) | 0.012-0.025 | 0.2 | NA | 1.10 |
| FV Leiden/prothrombin 20210 G>A (double heterozygotes) | 0.022-0.1 | 2-4.5 | 7-20 | 0.4-0.57 |

[a]VTE, venous thromboembolism; OR, odds ratio; NA, not available.
[b]Prevalences vary with the population studied.

## Screening and Counseling

*Screening:* Testing for thrombophilia is not routinely recommended for unselected patients with VTE. There is no evidence that testing reduces the risk for recurrent VTE or improves clinical outcomes in family members who undergo screening. Testing may be considered for individuals with the following:

- First unprovoked VTE at a young age
- Recurrent, especially unprovoked VTE
- VTE at an unusual site (eg, cerebral, mesenteric, portal veins)
- VTE during pregnancy or the puerperium
- VTE in a patient with a family history of recurrent VTE before age 50 years

The decision to test selected patients should be based on whether or not the results are likely to influence treatment. In the absence of evidence that early diagnosis of thrombophilia improves outcome, the decision to test asymptomatic at-risk family members should be made on an individual basis. Clarification of thrombophilia status may be useful in women considering hormonal contraception or pregnancy, and in families with a strong history of recurrent VTE at a young age.

*Counseling:* Hereditary thrombophilias are inherited in an autosomal dominant manner with incomplete penetrance. If one parent is heterozygous, each sibling is at 50% risk of being heterozygous for the mutation. If one parent is homozygous, each sibling has 100% chance of inheriting a heterozygous mutation. Although males and females are equally affected, women may have a greater risk of developing VTE at a young age because of exposures to estrogen and pregnancy.

Despite the increase in relative risk, the absolute risk of VTE is low in most asymptomatic individuals. The annual incidence of VTE in asymptomatic factor V Leiden or prothrombin 20210G>A heterozygotes ranges from 0.19% to 0.49% per year compared to 0.05% to 0.1% per year in relatives without thrombophilia. In the absence of a history of thrombosis, long-term anticoagulation is not recommended since the 3% per year risk of major bleeding

is greater than the less than 1% per year risk for thrombosis. The higher estimated absolute risks in asymptomatic individuals with AT, PC, or PS deficiency (1.0%-1.7% per year) and those homozygous for factor V Leiden or prothrombin 20210G>A (1.1%-1.3% per year) still do not exceed the major bleeding risk associated with long-term warfarin.

☞FAMILY HISTORY: For all inherited thrombophilias, the thrombotic risk is higher in individuals with a strong family history, particularly unprovoked VTE in multiple relatives at a young age. A positive family history increases the risk of VTE three- to four-fold among factor V Leiden and prothrombin 20210G>A heterozygotes. Additional coexisting thrombophilic mutations may explain the difference between symptomatic and asymptomatic families with a particular thrombophilia. For example, factor V Leiden was identified in 20% and 39% of thrombophilic families with deficiencies of PC and PS, respectively. Relatives with multiple thrombophilic disorders had a significantly higher incidence of VTE (72%) than those with PC deficiency (31%) or PS deficiency (19%) alone.

☞ENVIRONMENTAL FACTORS: The risk of VTE increases exponentially with advancing age. At least 50% of VTE events in individuals with inherited thrombophilia are provoked by one or more additional predisposing factors such as surgery, trauma, pregnancy, estrogen, malignancy, travel, immobility, and hospitalization.

☞GENOTYPE-PHENOTYPE CORRELATIONS: The clinical phenotype of inherited thrombophilia is highly variable, ranging from asymptomatic to recurrent severe VTE at an early age. The clinical presentation is influenced by the particular genotype, and coexisting genetic and environmental risk factors for VTE. Individuals with multiple thrombophilias have a higher risk of first and recurrent thrombosis, and tend to develop VTE at a younger age. Homozygous or compound heterozygous deficiencies of PC or PS are extremely rare and usually present at birth with massive VTE or neonatal purpura fulminans, characterized by widespread rapidly progressive hemorrhagic skin necrosis. Homozygous AT deficiency resulting in a complete protein deficiency is incompatible with life. Mutations which affect the heparin-binding site on the AT protein are less thrombophilic, and a small number of homozygous individuals with severe VTE have been reported. Individuals homozygous or compound heterozygous for factor V Leiden and prothrombin 20210G>A have a higher risk for thrombosis than heterozygotes for a single mutation. However, the clinical course of an acute thrombotic episode is not more severe or resistant to anticoagulation than in heterozygotes. The thrombotic risk in homozygotes is also substantially lower than the risk of homozygous PC or PS deficiency.

Pseudohomozygous factor V Leiden occurs in individuals who are doubly heterozygous for factor V Leiden and a factor V null mutation. Rather than attenuating the prothrombotic effect of a factor V allele, a coexisting factor V deficiency enhances it, resulting in an increased thrombotic risk and clinical phenotype similar to that of factor V Leiden homozygotes.

Because of the genetic diversity of mutations, the risk of VTE varies widely among individuals and families with an anticoagulant protein deficiency. PS mutations causing a severe quantitative protein deficiency confer a higher thrombotic risk than mutations resulting in a mild deficiency. Not all PS mutations are thrombophilic. The PS Heerlen (Ser460Pro) polymorphism results in a low free PS antigen, but no apparent increase in thrombotic risk. AT mutations affecting the thrombin-binding site are strongly prothrombotic with VTE occurring in 50% of affected individuals. Mutations affecting the heparin-binding site confer a much lower risk of VTE (<10% of heterozygotes).

## Management and Treatment

Prophylactic anticoagulation during high-risk circumstances may prevent some thrombotic episodes. However, consensus recommendations regarding prophylaxis are not based on thrombophilia status.

Initial management of VTE is the same as in individuals without thrombophilia. Acute VTE is treated with a course of low molecular weight or standard heparin or fondaparinux and initiation of warfarin. Resistance to heparin occurs rarely in patients with AT deficiency. Warfarin is started concurrently with heparin or fondaparinux and overlapped for at least 5 days and until the INR has been within the therapeutic range for at least 24 hours. High initial warfarin doses should be avoided, particularly in patients with PC and PS deficiency who have a higher risk of warfarin skin necrosis. There is no evidence that patients with inherited thrombophilia require a higher intensity of anticoagulation with heparin or warfarin.

Anticoagulation for at least 3 months is required after a provoked VTE associated with a reversible risk factor. Long-term anticoagulation is suggested for individuals with a first or recurrent unprovoked VTE, good anticoagulation monitoring, and a low bleeding risk. The presence of thrombophilia was not a major factor affecting consensus guidelines on duration of antithrombotic therapy, because these disorders are not strong determinants of recurrence risk. Identification of heterozygous factor V Leiden or prothrombin 20210G>A alone does not justify an extended duration of therapy. Patients with AT, PC, or PS deficiency may benefit from long-term anticoagulation, particularly those with a strong family history of VTE before age 50 years.

Dabigatran, a direct thrombin inhibitor and apixaban a direct anti-FXa inhibitor are approved for the prevention of stroke and thromboembolism in patients with atrial fibrillation. Rivaroxaban, an oral direct factor Xa inhibitor is approved for prevention of DVT in patients undergoing orthopedic surgery. It is also approved for the treatment of acute pulmonary embolism and long term prevention of recurrent VTE. The role of these new antithrombotic agents in the management of VTE is evolving.

Plasma-derived and recombinant AT products are approved for treatment and prophylaxis of VTE in hereditary AT deficiency. Accepted indications for AT replacement include refractory thrombosis, heparin resistance, and short-term thromboprophylaxis in high-risk circumstances when anticoagulation cannot be safely given, such as surgery and childbirth. A plasma-derived PC concentrate is approved for the treatment and prevention of VTE and purpura fulminans in patients with severe hereditary PC deficiency.

## Molecular Genetics and Molecular Mechanism

*Pathogenic Mechanisms and Molecular Basis:* AT, PC, and PS are natural anticoagulant proteins which regulate blood coagulation. AT inhibits thrombin and factor Xa and to a lesser extent, the other coagulation enzymes (factors IXa, XIa, XIIa, tissue plasminogen activator [tPA], and plasmin). The anticoagulant activity of AT is accelerated at least 1000-fold by binding to heparan sulfate on endothelial cells and all types of heparin.

More than 200 reported mutations in the *SERPINC1* gene encoding AT result in low plasma levels or functional defects. Mutations that affect the reactive (thrombin-binding) or heparin-binding sites on AT result in production of a dysfunctional protein.

PC is activated by thrombin bound to thrombomodulin on endothelial cells. APC cleaves and inactivates procoagulant factors Va and VIIIa, downregulating further thrombin generation. PS is a cofactor for APC and also has direct anticoagulant activity. At least 160 mutations in the PC gene (*PROC*) and nearly 300 mutations in the PS gene (*PROS1*) cause a quantitative deficiency or a dysfunctional protein.

Factor V Leiden refers to the specific point mutation (guanine to adenine substitution) at nucleotide 1691 in the factor V gene that results in an Arg506Gln substitution which eliminates one of the three APC cleavage sites. Because of this single amino acid change, factor Va is resistant to APC and is inactivated at a 10-fold slower rate than normal, which increases thrombin generation and the potential for thrombosis.

The 20210G>A mutation located in the 3' untranslated region of the prothrombin gene, increases the efficiency and accuracy of processing of the 3' end of the mRNA. The resulting accumulation of mRNA and increased prothrombin protein synthesis may enhance thrombin generation, promoting a prothrombotic state.

**BIBLIOGRAPHY:**

1. Recommendations from the EGAPP Working Group: routine testing for Factor V Leiden (R506Q) and prothrombin (20210G>A) mutations in adults with a history of idiopathic venous thromboembolism and their adult family members. *Genet Med.* 2011;13(1):67-76.

2. Lijfering WM, Brouwer JL, Veeger NJ, et al. Selective testing for thrombophilia in patients with first venous thrombosis: results from a retrospective family cohort study on absolute thrombotic risk for currently known thrombophilic defects in 2479 relatives. *Blood.* 2009;113(21):5314-5322.

3. Baglin T, Gray E, Greaves M, et al. Clinical guidelines for testing for heritable thrombophilia. *Br J Haematol.* 2010;149(2):209-220.

4. Marlar RA, Gausman JN. Protein S abnormalities: a diagnostic nightmare. *Am J Hematol.* 2011;86(5):418-421.

5. Segal JB, Brotman DJ, Necochea AJ, et al. Predictive value of factor V Leiden and prothrombin G20210A in adults with venous thromboembolism and in family members of those with a mutation: a systematic review. *JAMA.* 2009;301(23):2472-2485.

6. Mahmoodi BK, Brouwer JL, Ten Kate MK, et al. A prospective cohort study on the absolute risks of venous thromboembolism and predictive value of screening asymptomatic relatives of patients with hereditary deficiencies of protein S, protein C or antithrombin. *J Thromb Haemos.* 2010;8(6):1193-1200.

7. Zoller B, Berntsdotter A, Garcia de Frutos P, Dahlback B. Resistance to activated protein C as an additional genetic risk factor in hereditary deficiency of protein S. *Blood.* 1995;85(12):3518-3523.

8. Varga E, Kujovich J. Management of inherited thrombophilia: guide for genetics professionals. *Clin Genet.* Jan 2012;81(1):7-17.

9. Goldenberg NA, Manco-Johnson MJ. Protein C deficiency. *Haemophilia.* 2008;14(6):1214-1221.

10. Patnaik MM, Moll S. Inherited antithrombin deficiency: a review. *Haemophilia.* 2008;14(6):1229-1239.

11. Kujovich JL. Factor V Leiden thrombophilia. *Genet Med.* 2011;13(1):1-16.

12. Brouwer JL, Veeger NJ, van der Schaaf W, Kluin-Nelemans HC, van der Meer J. Difference in absolute risk of venous and arterial thrombosis between familial protein S deficiency type I and type III. Results from a family cohort study to assess the clinical impact of a laboratory test-based classification. *Br J Haematol.* 2005;128(5):703-710.

13. ten Kate MK, van der Meer J. Protein S deficiency: a clinical perspective. *Haemophilia.* 2008;14(6):1222-1228.

14. Guyatt GH, Akl EA, Crowther M, et al. Executive Summary: Antithrombotic therapy and prevention of thrombosis, 9th ed: American College of Chest Physicians Evidence-Based Clinical Practice Guidelines. *Chest.* 2012;141(2):7S-47S.

15. Dahlback B. Advances in understanding pathogenic mechanisms of thrombophilic disorders. *Blood.* 2008;112(1):19-27.

## Supplementary Information

**OMIM REFERENCES:**

[1] Thrombophilia due to Activated Protein C Resistance (OMIM #188055)

[2] Thrombophilia due to Protein C Deficiency (OMIM #612304 and #176860)

[3] Thrombophilia due to Protein S Deficiency (OMIM #612336 and #614514)

[4] Thrombophilia due to Antithrombin III Deficiency (OMIM #613118)

*Key Words:* Protein C, protein S, antithrombin III, factor V Leiden, prothrombin, anticoagulant, thrombosis

# 19 Pulmonary Embolism and Deep Vein Thrombosis

Fatima Donia Mili and W. Craig Hooper

## KEY POINTS

- *Disease summary:*
  - Pulmonary embolism (PE) and deep vein thrombosis (DVT) are a disease continuum of venous thromboembolism (VTE), a complex and serious multifactorial disorder of blood coagulation influenced by genetic and environmental risk factors, and their interactions.
  - Clinical presentations:
    - **DVT** is the formation of a thrombus in one of the deep veins, most commonly the lower extremities; occasionally, DVT can occur in the deep veins of the upper extremity, or in other locations.
    - **PE** is blockage in one or more pulmonary arteries occurring most commonly as a complication of DVT.
- *Differential diagnosis:*
  - **DVT**: cardiovascular disorders, septic arthritis, cellulitis, ruptured popliteal cyst, traumatic injury to a vein or artery
  - **PE:** any condition with clinical presentation characterized by chest pain, dyspnea, hemoptysis, or syncope
- *Monogenic forms:*
  - The well-established susceptibility genes for DVT/PE are factor V Leiden, factor II (or prothrombin), *SERPINC1* gene (in antithrombin deficiency), *PROC* gene (in protein C deficiency), *PROS1* gene (in protein S deficiency), A1 and B blood groups, and fibrinogen gamma gene.
- *Family history:*
  - Family history reflects inherited genetic susceptibilities, environmental, cultural, and behavioral factors in VTE. A positive family history is an independent risk factor for VTE, similarly among whites and African Americans, with an almost three times increased risk of VTE for both races. The risk of VTE is even higher among individuals who have a strong family history of VTE, that is, a first-degree relative with a history of VTE before the age of 50 years or a history of VTE among multiple relatives regardless of age. In addition, certain comorbid conditions, such as obesity, diabetes mellitus, hypertension, and cancer, could further increase the risk of VTE associated with a positive family history. Furthermore, there is evidence that only one-third of patients with a positive family history of VTE carry factor V Leiden variants among whites.
- *Twin studies:*
  - Among white monozygotic twins, the concordance rate with DVT or PE is 22% in males and 0.02% in females.
- *Environmental and clinical factors:*
  - Advanced age, race (whites and African Americans), previous episodes of VTE, prolonged immobilization, major trauma, spinal cord injury, burns, surgery, central venous catheterization, presence of a pacemaker
  - Female risk factors: pregnancy and postpartum period, estrogen-containing hormonal contraception, hormone replacement therapy
  - Obesity, diabetes mellitus
  - Cancer, myeloproliferative disorders, polycythemia vera, essential thrombocythemia, antiphospholipid syndrome, systemic lupus erythematosus, sickle cell disease
  - Endocrine disorders: thyroid dysfunction, Cushing syndrome, hyperprolactinemia
  - Major medical illness: nephrotic syndrome, inflammatory bowel disease, congestive heart failure, chronic obstructive pulmonary disease, paroxysmal nocturnal hemoglobinuria, disseminated intravascular coagulopathy
- *Pharmacogenomics:*
  - Although the US Food and Drug Administration (FDA) adapted guidelines for the clinical use of warfarin therapy when genotype information on cytochrome P450-2C9 complex (*CYP2C9*) and vitamin K-epoxide reductase complex subunit 1 (*VKORC1*) genes is available, the current recommendations for standard clinical practice do not include genetic testing.

## Diagnostic Criteria and Clinical Characteristics

PE and DVT are a disease continuum of VTE, a complex and serious multifactorial disorder of blood coagulation influenced by genetic and environmental risk factors, and their interactions. The updated paradigm for causal mechanisms of venous thrombosis is supported by the concept that inflammation and coagulation are interrelated, and incorporates the contributing factors of thrombosis initially postulated in the Virchow triad—abnormal blood flow, endothelial injury followed by accumulation of inflammatory markers, and increased hypercoagulability (also known as thrombophilia) characterized by activation of clotting factors. In 2008, the US Surgeon General called to action to prevent DVT and PE and urged all Americans to be aware of the risk factors, triggering events, and symptoms of DVT and PE, because these conditions represent a major public health problem associated with high morbidity and mortality rates, and substantial societal burden and economic costs. VTE is a common complication of hospitalization in medical and surgical patients. Guidelines for diagnosing VTE have been developed because of the lack of sensitivity and specificity of the clinical presentation of DVT and PE, and the low predictive value of their clinical symptoms, signs, and abnormalities of blood gases, chest radiograph, and electrocardiogram.

## Deep vein Thrombosis

*Diagnostic Criteria for DVT:*
* Pretest probability assessment of DVT using the Wells score.
* D-dimer test (measures plasma levels of a degradation product of cross-linked fibrin) or enzyme-linked immunosorbent assay (ELISA)-based D-dimer tests are used to rule out DVT.
* Venous compression ultrasonography is the imaging test of choice to diagnose DVT.

*Clinical Characteristics of DVT:* When DVT is symptomatic, the clinical presentation is nonspecific. Signs and symptoms include pain, tenderness along the distribution of the veins, edema, and erythema. DVT can be asymptomatic or recurrent, or result in emboli to the pulmonary arteries. Long-term complication of DVT is post-thrombotic syndrome (PTS), and even ulceration. DVT can be asymptomatic in almost 50% of the cases; 30% of patients with DVT will have a recurrent episode within the next 10 years. If DVT remains unrecognized and untreated, it could result in emboli to the pulmonary arteries and the development of PE, the most life-threatening complication of DVT. Much less commonly, DVT could result in phlegmasia alba dolens, a rare complication of DVT during pregnancy, or in phlegmasia cerulean dolens, a near-total venous occlusion caused by massive iliofemoral venous thrombosis.

## Pulmonary Embolism

*Diagnostic Criteria for PE:*
* Pretest probability assessment of PE using the Wells score or the revised Geneva score.
* D-dimer test or ELISA-based D-dimer test are used to rule out PE.
* Contrast-enhanced computed tomography (CT) arteriography and multi-detector computed tomography angiography (MDCTA) are considered the first-line imaging techniques to diagnose PE.

*Clinical Characteristics of PE:* PE is a life-threatening condition occurring most commonly (70%) as a complication of proximal vein thrombosis in approximately 50% of patients with documented proximal DVT. PE is characterized by an embolus which originates in the deep veins of the leg or pelvis, travels through the right side of the heart, and reaches the lung causing partial or complete blockage of the pulmonary arteries. PE is, however, most commonly asymptomatic, and its first diagnosis is often made until autopsy. Symptoms and signs of PE are nonspecific, and characterized by dyspnea, pleuritic chest pain, hemoptysis, and tachypnea. Chronic thromboembolic pulmonary hypertension is a long-term complication of PE resulting in chronic right heart failure. Severe cases with massive PE can lead to sudden death from right ventricular failure one in five individuals. It is estimated that about 30% of patients who develop clinically apparent PE die, although a large proportion of these patients die from other causes.

## Screening and Counseling

VTE is a complex trait with a multifactorial non-Mendelian mode of inheritance that involves multiple genes—thrombosis-susceptibility genes, environmental risk factors, as well as gene-gene and gene-environment interactions. Genetics factors are estimated to explain at least 60% of the heritability of VTE. Inherited thrombophilia is a genetic predisposition to venous thrombosis, and when associated with a DVT or PE event occurring in the absence of a known precipitating environmental factor, is referred to as idiopathic or unprovoked VTE. Inherited thrombophilia should be suspected when a patient has recurrent VTE, has a family history of relatives with DVT or PE, has an early-onset episode of VTE occurring before the age of 45 years, has DVT at an unusual site, or has no other obvious acquired risk factors, or if the patient is a woman who has a history of early pregnancy loss, late pregnancy loss, or severe pre-eclampsia.

*Screening:* The objective of screening for inherited thrombophilia is to identify individuals at risk for VTE. There is a strong evidence, however, that screening for thrombophilic disorders in the general population is not cost-effective because the incidence rate of symptomatic VTE in the general population is low, the clinical penetrance of symptomatic VTE among carriers of the most common thrombophilic conditions is incomplete, and there is no available long-term prophylactic therapy which is safe and cost-effective. Screening for primary prevention is recommended only for selected groups at high risk for VTE such as women considering oral contraceptives or hormone replacement therapy if they have a positive family history of VTE in a first-degree relative. Selective screening is also recommended, for example, during pregnancy or the puerperium for women with previous VTE history.

*Counseling:* The inheritance pattern of most inherited thrombophilic conditions is autosomal dominant. The clinical expression of thrombophilia is variable and influenced by the type of genetic factors, the number of risk alleles, and the interaction between genetic and environmental risk factors. In addition, family history of VTE is an independent risk factor for VTE. There is a significant genotype-phenotype correlation in VTE as suggested by the association between the severity of the disease and the type of thrombophilic mutations. Individuals referred for genetic counseling and their family members might be informed on advantages and disadvantages of genetic testing for thrombophilia, inheritance pattern of VTE, the risk of developing venous thrombosis, risk factors associated with VTE such as oral contraceptive use or obesity, and available prophylactic modalities for the prevention of VTE.

## Management and Treatment

The American College of Chest Physicians (ACCP), the American College of Physicians (ACP), and the American Academy of Family Physicians (AAFP) have recommended guidelines with the use of pharmacologic and nonpharmacologic interventions alone or in combination for the treatment of DVT or PE. Management of PE is also guided by the PE severity index (PESI), a scoring tool which stratifies patients with acute PE to predict both 30- and 90-day mortality.

**Anticoagulant therapy** is the treatment of choice for patients with proximal DVT or PE, and should be administered promptly in the absence of contraindications. The duration of the therapy depends on the procedure and the risk of the individual patient.

- **Heparin** exists in several forms, and is administrated immediately as the initial treatment of acute DVT and PE. Side effects of heparin include bleeding, heparin-induced thrombocytopenia (HIT), osteoporosis, and liver enzyme elevations.
  - **Unfractionated heparin (UFH)** is administered intravenously (IV) and requires laboratory monitoring with an activated partial thromboplastin time (aPTT) to maintain an effective therapeutic level and minimize the risk of excessive bleeding. Low-dose UFH (LDUFH) can be used in prevention of DVT.
  - **Low molecular weight heparin (LMWH)** (such as enoxaparin, dalteparin, tinzaparin) is safer than UFH. It is administered subcutaneously (SC) in a standard weight-based dose, and can be given on an outpatient basis. LMWH is the drug of choice in pregnant women with acute VTE because it does not cross the placenta.
- **Factor Xa inhibitors** is a new class of anticoagulant agents with anti-Xa activity and a more stable anticoagulant effect than heparin. *Fondaparinux* is administered parenterally (SC or IV) once daily. It received FDA approval and can be a good alternative to UFH or LMWH in the initial treatment or the prevention of DVT or PE. It has the advantage of fixed dosing and low risk of thrombocytopenia. Other compounds include *rivaroxaban*, *apixaban*, and *idraparinux*.
- **Vitamin K antagonists (VKAs):** Warfarin is a synthetic coumarin compound which inhibits the hepatic synthesis of vitamin K-dependent proteins. It is an equal mixture of two enantiomers, S-warfarin and R-warfarin, with S-warfarin having three to five times the potency of the R-isomer. Warfarin has anticoagulant and antithrombotic effects and is considered the prototype of VKAs. It is the most common oral anticoagulant for the primary and secondary prevention of VTE, and is indicated for long-term anticoagulation in all patients, except in pregnant women because it does cross the placenta and is teratogenic. Advantages of warfarin therapy are oral administration and low cost. Warfarin has, however, several disadvantages, including a slow onset of action, a narrow therapeutic index for both safety and effectiveness, and a large inter-patient variability in the dose-response relationship. Inter-patient variability response to warfarin is multifactorial, and is influenced by age, gender, genetic variations, body mass index (BMI), medications, as well as certain foods and dietary supplements. Frequent coagulation monitoring by international normalized ratio (INR) measurement and dosage adjustments are necessary to prevent severe bleeding events.

    **Thrombolytic therapy** includes fibrinolytic agents (such as streptokinase, urokinase, and recombinant tissue plasminogen activator [tPA]) that act by dissolving clots.

    **Surgical procedures** include thrombectomy and pulmonary embolectomy.

    **Mechanical interventions** are nonpharmacologic methods and include inferior vena cava filter (IVCF), intermittent pneumatic compression (IPC) devices, and elastic compression stockings.

*Prevention of VTE and Hospital-Acquired VTE:* VTE is a highly preventable disease. ACCP has recommended evidence-based guidelines for thromboprophylaxis to reduce the incidence of VTE. Prevention measures include pharmacologic interventions and are recommended for the following patients:

- **Nonorthopedic surgery or acute medical condition:** LMWH, low-dose heparin (LDH), or *fondaparinux* at least until discharge

- **Hip or knee arthroplasty or hip fracture surgery:** LMWH, *fondaparinux*, or warfarin for 10 to 35 days
- **Major trauma:** LMWH at least until discharge

    Despite widespread dissemination and implementation efforts of ACCP guidelines for the prevention of VTE among hospitalized patients, preventive methods are underutilized, particularly in patients with medical conditions. There is evidence that only 50% of inpatients with an acute medical illness receive VTE prophylaxis. When thromboprophylaxis is used, physicians' adherence to the guidelines is low. Barriers to adherence to guideline recommendations include a lack of familiarity with the guidelines, the perception that VTE is not a serious and potentially fatal disease, concern about risks of bleeding, and the perception that the guidelines are difficult to apply on a routine basis. A global initiative for the prevention of hospital-acquired VTE is currently underway, such as the recent validation of a VTE risk assessment and prevention protocol.

*Pharmacogenetics:* The goal of pharmacogenetics-based warfarin therapy is to improve the safety and the effectiveness of anticoagulation therapy. It is well established that genetic variability among patients plays an important role in determining the dose of warfarin and in minimizing the risk of over- or underdose during the induction phase. The primary genetic determinants that significantly influence the metabolism of warfarin are CYP2C9 and VKORC1 (Table 19-1). The CYP2C9 enzyme plays a role in the pharmacokinetics of warfarin and the metabolism of S-warfarin during warfarin induction. The *CYP2C9* gene has more than 30 known variant alleles. Patients who are homozygous for the reference allele *CYP2C9*1* metabolize warfarin normally. Patients with CYP2C9 polymorphisms have a reduced enzymatic activity and, consequently, a reduced warfarin metabolism. On the other hand, *VKORC1* plays a role in the pharmacodynamics of warfarin and correlates with its sensitivity. *VKORC1* encodes the vitamin K-epoxide reductase protein, the enzyme which catalyzes the conversion of vitamin K-epoxide to vitamin K. Warfarin inhibits epoxide reductase, leading to a reduced vitamin K and, consequently, to the decreased function of functionally active clotting factors. The frequencies of the *CYP2C9* and *VKORC1* variant alleles vary between racial and ethnic groups. Several other genes have a small but significant effect on warfarin dose requirements (Table 19-1): cytochrome P450 4F2 (CYP4F2) is a vitamin $K_1$ oxidase that catalyzes reduced vitamin K to hydroxyvitamin $K_1$ and removes vitamin K from the vitamin K cycle; the endothelium reticulum chaperone calumenin (CALU) and gamma-glutamyl carboxylase (GGCX) are implicated in the functional activation of clotting factors. Furthermore, although many genetic and nongenetic factors are implicated in the variation in warfarin dose requirements, there is evidence that variants of *CYP2C9* and *VKORC1* genes account for approximately 40% of individual warfarin dose variation. Numerous dosing algorithms for warfarin have been derived from multiple regression models to predict the stable therapeutic dose of warfarin. For example, the International Warfarin Pharmacogenetics Consortium (IWPC) has derived dosing algorithms using data from geographically diverse patients, and included clinical factors (warfarin indication, target INR, interacting drugs), demographic variables (age, race, weight, and height), and genetic variables (CYP2C9 and VKORC1 genotypes). IWPC concluded that incorporating genotype information improved clinical outcomes, especially for patients who required much higher or lower warfarin doses. Nevertheless, despite advances in pharmacogenetics-based warfarin therapy providing clinicians with a personalized approach

*Table 19-1 Pharmacogenetic Considerations in VTE*

| Gene | Associated Medications | Goal of Testing | Variants | Effect |
|------|------------------------|-----------------|----------|--------|
| CYP2C9 | Warfarin | Safety and effectiveness | *1 <br> *2, *3, *4, *5, *8, *11, *12, *13, *14, *16, *17, *18, *33 <br> *6, *15, *25 | Referent—normal dose <br> Variants—lower dose <br><br> Null genotype—life-threatening bleeding |
| VKORC1 1639 | Warfarin | Safety and effectiveness | G>A 3673 | Variant—lower dose |
| CYP4F2 | Warfarin | Safety and effectiveness | C>T | Variant—higher dose |
| CALU | Warfarin | Safety and effectiveness | A>G | Variant—higher dose |
| GGCX | Warfarin | Safety and effectiveness | C>G | Variant—lower dose |

to estimate the initial therapeutic dose of warfarin, and the availability of guidelines adapted from the FDA for the clinical use of warfarin therapy when genotype information is available (http://warfarindosing.org), there is currently no consensus for standard practice of genetic testing in clinical medical care. Indeed, genetic testing is not widely available, not cost-effective, DNA genotyping results require prolonged wait times, and the clinical benefits of genetic testing seem marginal compared with the standard of clinical care based on frequent INR monitoring.

## Molecular Genetics and Molecular Mechanism

Although the familial aggregation of VTE was recognized in the beginning of the 20th century, it was not until the late 1970s that the advances in the physiology of hemostatic and fibrinolytic systems were made and led to research on genetic defects associated with familial thrombosis. Genetic risk factors implicated in inherited thrombophilia and, therefore, in the pathogenesis of idiopathic VTE, play a role in the mechanisms leading to a hypercoagulable state due to a disrupted balance between procoagulant and anticoagulant determinants (Table 19-2).

From a historical perspective, in 1965, antithrombin deficiency was the first inherited thrombophilia to be reported and was identified in a Norwegian family with several members affected by venous thrombosis. Additional studies described similar phenotypes in families, providing further evidence that antithrombin deficiency is a risk factor for thrombosis. Antithrombin is one of the anticoagulant determinants responsible for the control of blood fluidity, and is a multifunctional serine protease inhibitor (serpin) that inactivates enzymes of the coagulation pathway, in particular thrombin and factor Xa, and less significantly factors IXa, XIa, XIIa. The molecular basis of antithrombin deficiency is characterized by a tremendous heterogeneity, with at least 220 mutations identified in the *SERPINC1* gene, the gene encoding for antithrombin. For example, most mutations altering the heparin-binding capacity of antithrombin are missense mutations, and frequently involve amino acid residues 41, 47, 99, and 129. Two decades after

the discovery of antithrombin deficiency, deficiencies of protein C and its cofactor protein S were identified as causes of inherited thrombophilia. Protein C and protein S deficiencies result in defects in the activated protein C anticoagulant system. Protein C is a vitamin K-dependent plasma glycoprotein that is cleaved to its activated form, activated protein C, and then acts as a serine protease to inactivate factors Va and VIIIa. *PROC* gene is the gene encoding for protein C. At least 270 mutations have been identified in the *PROC* gene, mainly missense, nonsense, and slicing mutations. Protein S is a potent anticoagulant protein that has a negative regulation effect on thrombin formation—it stimulates the proteolytic inactivation of factors Va and VIIIa by activated protein C. *PROS1* gene is the gene encoding for protein S. At least 220 mutations have been identified in the *PROS1* gene, commonly large deletions or duplications. Deficiencies in antithrombin, protein C, or protein S are rare and occur in only 5% to 20% of patients with idiopathic VTE. They are characterized by high penetrance of phenotype and a risk of recurrent VT and PE occurring at a young age. In addition, most of the cases of venous thrombosis associated with these deficiencies are heterozygous, while homozygous cases are rare and most frequently die in utero, or have neonatal purpura fulminans at birth. Few years after the association between antithrombin deficiency and VTE was established, ABO blood groups were reported to be involved in the risk of VTE. A1 and B blood groups are associated with higher risk of VTE than the OO-blood group, probably in part through mechanisms linked to higher plasma levels of von Willebrand and factor VIII factors. The A2 blood group (A2O1/A2O2/A2A2) is independently associated with lower risk of VTE.

In 1993, the most significant progress in understanding the genetics of hereditary thrombophilia was the discovery of resistance to the action of activated protein C which led to more advancement in research related to venous thrombosis. The phenotype of activated protein C resistance is the result of a gain-of-function point mutation in the coagulation factor V gene with the substitution of adenine for guanine at nucleotide position 1691, which causes the arginine in residue 506 to be replaced by glutamine in one of the protein's cleavage sites of the factor V protein (called factor V Leiden). This missense mutation converts factor Va to a molecule relatively resistant to cleavage, and consequently, to inactivation by activated protein C. Factor V Leiden is the most common genetic defect involved in the etiology of VTE. The second most common genetic cause of venous thrombosis is a mutation located in the prothrombin gene. A gain-of-function mutation with a guanine to adenine transition at nucleotide position 20210 in the 3' untranslated region of the prothrombin gene (also called prothrombin G20210A) is associated with increased levels of circulating prothrombin (or factor II). Plasma prothrombin is the precursor molecule of thrombin, a vitamin K-dependent protein which activates factors V and VIII and converts fibrinogen to fibrin. Although factor V Leiden and prothrombin G20210A mutations are common among whites, they are very rare among Africans, Asians, Native Americans, and Pacific Islanders. Furthermore, plasma fibrinogen has been recently reported to play a role in the risk of DVT among African Americans and whites. Fibrinogen (or factor I) is a glycoprotein containing three nonidentical chains (alpha, beta, and gamma). This clotting factor is the inactive precursor of fibrin, and is converted into fibrin through the action of thrombin and in the presence of calcium ions. Fibrinogen also acts as a cofactor in platelet aggregation. The mutation responsible for venous thrombosis is in the fibrinogen gamma gene (*FGG*) and involves a haplotype-tagging single-nucleotide polymorphism (SNP) characterized by a cytosine to thiamine substitution at nucleotide position 10034 (FGG 10034C>T). The mechanism implicated in the risk of DVT seems to be a reduction in the ratio of fibrinogen gamma' to total fibrinogen.

During the last decade, despite the large number of genome-wide association studies (GWAS) performed on venous thrombosis, progress in the understanding of the genetics of DVT and PE has been slow. Several new susceptibility loci for VTE with minor allele frequency (MAF) greater than 0.05 have been identified using GWAS methods, such as *GP6, F11, HIVEP1, C4BP4, TC2N,* and *STXBP5*. These loci, however, were associated with only a modest increased risk of VTE, with statistical significant odds ratios ranging from 1.1 to 1.35.

*Genetic Testing:* Although genetic testing for inherited thrombophilia is routinely available, its clinical utility has been estimated low. The Evaluation of Genomic Applications in Practice and Prevention (EGAPP) Working Group found convincing evidence to recommend against routine testing for factor V Leiden and prothrombin G20210A

*Table 19-2 Thrombophilia-Associated Susceptibility Variants*

| Candidate Gene (Chromosome Location) | Associated Variant [effect on protein] | Relative Risk | Frequency of Risk Allele (%) | Putative Functional Significance | Associated Disease Phenotype |
|---|---|---|---|---|---|
| *SERPINC1* (1q23-25) (heterozygote) | Multiple mutations [antithrombin deficiency] | 10-20 | 0.02%-0.17% | Inactivation of thrombin and factor Xa | DVT, PE |
| *PROC* (2q13-14) (heterozygote) | Multiple mutations [protein C deficiency] | 7-20 | 0.14%-0.50% | Defects in inactivation of factor Va and VIIIa | DVT, PE |
| *PROS1* (3q11.1) (heterozygote) | Multiple mutations [protein S deficiency] | 5-20 | 0.10%-1% | Defects in inactivation of factor Va and VIIIa | DVT, PE |
| Factor V (1q21) | *R506Q* (or *G1691A*) [substitution of arginine to glutamine at nucleotide 506] (rs6025) | Heterozygote: 3-10 | Heterozygote: 3%-5% whites, 2.2% Hispanics, 1.2% African Americans, 0.45% Asians, 1.25% Native Americans | Resistance of factor Va to inactivation by activated protein C | DVT |
| | | Homozygote: 9-80 | Homozygote: 0.004%-0.065% | | |
| Factor II (prothrombin) (11p11) | G20210A [guanine to adenine transition at nucleotide 20210] (rs1799963) | Heterozygote: 2-5 | Heterozygote: 1%-3% of whites, and 0.6% of African Americans | Defects in activation of factor V and VIII | DVT |
| | | Homozygote: NA | Homozygote: 0.001%-0.012% | | |
| A1 and B blood groups (9q34) | A1A1, A1A2, A1O1/ A1O2, BB/BO1/ BO2, A1B/A2B | 1.5-1.8 | 30% | Increased plasma levels of von Willebrand factor and factor VIII | DVT, PE |
| Fibrinogen gamma (4q31.3) | C10034T [substitution of cytosine to thiamin at nucleotide 10034] (rs2066865) | >2.0 among whites | 6% of whites, and >25% of African Americans | Reduction of plasma gamma' fibrinogen levels | DVT |

among adults with idiopathic VTE, as well as among asymptomatic adult family members of patients with VTE. These recommendations, however, do not apply to patients with other known risk factors, such as patients younger than 50 years with first unprovoked VTE, patients with recurrent VTE, patients with DVT at an unusual site, VTE during pregnancy or the puerperium, VTE associated with the use of oral contraceptive or hormone replacement therapy, patients with antiphospholipid syndrome, and patients with a family history of VTE in a first-degree relative younger than 50 years of age. Blood tests for thrombophilia include antithrombin, protein C and protein S functional assay, activated protein C resistance, factor V Leiden and prothrombin G20210A genotype, and fibrinogen tests.

*Future Directions:* New approaches in research are needed to identify additional genetic risk factors of VTE among different ethnic groups and explore new molecular and pathogenic mechanisms which will help better understand the incomplete penetrance and clinical heterogeneity of venous thrombosis, and predict VTE recurrence. For example, GWAS could be conducted using much larger sample size and novel analytic methods developed for rare variants with MAF less than or equal to 5. Current clinical trials that are evaluating new compounds might provide insight into anticoagulant therapy for VTE to potentially replace conventional anticoagulants such as heparin and VKAs. Basic research and drug development are needed to identify new drugs for VTE with low risk of bleeding. In addition, prospective studies would be helpful to define the role of thrombophilia testing in individuals with VTE.

### BIBLIOGRAPHY:

1. U.S. Department of Health and Human Services. The Surgeon General's call to action to prevent deep vein thrombosis and pulmonary embolism. 2008. http://www.surgeongeneral.gov/topics/deepvein. Accessed June, 2009.

2. Dahlbäck B. Advances in understanding pathogenic mechanisms of thrombophilic disorders. *Blood.* 2008;112:19-27.

3. Rosendaal FR, Reitsma PH. Genetics of venous thrombosis. *J Thromb Haemost.* 2009;7(suppl 1):301-304.

4. Gohil R, Peck G, Sharma P. The genetics of venous thromboembolism. *Thromb Haemost.* 2009;102:360-370.

5. Hooper WC. Venous thromboembolism in African Americans: a literature-based commentary. *Thromb Res.* 2010;125:12-18.

6. Varga EA, Kujovich JL. Management of inherited thrombophilia: guide for genetics professionals. *Clin Genet.* 2012;81:7-17.

7. Heit JA, Phelps MA, Ward SA, et al. Familial segregation of venous thromboembolism. *J Thromb Haemost.* 2004;2:731-736.

8. Mili FD, Hooper WC, Lally C, Austin H. The impact of co-morbid conditions on family history of venous thromboembolism in Whites and Blacks. *Thromb Res.* 2011;127:309-316.

9. Larsen TB, Sorensen HT, Skytthe A, et al. Major genetic susceptibility for venous thromboembolism in men: a study of Danish twins. *Epidemiology.* 2003;14:328-332.

10. Johnson JA, Gong L, Whirl-Carillo M, et al. Clinical pharmacogenetics implementation consortium guidelines for *CYP2C9* and *VKORC1* genotypes and warfarin dosing. *Clin Pharmacol Ther.* 2011;90:625-629. Online supplement available from www.pharmgkb.org.

11. Maynard G, Stein J. Preventing hospital-acquired venous thromboembolism: a guide for effective quality improvement. Prepared by the Society of Hospital Medicine. AHRQ publication no. 08-0075. Agency for Healthcare Research and Quality. 2009.

12. Recommendations from the EGAPP Working Group: routine testing for factor V Leiden (R506Q) and prothrombin (20210G>A) mutation in adults with a history of idiopathic venous thromboembolism and their adult family members. *Genetics Med.* 2011;13:67-76.

## Supplementary Information

**OMIM REFERENCES:**

[1] Hereditary Thrombophilia or Resistance to Activated Protein C; Factor V Leiden (#612309)

[2] Prothrombin Thrombophilia; Prothrombin 20210G-A (#176930)

[3] Antithrombin Deficiency; SERPINC1 (#613118)

[4] Protein C Deficiency; PROC (#176860)

[5] Protein S Deficiency; PROS1 (#176880)

[6] Dysfibrinogenemic Thrombophilia; FGG (#134850)

**Alternative Names:**
- Deep Venous Thrombosis
- Economy Class Syndrome
- Prothrombotic State

*Key Words:* Anticoagulant, deep vein thrombosis, family history, genetics, hypercoagulability, prophylaxis, pulmonary embolism, risk factors, thrombophilia

# 20 Arrhythmogenic Right Ventricular Cardiomyopathy

Carl Barnes and Matthew RG Taylor

## KEY POINTS

- *Disease summary:*
  - Arrhythmogenic right ventricular cardiomyopathy (ARVC), formerly referred to as arrhythmogenic right ventricular dysplasia (ARVD), is a heart muscle disease predominantly affecting the right ventricle.
  - Pathologically, the central feature is a progressive replacement of right ventricular myocardium with fibrofatty tissue.
  - Clinically, affected individuals present with palpitations, syncope, or sudden death as a result of ventricular arrhythmias, such as ventricular tachycardia or fibrillation, with symptomatic heart failure usually only in later stages.
  - While the majority of patients do not present with sudden cardiac death, ARVC may account for 10% to 20% of sudden cardiac death in individuals younger than age 35.
  - The prevalence of ARVC is estimated to be 1 case per 1000 to 5000 of the general population.

- *Hereditary basis:*
  - ARVC is familial in 30% to 50% of cases with onset usually in the second to fifth decades of life with males being three times more likely than females to manifest the phenotype.
  - The disease most commonly exhibits an autosomal dominant pattern of inheritance with reduced penetrance; however, rare autosomal recessive forms have also been described.
  - ARVC is a genetically heterogeneous condition with eight genes and four additional genetic loci have been identified thus far. A large proportion of known mutations occur in genes encoding structural proteins of the desmosome.

- *Differential diagnosis:*
  - When arrhythmias or sudden death are present, other inherited cardiac rhythm disorders should be considered including catecholaminergic polymorphic ventricular tachycardia, hereditary idiopathic ventricular tachycardia, Brugada syndrome, long QT syndrome, and short QT syndrome (Table 20-1).
  - When heart failure is present, other inherited cardiomyopathies should be considered including: dilated cardiomyopathy, hypertrophic cardiomyopathy, and left ventricular noncompaction.
  - A major nongenetic diagnosis to consider is idiopathic right ventricular outflow tract tachycardia, which can also cause the ventricular tachycardia with left bundle branch pattern seen in ARVC.
  - Naxos syndrome, a rare autosomal recessive condition includes palmoplantar keratosis and wooly hair in addition to ARVC.

## Diagnostic Criteria and Clinical Characteristics

The diagnosis of ARVC is based on 1994 guidelines from an international ARVC task force and are based on the presence or absence of major and minor criteria (Table 20-2)

The diagnosis of ARVC in individuals is made when the following are present:

- Two major criteria, or
- One major criteria plus two minor criteria, or
- Four minor criteria from different categories or systems

Some have argued that the above criteria may be too rigid for the evaluation of first-degree relatives in a family where ARVC has been confirmed. Under a modification proposed to the Task Force criteria, the diagnosis of ARVC is considered highly probable in a first-degree relative older than 14 years if any one minor criteria is present in the following categories: cardiac dysfunction, cardiac conduction or depolarization, cardiac repolarization, arrhythmias.

*Clinical Characteristics:* Individuals with ARVC will typically develop symptoms in the second to fifth decade, with males more likely than females to manifest the ARVC phenotype. Symptomatic presentation is fairly evenly split between palpitation, syncope, and sudden death. Abnormal electrocardiograms are present in up to 85% of cases and will often represent the first objective diagnostic abnormality that will then prompt additional testing.

Since sudden death is common and can occur without a diagnosis being made (if an autopsy is not done or the heart is incompletely evaluated) a careful family history is indicated in any young individual presenting with palpitations or syncope. Vigorous exercise can bring out dangerous arrhythmias and appears to be a risk factor for sudden death.

## Screening and Counseling

*Screening:* The assessment of individuals suspected of having ARVC should typically include

- Medical history
- Family history
- Physical examination
- Chest x-ray
- Electrocardiogram
- 24-hour ambulatory electrocardiogram
- Signal-averaged electrocardiogram (SAECG)
- Stress testing
- Two-dimensional echocardiography and/or cardiac magnetic resonance imaging (MRI) (echocardiography is typically the first-line imaging modality)

*Table 20-1  System Involvement*

| System | Manifestation | Comments |
|---|---|---|
| Cardiac (arrhythmia) | • Ventricular tachycardia with left bundle branch pattern, ventricular fibrillation; may be precipitated by vigorous exercise | • Median age of presentation is 26 years<br>• Electrocardiogram abnormalities present in up to 85% of patients<br>• Approximately 25% of patients present with palpitations<br>• Approximately 25% of patients present with syncope |
| Cardiac (heart failure) | • Right ventricular heart failure; some patients will develop left ventricular or biventricular heart failure | • Right ventricular wall motion abnormalities present in approximately 70% of patients |
| Sudden death | • May be brought on by vigorous exercise in competitive athletes | • Approximately 25% of patients present with sudden cardiac death |
| Dermatologic | • Palmoplantar keratosis and wooly hair in Naxos syndrome | • Minority of cases<br>• Autosomal recessive |

In selected cases, invasive studies including right ventricular angiography and endomyocardial biopsy should be considered.

Genetic testing is increasingly available. When genetic testing has identified an ARVC mutation in a family, genetic testing of at-risk family members can be done to determine which at-risk relatives will need longitudinal screening for the development of ARVC. Interpretation of ARVC studies and genetic testing results may be optimal in a center experienced with the diagnosis and management of ARVC.

At-risk individuals should be monitored periodically, perhaps on an annual basis to determine if they develop signs of the ARVC phenotype.

**Counseling:** The typical inheritance pattern is autosomal dominant and at a minimum a three-generation pedigree should be obtained for each family.

Families should be counseled that penetrance is age dependent and that the typical onset of observable symptoms is between the second and fifth decade. Some individuals with ARVC gene

*Table 20-2  Diagnostic Criteria for ARVC*

| Category/System | Diagnostic Modality | Major Criteria | Minor Criteria |
|---|---|---|---|
| Cardiac dysfunction | ECG or cardiac MRI | • Severe dilatation and reduction of RV ejection fraction with no (or only mild) LV involvement<br>• Localized RV aneurysms (akinetic or dyskinetic areas with diastolic bulging)<br>• Severe segmental dilatation of the RV | • Mild global RV dilatation and/or reduced ejection fraction with normal LV<br>• Mild segmental dilatation of the RV<br>• Regional RV hypokinesia |
| Cardiac conduction or depolarization | ECG and SAECG | • Epsilon waves or localized prolongation (>110 ms) of the QRS complex in the right precordial leads (V1-V3) | • Late potentials on SAECG |
| Cardiac repolarization | ECG | • None | • Inverted T waves in V2-V3 in persons >12 years and in the absence of RBB |
| Arrhythmias | ECG and Holter monitoring | • None | • LBB-type ventricular tachycardia on ECG, Holter monitor, or ETT<br>• Frequent (>1000/24 h) extrasystoles |
| Histopathology | Endomyocardial biopsy and autopsy | • Fibrofatty replacement of myocardium | • None |
| Family history | Pedigree analysis | • Familial disease confirmed at autopsy or surgery | • Family history of premature sudden death (<35 years) due to suspected ARVC<br>• Family history (clinical diagnosis based on present criteria) |

MRI, magnetic resonance imaging; RV, right ventricle or right ventricular; LV, left ventricle or left ventricular; ECG, electrocardiogram; SAECG, signal-averaged ECG; LBB, left bundle branch; ETT, exercise treadmill test; ARVC, arrhythmogenic right ventricular cardiomyopathy.

mutations may never develop overt symptoms giving the appearance that the condition may skip a generation. Males are also more likely to develop the phenotype than females.

Given the incomplete sensitivity of medical history and of various diagnostic testing modalities, genetic testing may be considered in a known case of ARVC in a family to allow for identification of other mutation carriers within the family. Current genetic testing appears to have a sensitivity of 40% to 50% for detecting pathogenic mutations.

## Management and Treatment

Management of an individual with known ARVC involves serial cardiology care, treatment of arrhythmias and heart failure, and consideration for implantable defibrillators, which appear to be effective in significantly reducing the incidence of sudden cardiac death. In cases where heart failure is severe and progressive, cardiac transplantation may be indicated.

Clinical predictors of worse prognosis and sudden cardiac death include young age, poorly tolerated ventricular tachycardia, syncope, severe right ventricular dysfunction, left ventricular heart failure, prior cardiac arrest, participation in competitive athletics, and a family history of early sudden death.

At-risk individuals who are asymptomatic probably do not need prophylactic treatment but should be monitored with regular cardiac evaluations as outlined in the screening section. If competitive sports are being pursued it is important to determine that no abnormalities are present since sports activity may increase the risk of sudden death fivefold in persons with ARVC due to sympathetic stimulation and volume overload. Some have suggested that asymptomatic individuals with normal cardiac studies but possessing known ARVC mutations be advised to restrict or limit physical activity, especially if a family history of sudden cardiac death due to ARVC is present.

## Molecular Genetics and Molecular Mechanism

*Syndrome/Gene/Locus:* The majority of genes identified thus far encode structural proteins of the desmosome (*JUP, PKP2, DSP, DSG2, DSC2*), an intercellular junction found in myocardium and epidermis involved in cell-cell adhesion as well as intracellular signaling pathways. Current pathogenesis models implicate abnormal cell-cell biomechanics as being important in the development of the disease.

The other known genes include *RYR2*, the cardiac ryanodine receptor, important in regulating intracellular calcium homeostasis. Transforming growth factor beta-3 (TGF-B3) is a regulatory cytokine involved in differentiation and cell proliferation in a variety of tissues. Its exact role in ARVC is unknown. The mechanism by which transmembrane protein 43 (TMEM43) causes ARVC is also unknown but it has been postulated that it may play a role in the peroxisome proliferator-activated receptor (PPAR)-gamma pathway.

*Genetic Testing: Clinical availability of testing:* Molecular genetic testing is increasingly available for ARVC genes through clinical laboratories in the United States and Europe. The clinical sensitivity for this testing is estimated to be 30% to 50% based on the research literature. It is possible that these data are biased toward mutation detection rates in large families where the evidence for a

**Table 20-3 *Molecular Genetic Testing***

| Locus | Gene | Genetic Testing Available | Mutation Prevalence in ARVC Cases |
|---|---|---|---|
| ARVD1 | *TGFB3* | Yes | Rare |
| ARVD2 | *RYR2* | Yes | Rare |
| ARVD3 | Unknown | No | Unknown |
| ARVD4 | Unknown | No | Unknown |
| ARVD5 | *TMEM43* | Yes | Rare |
| ARVD6 | Unknown | No | Unknown |
| ARVD7 | Unknown | No | Unknown |
| ARVD8 | *DSP* | Yes | 10% |
| ARVD9 | *PKP2* | Yes | 25% |
| ARVD10 | *DSG2* | Yes | 10% |
| ARVD11 | *DSC2* | Yes | 3% |
| ARVD12 | *JUP* | Yes | Rare |
| Naxos | *JUP* | Yes | Most cases of Naxos |

genetic etiology is greater than in isolated cases of ARVC with no family history.

Recently a database of ARVC genetic variants was developed that catalogues the effects of reported genetic variants as pathogenic, unknown, or nonpathogenic. (www.arvcdatabase.info)

*Utility of testing:* Guidelines for the use of ARVC genetic testing (Table 20-3) in patients and at-risk family members have only recently been proposed. In families with known ARVC pathogenic mutations, at-risk family members can be tested to help guide presymptomatic screening for the ARVC phenotype.

**BIBLIOGRAPHY:**

1. Thiene G, Nava A, Corrado D, Rossi L, Pennelli N. Right ventricular cardiomyopathy and sudden death in young people. *N Engl J Med.* 1988;318(3):129-133.

2. Basso C, Corrado D, Marcus FI, Nava A, Thiene G. Arrhythmogenic right ventricular cardiomyopathy. *Lancet.* 2009;373(9671):1289-1300.

3. Corrado D, Basso C, Thiene G. Arrhythmogenic right ventricular cardiomyopathy: an update. *Heart.* 2009;95(9):766-773.

4. Tsatsopoulou AA, Protonotarios NI, McKenna WJ. Arrhythmogenic right ventricular dysplasia, a cell adhesion cardiomyopathy: insights into disease pathogenesis from preliminary genotype–phenotype assessment. *Heart.* 2006;92(12):1720-1723.

5. Dalal D, Nasir K, Bomma C, et al. Arrhythmogenic right ventricular dysplasia: a United States experience. *Circulation.* 2005;112(25):3823-3832.

6. Nasir K, Bomma C, Tandri H, et al. Electrocardiographic features of arrhythmogenic right ventricular dysplasia/cardiomyopathy according to disease severity: a need to broaden diagnostic criteria. *Circulation.* 2004;110(12):1527-1534.

7. Lindstrom L, Wilkenshoff UM, Larsson H, Wranne B. Echocardiographic assessment of arrhythmogenic right ventricular cardiomyopathy. *Heart.* 2001;86(1):31-38.

8. McKenna, WJ, Thiene G, Nava A, et al. Diagnosis of arrhythmogenic right ventricular dysplasia/cardiomyopathy. Task Force of the Working Group Myocardial and Pericardial Disease of the European Society of Cardiology and of the Scientific Council on Cardiomyopathies of the International Society and Federation of Cardiology. *Br Heart J.* 1994;71(3):215-218.

9. Marcus FI, Zareba W, Calkins H, et al. Arrhythmogenic right ventricular cardiomyopathy/dysplasia clinical presentation and diagnostic evaluation: results from the North American Multidisciplinary Study. *Heart Rhythm.* 2009;6(7):984-992.

10. Hershberger RE, Lindenfeld J, Mestroni L, et al. Genetic evaluation of cardiomyopathy—a Heart Failure Society of America practice guideline. *J Card Fail.* 2009;15(2):83-97.

## Supplementary Information

**OMIM REFERENCE:**

[1] Arrhythmogenic Right Ventricular Cardiomyopathy (OMIM #107970)

| | |
|---|---|
| ARVD1 | (OMIM #107970) |
| ARVD2 | (OMIM #600996) |
| ARVD3 | (OMIM #602086) |
| ARVD4 | (OMIM #602087) |
| ARVD5 | (OMIM #604400) |
| ARVD6 | (OMIM #604401) |
| ARVD7 | (OMIM #609160) |
| ARVD8 | (OMIM #607450) |
| ARVD9 | (OMIM #609040) |
| ARVD10 | (OMIM #610193) |
| ARVD11 | (OMIM #610476) |
| ARVD12 | (OMIM #611528) |
| Naxos | (OMIM #601214) |

**Key Words:** Arrhythmogenic right ventricular cardiomyopathy or dysplasia, sudden cardiac death, arrhythmia

# 21 Atrial Fibrillation

Sunil Kapur and Calum A. MacRae

## KEY POINTS

- *Disease summary:*
  - Atrial fibrillation (AF) is the most common clinical arrhythmia (affecting ~10% of those in the seventh decade of life) and is a major cause of morbidity and mortality. AF is traditionally regarded as a sporadic, nongenetic disorder, but the ability to sustain the arrhythmia has long been known to require some underlying diathesis. There is growing evidence of an important heritable basis for many forms of AF, with the recent identification of several genetic determinants.
  - In AF the normal electrical impulses that are generated by sinoatrial node are replaced by waves of disorganized electrical activity that result from a combination of very rapidly firing triggers and abnormal conduction within local atrial re-entry circuits. This prevents co-ordinated contraction of the muscle which instead fibrillates in an uncontrolled manner (this leads to the arrhythmia's name). As a result the impulses reaching the ventricle to generate the hemodynamically important contracile activity are also highly irregular.
  - The arrhythmia involves the two upper chambers (right and left atria) of the heart, though in some instances the origins of the rapid electrical triggers may be in bands of cardiac muscle that envelop the ends of the pulmonary veins as they insert into the posterior aspect of the left atrium.
  - Clinical presentation: AF most often arises in the setting of other forms of heart disease, though there is evidence of shared mechanisms across these different contexts. AF may also arise in the absence of evidence of any associated cardiac disorder, so called lone AF. AF is often asymptomatic, but it may result in palpitations, dyspnea, chest tightness or pain, and even congestive heart failure (HF) in those predisposed. Individuals with AF have an increased risk of stroke both embolic and hemorrhagic. There may be typical precipitants for AF episodes including exercise or sleep.

- *Differential diagnosis:*
  - There are few other arrhythmias which exhibit the rapid irregular rhythm seen in AF. One arrhythmia that may be confused with AF is atrial flutter which results from a more organized macroreentry circuit, most commonly in the right atrium. As a result of the anatomic nature of the flutter circuit the atrial electrical activity is much more regular in nature, and AF can be distinguished from atrial flutter as the latter exhibits characteristic saw-toothed flutter waves of constant amplitude and frequency on a standard electrocardiogram. Importantly, there is no evidence of organized atrial activity on the electrocardiogram in AF, but both rhythms may result in irregular ventricular rhythm because of the nature of conduction between the atrium and the ventricle.

- *Monogenic forms:*
  - There are several genetic loci that have been reported in large kindreds with Mendelian AF (Table 21-1).

- *Family history:*
  - Estimates of the sibling recurrence risks range from 1.5- to 70-fold depending on the population that has been studied and the intensity of ascertainment. In a chart review of more than 2000 patients referred to arrhythmia specialists for managment of AF, investigators at the Mayo Clinic found that 5% had a family history of AF. This number was as high as 15% among patients with lone AF. Nearly 40% of individuals with lone AF referred to an electrophysiologist had at least one relative with the arrhythmia, and a substantial number reported having multiple relatives with AF.

- *Twin studies:*
  - In a representative study, concordance rates were twice as high for monozygotic pairs than for dizygotic pairs regardless of gender, 22.0% versus 11.6% ($p < .0001$). Estimates of the heritability of AF are approximately 62% (55%-68%) under an additive model.

- *Environmental factors:*
  - Numerous environmental factors have been associated with AF. The most obvious such factors include a wide range of acquired cardiac disorders: hypertension, coronary artery disease, some forms of valvular heart disease, congestive HF, and prior cardiac surgery. In some of these there may be shared heritable contributions to both AF and the underlying condition. AF is also associated with other acquired disorders including a number of pulmonary diseases such as pneumonia, lung cancer and pulmonary embolism, thyroid disorders, and systemic inflammation or infection. Other well-substantiated stimuli for AF are obesity, diabetes, and excessive alcohol consumption.

- *Genome-wide associations:*
  - Multiple associations exist including a major locus on 4q25 that exhibits one of the largest effect sizes observed in genetic association studies to date. Interestingly, this locus is also associated with atrial flutter.

- *Pharmacogenomics:*
  - There are currently no specific pharmacogenetic management strategies for AF, however, there is an emerging literature on the pharmacogenetics of warfarin use (see Chap. 6).

*Table 21-1 Mendelian Loci Associated With AF*

| Locus | Causative Gene | Associated Phenotypes |
| --- | --- | --- |
| 1p35-36 | NPPA | Elevated NPPA concentrations |
| 3p22.2 | SCN5A | Dilated cardiomyopathy |
| 4q25-26 | ANKB | Long QT syndrome, sudden death |
| 5p13 | NUP155 | Sudden death, fetal ventricular tachyarrhythmia, prolonged P-wave duration |
| 6q14-16 | Unknown | |
| 10q22-24 | Unknown | Mild cardiomyopathy |
| 11p15.5 | KCNQ1 | Prolonged QT interval |
| 17q23-24 | KCNJ2 | |

# Diagnostic Criteria and Clinical Characteristics

*Diagnostic Criteria for Atrial Fibrillation:* The fundamental diagnostic criteria for AF are

- Absence of an organized atrial rhythm
- Irregular conduction of electrical impulses to the ventricle

Diagnostic evaluation should include

- History and physical examination
  - Characterization of the presence and extent of symptoms
  - Definition of the type of AF (newly diagnosed, paroxysmal, persistent, or permanent); see Table 21-1
  - Possible precipitating factors including exercise, sleep apnoea, alcohol, or other known environmental contributors
  - Response to pharmacologic agents (if any)
  - History of underlying heart disease or precipitating factors for AF (eg, hyperthyroidism, alcohol)
- Electrocardiography to define other cardiac conditions. Importantly, ventricular pre-excitation should be excluded as this impacts therapy directly. In addition, in paroxysmal cases Holter monitoring may allow the burden of AF to be assessed independently from any symptoms.
- Transthoracic echocardiogram to assess for structural heart disease, to define cardiac chamber sizes, and to exclude pericardial disease or other rare contributors such as cardiac tumors.
- Chest radiograph to evaluate lung parenchyma and pulmonary vasculature.
- Laboratory evaluation should include baseline assessment of thyroid, renal and hepatic function, as well as markers of any clinically suspected contributing conditions. In addition, it is important to define baseline coagulation parameters.

*Clinical Characteristics:* AF often presents with isolated self-terminating episodes in its earliest stages, but these transient manifestations are themselves evidence of an underlying diathesis, in particular if they occur in the absence of any other cardiac disease. The natural history of such paroxysmal AF is that the episodes will tend to become more frequent and prolonged, often

requiring intervention in the form of direct current cardioversion to revert to sinus rhythm. Where AF is associated with other cardiac or medical problems, the natural history parallels that of the underlying disorder. Ultimately, a substantial proportion of those with AF will develop persistent or permanent AF. While this is typically in old age, in those where the inherited contribution is greatest permanent AF may supervene earlier in life.

Many different triggers are recognized by patients and their physicians including exercise, alcohol, sleep, or fevers. While these triggers may act in a very precise manner, such as onset of AF at a specific heart rate during exercise, they do not appear to discriminate distinctive natural histories. Different triggers will often segregate within the same extended kindreds with AF, where presumably the same primary underlying mechanism is shared. There is also considerable variation in the extent of symptoms in paroxysmal AF, which is associated with different success rates for management and may reflect intrinsic differences in the biology.

☞**HEART FAILURE RISK:** Even in lone AF, there may be the concurrent development of subtle evidence of a more generalized cardiac disease, as in many instances AF is an early symptom of a more generalized heart muscle disorder. Indeed, there is epidemiologic evidence that AF and HF are powerful risk factors for each other. In addition, HF, or any other acute change in hemodynamic loading conditions may also trigger episodes of AF through atrial stretch or other mechanisms.

☞**STROKE RISK:** AF is associated with an increased risk of both embolic and paradoxically hemorrhagic stroke. The mechanisms of thrombosis in AF are thought to be largely dependent on stasis, as a result of the incoordinate contraction and flow abnormalities in AF and any underlying structural heart disease. However, while the risk of stroke is generally related to the presence of structural heart disease, it may occur in individuals with lone AF. Together, these observations suggest that the endothelial or endocardial defects in AF are more complex than is currently understood.

## Screening and Counseling

*Screening:* No evidence exists at present for the screening of family members. There are no data to support screening at-risk family members even in kindreds in which multiple affected individuals have been identified. Screening may be feasible on the basis of nonparoxysmal components of the underlying heart disorders (ie, subtle structural cardiac defects), and it is important to remember that AF in one family member may be the first manifestation within a kindred of a more obvious form of heart muscle disease which independently may have more specific screening requirements.

In the setting of prior AF it is not uncommon to undertake Holter monitoring to detect potentially silent episodes of the arrhythmia. This may also be performed after a single episode when decisions are to be made regarding longer-term anticoagulation. There are few data on the sensitivity and specificity of such testing, which is largely driven by physician and patient preference. In individuals who present with conditions in which there is a high index of suspicion for AF, including embolic stroke, documented arterial embolism, or symptomatic palpitations suggestive of an irregular rhythm, electrocardiographic screening may be worthwhile, but here again data are limited. Biomarkers which identify the underlying diathesis toward AF would be extremely useful, and to date several sensitive biomarkers have been identified, but their specificity in family members is untested as a prospective tool.

*Counseling:* Familial aggregation of AF is common, in particular, in early onset lone AF cohorts that are enriched for inherited forms of the arrhythmia. Nevertheless, the majority of AF is not currently appreciated to have an inherited contribution. In addition, given the high population prevalence in older generations, phenocopies are likely to be encountered and counseling should only be undertaken after careful assessment of the entire extended kindred. Genetic results to date suggest that AF is highly heterogeneous with a wide range of cosegregating or acquired comorbidities such as HF, hypertension, or endocrine abnormalities. Therefore, generic counseling for individuals or families with AF patients is difficult.

## Management and Treatment

*Management:* The management of AF is focused on three broad areas: control of the ventricular rate, the maintenance of sinus rhythm, and anticoagulation.

**Rate control** has traditionally been the major focus of the acute management of AF. This should be undertaken after a careful analysis of the associated factors likely to be contributing to adrenergically mediated increases in the rate of atrioventricular (AV) conduction (eg, anxiety, fever, hypoxia, pain, pulmonary edema) as in most cases AV conduction is still physiologically regulated. In most cases the treatment of upstream drivers will lead to a rapid and significant reduction in the rate.

*Nodal agents* such as beta-blockers and calcium channel blockers are highly effective for graded control of the ventricular response, but in some individuals *class I or class III antiarrhythmic* agents may be necessary. *Digoxin*, which was classically used as an agent for rate control, is now used largely in conjunction with a beta-blocker or a calcium channel blocker to allow some residual rate response with exercise. In the setting of ventricular pre-excitation, pure nodal blockers should be avoided as they may increase the risk of 1:1 AV conduction and thus of malignant ventricular arrhythmia.

**Rhythm control** is often the preference of individual patients and physicians, especially if symptoms are disruptive. In randomized controlled trials the efficacy of most antiarrhythmic drugs for cardioversion is limited, though several class I agents have been used as a "pill in the pocket" solution for short-term outpatient management in low-risk subjects. In acutely unwell inpatients amiodarone is the drug of choice, though other drugs including procainamide, sotalol, and most recently ibutilide have been used.

For the maintenance of sinus rhythm, large drug trials are relatively sparse, but amiodarone and sotalol have both been successful in this context. Newer agents including dofetilide and dronedarone continue to be explored, but identifying those groups where the benefit outweighs the risks of these medications can be difficult.

The overall strategies of rate control versus rhythm control have been tested against each other and appear to be largely in equipoise with no objective effect of either strategy on mortality, cardiovascular end points, or quality of life. Rhythm control is associated with more drug side effects. However, some individuals are so symptomatic (often discordant with their objective hemodynamic findings) that they require an aggressive approach to rhythm control. Rate control is associated with trends to increases in hemodynamic tolerability, the relief of HF symptoms, and exercise tolerance.

*Pulmonary vein isolation* was developed as a therapy for AF when a subset of individuals were noted to have AF that appeared to be driven by rapid ectopic discharge of electrical foci in the pulmonary veins. Since these original observations, empiric electrical isolation of the pulmonary veins using percutaneous catheters has emerged as a common approach to rhythm control. Notably, there are small but significant short-term risks associated with these invasive procedures and long-term efficacy trials have not yet been completed to establish this as a primary strategy. The classic *surgical approach* to the treatment of AF is a "MAZE" operation that involves making several linear incisions to isolate the pulmonary veins and interrupt potential re-entry pathways that are thought to be required for the maintenance of AF.

**Anticoagulation** has been extensively studied in AF as the arrhythmia is such a significant risk factor for stroke and for other forms of thromboembolism. The rate of thromboembolic stroke is generally correlated with several key patient factors including age, gender, prior history of stroke or transient ischemic attack (TIA), and presence of other comorbidities such as valvular or myocardial disease. Patients with a stroke risk of less than 3% per year are considered low risk and benefit from aspirin therapy. The risks associated with warfarin, such as bleeding and inconvenience, outweigh the benefits in these low-risk patients, particularly in older age groups. High-risk individuals can be identified by a number of different scoring systems and there are extensive randomized controlled clinical trials that demonstrate net benefit for Coumadin in these populations. Clinicians may give individualized treatment to those who fall in intermediate-risk categories individually weighting bleeding risk and patient preference. The arrival of oral direct thrombin inhibitors promises to change this field dramatically, though to date data exist for the use of these agents only in those with nonvalvular AF.

**Pharmacogenetics** in modern AF management is mainly limited to the use of Coumadin where the narrow therapeutic index has long been a major problem, leading to excess bleeding or therapeutic failure in those patients with variable international normalized ratio (INR). Polymorphism in the cytochrome P4502C9 gene (*CYP2C9*) and the vitamin K epoxide reductase complex subunit 1 gene (*VKORC1*) has been demonstrated to influence the time to achieve steady state dose, the final dose, and subsequent variation in INR. However, there are also substantial environmental contributions to these parameters and the role of genetic testing for alleles at these loci or others in guiding anticoagulation management remains unproven.

## Molecular Genetics and Molecular Mechanism

The current mechanistic framework for AF is based on three overlapping concepts: increased automaticity in some cells, multiple re-entry circuits and fibrillatory conduction. It is thought that each of these contributes, to a varying degree, to the genesis and maintenance of AF in most individuals. However, in all animal models studied to date, AF will usually revert to normal sinus rhythm within hours of the removal of exogenous stimuli. These findings support a discrete diathesis in patients with AF, but the nature of this AF diathesis remains obscure.

The identification of genetic loci for Mendelian forms of AF has raised the possibility that the causal genes for AF may be accessible to positional cloning. The earliest descriptions of familial AF were followed by occasional examples of small monogenic kindreds until Brugada et al. described three extended families in which 10 of 26 at-risk individuals had AF. A genetic locus for the arrhythmia was identified on the long arm of chromosome 10. Subsequently, investigators have mapped and reported a locus on chromosome 6q 14-16 in a family with autosomal dominant lone AF. Interestingly, these genetic loci each overlap known dilated cardiomyopathy loci where the causal genes also remain uncloned. The identification of the causal mutations in these families will discern whether AF and cardiomyopathy result from different alleles in the same genes or from distinct genes.

AF, long QT syndrome, and dilated cardiomyopathy have now been observed to cosegregate in several kindreds. Several other loci for such atypical forms of AF have been identified and in some cases the responsible genes have been cloned (see Table 21-1 for complete list). In one example, investigators identified an activating mutation in the *KCNQ1* gene in a large Chinese family. This gene encodes the alpha subunit of the potassium channel responsible for the slow repolarizing current $I_{Ks}$ in myocytes. When *KCNE1* (the potassium channel beta subunit) was coexpressed in oocytes, the current density was noted to substantially increase and channel activation and deactivation were noted to be faster. Mutations in *KCNQ1* are typically associated with the long QT syndrome where the causal mutations have been thought to result in loss of channel function. The activation of conductance observed with the mutations identified in AF families would be predicted to render the atrial myocytes vulnerable to re-entry and result in AF through shortening the action potential and the effective refractory period. However, in these very families some of the affected members paradoxically exhibited prolonged QT. These findings suggest that the behavior of the mutant KCNQ1 protein is either context dependent with very distinct effects on atrial and ventricular physiology, or that our electrophysiologic understanding of the genesis of AF is incomplete. Similar activating mutations in the *KCNQ1* gene have now been observed in several families with AF and long QT. Finally, one must note that mutations in *KCNQ1* are only very rarely encountered in familial AF and have not been found on resequencing in large cohorts with lone AF.

Mutations in other genes encoding members of potassium channel complexes have been reported in the setting of familial AF, but the evidence supporting a causal role for these in AF is considerably less robust than for *KCNQ1*. Mutations of the *KCNE2* gene that code for the beta subunit responsible for the $I_{Kr}$ current were found in two Chinese probands with familial AF. In another distinct kindred with familial AF investigators reported a variant of the *KCJN2* gene that causes a gain of function at the potassium channel responsible for $I_{K1}$, the inwardly rectifying current in cardiac myocytes. Subsequent studies have demonstrated rare variants in potassium channel subunit genes in cohorts of individuals with AF, but rigorous genetic data supporting a causal role for these in AF does not exist and large-scale sequencing confirms that channel mutations are not a major cause of AF.

Two unique families with even more unusual features have contributed potentially tantalizing insights into the biology of AF. In one such family AF was associated with early childhood, sudden death, as well as cardiomyopathy, transmitted in a recessive manner. The gene was mapped to a single locus on chromosome 5p13 and homozygous mutations in *NUP155*, a gene encoding a member of the nuclear pore protein complex, were later identified to be responsible for the condition segregating within the family. The mutant protein appears to localize aberrantly and to reduce nuclear envelope permeability. Specific effects on both intranuclear import

of protein and extranuclear export of mRNA were observed, but their generalizability is unclear. How such a defect in a core cellular process leads to the cardiac specific phenotypes seen in this family remains obscure, but potential links with the atrial phenotypes seen in the Emery-Dreifuss muscular dystrophy syndromes caused by mutations in the nuclear laminar proteins emerin and lamin A/C deserve exploration. In a second unusual family with 11 clinical cases of AF, linkage analysis was again used to map an AF locus this time to chromosome 1p36-p35. In this instance, a novel heterozygous frameshift mutation in the natriuretic peptide precursor A gene, encoding the atrial natriuretic peptide (NPPA), was identified. High concentrations of NPPA secreted from the atrium were found circulating in the blood and are thought to result from a processing defect in the mutant isoform. This finding has uncovered a previously unforeseen link between alteration in a circulating hormone and the lowering of the arrhythmia threshold. Recent work suggests that there may be an effect of exogenous wild-type NPPA also appears to activate the $I_{Ks}$ potassium current, at least in vitro, which might link these apparently disparate mechanisms. This potential link between humoral signaling and atrial electrophysiology remains to be confirmed in vivo, and its broader relevance is unclear but implications are fascinating given the links between AF, HF, and obesity.

Finally somatic mutations in several cardiac connexin isoforms have been identified in the atria of individuals with AF. These results are intriguing, but the results are dependent on amplification methods that are difficult to completely control for and to date these findings are hypothesis generating.

Genome-wide association studies (GWAS) have identified multiple common variants that are associated with AF (Table 21-2). The largest effect size is associated with an area on chromosome 4q25 that is close to the gene encoding the paired-like homeodomain transcription factor 2 (*PITX2*). This gene appears to regulate pulmonary venous and atrial patterning, but it remains difficult to establish the chain of causality between the genetic variation and the AF phenotype. Other loci contain equally attractive candidates, but to date there are no mechanistic insights. It should also be noted that these common loci explain less than 10% of the inherited variance in cohorts where the inherited contribution has been rigorously estimated.

**Table 21-2 AF-Associated Susceptibility Variants (All Noncoding)**

| Locus | Associated Variant | Relative Risk | Possible Genes |
|---|---|---|---|
| 1p36 | rs17375901-T | 1.26 | *MTHFR, NPPA* |
| 1q21 | rs13376333-T | 1.52 | *KCNN3* |
| 1q24 | rs3903239-G | 1.14 | *PRRX1* |
| 4q25 | rs6843082-G | 2.03 | *PITX2* |
| 5q31 | rs2040862-G | 1.15 | *WNT8A* |
| 7q31 | rs3807989-A | 0.88 | *CAV1* |
| 9q22 | rs10821415-A | 1.13 | *C9ORF3* |
| 10q22 | rs10824026-G | 0.85 | *SYNPO2L* |
| 14q23 | rs1152591-A | 1.13 | *SYNE1* |
| 15q24 | rs7164883-G | 1.16 | *HCN4* |
| 16q22 | rs2106261-T | 1.25 | *ZFHX3* |
| 20q13 | rs13038095 | 1.47 | *SULF2-SRMP1* |

**Genetic Testing:** No role yet exists for genetic testing in the diagnosis or management of AF.

**Future Directions:** The identification of the major biologic pathways underlying AF, likely though the cloning of the major AF Mendelian genes, will accelerate the development of new tools to identify the clinical substrate for AF, as well as the mechanisms of the major associated disorders such as HF and stroke. Improved clinical phenotypes will also allow the identification of discrete subsets of AF and improve the resolution of genetic and clinical studies.

## BIBLIOGRAPHY:

1. Darbar D, Herron KJ, Ballew JD, et al. Familial atrial fibrillation is a genetically heterogeneous disorder. *J Am Coll Cardiol.* 2003;41(12):2185-2192.

2. Ellinor PT, Yoerger DM, Ruskin JN, MacRae CA. Familial aggregation in lone atrial fibrillation. *Hum Genet.* 2005;118(2):179-184.

3. Christophersen IE, Ravn LS, Budtz-Joergensen E, et al. Familial aggregation of atrial fibrillation: a study in Danish twins. *Circ Arrhythm Electrophysiol.* 2009;2(4):378-383. PMCID: 2760022.

4. Wolff L. Familial auricular fibrillation. *N Engl J Med.* 1943;229: 396-398.

5. Brugada R, Tapscott T, Czernuszewicz GZ, et al. Identification of a genetic locus for familial atrial fibrillation. *N Engl J Med.* 1997;336(13):905-911.

6. Ellinor PT, Shin JT, Moore RK, Yoerger DM, MacRae CA. Locus for atrial fibrillation maps to chromosome 6q14-16. *Circulation.* 2003;107(23):2880-2883.

7. Chen YH, Xu SJ, Bendahhou S, et al. KCNQ1 gain-of-function mutation in familial atrial fibrillation. *Science.* 2003;299(5604): 251-254.

8. Ellinor PT, Moore RK, Patton KK, Ruskin JN, Pollak MR, Macrae CA. Mutations in the long QT gene, KCNQ1, are an uncommon cause of atrial fibrillation. *Heart.* 2004;90(12):1487-1488.

9. Yang Y, Xia M, Jin Q, et al. Identification of a KCNE2 gain-of-function mutation in patients with familial atrial fibrillation. *Am J Hum Genet.* 2004;75(5):899-905.

10. Xia M, Jin Q, Bendahhou S, et al. A Kir2.1 gain-of-function mutation underlies familial atrial fibrillation. *Biochem Biophys Res Commun.* 2005;332(4):1012-1019.

11. Zhang C, Yuan GH, Cheng ZF, Xu MW, Hou LF, Wei FP. The single nucleotide polymorphisms of Kir3.4 gene and their correlation with lone paroxysmal atrial fibrillation in Chinese Han population. *Heart Lung Circ.* 2009;18(4):257-261.

## Supplementary Information

### OMIM REFERENCES:

[1] Atrial Fibrillation, Familial 1; ATFB1 (#060853)

[2] Atrial Fibrillation, Familial 2; ATFB2 (#608988)

[3] Atrial Fibrillation, Familial 3; ATFB3 (#607544)

[4] Atrial Fibrillation, Familial 4; ATFB4 (#611493)

[5] Atrial Fibrillation, Familial 5; ATFB5 (#611494)

[6] Atrial Fibrillation, Familial 6; ATFB6 (#612201)

[7] Atrial Fibrillation, Familial 7; ATFB7 (#613980)

[8] Atrial Fibrillation, Familial 8; ATFB8 (#613055)

[9] Atrial Fibrillation, Familial 9; ATFB9 (#613980)

[10] Atrial Fibrillation, Familial 10; ATFB10 (#614022)

[11] Atrial Fibrillation, Familial 11; ATFB11 (#614049)

[12] Atrial Fibrillation, Familial 12; ATFB12 (#614050)

[13] Sick Sinus Syndrome 1; SSS1 (#608567)

[14] Sick Sinus Syndrome 2; SSS2 (#163800)

### Alternative Names:

- Atrial Flutter
- Sinoatrial Disease
- Sick Sinus Syndrome

# 22 Brugada Syndrome and Related Cardiac Diseases

Ramon Brugada and Oscar Campuzano Larrea

## KEY POINTS

- *Disease summary:*
  - Brugada syndrome (BrS) was described in 1992. It is characterized by the presence of a typical electrocardiographic (ECG) pattern (right bundle branch block and persistent ST-segment elevation in right precordial leads) and it is associated with sudden cardiac death (SCD). To date, it is supposed to be responsible for 4% to 12% of total SCD cases, and 20% of SCD in patients with structurally normal hearts. The prevalence of the disease is difficult to estimate because the pattern is not always recognized or because it may transiently normalize. Nevertheless it is believed to be in the range of 1 to 5 in 10,000, being higher in Southeast Asia where the disease occurs endemically. The average age of diagnosis is usually around age 40, however, there has been description of affected individuals from age 1 to 84, and is more common in males than in females (8:1). BrS has also been described as responsible for sudden infant death syndrome (SIDS).

- *Hereditary basis:*
  - The BrS is a familial disease inherited with an autosomal dominant pattern of transmission and variable penetrance. In up to 60% of patients the disease can be sporadic, that is, absent in parents and other relatives. The BrS was classified as genetically determined with the identification in 1998 of the first mutations in *SCN5A*. Since then, more than 200 BrS-associated mutations have been described in *SCN5A*. Conversely, though, only 15% to 30% of patients with the clinical phenotype currently have a causative mutation identified at the *SCN5A* locus. Other 15 genes have been associated to BrS but with minor incidence: *GPD1L, SCN1B, SCN2B, SCN3B, RANGRF, SLMAP, KCNE3, KCNj8, HCN4, KCNE5, KCND3, CACNA1C, CACNB2, CACNA2D1,* and *TRPM4*.

- *Differential diagnosis:*
  - The ECG pattern is the *sine qua non* of BrS diagnosis. Of importance is the fact that the specific morphology of the precordial QRST pattern is critical for establishing the diagnosis of the syndrome. Only the type 1 ECG pattern—J-point elevation of greater than 2 mm with a coved (downward convex) ST segment—is diagnostic of BrS, with type 2 and type 3 "saddleback" patterns being less specific.

## Diagnostic Criteria and Clinical Characteristics

***Diagnostic Criteria:*** Sometimes, the diagnosis of BrS is difficult because of incomplete penetrance and dynamic ECG manifestations. Three repolarization patterns have been described: (a) type-1 ECG pattern, in which a coved ST-segment elevation greater than or equal to 2 mm is followed by a negative T wave, with little or no isoelectric separation, being this feature present in greater than one right precordial lead (from V1-V3); (b) type-2 ECG pattern, also characterized by a ST-segment elevation but followed by a positive or biphasic T wave that results in a saddle back configuration; (c) type-3 ECG pattern, a right precordial ST-segment elevation less than or equal to 1 mm either with a coved-type or a saddle-back morphology. Only the ECG type 1 would be considered as diagnostic of BrS. This ECG pattern type 1 may be spontaneously evident or it may be induced by a provocative drug challenge test using intravenous application of class 1A or 1C antiarrhythmic drugs (eg, ajmaline, flecainide), which block the cardiac sodium channel.

Cardiac events typically occur at rest, during sleep. The occurrence of arrhythmias during sleep may be due to an increased vagal activity and/or decreased sympathetic activity. This has been suggested in BrS patients by right precordial ST-segment elevation following intracoronary injection of acetylcholine, and decreased levels of norepinephrine in the synaptic cleft on positron emission tomography (PET). Some episodes of syncope or SCD may be triggered by hyperpyrexia, large meals (even leading to the suggestion of a full stomach test as a diagnostic test in the BrS), cocaine, and excessive alcohol consumption and sodium blockers. In some of these induced cases a genetic predisposition has been identified, indicating that some of these are acquired BrS, genetically predisposed.

Risk stratification in BrS is a matter of continuous controversy in these last years. In the medical and research community it is well accepted that symptoms (syncope or SCD) and male gender are associated with a higher risk or events. In these instances all agree that these patients should be protected with an implantable cardioverter-defibrillator (ICD). The controversy is most important in the approach to the asymptomatic patient, the individual who presents with a typical ECG pattern and who has no history of previous syncopal episodes. In this instance some experts will advocate for a close follow-up while others will propose the use of the electrophysiologic study as a risk stratifier to predict prognosis and to decide on the implantation of the ICD.

***Clinical Characteristics:*** Patients with BrS may remain asymptomatic although syncope or cardiac arrest has been described in 17% to 42% of diagnosed individuals. The age of symptom occurrence is consistently around the fourth decade of life in all the series (especially cardiac arrest), with no definite explanation for this observation thus far. Previous syncope may be present in up to 23% of patients who present with cardiac arrest. Up to 20% of patients with BrS may present supraventricular arrhythmias, and thus complain of palpitations and/or dizziness. An increased atrial vulnerability to both spontaneous and induced AF has been reported in patients with BrS. The electrophysiologic basis could be an abnormal atrial conduction. Whether atrial vulnerability is correlated to an increased susceptibility for ventricular arrhythmias is thus far unknown. Moreover, the typical ECG changes and arrhythmias in BrS may also be triggered by fever. Although the mechanism is not fully understood, some *SCN5A* mutations have been shown to alter the gating properties of cardiac sodium channels in a temperature-dependent manner, for example, more slow inactivation at higher temperatures. It has also been reported worst BrS ECG changes during exercise. This may be partially attributed to an enhanced slow inactivation in mutant channels, leading to an accumulation of the mutant channels in the slow inactivation state at fast heart rates. Other symptoms, such as neurally mediated syncope have been also recently associated to the BrS, but their implications for prognosis have not yet been established. As in the case of other Na⁺ channel–related disorders as type-3 long QT syndrome (LQTS), ventricular arrhythmias in the BrS typically occur at rest, especially during sleep, suggesting that vagal activity may play an important role in the arrhythmogenesis of BrS. In fact, published data on cardiac autonomic nervous system assessed by PET confirm that BrS patients display a certain degree of sympathetic autonomic dysfunction.

***Genotype-Phenotype Correlation:*** In a comparison between the ECG morphology of *SCN5A* mutation carriers versus patients where mutations in *SCN5A* had been excluded with the mutation-screening techniques currently available, it was described that *SCN5A* mutation carriers had significantly longer PQ intervals on the ECG and prolonged His-to-ventricle time during electrical programmed stimulation. Additionally, no significant differences have been described in QT time, QRS duration, and the magnitude of ST elevation. No significant difference with respect to prognosis has been published between *SCN5A*-positive BrS patients and non-*SCN5A* carriers. Among carriers of genetic mutations in *SCN5A*, patients and relatives with a mutation causing a truncated protein had a more severe phenotype and more severe conduction disorders than patients with missense mutations. In addition, identification of *SCN5A* mutations in combination with common variations can increase the risk of SCD.

## Management and Treatment

**Symptomatic patients:** There is no disagreement that patients with the typical ECG pattern who present with cardiac arrest or syncope of suspected cardiac origin should be protected with a defibrillator. Those patients who are highly symptomatic are recommended to be treated with quinidine to reduce the number of shocks.

    **Asymptomatic patients:** The controversy still remains as what to do with these patients. Some will advocate for follow-up until the patient develops a syncopal episode. It has to be though clear that not all patients will develop syncope as a first symptom and that this may actually be SCD. All symptomatic patients have been asymptomatic for several years, even decades prior to the first event. Other investigators will risk stratify these individuals according to the results of programmed electrical stimulation (PES). The use of PES is a matter of strong controversy. Several investigators will claim that it is of limited benefit in the identification of individuals at risk, while others will find it highly valuable, especially when inducing arrhythmias in a nonaggressive protocol.

## Molecular Genetics and Molecular Mechanism

***Molecular Mechanism:*** The right precordial ST-segment elevation is not well understood yet and the mechanisms for ST elevation in BrS are presumed to be multifactorial, including discrete

morphologic changes in the right ventricle of affected patients. There are two proposed mechanisms which may explain the ST-segment elevation in the right precordial leads in BrS: 1. The first hypothesis focuses on the presence of transmural voltage gradients due to heterogeneity in action potential duration between the right ventricular epicardium and endocardium. The cellular basis for this phenomenon is thought to be the result of a loss-of-function Na⁺ channel that differentially alters the activator protein (AP) morphology in epicardial versus endocardial cells. In fact, action potential durations are shorter in the epicardium, where the repolarizing transient outward potassium current ($I_{to}$) is more prominently expressed. This K⁺ current is quickly activated by membrane depolarization. It opposes and exceeds the depolarizing effect of the Na⁺ inward flux during the early phase of the AP plateau resulting in a pronounced AP notch and, in combination with depolarizing Ca²⁺ currents, in a "spike-and-dome" morphology. Consequently $I_{Na}$ reduction would further shorten epicardial action potential durations, and facilitate re-entrant excitation waves between depolarized endocardium and prematurely repolarized epicardium. In contrast, endocardial cells display a much smaller $I_{to}$ and consequently, Na⁺ current reduction would not affect significantly AP morphology and duration. The transmural in homogeneity of the cellular membrane voltage finally causes ST-segment elevation. 2. The second hypothesis involves preferential conduction slowing in the right ventricular outflow tract, leading to ST-segment elevation in right precordial leads. Regional differences in conduction velocity in the right ventricular epicardium would be aggravated by $I_{Na}$ reduction, and trigger the occurrence of epicardial re-entrant excitation waves.

***Genetic Testing:*** To date, 16 genes associated to BrS have been identified, however, most account for a small portion of the total cases. Given our limited knowledge on the genetic determinants of this syndrome, the management and risk stratification of BrS patients should be performed on a clinical basis. Nonetheless, genetic testing, when successful, allows confirmation of the diagnosis in borderline cases and identification of silent carriers. Nowadays, it is accepted that the etiology of the BrS is likely multifactorial, with genetic, environmental, and hormonal components contributing to its presentation and playing a role in the predisposition to arrhythmias and in the modulation of the phenotype. See Table 22-1.

## Molecular Genetic Testing

*SCN5A >300 pathogenic mutations*
*GPD1L <5 pathogenic mutations*
*SCN1B <5 pathogenic mutations*
*SCN2B <5 pathogenic mutations*
*SCN3B <5 pathogenic mutations*
*RANGRF <5 pathogenic mutations*
*SLMAP <5 pathogenic mutations*
*KCNE3 <5 pathogenic mutations*
*KCNj8 <5 pathogenic mutations*
*HCN4 <5 pathogenic mutations*
*KCNE5 <5 pathogenic mutations*
*KCND3 <5 pathogenic mutations*
*CACNA1C <10 pathogenic mutations*
*CACNB2B <10 pathogenic mutations*
*CACNA2D1 <5 pathogenic mutations*
*TRPM4 <10 pathogenic mutations*

**Table 22-1 Genes Associated With Brugada Syndrome**

| Channel | Function | Inheritance | Locus | Gene | Protein |
|---|---|---|---|---|---|
| Sodium | Loss | AD | 3p21-p24 | SCN5A | Nav1.5 |
| | Loss | AD | 3p22.3 | GPD1-L | glycerol-3-P-DH-1 |
| | Loss | AD | 19q13.1 | SCN1B | Navβ1 |
| | Loss | AD | 11q24.1 | SCN3B | Navβ3 |
| | Loss | AD | 11q23.3 | SCN2B | Navβ2 |
| | Loss | AD | 17p13.1 | RANGRF | RAN-G-release factor |
| | Loss | AD | 3p14.3 | SLMAP | sarcolemma associated protein |
| Potassium | Gain | AD | 11q13-q14 | KCNE3 | MiRP2 |
| | Gain | AD | 12p12.1 | KCNj8 | Kv6.1 Kir6.1 |
| | ? | AD | 15q24.1 | HCN4 | hyperpolarization cyclic nucleotide-gated 4 |
| | Gain | Sex-related | Xq22.3 | KCNE5 | potassium voltage-gated channel subfamily E member 1 like |
| | Gain | AD | 1p13.2 | KCND3 | Kv4.3 Kir4.3 |
| Calcium | Loss | AD | 2p13.3 | CACNA1C | Cav1.2 |
| | Loss | AD | 10p12.33 | CACNB2B | voltage-dependent β-2 |
| | ? | AD | 7q21-q22 | CACNA2D1 | voltage-dependent α2/δ1 |
| | Loss/Gain | AD | 19q13.33 | TRPM4 | transient receptor potential M4 |

AD, Autosomal Dominant

**BIBLIOGRAPHY:**

1. Brugada P, Brugada J. Right bundle branch block, persistent ST segment elevation and sudden cardiac death: a distinct clinical and electrocardiographic syndrome: a multicenter report. *J Am Coll Cardiol.* Nov 15 1992;20(6):1391-1396.

2. Brugada J, Brugada P. Further characterization of the syndrome of right bundle branch block, ST segment elevation, and sudden cardiac death. *J Cardiovasc Electrophysiol.* Mar 1997;8(3):325-331.

3. Brugada J, Brugada R, Brugada P. Right bundle-branch block and ST-segment elevation in leads V1 through V3: a marker for sudden death in patients without demonstrable structural heart disease. *Circulation.* Feb 10 1998;97(5):457-460.

4. Brugada R, Brugada J, Antzelevitch C, et al. Sodium channel blockers identify risk for sudden death in patients with ST-segment elevation and right bundle branch block but structurally normal hearts. *Circulation.* Feb 8 2000;101(5):510-515.

5. Chen Q, Kirsch GE, Zhang D, et al. Genetic basis and molecular mechanism for idiopathic ventricular fibrillation. *Nature.* Mar 19 1998;392(6673):293-296.

6. Yan GX, Antzelevitch C. Cellular basis for the Brugada syndrome and other mechanisms of arrhythmogenesis associated with ST-segment elevation. *Circulation.* Oct 12 1999;100(15):1660-1666.

7. Postema PG, Wolpert C, Amin AS, et al. Drugs and Brugada syndrome patients: review of the literature, recommendations, and an up-to-date website (www.brugadadrugs.org). *Heart Rhythm.* Sep 2009;6(9):1335-1341. Epub 2009 Jul 8 review.

8. Kapplinger JD, Tester DJ, Alders M, et al. An international compendium of mutations in the SCN5A-encoded cardiac sodium channel in patients referred for Brugada syndrome genetic testing. *Heart Rhythm.* Jan 2010;7(1):33-46.

9. Brugada J, Brugada R, Brugada P. Determinants of sudden cardiac death in individuals with the electrocardiographic pattern of Brugada syndrome and no previous cardiac arrest. *Circulation.* Dec 23 2003;108(25):3092-3096.

10. London B, Michalec M, Mehdi H, et al. Mutation in glycerol-3-phosphate dehydrogenase 1 like gene (GPD1-L) decreases cardiac Na+ current and causes inherited arrhythmias. *Circulation.* Nov 13 2007;116(20):2260-2268.

11. Brugada P, Brugada R, Brugada J. Should patients with an asymptomatic Brugada electrocardiogram undergo pharmacological and electrophysiological testing? *Circulation.* Jul 12 2005;112(2):279-292.

12. Watanabe H, Koopmann TT, Le Scouarnec S, et al. Sodium channel beta1 subunit mutations associated with Brugada syndrome and cardiac conduction disease in humans. *J Clin Invest.* Jun 2008;118(6):2260-2268.

13. Hu D, Barajas-Martinez H, Burashnikov E, et al. A mutation in the beta 3 subunit of the cardiac sodium channel associated with Brugada ECG phenotype. *Circ Cardiovasc Genet.* Jun 2009;2(3):270-278.

14. Cordeiro JM, Marieb M, Pfeiffer R, et al. Accelerated inactivation of the L-type calcium current due to a mutation in CACNB2b underlies Brugada syndrome. *J Mol Cell Cardiol.* May 2009;46(5):695-703.

15. Antzelevitch C, Pollevick GD, Cordeiro JM, et al. Loss-of-function mutations in the cardiac calcium channel underlie a new clinical entity characterized by ST-segment elevation, short QT intervals, and sudden cardiac death. *Circulation.* Jan 30 2007;115(4):442-449.

## Supplementary Information

**OMIM REFERENCES:**

[1] *SCN5A* OMIM: 600163

[2] *GPD1L* OMIM: 611778

[3] *SCN1B* OMIM: 612838

[4] *SCN2B* OMIM: 601327

[5] *SCN3B* OMIM: 608214

[6] *RANGRF* OMIM: 607954

[7] *SLMAP* OMIM: 602701

[8] *KCNE3* OMIM: 613119

[9] *KCNj8* OMIM: 600935

[10] *HCN4* OMIM: 613123

[11] *KCNE5* OMIM: 300328

[12] *KCND3* OMIM: 605411

[13] *CACNA1C* OMIM: 611875

[14] *CACNB2B* OMIM: 611876

[15] *CACNA2D1* OMIM: 114204

[16] *TRPM4* OMIM: 604559

***Key Words:*** Brugada syndrome, sudden cardiac death, channelopathy, arrhythmia

# 23 Long QT Syndrome

Shelly Weiss and Peter Hulick

## KEY POINTS

- *Disease summary:*
  - Inherited channelopathy characterized by elongated QT intervals on electrocardiogram (ECG), caused by delayed ventricular repolarization in the myocyte.
  - Increased propensity to syncope, polymorphous ventricular tachycardia (torsade de pointes), T-wave abnormalities, and sudden death. Unexplained seizures can also be an atypical presentation.
- *Family history (in addition to above characteristics):*
  - Sudden cardiac death
  - Sudden infant death syndrome
  - Congenital deafness
- *Hereditary basis:*
  - LQTS exhibits predominantly autosomal dominant inheritance, meaning there is a 50% chance of a child inheriting the disease causing mutation from a parent.
  - At least 12 genes have been implicated in LQTS, though the majority families have a mutation in *KCNQ1, KCNH2* and *SCN5A* which cause LQT1, LQT2, and LQT3, respectively.
  - There is variability of expression, even amongst family members with the same mutation.
- *Differential diagnosis:*
  - It is important to distinguish the hereditary forms of the syndrome from environmental (acquired) causes including QT interval prolonging therapies (ie, antiarrhythmic agents), myocardial ischemia, alternative cardiomyopathies, hypocalcemia and hypothyroidism.

## Diagnostic Criteria and Clinical Characteristics

### Diagnostic Criteria for Long QT Syndrome:

| EGC features | Points |
|---|---|
| QTc >450 ms (males), >470 ms (females)[a] | 3 |
| Torsade de pointes | 2 |
| T-wave alternans | 1 |
| Notched T wave in three leads | 1 |
| Decreased heart rate for age (below second percentile) | 0.5 |
| **Clinical history** | |
| Syncope | |
|   With stress | 2 |
|   Without stress | 1 |
| Congenital deafness | 0.5 |
| **Family history** | |
| Family members with definite LQTS | 1 |
|   Unexplained sudden cardiac death <30 years among immediate family members | 0.5 |

**And the absence of**
- Medications or disorders known to affect electrocardiographic findings

**Probability of LQTS**
| | |
|---|---|
| - Low | ≤1 |
| - Intermediate | 2-3 |
| - High | ≥4 |

[a]Calculated with Bazett's formula

### Allelic Differential Diagnosis:

- **Jervell and Lange-Nielsen syndrome (JNLS):** characterized by congenital sensorineural hearing loss and long QTc interval, inherited in an autosomal recessive manner (*KCNQ1* or *KCNE1*)
- **Brugada syndrome:** characterized by rapid polymorphic ventricular tachycardia or ventricular fibrillation and sudden death, inherited in an autosomal dominant manner (*SCN5A*).

### Differential Diagnosis:

- **Timothy syndrome (LQTS with syndactyly):** characterized by cardiac abnormalities (LQTS and/or structural defects), variable syndactyly of fingers or toes, facial anomalies and neurologic symptoms (autism, seizures, mental retardation), caused by de novo alterations in *CACNA1C*.
- **Andersen-Tawil syndrome (ATS):** characterized by muscle weakness, ventricular arrhythmias, prolonged QT interval, facial and limb anomalies, caused by alterations in *KCNJ2*.

## Screening and Counseling

**Screening:** The hallmark for screening patients for LQTS is the ECG by establishing evidence for QTc prolongation and examining the T-wave morphology (LQT1 broad T waves, LQT2 bifid T waves, LQT3 peaked and biphasic T waves). It is important to recognize that a normal ECG does not rule out the possibility of LQTS. If the clinical suspicion is strong, either because of a family history or consistent clinical symptoms, repeat ECG should be considered. Some individuals can have a normal resting ECG which makes identification of at-risk individuals challenging.

Normal QTc values vary with age and gender. For adult males, normal, borderline, and prolonged values are less than 430 ms, 430 to 450 ms, and greater than 450 ms, respectively, and for adult

**Table 23-1 Genetic Bases of Long QT Syndrome**

| Type | Gene | Trigger | Prevalence (%) |
|------|------|---------|----------------|
| LQT1 | KCNQ1 | Exercise, swimming, sudden emotion | 40-55 |
| LQT2 | KCNH2 | Sudden loud sound, sudden emotion | 35-45 |
| LQT3 | SCN5A | Sleep, rest, sudden emotion | 2-8 |
| LQT4 | ANK2 | Exercise | <1 |
| LQT5 | KCNE1 | Exercise, sudden emotion | <1 |
| LQT6 | KCNE2 | Rest, exercise | <1 |
| LQT7 | KCNJ2 | Syndromic, rest, exercise | <1 |
| LQT8 | CACNA1C | Syndromic | <1 |
| LQT9 | CAV3 | Rest, sleep | <1 |
| LQT10 | SCN4B | Exercise | <0.1 |
| LQT11 | AKAP9 | Exercise | <0.1 |
| LQT12 | SNTA1 | Rest | <0.1 |

females less than 450 ms, 450 to 470 ms, and greater than 470 ms. When the diagnosis is not clear based on ECG, the scoring system describe earlier, can be used to assess the likelihood of LQTS. Sometimes, QT prolongation can be identified with exercise or epinephrine challenges, particularly in LQT1 and LQT2. On occasion, prolongation is identified via Holter monitoring.

If a causative mutation has been identified in the family, genetic testing of family members can help screen for at-risk patients. It can be useful for uncovering concealed LQTS, that is, those who have normal QTc, however, testing cannot rule out LQTS due to the sensitivity of current clinical testing.

**Counseling:** LQT1-12 are inherited in an autosomal dominant manner, with variable expressivity. Each child of an affected individual has a 50% risk of inheriting the disease-causing mutation.

Predictive testing for at-risk family members can be performed through QTc analysis on resting and exercise, ECGs or specific mutation testing when the disease-causing mutation has been previously identified in the family. Molecular genetic testing for the family-specific mutation allows for early identification of at-risk family members, allowing the opportunity for appropriate screening and prophylactic treatment (ie, beta-blockers). Presymptomatic testing should be offered to all first-degree relatives of an affected individual. De novo mutations are relatively uncommon.

**Genotype-Phenotype Correlation:** The correlation between mutation type and location (specifically in LQT1-3) has been contributory to increased personalized risk assessment in LQT families (risk of cardiac event or sudden death, treatment response, physiologic triggers, and ECG analysis).

## Management and Treatment

**Management:**
- The mainstay of therapy in patients with LQTS remains beta-blockers, particularly in LQT1 and LQT2 patients. The role

of beta-blockers in LQT3 patients is more controversial. It is important to ensure adequate dosage, compliance, and avoidance of QT-prolonging drugs (www.qtdrugs.org).
- Implantable cardioverter-defibrillator (ICD) use is generally reserved for secondary prevention after a previous cardiac event or for primary prevention in individuals deemed high risk for an event and for those patients who continue to have symptoms despite adequate beta-blocker therapy.
- Minimally invasive video-assisted thoracic left cardiac sympathetic denervation (LCSD) procedures are under investigation and eventually may be a replacement for or serve as a bridge to ICD placement.

**Risk Assessment:**
- Five-year event risks (cardiac arrest or sudden cardiac death) are predominantly based on clinical parameters but genotype data is emerging that allows for a more personalized risk assessment. Gender and age are additional important parameters. Risk should be periodically revaluated as it is time dependent. When considering QTc values, the longest documented value has the best prognostic value, not necessarily the most recent QTc value.
  - Low risk = QTc ≤500 ms and nor prior syncope (0.5% 5-year risk)
  - Intermediate risk = QTc >500 ms or prior syncope (3% 5-year risk)
  - High risk = previous arrest history or spontaneous torsade de pointes (14% 5-year risk)
- Using genotype data for risk assessment that is reserved for LQT1, LQT2, and LQT3 where the data is more robust.
  - Cumulative survival rates are higher for LQT1 patients
  - Beta-blockers are most effective for LQT1 patients
  - In LQT1, a dominant negative conferred a twofold higher risk of cardiac events when compared to mutations causing haploinsufficiency of the proteinLQT3 generally confers a higher risk than LQT1 and LQT2 patients with similar QTc values

**Pharmacogenetics:** Targeted therapy is being explored based on genotype and the particular ion channel affected. For example, in LQT3 patients, the cardiac sodium channel is affected which results in a late inward sodium current thus prolonging repolarization. Medications that target the sodium channel (flecainide and mexiletine) and shorten this interval can normalize the QT. Whether shortening the QT with targeted pharmacologic agents based on genotype data offers a survival benefit remains to be determined.

**Genetic Testing:** DNA sequence analysis is clinically available for LQT1-12 (see Gene Tests http://www.genetests.org). Deletion or duplication studies are clinically available for approximately half of the associated loci, however, specific sensitivities are not known.

**Utility of testing:** A causative mutation can be detected in approximately 70% of high probability patients.

**BIBLIOGRAPHY:**

1. Goldenberg I, Moss, A. Long QT syndrome. *J Am Coll Cardiol.* 2008;51:2291-2300.
2. Goldenberg I, Moss AJ, Bradley J, et al. Long-QT syndrome after Age 40. *Circulation.* 2008;117:2192-2201.
3. Hedley PL, Jørgensen P, Schlamowitz S, et al. The genetic basis of long QT and short QT syndromes: a mutation update. *Hum Mutat.* 2009;30(11):1486-1511.
4. Roden DM. Long-QT syndrome. *N Engl J Med.* 2008;398(2): 169-176.

5.  Sauer BS, Moss AJ, McNitt S, et al. Long QT syndrome in adults. *J Am Coll of Cardiol.* 2007;49:329-337.

6.  Schwartz PJ, Moss AJ, Vincent GM, Crampton RS. Diagnostic criteria for the long QT syndrome: an update. *Circulation.* 1993;88:782-784.

7.  Vincent GM, Schwartz PJ, Denjoy I, et al. High efficacy of β-blockers in long-QT syndrome type 1; contribution of noncompliance and QT-prolonging drugs to the occurrence of β-blocker treatment "failures." *Circulation.* 2009;119:215-221.

## Supplementary Information

**OMIM** REFERENCES:

[1] Long QT Syndrome 1; KCNQ1 (#192500)

[2] Potassium Channel, Voltage-Gated, Subfamily H, Member 2; KCNH2 (+152427)

[3] Long QT Syndrome 3; SCN5A (#603830)

[4] Cardiac Arrhythmia, Ankyrin-B-Related; ANK2 (#600919)

[5] Potassium Channel, Voltage-Gated, ISK-Related Subfamily, Member 1; KCNE1 (+176261)

[6] Potassium Channel, Voltage-Gated, ISK-Related Subfamily, Member 2; KCNE2 (+603796)

[7] Potassium Channel, Inwardly Rectifying, Subfamily J, Member 2; KCNJ2 (*600681)

[8] Calcium Channel, Voltage-Dependent, L Type, Alpha-1C Subunit; CACNA1C (*114205)

[9] Long QT Syndrome 9; CAV3 (#611818)

[10] Long QT Syndrome 10; SCN4B (#611819)

[11] Long QT Syndrome 11; AKAP9 (#611820)

[12] Long QT Syndrome 12; SNTA1 (#612955)

*Key Words:* Prolonged QT interval, arrhythmia, syncope, sudden death

# 24 Dilated Cardiomyopathy

Solomon Sager, Jill S. Dolinsky, and Ray E. Hershberger

## KEY POINTS

- *Disease summary:*
  - Dilated cardiomyopathy (DCM) is characterized by left ventricular (LV) enlargement and systolic dysfunction.
  - The prevalence of DCM is 1 in 2700, however, this is undoubtedly an underestimate.
  - Histologic findings include myocyte hypertrophy, myocyte loss, and interstitial fibrosis.
  - Approximately 35% of DCM cases are deemed *idiopathic dilated cardiomyopathy (IDC)* after detectable causes have been excluded (Fig. 24-1).
  - 20% to 50% of IDC may be found in one or more family members, and if so, is termed *familial dilated cardiomyopathy (FDC)*. Of these cases, approximately 20% to 25% have identifiable genetic mutations correlating with disease phenotype.
- *Hereditary basis:*
  - A majority of heritable DCM is nonsyndromic disease isolated to the heart and can be divided into two subsets:
    - FDC, as defined above.
    - IDC with a known genetic mutation but no known familial penetrance. Because of the availability of genetic testing, some patients with IDC are sent for testing and have positive results.
  - Less commonly, heritable DCM can occur as part of a genetic syndrome; causes from autosomal and X-linked genes are shown (Table 24-1).
  - *Differential diagnosis:*
    - Differential includes all detectable causes of dilated cardiomyopathy: ischemic, congenital, primary valvular, toxin-induced, metabolic abnormalities, and infectious (Fig. 24-1).

## Diagnostic Criteria and Clinical Characteristics

### Diagnostic Criteria, DCM:
- Fractional shortening less than 25% (>2 SD) and/or ejection fraction less than 45% (>2 SD)
- LV enlargement

### Diagnostic Criteria Compatible With IDC:
- DCM with no evidence of a detectable cause (Fig. 24-1).

### Diagnostic Criteria, FDC:
- IDC occurring in at least two closely related family members.

### Clinical Characteristics:
- **Clinical presentation:** Patients usually present with advanced disease, including heart failure, arrhythmia, or stroke or other embolic phenomena from mural thrombus.
- **Asymptomatic disease:** It is occasionally diagnosed by serendipity with medical evaluation for other reasons; can be present by presymptomatic for years, emphasizing the importance of screening of family members.

## Screening and Counseling

### Screening:
☞**FAMILY HISTORY:** A careful family history of at least three generations should be obtained for all index patients with cardiomyopathy.

- **First goal:** Ascertain if cardiomyopathy is familial.
  - Due to reduced penetrance reported in some cases of FDC, a family history should extend to at least three generations to improve disease recognition.

- When the diagnosis of cardiomyopathy is suggested in a first-degree relative, the practitioner should request that the patient obtain additional information to confirm or exclude the diagnosis.
- **Second goal:** Ascertain inheritance pattern.
  - Majority of genetic cardiomyopathies are transmitted in an autosomal dominant pattern.

*Counseling:* As per guidelines, genetic and family counseling is recommended for all patients and families with cardiomyopathy.
- Multidisciplinary medical care involving genetic counselors is essential for DCM patients and families.
- Genetic counselors involvement includes obtaining a careful and comprehensive family history, education regarding disease transmission, advice on potential risks and benefits of genetic testing, and assistance in interpreting genetic test results.

## Management and Treatment

*Management and Treatment of Patients With DCM Phenotype:* Treatment of symptomatic individuals should be recommended as per guidelines for DCM and heart failure: angiotensin-converting enzyme inhibitors (ACEIs), beta-blockers, and implantable cardiac defibrillators (ICDs) when indicated; for patients with advanced heart failure, the above measures in addition to diuretics and inotropes, as indicated, and for end-stage disease, consideration of ventricular assist devices and/or cardiac transplantation.

*Management of Asymptomatic Family Members:* Asymptomatic, mutation-positive family members: close surveillance with clinical screening as discussed above (Fig. 24-2).

Asymptomatic LV dysfunction: treatment of asymptomatic LV dysfunction with beta-blockers and ACEIs will delay onset of symptoms, improve LV function, and may improve mortality.

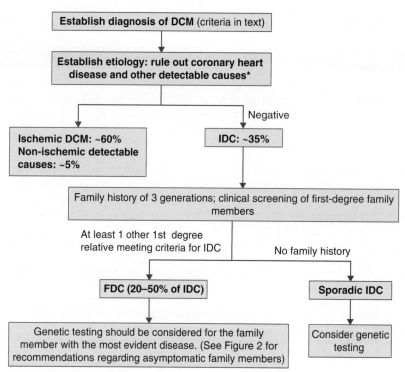

*Figure 24-1* Diagnostic Algorithm for Dilated Cardiomyopathy (DCM).

*Table 24-1 Syndromic Dilated Cardiomyopathy*

| Syndrome | Gene Symbol | Gene Product | Inheritance Pattern[a] | Additional Clinical Features |
|---|---|---|---|---|
| Emery-Dreifuss muscular dystrophy types 2 and 3 (EDMD2 and EDMD3), limb girdle muscular dystrophy (LGMD1B) | *LMNA* | Lamin A/C | EMD 2: AD<br>EMD3: AR<br>LGMD1B: AD | Joint contractures (more severe in EDMD), arrhythmias, childhood muscle weakness (shoulder or hip girdle in LGMD1B) |
| Hemochromatosis | *HFE* | Hereditary hemochromatosis | AR | Cirrhosis, diabetes, hypermelanotic pigmentation, increased serum iron and ferritin |
| Laing distal myopathy | *MYH7* | Beta-myosin heavy chain | AD | Childhood-onset weakness of ankles and great toes, then finger extensors. Neck flexors and facial weakness |
| Duchenne muscular dystrophy (DMD), Becker muscular dystrophy (BMD) | *DMD* | Dystrophin | XL | DMD: males: elevated CK, childhood muscle weakness, wheelchair bound by age 12, DCM after age 18; BMD: elevated CK, skeletal muscle weakness in 20s or lager; females can be affected with milder phenotype or DCM alone |
| Barth syndrome | *TAZ/G4.5* | Tafazzin | XL | Growth retardation, intermittent lactic academia, granulocytopenia, recurrent infections |

[a]AD, autosomal dominant; AR, autosomal recessive; XL, X-linked; CK, creatine kinase.

Adapted from Hershberger RE, Cowan J, Morales A, Siegfried JD. Progress with genetic cardiomyopathies: screening, counseling, and testing in dilated, hypertrophic, and arrhythmogenic right ventricular dysplasia/cardiomyopathy. *Circ Heart Fail.* 2009;2:253-261.

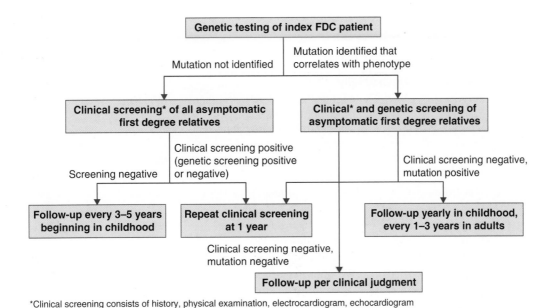

**Figure 24-2** Management of Asymptomatic Family Members

Asymptomatic conduction system disease: close surveillance; at times progressive but asymptomatic conduction system disease (CSD) in family members harboring mutations in *LMNA* may require prophylactic pacemaker or ICD placement. This important issue has been noted in the 2009 Heart Failure Society of America guideline document.

# Molecular Genetics and Molecular Mechanism

**Inheritance Pattern:** DCM with a known genetic cause (including FDC and genetic syndromes) is most commonly reported with autosomal dominant inheritance (~90% or greater). About 5% to 10% of cases are X-linked, and about 1% to 2% are autosomal recessive.

**Penetrance:** FDC demonstrates incomplete, age-dependent penetrance.

- In autosomal dominant forms, penetrance has been estimated to be approximately 10% at 20 years, 34% at 20 to 30 years, 60% at 30 to 40 years, and 90% at greater than 40 years of age, although gene-specific penetrance estimates are generally not yet available.
- Penetrance varies with genotype. For example, in DCM from *LMNA* mutations encoding lamin A/C, penetrance is reported as high as 100% in patients greater than 30 years of age, although for most genes penetrance estimates are not available.

FDC demonstrates variable expression.

- Within a single affected family, clinical symptoms in individual members may range from subtle (mild arrhythmias, asymptomatic LV dysfunction) to severe (sudden cardiac death, fulminant heart failure requiring transplantation).

- Expression varies for each genotype; between families carrying the same gene mutation, clinical manifestations commonly differ.

**Genotype:** Mutations associated with DCM have been identified in more than 30 genes (Table 24-2); tests are available for many of these and are catalogued at www.genetests.org.

**Phenotype:** There are three phenotypes of genetic DCM: DCM only, DCM with CSD, or DCM with skeletal muscle disease.

- Significant overlap exists between DCM only and DCM with CSD; the latter usually refers to DCM phenotypes that present with significant CSD and/or arrhythmia early in the course of DCM, that is, with minimal LV dilatation or systolic dysfunction. This is in contrast to the many cases of DCM with long-standing disease that eventually progress to develop significant CSD and/or arrhythmia, especially with advancing heart failure.

**Genotype-Phenotype Correlation:** Identifying a disease genotype in DCM is primarily to assist in the screening of asymptomatic family members (see Management and Treatment earlier). However, disease-causing mutations from some genes are associated with predictable clinical findings.

- *LMNA:* associated with prominent CSD and arrhythmias followed by onset of DCM and heart failure.
- *SCN5A:* case reports of CSD starting in adolescence and eventually progressing to LV dysfunction in adulthood.
- Importantly, there is genotype-phenotype overlap with other forms of cardiomyopathy; for example, a few mutations in the genes encoding sarcomeric proteins associated with DCM (eg, cardiac troponin T, beta-myosin heavy chain) have also been shown to cause hypertrophic or restrictive cardiomyopathy phenotypes even in the same kindred.

*Table 24-2  Genes Associated With DCM<sup>a</sup>*

| Gene | Protein | Function | OMIM | Mutation Detection Rate[b] |
|------|---------|----------|------|----------------------------|
| **Autosomal dominant dilated cardiomyopathy** | | | | |
| LMNA | Lamin A/C | Inner leaflet, nuclear membrane protein; confers stability to nuclear membrane; gene expression | 150330 | 5.5% overall, 7.3% FDC |
| MYH7 | Beta-myosin heavy chain | Sarcomeric protein; muscle contraction | 160760 | 4.8% overall, 6.3% FDC |
| TNNT2 | Cardiac troponin T | Sarcomeric protein; muscle contraction | 191045 | 2.3% overall, 2.9% FDC |
| MYH6 | Alpha-myosin heavy chain | Sarcomeric protein; muscle contraction | 160710 | 4.3% |
| SCN5A | Sodium channel | Controls sodium ion flux | 600163 | 2.6% |
| DES | Desmin | Dystrophin-associated glycoprotein complex; transduces contractile forces | 125660 | rare |
| MYBPC3 | Myosin-binding protein C | Sarcomeric protein; muscle contraction | 600958 | 2% |
| TPMI | Tropomyosin alpha-1 chain | Sarcomeric protein; muscle contraction | 191010 | rare |
| ACTC | Actin, alpha cardiac muscle 1 | Sarcomeric protein; muscle contraction | 102540 | rare |
| PLN | Cardiac phospholamban | Sarcoplasmic reticulum calcium regulator; inhibits SERCA2 pump | 172405 | ? |
| ZASP/LDB3 | LIM-binding domain 3 | Cytoskeletal assembly; involved in targeting and clustering of membrane proteins | 605906 | 1% |
| VCL | Metavinculin | Sarcomere structure; intercalated discs | 193065 | 1% |
| TCAP | Titin-cap or telethonin | Z-disc protein that associates with titin; aids sarcomere assembly | 604488 | rare |
| SGCD | Delta-sarcoglycan | Dystrophin-associated glyco-protein complex; transduces contractile forces | 601411 | rare |
| TTN | Titin | Sarcomere structure; extensible scaffold for other proteins | 188840 | ? |
| ACTN2 | Alpha-actinin-2 | Sarcomeric protein; muscle contraction | 102573 | rare |
| MLP/CSRP3 | Muscle LIP protein | Sarcomere stretch sensor/Z discs | 600824 | rare |
| ABCC9 | ATP-binding cassette transporter subfamily C member 9 | Regulatory subunit of inwardly rectifying cardiac potassium-ATP channel | 601439 | rare |
| TNNC1 | Cardiac troponin C | Sarcomeric protein; muscle contraction | 191040 | rare |
| EYA4 | Eyes-absent 4 | Transcriptional coactivators (six and dach) | 603550 | ? |
| TMPO | Thymopoietin | Lamin-associated nuclear protein | 188380 | 1.1% |
| PSEN 1/2 | Presenilin 1, presenilin 2 | Transmembrane proteins, gamma secretase activity | 104311/600759 | 1% |

**Table 24-2  Genes Associated With DCM[a] (Continued)**

| Gene | Protein | Function | OMIM | Mutation Detection Rate[b] |
|------|---------|----------|------|---------------------------|
| CRYAB | Alpha B crystallin | Cytoskeletal protein | 123590 | rare |
| PDLIM3 | PDZ LIM domain protein 3 | Cytoskeletal protein | 605889 | rare |
| MYPN | Myopalladin | Sarcomeric protein, Z disc | 608517 | 3.5% |
| LAMA4 | Laminin a-4 | Extracellular matrix protein | 600133 | 1.1% |
| ILK | Integrin-linked kinase | Intracellular serine-threonine kinase; interacts with integrins | 602366 | rare |
| ANKRD1 | Ankyrin repeat domain-containing protein 1 | Cardiac ankyrin repeat protein (CARP); localized to myopalladin/titin complex | 609599 | ? |
| RBM20 | RNA-binding protein 20 | RNA-binding protein of the spliceosome | | ? |
| **X-linked dilated cardiomyopathy** | | | | |
| TAZ/G4.5 | Tafazzin | Unknown | 300394 | ? |
| DMD | Dystrophin | Transduces contractile force | 300377 | ? |
| **Autosomal recessive dilated cardiomyopathy** | | | | |
| TNNI3 | Cardiac troponin I | Sarcomeric protein; muscle contraction | 191044 | Rare |

[a]For details on the laboratories performing genetic testing, please refer to www.genetests.org.
[b]Rare implies an estimated mutation frequency <1%; "?" implies little or no data to estimate mutation frequency.
Adapted from Dilated Cardiomyopathy Overview. Copyright, University of Washington, Seattle. 1997-2008, 2007. http://www.genetests.org; Burkett EL, Hershberger RE. Clinical and genetic issues in familial dilated cardiomyopathy. *J Am Coll Cardiol.* 2005;45:969-981.

**Genetic Testing:** Genetic testing should be considered for the one most clearly affected person in a family to facilitate family screening and management.

- Testing may begin with *LMNA*, *MYH7*, and *TNNT2* because of their higher mutation detection rates in people with DCM. However, rapidly evolving technologies are increasing the availability of testing for larger panels of genes associated with DCM at affordable rates.
- The principal rationale for genetic testing at this time is to identify disease-causing mutations in at-risk family members with minimal or no evidence of disease so that heightened clinical surveillance, more informed medical management, and/or reproductive decision making can be undertaken. In the future, with much more extensive gene mutation databases, specific genotypes may provide relevant genotype or phenotype information that may impact the medical management of individuals with a pre-existing diagnosis of DCM.
- If the patient selected for testing is found to have a mutation that correlates with DCM, the testing of asymptomatic family members should be considered (Fig. 24-2).
- It is important to discuss the risks and benefits of genetic testing with all affected and asymptomatic individuals, and to include a genetic counselor in these discussions.

☞**FAMILY MEMBERS (FIG. 24-2):**
- All asymptomatic first-degree relatives should undergo clinical screening for cardiomyopathy in both FDC and apparently sporadic cases of IDC (Fig. 24-2).
- Clinical screening should consist of history, physical examination, electrocardiogram (ECG), and echocardiogram.

- Common findings in asymptomatic affected family members include subtle left ventricular enlargement and/or mild decreases in LV function on echocardiogram; and first- or second-degree heart block, intraventricular conduction delays, and arrhythmias on ECG.

**BIBLIOGRAPHY:**

1. Dilated Cardiomyopathy Overview. Copyright, University of Washington, Seattle. 1997-2008, 2007. http://www.genetests.org.
2. Richard P, Villard E, Charron P, Isnard R. The genetic bases of cardiomyopathies. *J Am Coll Cardiol.* 2006;48(suppl A):A79-A89.
3. Hershberger R, Lindenfeld J, Mestroni L, Seidman C, Taylor M, Towbin J. Genetic evaluation of cardiomyopathy: a HFSA Comprehensive Heart Failure Practice Guideline. *J Card Fail.* 2009;15:83-97.
4. Mestroni L, Maisch B, McKenna WJ, et al. Guidelines for the study of familial dilated cardiomyopathies. Collaborative Research Group of the European Human and Capital Mobility Project on Familial Dilated Cardiomyopathy. *Eur Heart J.* 1999;20:93-102.
5. Mestroni L, Rocco C, Gregori D, et al. Familial dilated cardiomyopathy: evidence for genetic and phenotypic heterogeneity. *J Am Coll Cardiol.* 1999;34:181-190.
6. Hershberger R. Familial dilated cardiomyopathy. *Prog Pediatr Cardiol.* 2005;20:161-168.
7. Burkett EL, Hershberger RE. Clinical and genetic issues in familial dilated cardiomyopathy. *J Am Coll Cardiol.* 2005;45:969-981.
8. Taylor MR, Fain PR, Sinagra G, et al. Natural history of dilated cardiomyopathy due to lamin A/C gene mutations. *J Am Coll Cardiol.* 2003;41:771-780.

9.  McNair WP, Ku L, Taylor MR, et al. SCN5A mutation associated with dilated cardiomyopathy, conduction disorder, and arrhythmia. *Circulation.* 2004;110:2163-2167.

10. Parks SB, Kushner JD, Nauman D, et al. Lamin A/C mutation analysis in a cohort of 324 unrelated patients with idiopathic or familial dilated cardiomyopathy. *Am Heart J.* 2008;156:161-169.

11. Hershberger RE, Cowan J, Morales A, Siegfried JD. Progress with genetic cardiomyopathies: screening, counseling, and testing in dilated, hypertrophic, and arrhythmogenic right ventricular dysplasia/cardiomyopathy. *Circ Heart Fail.* 2009;2:253-261.

## Supplementary Information

For details on laboratories performing genetic testing discussed in this chapter and other general information, please refer to www .genetests.org, which maintains an updated directory of genetic testing laboratories.

**Alternative Names:**
• Familial Dilated Cardiomyopathy
• Idiopathic Dilated Cardiomyopathy

***Key Words:*** Dilated cardiomyopathy, familial dilated cardiomyopathy, idiopathic dilated cardiomyopathy, genetics, congestive heart failure

# 25 Hypertrophic Cardiomyopathy

Polakit Teekakirikul, Christine E. Seidman, and Carolyn Y. Ho

## KEY POINTS

- *Disease summary:*
  - Hypertrophic cardiomyopathy (HCM) is an inherited disorder of cardiac muscle characterized by left ventricular hypertrophy (LVH) in the absence of other cardiovascular or systemic conditions (eg, valvular heart diseases or long-standing hypertension).
  - The histopathologic hallmarks include myocyte hypertrophy, myocardial disarray, and fibrosis.
  - The prevalence of HCM is 1:500 in the general population, with at least 60% caused by mutation in one of the genes encoding different components of the sarcomere protein (see Molecular Genetics section).
- *Hereditary basis:*
  - HCM is inherited in an autosomal dominant manner with age-dependent penetrance and variable expressivity.
- *Differential diagnosis:*
  - It is clinically important to distinguish HCM from acquired LVH (eg, physiologic hypertrophy from athletic training, hypertensive heart disease), inherited LVH with multisystem involvement (eg, metabolic cardiomyopathy, cardiac amyloidosis) and syndromes with LVH as a presenting feature. Such diseases with similar cardiac morphologic finding can have different modes of inheritance, natural histories, and therapeutic strategies (Table 25-1).

## Diagnostic Criteria and Clinical Characteristics

### Diagnostic Criteria for Hypertrophic Cardiomyopathy:

**Presence of the following**

- Unexplained LVH with nondilated left ventricular chamber
  - Although asymmetric septal hypertrophy is most common, the patterns of hypertrophy are variable and can include concentric and apical hypertrophy.
  - Most often diagnosed by echocardiography; cardiac MRI may be used to further evaluate left ventricular morphology and to assess for myocardial scar.
  - Additional findings may include systolic anterior motion (SAM) of the mitral valve with associated left ventricular outflow tract obstruction and mitral regurgitation, mid ventricular obstruction, and diastolic dysfunction.
  - Less than 10% of patients may develop a burnt-out or end-stage phase characterized by systolic dysfunction, occasionally with regression of LVH and left ventricular dilatation.
- Pathognomonic histopathologic features: myocyte disarray, hypertrophy, and cardiac fibrosis

**Other findings associated with HCM include**

- Prominent apical impulse or lift
- Brisk, occasionally bifid carotid upstroke
- A harsh crescendo-decrescendo systolic murmur from dynamic obstruction, best heard at the lower left sternal border and apex, radiating to the axilla and base
- Abnormal electrocardiogram (ECG) patterns
  - LVH with repolarization abnormalities
  - Q waves
  - T-wave inversions

**And the absence of**

- Other cardiovascular conditions or systemic diseases (such as long-standing hypertension, valvular heart diseases, etc) that could account for the degree of LVH seen

**Clinical Characteristics:** The clinical spectrum of HCM varies widely from individual to individual, even within the same family, ranging from asymptomatic to progressive heart failure and sudden cardiac death. Common symptoms include shortness of breath particularly on exertion, chest pain, palpitations, orthostatic light-headedness, presyncope, and syncope. Diastolic dysfunction is a common finding preceding the development of both hypertrophy and symptoms in sarcomere mutation carriers. Individuals with HCM are at an increased risk for arrhythmias. Atrial fibrillation (AF) is common and associated with increased thromboembolic risk. Sudden cardiac death (SCD) risk is also increased and HCM is the leading cause of SCD in competitive athletes and young individuals in the United States.

## Screening and Counseling

**Screening:** The diagnosis of HCM is suggested by an autosomal dominant pattern of inheritance of unexplained LVH without systemic disease involvement. A family history of the following should be explored in relatives: HCM, LVH, heart failure, cardiac transplantation, SCD or unexplained premature death, conduction disease (eg, need for pacemakers) or arrhythmias, and thromboembolic disease.

In probands, the identification of unexplained LVH is the traditional basis for diagnosing HCM. However, LVH is a sign of established disease only and cannot identify at-risk mutation carriers in the family. It is also nonspecific and cannot differentiate HCM from other forms of cardiac hypertrophy (either genetic or acquired). Incorporating genetic screening of sarcomere genes into clinical evaluation allows confirmation of diagnosis and age-independent identification of relatives at risk for developing HCM. Sarcomere mutations can be identified in approximately 60% of patients with familial HCM and approximately 40% of patients without family history of disease including patients with childhood onset. If a pathogenic mutation is found, confirmatory (predictive) genetic testing can be performed in relatives to identify those definitively at risk for disease. However, sarcomere mutations will not be detected

*Table 25-1 Genetic Differential Diagnosis*

| Syndrome | Symbol of Associated Gene | Associated Findings |
|---|---|---|
| Hypertrophic cardiomyopathy | see Molecular Genetics section | Isolated cardiac hypertrophy |
| Fabry disease | GLA | LVH, acroparesthesias, angiokeratomas, hypohidrosis, ocular involvement, renal insufficiency (proteinuria to end-stage renal disease), cerebrovascular disease |
| Danon disease | LAMP2 (X-linked) | LVH, ventricular pre-excitation and arrhythmias, rapid progression of heart failure, extracardiac manifestations (skeletal and neurologic) |
| PRKAG2 cardiomyopathy | PRKAG2 | LVH and cardiac conduction system defects (including pre-excitation) due to excessive glycogen accumulation |
| Cardiac amyloidosis (Familial) | TTR | LVH, sensorimotor neuropathy, autonomic neuropathy, due to amyloid infiltration |
| Friedreich ataxia (FRDA) | FXN | Slowly progressive ataxia of gait and limbs, depressed tendon reflexes, dysarthria, muscle weakness, spasticity, optic nerve atrophy, scoliosis, bladder dysfunction, loss of position, and vibration sense. Two-thirds of patients have cardiomyopathy |

Gene names: *GLA*, alpha-galactosidase A; *LAMP2*, lysosomal-associated membrane protein 2; *PRKAG2*, gamma-2 regulatory subunit of AMP-activated protein kinase (AMPK); *TTR*, transthyretin; *FXA*, frataxin.

in all individuals with unexplained LVH. A negative result from the genetic testing only eliminates sarcomere gene mutations from the list but does not exclude a genetic cause of LVH. Clinical screening of at-risk relatives may still be appropriate. A diagnostic algorithm for the evaluation of patients presenting with unexplained LVH is summarized in Table 25-2.

***Counseling:*** HCM is caused by mutations in genes encoding sarcomere proteins and is inherited in an autosomal dominant manner with age-dependent penetrance and variable expressivity. Each child of an affected parent has a 50% risk of inheriting the condition. In approximately 5% of patients with HCM, more than one sarcomere mutation is identified. In such cases, it is important to determine the inheritance patterns (*cis* or *trans*) to allow appropriate family evaluation. A proband with HCM may also have disease resulting from a de novo mutation. The proportion of HCM cases with de novo mutations has not been precisely determined.

Genetic testing of at-risk relatives can be performed if a disease-causing (pathogenic) mutation has been identified in the proband. Such testing should be performed in the context of formal genetic counseling. This testing will help identify relatives at risk for developing HCM at an early stage but typically does not provide additional information to predict symptoms, age of onset, clinical severity, and progression rate. Longitudinal clinical follow-up to assess for phenotypic conversion can be focused on pathogenic mutation carriers. Relatives who have not inherited the family's pathogenic mutation can be reassured because neither they nor their offspring are at risk for HCM development. Predictive genetic testing in HCM families with a disease-causing mutation is also available as part of reproductive planning through preimplantation genetic diagnosis (PGD) to attempt pregnancy that does not carry the disease-causing mutation. If a variant of unclear significance (VUS) is identified, segregation studies with combined clinical and genetic testing in other relatives can be valuable to assist in determining the variant's pathogenicity. If clinical significance cannot be more clearly established, VUS results cannot be used in predictive genetic testing for the family.

*Genotype-phenotype correlation*: Genotype-phenotype correlations are not yet robust and are of limited usefulness for clinical management of patients with HCM.

## Management and Treatment

Three major aspects for managing HCM include risk assessment for SCD, treatment of symptoms, and family evaluation or management.

***Risk Assessment for SCD:*** A subset of patients with HCM is at significantly increased risk for sudden death and clinical risk assessment remains challenging. The traditional parameters used to assess an individual's risk for SCD include the following:

- Prior history of cardiac arrest, resuscitated sudden death or significant ventricular tachycardia
- Nonsustained ventricular tachycardia on ambulatory monitoring
- Massive LVH (>30 mm)
- Hypotensive response to exercise
- Family history of SCD
  - Identification of a mutation that has been consistently associated with increased SCD risk
- Unexplained syncope

Echocardiogram, exercise testing and Holter monitoring are used for a complete risk assessment. However, accurate estimation of an individuals' risk is difficult. The positive predictive value of each parameter individually is low. However, the presence of two or more risk factors has been associated with an increased risk of SCD. In contrast, the individual without any risk indicators is likely at low risk for SCD. Individuals with a history of prior cardiac arrest or aborted sudden death are advised to undergo placement of a secondary prevention implantable cardioverter-defibrillator (ICD) as they are at highest risk of SCD. Patients with one or more risk factors may appropriately consider having an ICD placed for primary prevention.

**Table 25-2 Algorithm for Diagnostic Evaluation of Patients With Hypertrophic Cardiomyopathy**

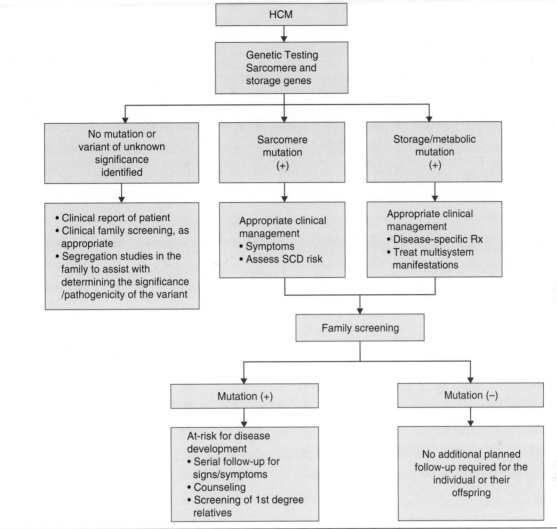

Due to the association between HCM and sudden death in competitive athletes, patients with HCM are advised to avoid intense, competitive training, heavy isometric exercise, and burst activities. Moderate recreational activity is typically acceptable.

**Management of Symptoms:** Medical therapy used for alleviation of symptoms typically include beta-adrenergic and L-type calcium channel antagonists to slow heart rate, increase diastolic filling time, reduce contractility, and blunt dynamic intracavitary gradients. Diuretics may be used judiciously to reduce symptomatic volume overload; however, excessive diuresis may not be well tolerated, particularly if there is preload dependence from severe obstruction or decreased LV compliance. Disopyramide may also be administered to relieve outflow tract obstruction due to its negative inotropic effects. Afterload reduction should be avoided in patients with obstructive physiology because it can increase gradients.

For medically refractory patients with symptomatic obstruction, alcohol septal ablation or surgical myectomy may be performed to mechanically reduce septal thickness, ameliorate obstruction, and alleviate symptoms. Anticoagulation is also required for patients with paroxysmal or persistent atrial fibrillation because of an increased risk of thromboembolic complications. Cardiac transplantation may be necessary for those individuals who progress to end-stage heart failure, once medical treatment options have been exhausted.

**Family Screening:** Screening guidelines have been proposed for the serial clinical evaluation of apparently unaffected at-risk relatives, using physical examination, echocardiography, and ECG (Table 25-3). Clinical manifestations typically develop during adolescence and early adulthood but may also present later in life. Therefore, the absence of clinical findings on initial assessment does not exclude the possibility of future disease development and associated risks. As such, serial screening and follow-up is required.

If a pathogenic mutation is identified in the family, predictive genetic testing can be used to definitively determine which relatives are at risk for disease development. Longitudinal clinical follow-up can then be focused only on mutation carriers.

**Table 25-3** *Guidelines for Clinical Screening of Clinically Unaffected At-Risk Family Members*

| Age | Screening Guideline |
|---|---|
| <12 years | Optional but recommended if any of the following is present:<br>1. Symptoms or signs suggestive of HCM<br>2. A malignant family history of premature HCM-related death, early onset of hypertrophy or other serious complications<br>3. Competitive athletic participation |
| 12-18 years | Serial screening every 12 to 18 months |
| >18-21 years | At the onset of symptoms or at least every 3 to 5 years. More frequent intervals are appropriate in families with malignant clinical courses. |

Adapted from Maron BJ, Seidman JG, Seidman CE. Proposal for contemporary screening strategies in families with hypertrophic cardiomyopathy. *J Am Coll Cardiol.* 2004b;44:2125-2132.

# Molecular Genetics and Molecular Mechanism

## Syndrome/Gene/Locus

### ☞SARCOMERE GENES ASSOCIATED WITH HCM:

Familial hypertrophic cardiomyopathy (CMH1)/cardiac beta-myosin heavy chain (MYH7)/14q12

Familial hypertrophic cardiomyopathy (CMH2)/cardiac troponin T (TNNT2)/1q32

Familial hypertrophic cardiomyopathy (CMH3)/tropomyosin 1 alpha chain (TPM1)/15q22.1

Familial hypertrophic cardiomyopathy (CMH4)/cardiac myosin-binding protein C (MYBPC3)/11q11.2

Familial hypertrophic cardiomyopathy (CMH7)/cardiac troponin (TNNI3)/19q13.4

Familial hypertrophic cardiomyopathy (CMH8)/myosin light polypeptide 3 (MYL3)/3p

Familial hypertrophic cardiomyopathy (CMH10)/myosin regulatory light chain 2 (MYL2)/12q23-q24.3

Familial hypertrophic cardiomyopathy (CMH11)/alpha cardiac actin (ACTC1)/15q14

The sarcomere is the basic functional contractile unit of the cardiac myocyte. Proteins are organized into thick (myosin heavy and light chains) and thin filaments (actin, troponins, and alpha-tropomyosin) that slide past one another and generate contractile force. The detachment and attachment of actin and myosin head contribute to contraction and relaxation at the molecular level. ATP hydrolysis provides energy for this motor, both for force generation and relaxation. Well-orchestrated fluxes in intracellular calcium concentration coordinate thick and thin filament interaction.

Mutations in the sarcomere apparatus may alter actin-myosin interaction, calcium handling, force generation, and force transmission, leading to the characteristic features of HCM via perturbations in important signaling pathways (eg, NFAT, Mef2, CaMKII, and TGFbeta). However, the precise mechanisms leading from sarcomere mutation to clinical disease are not yet known. To date, more than 1000 distinct mutations in genes encoding different components of the sarcomere have been identified. Mutations in MYH7 and MYBPC3 are the most common. A variety of mutation types have been found, including missense, truncations, insertion or deletions and splice site mutations.

***Genetic Testing:*** Molecular genetic testing for HCM typically analyzes all genes encoding different components of the sarcomere apparatus and a variety of metabolic and mitochondrial genes that may produce phenocopies (Table 25-4). Genetic testing is clinically available for HCM. Information regarding clinical testing laboratories can be obtained at Gene Tests website (http://www.genetests.org). Genetic testing can be considered in all individuals with a clinical diagnosis of HCM, regardless of age. If a pathogenic mutation is identified, predictive genetic testing can be offered for all relatives to assist in definitive determination of their risk.

## BIBLIOGRAPHY:

1. McKenna WJ, Behr ER. Hypertrophic cardiomyopathy: management, risk stratification, and prevention of sudden death. *Heart.* 2002;87(2):169-176.

2. Maron BJ. Hypertrophic cardiomyopathy: a systematic review. *JAMA.* 2002;287(10):1308-1320.

3. Elliott P, McKenna WJ. Hypertrophic cardiomyopathy. *Lancet.* 2004;363(9424):1881-1891.

4. Nishimura RA, Holmes DR Jr. Clinical practice. Hypertrophic obstructive cardiomyopathy. *N Engl J Med.* 2004;350(13): 1320-1327.

5. Nagueh SF, Bachinski LL, Meyer D, et al. Tissue Doppler imaging consistently detects myocardial abnormalities in patients with hypertrophic cardiomyopathy and provides a novel means for an early diagnosis before and independently of hypertrophy. *Circulation.* 2001;104(2):128-130.

6. Ho CY, Sweitzer NK, McDonough B, et al. Assessment of diastolic function with Doppler tissue imaging to predict genotype in preclinical hypertrophic cardiomyopathy. *Circulation.* 2002;105(25):2992-2997.

7. Ho CY. Genetics and clinical destiny: improving care in hypertrophic cardiomyopathy. *Circulation.* 2010;122(23):2430-2440; discussion 2440.

8. Morita H, Rehm HL, Menesses A, et al. Shared genetic causes of cardiac hypertrophy in children and adults. *N Engl J Med.* 2008;358(18):1899-1908.

9. Girolami F, Ho CY, Semsarian C, et al. Clinical features and outcome of hypertrophic cardiomyopathy associated with triple sarcomere protein gene mutations. *J Am Coll Cardiol.* 2010;55(14): 1444-1453.

*Table 25-4 Molecular Genetic Testing*

| Gene | Prevalence (%) | Allelic Disorders |
|---|---|---|
| **HCM sarcomere proteins** | | |
| *MYH7* | 35 | DCM, laing distal myopathy |
| *MYBPC3* | 40 | DCM |
| *TNNT2* | 8 | DCM |
| *TNNI3* | 10 | DCM, restrictive cardiomyopathy |
| *TPM1* | 5 | DCM |
| *MYL2* | <1 | |
| *MYL3* | <1 | |
| *ACTC1* | Rare | DCM |
| **Inherited LVH** | | |
| *PRKAG2* | Unknown | Glucose metabolism; pre-excitation and conduction disease; CPMVT |
| *LAMP2* | Unknown | |
| *CSRP3* | Unknown | |
| *GLA* | Unknown | |
| *TTR* | Unknown | |
| **Other genes implicated in HCM** | | |
| *TNNC1* | Unknown | DCM |
| *ACTN2* | Unknown | DCM |
| *CAV3* | Unknown | |
| *MYOZ2* | Unknown | |
| *NEXN* | Unknown | |
| *PLN* | Unknown | |
| Mitochondrial genes | Unknown | |

DCM, dilated cardiomyopathy; CPMVT, catecholaminergic polymorphic ventricular tachycardia.

Adapted from Ho CY. New paradigms in hypertrophic cardiomyopathy: insights from genetics. *Prog Pediatr Cardiol*. May 2011;31(2): 93-98; Cirino AL, Ho CY. Familial hypertrophic cardiomyopathy overview. In: Pagon RA, Bird TD, Dolan CR, Stephens K, eds. GeneReviews [Internet].

10. Ingles J, Doolan A, Chiu C, Seidman J, Seidman C, Semsarian C. Compound and double mutations in patients with hypertrophic cardiomyopathy: implications for genetic testing and counselling. *J Med Genet*. 2005;42(10):e59.

11. Elliott PM, Poloniecki J, Dickie S, et al. Sudden death in hypertrophic cardiomyopathy: identification of high risk patients. *J Am Coll Cardiol*. 2000;36(7):2212-2218.

12. Fatkin D, Graham RM. Molecular mechanisms of inherited cardiomyopathies. *Physiol Rev*. 2002;82(4):945-980.

13. Wang L, Seidman JG, Seidman CE. Narrative review: harnessing molecular genetics for the diagnosis and management of hypertrophic cardiomyopathy. *Ann Intern Med*. 2010;152(8):513-520, W181.

14. Teekakirikul P, Eminaga S, Toka O, et al. Cardiac fibrosis in mice with hypertrophic cardiomyopathy is mediated by non-myocyte proliferation and requires Tgf-beta. *J Clin Invest*. 2010;120(10):3520-3529.

15. Konno T, Chen D, Wang L, et al. Heterogeneous myocyte enhancer factor-2 (Mef2) activation in myocytes predicts focal scarring in hypertrophic cardiomyopathy. *Proc Natl Acad Sci U S A*. 2010;107(42):18097-18102.

16. Bers DM, Guo T. Calcium signaling in cardiac ventricular myocytes. *Ann N Y Acad Sci*. 2005;1047:86-98.

## Supplementary Information

**OMIM REFERENCES:**

[1] Familial Hypertrophic Cardiomyopathy (CMH1); MYH7 (#192600)

[2] Familial Hypertrophic Cardiomyopathy (CMH2); TNNT2 (#115195)

[3] Familial Hypertrophic Cardiomyopathy (CMH3); TPM1 (#115196)

[4] Familial Hypertrophic Cardiomyopathy (CMH4); MYBPC3 (#600958)

[5] Familial Hypertrophic Cardiomyopathy (CMH7); TNNI3 (#613690)

[6] Familial Hypertrophic Cardiomyopathy (CMH8); MYL3 (#608751)

[7] Familial Hypertrophic Cardiomyopathy (CMH10); MYL2 (#608758)

[8] Familial Hypertrophic Cardiomyopathy (CMH11); ACTC1 (#612098)

**Alternative Names:**
- Hereditary Ventricular Hypertrophy
- Asymmetric Septal Hypertrophy (ASH)
- Idiopathic Hypertrophic Subaortic Stenosis

***Key Words:*** Hypertrophic cardiomyopathy, cardiomyopathy, left ventricular hypertrophy, myocyte disarray, cardiac fibrosis, sarcomere, shortness of breath, palpitations, syncope, sudden cardiac death, arrhythmias

# 26 Bicuspid Aortic Valve Disease

Neal K. Lakdawala, Elizabeth A. Sparks, and Alexander R. Opotowsky

## KEY POINTS

- *Disease summary:*
  - Bicuspid aortic valve (BAV) disease is the commonest congenital heart lesion, affecting approximately 1% to 2% of the population and is approximately three times more common in men.
  - BAV is typically nonsyndromic, but is seen with increased frequency in the Turner and potentially Loeys-Dietz syndromes.
  - BAV is usually an isolated cardiac lesion but is often seen in conjunction with coarctation of the aorta and other obstructive left-sided lesions (Shone complex, hypoplastic left heart syndrome).
  - Aortic stenosis (AS) develops in most patients with BAV. The incidence of AS increases with age and BAV is the commonest indication for aortic valve replacement in patients under 70 years old.
  - Aortic regurgitation (AI) and infective endocarditis are also more prevalent in BAV.
  - BAV is associated with an elevated risk of developing thoracic aortic dilation and aneurysms (TADA) and subsequent aortic dissection and rupture. In children, the risk of aortic aneurysm increases with age, indicating the progressive nature of aortic dilation.
  - Longitudinal echocardiographic monitoring is recommended for patients with BAV, both for development or progression of valvular stenosis or regurgitation, and also for ascending aortic dilation. If the ascending aorta cannot be well visualized with transthoracic echocardiography (TTE), either computed tomography (CT) or magnetic resonance angiography (MRA) should be performed.
- *Family history:*
  - Familial involvement has been reported in 37% of patients with BAV. When familial disease is present, inheritance is autosomal dominant with variable penetrance.
  - There is an increased risk of aortic dilation in individuals with apparently normal tricuspid aortic valve who are first-degree relatives of patients with BAV.
  - Screening of first-degree relatives of probands with BAV is recommended and this is most commonly accomplished by transthoracic echocardiography.
- *Genetic factors:*
  - Mutations in *NOTCH1* have been identified in limited kindreds with BAV and aortic calcification.
  - Mutations in *ACTA2* have been identified in kindreds with TADA, livedo reticularis, and BAV.
  - In the vast majority of cases, the genetic etiology of BAV has not been identified.

## Diagnostic Criteria and Clinical Characteristics

***Diagnosis:*** The cusps or leaflets of the normally tricuspid aortic valve are named after the adjacent coronary ostia, right coronary cusp, left coronary cusp, and noncoronary cusp. Fusion of two cusps causes BAV. The most common BAV morphology involves fusion of the right and left coronary cusps (R-L fusion), followed by right and noncoronary cusp fusion (R-N fusion), whereas fusion of the left and noncoronary cusps is exceedingly rare.

Physical examination provides clues to the diagnosis, but BAV is usually diagnosed by TTE. Notably, a prominent raphe, or ridge, at the site of leaflet fusion may provide the false impression of three distinct leaflets when the aortic valve is visualized *during diastole*. Accordingly diagnosis rests on visualizing two, instead of three aortic leaflets *during systole*. Supporting features are systolic doming or diastolic prolapse of the aortic valve and an abnormal leaflet coaptation plane. Not infrequently, limited image quality can limit visualization of the aortic leaflets and obscure the diagnosis. Diagnosis may also be confirmed with transesophageal echocardiography, cardiac CT, or cardiac MRI.

***Clinical Characteristics:***

☞ THE DEVELOPMENT OF AORTIC VALVE DYSFUNCTION: AS is the most common manifestation of valvular dysfunction with BAV, with the majority of patients developing clinically relevant AS at some point. AS may be congenital (small valve orifice at birth) or, more commonly, develop due to an active process leading to valvular calcification and decreased mobility. AR is less common than stenosis and may result from redundant valve tissue, aortic root dilation, or infective endocarditis. There is an increased risk for development of infective endocarditis, likely related to turbulent flow and the consequent presence of a denuded valve surface allowing bacterial seeding.

☞ ASSOCIATED ANOMALIES: TADA is an important manifestation of BAV. Even in the absence of aortic dilation, there is evidence of abnormal aortic wall histology associated with BAV including increased apoptosis of vascular smooth muscle cells. Aortic pathology in patients with BAV and aortic aneurysms demonstrate findings consistent with what has historically been termed as "cystic medial necrosis," namely fragmented elastic lamellae with increased basophilic ground substance with a paucity of vascular smooth muscle cells without evidence of inflammation. Similar to that seen with Marfan disease, there is altered matrix metalloproteinase activity, in a pattern different than what is seen with aortic aneurysms associated with tricuspid aortic valve. The prevalence of aortic disease varies by age group, anatomic aortic position, and definition of aortic dilation and aneurysm. Aortic dilation occurs most frequently at the ascending aorta (between the sinotubular junction and the right brachiocephalic artery), but also can affect the sinuses of Valsalva. The aortic arch, descending thoracic aorta, and abdominal aorta are typically spared.

There is a 6% lifetime risk of thoracic aorta dissection or rupture in BAV; ninefold greater than age matched individuals without BAV. The main risk factors for dissection are aortic size and rate of growth. Given the relative rarity of dissection, there are limited data on other independent predictors. Dissection related to BAV is associated with the same signs and symptoms as other causes of dissection and dissection appears to occur at similar aortic size on average as other causes of dissection. There are few data comparing outcomes between BAV and other causes of dissection.

While still relatively uncommon, there is an increased prevalence of coarctation of the aorta and hypoplastic left heart syndrome in patients with BAV. Conversely, approximately 50% of patients with coarctation of the aorta have BAV. There is also an increased prevalence of left dominant coronary circulation in BAV.

Dilation of the proximal pulmonary trunk and abnormalities of the pulmonary arterial wall are seen in patients with BAV, even those with a structurally normal pulmonary valve. This is of clinical significance when surgical repair with a Ross procedure (using the native pulmonary root and valve as a neoaorta/aortic valve) is considered; as these patients may be at increased risk for neoaortic dilation.

Emerging evidence suggests a risk of intracranial arterial aneurysms in BAV. Leaflet morphology is a predictor of associated anomalies and outcomes.

As shown in Fig. 26-1, the frequency of associated cardiac anomalies and major clinical outcomes appears to be influenced by leaflet morphology. Right noncoronary fusion (~25% of cases) is associated with a greater burden of valvular dysfunction, while fusion of the right and left coronary cusps (~75% of cases) is more

highly associated with dilation of the aorta at the sinuses of Valsalva and coarctation of the aorta.

## Screening and Counseling

***Screening:*** In nonsyndromic BAV, first-degree relatives should undergo TTE-based screening for both BAV and thoracic aortic aneurysm (TAA). Definitive evidence of familial involvement is present in approximately 37% of probands with BAV. Moreover, the prevalence of aortic dilation may be increased in individuals with tricuspid aortic valve who have first-degree relatives with BAV. The clinical significance of this finding is as yet unknown, and recommendations for monitoring aortic size in first-degree relatives of patients with BAV are not available.

***Counseling:*** BAV likely has autosomal dominant inheritance with incomplete penetrance with approximately 3:1 male-female preponderance. In some kindreds, BAV appears to represent one end of a spectrum of left-sided obstructive lesions including hypoplastic left heart syndrome. A detailed family history may provide a better basis for estimating the likelihood that a prospective parent with isolated BAV may have offspring with more severe disease. Fetal echocardiography is usually recommended if the mother or father has isolated BAV.

## Management and Treatment

***BAV Without Valvular Dysfunction or Aortic Dilation:*** Asymptomatic patients without aortic dilation require interval follow-up. This should include a clinical examination and TTE

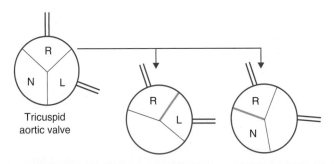

| | Right-left fusion | Right-non fusion |
|---|---|---|
| Proportion of bicuspid valves | ~75% | ~25% |
| Terminology (Valve orientation) | Anterior posterior | Right-left |
| Terminology (Commissure orientation) | Horizontal | Vertical |
| Coarctation | ↑↑↑ | ↑ |
| Stenosis & regurgitation | ↑ | ↑↑↑ |
| Dilation, aortic root | ↑↑↑ | ↑ |
| Dilation, ascending | ↑↑ | ↑↑ |
| Left dominant coronary circulation | ↑↑↑ | = |

*Other morphologies, including fusion of the left coronary and non-coronary cusps, are extremely rare

***Figure 26-1*** Leaflet Morphology is a Predictor of Associated Anomalies and Outcomes in Bicuspid Aortic Valve Disease.

screening to detect valvular or aortic pathology. The timing of repeat TTE is not defined for patients without AS, AI, or aortic dilation, though some recommend repeat TTE monitoring every 3 to 5 years (or with the onset of symptoms). If the ascending aorta is inadequately imaged with TTE, CT, or MRA can be performed. Screening for cerebral aneurysms with head and neck CT angiography or MRA may be reasonable, but consensus guidelines have not yet addressed this topic.

**BAV With Aortic Valve Dysfunction:** Patients with asymptomatic AS (mild, moderate, or severe) should undergo regular follow-up echocardiography to identify progression of valve disease every year for severe AS, every 1-2 years for moderate AS, and every 3 to 5 years for mild AS. In general, only severe AS causes symptoms. As with tricuspid aortic valve stenosis, valve replacement is indicated at the onset of symptoms. There is no effective medical therapy for AS.

As is the case with AS, patients with asymptomatic AR should undergo longitudinal clinical evaluation including TTE. The frequency of follow-up is determined by the severity of AR and the presence of associated left ventricular (LV) enlargement. Vasodilators (eg, dihydropyridines) are recommended for patients with uncontrolled hypertension or for patients with symptomatic AR who are not surgical candidates. Aortic valve replacement or repair is indicated for the development of symptoms or reduced LV ejection fraction (<50%). As in the case of AS, typically only severe AR is responsible for symptoms or ventricular remodeling.

**BAV With TADA:** The presence of TADA should prompt increased frequency of aortic imaging, lifestyle recommendations, and potentially medical and/or surgical intervention. Depending on the size of the aorta and rate of enlargement, repeat imaging should be performed to detect further dilation every 6 to 12 months. Imaging can be performed with TTE, CT or MRA, and ideally the same imaging modality would be repeated in the future to avoid intermodality measurement differences.

Patients with TADA should be counseled to avoid heavy lifting and contact sports as outlined in the 36th Bethesda Conference recommendations. Although medical therapy for TADA has not been studied in BAV, based on experience with TADA in Marfan syndrome (MFS), beta-blocker therapy is often used and angiotensin receptor blockers or angiotensin-converting enzyme inhibitors may be considered. Prophylactic replacement of the aorta is usually recommended when the thoracic aortic diameter is greater than 5 cm, or between 4 and 5 cm with any of the following: increase

in diameter greater than 0.5 cm/y, family history of dissection at smaller diameter, independent need for aortic valve surgery, and aortic diameter greater than 4 cm or if the ratio of the maximal ascending or aortic root area in $cm^2$ divided by the patient's height in meters exceeds 10.

## Molecular Genetics and Molecular Mechanism

**Gene/Locus:**

*NOTCH1*/9q34

Vascular smooth muscle cell alpha- actin (*ACTC2*)/10q23

*NOTCH1* encodes a signaling and transcriptional regulator that is critical for development (Table 26-1). Nonsense and frameshift mutations in *NOTCH* have been shown to cause BAV and associated cardiac features in select kindreds. Mutations in *ACTA2* account for approximately 14% of familial TAAs and are sometimes also associated with BAV.

Additionally, genome-wide linkage studies of kindreds affected by BAV have identified three other disease loci on chromosomes 18, 5, and 73 with LOD score of 3.8, 2.7, and 2.7, respectively. Nevertheless, a precise genetic etiology has not been described for the majority of patients with BAV. Syndromic presentation of BAV is uncommon, although it is a recognized manifestation of Turner syndrome and several other disorders (Table 26-2).

**Genetic Testing:** Genetic testing for BAV is not currently advised. The genetic basis of BAV remains poorly understood and previously described mutations likely account for less than 10% of cases. In the future, testing is expected to be of value, as it may assist in the identification of family members without BAV, but who are at risk of developing aortic dilation or having offspring with BAV and associated defects.

Clinical genetic testing for *NOTCH1* mutations is not currently available. DNA sequence analysis is clinically available for *ACTA2*, but given the circumscribed associations of *ACTA2* mutations with aortic aneurysms and livedo reticularis, it is not advised that sequencing be performed in the absence of these features.

**Future Directions:** Discovery of novel genetic pathways and mechanisms of aortic valve dysfunction and aortic aneurysm development may usher in an era of improved screening of family members and therapies to prevent complications of BAV.

*Table 26-1 Genetic Causes of Nonsyndromic BAV*

| Gene Symbol | Frequency of BAV Among Mutation Carriers | Associated Findings |
|---|---|---|
| *NOTCH1* | >50% | Calcific degeneration of both bicuspid *and tricuspid* aortic valves in mutation carriers with associated aortic stenosis. Other congenital cardiac anomalies are common. |
| *ACTA2* | <10% | Persistent livedo reticularis, thoracic aortic aneurysms, patent ductus arteriosum, and iris flocculi; all more common in mutation carriers than BAV. |

*Table 26-2 Syndromes Associated With an Increased Risk of BAV*

| Syndrome | Genetic Etiology | Frequency of BAV | Associated Cardiac Involvement | Key Clinical Features |
|---|---|---|---|---|
| Turner | 45, X | ~30% | Coarctation of the aorta, pulmonic stenosis | Chap. 10 |
| Shone complex | Unknown | <50% | Supravalvular mitral ring, parachute mitral valve, subaortic stenosis, coarctation of the aorta | Multiple left-sided obstructive lesions |
| Hypoplastic left heart syndrome | Unknown | ~38% (when aortic atresia absent) | Mitral stenosis and atresia | Mitral and aortic valvular atresia or severe stenosis with consequent hypoplastic left ventricular and ascending aorta/aortic arch |
| Loeys-Dietz | *TGFBR1* and *TGFBR2* mutations | Likely ~10%-20% | Aneurysm, dissection and rupture of the aorta and great vessels; patent ductus | Chap. 10 |

**BIBLIOGRAPHY:**

1. Tadros TM, Klein MD, Shapira OM. Ascending aortic dilatation associated with bicuspid aortic valve: pathophysiology, molecular biology, and clinical implications. *Circulation.* 2009;119:880-890.

2. Fernandes SM, Sanders SP, Khairy P, et al. Morphology of bicuspid aortic valve in children and adolescents. *J Am Coll Cardiol.* 2004;44:1648-1651.

3. Schievink WI, Raissi SS, Maya MM, Velebir A. Screening for intracranial aneurysms in patients with bicuspid aortic valve. *Neurology.* 2010;74:1430-1433.

4. Huntington K, Hunter AGW, Chan KL. A prospective study to assess the frequency of familial clustering of congenital bicuspid aortic valve. *J Am Coll Cardiol.* 1997;30:1809-1812.

5. Biner S, Rafique AM, Ray I, Cuk O, Siegel RJ, Tolstrup K. Aortopathy is prevalent in relatives of bicuspid aortic valve patients. *J Am Coll Cardiol.* 2009;53:2288-2295.

6. Writing Committee M, Bonow RO, Carabello BA, et al. 2008 focused update incorporated into the ACC/AHA 2006 guidelines for the management of patients with valvular heart disease: a report of the American College of Cardiology/American Heart Association Task Force on Practice Guidelines (Writing Committee to revise the 1998 guidelines for the management of patients with valvular heart disease): endorsed by the Society of Cardiovascular Anesthesiologists, Society for Cardiovascular Angiography and Interventions, and Society of Thoracic Surgeons. *Circulation.* 2008;118:e523-e661.

7. Bonow RO, Cheitlin MD, Crawford MH, Douglas PS. Task Force 3: valvular heart disease. *J Am Coll Cardiol.* 2005;45:1334-1340.

8. Writing Group M, Hiratzka LF, Bakris GL, et al. 2010 ACCF/AHA/AATS/ACR/ASA/SCA/SCAI/SIR/STS/SVM guidelines for the diagnosis and management of patients with thoracic aortic disease: a report of the American College of Cardiology Foundation/American Heart Association Task Force on Practice Guidelines, American Association for Thoracic Surgery, American College of Radiology, American Stroke Association, Society of Cardiovascular Anesthesiologists, Society for Cardiovascular Angiography and Interventions, Society of Interventional Radiology, Society of Thoracic Surgeons, and Society for Vascular Medicine. *Circulation.* 2010;121:e266-e369.

9. Garg V, Muth AN, Ransom JF, et al. Mutations in NOTCH1 cause aortic valve disease. *Nature.* 2005;437:270-274.

10. Guo DC, Pannu H, Tran-Fadulu V, et al. Mutations in smooth muscle [alpha]-actin (ACTA2) lead to thoracic aortic aneurysms and dissections. *Nat Genet.* 2007;39:1488-1493.

11. Martin LJ, Ramachandran V, Cripe LH, et al. Evidence in favor of linkage to human chromosomal regions 18q, 5q, and 13q for bicuspid aortic valve and associated cardiovascular malformations. *Hum Genet.* 2007;121:275-284.

## Supplementary Information

**OMIM REFERENCES:**

[1] Bicuspid Aortic Valve Disease; NOTCH1 (#190198)

[2] Familial Thoracic Aortic Aneurysms 6; ACTA2 (#611788)

[3] Hypoplastic Left Heart Syndrome (#241550)

[4] Loeys-Dietz Syndrome: TGFBR1 (#190181) and TGFBR2 (#190182)

*Key Words:* Bicuspid aortic valve, aortic stenosis, aortic regurgitation, endocarditis, thoracic aortic aneurysm, aortic dissection, coarctation of the aorta, Turner syndrome

# 27 Thoracic Aortic Aneurysms and Acute Aortic Dissections

Ellen S. Regalado, Dong-Chuan Guo, and Dianna M. Milewicz

## KEY POINTS

- *Disease summary:*
  - Thoracic aortic aneurysms (TAAs) are an enlargement of the aortic root, ascending aorta, or both; thoracic aneurysms can also involve the descending thoracic aorta but are not the focus of this chapter. Thoracic aortic dissections can originate at the ascending aorta (termed as type A dissection by the Stanford classification) or at the descending aorta just distal to the origin of the left subclavian artery (termed as type B dissection). This chapter reviews the heritable bases of thoracic aortic aneurysms and aortic dissections (TAAD), which are typically considered as a single genetic entity.
  - Approximately 20% of individuals with TAAD but without an identified genetic syndrome also have a first-degree relative with TAAD (termed familial thoracic aortic aneurysm and dissection or FTAAD).
  - FTAAD is primarily inherited in an autosomal dominant pattern with reduced penetrance and variable expressivity.
  - The clinical presentation of FTAAD is variable in terms of age of onset, aortic disease presentation, and associated features such as bicuspid aortic valve, patent ductus arteriosus, other arterial aneurysms, and occlusive vascular disease leading to early-onset stroke and coronary artery disease (CAD).
  - The clinical heterogeneity is due to underlying genetic heterogeneity, with seven genes identified to date for FTAAD.

- *Differential diagnosis:*
  - Marfan syndrome, Loeys-Dietz syndrome, vascular Ehlers-Danlos syndrome, Turner syndrome, aneurysms-osteoarthritis syndrome (AOS)

- *Monogenic forms:*
  - Mutations in the *ACTA2, MYH11, MYLK, TGFBR1, TGFBR2, SMAD3,* and *FBN1* genes have been identified to cause FTAAD. Approximately 25% of FTAAD families have mutations in one of these genes. The identification of large families with FTAAD in which the phenotype is not linked to these genes confirms further genetic heterogeneity for this condition.

- *Family history:*
  - Approximately 20% of individuals with TAAD have a first-degree relative with TAAD. The 80% of patients without a family history are classified as "sporadic" TAAD.

- *Twin studies:*
  - No twin studies have been published for this disease.

- *Environmental factors:*
  - Hypertension and the presence of a bicuspid aortic valve (BAV) are the major risk factors for this disease. Other environmental risk factors include cocaine or other stimulant use, trauma, weight lifting, infections of the aortic wall. Pheochromocytoma, aortic coarctation, inflammatory vasculitis, and polycystic kidney disease are other conditions associated with thoracic aortic dissection.

- *Genome-wide associations and copy number variant analysis:*
  - Single-nucleotide polymorphisms (SNPs) in the linkage disequilibrium block at chromosome 15q21.1 are associated with sporadic TAAD. This block encompasses *FBN1*, the gene that causes Marfan syndrome. Recurrent duplications of 16p13.1 confer an 11-fold increased risk for TAAD.

## Diagnostic Criteria and Clinical Characteristics

### Diagnostic Criteria for TAAD:

**Diagnostic evaluation should include at least one of the following:**

- Enlargement of the aortic root at the sinuses of Valsalva and/or the ascending aorta based on age, gender and body surface area.
- Aortic dissection involving the ascending and/or the descending thoracic aorta.

Familial TAAD is based on the diagnosis of TAAD in at least two first- or second-degree members of a family in which the affected members do not have the features of a known syndrome.

**The presence of syndromic features may be diagnostic for the following conditions:**

- Marfan syndrome, vascular Ehlers-Danlos syndrome, Loeys-Dietz syndrome, Turner syndrome, Aneurysms-osteoarthritis syndrome (AOS)

*Clinical Characteristics:* The major diseases affecting the ascending thoracic aorta are aortic aneurysms (defined as a localized, permanent dilatation of an artery) and acute aortic dissections, collectively designated as TAAD. TAAs may involve the aortic root at the level of the sinuses of Valsalva, the ascending thoracic aorta, or both. The natural history of TAAs is to asymptomatically enlarge over time until an acute tear in the intimal layer leads to an ascending aortic dissection (termed as Stanford type A dissections). With dissection, blood penetrates into the aortic wall and separates the aortic layers, which can lead to aortic rupture and other complications. Type A aortic dissections cause sudden death in up to 40% of individuals, while survivors have a 1% per hour death rate until they undergo emergent surgical repair. Less-deadly aortic dissections originate in the descending thoracic aorta just distal to the branching of the subclavian artery (Stanford type B dissections) and are also part of the TAAD disease spectrum. Therefore, clinical and genetic predictors are needed to identify who is at risk for TAAD.

It has been recognized for many years that there are genetic syndromes that predispose individuals to TAAs and dissections. Most prominent among these syndromes is Marfan syndrome where virtually every affected patient will have a TAA primarily involving the aortic root during their lifetime. Marfan syndrome arises from mutations in the *FBN1* gene encoding fibrillin and is characterized by ocular, musculoskeletal, integumentary, and other cardiovascular features. More recently, Loeys-Dietz syndrome due to mutations in the genes for the transforming growth factor receptors type I and II, *TGFBR1* and *TGFBR2*, respectively, has been described with musculoskeletal, cutaneous, and craniofacial features, along with arterial tortuosity, aneurysms, and dissections. Additionally, mutations in *TGFBR2* confer a high risk for aortic dissections at smaller aortic diameters; some reports indicate that *TGFBR1* mutations confer a similar risk. Recently a new syndromic form of TAAD due to *SMAD3* mutations, referred to as AOS, and characterized by arterial aneurysms and tortuosity, early-onset joint disease such as osteoarthritis, and mild craniofacial abnormalities including hypertelorism and abnormal uvula has been described.

A majority of individuals with TAAD do not have a characterized genetic syndrome and approximately 20% of these individuals have a first-degree relative with TAAD. A predisposition to TAAD in the absence of syndromic features can be inherited in an autosomal dominant manner with decreased penetrance and variable expression, termed as FTAAD. FTAAD exhibits clinical heterogeneity which is apparent in the variation observed within and among families in the following areas: age of onset, location of the TAAs, aortic disease presentation, and progression, risk for early dissection, and associated features, such as BAV, patent ductus arteriosus, abdominal aortic aneurysms, aneurysms, and/or dissections of other arteries (including intracranial aneurysms), and occlusive vascular diseases including early-onset stroke and CAD. Mutations in seven genes have been identified to cause nonsyndromic familial TAAD: *ACTA2, MYH11, MYLK, TGFBR1, TGFBR2, SMAD3,* and *FBN1,* which are responsible for approximately 25% of families with FTAAD. The clinical variability of FTAAD and the identification of multiple genes and loci associated with the disease confirm the genetic heterogeneity of FTAAD.

## Screening and Counseling

*Screening:* In FTAAD families, individuals at risk for inheriting the presumed defective gene predisposing to TAAD should be imaged for aortic disease. If TAAD in the family is associated with only aortic root aneurysms involving the sinuses of Valsalva, echocardiography may be sufficient to screen and monitor aortic disease in at-risk individuals. If the aneurysms involve the ascending aorta, computed tomography (CT), or magnetic resonance (MR) imaging may be necessary to adequately visualize on the ascending aorta. If there are associated features present in the family, such as

intracranial and other arterial aneurysms or BAV, then at-risk family members need to be screened for these diseases also.

The relatives of individuals presenting with sporadic TAAD who do not have a family history or syndromic features are also at an increased risk for TAAD. Current recommendations are to screen the first-degree relatives of these patients for aortic disease, especially in patients presenting with TAAD under the age of 55 years.

Molecular genetic testing for *ACTA2* mutations, which are responsible for 10% to 14% of familial aortic disease, is recommended in patients with FTAAD. Sequencing of the other six genes (*TGFBR1, TGFBR2, MYH11, FBN1, MYLK,* and *SMAD3*) may be considered in individuals with TAAD and other clinical findings associated with mutations in these genes. Genetic testing should also be considered for patients with early-onset sporadic TAAD without other predisposing factors.

*Counseling:* FTAAD is inherited in an autosomal dominant manner with variable expression and reduced penetrance. Each child of an affected parent has up to 50% chance of inheriting the genetic predisposition to TAAD and should undergo aortic imaging. If the causative gene mutation is identified, at-risk relatives should undergo genetic counseling and testing and only the relatives who carry the mutation need to undergo routine aortic and other vascular imaging.

Genotype-phenotype correlations have not been delineated for most of the genes causing FTAAD; however, genotype-phenotype correlation has emerged based on initial data on *ACTA2*. The *ACTA2* p.R258C and p.R258H mutations predispose to TAAD and premature ischemic stroke, whereas the p.R149C mutation predisposes to TAAD and CAD. A recurrent de novo *ACTA2* mutation, p.R179H, causes dysfunction of smooth muscle cells throughout the body, leading to a severe and early-onset vascular disease that includes aortic aneurysms, diffuse cerebrovascular disease characterized by stenosis and fusiform dilatation of cerebral vessels and periventricular white matter hyperintensities on MRI, as well as fixed dilated pupils, hypotonic bladder, malrotation and hypoperistalsis of the gut, and pulmonary hypertension.

## Management and Treatment

*Management:* At-risk individuals need to undergo surveillance for aortic disease and associated vascular disease. Imaging of the thoracic aorta by echocardiography, CT, or MR imaging should be performed at regular intervals for affected and at-risk individuals. Treatment with beta-adrenergic blocking agents that have been shown to slow the growth of aortic aneurysms in patients with Marfan syndrome are recommended. Although medical treatments can slow the enlargement of an aneurysm, the mainstay of treatment to prevent premature deaths due to dissections is surgical repair of the TAA. This is typically recommended when the aneurysm's diameter reaches 5 to 5.5 cm; however, studies on patients presenting with acute type A dissections indicate that up to 60% present with aneurysms smaller than 5.5 cm in diameter. Elective surgical repair of a thoracic aortic aneurysm at smaller diameters (4-5 cm depending on the gene altered) should be considered for patients with a genetic syndrome or other predisposition to acute aortic dissection. Early aortic repair should also be considered for individuals with a documented family history of aortic dissection with minimal aortic enlargement but no causative mutation is identified. Affected individuals and at-risk individuals should also be counseled against smoking, drug abuse, isometric exercises, including heavy weight lifting, and contact sports that could lead to traumatic injury to the chest. Pregnant women with aortic dilatation or genetic predisposition to TAAD should be counseled regarding risk of aortic dissection and/or rupture with pregnancy and the heritable nature of TAAD. Pregnant women should be closely monitored by a cardiologist and a high-risk obstetrician throughout the pregnancy and the postpartum period.

Once a causative gene is identified in a FTAAD family, gene-based management should be pursued. Patients with *TGFBR1* and *TGFBR2* mutations are at risk for aneurysms of the aorta and its branches, along with intracranial aneurysms, and screening for vascular diseases beyond the thoracic aorta is recommended. Prophylactic repair of the aorta when the diameter reaches 4.2 cm by echocardiography should be considered in individuals with *TGFBR2* mutations due to the risk of early acute aortic dissection; some reports indicate that patients with *TGFBR1* mutations are at a similar risk for early dissections. *SMAD3* mutation carriers can present with TAAD and other arterial aneurysms, therefore imaging of the entire aorta, branch vessels, and the cerebrovascular circulation is also recommended in these patients. In addition, aortic dissection in individuals with mildly dilated aortas has been reported for *SMAD3* and so early surgical repair is recommended. Similarly, aortic dissections with minimal enlargement of the ascending aorta have been reported in patients with *MYLK* mutations. *ACTA2* mutations cause early-onset stroke and CAD, and screening for these diseases is recommended, especially for some recurrent mutations in these genes. *MYH11* mutations are identified in families with TAAD associated with patent ductus arteriosus (PDA); in these families, ascending aortic dissections at diameters less than 5 cm are common, leading to the recommendation of repair when the ascending aorta reaches 4.5 cm.

**Surveillance:** Individuals with known aortic disease should be monitored with serial imaging and aortic measurements obtained at reproducible anatomic landmarks. Individuals with a known mutation in a TAAD-associated gene need gene-guided surveillance for aortic disease and associated conditions (eg, intracranial and other arterial aneurysms, CAD, and cerebrovascular disease). In the absence of a genetic marker to identify at-risk individuals, aortic imaging is recommended for first-degree relatives of individuals with TAAD. Because of the variability of age of onset of TAAD, aortic imaging of at-risk relatives in every 2 years is warranted.

**Therapeutics:** Beta-adrenergic blocking agents and other drugs that reduce hemodynamic stress on the aorta and reduce the rate of dilatation should be considered.

## Molecular Genetics and Molecular Mechanism

**ACTA2:** *ACTA2* encodes the smooth muscle-specific alpha-actin, which is a major contractile protein in aortic smooth muscle cells. Missense mutations in *ACTA2* are predicted to affect the structure and assembly of actin filaments as well as its ability to bind to regulatory proteins or the nucleotide. Several *ACTA2* missense mutations have been described and explain 10% to 14% of FTAAD. The ACTA2 protein sequence is highly conserved from human to zebrafish and the *ACTA2* gene is relatively invariant in the general population so all mutations that disrupt amino acids in the protein should be considered as disease causing.

**MYH11:** *MYH11* encodes the smooth muscle-specific isoform of the beta-myosin heavy chain protein, which forms the thick filaments of contractile units in smooth muscle cells. Evidence suggests that mutant MYH11 acts in a dominant-negative manner by altering the stability of the coiled-coil structure in the rod region of the protein through its interaction with wild-type MYH11. A variety of deletions and splice-donor site and missense mutations in *MYH11* predicted to affect the structure and assembly of myosin thick filaments have been identified in families with TAAD associated with PDA. *MYH11* mutations are a rare cause TAAD associated with PDA and responsible for approximately 2% of FTAAD.

**MYLK:** *MYLK* encodes the myosin light chain kinase (MLCK), which is a ubiquitously expressed kinase whose only target of phosphorylation is the 20 kDa regulatory light chain (RLC) of smooth and nonmuscle myosin. MLCK is highly expressed in smooth muscle cells, where phosphorylation of RLC by MLCK initiates the physiologic contraction of smooth muscle cells. A p.R1480X mutation located in the MLCK domain and a variant in the calmodulin (CaM)-binding sequence (p.S1759P) segregated with the disease in two FTAAD families (2%) and are predicted to affect the kinase activity.

**TGFBR1, TGFBR2:** *TGFBR1* and *TGFBR2* are ubiquitously expressed transmembrane receptor proteins with serine-threonine kinase activity in the transforming growth factor beta (TGFβ) signaling pathway responsible for cellular proliferation, differentiation, and extracellular matrix production. TGFBR1 is recruited by TGFBR2 in response to TGFβ-binding which transduces the TGFβ signal intracellularly by recruitment and phosphorylation of SMAD proteins. *TGFBR1* mutations leading to TAAD occur predominantly in the functionally important kinase domain and are predicted to cause loss of function. However, evidence also suggests that the TGFβ pathway may be upregulated in aortic tissue from individuals with *TGFBR2* mutations. The precise function of the abnormal gene products is currently under investigation. Missense mutations that affect the kinase domain of *TGFBR1 and TGFBR2* causing TAA and aortic dissections and other arterial aneurysms have been described in families with and without the syndromic features of Loeys-Dietz syndrome.

**SMAD3:** The SMAD3 protein is a direct mediator of the TGFβ signaling pathway. SMAD3 and SMAD2 proteins form homomeric and heteromeric complexes with SMAD4, which accumulate in the nucleus and regulate expression of target genes. Four *SMAD3* mutations have been identified in FTAAD families: a frameshift mutation (p.N218fs) leading to premature termination of protein translation and three missense mutations, p.E239K, p.R279K, and p.A112V that disrupt highly conserved amino acids and are predicted to disrupt protein function. *SMAD3* frameshift and missense mutations located in exon 6 have also been identified in individuals with the AOS.

**FBN1:** Fibrillin-1 is an extracellular matrix protein that contributes to large structures called microfibrils that participate in the formation and homeostasis of the elastic matrix, in matrix-cell attachments, and possibly in the regulation of selected growth factors. More than 600 *FBN1* mutations that cause Marfan syndrome or related phenotypes have been described. *FBN1* mutations have been identified in patients without Marfan syndrome with both FTAAD and sporadic TAAD.

**Sporadic TAAD:** Genome-wide association analysis identified copy number variants (CNVs) including a recurrent duplication of chromosome 16p13.1 that were enriched in patients with sporadic TAAD compared to population controls. The duplicated 16p13.1 region, which encompasses nine genes including *MYH11*, confers

*Table 27-1 Thoracic Aortic Aneurysm and Dissection-Associated Susceptibility Variants*

| Candidate Gene (Chromosome Location) | Odds Ratio | Frequency of Risk Allele | Associated Disease Phenotype |
|---|---|---|---|
| *FBN1* (15q21.1) | 1.6-1.8 | Various | Sporadic TAAD |
| 16p13.1 duplication | 10.7 | 0.01% among Caucasians | Sporadic TAAD[a] |

[a]Genomic CNVs at 16p13.1 locus were also associated with autism, mental retardation, schizophrenia, attention-deficit hyperactivity disorder.

a 10.7-fold risk for TAAD (Table 27-1). The genome-wide association study (GWAS) also identified various SNPs at the 15q21.1 locus associated with an increased risk for sporadic TAAD with an odds ratio of 1.6 to 1.8. This locus spans the *FBN1* gene suggesting that rare and common genetic variants in this region lead to thoracic aortic disease in patients with Marfan syndrome and sporadic TAAD.

**Genetic Testing:** DNA sequencing analysis is available as a clinical test for all of these genes. Deletion-duplication analysis as well as multigene panels in which some or all of the genes causing Marfan syndrome, Loeys-Dietz syndrome, and FTAAD are sequenced simultaneously are also available. See Gene Reviews for current listing of laboratories offering testing for these genes.

Identification of the disease-causing gene mutation informs timing of aortic repair and need for surveillance for associated features and complications. Genetic testing allows for identification of at-risk relatives needing surveillance and exclusion of increased risk for TAAD in relatives who do not carry the gene mutation.

**Future Directions:** Although the causative gene has been identified in 25% of FTAAD families, there are clearly more genes to be identified for FTAAD. The advent of whole exome and genome sequencing should rapidly increase the rate of novel gene identification for FTAAD.

Further studies need to be pursued to further understand the genetic basis of sporadic TAAD. Ideally, identification of the genes predisposing to nonfamilial disease would be defined so that such variants could be used to identify individuals at risk for TAAD in the general population.

**BIBLIOGRAPHY:**

1. LeMaire SA, McDonald ML, Guo DC, et al. Genome-wide association study identifies a susceptibility locus for thoracic aortic aneurysms and aortic dissections spanning FBN1 at 15q21.1. *Nat Genet.* 2011;43(10):996-1000.
2. Kuang SQ, Guo DC, Prakash SK, et al. Recurrent chromosome 16p13.1 duplications are a risk factor for aortic dissections. *PLoS Genet.* 2011;7(6):e1002118.
3. Roman MJ, Devereux RB, Kramer-Fox R, O'Loughlin J. Two-dimensional echocardiographic aortic root dimensions in normal children and adults. *Am J Cardiol.* 1989;64(8):507-512.
4. Hiratzka LF, Bakris GL, Beckman JA, et al. 2010 ACCF/AHA/AATS/ACR/ASA/SCA/SCAI/SIR/STS/SVM guidelines for the diagnosis and management of patients with thoracic aortic disease: executive summary. A Report of the American College of Cardiology Foundation/American Heart Association Task Force on Practice Guidelines, American Association for Thoracic Surgery, American College of Radiology, American Stroke Association, Society of Cardiovascular Anesthesiologists, Society for Cardiovascular Angiography and Interventions, Society of Interventional Radiology, Society of Thoracic Surgeons, and Society for Vascular Medicine. *Circulation.* 2010.
5. Loeys BL, Schwarze U, Holm T, et al. Aneurysm syndromes caused by mutations in the TGF-beta receptor. *N Engl J Med.* 2006;355(8):788-798.
6. Tran-Fadulu V, Pannu H, Kim DH, et al. Analysis of multigenerational families with thoracic aortic aneurysms and dissections due to TGFBR1 or TGFBR2 mutations. *J Med Genet.* 2009;46(9):607-613.
7. van de Laar IM, Oldenburg RA, Pals G, et al. Mutations in SMAD3 cause a syndromic form of aortic aneurysms and dissections with early-onset osteoarthritis. *Nat Genet.* 2011;43(2):121-126.
8. van de Laar IM, van der Linde D, Oei EH, et al. Phenotypic spectrum of the SMAD3-related aneurysms-osteoarthritis syndrome. *J Med Genet.* 2012;49(1):47-57.
9. Biddinger A, Rocklin M, Coselli J, Milewicz DM. Familial thoracic aortic dilatations and dissections: a case control study. *J Vasc Surg.* 1997;25(3):506-511.
10. Albornoz G, Coady MA, Roberts M, et al. Familial thoracic aortic aneurysms and dissections—incidence, modes of inheritance, and phenotypic patterns. *Ann Thorac Surg.* 2006;82(4):1400-1405.
11. Pannu H, Tran-Fadulu V, Papke CL, et al. MYH11 mutations result in a distinct vascular pathology driven by insulin-like growth factor 1 and angiotensin II. *Hum Mol Genet.* 2007;16(20):3453-3462.
12. Zhu L, Vranckx R, Khau Van KP, et al. Mutations in myosin heavy chain 11 cause a syndrome associating thoracic aortic aneurysm/aortic dissection and patent ductus arteriosus. *Nat Genet.* 2006;38(3):343-349.
13. Guo DC, Pannu H, Papke CL, et al. Mutations in smooth muscle alpha-actin (*ACTA2*) lead to thoracic aortic aneurysms and dissections. *Nat Genet.* 2007;39:1488-1493.
14. Wang L, Guo DC, Cao J, et al. Mutations in myosin light chain kinase cause familial aortic dissections. *Am J Hum Genet.* 2010;87(5):701-707.
15. Regalado ES, Guo DC, Villamizar C, et al. Exome sequencing identifies SMAD3 mutations as a cause of familial thoracic aortic aneurysm and dissection with intracranial and other arterial aneurysms. *Circ Res.* 2011;109(6):680-686.
16. Guo DC, Papke CL, Tran-Fadulu V, et al. Mutations in smooth muscle alpha-actin (ACTA2) cause coronary artery disease, stroke, and Moyamoya disease, along with thoracic aortic disease. *Am J Hum Genet.* 2009;84(5):617-627.
17. Milewicz DM, Ostergaard JR, la-Kokko LM, et al. De novo ACTA2 mutation causes a novel syndrome of multisystemic smooth muscle dysfunction. *Am J Med Genet A.* 2010;152A(10):2437-2443.
18. Pape LA, Tsai TT, Isselbacher EM, et al. Aortic diameter >or = 5.5 cm is not a good predictor of type A aortic dissection: observations from the International Registry of Acute Aortic Dissection (IRAD). *Circulation.* 2007;116(10):1120-1127.
19. Loeys BL, Chen J, Neptune ER, et al. A syndrome of altered cardiovascular, craniofacial, neurocognitive and skeletal development caused by mutations in TGFBR1 or TGFBR2. *Nat Genet.* 2005;37(3):275-281.
20. Beroud C, Collod-Beroud G, Boileau C, Soussi T, Junien C. UMD (Universal mutation database): a generic software to build and analyze locus-specific databases. *Hum Mutat.* 2000;15(1):86-94.
21. Francke U, Berg MA, Tynan K, et al. A Gly1127Ser mutation in an EGF-like domain of the fibrillin-1 gene is a risk factor for ascending aortic aneurysm and dissection. *Am J Hum Genet.* 1995;56(6):1287-1296.

22. Milewicz DM, Michael K, Fisher N, Coselli JS, Markello T, Biddinger A. Fibrillin-1 (FBN1) mutations in patients with thoracic aortic aneurysms. *Circulation*. 1996;94(11):2708-2711.

23. Brautbar A, LeMaire SA, Franco LM, Coselli JS, Milewicz DM, Belmont JW. FBN1 mutations in patients with descending thoracic aortic dissections. *Am J Med Genet A*. 2010;152A(2):413-416.

## Supplementary Information

**OMIM REFERENCES:** will need to limit to relevant OMIM references condition; Gene Name (OMIM#)

[1] Aortic Aneurysm, Familial Thoracic 6; AAT6; Actin, Alpha-2, Smooth Muscle, Aorta; ACTA2 (#102620)

[2] Aortic Aneurysm, Familial Thoracic 4; AAT4; Myosin, Heavy Chain 11, Smooth Muscle; MYH11 (#160745)

[3] Aortic Aneurysm, Familial Thoracic 7; AAT7; Myosin Light Chain Kinase; MYLK (#600922)

[4] Aortic Aneurysm, Familial Thoracic 3; AAT3; Transforming Growth Factor-Beta Receptor, Type II; TGFBR2 (#190182)

[5] Aortic Aneurysm, Familial Thoracic 5; AAT5; Transforming Growth Factor-Beta Receptor, Type I; TGFBR1 (#190181)

[6] Mothers Against Decapentaplegic, Drosophila, Homolog of, 3; SMAD3 (#603109)

[7] Fibrillin 1; FBN1 (#134797)

**Alternative Name:**
- Aortic Aneurysm, Familial Thoracic

*Key Words:* Thoracic aortic aneurysm, thoracic aortic dissection, *ACTA2, MYH11, TGFBR1, TGFBR2, MYLK, SMAD3, FBN1*

# 28 Marfan Syndrome

Reed E. Pyeritz

## KEY POINTS

- *Disease summary:*
  - Marfan syndrome (MFS) is a relatively common heritable disorder of connective tissue that affects many tissues and organs, most prominently the ocular, cardiovascular, and musculoskeletal systems. The natural history predicts early demise, typically from aortic dissection. However, advances in medical and surgical management over the past three decades have extended life expectancy to near normal.

- *Hereditary basis:*
  - MFS is an autosomal dominant condition found in all populations. Reproduction is affected in the most severe cases, so sporadic cases represent one-quarter to one-third of all cases. Most cases (>95%) are due to mutations in *FBN1*, the product of which is a large glycoprotein in the extracellular matrix, especially elastic fibers. The molecule also functions to stabilize the latent transforming growth factor beta (TGFβ) complex, so the pathogenesis to an important extent involves excess canonical and noncanonical signaling.
  - MFS shows no ethnic predilection and occurs at a prevalence of at least 1 per 3 to 5000.

- *Differential diagnosis:*
  - A number of syndromes include ectopia lentis, including an autosomal dominant form due to mutations in *FBN1* with mild MFS-like skeletal features but no involvement of the aorta.
  - Isolated dilatation of the aortic root can occur in the absence of other features of MFS. Dilatation of the ascending aorta, typically of the mid portion more than the sinuses, often accompanies a bicuspid aortic valve. Dilatation, dissection, or both of any portion of the aorta can be inherited as an autosomal dominant trait and can be due to mutations in a growing list of genes (*FBN1, TGFBR1, TGFBR2, ACTA2, MY11, SMAD3, COL3A1*).
  - Many individuals have some features of MFS but fail to meet the revised Ghent criteria. If the individual is a child, then features sufficient to diagnose MFS may emerge with time, and a diagnosis of emerging MFS is useful to ensure that routine follow-up is maintained. Other individuals never warrant a diagnosis of MFS, despite having numerous, mild features. A diagnosis of MASS phenotype is appropriate for the individual with several of the following: mitral valve prolapse (MVP), myopia, an aortic root at the upper limits of normal, mild skeletal features, and striae distensae. This phenotype is of unclear molecular cause, can be inherited as an autosomal dominant trait, and, importantly, is not generally associated with progressive aortic dilatation or dissection.
  - In the Loeys-Dietz syndrome (LDS), the aorta and its branches are tortuous from an early age and the aorta tends to dissect at a smaller diameter than in MFS. The craniofacial characteristics include cleft palate or bifid uvula, craniosynostosis, and increased head circumference. The lens of the eye does not dislocate in LDS. Molecular testing for mutations in *TGFBR1* and *TGFBR2* can distinguish LDS from MFS.

## Diagnostic Criteria and Clinical Characteristics

***Diagnostic Criteria for MFS:*** The revised Ghent criteria have been expanded to include molecular genetic testing. MFS can be diagnosed by

- A family history of documented MFS and presence of ectopia lentis or dilatation of the aortic root.
- In the absence of a family history, presence of ectopia lentis, and dilatation of the aortic root.
- Presence of either ectopia lentis or dilatation of the aortic root and a positive systemic score (a combination of multiple features, including elongated limbs, anterior chest deformity, dural ectasia, pneumothorax, craniofacial features, and MVP: see Management and Treatment section).
- Having a pathogenic mutation in *FBN1* known to cause MFS in either the patient's family of another individual with documented MFS qualifies for a diagnosis of MFS.

***Clinical Characteristics:*** Patients present to medical attention with any of a variety of clinical issues. Occasionally infants are diagnosed because of severe skeletal features; they typically have severe mitral regurgitation as their major cardiovascular issue. At the other end of the phenotypic spectrum, adults with MFS can first present with acute aortic dissection. An ophthalmologist may suggest the diagnosis based on detection of lens subluxation.

Children with the most severe forms of MFS have poorly developed skeletal muscle and a paucity of subcutaneous adipose tissue. However, some people with MFS are robust, and there is a propensity for developing central adiposity in adulthood.

## Screening and Counseling

***Screening:*** When MFS is suspected, such as in a relative of a person with documented MFS or in a person with one, a protocol for establishing or discarding the diagnosis of MFS is as follows:

- In a family in which the pathogenic mutation is known, DNA testing is the most effective and most economic method of screening.

- Echocardiography to detect MVP, mitral regurgitation, dilatation of the sinuses of Valsalva, and aortic regurgitation.
- Detailed ophthalmologic examination with the pupils dilated to detect ectopia lentis.

**Counseling:** MFS is an autosomal dominant syndrome with age dependency and variable expression. True nonpenetrance is uncommon. Males and females are equally frequently and severely affected.

Presymptomatic testing can be performed based on a familial mutation. This is important to reassure those unaffected relatives who can then be spared clinical screening. If the familial mutation is not known or if a person is mutation-positive, then the individual should undergo the clinical screening protocol detailed earlier.

Women with MFS of childbearing age should have their clinical status evaluated carefully before undertaking a pregnancy. An aortic root dimension greater than 40 mm should prompt consideration of valve-sparing aortic root repair to prevent type A aortic dissection in the peripartum period.

☞**GENOTYPE-PHENOTYPE CORRELATION:** Mutations in *FBN1* cause a wide range of conditions that seemingly bear little phenotypic relationship (eg, MFS and Weill-Marchesani syndrome or geleophysic dysplasia). Mutations in the mid portion of the gene that substitute a cysteine residue in a calcium-binding EGF-like motif often produce a more severe, classic form of MFS.

## Management and Treatment

**Ocular Features:** The frequency of ophthalmologic evaluation depends on the nature and severity of the features but should begin as soon as the diagnosis of MFS is suspected. Early correction on visual acuity is crucial to preventing amblyopia. A dislocated lens that severely interferes with vision can be removed and replaced with an implant. This should only be performed by an ocular surgeon well versed in MFS because of the risk of retinal detachment. Long-term evaluation is essential because of the increased risks of cataract and glaucoma. In general, surgery to improve myopia by reshaping the cornea is contraindicated because the cornea is naturally abnormally flat.

**Aortic Dilatation:** Transthoracic echocardiography, begun as soon as the diagnosis of MFS is suspected, is ideal for following the risk of dilatation of the sinuses of Valsalva. The frequency of examination is dictated by the degree of enlargement and its rate of change, but no less than annually is routine. Chronic beta-adrenergic blockade reduces the rate of dilatation and the risk of dissection. Trials of the effectiveness of angiotensin receptor blockade to reduce the rate of, or even reverse, dilatation are ongoing. Factors that determine when to perform prophylactic surgery include the absolute diameter (50 mm or greater in an adult), the rate of change (>5 mm in 6 months), the severity of aortic regurgitation, and a history of aortic dissection in a relative with MFS. Although replacement of the aortic root with a composite graft that includes a mechanical valve is the gold standard, it does require lifelong anticoagulation. Insertion of a conduit that preserves the native aortic valve holds great promise for avoiding the need for anticoagulation, but must be performed before the valve cusps are stretched or fenestrated (typically before moderate aortic regurgitation develops).

**Mitral Valve Prolapse:** Because MVP frequently progresses, regular monitoring is important. Mitral valve repair can lead to an excellent long-term solution to severe mitral regurgitation.

**Aortic Dissection:** Since most acute aortic dissection in MFS involves the root (type A), the best management is preventive, using a combination of beta-blockade and prophylactic root repair. Acute type A dissection is a surgical emergency. Dissection involving the descending thoracic aorta, either acute type B or residual from a type A, can be managed with medication to control blood pressure to the low-normal range. Development of symptoms of further dissection or branch arterial hypoperfusion, or expansion beyond 6 cm should prompt surgical repair. The use of intravascular stents in MFS is generally avoided.

**Skeletal Features:** The indications for repair of pectus excavatum are compromise of either venous return or severe restriction of vital capacity. If possible, repair should be done after the pubertal growth spurt to minimize the chance of recurrence. Scoliosis can progress at any time, even adulthood, but the risk is greatest during skeletal growth. Therefore, regular monitoring by an orthopedist skilled in MFS is essential. Bracing has a role during growth, but often is ineffective for thoracic curvature. While surgical stabilization used to be delayed until growth was nearly complete, new techniques that permit expansion of stabilizing rods enable earlier intervention.

**Pneumothorax:** While a chest tube might be effective initially, pneumothoraces in MFS have a high recurrence risk. Therefore, early consideration of an operative procedure, including pleurodesis, is warranted.

**Pregnancy:** In addition to the 50-50 risk that the offspring of an affected woman will also have MFS, there is an increased risk of aortic dissection during the third trimester of pregnancy, delivery, and even for several months after delivery. The risk of dissection is strongly correlated with aortic root diameter. Any woman with an aortic root greater than 40 mm should consider either not becoming pregnant or undergoing a prophylactic valve-sparing root repair first.

## Molecular Genetics and Molecular Mechanism

**Genes/Loci:**

☞**FIBRILLIN-1/FBN1/15Q21:** Defects in the large extracellular glycoprotein fibrillin-1 cause virtually all cases of classic MFS. A proband with classic MFS has a 95% chance of having a mutation detected in *FBN1*. Fibrillin-1 is an integral component of elastic fibers but also exists in microfibrils unassociated with elastin, such as in the ocular zonules. An important role for fibrillin is modulation of activity of TGFβ signaling through binding of the latent TGFβ binding complex. Mutations in *FBN1* that cause MFS typically result in overactivity of TGFβ. Currently, off-label treatment with agents that interfere with TGFβ synthesis or activity through either its canonical or noncanonical pathways are being studied.

**Genetic Testing:** DNA sequencing and deletion or duplication analyses of *FBN1* are available from number of laboratories in North America and around the world (see Gene Tests http://www.ncbi.nlm.nih.gov/sites/GeneTests/lab/clinical_disease_id/2104?db=genetests).

## Bibliography:

1. David TE, Armstrong S, Maganti M, Colman J, Bradley TJ. Long-term results of aortic valve-sparing operations in patients with Marfan syndrome. *J Thorac Cardiovasc Surg*. 2009;138(4):859-864; discussion 863-864.
2. Dietz HC. Marfan syndrome. http://www.ncbi.nlm.nih.gov/books/NBK1335/. Accessed Dec 1, 2011.
3. Glesby M, Pyeritz R. Association of mitral valve prolapse and systemic abnormalities of connective tissue. *JAMA*. 1989;262:523-528.
4. Lacro RV, Dietz HC, Wruck LM, et al. Rationale and design of a randomized clinical trial of beta blocker therapy (atenolol) vs. angiotensin II receptor blocker therapy (losartan) in individuals with Marfan syndrome. *Am Heart J*. 2007;154:624-631.
5. Loeys B, De Backer J, Van Acker P, et al. Comprehensive molecular screening of the FBN1 gene favors locus homogeneity of classical Marfan syndrome. *Hum Mutat*. 2004;24:140-146.
6. Loeys BL, Dietz HC, Braverman AC, et al. The revised Ghent nosology for the Marfan syndrome. *J Med Genet*. 2010;47:476-485.
7. Pyeritz RE, Loeys B. The 8th international research symposium on the Marfan syndrome and related conditions. *Am J Med Genet*. 2012 Jan;158A(1):42-49.
8. Pyeritz RE. Evaluation of the tall adolescent with some features of Marfan syndrome. *Genet Med*. 2012;14(1):171-177.
9. Pyeritz RE. Marfan syndrome and related disorders. In: Rimoin DL, Pyeritz RE, Korf BR (eds). *Emery and Rimoin's Essential Medical Genetics*. Oxford: Academic Press, 2013;567-74.
10. Rossiter JP, Repke JT, Morales AJ, et al. A prospective longitudinal evaluation of pregnancy in the Marfan syndrome. *Am J Obstet Gynecol*. 1995;173:1599-1606.
11. Shores J, Berger KR, Murphy EA, Pyeritz RE. Chronic β-adrenergic blockade protects the aorta in the Marfan syndrome: a prospective, randomized trial of propranolol. *N Engl J Med*. 1994;330:1335-1341.


## Supplementary Information

### OMIM References:

[1] 154700

[2] 134797

### URLs:

1. National Marfan Foundation: Marfan.org
2. Canadian Marfan Association: Marfan.ca

***Key Words:*** Aortic aneurysm, aortic dissection, mitral valve prolapse, ectopia lentis, dolichostenomelia, arachnodactyly, dural ectasia

# 29 Loeys-Dietz Syndrome

Gretchen Oswald and Harold C. Dietz

## KEY POINTS

- *Disease summary:*
  - Loeys-Dietz syndrome (LDS) is a connective tissue disorder characterized by vascular features (aortic aneurysm or dissection and arterial tortuosity with risk of aneurysm throughout the arterial tree) in addition to a variety of skeletal (scoliosis, pectus deformity, joint laxity, clubfoot or varus deformities, cervical spine instability) and cutaneous features (skin translucency, hernias, abnormal scarring). A proportion of individuals who come to medical attention at young ages have severe craniofacial anomalies (craniosynostosis, cleft palate, hypertelorism) typically associated with more severe vascular disease. The spectrum of physical manifestations is broad.
  - LDS is caused by mutations in *TGFBR1*, *TGFBR2*, *SMAD3*, and *TGFB2* genes.
- *Hereditary basis:*
  - LDS is an autosomal dominant disorder.
- *Differential diagnosis:*
  - It is important to differentiate between LDS and other aortic aneurysm syndromes as systemic manifestations, imaging management, and surgical intervention guidelines differ according to diagnosis.

## Diagnostic Criteria and Clinical Characteristics

**Diagnostic Criteria:** Diagnostic criteria have not been established. Molecular genetic testing plays an important role in distinguishing LDS from other aortic aneurysm syndromes. For the differential diagnosis for LDS, see Table 29-1.

**Clinical Characteristics:** The majority of individuals with LDS will present with aortic root aneurysm or dissection. With three-dimensional computed tomography angiography or magnetic resonance angiography, arterial tortuosity can be a diagnostic clue. The presence of additional skeletal, cutaneous, or allergy findings should prompt genetic evaluation and testing. The first cohort of patients described in 2005 had more severe craniofacial features (LDS1), while other patients presented with more prominent cutaneous features (LDS2). *SMAD3* mutations were described in 2011 and *TGFB2* mutations in 2012, leading to renaming of subtypes of LDS based on genotype (mutations in *TGFBR1*, *TGFBR2*, *SMAD3* and *TGFB2* causing LDS 1, 2, 3, and 4, respectively). All four types of LDS show a broad continuum of associated features. Unless noted, percentages noted in Table 29-2 are reported in individuals with *TGFBR1/2* mutations.

## Screening and Counseling

**Screening:** Consider *TGFBR1/2*, *SMAD3* and *TGFB2* testing in any individual with aortic root aneurysm plus craniofacial, skeletal, and/or the cutaneous features.

Absence of craniofacial, skeletal, or cutaneous features should prompt *ACTA2* and *MYH11* testing (for FTAAD), especially in the presence of vascular occlusive disease or patent ductus arteriosus (PDA). Absence of aortic root aneurysm with aortic or arterial dissection should first prompt *COL3A1* testing (for Ehlers-Danlos, vascular type). Presence of lens dislocation should prompt *FBN1* testing (for Marfan). Absence of any craniofacial, skeletal, or cutaneous features with distal ascending aortic aneurysm may suggest BAV with ascending aneurysm (genes largely unknown).

**Counseling:** LDS is an autosomal dominant disorder. Approximately 25% of individuals with LDS have an affected parent; approximately 75% of individuals represent de novo gene mutations. Individuals with *SMAD3* gene mutations have been reported to have osteoarthritis as an additionally recognized feature, although this is seen in many connective tissue disorders including other etiologies of LDS. Reduced penetrance has rarely been seen and both intrafamilial and interfamilial variability occurs.

## Management and Treatment

Cardiovascular management includes routine echocardiograms to assess for aneurysms; surgical intervention should be considered at smaller dimensions than in other aneurysm syndromes because aortic dissection has been observed with aortic dimensions in the 4-cm range in adults in LDS.

Imaging of the entire vascular tree (head through pelvis) should be performed at baseline and every 12 to 24 months as indicated based on aneurysm detection. Surgical intervention is usually well tolerated as blood vessels are not typically friable.

Blood pressure-lowering medications should be implemented to reduce hemodynamic stress on aorta or arteries. There is mouse model evidence that the angiotensin-receptor-blocker class of medications at optimal dosage may provide enhanced benefit in this patient population.

Lifestyle modifications to reduce stress on vasculature should be encouraged such as avoiding contact or competitive sports and isometric exercises. Agents such as decongestants that stimulate the cardiovascular system should be avoided. Vasoconstrictors (eg, triptans) as management for headaches should also be avoided. Baseline cervical spine imaging (x-rays of neck in the flexion and extension positions) should be performed.

Individuals should be referred to Orthopedics, General Surgery, Gastrointestinal, and Allergy specialists as needed for specific treatment and intervention.

**Table 29-1 Genetic Differential Diagnosis**

| Syndrome | Gene | Associated Features |
|---|---|---|
| Marfan syndrome | *FBN1* | Cardiovascular: aortic root aneurysm<br>Skeletal: scoliosis, pectus deformity, flat feet, arachnodactyly, tall stature<br>Other: ocular lens dislocation |
| Familial thoracic aortic aneurysm disease (FTAAD) | *ACTA2, MYH11, MYLCK(TGFBR1, TGFBR2, SMAD3, TGFB2)*[a] | Cardiovascular: aortic root aneurysm, bicuspid aortic valve (BAV) or patent ductus arteriosus (PDA), vascular occlusive disease<br>Skeletal: none<br>Other: livedo reticularis, iris flocculi |
| Ehlers-Danlos syndrome, vascular type | *COL3A1, TGFB2* | Cardiovascular: typically lack aortic root aneurysm; aneurysm or dissection throughout arterial tree<br>Skeletal: finger joint hypermobility<br>Cutaneous: abnormal scarring, translucent skin, easy bruising<br>Other: bowel or uterine rupture |
| Arterial tortuosity syndrome | *SLC2A10* | Cardiovascular: significant and widespread arterial tortuosity, pulmonary artery and other arterial stenosis; rare aortic aneurysm<br>Skeletal: joint hypermobility<br>Cutaneous: soft, doughy or hyperextensible skin<br>Other: hernias |
| BAV and ascending aneurysm | *NOTCH1* (rare); largely unknown | Cardiovascular: family or personal history of BAV, aortic coarctation, left-sided heart defects, ascending aortic aneurysm<br>Skeletal: none<br>Cutaneous: none |
| Shprintzen-Goldberg syndrome | Unknown *SKI* | Cardiovascular: mitral valve prolapse, rare aortic aneurysm<br>-Skeletal: scoliosis, pectus deformity, arachnodactyly, contractures, joint hypermobility<br>-Other: craniosynostosis, prominent lateral palantine edge, intellectual disability |

[a]Gene mutations in these genes have been reported in both LDS and FTAAD.

Gene names: *FBN1*, fibrillin 1; *COL3A1*, collagen, type 3, alpha-1; *ACTA2*, smooth muscle aortic alpha-actin; *MYH11*, myosin, heavy chain 11, smooth muscle; *TGFBR1*, transforming growth factor beta receptor 1; *TGFBR2*, transforming growth factor beta receptor 2, *SMAD3*, mothers against decapentaplegic, Drosophila, homolog of, 3; *SKI*, SK oncogene; *SLC2a10*, solute carrier family 2, member 10; *NOTCH1*, notch, Drosophila, homolog of, 1.

## Molecular Genetics and Molecular Mechanism

**Syndrome/Gene/Locus:**

LDS1a/1b/transforming growth factor beta receptor 1 (*TGFBR1*)/9q22.33

LDS2a/2b/transforming growth factor beta receptor 2 (*TGFBR2*)/3p24.1

LDS 3/mothers against decapentaplegic, Drosophila, homolog of, 3 (*SMAD3*)/15q22.33

LDS 4/transforming growth factor beta 2

In initial reports, LDS1 referred to individuals with more severe craniofacial features (hypertelorism and cleft palate or bifid uvula) that typically presented with more aggressive aortic root aneurysm growth in childhood (1a for those with *TGFBR1* mutations and 1b for those with *TGFBR2* mutations). LDS2 referred to individuals that typically lacked the craniofacial or skeletal features, but

presented with prominent cutaneous features. Evolving identification of genetic etiologies of LDS and an appreciation for the broad spectrum of clinical variability prompted renaming of LDS subtypes based on genotype.

Importantly, aortic and arterial aneurysm, dissection, and tortuosity are common in all patients with LDS regardless of craniofacial features.

TGFB signaling regulates fundamental cell processes including proliferation, migration, and apoptosis across a wide variety of cell types. TGFBR1 and TGFBR2 are cell-surface receptors that are activated by the binding of the TGFB ligand. Once activated, the receptors phosphorylate SMAD2 and SMAD3 proteins to allow association with SMAD4 and subsequent translocation into the nucleus to regulate transcription of TGFB responsive genes that control cell responses. Mutations in these genes result in paradoxically enhanced TGFB signaling in at least some cell types and tissues.

***Genetic Testing:*** Multiple laboratories throughout the United States offer clinical testing for LDS; some laboratories offer aortic

Table 29-2 **System Involvement**

| System | Manifestation | Incidence |
|---|---|---|
| Cardiovascular or vascular | Aortic root aneurysm or dissection | 95% |
| | Congenital heart defect (PDA, ASD, VSD, BAV) | 9% (LDS3), 35% (LDS1), rare (LDS2) |
| | Arterial tortuosity | 95% |
| | Arterial or nonroot aortic aneurysm | 50% |
| Craniofacial | Broad or bifid uvula | 58% (LDS3), 90% (LDS1), 25% (LDS2) |
| | Hypertelorism | 37% (LDS3), 90% (LDS1), rare (LDS2) |
| | Craniosynostosis | 48% (LDS1) |
| Skeletal | Scoliosis | 55% |
| | Pectus deformity | 16% (LDS3), 68% (LDS1), rare (LDS2) |
| | Joint laxity | 19% (LDS3), 68% (LDS1), 100% (LDS2) |
| | Clubfoot | Common in childhood diagnoses (23%) |
| | Forefoot varus deformity | 39% |
| | Cervical spine instability or cervical abnormalities | 51% |
| Cutaneous | Translucent skin | Very common in diagnoses of all ages |
| | Easy bruising | |
| | Dystrophic scars | |
| | Hernias | |
| Gastrointestinal or allergy | Asthma | 45% |
| | Allergic rhinitis | 48% (*percentages based on pediatric population; less frequent in adulthood*) |
| | Eczema | |
| | Food allergy | 38% |
| | Eosinophilic gastrointestinal disease | 31% |
| | | 10% |

Table 29-3 **Molecular Genetic Testing**

| Gene | Testing Modality | Mutation Type | Proportion of LDS Attributed to Mutations in This Gene |
|---|---|---|---|
| *TGFBR1* | Sequence analysis Deletion analysis | Missense, nonsense, splice-site | ~25% |
| *TGFBR2* | Sequence analysis Deletion analysis | Missense, nonsense, splice-site | ~75% |
| *SMAD3* | Sequence analysis | Missense, nonsense | Rare |
| *TGFB2* | Sequence analysis Deletion analysis | Missense, nonsense | Unknown |

aneurysm panels (see Table 29-3). There is high utility in obtaining a molecular diagnosis for LDS because although there is significant clinical overlap with Marfan syndrome, vascular disease can be more aggressive. Other manifestations including cervical instability and gastrointestinal or allergic disease appear specific to LDS.

## BIBLIOGRAPHY:

1. In: Gene Tests: Medical Genetics Information Resource (database online). Educational Materials: [Loeys-Dietz Syndrome]. Copyright, University of Washington, Seattle. 1993-2011. http://www.genetests.org. Accessed October 31, 2011.

2. Loeys BL, Chen J, Neptune ER, et al. A syndrome of altered cardiovascular, craniofacial, neurocognitive and skeletal development caused by mutations in *TGFBR1* or *TGFBR2*. *Nature Genet.* 2005;37:275-281.

3. van de Laar IMBH, Oldenburg RA, Pals G, et al. Mutations in *SMAD3* cause a syndrome form of aortic aneurysms and dissections with early-onset osteoarthritis. *Nature Genet.* 2011;43:121-126.

4. Lindsay ME, Schepers D, Bolar NA, et al. Loss-of-function mutations in TGFB2 cause a syndromic presentation of thoracic aortic aneurysm. *Nat Genet.* 2012;44(8):922-927.

5. Tran-Fadulu V, Pannu H, Kim DH, et al. Analysis of multigenerational families with thoracic aortic aneurysms and dissections due to *TGFBR1* or *TGFBR2* mutations. *J Med Genet.* 2009;46:607-613.

6. Regalado ES, Guo DC, Villamizar C, et al. Exome sequencing identifies *SMAD3* mutations as a cause of familial thoracic aortic aneurysm and dissection with intracranial and other arterial aneurysms. *Circ Res.* 2011;109(6):680-686.

7.  Loeys BL, Schwarze U, Holm T, et al. Aneurysm syndromes caused by mutations in the TGF-beta receptor. *New Eng J Med.* 2006;355:788-798.

8.  Frischmeyer-Guerrerio PA, et al. A Mendelian Presentation of and Mechanism for Multiple T$_H$2-Mediated Allergic Diseases (submitted).

9.  Erkula G, Sponseller PD, Paulsen LC, Oswald GL, Loeys BL, Dietz HC. Musculoskeletal findings of Loeys-Dietz syndrome. *J Bone Joint Surg Am.* 2010;92(9):1876-1883.

## Supplementary Information

**OMIM REFERENCES:**

[1] Loeys-Dietz Syndrome, Type 1A (#609192)

[2] Loeys-Dietz Syndrome, Type 1B (#610168)

[3] Loeys-Dietz Syndrome, Type 2A (#608967)

[4] Loeys-Dietz Syndrome, Type 2B (#610380)

[5] Loeys-Dietz Syndrome, Type 3; LDS1C (#613795)

[6] Loeys-Dietz Syndrome, Type 4; (#614816)

**Alternative Name:**
•  Marfan Syndrome, Type 2

*Key Words:* Aortic aneurysm, dissection, arterial tortuosity, *TGFBR1*, *TGFBR2*, *SMAD3*, *TGFB2*, connective tissue

# 30 Abdominal Aortic Aneurysm

S. Helena Kuivaniemi, Gerard C. Tromp, Irene Hinterseher, and David J. Carey

## KEY POINTS

- *Disease summary:*
  - Abdominal aortic aneurysms (AAAs), defined as dilatations of the aorta, are a complex disease with both genetic and environmental risk factors.
  - Prevalence: 1% to 2% of Caucasian populations harbor AAAs in industrialized countries. Prevalence increases with age to about 10% among men over 65 years of age.
  - AAA is the 17th leading cause of death in the United States, with approximately 15,000 deaths per year.
  - Risk factors: The most important known risk factors are smoking, positive family history, advanced age, and male sex. Elevated cholesterol levels and hypertension are mild risk factors. Diabetes, African-American ethnicity, and female sex are protective factors.
  - AAAs have a complex, poorly understood pathophysiology, in which inflammation, smooth muscle cell apoptosis, reactive oxygen species, extracellular matrix degradation, and activation of matrix metalloproteinases play a role.

- *Differential diagnosis:*
  - Diverticulitis, renal colic, and gastrointestinal hemorrhage belong to the differential diagnosis of ruptured AAA.

- *Monogenic forms:*
  - Aortic aneurysms can be found in patients with the Ehlers-Danlos syndrome type IV, the Marfan syndrome, and fibromuscular dysplasia. These Mendelian diseases are far less common than AAA and patients with these diseases constitute only a very small fraction of AAA patients, representing a rare form of AAA.

- *Family history:*
  - Family history of AAA is an important risk factor for AAA with an odds ratio (OR) = 1.96 (95% CI: 1.68-2.28) determined in population-based screening studies. Two formal segregation analyses have been published for AAA. Both studies demonstrated statistically significant evidence for a genetic model. In one study an autosomal recessive model for a major gene had the best fit, whereas in the other study an autosomal dominant model for a major gene was the best fit for the familial aggregation of AAA in their sample. A third report, in which a large collection of AAA families with 233 multiplex families was described, found that 72% of the AAA families were consistent with an autosomal recessive pattern, while 25% showed an autosomal dominant pattern of inheritance. Not finding a single mode of inheritance is consistent with AAA being a multifactorial disease where different loci can have distinct modes of inheritance.

- *Twin studies:*
  - Only four case reports on twins with AAA have been published.

- *Environmental factors:*
  - Smoking is the most important identified risk factor with an OR = 3.34 (95% CI: 3.04-3.67) for men and 3.80 (95% CI: 1.57-9.20) for women with a history of smoking.

- *DNA linkage studies:*
  - Shibamura and colleagues studied 119 AAA families using an affected relative pair (ARP) approach with sex and number of affected relatives, and their interactions as covariates, allowing for genetic heterogeneity. Using a two-phase, two-stage study design, a whole genome scan was completed using approximately 400 microsatellite markers. The first phase analyzed 36 multiplex families with 78 ARPs using sex and the number of first-degree relatives as covariates. Twelve regions on eight chromosomes (3, 4, 5, 6, 9, 14, 19, 21) were identified as being worthy of follow-up with $p$ less than 0.05. The second stage of phase 1 was to genotype additional markers in regions giving positive results. Phase 2 included testing of positive markers in 83 new multiplex families, which included 157 ARPs. After detailed follow-up analysis with a combined set of 235 ARPs, significant linkage was found on chromosomes 4q31 (LOD score = 3.73, $p$ = .0012) and 19q13 (LOD score = 4.75, $p$ = .00014). These genomic regions have been designated as AAA2 and AAA1 susceptibility loci, respectively, in Online Mendelian Inheritance in Man (OMIM). In addition, a second locus on chromosome 4, at 4q12, had a LOD of 3.13 ($p$ = .0042).

- *Genome-wide associations:*
  - Elmore and colleagues carried out a genome-wide genetic association study (GWAS) for AAAs using pooled DNA samples and a case-control design. They found a haplotype on chromosome 3p12.3 associated with AAA. One single-nucleotide polymorphism (SNP) in this region (rs7635818) was genotyped in a total of 502 cases and 736 controls from the original study population ($p$ = .017) and 448 cases and 410 controls from an independent replication sample ($p$ = .013; combined $p$ = .0028; combined OR = 1.33). An even stronger association with AAA was observed in a subset of smokers (391 cases, 241 controls, $p$ = .00041, OR = 1.80), which represent the highest-risk group for AAA. The AAA-associated haplotype is located 200 kbp upstream of the *CNTN3* gene transcription start site.

- *Other significant genetic studies:*
  - Using 2836 AAA cases and 16,732 controls, a large consortium tested a variant, rs10757278, discovered from another GWAS on coronary artery disease, in five different vascular phenotypes: coronary artery disease, peripheral arterial disease, atherosclerotic stroke, intracranial aneurysms, and AAA. The SNP rs10757278 was associated with AAA ($p = 1.2 \times 10^{-12}$; OR = 1.31, 95% CI: 1.22-1.42). This is the first genetic variant associated with AAA, intracranial aneurysms and other cardiovascular diseases and it suggests a common pathway in vascular disease etiology. The SNP rs10757278 is located on chromosome 9p21 in a gene called *ANRIL*, a noncoding RNA. It is of interest that another SNP, rs10811661, known to be associated with type 2 diabetes and located 10 kb away from rs10757278, was not associated with AAA. This finding is in agreement with epidemiologic data demonstrating that diabetes is not a risk factor for AAA.

# Diagnostic Criteria and Clinical Characteristics

### *Diagnostic Criteria for AAA:*
**Diagnostic evaluation should include at least one of the following:**

- **Physical examination:** feeling for pulsatile abdominal mass and auscultation to detect bruit. Physical examination will miss AAA in about 50% of the time. Examination should, therefore, always include abdominal ultrasonography.
- Abdominal ultrasonography examination includes measurement of the aorta in anterior-posterior, transverse, and longitudinal dimensions. Once AAA is diagnosed, imaging should be repeated every 3 to 12 months until the AAA grows greater than 1 cm/y or it has reached 5.5 cm and surgical intervention is warranted.
- Computed tomographic angiography should be done before repair operation.

### *Clinical Characteristics:*
- **Definition:** AAA is defined as a dilatation of infrarenal aorta to a diameter greater than 3 cm.
- **Symptoms and signs:** Most AAAs are asymptomatic and silent until rupture and sudden death. Patients might experience abdominal discomfort; back pain; feel abdominal pulsation; pain in legs, chest or groin; anorexia nausea and vomiting; constipation; and dyspnea.
- **Rupture of AAA:** Mortality associated with ruptured AAA is greater than 60%. About half of patients with ruptured AAA have a triad of hypotension, back pain, and pulsatile abdominal mass.

# Screening and Counseling

***Screening:*** Abdominal ultrasonography examination is a cheap, noninvasive, and effective method for finding AAAs. Ultrasonography usually underestimates the size of an AAA by about 0.3 cm. Patients who should definitively undergo screening for AAA include

- Male smokers who are greater than 60 years of age
- Individuals who have positive family history for AAA and are greater than 50 years of age
- Individuals with a connective tissue disorder (Marfan syndrome, Ehlers-Danlos syndrome type IV, and fibromuscular dysplasia)
- Individuals with arteritis, for example Takayasu and giant cell arteritis

***Counseling:*** Individuals with positive family history for AAA and greater than 50 years of age should be encouraged to have abdominal ultrasonography examination to find aortic dilatation. Patients with positive family history for AAA often have a more aggressive disease in that the AAA develops at earlier age, grows faster, and is more prone to rupture.

# Management and Treatment

***Management:*** Presently, the only option available for AAA patients is open or endovascular surgical repair. These types of procedures are only recommended, however, when patients have AAAs *greater than or equal to* 5.5 cm in diameter, where risk of rupture outweighs risk of procedure.

# Molecular Genetics and Molecular Mechanism

***Genetic Testing:*** None currently available
***Future Directions:*** AAAs are a chronic disease whose pathogenesis is poorly understood. The lack of knowledge about the underlying molecular mechanisms is hampering the development of treatment modalities. Currently surgical intervention is successful, but is used at a late stage of the disease leaving patients with small AAAs in the unpleasant situation of having to "wait and see" until the AAA has grown large enough for the risk of rupture and its attendant morbidity and mortality to outweigh the interventional risk. Development of methods to slow down the growth of small AAAs requires better understanding of the molecular pathways involved in this process.

Unraveling the pathophysiology of AAA and identifying the specific risk factors for AAA will require interdisciplinary approaches. Identification of susceptibility genes, in which sequence variants confer risk to the AAA phenotype, can be accomplished through the integration of expression, linkage, and genetic association analyses. Risk loci have been identified through linkage studies as well as GWAS, see Table 30-1. Furthermore, genome-wide studies with large sample sizes are needed to identify additional genetic factors which contribute to the development, growth, and rupture of AAA. The identified risk factors could provide the basis for genetic testing to identify individuals harboring AAA before the rupture occurs and leads to sudden death. Identification of the AAA susceptibility

*Table 30-1 **Genomic Regions Harboring Susceptibility Variants***

| Approach Used | Chromosomal Region | Marker | LOD Score | Frequency of Risk Allele |
|---|---|---|---|---|
| DNA linkage study | 19q13 | D19S416 | 4.75 | NA |
| DNA linkage study | 4q31 | D4S1644 | 3.73 | NA |
| GWAS | 3p12.3 | rs7635818 | NA | 0.42 |
| Candidate SNP study | 9p21 | rs10757278 | NA | 0.48 |

gene(s) will also allow us to develop animal models for testing new therapies.

## BIBLIOGRAPHY:

1. Beckman JA, Creager MA. Aortic aneurysms: clinical evaluation. In: Creager MA, Dzau VJ, Loscalzo J, eds. *Vasc Med.* Philadelphia, PA: Saunders Elsevier, Inc.; 2006:560-569.

2. Lederle FA, Johnson GR, Wilson SE, et al. Prevalence and associations of abdominal aortic aneurysm detected through screening. Aneurysm Detection and Management (ADAM) Veterans Affairs Cooperative Study Group. *Ann Intern Med.* 1997;126:441-449.

3. Boddy AM, Lenk GM, Lillvis JH, Nischan J, Kyo Y, Kuivaniemi H. Basic research studies to understand aneurysm disease. *Drug News Perspect.* 2008;21:142-148.

4. Kuivaniemi H, Shibamura H, Arthur C, et al. Familial abdominal aortic aneurysms: collection of 233 multiplex families. *J Vasc Surg.* 2003;37:340-345.

5. Lederle FA, Johnson GR, Wilson SE. Abdominal aortic aneurysm in women. *J Vasc Surg.* 2001;34:122-126.

6. Shibamura H, Olson JM, van Vlijmen-van Keulen C, et al. Genome scan for familial abdominal aortic aneurysm using sex and family history as covariates suggests genetic heterogeneity and identifies linkage to chromosome 19q13. *Circulation.* 2004;109:2103-2108.

7. Elmore JR, Obmann MA, Kuivaniemi H, et al. Identification of a genetic variant associated with abdominal aortic aneurysms on chromosome 3p12.3 by genome wide association. *J Vasc Surg.* 2009;49:1525-1531.

8. Helgadottir A, Thorleifsson G, Magnusson KP, et al. A sequence variant on chromosome 9p21 confers risk of both abdominal aortic aneurysm and intracranial aneurysm in addition to coronary artery disease. *Nat Genet.* 2008;40:217-224.

9. Ogata T, MacKean GL, Cole CW, et al. The life-time prevalence of abdominal aortic aneurysms among siblings of aneurysm patients is eight-fold higher than among siblings of spouses; an analysis of 187 aneurysm families in Nova Scotia, Canada. *J Vasc Surg.* 2005;42:891-897.

10. Lenk GM, Tromp G, Weinsheimer S, Gatalica Z, Berguer R, Kuivaniemi H. Whole genome expression profiling reveals a significant role for immune function in human abdominal aortic aneurysms. *BMC Genomics.* 2007;8:237.

11. Nischan J, Gatalica Z, Curtis M, Lenk GM, Tromp G, Kuivaniemi H. Binding sites for Ets family of transcription factors dominate the promoter regions of differentially expressed genes in abdominal aortic aneurysms. *Circ Cardiovasc Genet.* 2009;2(6):565-572.

## Supplementary Information

### OMIM REFERENCES:

[1] Aortic Aneurysm, Abdominal (# 100070)

[2] Aortic Aneurysm, Familial Abdominal 1 (# %609781)

[3] Aortic Aneurysm, Familial Abdominal 2 (#%609782)

[4] Aortic Aneurysm, Familial Abdominal 3 (# %611891)

### Alternative Names:

- AAA
- AAA1
- Aneurysm, Abdominal Aortic
- Abdominal Aortic Aneurysm
- Arteriomegaly, Included
- Aneurysms, Peripheral, Included

*Key Words:* 19q13, 4q31, 3p12.3, 9p21, inflammation, ultrasonography screening, contactin-3, extracellular matrix

# 31 Sickle Cell Anemia

Abdulrahman Alsultan and Martin H. Steinberg

## KEY POINTS

- *Disease summary:*
  - Sickle cell anemia (HbSS) is caused by homozygosity for a point mutation in the β-globin gene (*HBB*) that leads to replacement of glutamic acid by valine at position six of the β-globin chain of hemoglobin (β6 Glu>Val) leading to the synthesis of abnormal β-globin chains. The HbS β-globin chain pairs with normal α-globin chains to produce sickle hemoglobin or HbS ($\alpha2\beta^S2$).
  - Clinical presentation of HbSS is heterogeneous among patients even though all cases have the identical HbS mutation suggesting modification of the disease phenotype by other genes and the environment.
  - Complications can be related to sickle vaso-occlusion, for example, acute painful episodes, osteonecrosis, and acute chest syndrome and also be associated with the degree of hemolysis, for example, gallbladder disease, stroke, priapism, leg ulcers, and pulmonary hypertension.
  - The major treatment modalities include blood transfusion for severe anemia, stem cell transplantation for selected cases and administration of hydroxyurea (hydroxycarbamide) to stimulate the production of fetal hemoglobin (HbF) that by virtue of its effects on HbS polymerization, can decrease most complications of disease and extend lifespan.

- *Hereditary basis:*
  - HbSS is inherited in an autosomal recessive fashion. If both parents are carriers, each child has a 25% risk of inheriting the disease.
  - HbSS can be seen in successive generations given the high carrier rates in some populations.

- *Differential diagnosis:*
  - It is important to distinguish HbSS from other forms of sickle cell disease that are shown in Table 31-1, especially in genetic counseling.

## Diagnostic Criteria and Clinical Characteristics

***Diagnostic Criteria for Sickle Cell Anemia:*** HbSS is a monogenic disease caused by homozygosity for a point mutation in the *HBB* that leads to replacement of glutamic acid by valine at position six of β-globin (β6 Glu>Val). Diagnosis of HbSS can be established based on family studies, history and physical examination, hematologic studies and by separating the hemoglobin fractions present in red blood cells by high-performance liquid chromatography (HPLC) or some other similarly sensitive and rapid method (Table 31-1). The definitive method of ascertaining the presence of HbS and/or identifying homozygosity or heterozygosity for the HbS ($\beta^S$) mutation is based on DNA testing. The term sickle cell disease includes HbSS and other genotypes as shown in Table 31-1. The large range of HbF levels reflects different haplotypes of the HbS-globin gene.

***Clinical Characteristics:*** Clinical presentation of HbSS is widely heterogeneous among patients and the severity and extent of HbSS-related complications are difficult to predict in any individual patient. HbSS-related complications include acute painful episodes, osteonecrosis, acute chest syndrome, gallbladder disease, splenic dysfunction, splenic sequestration, stroke, priapism, leg ulcers, pulmonary hypertension, renal failure, proliferative retinopathy, and predisposition to infections, for example, osteomyelitis. The rate of complications in HbSC disease and HbS-β⁺ thalassemia is about half of that seen in HbSS, HbSS-∝ thalassemia, and HbS-β⁰ thalassemia.

## Screening and Counseling

***Screening:*** Neonatal screening for HbSS is now universal in the United States and many other parts of the world and was shown to decrease HbSS-related fatality in infancy. Early diagnosis allows prompt initiation of comprehensive clinical care that includes starting prophylactic penicillin to prevent serious pneumococcal infections and educating parents about other potential complications in HbSS. Children with HbSS are also screened using transcranial Doppler ultrasound to measure flow rate in the major cerebral arteries. Randomized controlled studies showed that a high flow rate was predictive of a future stroke and that prophylactic transfusion could prevent most new and recurrent strokes.

Newborn screening also detects carriers of sickle cell trait. Parents of these individuals are usually notified and in some states, counseling is provided. Outside of newborn screening programs, general population screening for sickle cell trait is not indicated,

*Table 31-1 Types of Sickle Cell Disease*

| Type | Hemoglobin HPLC | | | | | Severity |
| | HbA | HbA2 | HbF | HbS | Other | |
| --- | --- | --- | --- | --- | --- | --- |
| HbSS (sickle cell anemia) | 0 | <3.6 | <10 | 90-95 | | Severe |
| HbSS-α thalassemia | 0 | <3.6 | <10 | 90-95 | Low MCV | Severe |
| HbS-β⁰ thalassemia | 0 | ≥3.6 | <10 | 90-95 | | Severe |
| HbS-β⁺ thalassemia | 5-30 | ≥3.6 | <10 | 60-90 | | Moderate |
| HbSC disease | 0 | <3.6 | <3 | 45-50 | HbC 45-50 | Moderate |
| HbS-O_Arab | 0 | <3.6 | <3 | 45-50 | Hb O_Arab 45-50 | Severe |
| HbS-HPFH | 0 | <3.6 | 20-40 | 60-80 | | Mild |

HPFH, hereditary persistence of fetal hemoglobin.

but instead should be limited to individuals from at-risk populations who are pregnant or are planning a pregnancy, who are in need of cardiothoracic surgery, are blood donors or who have bleeding into the anterior chamber of the eye, or hematuria.

**Counseling:** HbSS is inherited in an autosomal recessive fashion. If both parents are carriers, each child has a 25% risk of inheriting the disease. Antenatal diagnosis of sickle cell disease is available. Before considering prenatal diagnosis, parents should be counseled about the risks of the procedure, the consequences of a positive diagnosis, the likelihood of an affected fetus, and options for termination. Establishing the parental globin gene mutations by DNA-based testing is a prerequisite. DNA testing of chorionic villus samples or amniotic fluid cells is available.

☞GENOTYPE-PHENOTYPE CORRELATION: HbSS phenotype is widely variable. HbF level and coinheritance of α-thalassemia are known modifiers of the severity of HbSS. High HbF ameliorates complications related to sickle vaso-occlusion like pain crisis and acute chest syndrome. Coinheritance of α-thalassemia decreases the degree of hemolysis and increases baseline hemoglobin so it minimizes the frequency of complications related to the hemolytic process like leg ulcers, stroke, and cholelithiasis. Polymorphisms in genes involved in inflammation, for example, TGF-β or BMP pathway might also influence the severity of HbSS.

## Management and Treatment

**Prophylactic Measures:** Penicillin prophylaxis needs to be started as soon as the diagnosis of HbSS is established. Penicillin has to be continued at least for the first 5 years of life to prevent life-threatening infections. Folic acid supplementation is often used as chronic hemolysis increases its requirements and some diets lack sufficient folate. HbSS patients need to be vaccinated against encapsulated organisms, for example, *Streptococcus pneumoniae* and receive yearly influenza vaccine.

**Hydroxyurea:** It is a chemotherapeutic agent that has been shown to increase HbF level in HbSS and lessen the frequency and severity of pain crisis and acute chest syndrome and increase baseline hemoglobin level. Side effects are mainly related to bone marrow suppression. Concerns about risk of infertility or increased risk of secondary malignancy may have limited its use, however, there is no evidence of such complications among HbSS patients

on hydroxyurea. Most adults should take hydroxyurea and recently completed studies in babies suggest that it is reasonable to start this drug at an early age, however long-term studies are needed. In adults, in addition to reducing the morbidity of disease, it is likely that the lifespan of patients taking this drug is increased.

**Blood Transfusion:**
- **Indications for acute blood transfusion:** acute splenic sequestration, aplastic crisis, hyperhemolysis, acute chest syndrome, stroke, and preparation for surgery
- **Indications for chronic blood transfusion:** stroke, recurrent acute chest syndrome, recurrent splenic sequestration, and severe anemia from renal disease

**Hematopoietic Stem Cell Transplant:** It is the only available cure for HbSS. However, treatment-related complications and lack of human leukocyte antigen (HLA)-matched related donors limit the use of such modality of treatment.

**Gene Therapy:** No patient has yet been treated. Therapeutic trials are planned and a single patient with HbE-β thalassemia has responded well to gene therapy.

## Molecular Genetics and Molecular Mechanism

**Syndrome/Gene/Locus:**

Sickle cell anemia/β-globin (HBB)/11p15.4

The most predominant type of hemoglobin present beyond 6 months of age is the adult hemoglobin (HbA). HbA consists of two α- and two β-globin chains. Mutations in *HBB* can cause either an abnormal β-globin like HbS or a decrease or absence of β-globin that is known as β-thalassemia. Polymerization of deoxy sickle hemoglobin (deoxy HbS) injures the sickle erythrocyte. Damaged sickle cells die prematurely (hemolytic anemia), mainly by being trapped in the reticuloendothelial system but some hemolyze intravascularly. Sickle erythrocytes occlude blood vessels of all sizes. The complex pathophysiology resulting from sickle vaso-occlusion and hemolytic anemia includes at a minimum: abnormal erythrocyte volume regulation, impaired nitric oxide bioavailability, reperfusion injury, inflammation and oxidant damage, abnormal intercellular interactions, endothelial injury and leukocyte and platelet activation. In sickle cell trait,

HbS levels are less than 40% of total hemoglobin so in normoxic conditions, these cells do not deform when deoxygenated except in the renal medulla where pH and oxygen levels are low and the solute concentration is high. As a result sickle cell trait is not considered a form of sickle cell disease.

*Genetic Testing:* DNA analysis is clinically available for sickle cell anemia (see Gene Tests http://www.ncbi.nlm.nih.gov/sites/GeneTests/lab/mim/603903).

## BIBLIOGRAPHY:

1. Steinberg MH. Predicting clinical severity in sickle cell anaemia. *Br J Haematol.* 2005;129:465-481.

2. Consensus conference. Newborn screening for sickle cell disease and other hemoglobinopathies. *JAMA.* 1987;258:1205-1209.

3. Adams RJ, McKie VC, Hsu L, et al. Prevention of a first stroke by transfusions in children with sickle cell anemia and abnormal results on transcranial Doppler ultrasonography. *N Engl J Med.* 1998;339:5-11.

4. Gaston MH, Verter JI, Woods G, et al. Prophylaxis with oral penicillin in children with sickle cell anemia. A randomized trial. *N Engl J Med.* 1986;314:1593-1599.

5. Charache S, Terrin ML, Moore RD, et al. Effect of hydroxyurea on the frequency of painful crises in sickle cell anemia. Investigators of the Multicenter Study of Hydroxyurea in Sickle Cell Anemia. *N Engl J Med.* 1995;332:1317-1322.

6. Charache S, Barton FB, Moore RD, et al. Hydroxyurea and sickle cell anemia. Clinical utility of a myelosuppressive "switching" agent. The Multicenter Study of Hydroxyurea in Sickle Cell Anemia. *Medicine (Baltimore).* 1996;75:300-326.

7. Steinberg MH, McCarthy WF, Castro O, et al. The risks and benefits of long-term use of hydroxyurea in sickle cell anemia: a 17.5 year follow-up. *Am J Hematol.* 2010;85:403-408.

8. Steinberg MH, Barton F, Castro O, et al. Effect of hydroxyurea on mortality and morbidity in adult sickle cell anemia: risks and benefits up to 9 years of treatment. *JAMA.* 2003;289:1645-1651.

9. Hsieh MM, Fitzhugh CD, Tisdale JF. Allogeneic hematopoietic stem cell transplantation for sickle cell disease: the time is now. *Blood.* 2011;118:1197-1207.

10. Kato GJ, Gladwin MT, Steinberg MH. Deconstructing sickle cell disease: reappraisal of the role of hemolysis in the development of clinical subphenotypes. *Blood Rev.* 2007;21:37-47.

11. Kato GJ, Hebbel RP, Steinberg MH, Gladwin MT. Vasculopathy in sickle cell disease: biology, pathophysiology, genetics, translational medicine, and new research directions. *Am J Hematol.* 2009;84: 618-625.

## Supplementary Information

### OMIM REFERENCE:

[1] Sickle Cell Anemia; HBB (#603903)

### Alternative Name:

• Sickle Cell Disease

*Key Words:* Sickle cell anemia, acute painful episodes, osteonecrosis, acute chest syndrome, gallbladder disease, splenic dysfunction, splenic sequestration, stroke, priapism, leg ulcers, pulmonary hypertension, renal failure, proliferative retinopathy, hydroxyurea

# 32 Hemophilia

Christopher E. Walsh

## KEY POINTS

- *Disease summary:*
  - The hemophilia A and B are sex-linked disorders leading to deficiencies of coagulation factor VIII (FVIII) and FIX, respectively. Bleeding is the hallmark of the disease, principally joint and soft tissue bleeding. The level of factor is directly related to the clinical severity of the disease where severe disease is less than 1% activity, moderate disease is 1% to 5%, and mild disease is greater than 5%. FXI deficiency (also known as hemophilia C), bleeding classically is not directly related to factor level and occurs several days after initial trauma or surgery. Antibodies to factor proteins termed inhibitors occur in 20% to 30% of FVIII patients and 2% to 4% of FIX patients. Inhibitor levels greater than 5 Bethesda units (BUI) require the use of bypassing agents such as Novoseven (FVIIa) and/or FVIII inhibitor bypassing activity (FEIBA).

- *Differential diagnosis:*
  - Bleeding disorders such as von Willebrand disease, disseminated intravascular coagulopathy (DIC), liver disease, and acquired hemophilia may manifest clinically in a similar fashion.

- *Monogenic forms:*
  - See above.

- *Family history:*
  - 30% of sex-linked disorders occur de novo, however, family history of hemophilia and inhibitor is important.

- *Twin studies:*
  - Approximately 88% concordance rate of phenotype and inhibitor risk.

- *Environmental factors:*
  - Involved with development of inhibitor such as time of factor infusion with coexisting inflammatory insult, high frequency of factor (time of surgery).

- *Genome-wide associations:*
  - Modifier genes may affect predisposition for inhibitor development.

- *Pharmacogenomics:*
  - The half-lives of FVIII and FIX are 12 and 20 hours, respectively. Intravenous infusions of recombinant or plasma-purified factors are the standard of care. New long-acting factors are in phase II or III of clinical trials.

## Diagnostic Criteria and Clinical Characteristics

***Diagnostic Criteria for Hemophilia:*** **Diagnostic evaluation should include at least one of the following (see Figure 32-1 algorithm):**

- Bleeding phenotype
  - Prolonged partial thromboplastin time (PTT) with normal prothrombin time (PT), normal platelet count
  - FVIII or FIX levels measured lower than normal (normal range 50%-150%)
  - FVIII and FIX inhibitor levels measured (normal <0.6 BUI)
- Gold standard—mutational analysis of FVIII and FIX genes

***Clinical Characteristics:*** Joint bleeding (spontaneous), muscle bleeding (spontaneous), epistaxis or gum bleeding, intracranial/subdural/epidural/subarachnoid bleeding, hematuria; circumcision bleeding

## Screening and Counseling

***Screening:*** Screening tests include PTT, PT, complete blood count (CBC) or different factor levels, von Willebrand levels, Bethesda titer.

***Counseling:***
- Inheritance, penetrance
- Sex-linked recessive and with maternal transmission to male offspring who are affected. Female carriers may be affected due to lyonization and can have severe disease. Female offspring can rarely carry mutations in each allele and become severely affected.
- Penetrance—100%

☞**GENOTYPE-PHENOTYPE CORRELATION:** FVIII mutations by percentage include inversion 22 translocation, large deletions, splice mutations, and nonsense and missense mutations. The majority of mutations lead to severe phenotype and in general a higher risk of inhibitor formation. FIX mutations are predominantly missense mutations with a significantly lower risk of inhibitor.

## Management and Treatment

***Management:***
- Infusion of factor is performed either on demand after bleeding has occurred or prophylactic infusions used to prevent bleeding. On demand therapy is typically used for patients with mild disease (0-3 bleeding episodes/y). Factor is administered after bleeding has occurred.

**Diagnosis of Hemophilia**

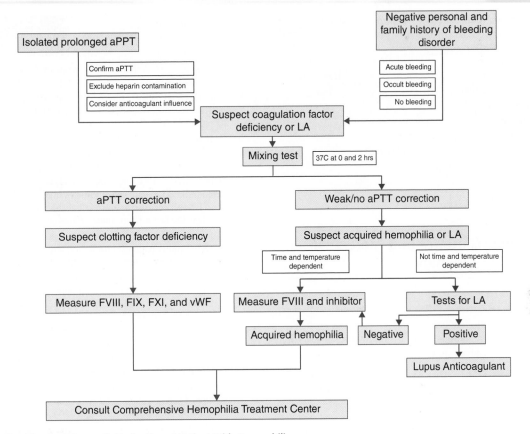

*Figure 32-1* Algorithm for Diagnostic Evaluation of Patient With Hemophilia.

- While factor prophylaxis for children is the standard of care (estimated at 80% of hemophilic children on prophylaxis), prophylaxis in adolescents and adults has not been embraced (prophylaxis estimated at 30%-50%). In children with severe hemophilia prophylaxis has been demonstrated to significantly reduce joint bleeding that correlates with near-normal joint outcomes. Prophylaxis dosing is typically three times a week for FVIII patients (30-50 U/kg) and twice a week for FIX (30-50 U/kg). Maintaining trough levels of factor greater than 1% significantly reduces bleeding, therefore dosing of factor is performed with this goal in mind. The relatively short half-life of FVIII (10-12 hours) and FIX (18-22 hours) requires multiple weekly infusions to maintain a trough level greater than 1%.

- Inhibitors or antibodies directed against FVIII occur in approximately 20% of patients; the risk is twice as great in African American and Hispanic patients than Caucasians. Treatment of inhibitors is to eradicate the antibody using immune tolerance therapy (ITT). Daily infusions of FVIII are given over a period of months to eradicate anti-FVIII antibodies. ITT is effective in approximately 70% of patients treated. For those patients who fail ITT or who bleed infrequently, two drugs, Novoseven (FVIIa) and FEIBA are administered. Recent studies show an effectiveness of 60% to 70% in preventing or reducing bleeding episodes. The risk of thrombosis is approximately less than 1% with either product and a head-to-head comparison showed equal efficacy of these drugs. Bethesda titers (BUI) are the inverse of the dilution of patient plasma that produces a 50% reduction of FVIII. For patients with a Bethesda titer less than 5, higher than normal doses of FVIII may be given to patients for bleeding. However, patients with BUI greater than 5, FVIIa or FEIBA must be used to treat acute bleeding. Inhibitors to FIX do occur a rate of 2% to 4% of patients. Typically many of these patients also develop severe allergic or anaphylactic reactions to FIX and are extremely difficult to tolerize. Novoseven is typically used as FEIBA contains FIX.

*Therapeutics:*
- A number of FDA products are available for patients that are derived from recombinant technology or plasma.
- Recombinant factor products—generated by genetically engineered cell lines, free of infectious virus, examples—Advate (FVIII), Kogenate (FVIII), Xyntha (FVIII), Benefix (FIX).
- Plasma-derived products—purified from US source plasma, examples—Mononine (FIX), Hemofil M (FVIII)

*Pharmacogenetics:* See Table 32-1.

**Table 32-1 Pharmacogenetic Considerations Hemophilia**

| Gene | Associated Medications | Goal of Testing | Effect |
|------|------------------------|-----------------|--------|
| FVIII | Recombinant FVIII (Advate, Kogenate, Xyntha), Plasma-derived FVIII (Hemofil M, Alphanate) | FVIII levels | Prevention of bleeding if level >1% |
| FIX | Recombinant FIX (Benefix), Plasma-derived FIX (Alphanine, Mononine) | FIX levels | |

## Molecular Genetics and Molecular Mechanism

**Genetic Testing:**
- The most comprehensive FVIII mutation database (~1492) is located on line at http://hadb.org.uk.
- A number of FIX mutations exist at http://www.kcl.ac.uk/ip/petergreen/haemBdatabase.html.

☞**CLINICAL AVAILABILITY OF TESTING:** Mutational analysis is available (City of Hope)—insurance does not cover costs; therefore, many patients not tested unless on clinical study.

**Future Directions:**
- Long-acting factors—several companies are developing FVIII and FIX that have prolonged half-life (1.8 × existing FVIII, 5 × existing FIX)
- Gene therapy—In a phase I or II trial, six severe FIX patients were treated with an adeno-associated virus (AAV) vector; they maintained FIX levels from 2% to 10% for several years after receiving one dose of virus. No spontaneous bleeding episodes were reported during this period. At the highest vector dose used, patients developed immune hepatitis.

**BIBLIOGRAPHY:**

1. Srivastava A, Brewer AK, Mauser-Bunschoten EP, et al. Guidelines for management of hemophilia. *Haemophilia*, 2012.
2. Roberts HR, Hoffman M. Hemophilia A and hemophilia B. In: Beutler E, Lichtman MA, Coller BS, et al, eds. *Williams Hematology*. 7th ed. New York, NY: McGraw-Hill. 2006;1867-1886.
3. Jones PK, Ratnoff OD. The changing prognosis of classic hemophilia (factor VIII "deficiency"). *Ann Intern Med.* 1991;114:641-648.
4. Darby SC, Kan SW, Spooner RJ, et al. Mortality rates, life expectancy, and causes of death in people with hemophilia A or B in the United Kingdom who were not infected with HIV. *Blood.* 2007;110:815-825.
5. Rosner F. Hemophilia in the Talmud and rabbinic writings. *Ann Intern Med.* 1969;70:833-837.
6. Jayandharan GR, Srivastava A, Srivastava A. *Semin Thromb Hemost.* 2012;38(1):64-78.
7. Hedner U, Ginsburg D, Lusher JM, High KA. Congenital Hemorrhagic Disorders: New Insights into the Pathophysiology and Treatment of Hemophilia. *Hematology Am Soc Hematol Educ Prog.* 2000;241-265.
8. Belvini D, Salviato R, Radossi P, et al. Molecular genotyping of the Italian cohort of patients with hemophilia B. *Haematologica.* 2005;90:635-642.
9. Andrikovics H, Klein I, Bors A, et al. Analysis of large structural changes of the factor VIII gene, involving intron 1 and 22, in severe hemophilia A. *Haematologica.* 2003;88:778-784.
10. Reijnen MJ, Peerlinck K, Maasdam D, Bertina RM, Reitsma PH. Hemophilia B Leyden: substitution of thymine for guanine at position-21 results in a disruption of a hepatocyte nuclear factor 4 binding site in the factor IX promoter. *Blood.* Jul 1 1993;82(1):151-158.
11. Miller CH, Benson J, Ellingsen D, et al. F8 and F9 mutations in US haemophilia patients: correlation with history of inhibitor and race/ethnicity. *Haemophilia.* May 2012;18(3):375-382.
12. Gouw SC, van den Berg HM, Oldenburg J, et al. F8 gene mutation type and inhibitor development in patients with severe hemophilia A: systematic review and meta-analysis. *Blood.* 2012;119:2922-2934.
13. Astermark J, Berntorp E, White GC, Kroner BL; MIBS Study Group. The Malmö International Brother Study (MIBS): further support for genetic predisposition to inhibitor development in hemophilia patients. *Haemophilia.* May 2001;7(3):267-272.
14. Nathwani AC, Tuddenham EG, Rangarajan S, et al. Adenovirus-associated virus vector—mediated gene transfer in hemophilia B. *N Engl J Med.* 2011;365(25):2357-2365.
15. Li H, Haurigot V, Doyon Y, et al. In vivo genome editing restores hemostasis in a mouse model of hemophilia. *Nature.* 2011;475(7355):217-221.

## Supplementary Information

**OMIM REFERENCES:** [will need to limit to relevant OMIM references]
**Official Symbol:** F8
**Name:** Coagulation Factor VIII, procoagulant component [*Homo sapiens*]
**Other Aliases:** RP11-115M6.7, AHF, DXS1253E, F8B, F8C, FVIII, HEMA
**Other Designations:** Antihemophilic Factor; Coagulation Factor VIII; Coagulation Factor VIIIc; Factor VIII F8B
**Chromosome:** X
**Location:** Xq28
**Annotation:** Chromosome X, NC_000023.10 (154064063.154250998, complement)
**MIM:** 300841

# 33 Aplastic Anemia, Bone Marrow Failure Syndromes

Rodrigo Calado

## KEY POINTS

- *Disease summary:*
  - Aplastic anemia (AA) is the prototypic disease of hematopoietic stem cell failure. It is characterized by an empty bone marrow resulting in low peripheral blood cell counts (pancytopenia).
  - AA can be acquired or inherited. Most common types of inherited AA are Fanconi anemia, dyskeratosiscongenita, and Shwachman-Diamond syndrome.
  - Acquired AA is an immune-mediated condition in which activated type-1 cytotoxic T cells target hematopoietic stem and progenitor cells in the marrow.
  - Whereas congenital AA is more frequent in the first and second decades of life and is associated with physical abnormalities (café-au-lait spots, hyperpigmentation, short stature, abnormal thumbs in Fanconi anemia; nail dystrophy, leukoplakia, and reticular hyperpigmentation in dyskeratosiscongenita; and exocrine pancreatic insufficiency in Shwachman-Diamond syndrome), the incidence of acquired AA is bimodal, peaking in adolescence (15 years) and greater than 50 years and physical anomalies are absent.

- *Differential diagnosis:*
  - Other causes of pancytopenia must be excluded: acute leukemia, myelodysplastic syndrome, pernicious anemia, bone marrow infiltration by other neoplasias.
  - It is not uncommon that a constitutional type of aplastic anemia to manifest without the usual clinical findings. Thus, it is necessary to perform ancillary diagnostic tests for the differential diagnosis of inherited bone marrow failure syndromes (Table 33-1), especially in children. Chromosome breakage test is routinely performed for the diagnosis of Fanconi anemia and telomere length measurement for the diagnosis of dyskeratosis congenita.

- *Monogenic forms:*
  - Fanconi anemia, dyskeratosis congenita, and Shwachman-Diamond syndrome are monogenic forms of constitutional aplastic anemia (Table 33-1).
  - Fanconi anemia: biallelic mutations in one of the at least complementation groups (FANC) (A, B, C, D1 [BRCA2], D2, E, F, G, I, J [BRIP1/BACH1], L, M, N [PALB2], O [RAD51C], and P [SLX4]) are necessary for disease, except for the *FANCB* gene, which is located in the X chromosome. Mutations in *FANCA* are etiologic in up to 70% of cases; mutations in *FANCC* are found in approximately 14% of patients; mutations in *FANCG* are found in 10% of cases; and mutations in each of the other complementation groups are observed in less than 3% of cases.
  - Dyskeratosiscongenita: the X-linked form is caused by mutations in the *DKC1* gene (~30% of cases); the autosomal dominant form may be caused by mutations in *TINF2* (~15%), *TERC* (~10%), or *TERT* (~10%); the autosomal recessive form is rare and mutations in *TERT*, *TERC*, *NHP2* (<1%), *NOP10* (<1%), or *TCAB1* (<1%) are etiologic.
  - Shwachman-Diamond syndrome: biallelic mutations in the *SBDS* gene are found in approximately 90% of patients.
  - Acquired AA: although the vast majority of cases are immune mediated, heterozygous mutations in *TERT*, *TERC*, or *SBDS* are found in approximately 10% of cases and are considered genetic risk factors for disease.

- *Family history:*
  - Patients with constitutional aplastic anemia usually have a positive family history for aplastic anemia, but also for leukemia or other types of cancer. Of clinical significance, in "acquired"AA, a family history for leukemia, pulmonary fibrosis, or hepatic disease may suggest the presence of a telomerase mutation.

- *Environmental factors:*
  - Acquired AA is an immune-mediated disease and some environmental factors may play a role, such as viruses in hepatitis-associated AA.

## Diagnostic Criteria and Clinical Characteristics

**Diagnostic evaluation should include**

- Complete blood counts (CBC) with reticulocyte count peripheral blood smear. CBC will show marked reduction in three or less commonly two of the three cell lines. Peripheral blood smear will demonstrate reduction in cell counts with normal morphology, but usually macrocytosis is present. For severe AA, at least two of the three following criteria are necessary: (1) absolute neutrophil count less than 500/µL; (2) platelet count less than 20,000/µL; (3) reticulocyte count (automated) less than 60,000/µL.
- Bone marrow aspirate and biopsy, including cytogenetic analysis. Overall marrow cellularity should be less than 30% (excluding lymphocytes).
- Peripheral blood flow cytometry for GPI-anchored proteins to detect associated paroxysmal nocturnal hemoglobinuria (PNH).
- Chromosome breakage test with diepoxybutane (DEB) or mitomycin C (MMC) for the diagnosis of Fanconi anemia.

*Table 33-1 Genetic Differential Diagnosis*

| Syndrome | Gene(s) Involved | Function | Ancillary Diagnostic Testing |
|---|---|---|---|
| Dyskeratosis congenita<br>X-linked<br>Autosomal dominant<br>Autosomal recessive | *DKC1*<br>*TERC, TERT, TINF2*<br>*NHP2, NOP10, TCAB1* | Telomere maintenance | Telomere length measurement<br>Mutation screening |
| Fanconi anemia | At least 15 genes<br>*FANC-A* to *FANC-P* | DNA repair<br>FA pathway for DNA damage response | Chromosome breakage test with cross-linking agents (diepoxybutane [DEB] or mitomycin C [MMC]) |
| Shwachman-Diamond syndrome | *SBDS* | Putative RNA processing | Mutation screening |
| Acquired aplastic anemia | *TERT, TERC, SBDS* in ~10% of cases | - | Telomere length measurement<br>Mutation screening |

Gene names: *DKC1*, dyskeratosis congenita 1; *TERC*, telomerase RNA component; *TERT*, telomerase reverse transcriptase; *TINF2*, TERF1-interacting nuclear factor 2; *NHP2*, NHP2 ribonucleoprotein homolog; *NOP10*, NOP10 ribonucleoprotein homolog; *TCAB1*, telomerase Cajal body protein 1; *FANC-X*, Fanconi anemia complementation group; *SBDS*, Shwachman-Bodian-Diamond syndrome.

- Telomere length measurement may be helpful for overall prognosis and to diagnose a telomere disease when telomere length is less than first percentile (cryptic dyskeratosis congenita or dyskeratosis congenita-like disease).
- Serum amylase and lipase and fat in the stool may be helpful and Shwachman-Diamond syndrome is suspected in children.

**And the absence of**
- Giant platelets, microspherocytes, schistocytes (fragmented red cells), all indicative of peripheral destruction should not be present.
- Biopsy and aspirate should rule out significant dysplasia of the three lineages, increased number of blasts, abnormal karyotype (all indicating myelodysplasia), and fibrosis.

*Clinical Characteristics:* The clinical presentation derives from low peripheral blood cell counts. Patients may present with symptoms of anemia such as fatigue, weakness, headache, and dyspnea are common and in older patients anemia may also manifest as chest pain. Thrombocytopenia results in mucosal and cutaneous bleeding: petechiae, bruises, epistaxis, and gum bleeding are more frequently observed. The most severe complication of thrombocytopenia is intracranial hemorrhage. Neutropenia clinically manifests as infection, mainly bacterial infection at presentation with fever. Chronic neutropenia is an important risk factor for fungal infections.

Physical findings relate to anemia (palor) and bleeding (petechiae and bruises). Infection sites may have little signs of inflammation due to neutropenia. Adenopathy and splenomegaly should not be present.

For constitutional AA, café-au-lait spots, hyperpigmentation, short stature, abnormal thumbs are suggestive of Fanconi anemia; nail dystrophy, reticular skin hyperpigmentation, and leukoplakia are characteristic of dyskeratosis congenita.

## Screening and Counseling

*Screening:* In patients with acquired AA, approximately 10% will carry a telomerase or *SBDS* gene mutation. Screening for Fanconi anemia is regularly performed in most patients with AA (especially in the first three decades of life) by the chromosome breakage test (Table 33-1). It is becoming more common to measure the telomere length of peripheral blood leukocytes of patients with AA, which can detect a telomere disease and indicate a telomerase mutation with telomere lengths less than first percentile, but also predict chances of relapse and malignant clonal evolution (Table 33-1). When very short telomeres are detected, family members should be screening for telomere length and also for gene lesions, if a specific mutation is detected. Potential matched sibling donors for bone marrow transplantation should be screening, since they may be silent carriers and poor donors.

*Counseling:* If Fanconi anemia is diagnosed in a patient, each sibling has a 25% chance of inheriting both mutated genes, 50% of being a carrier, and 25% of not being a carrier. Carriers are asymptomatic.

The pattern of inheritance in dyskeratosis congenita is complex. Mutations in *DKC1* usually have high penetrance and male siblings have a 50% chance of inheriting the mutated gene. For mutations in *TERT* or *TERC*, penetrance is lower and silent carriers are commonly observed in family members. The risk of developing disease is not well known yet. However, disease anticipation occurs in families with *TERT* or *TERC* mutations with disease being more severe and/or earlier age of onset with generation. This is due to the fact that patients inherit both the mutation and short telomeres from the affected parent, and telomeres are shorter at each generation.

## Management and Treatment

Hematopoietic stem cell transplant (HSCT) and immunosuppressive therapy are the main treatment modalities for acquired AA.

*HSCT:* Allogeneic human leukocyte antigen (HLA)-matched sibling donor transplant is indicated for patients with severe AA with an 85%-95% 5-year overall survival. HSCT replaces hematopoiesis and resets the immune system. However, a matched sibling donor is not available for many patients and alternative HSC sources for transplant (haploidentical, matched unrelated, umbilical cord) are not regularly used as frontline therapy yet, and should be reserved for patients who failed other therapies. Bone marrow failure in Fanconi anemia, dyskeratosis congenita, and Shwachman-Diamond syndrome also may be cured with HSCT. However, the other phenotypes associated with disease cannot be prevented with HSCT. Patients with dyskeratosis congenita have a higher risk of lung and liver complications after HSCT.

***Immunosuppressive Therapy:*** Patients with nonsevere acquired AA or with severe acquired AA without a matched sibling donor may be effectively treated with immunosuppression. The most effective modality of immunosuppression is based on antithymocyte globulin and cyclosporine; two-thirds of patients respond with an 80% 5-year overall survival. The major complications of immunosuppression are relapse and clonal evolution to myelodysplasia and acute leukemia.

***Androgens:*** Patients with constitutional AA may have their blood counts ameliorated and reach transfusion independence with androgen therapy. Androgens are known to increase the red blood cell mass and specifically in patients with telomerase mutations; androgens increase telomerase activity in hematopoietic progenitors.

***Supportive Care:*** Patients should receive blood transfusions for cytopenias with irradiated and filtrated blood components, as blood counts are not expected to increase fast after HSCT or immunosuppression. Broad-spectrum antibiotics are necessary for patients with febrile neutropenia and fungal infections must be investigated in patients with more chronic neutropenia. Growth factors (erythropoietin, granulocyte colony-stimulating factor [G-CSF], thrombopoietin) may be helpful in selected cases in the management of cytopenias.

## Molecular Genetics and Molecular Mechanism

In Fanconi anemia, mutations result in defects in the DNA-damage repair machinery, ultimately resulting in increased risk of cancer and marrow failure. The exact mechanism by which abnormal DNA repair causes marrow failure is not completely understood.

In dyskeratosis congenita, mutations cause excessive telomere shortening of hematopoietic stem and progenitor cells, activating senescence and apoptosis, clinically translating in HSC to maintain the blood cell counts. Short telomeres also increase chromosomal instability, explaining the higher incidence of cancer.

In Shwachman-Diamond syndrome, SBDS protein is thought to play a role in RNA processing. SBDS also appears to play a role in stabilization of the mitotic spindle.

***Genetic Testing:***

- **Fanconi anemia:** Diagnosis is based on chromosomal breakage studies. Sequence analysis of the 15 genes involved in Fanconi anemia is clinically available, but its clinical relevance is limited.
- **Dyskeratosis congenita:** Telomere length measurement is very helpful in the diagnosis of dyskeratosis congenita, which is highly suspected with telomere lengths less than first percentile. Genetic sequencing of *DKC1*, *TERT*, *TERC*, and *TINF2* are clinically available and may be helpful in the selection of sibling donors for transplant and for genetic screening and counseling.
- **Shwachman-Diamond syndrome:** Sequence analysis for SBDS is clinically available and is helpful to confirm diagnosis and for genetic counseling.

***Future Directions:*** The recent identification of mutations in telomerase complex and telomere-protecting genes elucidated the mechanisms of marrow failure in dyskeratosis congenita and some cases of acquired AA. That telomere shortening causes cell senescence, apoptosis, and chromosomal instability provides a mechanism for HSC failure and proclivity to cancer. The mechanisms that regulate telomerase expression and telomere elongation are elusive and their understanding may help identify potential therapeutic targets.

The function of SBDS protein is poorly understood. Although there is evidence that this protein plays a role in ribosomal biogenesis, the link to marrow failure is elusive. The comprehension of SBDS function may help understand the mechanisms of disease in Shwachman-Diamond syndrome.

**BIBLIOGRAPHY:**

1. Alter BP, Baerlocher GM, Savage SA, et al. Very short telomere length by flow fluorescence in situ hybridization identifies patients with dyskeratosis congenita. *Blood.* Sep 1 2007;110(5):1439-1447.

2. Bagby GC, Alter BP. Fanconi anemia. *Semin Hematol.* 2006;43: 147-156.

3. Burwick N, Shimamura A, Liu JM. Non-Diamond Blackfan anemia disorders of ribosome function: Shwachman Diamond syndrome and 5q-syndrome. *Semin Hematol.* Apr 2011;48(2):136-143.

4. Calado RT. Telomeres and marrow failure. *Hematology Am Soc Hematol Educ Program.* 2009;338-343.

5. Calado RT, Young NS. Telomere diseases. *N Engl J Med.* Dec 10 2009;361(24):2353-2365.

6. Scheinberg P, Cooper JN, Sloand EM, Wu CO, Calado RT, Young NS. Association of telomere length of peripheral blood leukocytes with hematopoietic relapse, malignant transformation, and survival in severe aplastic anemia. *JAMA.* Sep 22 2010;304(12):1358-1364.

7. Scheinberg P, Nunez O, Weinstein B, et al. Horse versus rabbit antithymocyte globulin in acquired aplastic anemia. *N Engl J Med.* Aug 4 2011;365(5):430-438.

8. Shimamura A. Clinical approach to marrow failure. *Hematology Am Soc Hematol Educ Program.* 2009;329-337.

9. Young NS, Calado RT, Scheinberg P. Current concepts in the pathophysiology and treatment of aplastic anemia. *Blood.* Oct 15 2006;108(8):2509-2519.

## Supplementary Information

**OMIM REFERENCES:**

Condition; Gene Name (OMIM#)

[1] Fanconi Anemia, Complementation Group A; FANCA (#227650)

[2] Fanconi Anemia, Complementation Group B; FANCB (#300514)

[3] Fanconi Anemia, Complementation Group C; FANCC (#227645)

[4] Fanconi Anemia, Complementation Group D1; FANCD1 (#605724)

[5] Fanconi Anemia, Complementation Group D2; FANCD2 (#227646)

[6] Fanconi Anemia, Complementation Group E; FANCE (#600901)

[7] Fanconi Anemia, Complementation Group F; FANCF (#603467)

[8] Fanconi Anemia, Complementation Group G; FANCG (#614082)

[9] Fanconi Anemia, Complementation Group I; FANCI (#609053)

[10] Fanconi Anemia, Complementation Group J; FANCJ (#609054)

[11] Fanconi Anemia, Complementation Group L; FANCL (#614083)

[12] Fanconi Anemia, Complementation Group M; FANCM (#614087)

[13] Fanconi Anemia, Complementation Group N; FANCN (#610832)

[14] Fanconi Anemia, Complementation Group O; FANCO (#613390)

[15] Fanconi Anemia, Complementation Group P; FANCP (#613951)

[16] Dyskeratosis Congenita, X-Linked; DKC1 (#305000)

[17] Dyskeratosis Congenita, Autosomal Dominant; TERC (#127550)

[18] Dyskeratosis Congenita, Autosomal Dominant; TERT (#613989)

[19] Dyskeratosis Congenita, Autosomal Dominant; TINF2 (#613990)

[20] Dyskeratosis Congenita, Autosomal Recessive; NHP2 (#613987)

[21] Dyskeratosis Congenita, Autosomal Recessive; NOP10 (#224230)

[22] Dyskeratosis Congenita, Autosomal Recessive; TCAB1 (#613988)

[23] Shwachman-Diamond Syndrome; SBDS (#260400)

# 34 Myeloproliferative Disorders

John O. Mascarehas and Ronald Hoffman

## KEY POINTS

- *Disease summary:*
  - The classic myeloproliferative neoplasms (MPNs) are a group of clonal hematopoietic stem cell disorders associated with an increased thrombotic tendency and the potential to evolve into acute myeloid leukemia. The central and shared feature in MPNs is effective clonal myeloproliferation with resultant peripheral blood granulocytosis, thrombocytosis, or erythrocytosis that is devoid of dyserythropoiesis, or granulocytic dysplasia. For the sake of this chapter, only the four classic MPNs will be discussed.
  - Chronic myelogenous leukemia (CML) is characterized by a pathogenic reciprocal chromosomal translocation involving chromosomes 9 and 22, t(9;22).
  - Polycythemia vera (PV) is a characterized by an absolute increase in red cell mass and often accompanied by leukocytosis, thrombocytosis, and splenomegaly.
  - Essential thrombocythemia (ET) is characterized primarily by thrombocytosis and an elevated risk for both thrombotic and hemorrhagic consequences.
  - Primary myelofibrosis (PMF) is characterized by progressive symptomatic splenomegaly, cytopenias, peripheral blood leukoerythroblastosis and dacrocytes, bone marrow fibrosis, and extramedullary hematopoiesis.

- *Differential diagnosis:*
  - Myelodysplastic syndrome (MDS), acute myeloid leukemia, juvenile and chronic myelomonocytic leukemia, secondary causes of thrombocytosis, erythrocytosis and marrow fibrosis, leukemoid reaction, chronic eosinophilic leukemia, chronic neutrophilic leukemia

- *Monogenic forms:*
  - CML is believed to be the result of a fusion oncogene involving breakpoint cluster region (chromosome 22) and Abelson leukemia virus (chromosome 9)—t(9;22)(q34;q11). This p210 *BCR-ABL* oncogene encodes for a constitutively active cytoplasmic tyrosine kinase.

- *Family history:*
  - A large population-based case-control study conducted in Sweden identified a five- to sevenfold elevated risk of MPNs in first-degree relatives of patients with MPNs supporting the theory of shared susceptibility genes.

- *Twin studies:*
  - Concordance of disease is not observed between twins.

- *Environmental factors:*
  - Radiation may play a causative role in some patients as high-dose irradiation after atomic bomb exposure has been linked to an increased risk of developing chronic myeloid leukemia and in vitro exposure to high-dose irradiation can induce *BCR-ABL* expression in myeloid cell lines. Recently, a statistically significant cluster of cases of PV have been identified in a tri-county area in Eastern Pennsylvania and ongoing investigation of potential toxins present in this area is an area of research.

- *Genome-wide associations:*
  - There are susceptibility haplotypes that have been identified that increase the risk of developing an MPN. For example, single-marker analysis and haplotype analysis have identified a *BCL2* single-nucleotide polymorphism (SNP) that increase the risk for developing CML by an odds ratio (OR) of 1.84 for three to four risk alleles versus zero to one risk alleles. See Table 34-1 for more information.

- *Pharmacogenomics:*
  - Although not routinely done in clinical practice, OCT-1 activity can be measured in CML CD34+ cells and decreased activity is associated with reduced uptake of imatinib and poor response to therapy. SNPs have been identified in the *OCT-1* gene that will likely explain the interperson variability of transporter activity.

## Diagnostic Criteria and Clinical Characteristics

*Diagnostic Criteria:* See Fig. 34-1 for both a genetic- and histology-based diagnostic algorithm for classic chronic MPNs. Below are the World Health Organization (WHO) diagnostic criteria for CML and the classic Ph⁻ MPNs.

**2008 WHO diagnostic criteria for CML**

The presence of Philadelphia chromosome by conventional cytogenetics (karyotyping) or fluorescence in situ hybridization (FISH) analysis, or *BCR-ABL1* fusion mRNA by reverse transcription polymerase chain reaction (RT-PCR) in the setting of neutrophilia in all stages of maturation.

**2008 WHO diagnostic criteria for PV***

**Table 34-1 MPN-Associated Susceptibility Variants**

| Candidate Gene (Chromosome Location) | Associated Variant [effect on protein] (assayed by affymetrix/ illumina) | Risk | Frequency of Risk Allele | Putative Functional Significance | Associated Disease Phenotype |
|---|---|---|---|---|---|
| JAK2 (9p24) | JAK2 exon 12 (rs10974944) | 2.1 OR | 64% | EPOR signaling | PV |
| JAK2 (9p24) | JAK2 V617F (rs12343867) | 1.9 OR | | Cytokine receptor signaling | ET, PV, MF |
| BCL2 (18) | rs1801018 | 2.16 OR | | Regulation of apoptosis pathway | CML |

**Major Criteria**

1. Hgb greater than 18.5 g/dL (men), greater than 16.5 g/dL (women) *or* Hgb greater than 17 g/dL(men), greater than 15 g/dL (women) if associated with a sustained increase of at least 2 g/dL from baseline value that cannot be attributed to correction of iron deficiency *or* Hgb or hematocrit greater than the 99th percentile of reference range for age, sex, or altitude of residence *or* red cell mass greater than 25% above the mean normal predicted
2. Presence of *JAK2*V617F or similar mutation such as *JAK2* exon 12

**Minor Criteria**

1. Bone marrow trilineage myeloproliferation
2. Subnormal serum erythropoietin (Epo) level
3. Endogenous erythroid colony (EEC) growth

*The diagnosis of PV requires meeting either both major criteria and one minor criterion or the first major criterion and two minor criteria.

**2008 WHO diagnostic criteria for ET***

**Major Criteria**

1. Platelet count greater than or equal to $450 \times 10^9$/L
2. Megakaryocyte proliferation with large and mature morphology, no or little granulocyte or erythroid proliferation
3. Not meeting WHO criteria for CML, PV, PMF, MDS, or other myeloid neoplasm
4. Demonstration of *JAK2*V617F *or* other clonal marker *or* no evidence of reactive thrombocytosis

*The diagnosis of ET requires meeting all 4 major criteria.

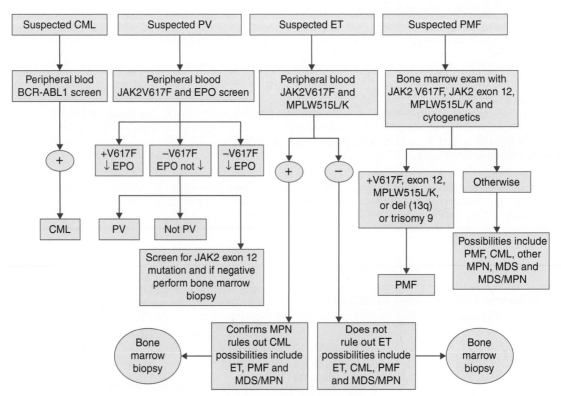

**Figure 34-1** A Genetic- and Histology-Based Diagnostic Algorithm for CML, PV, ET, and PMF.
Modified from: Teffreri, A. *et al*. (2009) Myeloproliferative neoplasms: contemporary diagnosis using histology and genetics *Nat Rev. Clin. Oncol.* doi: 10.1038/nrclinonc. 2009.149

**2008 WHO diagnostic criteria for PMF\***

**Major Criteria**

1. Megakaryocyte proliferation and atypia[γ] accompanied by either reticulin and/or collagen fibrosis, or in the absence of reticulin fibrosis, the megakaryocyte changes must be accompanied by increased bone marrow cellularity, granulocytic proliferation, and often decreased erythropoiesis (ie, prefibrotic PMF).
2. Not meeting WHO criteria for CML, PV, MDS, or other myeloid neoplasm.
3. Demonstration of *JAK2*V617F or other clonal marker or no evidence of reactive bone marrow fibrosis.

**Minor Criteria**

1. Leukoerythroblastosis
2. Increased serum lactate dehydrogenase (LDH)
3. Anemia
4. Palpable splenomegaly

\*The diagnosis of PMF requires meeting all three major criteria and two minor criteria.

[γ]Small to large megakaryocytes with an aberrant nuclear or cytoplasmic ratio and hyperchromatic and irregularly folded nuclei and dense clustering.

*Clinical Characteristics of CML, PV, ET, and MF:*

☞**GENOTYPE-PHENOTYPE CORRELATION:** Much interest is in how a single gene mutation can be identified in several MPNs displaying both diverse and overlapping clinical phenotypes. The clinical phenotype in the Ph⁻ MPNs is in part a function of *JAK2*V617F gene dose. Acquired uniparental disomy of chromosome 9p in many PV and MF cases leads to homozygosity of the *JAK2*V617F allele and higher burden disease is associated with a PV phenotype and lower burden with an ET phenotype. Additionally, various SNPs that have been identified in *JAK2* show strong association with PV and ET but not MF. Although, a single erythropoietin receptor (EPOR) SNP (rs 318699) appears to be associated with a PV phenotype, genetic variation in *GCSFR* and *MPL* genes does not seem to add to the phenotypic diversity observed in MPNs.

## Management and Treatment

*Management:* CML is treated with oral small molecule tyrosine kinase inhibitors (TKIs): imatinib, dasatinib or nilotinib in the chronic phase. The accelerated and blast phase of the disease are often either unresponsive to or highly likely to relapse after TKI therapy alone and require hematopoietic stem cell transplantation (SCT). Disease response is monitored by the presence

| MPN | Symptoms | Signs | Complications |
|---|---|---|---|
| CML | Asymptomatic, fatigue, weight loss, bony pains, anorexia | Splenomegaly, gout | Progression to accelerated (AP) or blast phase (BP). |
| PV/ET | Asymptomatic, night sweats, pruritus, fatigue, global weakness, bony pains, muscle aches, dizziness, headache, paresthesias, visual disturbances, anorexia, early satiety, epigastric distress, erythromelalgia, Raynaud, digital ischemia/gangrene, joint pain | Hypertension, cyanosis, conjunctival plethora, hepatosplenomegaly, ascites, gout | Arterial and venous thrombotic events, transformation to MF and acute leukemia |
| PMF | Weight loss, night sweats, fevers, pruritus, fatigue, global weakness, malaise, early satiety, anorexia, abdominal pain, constipation, diarrhea, joint pain | Cachexia, conjunctival pallor, hepatosplenomegaly, ascites, edema, gout | Transformation to acute leukemia, transfusion dependence and iron overload |

## Screening and Counseling

*Screening:* Genetic screening is not routinely recommended, however testing for *JAK2*V617F, *JAK2* exon 12, or *MPL* mutations in peripheral blood granulocytes in cases of Budd-Chiari syndrome without obvious etiology is warranted. This is especially true in young females despite a normal hematologic profile.

*Counseling:* Studies involving cases of familial MPNs suggest an inheritance with incomplete penetrance. *JAK2*V617F is believed to be an acquired somatic mutation in familial cases as it is in sporadic cases. No formal recommendation on screening first-degree relatives of patients with MPN exist.

in the peripheral blood or bone marrow of the Philadelphia chromosome, t(9;22), or *BCR-ABL1* molecular transcript by conventional cytogenetics, FISH, or quantitative RT-PCR, respectively. The detection of the presence of *BCR-ABL1* mRNA transcript by PCR in either the peripheral blood or bone marrow is the most sensitive tool to determine depth of clinical response. Achieving a major molecular response (>threefold log reduction in baseline BCR-ABL transcript) is highly predictive of a favorable clinical outcome and disease-free survival. TKI therapy is continued indefinitely since a 50% relapse rate has been reported in patients stopping TKI despite obtaining a molecular response. Interferon is rarely used in clinical practice with the advent of TKIs. SCT is reserved for those patients that acquire

**Table 34-2** *Pharmacogenetic Considerations in MPN*

| Gene | Associated Medications | Goal of Testing | Variants | Effect |
|------|------------------------|-----------------|----------|--------|
| *OCT-1* (organic cation transporter 1) | Imatinib | Efficacy | *P283L* *R287G* | Decreased uptake of imatinib due to low OCT-1 activity |

TKI-resistant ABL kinase domain mutations such as T315I or develop blast phase disease.

ET and PV are managed with a risk-adapted therapy approach. These patients are at elevated risk for venous and arterial thrombosis, hemorrhage, transformation to MF and acute leukemia. Low-risk ET and PV patients (age <60 and without a history of major thrombosis) can be managed with low-dose daily aspirin. Phlebotomy is employed for low-risk PV patients to maintain a hematocrit less than 45% for a man and less than 42% for a woman. High-risk ET and PV patients (age >60, history of thrombosis) or symptomatic patients are treated with cytoreductive therapy with hydroxyurea or anagrelide. Hydroxyurea plus aspirin has been shown in a large study to be superior to anagrelide plus aspirin in reducing the risk of arterial thrombotic events, bleeding, and transformation to MF. Peginterferon alfa-2a has also shown promise as an agent with the potential to modulate blood counts, decrease spleen size, and even reduce molecular markers of disease.

PMF is classified by various risk stratification systems based on prognosis. Low, intermediate-1 (int-1), intermediate-2, and high-risk disease by International Working Group for Myelofibrosis Research and Treatment is a recent system based on five validated risk factors (age, hemoglobin, constitutional symptoms, leukocytosis, and circulating blasts) that predicts median survivals of 135, 95, 48, and 27 months, respectively. Low-risk and int-1 MF patients can be treated with supportive care only and watched for progression of disease before moving to conventional therapies such as thalidomide, lenalidomide, danazol, and melphalan. Patients with int-2 and high-risk disease are eligible for experimental therapies with JAK2 inhibitors, histone deacetylase inhibitors (HDACIs), inhibitors of angiogenesis, mammalian target of rapamycin (mTOR) inhibitors, and newer-generation immunomodulatory drugs (IMiDs). Patients under the age of 65 and with an human leukocyte antigen (HLA)-matched sibling or unrelated donor are considered candidates for SCT. SCT is the only treatment modality available that offers the potential for cure.

☞**THERAPEUTICS:**

- **Anagrelide:** Selectively reduces platelet count and used as second line to hydroxyurea in high-risk ET.
- **Androgens:** Effective in a subset of MF patients in alleviating anemia. Virilizing effects can be an issue in women.
- **Aspirin:** Antiplatelet agent integral for reducing thrombotic risk in ET and PV.
- **Hydroxyurea:** Nonselective cytoreductive agent of choice in high-risk ET, PV, and MF. Also effective in reducing the size of symptomatic spleen.
- **IMiDs:** Immunomodulatory agents such as thalidomide, lenalidomide, and pomalidomide have the ability to improve the anemia associated with MF and reduce splenomegaly in a subset of patients.
- **JAK2 inhibitors:** Still in various phase I, II, and III clinical trials have demonstrated potential in rapidly and dramatically reducing splenomegaly, and improving constitutional

symptoms in both *JAK2* wild type and V617F-positive MPN patients. Unclear if these experimental agents can decrease clonal markers of disease, as measured by *JAK2*V617F allele burden.

- **Interferon alfa:** Pegylated interferon alfa-2b was the gold standard treatment for CML before 2000 and is now being investigated as part of combination therapy with imatinib in CML. Pegylated interferon alfa-2a is a nonleukemogenic injectable given weekly and is the only agent known to induce complete molecular remission in patients with PV. Interferon alfa may have a role in treating some patients with the prefibrotic form of MF. This therapy is mostly tolerable with a mild toxicity profile.

☞**PHARMACOGENETICS:** Personalized medicine will become important as the metabolism of newer experimental agents is better characterized. Currently *OCT-1* has been recognized as a gene of interest since this encodes for a protein that is integral in allowing various drugs to enter into a cell. Lower levels of OCT-1 activity in CML CD34+ cells are associated with reduced influx of imatinib. Variants of *OCT-1* gene have already been identified and likely influence transporter activity and may help explain differences in response to therapy in people. See Table 34-2.

## Molecular Genetics and Molecular Mechanism

The pathogenetic mechanism underlying the MPNs is complex and not yet fully elucidated. The identification of loss of heterozygosity (LOH) on the short arm of chromosome 9 in a proportion of MPN patients via genome-wide microsatellite screening leads to the realization that 9p may hold a pathogenic mutation and focused much attention to this region of the genome. The gain-of-function point mutation at position1849 in exon 14 of the Janus kinase 2 gene (*JAK2*), results in a G>T switch causing phenylalanine to be substituted for valine at codon 617. This interrupts the auto-inhibitory function of the JH2 pseudokinase domain of *JAK2*, allowing for constitutive tyrosine kinase activity. *JAK2*V617F has been identified in not only myeloid cells, but also B, T, and NK cells indicating the clonal cell of origin is a multipotent hematopoietic stem cell with the potential to give rise to both myeloid and lymphoid progenitors. Hematopoietic cells expressing *JAK2*V617F are characterized by constitutive cytokine independent cell growth, survival, and differentiation. The presence of *JAK2*V617F is not sufficient to cause ET (50%) or MF (50%) but appears nearly essential for PV (97%). The *JAK2*V617F allele burden influences MPN phenotype with low burden (<50%) associated with ET and high burden (>50%) associated with PV and MF. Mutations in exon 12 of *JAK2* as well as MPLW515L/K (encoding the thrombopoietin receptor) have also been identified in MPN patients and although do not appear to be initiating events either, do influence clinical phenotype. The presence of *JAK2* exon 12 mutation also favors erythropoiesis and a PV-like phenotype and is found in approximately 15% and 1.5% of *JAK2*617F-negative PV and MF cases, respectively. Additionally, the coexpression of *MPL*W515L/K in *JAK2*V617F-positive MF patients also influences the clinical phenotype and this may in part be due to the relative high MPL allele burden. It is not yet clear if the MPL mutation represents an earlier event and the *JAK2*V617F a latter acquired mutation. Ten-Eleven translocation (TET2) have been identified in both familial MPNs as well as sporadic cases. *TET2* mutations are seen mostly in older *JAK2*V617F-positive and -negative MPN patients and do not appear to hold clinical prognostic significance. The *TET2* gene encodes a putative tumor suppressor gene located on a region of chromosome 4q24 that is breakpoint involved in acute myeloid leukemia (AML)-associated chromosomal translocations, as well as frequently mutated in cases of MDS, and systemic mastocytosis. Analysis of *TET2* gene mutations in familial MPNs have demonstrated that this is an acquired mutation and not associated with enhanced susceptibility to developing an MPN.

Oncogenic mutations are rare in Ph⁻ MPNs and include mutations involving EPOR, Ras, c-KIT, and p53. The identification of these mutations have not provided significant insight into the pathogenesis of MPNs. However, noted epigenetic modifications in MF have exposed a whole new array of therapeutic targets. DNA promoter site methylation and histone acetylation are known epigenetic phenomena that ultimately influence tumor suppressor gene expression. Promotion of histone acetylation by HDACI can lead to the upregulation of silenced genes responsible for cell growth, differentiation and survival, as well as preferentially direct JAK2V617F to proteasomal degradation.

Bone marrow transplant mouse models expressing JAK2V617F in bone marrow hematopoietic cells of different mouse strains results in different MPN phenotypes and provided evidence that a single gene mutation can lead to different clinical pictures underscoring the influence of an individual's germline genetic variation. Although several JAK2 SNPs have been discovered to influence phenotypic diversity within the MPNs, only one germline SNP has been shown to predispose to the development of both *JAK2*V617F+ and *JAK2* exon 12+ MPN (Table 34-1). SNPs genome-wide association studies (GWAS) have revealed a clear association between the *JAK2* SNP rs10974944 and increased risk for developing an MPN, stressing the importance of *JAK2* germline gene variation as a potential contributing factor to the development of a *JAK2*V617F+ MPN.

***Genetic Testing:*** BCR-ABL1, *JAK2*V617F, *JAK2* exon 12, and *MPL*W515L/K testing is recommended as part of the MPN diagnostic algorithm (Fig. 34-1) and is now incorporated into the revised 2008 WHO diagnostic criteria. *JAK2*V617F, *JAK2* exon 12, and *MPL*W515L/K are detected in peripheral blood or bone marrow by qualitative PCR and allele burden quantified by allele-specific PCR. *BCR-ABL* can be tested in cases of suspected CML from peripheral blood granulocytes or bone marrow cells by conventional cytogenetics, FISH techniques or RT-PCR.

***Future Directions:*** Imatinib is the prototype of targeted therapy based on the understanding of the molecular mechanism underlying CML and has dramatically improved response rates and survival. Importantly, this has also provided a model in which drugs for the other MPNs are designed in order to target the aberrant expression of enzymes and receptors particular to the malignant clones. Continued research and attention to the identification of

specific SNPs and haplotypes that increase susceptibility to developing MPNs will hopefully yield more insight into the exact pathogenesis of MPNs. Intense laboratory research continues to search for other yet unknown genetic lesions that likely precede *JAK2* or *MPL* mutations and determine the initiating event that causes these myeloid malignancies. The emergence of high-throughput genomic testing will undoubtedly assist in the identification of genetic causes in MPNs and allow for the design of novel therapies.

In the near future, combination therapy exploiting distinct therapeutic mechanisms and non-overlapping toxicities utilizing agents such as peginterferon alfa-2a, JAK2 inhibitors, HDACIs and other epigenetic targeted therapies, and inhibitors of cytokine activity in Ph⁻ MPNs. Combination interferon alfa and imatinib induction followed by maintenance interferon alfa is also being evaluated in CML. Newer more selective and potent BCR-ABL inhibitors are being designed and tested in the clinic as well. Lastly, exploiting the expansion of specific downregulated leukemia-specific cytotoxic T cells in patients with CML offers an entirely different therapeutic strategy directed toward deleting the malignant clone.

## BIBLIOGRAPHY:

1. Engler JR, Frede A, Saunders VA, Zannettino AC, Hughes TP, White DL. Chronic myeloid leukemia CD34+ cells have reduced uptake of imatinib due to low OCT-1 Activity. *Leukemia.* Apr 2010;24(4):765-770.

2. Kim DH, Xu W, Ma C, et al. Genetic variants in the candidate genes of the apoptosis pathway and susceptibility to chronic myeloid leukemia. *Blood.* Mar 12 2009;113(11):2517-2525.

3. Kralovics R, Teo SS, Buser AS, et al. Altered gene expression in myeloproliferative disorders correlates with activation of signaling by the V617F mutation of Jak2. *Blood.* Nov 15 2005;106(10):3374-3376.

4. Landgren O, Goldin LR, Kristinsson SY, Helgadottir EA, Samuelsson J, Bjorkholm M. Increased risks of polycythemia vera, essential thrombocythemia, and myelofibrosis among 24,577 first-degree relatives of 11,039 patients with myeloproliferative neoplasms in Sweden. *Blood.* Sep 15 2008;112(6):2199-2204.

5. Lasho TL, Pardanani A, McClure RF, et al. Concurrent MPL515 and JAK2V617F mutations in myelofibrosis: chronology of clonal emergence and changes in mutant allele burden over time. *Br J Haematol.* Dec 2006;135(5):683-687.

6. Olcaydu D, Harutyunyan A, Jager R, et al. A common JAK2 haplotype confers susceptibility to myeloproliferative neoplasms. *Nat Genet.* Apr 2009;41(4):450-454.

7. Olcaydu D, Skoda RC, Looser R, et al. The 'GGCC' haplotype of JAK2 confers susceptibility to JAK2 exon 12 mutation-positive polycythemia vera. *Leukemia.* Oct 2009;23(10):1924-1926.

8. Pardanani A, Fridley BL, Lasho TL, Gilliland DG, Tefferi A. Host genetic variation contributes to phenotypic diversity in myeloproliferative disorders. *Blood.* Mar 1 2008;111(5):2785-2789.

9. Seaman V, Jumaan A, Yanni E, et al. Use of molecular testing to identify a cluster of patients with polycythemia vera in eastern Pennsylvania. *Cancer Epidemiol Biomarkers Prev.* Feb 2009;18(2):534-540.

10. Tefferi A, Skoda R, Vardiman JW. Myeloproliferative neoplasms: contemporary diagnosis using histology and genetics. *Nat Rev Clin Oncol.* Nov 2009;6(11):627-637.

11. Tefferi A, Thiele J, Orazi A, et al. Proposals and rationale for revision of the World Health Organization diagnostic criteria for polycythemia vera, essential thrombocythemia, and primary myelofibrosis: recommendations from an ad hoc international expert panel. *Blood.* Aug 15 2007;110(4):1092-1097.

## Supplementary Information

**OMIM REFERENCES:** [will need to limit to relevant OMIM references]

[1] Polycythemia Vera; JAK2 (#263300)

[2] Thrombocythemia, Essential; MPL, THPO, JAK2 (#187950)

**Alternative Names:**
- Chronic Granulocytic Leukemia
- Agnogenic Myeloid Metaplasia
- Myelofibrosis With Myeloid Metaplasia
- Chronic Idiopathic Myelofibrosis
- Polycythemia Rubra Vera
- Primary Thrombocytosis
- Idiopatic Thrombocytosis

*Key Words:* Myeloproliferative neoplasm, chronic myeloid leukemia, polycythemia vera, essential thrombocythemia, myelofibrosis, JAK2, MPL

# 35 The Myelodysplastic Syndrome

Shyamala C. Navada and Lewis R. Silverman

- *Disease summary:*
  - The myelodysplastic syndrome (MDS), a primary bone marrow failure state, represents a heterogeneous hematopoietic stem cell disorder, which results in abnormal cellular maturation and peripheral blood cytopenias. Greater than 50% of patients with MDS have clonal cytogenetic abnormalities, which help to stratify the disease into poor, intermediate, and good prognostic groups. The identification of recurrent mutations in MDS has led to insights into the pathophysiology of the disease.
  - MDS is primarily a disease of older individuals with a median age of diagnosis over 70 years. It is more common in males than females.
  - Although the clinical presentation is nonspecific, symptoms are primarily related to the cytopenias. The most common cytopenia is anemia; therefore, patients often present with fatigue, weakness, dyspnea on exertion, and angina pectoris.
  - MDS is characterized by progressive bone marrow failure, and the most common causes of death in higher-risk patients are infection and bleeding.
  - Approximately 35% to 40% of patients with MDS progress to acute myeloid leukemia (AML), which confers a poor prognosis.
- *Differential diagnosis:*
  - Infections (including HIV, Epstein-Barr virus [EBV], cytomegalovirus [CMV], parvovirus B19), nutritional deficiencies ($B_{12}$ or folate), drug-induced myelosuppression, myeloproliferative neoplasms, and other hematologic malignancies affecting the bone marrow, such as lymphoma, leukemia, multiple myeloma, and paroxysmal nocturnal hemoglobinuria (PNH)
- *Monogenic forms:*
  - No single gene cause of MDS is known to exist.
- *Family history:*
  - There is no evidence that family members who have first-degree relatives with MDS are at higher risk of developing the disease. While the majority of MDS is sporadic, rare inherited bone marrow failure syndromes may predispose patients to myeloid malignancies, including MDS and AML. These include Fanconi anemia, dyskeratosis congenita, Shwachman-Diamond syndrome, and Diamond-Blackfan syndrome.
- *Twin studies:*
  - No increased risk in monozygotic twins has been reported in the literature.
- *Environmental factors:*
  - Although the etiologic agent cannot be identified in the majority of patients, exposure to ionizing radiation, chemicals, chemotherapy agents (particularly alkylating agents and topoisomerase II inhibitors), and other environmental agents can be implicated. Benzene exposure, in particular, has a strong association with the development of MDS and AML. In addition, there may be an increased risk of MDS with the use of permanent hair dyes and cigarette smoking.
- *Genome-wide associations:*
  - Genes involved in the regulation of histone function and DNA methylation are recurrently mutated in MDS, suggesting an important link between genetic and epigenetic mechanisms in this disease (Table 35-1). The mechanism by which these mutations contribute to disease pathogenesis and progression is currently under study. Testing for these mutations is not part of routine clinical practice at this time.
- *Pharmacogenomics:*
  - When available, testing for gene mutations can help to assess the prognosis of an individual patient's disease and guide in treatment approaches.

## Diagnostic Criteria and Clinical Characteristics

***Diagnostic Criteria for MDS:*** Diagnostic evaluation should include

- Complete blood count with differential and reticulocyte count.
- Examination of the peripheral blood smear.
- A bone marrow aspirate and biopsy, including studies for flow cytometry and cytogenetics. The diagnosis of MDS is based primarily on morphologic manifestations of dysplasia and aberrant maturation in the peripheral blood and bone marrow lineages.

These include but are not limited to megaloblastoid erythropoiesis, nucleocytoplasmic asynchrony in the myeloid and erythroid precursors, and dysmorphic megakaryocytes.
- Iron studies, $B_{12}$ or folate levels, serum erythropoietin level.
- Thyroid-stimulating hormone (TSH), T3 and T4 to rule out hypothyroidism.
- Documentation of transfusion history.

***Clinical Characteristics:*** The clinical presentation is variable. Symptoms often correlate with a patient's cytopenias, with those associated with anemia being the most common. These include fatigue, weakness, dyspnea, angina, and cardiac dysfunction.

*Table 35-1* **Genetic Abnormalities in MDS**

| Candidate Gene | Chromosome | Frequency in MDS (%) | Putative Functional Significance |
|---|---|---|---|
| ASXL1 | 20q | 11-15 | Unknown |
| CBL | 11q | 1 | Unknown |
| DNMT3A | 2p | 8 | Decreased survival |
| EZH2 | 7q | 2-6 | Decreased survival |
| FLT3 ITD | 13q | 0-2 | Decreased survival |
| IDH1/ IDH2 | 2q/15q | 4-11 | Decreased survival |
| JAK2 | 9p | 2 | Unknown |
| N/KRAS | 1p/12p | 3-6 | Increased risk of progression to AML |
| NPM1 | 5q | 2 | Unknown |
| RUNX1 | 21q | 4-14 | Decreased survival; more common in therapy-related MDS |
| TET2 | 4q | 11-26 | Unknown |
| TP53 | 17p | 10-18 | Decreased survival and increased risk of progression to AML |
| UTX | Xp | NA | Unknown |

Fatigue may be disproportionate to the degree of anemia. Patients may also present with signs and symptoms related to neutropenia, including bacterial infections, or thrombocytopenia, including easy bruising, ecchymosis, petechiae, epistaxis, gingival bleeding, or gastrointestinal bleeding. Physical findings are also nonspecific. Organomegaly is infrequently observed. Lymphadenopathy and skin infiltration may occur but are uncommon. The classic laboratory findings include peripheral blood cytopenias, anemia with macrocytosis, and functional abnormalities involving one or more cell lines. In most patients, the bone marrow is hypercellular, and there are dysplastic features in the progenitor cells.

## Screening and Counseling

**Screening:** Family members of patients with MDS are not routinely screened. There is no known genetic predisposition to development of the disease.

**Counseling:** There is an increased risk of developing MDS and AML in hereditary bone marrow failure syndromes, and counseling is warranted in these cases. These inherited syndromes include Fanconi anemia, dyskeratosis congenita, Shwachman-Diamond syndrome, and Diamond-Blackfan syndrome. Children with Down syndrome are at increased susceptibility for developing MDS and AML among other hematologic malignancies.

## Management and Treatment

Due to the heterogeneous nature of MDS, treatment depends on several factors, including a patient's age, comorbidities, symptoms, and stage of the disease. The International Prognostic Scoring System (IPSS) is often used to determine stage. The IPSS was developed based on the percentage of bone marrow blasts, cytogenetics, and degree of cytopenias and has predictive value for both survival and risk of transformation to leukemia in patients with untreated primary MDS. More recently, the IPSS has been revised (R-IPSS) to include additional cytogenetic subgroups, depth of cytopenias, and further classify the percentage of blasts. In addition, it was recognized that age, performance status, serum ferritin, and lactate dehydrogenase (LDH) were predictive of survival. Patients are divided into five groups: very low, low, intermediate, high, and very high risk.

Within the R-IPSS categories, MDS can be stratified in lower-risk and higher-risk subgroups when determining prognosis and making treatment decisions. "Lower risk" incorporates very low and low R-IPSS categories, and "higher risk" includes high and very high groups. Lower-risk patients can often be observed initially and once treatment is initiated, the goal is to improve hematologic parameters and symptoms. On the other hand, higher-risk patients require treatment with either hypomethylating agents or allogeneic stem cell transplantation (ASCT) in order to prolong survival and delay transformation to AML.

**Supportive Therapies:** Treatment with red cell transfusions, erythropoiesis-stimulating agents (ESAs), myeloid cytokines, thrombopoietic growth factors, and iron chelation therapy is used to support patients, with the goal of improving quality of life, reducing transfusion requirements, and reducing infectious risks.

**Red Cell Transfusions:** Over 50% of patients with newly diagnosed disease have a hemoglobin level less than 10 g/dL. Anemia in the elderly is associated with a worse performance status and decreased quality of life compared to healthy controls. Red cell transfusions are a common modality to treat anemia and may be the only effective therapy in patients who do not respond to or are not candidates for alternate interventions. Therapy should be based on individual symptoms, such as fatigue and dyspnea, as well as comorbid conditions.

**Erythropoiesis-Stimulating Agents:** Erythropoietin (Epo) and granulocyte colony-stimulating factor (G-CSF) are regulatory glycoproteins that control the proliferation and differentiation of bone marrow stem cells. Human recombinant erythropoietin has been used as monotherapy in patients with MDS and has induced erythroid responses in up to 50% to 60% of selected patients. Patients with serum Epo levels less than 500 IU/L and an absent or low transfusion requirement (<2 U/mo) are more likely to have favorable responses. The addition of G-CSF to Epo can improve erythroid responses in a subset of patients. Administration of ESAs alone or in combination with G-CSF is safe and effective and can help to palliate symptoms in lower-risk patients with anemia.

**Myeloid Growth Factors:** Several studies have evaluated the role of granulocyte-macrophage colony-stimulating factor (GM-CSF) in MDS. In one randomized controlled study, patients received either treatment with GM-CSF or underwent observation. Those treated with GM-CSF had a decrease in frequency of infections and an increase in their white blood cell counts components. There was no difference in platelet counts, hemoglobin, or transfusion requirements between the two groups. The risk of leukemic transformation appeared the highest in those patients with greater than

15% blasts in the bone marrow. The use of GM-CSF as maintenance therapy is controversial and not routinely used in patients with neutropenia. G-CSF has also been evaluated in randomized controlled trials in patients with higher-risk MDS. No difference was observed in time to progression to AML; however, in those patients with excess blasts, there was a decrease in overall survival, which led to early termination of the study. Myeloid growth factors are commonly used in the setting of neutropenic fever but otherwise not considered standard practice in patients with low white blood cell counts.

*Thrombopoietic Growth Factors:* Thrombocytopenia is common in MDS patients and over time can increase the risk of life-threatening bleeding. Platelet transfusions have short-term efficacy, but with their chronic use, there is the risk of development of alloantibodies, which can lead to refractory responses to transfusions. Platelets may also be dysfunctional, which can increase the risk of bleeding. MDS can be associated with autoimmune disorders, including immune thrombocytopenia purpura (ITP), which may respond to the combination of steroids and intravenous immunoglobulin. More recently, thrombopoietic receptor agonists, including eltrombopag and romiplostim have been evaluated. Their role and utility are still under study in clinical trials, and their use is not considered standard of care.

*Iron Chelation Therapy:* MDS patients who require chronic transfusions are at risk for iron overload, which can lead to organ damage, particularly cardiac dysfunction. Current National Comprehensive Cancer Network (NCCN) guidelines recommend consideration of iron chelation for lower-risk patients who receive 20 to 30 U of red cells over the course of their lifetime if ongoing transfusions are anticipated. For patients with serum ferritin greater than 2500 ng/mL, the recommendation is to decrease ferritin to less than 1000 ng/mL. The most commonly used chelation therapies include subcutaneous or intravenous deferoxamine or oral deferasirox.

*Immunosuppressive Therapies:* A subset of patients with MDS who present with pancytopenia and bone marrow hypoplasia may benefit from immunosuppressive therapy with antithymocyte globulin (ATG). These responses are mainly characterized by loss of transfusion requirements. Factors that predict a higher response to immunosuppressive therapy include age less than 60, low IPSS score, short duration of transfusion dependence, and presence of HLA-DR15 phenotype.

*Lenalidomide:* Lenalidomide is an immunomodulatory drug that can reduce red cell transfusion dependence and improve erythropoiesis, particularly in patients with lower-risk MDS with del(5q).

*Hypomethylating Agents:* Hypermethylation with aberrant silencing of tumor suppressor genes is thought to contribute to the pathogenesis of MDS. There are two hypomethylating agents, azacitidine and decitabine, that can re-express silenced genes and are used in the treatment of both lower-risk and higher-risk disease. Compared with supportive care in a phase III trial, azacitidine demonstrated significantly improved response rates, delay in transformation to AML, improved quality of life, and improved survival. This trial led to the approval of azacitidine by the US Food and Drug Administration as a first-line treatment for patients with MDS across all risk categories. In an international phase III trial, azacitidine was compared with conventional care regimens (including best supportive care, low-dose cytarabine, and induction chemotherapy) in higher-risk disease, and the group that received azacitidine had improved overall survival ($p < .0001$).

*Allogeneic Stem Cell Transplantation:* ASCT is the only curative therapy for MDS, although many patients are not candidates because of age, comorbidities, or lack of a suitable donor. Younger age, shorter duration of disease, female gender, and de novo MDS are predictors of improved disease-free survival. The exact timing and optimal conditioning regimen are under investigation. Lower-risk patients have better outcomes when transplantation is delayed until disease progression but prior to development of AML.

*Pharmacogenetics:* The incorporation of pharmacogenetics into the treatment of patients with MDS is an ongoing process. Since MDS is a complex and heterogeneous disease, targeted therapy is not available for the majority of abnormal karyotypes or gene mutations. However, it is well known that patients who present with an isolated del(5q) have a favorable prognosis and have a high response rate to lenalidomide. In addition, a subset of patients with MDS and isolated trisomy 8 respond well to immunosuppressive therapy. These patients are more likely to be young, have refractory anemia of short duration, and have the presence of HLA-DR15 phenotype. Testing for gene mutations in MDS is a relatively new phenomenon and therefore therapeutic targets are still under development. It has been postulated that certain mutations, including *DNMT3A*, *IDH1/IDH2*, and *TET2*, are associated with better responses to hypomethylating agents, such as azacitidine or decitabine (Table 35-2).

*Table 35-2 Pharmacogenetics in Myelodysplastic Syndromes*

| Genetic Abnormality | Associated Medications | Goal of Testing | Variants | Effect |
|---|---|---|---|---|
| Del(5q)—RPS14, mIR-145/146a | Lenalidomide | Efficacy | NA | Improved response rates and transfusion independence |
| Trisomy 8 | Immunosuppression | Efficacy | NA | Improved efficacy in a subset of younger patients with HLA-DR15 |
| Monosomy 7 | Azacitidine | Efficacy | NA | Improved response rates and overall survival |
| DNMT3A | Hypomethylating agents | Efficacy | NA | Improved efficacy from preliminary data |
| IDH1/IDH2 | Hypomethylating agents | Efficacy | NA | Improved efficacy from preliminary data |
| TET2 | Hypomethylating agents | Efficacy | NA | Improved efficacy from preliminary data |

# Molecular Genetics and Molecular Mechanism

*Cytogenetics:* Greater than 50% of patients with MDS have clonal cytogenetic abnormalities. The molecular effects of several of these abnormalities are still under investigation; however, they have helped stratify MDS into very good, good, intermediate, poor, and very poor prognostic groups. The most frequent abnormalities are either loss or gain of genetic material. The R-IPSS identifies five cytogenetic risk groups: Very good prognosis includes patients with −Y or del(11q); good prognosis includes a normal karyotype, del(5q), del(12p), or del(20q); intermediate prognosis includes del(7q), +8, +19, i(17q), or any other single or double independent clones; poor prognosis includes patients with monosomy 7, inv (3)/t (3q)/del(3q), −7/(del 7q), or three abnormalities; and very poor includes more than three chromosomal abnormalities.

Genetic instability as demonstrated by clonal evolution occurs in a substantial number of patients. Approximately 20% to 35% of patients will develop a chromosomal abnormality during the course of their disease. Clonal evolution is often associated with an adverse effect on survival and risk of leukemic transformation.

The gold standard for cytogenetic analysis is currently metaphase cytogenetics, which can detect balanced chromosomal changes such as translocations or inversions as well as unbalanced changes, such as trisomies or deletions. However, not all cytogenetic abnormalities can be detected with this technique since it has relatively low resolution and cells need to be dividing. Other techniques, such as fluorescence in situ hybridization (FISH) and single-nucleotide polymorphism (SNP) arrays can detect further chromosomal abnormalities in MDS patients. As newer techniques continue to develop such as microarray gene expression and methylation profiling, risk stratification will continue to improve.

*Somatic Point Mutations:* In recent years, genomic approaches, including next-generation sequencing and mass-spectrometry-based genotyping, have helped to identify recurrent mutations in MDS. The identification of recurrent mutations has led to insights into the pathophysiology of the disease. Genes involved in the regulation of histone function (*EZH2*, *ASXL1*, and *UTX*) and DNA methylation (*DNMT3A*, *IDH1/IDH2*, and *TET2*) are recurrently mutated in MDS, suggesting an important link between genetic and epigenetic mechanisms in this disease. Although single gene mutations are not currently used in prognostic scoring systems, they will likely become important predictors of clinical phenotypes and overall survival.

*Genetic Testing:* Although chromosomal analysis is a routine diagnostic tool in MDS, testing of gene mutations remains experimental. Chromosomal analysis is used to assist in prognostication but has limited value in decisions about therapy with the exception of del(5q).

*Future Directions:* While the genetics of MDS was previously characterized by cytogenetic abnormalities, the recent discovery of somatic mutations has provided new knowledge regarding the pathophysiology of the disease and has the promise to lead to novel therapeutic interventions. Mutations in genes encoding regulators of the epigenome represent an important new paradigm in MDS genetics. Further research is needed to define the prevalence of these mutations in various subtypes of MDS and understand the biologic consequences of these mutations. This, in turn, could help improve the ability to diagnose the disease, evaluate for progression, monitor response to treatment, and assess prognosis.

**BIBLIOGRAPHY:**

1. Bejar R, Stevenson K, Abdel-Wahab O, et al. Clinical effects of point mutations in myelodysplastic syndromes. *N Engl J Med.* 2011;364:2496-2506.
2. Bejar R, Levine R, Ebert BL. Unraveling the molecular pathophysiology of myelodysplastic syndromes. *J Clin Oncol.* 2011;29:504-515.
3. Fenaux P, Mufti GJ, Hellstrom-Lindberg E, et al. Efficacy of azacitidine compared with that of conventional care regimens in the treatment of higher-risk myelodysplastic syndromes: a randomized, open-label, phase III study. *Lancet Oncol.* 2009;10: 223-232.
4. Greenberg PL, Tuechler H, Schanz J, et al. Revised international prognostic scoring system (IPSS-R) for myelodysplastic syndromes. *Blood.* 2012;120(12):2454-2465.
5. Greenberg PL, Sun Z, Miller KB, et al. Treatment of myelodysplastic syndrome patients with erythropoietin with or without granulocyte colony-stimulating factor: results of a prospective randomized phase 3 trial by the Eastern Cooperative Oncology Group (E1996). *Blood.* 2009;114:2392-2400.
6. Graubert T, Walter MJ. Genetics of myelodysplastic syndromes: new insights. *Hematology Am Soc Hematol Educ Program.* 2011;2011:543-549.
7. List A, Dewald G, Bennett J, et al. Lenalidomide in the myelodysplastic syndrome with chromosome 5q deletion. *N Engl J Med.* 2006;355:1456-1465.
8. Mufti GJ, Gore SD, Santini V, et al. Influence of karyotype on overall survival in patients with higher-risk myelodysplastic syndrome treated with azacitidine or a conventional care regimen. *Blood.* 2009;114:Abstract 1755.
9. Silverman LR. The myelodysplastic syndrome. In: Hong WK, Bast RC Jr, Hait WN, et al, eds. *Cancer Medicine.* 8th ed. Shelton, CT: PMPH-USA; 2010:1544-1558.
10. Tiu R, Visconte V, Traina F, et al. Updates in cytogenetics and molecular markers in MDS. *Curr Hematol Malig Rep.* 2011;6:126-135.

## Supplementary Information

**OMIM REFERENCES:**

[1] Additional Sex Combs-Like 1; ASXL1 *612990
[2] CAS-BR-M murine ecotropic retroviral transforming sequence homolog; CBL*165360
[3] DNA methyltransferase 3A; DNMT3A*602769
[4] Enhancer of Zeste, Drosophila, homolog 2; EZH2*601573
[5] FMS-related tyrosine kinase 3; FLT3 ITD*136351
[6] Isocitrate dehydrogenase 1/Isocitrate dehydrogenase 2;IDH1/IDH2*147700/*147650
[7] Janus kinase 2; JAK2*147796
[8] Neuroblastoma RAS viral oncogene homolog/V-KI-RAS2 Kirsten rat sarcoma viral oncogene homolog; N/KRAS*164790/*190070
[9] Nucleophosmin/nucleoplasmin family, member 1; NPM1*164040
[10] RUNT-related transcription factor 1; RUNX1*151385
[11] TET oncogene family, member 2; TET2*612839
[12] Tumor protein p53; TP53*191170
[13] Ubiquitously transcribed tetratricopeptide repeat gene on X chromosomE; UTX*300128

*Key Words:* myelodysplastic syndrome, MDS, cytogenetics, pharmacogenetics, hypomethylating agents, azacitidine, decitabine, lenalidomide

# 36 Acute Myeloid Leukemia

Michael Heuser and Felicitas Thol

## KEY POINTS

- *Disease summary:*
  - Acute myeloid leukemia (AML) is a malignant disease originating from a hematopoietic cell that has acquired self-renewal properties. Hundreds of genetic aberrations have been described in AML cells, and recent evidence suggests that on average 13 genetic aberrations are present in AML cells.
  - Patients usually present with signs of anemia, infection, or bleeding.
  - The diagnosis is made if greater than or equal to 20 myeloid blasts are present in peripheral blood or bone marrow.
  - Conventional cytogenetics and molecular screening for fusion proteins PML-RARα, RUNX1-RUNX1T1, CBFB-MYH11, and for mutations of *NPM1*, *CEBPA*, and *FLT3* should be obtained at diagnosis.
  - Intensive chemotherapy should be given to all eligible patients consisting of cytarabine and an anthracycline.
  - Consolidation treatment consists of high-dose cytarabine or allogeneic hematopoietic stem cell transplantation depending on prognostic factors.
  - Acute promyelocytic leukemia (APL) is treated differently than other AML patients (including all-trans retinoic acid [ATRA] and an anthracycline) and has a good prognosis.

- *Differential diagnosis:*
  - Includes myelodysplastic syndromes (MDSs), aplastic anemia, other leukemias, or myeloproliferative neoplasms.

- *Monogenic forms:*
  - No monogenic form of AML is known. However, AML can be recapitulated in the xenotransplant model by overexpression of the fusion gene MLL-AF9 and MLL-ENL in human cord blood cells.

- *Family history:*
  - AML is considered as an acquired disease with no increased risk for family members. However, there are rare familial cases of AML in whom germline mutations in *RUNX1*, *CEBPA*, and *GATA2* have been found; 20% to 60% of carriers of these mutations develop myeloid malignancies.

- *Twin studies:*
  - Twin studies showed a high rate of concordance of AML between identical twins. However, the risk to develop AML for the twin of an AML patient is similar as in the normal population after the age of 6.

- *Environmental factors:*
  - Exposure to benzene, radiation, and chemotherapy (topoisomerase II inhibitors, alkylating agents) are known risk factors for AML.

- *Genome-wide associations:*
  - Three single-nucleotide polymorphisms (SNPs) have been identified to confer susceptibility to therapy-related AML (rs1394384, rs1381392, and rs1199098). They have not been prospectively tested to guide management of patients treated with chemotherapy.

- *Pharmacogenomics:*
  - SNPs in activating and inactivating enzymes of cytarabine have been shown to affect treatment toxicity and outcome, but are not routinely evaluated. Cytarabine dose is currently not adapted to the genotype of its metabolizing enzymes.

## Diagnostic Criteria and Clinical Characteristics

Diagnostic evaluation should include.
- Differential blood count.
- Wright-Giemsa stained blood or bone marrow smears evaluated by light microscopy to verify the presence of greater than or equal to 20% myeloid blasts.
- Myeloid lineage of blast cells is confirmed by cytochemical stains such as myeloperoxidase, Sudan black B (myeloid) or nonspecific esterase (monocytic), and/or by immunophenotyping for hematopoietic progenitor cells (CD34, HLA-DR, CD117), myeloid (MPO, CD13, CD33), monocytic (CD14, CD64), erythroid (CD71, glycophorin A), or megakaryoblastic (CD41, CD61) cell surface antigens.
- Conventional cytogenetic analysis of bone marrow cells using chromosome banding techniques is required for correct classification of AML according to the 2008 WHO classification.
- Reverse transcriptase-polymerase chain reaction (RT-PCR) and/or fluorescence in situ hybridization (FISH) are recommended for some recurrent translocations t(8;21)(q22;q22); inv(16) (p13q22) or t(16;16)(p13;q22); t(15;17)(q22;q12) and gene mutations (*NPM1*, *CEBPA*, *FLT3*) due to their impact on treatment decisions.
- Human lymphocyte antigen (HLA) typing of patients less than 70 to 75 years of age depending on the results of cytogenetic and molecular analyses.

*Clinical Characteristics:* Patients present with symptoms related to anemia, infection, and bleeding like fatigue, weakness, dyspnea on exertion, fever, abscess, mucosal bleeding or petechiae, and signs of extramedullary cell masses like gingival hyperplasia or skin lumps.

About 5% of cases are asymptomatic and are diagnosed based on differential blood counts. Severe anemia or thrombocytopenia may require blood transfusions and infections require antibiotic treatment. Patients with APL characterized by t(15;17)(q22;q12) may develop disseminated intravascular coagulation requiring treatment in the ICU. Historical data suggest that the median survival of untreated patients is 6 months.

## Screening and Counseling

*Screening:* The vast majority of AML cases are acquired during a lifetime, and no markers for early detection or for screening of family members have been established. For rare familial cases of AML, predisposing mutations in *RUNX1* (like in familial platelet disorder where constitutional microdeletions involving chromosomal region 21q22.12 leads to a deletion in *RUNX1*), *CEBPA,* or *GATA2* have been identified. Currently, screening for *RUNX1, CEBPA,* or *GATA2* mutations should only be offered to family members if a family member of the patient has been diagnosed with AML and also harbors a mutation in *RUNX1, CEBPA,* or *GATA2.*

Several genetic syndromes are associated with an increased risk to develop AML (eg, Fanconi anemia, congenital neutropenia). There are also several predisposing conditions for AML like myelodysplastic syndromes, myeloproliferative neoplasms, aplastic anemia, and paroxysmal nocturnal hemoglobinuria. AML may also develop secondary to chemotherapy. However, AML cases are genetically very heterogeneous and thus no genetic markers exist to date that could be used for screening for secondary AMLs. In AML patients in whom allogeneic hematopoietic stem cell transplantation (alloHSCT) is anticipated, siblings and in some cases also parents are screened for their HLA type to identify potential donors.

*Counseling:* Familial AML is very uncommon. Familial platelet disorder is an autosomal dominant disease associated with *RUNX1* mutations. A myeloid malignancy like myelodysplastic syndrome (MDS) or AML develops in 20% to 60% of patients (median 35%). In patients with chromosome 21q22 deletions AML developed in 25% (3 of 12 patients). Nearly all family members tested positive for CEBPA mutations developed AML. In family members with proven *GATA2* mutations MDS or AML developed in 53%.

As family members of AML patients may become stem cell donors, information on the risks of stem cell harvest will be required. Bone marrow hematopoietic stem cells are harvested from anesthesized patients by multiple punctures of both iliac crests. Alternatively, hematopoietic stem cells may be mobilized to the peripheral blood by subcutaneous administration of granulocyte colony-stimulating factor (G-CSF). These stem cells can then be harvested by leukapheresis. G-CSF administration in breast cancer patients treated with chemotherapy increased the risk to develop MDS or AML by threefold. However, registry data from the United States and Europe have not identified any increased risk of AML or MDS when G-CSF was administered to over 100,000 healthy individuals who donated peripheral blood stem cells, however, the median follow-up of these studies is less than 5 years.

## Management and Treatment

*Management:* AML is a heterogeneous group of diseases that are classified according to the World Health Organization (WHO) classification from 2008. Two-thirds of the patients can be classified according to cytogenetic or molecular aberrations. Patients should be offered the opportunity to participate in clinical trials. Some study groups have implemented a rapid molecular screening (within 48 hours) for patients with suspected AML to identify predictive markers that will guide the subsequent treatment. These aberrations include t(8;21)(q22;q22); inv(16)(p13q22) or t(16;16) (p13;q22); t(15;17)(q22;q12) and mutations of *NPM1* and *FLT3.* All patients should receive intensive induction and consolidation chemotherapy, however, as the median age at diagnosis is 70 years, several patients are not eligible for intensive chemotherapy.

*Therapeutics:*

☞INDUCTION CHEMOTHERAPY: Cytarabine in combination with daunorubicin or idarubicin is the standard treatment for induction chemotherapy. The first treatment cycle may be repeated after 3 to 4 weeks. About 70% to 80% of patients 60 years or younger and approximately 50% of patients older than 60 years achieve a complete remission (<5% blasts in bone marrow and normalized blood counts) after induction chemotherapy. Mortality during induction chemotherapy ranges from 5% to 10%. High remission rates are achieved in molecular subtypes with t(8;21)(q22;q22), inv(16)(p13q22) or t(16;16)(p13;q22), and mutations of *NPM1* independent of patient's age supporting the application of intensive chemotherapy also in elderly patients with these aberrations.

☞CONSOLIDATION TREATMENT: Current options include high-dose cytarabine ($3g/m^2$ every 12 hours on days 1, 3, and 5) and alloHSCT in medically fit patients. The choice of consolidation treatment is based on prognostic factors that include clinical, but importantly also cytogenetic and molecular characteristics. Poor risk prognostic markers that guide treatment of choice in favor of alloHSCT are listed in Table 36-1. Patients with low or intermediate relapse risk receive three to four cycles of high-dose cytarabine. Patients with high and intermediate relapse risk benefit from alloHSCT (27% and 17% risk reduction for death, respectively). Recent data indicate that alloHSCT from related and unrelated matched donors are equally effective. Intermediate risk patients without cytogenetic aberrations can be further characterized by their mutations in *NPM1* and *FLT3.* Only patients with *FLT3*-internal tandem duplication (ITD) and patients without *NPM1, FLT3,* and *CEBPA* mutations had improved relapse-free survival compared to all other patients. The development of reduced intensity conditioning regimens permits the performance of alloHSCT in patients up to 70 years.

☞TREATMENT OF ELDERLY PATIENTS NOT ELIGIBLE FOR INTENSIVE CHEMOTHERAPY Low-dose cytarabine treatment of patients not eligible for intensive chemotherapy because of comorbidities or poor general condition prolongs survival

*Table 36-1 Prognostic Factors in AML That May Influence the Choice of Consolidation Treatment (High-Dose Cytarabine vs AlloHSCT)*

| Prognostic Factor | Characteristic |
|---|---|
| Cytogenetic risk | Good, intermediate, poor |
| Age | Younger than 60 to 65 years vs older |
| FLT3-ITD | Absent vs present |
| Response to induction chemotherapy | CR or PR vs refractory |

compared to best supportive care. In patients with 20% to 30% blasts in bone marrow, treatment with the DNA methyltransferase inhibitor azacytidine has been approved and has been shown to improve overall survival. Another hypomethylating agent, decitabine, has been approved for the treatment of AML patients 65 years or older independent of blast count in Europe but not in the United States. However, long-term remissions are rarely seen in these patients, and best supportive care may remain the only option.

☞ **TREATMENT OF APL:** The hallmark of APL is the t(15;17) translocation leading to the PML-RARα fusion protein, whereas other translocations involving RARα are rare in APL. Poor prognostic factors include white blood cells greater than 10,000/μL, platelet count less than 40,000/μL, and age greater than 60 years. Induction and consolidation treatment uses an anthracycline combined with ATRA. The addition of ATRA to chemotherapy has improved event-free survival from approximately 20% to 75% at 5 years. Cytarabine does not improve outcome of APL patients and has been omitted from current treatment protocols. Maintenance treatment is currently performed with ATRA and 6-marcaptopurine and methotrexate for 1 to 2 years. Quantitative RT-PCR is used to monitor remission status and minimal residual disease (MRD) by quantifying PML or RARα transcripts. In case of molecular or clinical relapse treatment with arsenic trioxide is initiated and alloHSCT is recommended. Combination treatment of ATRA and arsenic trioxide without chemotherapy as upfront treatment has recently been shown to have excellent results with reduced toxicity and will become standard first-line treatment in APL.

☞ **ATRA TREATMENT IN NON-APL PATIENTS:** ATRA in combination with chemotherapy has been tested in patients with AML other than APL and has shown efficacy in elderly patients, especially in patients with mutations in *NPM1* or low levels of MN1 expression. Preliminary data of a randomized trial comparing chemotherapy with ATRA to chemotherapy alone in younger AML patients has shown a benefit of ATRA for event-free survival.

☞ **FLT3 INHIBITOR TREATMENT:** Mutations of *FLT3* are found in up to 30% of AML patients, and *FLT3*-ITDs confer a poor prognosis. Several FLT3 inhibitors, including monoclonal antibodies and tyrosine kinase inhibitors (TKIs), are under investigation as single agents and in combination with other therapies in relapsed and refractory populations as well as newly diagnosed patients. Single-agent studies showed that FLT3 inhibitors are well tolerated and inhibit their target; however, clinical activity was modest and transient. Thus, FLT3 inhibitors are currently evaluated in combination with chemotherapy. The most widely studied drugs are midostaurin (PKC412), AC220, lestaurtinib (CEP-701), sunitinib, and sorafenib.

☞ **TREATMENT OF RELAPSED OR REFRACTORY AML:** The most important adverse prognostic factors at relapse are length of first complete remission, cytogenetics, and in patients with normal karyotype, higher patient age, and presence of FLT3-ITD. AlloHSCT should be considered for all eligible patients. Reinduction treatment should be given before alloHSCT and should include intermediate-dose cytarabine.

☞ **MRD MONITORING:** Monitoring of MRD by qRT-PCR is routinely performed in APL patients to quantify transcript levels of the fusion protein PML-RARα every 3 to 6 months for 3 to 5 years. MRD monitoring has also been established for fusion proteins CBFB-MYH11 of inv(16) or t(16;16), RUNX1-RUNX1T1 (AML1-ETO) of translocation t(8;21), and for 95% of the known *NPM1* mutations.

☞ **PHARMACOGENETICS:** The most active drug in AML cells is cytarabine, which is activated by deoxycytidine kinase and is degraded by cytidine deaminase and deoxycytidylate deaminase. SNPs in these genes have been associated with treatment outcome. The TT genotype of SNP C-451T in the promoter of cytidine deaminase was associated with a relative risk of death of 1.56. Patients with -360CC/-201CC compound genotype of deoxycytidine kinase had a worse response to chemotherapy in another study. However, individual dosing of cytarabine according to SNP genotypes has not been tested and thus SNP genotyping is not routinely performed.

## Molecular Genetics and Molecular Mechanism

See Table 36-2.

***Cytogenetic Aberrations:*** A large number of cytogenetic aberrations have been identified in patients with AML. A minority of these aberrations result in a distinct molecular and clinical profile and are now integrated into the WHO 2008 classification. Important examples are t(8;21) and inv(16) which are the characteristic aberrations for core-binding factor (CBF) leukemias. Both cytogenetic rearrangements disrupt genes that encode subunits of CBF, a transcription factor that functions as an essential regulator of normal hematopoiesis.

**t(8;21):** This translocation leads to the fusion protein RUNX1-RUNX1T1. It can be found in 5% of AML patients (more frequently younger patients). More than 70% of patients with t(8;21) show additional cytogenetic aberrations. Patients with t(8;21) carry a good prognosis. However, mutations in KIT occur in 25% of patients, which is associated with an adverse prognosis. A splice variant of RUNX1-RUNX1T1 with an extra exon (exon 9a) is sufficient to induce AML in mice, and RUNX1-RUNX1T1 combined with FLT3-ITD can induce leukemia in mice.

**Inv16 and t(16;16):** This aberration leads to the fusion protein CBFB-MYH11. It occurs in a similar frequency as t(8;21) in AML patients and again affects younger adults more often. The prognosis is similarly favorable as for t(8;21). Mouse studies show that CBFB-MYH11 inhibits myeloid differentiation and collaborates with *MN1* and *PLAGL2* to induce AML in mice.

**t(15;17):** This translocation characterizes APL. It produces the PML-RARα fusion protein which leads to aberrant expression of retinoic acid receptor target genes thus inhibiting myeloid differentiation. In 30% of patients mutated FLT3-ITD is found. Transgenic mice expressing PML-RARα develop a long-latency leukemia that is accelerated by coexpression of FLT3-ITD.

***Gene Mutations:*** The number of known gene mutations occurring in AML is steadily increasing secondary to next-generation sequencing technologies. Some of these mutations have distinct prognostic and therapeutic implications. In all AML patients, at least one mutation can be identified and on average 13 genes are mutated per patient. This mutational diversity contributes to the heterogeneity of the disease. Given the prognostic implications of mutations, cytogenetic aberrations and gene expression profiles, treatments are developed that target specifically these mutated genes.

***NPM1:*** Nucleophosmin 1 (*NPM1*) encodes for a protein involved in the biogenesis of ribosomes and assisting small proteins

*Table 36-2  Common Gene Mutations and Aberrantly Expressed Genes in AML*

| Gene | Mutation Frequency | Biologic Function | Clinical Implications of Mutation |
|---|---|---|---|
| NPM1 | 25% | Transcription factor involved in differentiation of hematopoietic cells | Favorable prognosis in CN-AML patients without FLT3-ITD |
| FLT3 | 25% | Receptor tyrosine kinase | Inferior outcome in patients with CN-AML, treatment with FLT3 inhibitor currently under investigation |
| DNMT3A | 20% | DNA methyltransferase, involved in epigenetic regulation | Inferior outcome |
| CEBPA | 10%-15% of CN-AML | Transcription factor involved in differentiation of hematopoietic cells | Favorable impact on outcome if double mutated |
| IDH1/2 | 15%-20% | Enzyme that catalyzes the oxidative decarboxylation of isocitrate to $\alpha$-ketoglutarate | No consistent prognostic impact |
| NRAS | 10%-15% of CN-AML | Guanine nucleotide-binding protein involved in signal transduction of membrane receptors like FLT3 and c-KIT | No prognostic impact |
| TET2 | 10%-20% | Epigenetic regulation | No prognostic impact |
| ASXL1 | 10% | Polycomb gene, chromatin remodelling | No independent prognostic marker, possibly inferior impact |
| RUNX1 | 5%-10% | Transcription factor | Inferior outcome |
| MLL | 5%-10% of CN-AML | Histone methyltransferase involved in gene expression during hematopoiesis | Inferior outcome |
| WT1 | 10% of CN-AML | Transcription factor involved in regulation of apoptosis, proliferation and differentiation of hematopoietic progenitor cells | Controversial (possible inferior outcome might be overcome by higher doses of cytarabine) |
| c-KIT | 25% of patients with CBF leukemias | Receptor tyrosine kinase, whose ligand is the stem cell factor | Unfavorable outcome for patients with CBF-AML |

| Gene Expression | Biologic Function | Clinical Implications of Overexpression |
|---|---|---|
| MN1 | Transcription cofactor | Inferior outcome |
| ERG | Member of the ETS transcription factor family | Inferior outcome |
| BAALC | Unknown | Inferior outcome |
| EVI-1 | Transcription factor | Inferior outcome |

NPM1, nucleophosmin; FLT3, FMS-like tyrosine kinase 3; CN-AML, cytogenetically normal acute myeloid leukemia; CEBPA, CCAAT/enhancer binding protein alpha; ATRA, all-trans retinoic acid; IDH, isocitrate dehydrogenase; RAS, RAt sarcoma; MLL, mixed-lineage leukemia; WT1, Wilms tumor 1; CBF-AML, core-binding factor AML.

in their transport to the nucleolus. Mutations in *NPM1* are found in 25% to 35% of AML patients, with the largest number occurring in patients with cytogenetically normal (CN) AML. The mutated form leads to an abnormal cytoplasmic localization of the NPM1 protein. Patients with the mutation and without the FLT3-ITD have a favorable outcome. Transgenic mouse models show myeloproliferation in one-third of the mice. Insertional mutagenesis studies suggest that mutated *NPM1* interacts with activated *CSF2*, *FLT3*, and *RASGRP1*.

**FLT3:** The FMS-like tyrosine kinase 3 (*FLT3*) gene encodes for a tyrosine kinase receptor and is mutated in a quarter of patients with AML. Mutations in *FLT3* can be found in the juxtamembrane (JM) (20% of AML patients) as well as the

tyrosine kinase domain (TKD) (5% of AML patients). Mutations leading to an ITD of the JM domain result in a continuously activated tyrosine kinase. These mutations have adverse prognostic implications. The role of the prognostic implications of point mutations in the TKD domain remains controversial. FLT3-ITD transgenic mice develop a lethal myeloproliferation in BALBc mice and collaborate with several other genes to induce AML.

**CEBPA:** *CEBPA* (CCAAT/enhancer binding protein alpha) encodes for a transcription factor, which is involved in the differentiation of hematopoietic cells. Mutations in *CEBPA* can be found in 10% to 18% of patients with CN-AML (especially with a 9q deletion). Mutations can be monoallelic or biallelic.

Only biallelic mutations (not the monoallelic mutation) correlate with a favorable prognostic effect. Both N- and C-terminal mutations have a transforming effect in mouse bone marrow cells.

**DNMT3A:** DNA methyltransferase 3A (*DNMT3A*) belongs to the group of DNA methyltransferases that catalyze the addition of methyl groups to the cytosine residue of CpG dinucleotides. Mutations in *DNMT3A* occur in 15% to 20% of AML patients with the highest incidence in CN-AML patients. The majority of mutations affect codon R882. Mutations in *DNMT3A* are associated with an adverse outcome in AML patients.

**IDH1/IDH2:** NADP$^+$-dependent isocitrate dehydrogenase genes 1 and 2 (*IDH1* and *IDH2*) encode for enzymes that catalyze the oxidative decarboxylation of isocitrate to alpha-ketoglutarate. No consistent prognostic impact has been found. It has been suggested that IDH2R140Q mutations have a favorable prognostic impact. Mutant IDH1 and IDH2 can metabolize isocitrate into 2-hydroxyglutarate, unveiling a neomorphic enzyme function for these proteins. Recent evidence suggests that 2-hydroxyglutarate acts as an oncometabolite that competes with alpha ketoglutarate as a cofactor of hydroxylases like TET2, JMJD2C, or EGLN1. IDH1 mutant transgenic mice develop splenomegaly and increased hematopoietic stem cell numbers. Mutant IDH1 accelerates leukemogenesis in cooperation with HOXA9.

**TET2:** The ten-eleven-translocation 2 (*TET2*) gene encodes for an enzyme that catalyzes the conversion of methylcytosine to 5-hydroxymethylcytosine. Earlier studies have shown that *TET2* plays an important role in myelopoiesis through epigenetic regulation of genes. Mutations in *TET2* have been described to occur in 10% to 20% of AML patients. TET2 mutations have no clear prognostic impact in AML patients. Recent loss-of-function mouse models show that loss of *TET2* induces myeloproliferation in mice.

**RUNX1:** Runt-related transcription factor 1 (*RUNX1*) is critical for the earliest steps of hematopoiesis. Deregulation of *RUNX1* occurs in AML through chromosomal rearrangements as well as mutations. Mutations occur in about 4% to 10% of AML patients and are associated with inferior outcome. Loss of *RUNX1* is embryonically lethal.

**WT1:** Wilms tumor 1 gene (*WT1*) is a transcription factor involved in the regulation of apoptosis, proliferation and differentiation of hematopoietic progenitor cells. Mutations in *WT1* have been identified in approximately 10% of patients with CN-AML. The prognostic implications of the mutations are controversial. While some studies have found a negative prognostic impact others have found no prognostic implication. The SNP rs16754 located in the mutational hotspot of *WT1* can be identified in 25% of patients and appeared to be associated with an improved outcome in adult and pediatric patients with CN-AML.

**KIT:** The tyrosine-protein kinase *KIT* is expressed on the surface of hematopoietic stem cells. Mutations in *KIT* occur in a quarter of patients with CBF leukemias. They carry an adverse prognostic impact in this otherwise prognostically favorable cohort.

**NRAS and KRAS:** NRAS and KRAS belong to a family of guanine nucleotide-binding proteins involved in signal transduction of several membrane receptors like FLT3 and c-KIT. Heterozygous point mutations occur with a frequency of 10% to 15% (*NRAS*) and 5% (*KRAS*) in AML patients. These mutations cause constitutive activation of the RAS proteins and the downstream effectors like MAPK or ERK. However, the mutations do not influence outcome in patients with AML.

**MLL1:** Mixed-lineage leukemia (*MLL1*) encodes for a histone methyltransferase which regulates expression of multiple hematopoietic transcription factors. Partial tandem duplications (PTDs) of *MLL1* that duplicate the 5' part of the gene occur in 5% to 10% of CN-AML patients. This alteration correlates with an inferior relapse-free survival. *MLL1* is a frequent target of translocations involving chromosome 11q23.

**ASXL1:** Additional sex comb-like 1 (*ASXL1*) belongs to the enhancer of trithorax and polycomb (*ETP*) genes that can both activate or repress Hox genes. Depending on the cellular context *ASXL1* can act as a transcriptional activator or repressor of retinoic acid receptor (RAR) activity. Mutations in *ASXL1* occur in about 10% of AML patients. In univariate, but not multivariate analysis ASXL1 was an independent prognostic factor. *ASXL1* knockout mice exhibit defects in differentiation of lymphoid and myeloid progenitors but do not show evidence of myeloproliferation or leukemia.

**BCOR:** BCOR (BCL6 corepressor) encodes for a protein that interacts with BCL6. Mutations in *BCOR* were recently identified in 3.6% of AML patients and may implicate an adverse outcome.

Aberrant gene expression in AML has also been described to be an important prognostic factor. The most significant deregulated genes include *MN1, ERG, BAALC,* and *EVI1*. High expressions of all four genes are associated with a worse prognosis. Mouse models investigating ectopic expression of these genes in primary bone marrow demonstrate an oncogenic role in leukemogenesis for these genes.

Other less frequently mutated genes include *JAK2* and *CBL* as well as newly described genes involved in splicing and the cohesin complex (including *SF3B1, SRSF2, ZRSR2, U2AF1, STAG2, SMC1A, SMC3,* and *RAD21*). Future studies will clarify their prognostic as well as functional role in leukemogenesis and will evaluate their role as potential therapeutic targets.

*Genetic Testing:* Conventional cytogenetic analysis and FISH for selected targets are essential for the workup of AML. Rapid molecular screening for fusion proteins PML-RARα, RUNX1-RUNX1T1, and CBFB-MYH11 and for mutations in *NMP1* and *FLT3* has been introduced in several study groups to guide genotype-specific treatment. HLA typing is essential for patients and their siblings if they are eligible for allogeneic hematopoietic stem cell transplantation. During treatment and follow-up, minimal residual disease is monitored in patients with APL with the PML-RARα fusion protein. At relapse cytogenetic analysis has to be repeated in all patients.

*Future Directions:* AML has been a paradigmatic disease to show the success of genetic testing. Discovery of the t(15;17) translocation and the resulting fusion protein PML-RARα has led to the discovery of the first targeted therapy with ATRA leading to a dramatically improved survival rate. One of the first patient genomes that were completely sequenced also came from an AML patient. Results from whole genome sequencing suggest that there are approximately 13 mutations in the coding region of each AML genome. This relatively low complexity makes AML an ideal model disease also for the future to study interactions of these mutations and identify efficient drug targets. Whole genome or exome sequencing will further diversify the disease into even more genetic subgroups for which targeted therapies will be evaluated. Thus, it is expected that high throughput sequencing technologies will be introduced in the diagnostic workup, for selection of targeted therapies, and in monitoring of minimal residual disease.

## BIBLIOGRAPHY:

1. Dohner H, Estey EH, Amadori S, et al. Diagnosis and management of acute myeloid leukemia in adults: recommendations from an international expert panel, on behalf of the European Leukemia Net. *Blood.* 2010;115:453-474.

2. Vardiman JW, Thiele J, Arber DA, et al. The 2008 revision of the WHO classification of myeloid neoplasms and acute leukemia: rationale and important changes. *Blood.* 2009;114(5):937-951.

3. Arber DA, Vardiman JW, Brunning RD, et al. Acute myeloid leukaemia with recurrent genetic abnormalities. In: Swerdlow SH, Campo E, Harris NL, et al, eds. *WHO Classification of Tumours of Haematopoietic and Lymphoid Tissues.* 4th ed. Lyon, France: International Agency for Research on Cancer; 2008:110-123.

4. Owen C, Barnett M, Fitzgibbon J. Familial myelodysplasia and acute myeloid leukaemia—a review. *Br J Haematol.* 2008;140:123-132.

5. Ganly P, Walker LC, Morris CM. Familial mutations of the transcription factor RUNX1 (AML1, CBFA2) predispose to acute myeloid leukemia. *Leuk Lymphoma.* 2004;45:1-10.

6. Smith ML, Cavenagh JD, Lister TA, Fitzgibbon J. Mutation of CEBPA in familial acute myeloid leukemia. *N Engl J Med.* 2004;351:2403-2407.

7. Hahn CN, Chong CE, Carmichael CL, et al. Heritable GATA2 mutations associated with familial myelodysplastic syndrome and acute myeloid leukemia. *Nat Genet.* 2011;43:1012-1017.

8. Burnett A, Wetzler M, Lowenberg B. Therapeutic advances in acute myeloid leukemia. *J Clin Oncol.* 2011;29:487-494.

9. Schlenk RF, Dohner K, Krauter J, et al. Mutations and treatment outcome in cytogenetically normal acute myeloid leukemia. *N Engl J Med.* 2008;358:1909-1918.

10. Sanz MA, Grimwade D, Tallman MS, et al. Management of acute promyelocytic leukemia: recommendations from an expert panel on behalf of the European Leukemia Net. *Blood.* 2009;113:1875-1891.

11. Marcucci G, Haferlach T, Dohner H. Molecular genetics of adult acute myeloid leukemia: prognostic and therapeutic implications. *J Clin Oncol.* 2011;29:475-486.

## Supplementary Information

### OMIM REFERENCES:

[1] Acute Myeloid Leukemia; AML (#601626)

[2] Myelodysplastic Syndrome; MDS (#601626)

[3] Familial Platelet Disorder With Propensity to Myeloid Malignancy; FPD/AML(# 601399)

### Alternative Name:

• Acute Myelogenous Leukemia

*Key Words:* AML, MDS, APL, NPM1, FLT3, CEBPA, t(8;21), t(16;16), inv(16), t(15;17), AML1-ETO fusion, RUNX1/RUNX1T1 fusion, CBFB/MYH11 fusion, PML/RARA fusion

# 37 Multiple Myeloma and Other Plasma Cell Disorders

Esteban Braggio and Rafael Fonseca

## KEY POINTS

- *Disease summary:*
  - Multiple myeloma (MM) is a plasma cell malignancy characterized by accumulation of clonal antibody-secreting plasma cells.
  - MM accounts for 1% of all cancers and 10% of all hematologic malignancies.
  - Almost all MM evolves from an asymptomatic premalignant stage termed as monoclonal gammopathy of undetermined significance (MGUS).
  - MM is now believed to be curable in only a small fraction of cases, and has a median overall survival of 5 years.
  - The major clinical manifestations are bone lesions, anemia, hypercalcemia, renal failure, and an increased risk of infections.
  - Genetic abnormalities are used for disease risk stratification and therapeutic decision making.

- *Differential diagnosis:*
  - Other hematologic disorders associated with monoclonal gammopathies, such as amyloidosis, Waldenström macroglobulinemia (WM) and polyneuropathy, organomegaly, endocrinopathy, M protein, and skin lesions (POEMS). Both IgM MGUS and WM represent fundamentally different disorders that arise from clonal cells different from the plasma cells.

- *Monogenic forms:*
  - No single gene cause of MM is known to exist.

- *Family history:*
  - Reports have described families with affected members in two or more generations, with two or more affected members in a single generation. First-degree family members of an MGUS affected individual have elevated risks of MGUS and MM.

- *Twin studies:*
  - Few studies report the occurrence of MM in monozygotic or dizygotic twins.

- *Environmental factors:*
  - Several studies have pointed to links between MM and environmental exposure to certain kinds of chemicals and radiation, however, most have been limited and there is no major environmental agent identified. It is currently believed that most MM is sporadic and not driven by genetic susceptibility or environmental factors.

- *Genome-wide associations:*
  - First genome-wide association studies (GWAS) have been recently published in MM. One study suggested that MM patients could be classified based on the germline single-nucleotide polymorphism (SNP) profiles into two distinct groups of good prognosis (>3 year progression-free survival [PFS]) and bad prognosis (<1 year PFS). Another study proposed the correlation of several SNPs with the clinical extent of the bone disease. Further validations are needed to confirm these findings.

## Diagnostic Criteria and Clinical Characteristics

***Diagnostic Criteria for MM:*** The diagnosis of MM requires 10% or more clonal plasma cells (PCs) on bone marrow examination or a biopsy-proven plasmacytoma, plus evidence of end-organ damage related to the underlying disorder. Organ damage is usually identified by the acronym *CRAB*, which includes

- C—calcium elevation (>11.5 mg/dL)
- R—renal dysfunction (creatinine >2 mg/dL)
- A—anemia (hemoglobin <10 g/dL)
- B—bone disease (lytic lesions or osteoporosis)

When MM is suspected clinically, diagnostic evaluation should include

- **Blood and urine tests:** Patients should be tested for the presence of monoclonal proteins in blood and urine by serum or urine protein electrophoresis, serum immunofixation, and serum-free light-chain (SFLC) assays.
- If M proteins are present, additional blood tests are recommended to measure blood cell counts and levels of calcium, uric acid, creatinine, and beta-2 microglobulin.
- Bone marrow biopsy and aspirate.
- Imaging which may include plain x-rays (metastatic bone survey), computed tomography (CT) scan, and magnetic resonance imaging (MRI).

***Clinical Characteristics:*** The disease is systemic and can cause renal insufficiency, bone lesions and fractures, fatigue due to anemia, and degraded function of the marrow and the immune system.

☞**SYMPTOMS:** The disease is asymptomatic in early stages (MGUS and smoldering multiple myeloma [SMM]). Symptoms at the time of disease progression mainly include bone pain and fractures, fatigue due to anemia, and symptoms of hypercalcemia such as loss of appetite, nausea, thirst, constipation, and confusion.

Other symptoms may include weakness or numbness in the legs, weight loss, and repeated infections.

☞**RISK FACTORS:**

• **Age:** The median age of people who develop multiple myeloma is 65 years.
• **Sex:** It is slightly more common in men than in women.
• **Race:** Individuals of African origin have twofold risk to develop MM when compared with Caucasians.
• **History of MGUS:** Every year 1% of the people with MGUS develop MM.
• **Obesity:** The risk of MM is increased in obese individuals.

## Screening and Counseling

*Screening:* There are no specific genes or loci that confer increased susceptibility to myeloma. Therefore no genetic counseling is recommended on a routine basis. However, for families with more than one affected individual, counseling may be appropriate.

Regarding the genetic changes observed in the tumor cells, no specific genetic markers are required to make a MM diagnosis, as this can be solely made on the basis of morphologic changes in the bone marrow. However, significant advances have been made to identify genetic abnormalities and molecular signatures that can predict clinical outcome in MM patients and include them in the routine clinical tests. Several genetic classifications are used in MM, generating between five and eight disease subgroups depending on the classification used. A two-group classification (standard and high-risk categories) based on the presence of specific genetic abnormalities has been recently proposed by the Mayo Stratification of Myeloma and Risk-Adapted Therapy guidelines (Table 37-1).

*Counseling:* The identification of high-risk genetic features is key for the more appropriate counseling of the high-risk MM, since the management of this subgroup of patients remains very challenging.

## Management and Treatment

*Management:* Therapy should be initiated only for symptomatic disease. Given that for most patients MM is an incurable disease, the main goals of the therapy are to relieve symptoms, avoid disease-related complications, be well tolerated with minimal toxicity, improve quality of life, and prolong life. The ability for establishing risk-adapted therapeutic strategies is critical in the treatment of MM. While the value of a complete response (CR) is still debated

*Table 37-1 Genetic Abnormalities Used on the Risk-Based Stratification*

| Standard Risk (75%) | High Risk (25%) |
| --- | --- |
| Hyperdiploid | Deletion 17p13 |
| t(11;14)(q13;q32) | t(4;14)(p16;q32) |
| t(6;14)(p21;q32) | t(14;16)(q32;q23) |
| All other abnormalities not found in high-risk group | Metaphase deletion 13 |
| | Metaphase hypodiploid |

the ability of current treatment strategies to do that has been greatly enhanced and in most cases seems to correlate with clinical benefit. In one study it was shown that CR was important for patients with high-risk disease, but not for those with low-risk disease, as defined by gene expression profiling.

The management of MM is usually divided into those patients who are stem cell transplant candidates and those who are not. A second stratification further segregates these subgroups according to genetic risk status. For those candidates for transplant an active induction regimen (based on risk stratification) followed by stem cell transplant, and possibly with maintenance therapy will likely be the future standard of care. Effective, but well-tolerated therapy is important for the elderly, with regimens such as lenalidomide and low-dose dexamethasone being used in low-risk disease and melphalan, prednisone, and bortezomib for those with high-risk features.

*Therapeutics:* A variety of therapeutic options are available for treating MM. The recent incorporation of thalidomide, its analogous compounds known as immunomodulatory drugs (IMiDs) and the proteasome inhibitor bortezomib in the treatment of MM has significantly improved the outcome of the disease. Multiple clinical trials have confirmed the superior response rate and PFS rates for IMiDs and bortezomib compared with older therapeutic combinations. Additionally, the use of these novel compounds in combination shows a significant superior effect than single-agent therapy. The approach for treatment of symptomatic MM is based on the eligibility for autologous stem cell transplantation (ASCT) and the risk stratification. A summary of the most recent recommendations is outlined in Table 37-2.

## Genetics and Molecular Mechanism

Myeloma is characterized by a very complex karyotype. Genetic aberrations are observed from the very early stages of the disease and are key elements in the establishment of the clonal PC population. Several genetic abnormalities influence the disease course and are important tools in the risk stratification of the MM. Aneuploidy is frequently observed in MM and delineates the disease into two major subtypes, hyperdiploid and nonhyperdiploid myeloma.

Hyperdiploid MM exhibits extra copies of multiple chromosomes, especially of odd chromosomes 3, 5, 7, 9, 11, 15, 19, and 21. The nonhyperdiploid myeloma is mainly characterized by translocations involving the IgH locus on chromosome 14 with several chromosomal partners. Primary IgH translocations are the initiating event in MM pathogenesis. All these translocations lead to the activation of proto-oncogenes located in multiple partner chromosomes such as 11p13 (*CCND1*; found in 15% of patients), 4p16 (*MMSET* and *FGFR3*; 15%), 16q23 (*MAF*; 5%), 6p21 (*CCND3*; <5%), and 20q12 (*MAFB*; <5%). Each of these translocations is associated with a specific prognostic outcome. Each one of these groups (hyper- and nonhyperdiploid MM) comprises approximately half of patients with very low overlapping between the categories.

*Genomic Abnormalities With Prognostic Outcome:*

☞**t(4;14)(p16;q32):** The presence of t(4;14)(p16;q32) is associated with poor outcome and aggressive clinical features, both at diagnosis and after either standard or high-dose chemotherapy. It has been suggested that patients with this abnormality treated with bortezomib show better outcome than with previous treatments;

*Table 37-2  Treatment Recommendation for Patients Classified Based on Eligibility for ASCT and Risk-Stratification Groups*

|  | Risk Stratification | Initial Therapy | Consolidation | Maintenance |
|---|---|---|---|---|
| Transplant-eligible patients | Standard risk | Len and low-dex | ASCT or Len and low-dex | Len |
|  | High risk | CyBorD or Bor and low-dex | ASCT | Bortezomib based |
| Transplant-ineligible patients | Standard risk | MPT or Len |  | Not recommended |
|  | High risk | MPV or CyBorD |  | Not recommended |

Len, lenalidomide; low-dex: low-dose dexamethasone; ASCT, autologous stem cell transplantation; Bor, bortezomib; CyBorD, cyclophospha-mide/bortezomib/dexamethasone; MPT, melphalan/prednisone/thalidomide; MPV, melphalan/prednisone/bortezomib.

however, t(4;14)(p16;q32) still has prognostic implications in large groups of patients treated with this drug. It is now believed that bortezomib partially, but not totally, overcomes the negative prognostic effect of t(4;14)(p16;q32). Unbalanced translocations with loss of the der14 (*FGFR3*) are commonly observed, suggesting that *MMSET* and not *FGFR3* may play a critical role in the clonal expansion of t(4;14)(p16.3;q32) MM cells.

☞**t(14;16)(q32;q23) AND OTHER MAF TRANSLOCATIONS:** t(14;16)(q32;q23) and t(14;20)(q32;q12) are associated with aggressive disease and with a negative outcome in MM treated with conventional, alkylator-based, and high-dose chemotherapy. Patients with t(14;16)(q32;q23) had a high propensity to display circulating cells, a feature of aggressiveness. These translocations have not been completely incorporated in the clinical routine tests given their very low prevalence. One large study has recently questioned whether t(14;16)(q32;q23) is prognostic, but at least three other series have shown its prognostic effects.

☞**t(11;14)(q13;q32):** t(11;14)(q13;q32) is associated with low plasma cell proliferation, low levels of serum monoclonal proteins, and good prognosis. It is found in a high proportion of MM patients with the IgM variant and light-chain amyloidosis. Patients with this translocation more frequently express CD20 and have lymphoplasmacytic morphology.

☞**DELETION OF 17p:** Deletion of 17p13 is a rare event at diagnosis (~10% of MM patients), but it becomes more common with disease progression. This abnormality is currently the single most important genetic prognostic factor in MM, irrespective of the treatment received, suggesting that none of the therapies had a significant impact in patients with 17p13 deletion. Patients with deletion of 17p13 often have associated hypercalcemia, extramedullary disease, central nervous system (CNS) involvement, high serum creatinine levels, and plasmacytomas. The simultaneous presence of deletion 17p13 and t(4;14)(p16.3;q32) is unusual, suggesting they are mutually exclusive abnormalities. The gene responsible for the negative effect of this abnormality has not been completely identified, but evidences indicate *TP53* as the strongest candidate.

☞**DELETION OF CHROMOSOME 13:** Deletion of chromosome 13 is one of the most common abnormalities, found in approximately 50% of newly diagnosed MM patients. Some studies have shown a similar prevalence in MGUS, indicating that it is an initial event in the disease. The abnormality is associated with poor survival when exclusively identified in metaphase cells, whereas it has an intermediate survival when solely detected in interphase cells. The most likely explanation for the difference in prognostic value is that the deletion seen in metaphases is an indicator of a more proliferative clone and higher tumor burden. Chromosome 13 is associated with an inferior outcome as it is likely a surrogate markers of high-risk genetic categories such as t(4;14)(p16.3;q32).

☞**1q21 AMPLIFICATION:** Gain of 1q21 is seen in a third of MM cases. Although the gain of 1q21 has been associated with aggressive disease and poor prognosis, its prognostic effect is still under investigation and its analysis has not been implemented into routine clinical tests. The proposed target of this region is *CKS1B*.

☞**PLOIDY:** Hyperdiploid MM is associated with good prognosis.

### Genetic Testing:

☞**CLINICAL AVAILABILITY OF GENETIC TESTING:**

**Fluorescence in situ hybridization (FISH):** FISH has been successfully incorporated as a routine test in the clinical laboratory. FISH detects cryptic translocations and can be performed on interphase nuclei, thus overcoming the major limitations related with the conventional cytogenetics analysis in MM. Only PCs must be scored, which can be achieved by purifying PCs (using anti-CD138 beads) or identifying the PCs by performing FISH in combination with immunofluorescence detection of cytoplasmic immunoglobulin light chain (eg, cIg-FISH). A major limitation is that FISH asks specific questions, thus failing to provide a whole genome analysis. However, until high-throughput technologies become routinely used, FISH remains the standard tool for genetic abnormality detection.

**Gene expression profiling (GEP):** The use of GEP as a risk-stratification tool has been successfully implemented in MM. Different gene indices have been implemented in the patient's risk stratification. These indices show good correlation with other markers of disease aggressiveness such as tumor proliferation. As aforementioned, the sorting of PC is critical and the purity of the population obtained needs to be ascertained. A major weakness of GEP is that it cannot predict the presence of 17p13 deletion, one of the most powerful poor prognosis genetic factors in MM. If GEP becomes a more accepted tool it would likely replace FISH as the prognostic tool of choice in the clinic routine.

**aCGH/SNP arrays:** Array-based comparative genomic hybridization (aCGH)/SNP arrays simultaneously analyze the whole genome for copy number abnormalities (both arrays) and uniparental disomies (SNP arrays only) in higher resolution than FISH. These molecular tools are ideal for analyzing ploidy status more precisely than FISH. A major limitation of these tools is that they cannot be used in the identification of balanced translocations, which are commonly observed in MM. Their use has not been implemented in the clinical laboratory.

☞**UTILITY OF TESTING:** The accurate risk stratification of MM patients has profound consequences on clinical decisions and therapy selection. The main challenge is the reliable identification of high-risk patients, as better therapeutic strategies need to be formulated for that subgroup of patients.

☞**RECOMMENDED GENETIC TESTING IN MYELOMA:** The ideal genetic prognostic tools should be reliable in predicting outcome, have desirable features to be developed as standard clinical laboratory tests (ie, good reproducibility and accuracy), be widely available, and easy to interpret. Currently, the detection of either t(4;14)(p16.3;q32), t(14;16)(q32;q23) and deletion 17p13 by FISH, as well as deletion 13 by conventional cytogenetics defines the high-risk prognostic group (Table 37-1). Other high-risk translocations, such as t(14;20)(q32;q12) and t(8;20)(q24;q12) have a low prevalence (<2%) and merely for practical reasons their inclusion has not been made routine in clinical tests. In the absence of high-risk genetic abnormalities, MM patients are included in the low-risk group.

*Future Directions:* Comprehensive high-resolution approaches are very powerful tools in the analysis of MM genetics. They provide a complete analysis at DNA (aCGH or SNP arrays) or RNA level (GEP) of the already defined genetic risk factors and in the identification of potential novel disease markers. The incorporation of these approaches in the clinical laboratory is long anticipated, or at least markers derived from these genomic efforts that could be converted to more widespread prognostic tests. There is no doubt that these tests will become the standard of care in the near future of MM, once they overcome the main limitations related with the routinely implementation of PCs purification, the complexity of the analysis associated, and the cost of the assays.

## BIBLIOGRAPHY:

1. Landgren O, Kyle RA, Pfeiffer RM, et al. Monoclonal gammopathy of undetermined significance (MGUS) consistently precedes multiple myeloma: a prospective study. *Blood.* 2009;113:5412-5417.

2. Durie BG, Van Ness B, Ramos C, et al. Genetic polymorphisms of EPHX1, Gsk3beta, TNFSF8 and myeloma cell DKK-1 expression linked to bone disease in myeloma. *Leukemia.* 2009;23:1913-1919.

3. Bergsagel PL, Kuehl WM, Zhan F, Sawyer J, Barlogie B, Shaughnessy J Jr. Cyclin D dysregulation: an early and unifying pathogenic event in multiple myeloma. *Blood.* 2005;106:296-303.

4. Shaughnessy JD Jr., Zhan F, Burington BE, et al. A validated gene expression model of high-risk multiple myeloma is defined by deregulated expression of genes mapping to chromosome 1. *Blood.* 2007;109:2276-2284.

5. Kumar SK, Mikhael JR, Buadi FK, et al. Management of newly diagnosed symptomatic multiple myeloma: updated Mayo Stratification of Myeloma and Risk-Adapted Therapy (mSMART) consensus guidelines. *Mayo Clin Proc.* 2009;84:1095-1110.

6. Haessler J, Shaughnessy JD Jr., Zhan F, et al. Benefit of complete response in multiple myeloma limited to high-risk subgroup identified by gene expression profiling. *Clin Cancer Res.* 2007;13:7073-7079.

7. Rajkumar SV. Multiple myeloma: 2011 update on diagnosis, risk-stratification, and management. *Am J Hematol.* 2011;86:57-65.

8. Fonseca R, Barlogie B, Bataille R, et al. Genetics and cytogenetics of multiple myeloma: a workshop report. *Cancer Res.* 2004;64:1546-1558.

9. Fonseca R, Bergsagel PL, Drach J, et al. International Myeloma Working Group molecular classification of multiple myeloma: spotlight review. *Leukemia.* 2009;23:2210-2221.

10. Avet-Loiseau H, Attal M, Moreau P, et al. Genetic abnormalities and survival in multiple myeloma: the experience of the Intergroupe Francophone du Myelome. *Blood.* 2007;109:3489-3495.

11. Fonseca R, Blood E, Rue M, et al. Clinical and biologic implications of recurrent genomic aberrations in myeloma. *Blood.* 2003;101:4569-4575.

12. Reece D, Song KW, Fu T, et al. Influence of cytogenetics in patients with relapsed or refractory multiple myeloma treated with lenalidomide plus dexamethasone: adverse effect of deletion 17p13. *Blood.* 2009;114:522-525.

## Supplementary Information

### OMIM REFERENCE:

[1] Multiple Myeloma (#254500)

### Alternative Names:
- Plasma Cell Myeloma
- Plasma Cell Dyscrasia
- Plasmacytoma
- Plasmacytoma of Bone
- Plasma Cell Neoplasm
- Extraosseous Plasmacytoma

*Key Words:* Multiple myeloma, genetic abnormalities, clinical outcome, FISH, gene expression profiling, risk stratification

# 38 Alpha-Thalassemia

Renzo Galanello, Antonio Cao, and Raffaella Origa

## KEY POINTS

- *Disease summary:*
  - Alpha-thalassemia is one of the most common hemoglobin (Hb) genetic disorder, characterized by reduced or absent production of the alpha-globin chains, especially frequent in Mediterranean, South East Asia, Africa, India, and the Middle East.
  - Four main conditions resulting from deletion or inactivation (nondeletion mutants) of one, two, three, or all four alpha-globin genes are recognized. Carriers of alpha$^0$-thalassemia (two deleted alpha-globin genes, ie, alpha-thalassemia trait) show microcytosis, hypochromia, and normal percentages of HbA2 and HbF, carriers of alpha$^+$-thalassemia (one deleted or nonfunctional alpha-globin gene, ie, alpha-thalassemia silent carrier) have either a silent hematologic phenotype or present with a moderate thalassemia-like hematologic picture. Two are the alpha-thalassemia clinically significant forms: Hb Bart hydrops fetalis syndrome and HbH disease (four and three deleted or nonfunctional alpha-globin genes, respectively). Hb Bart hydrops fetalis syndrome is the most severe form, characterized by fetal onset of generalized edema, pleural and pericardial effusions, and severe hypochromic anemia, in the absence of ABO or Rh blood group incompatibility. Death usually occurs in the neonatal period. HbH disease is characterized by microcytic, hypochromic hemolytic anemia, hepatosplenomegaly, mild jaundice, and sometimes thalassemia-like bone changes. Detection of red blood cell inclusion bodies (precipitated HbH) with supravital stain and HbH by hemoglobin analysis with high-performance liquid chromatography (HPLC) or electrophoresis is diagnostic for HbH disease. Genetic testing is used to confirm hematologic and clinical diagnosis and is useful in carriers for genetic counseling. If both parents carry an alpha$^0$ mutation, they have a risk of 25% of having an offspring with Hb Bart syndrome at each conception. In patients with HbH, genetic testing has a prognostic value, as interactions between nondeletional molecular defects or between deletional and nondeletional defects result in more severe phenotypes than interactions with deletional molecular defects.

- *Hereditary basis:*
  - Alpha-thalassemia follows an autosomal recessive inheritance pattern.

- *Differential diagnosis (see Table 38-1):*
  - Hydrops fetalis is associated with many other conditions, including immune-related disorders, fetal cardiac anomalies, chromosomal abnormalities, fetal infections, genetic disorders, and maternal and placental disorders. However, the combination of a hydropic fetus with a very high Hb Bart, is not found in other conditions.
  - HbH disease may be distinguished from other hemolytic anemias by (1) microcytosis, which is uncommon in other forms of hemolytic anemia, (2) the fast-moving band (HbH) on Hb qualitative or quantitative analysis, (3) the presence of inclusion bodies (precipitated HbH) in red blood cells after vital stain, and (4) absence of morphologic or enzymatic changes characteristic of other forms of inherited hemolytic anemia (eg, hereditary spherocytosis or elliptocytosis, glucose-6-phosphate dehydrogenase deficiency [G6PD] deficiency, 5-pyridin-dinucleotidase deficiency).
  - Alpha$^+$-, alpha$^0$-thalassemia carriers and beta-thalassemia carriers both show microcytosis and hypochromia, but beta-thalassemia carriers are distinguished by increased HbA2 (>4%). Iron status determination (serum iron, transferrin, and sometimes serum ferritin) is used to identify the presence of iron deficiency anemia which is also characterized by microcytosis and hypochromia.

## Diagnostic Criteria and Clinical Characteristics

### Diagnostic Criteria:

#### ☞Hb Bart Hydrops Fetalis Syndrome:

- Very severe fetal macrocytic anemia
- Hb Bart (85%-90%)
- Absence of HbF and HbA at Hb analysis with electrophoresis or HPLC
- Molecular analysis (see Genetic Testing paragraph)

#### ☞HbH Disease:

- Microcytic hypochromic anemia and reduced (<2%) HbA2
- Presence of variable amounts (up to 30%) of HbH
- In the neonatal period, approximately 25% of Hb Bart
- Molecular analysis (see Genetic Testing paragraph)

#### ☞Alpha-Thalassemia Carrier:

- Reduced mean corpuscular volume (MCV) and mean cell volume (MCH) in --alpha/--alpha and -- --/alpha alpha carriers
- Normal red cell indices or only slightly reduced MCV and MCH in −alpha/alpha alpha carriers
- Normal or slightly reduced HbA2, normal HbF
- Inclusion bodies (precipitated beta-4 tetramers) after incubation of erythrocytes with 1% brilliant cresyl blue supravital stain
- Reduced alpha- or beta-globin chain ratio in vitro
- Molecular analysis (see Genetic Testing paragraph)

### Clinical Characteristics:

#### ☞Hb Bart Hydrops Fetalis Syndrome

- Marked hepatosplenomegaly, diffuse edema, heart failure, and extramedullary erythropoiesis
- Hydropic fetus

*Table 38-1* **Genetic Differential Diagnosis**

| Syndrome | Gene Symbol | Associated Findings |
|---|---|---|
| Beta-thalassemia carrier | *HBB* | Clinically asymptomatic, reduced MCV and MCH with increased HbA2 level, microcytosis, hypochromia, anisocytosis, and poikilocytosis in peripheral blood smear. |
| X-linked mental retardation syndrome associated with alpha-thalassemia | *ATRX* | Distinctive craniofacial features, genital anomalies, and severe developmental delays with hypotonia and intellectual disability. Hematologic picture of a mild alpha-thalassemia trait. An acquired form is associated with myelodysplasia. |
| Alpha-thalassemia or mental retardation 16 syndrome | *ATR16* | Relatively mild mental retardation, variety of facial and skeletal abnormalities and developmental delay. Hematologic picture of an alpha-thalassemia trait. |

Gene names: *HBB*, beta-globin gene; *ATRX*, alpha-thalassemia or mental retardation syndrome X-linked gene; *ATR16*, familial mental retardation syndrome ATR-16 gene

☞**HbH Disease:**
- Enlargement of the spleen and less commonly the liver, mild jaundice, sometimes mild-to-moderate thalassemia-like skeletal changes, hypersplenism and gallstones, acute episodes of hemolysis in response to oxidant drugs and infections, aplastic crises due to B19 parvovirus infection.

- Minor disability in the majority of individuals. However, some are severely affected, requiring regular blood transfusions; in very rare cases hydrops fetalis is present.
- Iron overload is uncommon but has been reported in older individuals, usually as a result of repeated blood transfusions or increased iron absorption.
- Pregnancy is possible; worsening of anemia requiring blood transfusion has been reported.

☞**Alpha-Thalassemia Carrier**
- Usually asymptomatic

## Screening and Counseling

*Screening:* The following screening tests can be used to detect alpha thalassemia:

- **Red blood cell indices:** microcytic anemia in HbH disease or alpha-thalassemia trait; indices are usually normal in silent carriers and macrocytosis is present in Hb Bart syndrome as a result of extreme reticulocytosis and megaloblastoid erythropoiesis (see Table 38-2).
- **Peripheral blood smear:**
  - **Hb Bart syndrome:** large, hypochromic red cells and severe anisopoikilocytosis.
  - **HbH disease:** microcytosis, hypochromia, anisocytosis, poikilocytosis (spiculated teardrop and elongated cells), and very rare erythroblasts.
  - **Carriers:** reduced MCV, MCH, and red blood cell morphologic changes that are less severe than those in affected individuals; erythroblasts are not seen.
- **Red blood cell supravital stain of peripheral blood:** HbH inclusions (beta-4 tetramers) can be demonstrated in 5% to 80% of the erythrocytes of individuals with HbH disease following incubation of fresh blood with 1% brilliant cresyl blue for 4 to 24 hours. Rare red blood cells with HbH inclusions can be detected in subjects with alpha-thalassemia trait and the silent carrier state.
- **Qualitative and quantitative Hb analysis:** (by cellulose acetate electrophoresis, weak-cation HPLC, and supplemental techniques such as isoelectric focusing and citrate agar electrophoresis) identifies the amount and type of Hb present.

*Table 38-2* **Red Blood Cell Indices in the Most Common Alpha-Thalassemia Genotypes**

| Genotype | Sex | Hb (g/dL) | MCV (fl) | MCH (pg) | HbA2 (%) |
|---|---|---|---|---|---|
| $-\alpha^{3.7}\,\alpha/\alpha\alpha$ [a] | M | $14.4 \pm 0.9$ | $75.4 \pm 4.8$ | $25.4 \pm 2.1$ | $2.5 \pm 0.3$ |
| | F | $12.0 \pm 1.0$ | | | |
| $-\alpha^{3.7}\,\alpha/-\alpha$ [b] | M | $13.6 \pm 0.8$ | $71.3 \pm 3.0$ | $23.8 \pm 2.0$ | $2.4 \pm 0.3$ |
| | F | $11.8 \pm 0.9$ | | | |
| $\alpha^{nondeletion}\alpha/\alpha\alpha$ [a] | M | $14.4 \pm 1.1$ | $75.7 \pm 3.0$ | $25.6 \pm 1.4$ | $2.5 \pm 0.3$ |
| | F | $12.2 \pm 0.8$ | | | |
| $--/\alpha\alpha$ [b] | M + F | $13.2 \pm 1.6$ | $65.0 \pm 3.3$ | $21.0 \pm 1.3$ | $2.4 \pm 0.1$ |
| $--/-\alpha$ [c] | M + F | $10.3 \pm 0.8$ | $61.0 \pm 4.0$ | $19.0 \pm 1.0$ | $<2.0$ |
| $--/\alpha^{nondeletion}\,\alpha$ [c] | M + F | $9.0 \pm 0.7$ | $64.0 \pm 6.0$ | $19.0 \pm 1.0$ | $<2.0$ |

[a]alpha-thalassemia silent carrier
[b]alpha-thalassemia trait
[c]HbH disease

*Counseling:* Alpha-thalassemia is an autosomal recessive inherited disease. At each conception, if both parents carry an alpha$^0$ mutation ($-$ $-$/alpha alpha), they are at risk of 25% of having an offspring with Hb Bart syndrome, a 50% chance of having a child with alpha-thalassemia trait and a 25% chance of having a normal child. When one parent carries an alpha$^0$ mutation ($-$ $-$/alpha alpha) and the other is an alpha$^+$-thalassemia carrier ($-$alpha/alpha alpha or alpha$^{nondeletion}$ alpha/alpha alpha), each offspring has a 25% chance of having HbH disease, a 25% chance of having alpha-thalassemia trait, a 25% chance of being an alpha-thalassemia carrier, and a 25% chance of being a noncarrier. Each child of an individual with HbH disease inherits the mutation for either alpha$^0$-thalassemia or alpha$^+$-thalassemia and is thus an obligate heterozygote.

Prenatal testing may be carried out for couples who are at high risk of having a fetus with Hb Bart syndrome not only for the severity of this syndrome and the absence of an effective treatment, but also to avoid the severe maternal toxemic complications during pregnancy. Hydrops fetalis due to nondeletional alpha-thalassemias (homozygosity for alpha-globin variants) or to the interaction of alpha$^0$-thalassemia with a nondeletional allele has been rarely reported and prenatal diagnosis should be considered in these cases.

☞**Genotype-Phenotype Correlation:** Alpha-thalassemia phenotype correlates very well with the degree of alpha-globin chain deficiency. In general, interactions between deletional and nondeletional molecular defects result in more severe phenotypes than interactions of deletional molecular defects. This is clearly evident in HbH disease in terms of age at presentation, degree of anemia, prevalence of jaundice, hepatosplenomegaly, bone changes, and need of red blood cell transfusions.

## Management and Treatment

Hb Bart syndrome currently has no effective treatment. In some cases, noninvasive monitoring by Doppler ultrasonography, intrauterine transfusions, and hematopoietic stem cell transplantation has improved the prognosis of individuals with this disorder. However, these neonates have marked cardiopulmonary problems and high frequency of congenital malformations (patent ductus arteriosus, limb and genital abnormalities) in addition to the hematopoietic failure and further human experimentation should be discouraged until more effective therapies (eg, somatic gene therapy) are available.

HbH disease is usually benign in the Mediterranean population. Affected patients need regular monitoring for early detection and treatment of possible complications, such as worsening of anemia, cholelithiasis and iron overload. Folic acid supplementation is recommended by some clinicians. Sporadic red blood cells transfusions can be requested in case of hemolytic or aplastic crises, and pregnancy. Repeated transfusions are to be considered in a subset of patients usually from South-East Asia and Middle East, who are severely anemic. Splenectomy should be performed only in case of massive splenomegaly or hypersplenism; however, the risk of severe, life-threatening venous thrombosis should be always considered. Other complications, such as gallstones and leg ulcers, require appropriate medical or surgical treatment.

Carriers of alpha$^0$- or alpha$^+$-thalassemia do not need treatment.

## Molecular Genetics and Molecular Mechanism

In normal individuals, alpha-globin genes encoding the alpha-globin chains are duplicated and localized in the telomeric region of chromosome 16 (16p 13.3). Expression of these genes is dependent on four remote regulatory elements (named multispecies conserved sequences or MCS R1 to R4) located about 40 kb upstream in the introns of a flanking gene. The relative level of transcription of the two alpha-globin loci differs, as the alpha-2 gene encodes two to three times more alpha globin than alpha-1 gene.

Alpha-thalassemia encompasses all of those conditions characterized by decrease in production of alpha-globin chains due more frequently to deletions and less commonly to nondeletional defects of one or more of the four alpha-globin genes.

The most common deletions remove a single alpha-globin gene, resulting in the mild alpha$^+$ thalassemia phenotype ($-$alpha/alpha alpha). The $-$alpha$^{3.7}$ and $-$alpha$^{4.2}$ deletions, due to reciprocal recombinational events between highly homologous regions, are the most common alpha$^+$-thalassemia defects. Other rare deletions totally or partially remove one of the two alpha-globin gene. When extended deletions remove both alpha-globin genes, the alpha-globin synthesis from a chromosome is completely abolished, resulting in alpha$^0$-thalassemia. Very rarely, alpha$^0$-thalassemia results from deletion of the MCS-R elements, with both alpha genes intact. Nondeletional defects include single-nucleotide substitutions or oligonucleotide deletions and insertions in regions critical for alpha gene expression. In general, nondeletion-thalassemia determinants give rise to a more severe reduction in alpha-chain synthesis than the deletion type. The most common nondeletional variants are the alpha$^{IVS1(-5nt)}$ in Mediterranean, polyadenilation site mutations in Mediterranean and Middle East, termination codon mutations resulting in elongated alpha-globin variants including Hb Constant Spring and Hb Koya Dora in South East Asia, Hb Icaria in Mediterranean, and Hb Seal Rock in American Black families. Moreover, hyperunstable globin variants such as Hb Quong Sze, Hb Suan Dok, and Hb Heraklion might produce the phenotype of alpha-thalassemia.

*Genetic Testing:* Polymerase chain reaction-based methods have been developed for the most common alpha-thalassemia mutations. GAP-polymerase chain reaction, using specific primers flanking the deletion break-points, detects deletions associated with alpha$^+$- or alpha$^0$-thalassemia. Single-tube multiplex polymerase chain reaction assays for detection of the most common and frequently observed determinants of alpha-thalassemia have been developed. Alpha-globin gene sequence analysis can be performed to identify nondeletional point mutations. For suspected rearrangements (deletions or duplications) of the alpha gene cluster or of the MCS-R regions, the recently available multiplex ligation-dependent probe amplification method (MLPA) can be used. Definition of alpha-globin genotype in carriers is useful for genetic counseling, whereas, in patients with HbH disease, is useful for prognosis, as the nondeletional forms are more severe than the deletional forms.

**Bibliography:**

1. Galanello R, Cao A. Alpha-thalassemia. Gene Reviews, available at http://www.ncbi.nlm.nih.gov/books/NBK1435/; last updated June 7, 2011.

2. Gibbons RJ, Pellagatti A, Garrick D, et al. Identification of acquired somatic mutations in the gene encoding chromatin-remodeling

factor ATRX in the alpha-thalassemia myelodysplasia syndrome (ATMDS). *Nat Genet.* 2003;34:446-449.

3. Gibson WT, Harvard C, Qiao Y, Somerville MJ, Lewis ME, Rajcan-Separovic E. Phenotype-genotype characterization of alpha-thalassemia mental retardation syndrome due to isolated monosomy of 16p13.3. *Am J Med Genet A.* 2008;146A:225-232.

4. Origa R, Sollaino MC, Giagu N, Barella S, Campus S. Clinical and molecular analysis of haemoglobin H disease in Sardinia: hematological, obstetric and cardiac aspects in patients with different genotypes. *Br J Haematol.* 2007;136:326-332.

5. Galanello R, Cao A. Gene test review. Alpha-thalassemia. *Genet Med.* Feb 2011;13(2):83-88.

6. Harteveld CL, Higgs DR. Alpha-thalassemia. *Orphanet J Rare Dis.* May 28 2010;5:13.

7. Vichinsky EP. Alpha thalassemia major—new mutations, intrauterine management, and outcomes. *Hematology Am Soc Hematol Educ Program.* 2009:35-41.

8. Chui DH, Fucharoen S, Chan V. Hemoglobin H disease: not necessarily a benign disorder. *Blood.* 2003;101:791-800.

9. Viprakasit V, Harteveld CL, Ayyub H, et al. A novel deletion causing alpha thalassemia clarifies the importance of the major human alpha globin regulatory element. *Blood.* May 1 2006;107(9):3811-3812.

10. Higgs DR. Molecular mechanisms of alpha thalassemia. In: Steinberg MH, Forget PG, Higgs DR, Nagel RL, eds. *Disorders of Hemoglobin: Genetics, Pathophysiology, and Clinical Management.* Cambridge, UK: Cambridge University Press; 2001:405-430.

11. Chong SS, Boehm CD, Higgs DR, Cutting GR. Single-tube multiplex-PCR screen for common deletional determinants of alpha-thalassemia. *Blood.* 2000;95:360-362.

12. Galanello R, Sollaino C, Paglietti E, et al. Alpha-thalassemia carrier identification by DNA analysis in the screening for thalassemia. *Am J Hematol.* 1998;59:273-278.

## Supplementary Information

**OMIM References:**

[1] Hemoglobin—Alpha Locus 1; HBA1 (#141800)

[2] Hemoglobin—Alpha Locus 2; HBA2 (#141850)

[3] Hemoglobin—Zeta Locus; HBZ (#142310)

[4] Thalassemias (#604131)

**Key Words:** Microcytic anemia, alpha-thalassemia, hydrops fetalis, Hemoglobin H syndrome, Hb Bart

# 39 Genetic Platelet Disorders

Beau Mitchell

## KEY POINTS

- *Disease summary:*
  - Genetic platelet disorders are an expanding group of platelet abnormalities caused by single gene mutations. The clinical manifestations are usually mucocutaneous bleeding and range from moderate post-traumatic bleeding to spontaneous life-threatening hemorrhage. Patients may have low-to-normal platelet counts depending on the specific defect. Several defects also cause associated syndromes.

- *Differential diagnosis:*
  - If platelet count low: immune thrombocytopenia, thrombotic thrombocytopenic purpura, if platelet count normal: use of antiplatelet agents

- *Monogenic forms:*
  - The most well-characterized syndromes are Glanzmann thrombasthenia (GT) and Bernard-Soulier (BS) syndrome, resulting from mutations of alphaIIbbeta3 (*ITGA2B* and *ITGB3*) and the GPIb-IX-V complex (*GP1BA*, *GP1BB*, and *GP9*), respectively. These are the primary surface receptors mediating aggregation and adhesion, respectively.
  - Platelet type, pseudo von Willebrand disease (VWD) results from a mutation in GP1b alpha (*GP1BA*), causing increased binding and clearance of von Willebrand factor.
  - Other known surface receptors defects: mutations in alpha2beta1 (*ITGA2* and *ITGB1*) and GPVI (*GP6*), cause reduced collagen adhesion; P2Y12 (*P2RY12*) mutations cause abnormal secretion and response to ADP.
  - Wiskott-Aldrich syndrome (WAS) results from mutation of WAS. Microthrombocytopenia with abnormal platelet function in the setting of global immune dysfunction, X-linked thrombocytopenia (XLT) is a milder form.
  - Defects in protein trafficking and granule formation
    - Alpha-granule defects—Gray platelet syndrome caused by mutations in *NBEAL2* (localized to 3p21.1-3p22.1), and Quebec platelet syndrome caused by tandem duplication of the urokinase plasminogen activator gene (PLAU)
    - Delta-granule defects—Hermansky-Pudlak syndrome: many genes identified so far (*HSPS1, HPS3, HPS4, HPS5, HPS6, HPS7, HSP8, HSP9, AP3B1, DTNBP1, BLOC1S3, BLOC1S4, BLOC1S5,* and *BLOC1S6*)
  - Scott syndrome results from defective regulation of phosphatidylserine on the platelet surface due to mutation of transmembrane protein 16F (*TMEM16F*), official gene name is *ANO6* (anoctamin 6)
  - Defects in transcription factors *FOXA2, HOXA11, GATA1, FLI1, RUNX1* cause familial thrombocytopenia and platelet dysfunction along with skeletal, immune, and other organ system defects.
  - Defects in platelet production: congenital amegakaryocytic thrombocytopenia (CAMT)—caused by mutations in thrombopoietin receptor gene (*MPL*); thrombocytopenia absent radius (TAR), caused by a mutation in *RBM8A* with a minimally deleted 200-kb region at chromosome band 1q21.1 that is necessary but not sufficient to cause TAR; *MHY9* mutations result in defective myosin function, thrombocytopenia, and giant platelets.

- *Family history:*
  - Majority of known mutations are autosomal dominant inheritance. GT, BS, CAMT, and TAR are autosomal recessive. WAS and GATA-I are X-linked.

- *Twin studies:*
  - Not reported for known mutations.

- *Environmental factors:*
  - Hemostatic challenges, such as menstruation, childbirth, and surgery, may unveil or worsen bleeding symptoms. Heat or humidity and illness may also affect bleeding symptoms.

- *Genome-wide associations:*
  - Many genes or single-nucleotide polymorphism (SNP) associations have been reported, correlating to platelet count (ATXN2, NAA25, C12orf51, and PTPN11), platelet function (GP6, PEAR1, ADRA2A, PIK3CG, JMJD1C, MRVI1, and SHH), platelet lifespan (BCLXL), and other parameters. However, thus far no clinically relevant association has been identified.

- *Pharmacogenomics:*
  - Polymorphisms of cytochrome p450 gene *CYP2C19* and COX-1 gene *PTGS1* modulate platelet response to clopidogrel and aspirin, respectively. However, no clinical relevance has been demonstrated.

## Diagnostic Criteria and Clinical Characteristics

*Diagnostic Criteria for Inherited Platelet Disorders:*

**Diagnostic evaluation should include at least one of the following (see Fig. 39-1 algorithm):**

- Complete blood count and peripheral smear review of all cell lines
- Examination of platelet morphology
- Platelet aggregation studies
- Detailed family bleeding history
- Detailed medication history

**And the absence of**

- Concurrent use of antiplatelet agents

*Clinical Characteristics:*

- Bleeding is generally mucosal. Patients may also have easy bruising and petechiae.
- Epistaxis and oral bleeding may be prolonged and life threatening.
- Menstruation, especially menarche, poses a high bleeding risk.
- Childbirth is a high-risk hemostatic challenge for both mother and baby.
- Generally, bleeding symptoms decline with age.
- Bleeding characteristics tend to run in families.

## Screening and Counseling

*Screening:* Screening is recommended for symptomatic patients' family members to identify those at risk for bleeding. Some undiagnosed individuals discover their bleeding risk only when hemostatically challenged. This is particularly true for young girls at menarche who may have a life-threatening first bleed. Screening may also be warranted for management of the nonhematologic manifestations of the defect, such as in Wiskott-Aldrich.

*Counseling:* The individual familial platelet disorders are inherited as indicated earlier. Genetic counseling is recommended for both family planning and the mother's/baby's safety during pregnancy. Many of the inherited defects have at least some laboratory manifestation which allows identification of carriers. Prenatal diagnosis has been performed in GT.

Genotype-phenotype correlation is consistent for the most severe platelet defects, such as GT, BS, TAR, and CAMT. The bleeding phenotypes in some of the storage pool defects and in WAS are more variable. In general, the family and personal bleeding history are more accurate predictors of bleeding risk than genotype, making an extensive family bleeding history critical.

## Management and Treatment

**Transfusion** during severe hemorrhage is primarily directed toward replacing the defective platelets with normal. Making the correct diagnosis is critical for directing therapy as well as avoiding inappropriate therapy, for example, giving immune globulin for an incorrect diagnosis of immune thrombocytopenia.

**Alloimmunization** is a severe complication in both GT and BS, with antibodies directed against GPIIbIIIa and GPIb, respectively, and is a dire occurrence since it limits therapeutic options.

**Hormonal therapy**: Oral contraceptives, depot medroxyprogesterone acetate (DMPA), or local treatments (such as levonorgestrel-releasing intrauterine system [IUS]) have been

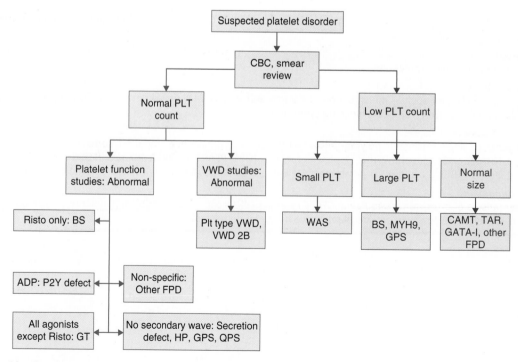

*Figure 39-1* Algorithm for Diagnostic Evaluation of Patient With Inherited Platelet Defect.

*Table 39-1* **Pharmacogenetic Considerations in Treatment With Antiplatelet Agents**

| Gene | Associated Medications | Goal of Testing | Variants | Effect |
|------|------------------------|-----------------|----------|--------|
| *CYP2C19* Cytochrome P450 system | Clopidogrel | Efficacy | *2 or *3 | Possible clopidogrel "resistance" |
| *COX-1* | Aspirin | Efficacy | >20 SNPs | Possible aspirin "resistance" |

helpful in controlling menorrhagia. These work by regulating endometrial growth and also by controlling the timing of the menstrual cycle.

**Antifibrinolytic agents** may be helpful in some of the milder platelet defects, such as Hermansky-Pudlak.

**Recombinant activated factor VIIa** has been used in both GT and BS, particularly those who have developed antiplatelet antibodies. FVIIa works in platelet defects because FVIIa can generate enough thrombin on the defective platelet surface to initiate coagulation. Also, GT and BS platelets still have a fibrin receptor which allows for some platelet agglutination in the presence of FVIIa.

**Thrombopoietin mimetics** are currently in clinical trials to determine their effect on bleeding and thrombocytopenia in inherited platelet disorders such as WAS.

**Hematopoietic stem cell transplantation** has been performed in several cases of GT. It is also recommended as treatment for some of the nonplatelet manifestations of diseases such as WAS and CAMT.

**Pharmacogenetics:** Several polymorphisms in the genes *CYP2C19* and *COX-1* reduce in vitro platelet sensitivity to clopidogrel and aspirin, respectively (Table 39-1), but so far no clinical relevance has been demonstrated. No genetics-driven tailoring of therapy is indicated at this time.

defects or functional polymorphisms will undoubtedly be uncovered and the list of inherited platelet disorders will continue to expand.

**BIBLIOGRAPHY:**

1. Nurden AT. Glanzmann thrombasthenia. *Orphanet J Rare Dis.* Apr 6 2006;1:10.
2. Lanza F. Bernard-Soulier syndrome. *Orphanet J Rare Dis.* Nov 16 2006;1:46.
3. Althaus K, Greinacher A. MYH9-related platelet disorders. *Semin Thromb Hemost.* Mar 2009;35(2):189-203.
4. Israels SJ, Kahr WH, Blanchette VS, Luban NL, Rivard GE, Rand ML. Platelet disorders in children: a diagnostic approach. *Pediatr Blood Cancer.* Jun 2011;56(6):975-983.
5. Gunay-Aygun M, Zivony-Elboum Y, Gumruk F, et al. Gray platelet syndrome: natural history of a large patient cohort and locus assignment to chromosome 3p. *Blood.* Dec 2 2010;116(23): 4990-5001.
6. Nurden AT, Fiore M, Pillois X, Nurden P. Genetic testing in the diagnostic evaluation of inherited platelet disorders. *Semin Thromb Hemost.* 2009;35(2):204-212.
7. Kunicki TJ, Nugent DJ. The genetics of normal platelet reactivity. *Blood.* Oct 14 2010;116(15):2627-2634.
8. Watkins NA, O'connor MN, Rankin A, et al. Definition of novel GP6 polymorphisms and major difference in haplotype frequencies between populations by a combination of in-depth exon resequencing and genotyping with tag single nucleotide polymorphisms. *J Thromb Haemost.* 2006;4(6):1197-1205.

## Molecular Genetics and Molecular Mechanism

Several genome-wide association studies (GWAS) have looked for associations with atherosclerotic disease. The majority of signals have been in noncoding regions, and thus far none of the identified polymorphisms have proven to be clinically significant.

*Genetic Testing:* Genetic testing is not generally commercially available for inherited platelet defects, although most known genes can be sequenced on a research basis.

Rapid genetic diagnosis using small blood volumes would be a useful tool in diagnosing genetic platelet disorders. Currently diagnosis rests on morphologic and functional analyses, and is made more difficult because the patients typically present in infancy or childhood. Prenatal genetic testing has been utilized for GT but required full sequencing and identification of the mutations in the parents' *ITGA2B* and *ITGB3* genes beforehand.

*Future Directions:* Gene therapy for inherited GT and other platelet disorders is on the horizon, and durable platelet response after gene therapy has been achieved in canines with GT. As the molecular function of the platelet continues to be unraveled, further genetic

## Supplementary Information

**OMIM REFERENCES:**

[1] Glanzmann Thrombasthenia; ITGA2B, ITGB3 (#273800)

[2] Bernard-Soulier; GP1BA, GP1BB, GP9 (#231200)

[3] Hermansky-Pudlak; HSPS1, HPS3, HPS4, HPS5, HPS6, AP3B1, DTNBP1, and BLOC1S3 (#203300)

[4] Wiskott-Aldrich Syndrome; WAS (#301000)

[5] Pseudo von Willebrand Disease; GP1BA (#177820)

[6] Thrombocytopenia Absent Radius; Chromosome 1q21.1 Deletion (#274000)

[7] Amegakaryocytic Thrombocytopenia; MPL (#604498)

[8] Scott Syndrome; TMEM16F (#608663)

[9] Paris-Trousseau; FLI1 (#188025)

[10] May-Hegglin, Fechtner, Sebastian, and Epstein Syndromes; MYH9 (#160775)

*Key Words:* Platelet, platelet disorder, thrombocytopenia

# 40 **Familial Cancer Syndromes**

Elizabeth A. Comen and Kenneth Offit

## KEY POINTS

- *Disease summary:*
  - Familial cancer syndromes are defined as cancers that arise in families with a genetic predisposition to develop cancer.
  - To date, up to 10% of all cancer diagnoses are in individuals with an inherited genetic mutation causing increased risk. Most of the common syndromes are a result of autosomal dominant mutations and result in earlier age at cancer diagnosis than those found in the general population.
  - Familial cancer predisposition may refer to syndromes where one or two types of cancer are dominant, such as breast and ovarian cancer in *BRCA1* mutation carriers. Alternatively, familial cancer syndromes may refer to syndromes which result in multiple affected organs, such as the case with HNPCC (Lynch syndrome) whereby mutations in DNA mismatch repair genes confer an increased risk to multiple types of cancers, for example, large and small bowel, uterus, stomach, ovaries, urinary tract, etc.
  - As the ability to identify and understand the genetic and genomic changes in an individual progresses, our understanding of inherited risk is likely to change. Models which incorporate multifactorial genetic and environmental influences will evolve to better assess familial risk.

- *Differential diagnosis:*
  - The differential diagnosis includes sporadic cancers and environmental or carcinogen risk-associated cancers. The differential must include careful consideration of a patient's family history and consideration of identifiable risk factors (such as tobacco use, asbestos exposure, etc). A careful assessment of familial and environmental risk factors is essential to determining whether to pursue genetic testing.

- *Monogenic forms:*
  - Several examples of a single gene causing cancer are known. The most common examples include but are not limited to *p53* (Li-Fraumeni syndrome), *BRCA1* or *BRCA2* (breast or ovarian syndromes), mismatch repair genes (Lynch syndrome), and the *APC* gene (familial adenomatous polyposis [FAP]).

- *Family history:*
  - Taking a detailed family history is critical for identifying a familial cancer syndrome. This includes obtaining information on first-, second-, and third-degree relatives. For many of the cancer syndromes, there are established diagnostic criteria for determining whether a family may harbor a predisposing gene.

- *Twin studies:*
  - To date, twin studies are limited by the challenge of differentiating common environmental factors from heritable risk. However, twin studies do suggest an increased risk among twins when one twin is affected. This is particularly true for colorectal, lung, breast, prostate, and stomach cancer and if the affected individual is young at the time of cancer diagnosis.

- *Environmental factors:*
  - There are numerous environmental factors (carcinogens) which are associated with an increased cancer risk. Carcinogens are identified as any substance (including radiation) with the capacity to perturb the cellular metabolic functions or genome directly. Furthermore, heritable risk is not independent of environmental risk. The environment can uniquely affect predisposing heritable risks, by tipping the balance toward the development of cancer in those patients with underlying risk factors.

- *Genome wide associations with common variants:*
  - With respect to cancer heritability, numerous genome-wide association studies (GWAS) have been conducted. GWAS studies have elucidated the complexity of heritable risk, illustrating that there may be numerable cancer susceptibility loci which individually confer only a modest increased risk of cancer. Efforts are underway to develop polygenic models which may account for the risks associated with multiple susceptibility loci. Currently, the use of GWAS associated risk factors is not clinically implemented.

- *Pharmacogenomics:*
  - Genetic testing for pharmacogenomic assays will likely to increase as the technology meets the necessity for clinical utility. Thus far, genetic testing for pharmacogenomic assessment is not routine with a few key examples summarized in Table 40-1.

- *Whole genome and exome sequencing:*
  - Recently it has become possible to analyze both common and rare genetic variants, as well as structural changes across entire genomes. The results of this work are defining new syndromes of disease predisposition, as well as uncovering unsuspected ones. Clinical translation of these technologies remains a central challenge of genomic medicine.

## Diagnostic Criteria and Clinical Characteristics

***Diagnostic Criteria for Familial Cancer Syndromes:*** There is no one diagnostic criterion for familial cancer syndromes. Specific criteria are largely dependent on the specific cancer syndrome and the patient population. In general, criteria for identifying a syndrome are based on noting the early onset of family members with specific cancers and the clustering of associated cancers with the involvement of multiple generations. Criteria may be qualified by the increased prevalence of certain cancers within a given population. For example, *BRCA*-associated breast and ovarian cancer syndromes are more common among those of Ashkenazi Jewish descent. As a result, genetic testing may be warranted in a young Ashkenazi Jewish woman with newly diagnosed breast cancer, even if she has no known relatives with breast cancer. For an extensive review of diagnostic criteria for specific cancer syndromes, please see the review by Garber and Offit and Weitzel and Offit.

***Clinical Characteristics:*** In general, early onset of diagnosis of multiple family members with cancer is suggestive of a number of familial cancer syndromes. For select familial syndromes, there are also clinical characteristics that may be specific to each syndrome. For example, in Cowden syndrome, an inherited breast and thyroid syndrome, afflicted probands may also have characteristic hamartomas, oral and skin papillomas, and other neurologic findings. Similarly, in Peutz-Jeghers syndrome, a syndrome associated with a number of cancers including pancreatic, liver, lung, and breast cancer, affected probands may have characteristic clubbing, mucocutaneous hyperpigmentation, and early childhood intussusception. The pathognomonic clinical characteristics for each of familial cancer syndromes are reviewed extensively elsewhere.

## Screening and Counseling

***Screening:*** When considering screening for a familial cancer syndrome, the most critical first step is an accurate assessment of family history. Furthermore, family history ought to be seen as an evolving part of a patient's record, as key changes may occur over time. When a familial cancer syndrome is suspected, the first person to genetically test is a family member with the affected cancer. Subsequent to identifying a known syndrome, genetic testing of potentially affected family members helps guide who may need additional cancer surveillance. Once a familial cancer syndrome is detected, all potentially affected family members should consider genetic testing after counseling with an appropriately trained physician or genetic counselor. Genetic testing ought to be considered only if the test in consideration can be adequately interpreted and will aid in the diagnosis or influence management of family members at increased risk.

Screening for specific cancers as part of a familial cancer syndrome ought to follow set guidelines for each particular syndrome. Very often, screening consists of routine clinical practices (magnetic resonance imaging [MRI], mammograms, colonoscopies etc) performed earlier than the guidelines set forth for the general population. In FAP syndrome, for example, at-risk family members should begin sigmoidoscopy as early as 10 to 12 years of age. Similarly, in *BRCA1* or *BRCA2* mutation carriers, women are eligible for early MRI screening (not routine practice).

***Counseling:*** Because of the significant ramifications of genetic testing, all patients considering genetic testing ought to receive counseling from appropriately trained physicians, genetic counselors or nurses, and cancer care providers. The American Society of Clinical Oncology (ASCO), the National Society of Genetic Counselors (NSGC), the Oncology Nursing Society (ONS), and other healthcare professional organizations have set forth guidelines

*Table 40-1* **Pharmacogenetic Considerations**

| Gene | Associated Medications | Goal of Testing | Key Variants | Effect |
|---|---|---|---|---|
| Enzyme UGT1A1 | Irinotecan (chemotherapy) | Chemotherapy metabolism | *UGT1A1\*28* | Decreased UGTA1 enzyme variability may result in high irinotecan levels and potentially lethal side effects |
| Enzyme TPMT | Thiopurine drugs (azathioprine, 6-mercaptopurine, 6-thioguanine) | Chemotherapy metabolism | *TPMT \*2,\*3A,\*3B, \*3C* | Genetic variations in TPMT affect the metabolism of chemotherapy used for a number of cancers including acute lymphoblastic leukemia |
| Enzyme DPD | 5-FU (chemotherapy) | Chemotherapy metabolism | *DPYD\*2A* | Genetic variation in the enzyme DPD may result in toxic levels of 5-FU |

*Table 40-2* **Notable Genes Associated With Hereditary Cancer Predispositions**

| Syndrome | Major Component Tumors | Associated Genes |
|---|---|---|
| Hereditary breast cancer syndromes | Breast cancer, ovarian cancer prostate cancer, pancreatic cancer, melanoma | BRCA1, BRCA2, PALB2 |
| Li-Fraumeni syndrome | Breast cancer, sarcomas, brain tumors, adrenocortical carcinomas | P53 |
| Cowden syndrome | Breast, thyroid, endometrial cancers | PTEN |
| Ataxia telangiectasia | Leukemias | ATM |
| Lynch syndrome | Colon, endometrial cancers, gastric, hepatobiliary, ovarian, pancreatic, renal, pelvis, small bowel, and ureteral cancers | MLH1, MSH2, MSH6, PMS2 |
| Familial adenomatous polyposis | Colon, gastric, duodenal, and ampullary cancers | APC |
| Mismatch repair cancer syndromes | Most commonly colon, CNS, hematologic cancers | MLH1, MSH2, MSH6, PMS2 |
| Hereditary diffuse gastric cancer | Gastric and lobular breast cancers | CHD1 |
| Peutz-Jeghers syndrome | Colon, small bowel, breast, ovarian, pancreatic cancers | STK11 |
| Hereditary pancreatic cancer | Pancreatic, breast, and ovarian cancers | BRCA2, PALB2 |
| Hereditary melanoma pancreatic syndrome | Pancreatic cancer, melanoma | CDKN2A (p16) |
| Melanoma syndromes | Melanoma | CDNK2 (p16), CDK4, CMM |
| Neurofibromatosis | Neurofibrosarcoma, pheochromocytoma, optic gliomas, meningiomas | NF1 |
| Tuberous sclerosis | Renal cancer, multiple bilateral renal angiomyolipoma, myocardial rhabdomyoma, ependymoma, giant cell astrocytoma | TSC1, TSC2 |
| Bloom syndrome | Leukemia, tongue carcinoma, squamous cancers, Wilms tumor | BLM |
| Fanconi anemia | Leukemia, squamous cancers, hepatoma, brain, skin, vulvar, cervical cancers, as well breast and ovarian cancers | FANCA, B, C, D2, E, F, G, I, L, M, N |
| Wiskott-Aldrich syndrome | Hematopoietic malignancies | WAS |
| Severe combined immune deficiency | B-cell lymphoma | IL2RG, ADA, JAK3, RAG1, RAG2, IL7R, CD45, Artemis |
| von Hippel-Lindau syndrome | Hemangioblastomas, renal cell cancers, pheochromocytomas, endolymphatic sac tumors | VHL |
| Beckwith-Wiedemann syndrome | Wilms tumor, hepatoblastoma, adrenal carcinoma, gonadoblastoma | CDKN1C, NSD1 |
| Wilms tumor syndrome | Wilms tumor, gonadoblastoma | WT1 |
| Retinoblastoma | Retinoblastoma, osteosarcoma | RB1 |
| MEN1 | Pancreatic islet cell tumors, pituitary adenomas, parathyroid adenomas | MEN1 |
| MEN2 | Medullary thyroid cancers, pheochromocytoma, parathyroid hyperplasia | RET |

Used with permission from Weitzel JN, Blazer KR, Macdonald DJ, Culver JO, Offit K. Genetics, genomics, and cancer risk assessment state of the art and future directions in the era of personalized medicine. *CA Cancer J. Clin.* 2011

for cancer risk counseling, risk assessment, and genetic testing. Counseling may include one or more sessions and ideally covers the consequences of genetic testing as well as a discussion of management options, including relevant surgical, chemoprevention, and screening options. As genetic testing becomes increasingly more prevalent, it will be especially important for all healthcare providers to be trained in adequate family history assessments so that at-risk individuals are appropriately identified.

## Management and Treatment

*Management:* As discussed earlier, management of individuals with select familial cancer syndromes is a function of the specific syndrome as well as the available genetic testing and screening.

*Therapeutics:* From a therapeutic perspective, treatment of individuals at risk for a familial cancer syndrome is divided into screening or surveillance, chemoprevention, and surgical options. For women at increased risk for breast cancer, for example, increased surveillance and screening with MRI and mammograms may be warranted. Chemoprevention with hormone modulating agents such as tamoxifen, raloxifene, and more recently exemestane are also potential options. Risk-reducing surgeries such as salpingo-oophorectomy may be required in some cases, while other approaches, such as prophylactic mastectomies may be offered in a more nondirective manner for *BRCA* mutation carriers who prefer active surveillance Any intervention, be it chemoprevention or risk-reducing surgery in an otherwise healthy individual, necessitates an ongoing discussion and realistic understanding of the risk of the disease, the consequences of surgery, and the potential benefit versus risk. For a more extensive review of the role of risk-reducing surgeries in the setting of hereditary cancers, please see the ASCO or SSO review of the role of risk-reducing surgery in hereditary cancer syndromes.

Lastly, as oncology moves toward more targeted, personalized therapies alongside an increased understanding of the genetic mechanisms underlying cancer, treatment may also be based on known hereditary genetic defects. In clinical trials now, PARP inhibitors are an example of a new class of medications aimed at treating *BRCA1* or *BRCA2* carriers with breast or ovarian cancer. PARP inhibitors work by leveraging an existing DNA repair defect inherent in cancers arising from *BRCA1* or *BRCA2* mutations.

*Pharmacogenetics:* There are a number of pharmacogenetic considerations with respect to specific cancer treatments. In particular, key examples of genes related to chemotherapy metabolism are outlined in Table 40-1 and reviewed more extensively elsewhere. While variants in these genes are not cancer predisposing, they may significantly affect chemotherapy metabolism.

## Molecular Genetics and Molecular Mechanism

*Genetic Testing:* (Table 40-2) As per the ASCO policy statement for genetic testing for cancer susceptibility, genetic testing ought to be considered if the following criteria are met:

1. The individual being tested has a personal or family history suggestive of genetic cancer susceptibility
2. The genetic test can be adequately interpreted
3. The test results have accepted clinical utility

Those in a position to offer genetic risk assessment are obliged to only offer those tests that are deemed safe and clinically appropriate. Thus far, the common genetic variants found by GWAS have not had sufficient effect size (level of risk) to be appropriate for clinical counseling. While a number of direct-to-consumer (DTC) tests for various single-nucleotide polymorphisms (SNPs) potentially associated with increased risk have recently become available, the clinical utility and relevance of these tests is uncertain to date. Recently next-generation sequencing has begun to provide panels of gene pathways for testing, including dozens of genes tested at one time. This poses challenges for genetic counseling. Soon, entire exomes and genomes will be screened, posing challenges for communication of incidental findings.

*Future Directions:* The future of medicine is undoubtedly moving toward an improved understanding of the genetic mechanisms underlying cancer. To this end, the identification of familial cancer syndromes for surveillance, screening, and prevention will become increasingly more important. In addition to the known genetic cancer risk factors, the unfolding of the genome will continue to elucidate additional genetic variations of varying significance. Effective risk models will likely incorporate multiple genetic risk factors (polygenic models) and epigenetic and other environmental contributions. The evolution of improved risk detection necessitates concomitant progress in our prevention and treatment strategies for at-risk populations.

### BIBLIOGRAPHY:

1. Lichtenstein P, Holm NV, Verkasalo PK, et al. Environmental and heritable factors in the causation of cancer—analyses of cohorts of twins from Sweden, Denmark, and Finland. *N Engl J Med.* 2000;343(2):78-85.

2. Stadler ZK, Vijai J, Thom P, et al. Genome-wide association studies of cancer predisposition. *Hematol Oncol Clin North Am.* 2010;24(5):973-996.

3. Garber JE, Offit K. Hereditary cancer predisposition syndromes. *J Clin Oncol.* 2005;23(2):276-292.

4. Ziogas A, Horick NK, Kinney AY, et al. Clinically relevant changes in family history of cancer over time. *JAMA.* 2011;306(2):172-178.

5. Robson ME, Storm CD, Weitzel J, Wollins DS, Offit K; American Society of Clinical Oncology. American Society of Clinical Oncology policy statement update: genetic and genomic testing for cancer susceptibility. *J Clin Oncol.* 2010;28(5):893-901.

6. Trepanier A, Ahrens M, McKinnon W, et al. Genetic cancer risk assessment and counseling: recommendations of the national society of genetic counselors. *J Genet Couns.* 2004;13(2):83-114.

7. Calzone KA, Jenkins J, Masny A. Core competencies in cancer genetics for advanced practice oncology nurses. *Oncol Nurs Forum.* 2002;29(9):1327-1333.

8. Fisher B, Costantino JP, Wickerham DL, et al. Tamoxifen for the prevention of breast cancer: current status of the National Surgical Adjuvant Breast and Bowel Project P-1 study. *J Natl Cancer Inst.* 2005;97(22):1652-1662.

9. Goss PE, Ingle JN, Alés-Martínez JE, et al. Exemestane for breast-cancer prevention in postmenopausal women. *N Engl J Med.* 2011;364(25):2381-2391.

10. Guillem JG, Wood WC, Moley JF, et al. ASCO/SSO review of current role of risk-reducing surgery in common hereditary cancer syndromes. *J Clin Oncol.* 2006;24(28):4642-4660.

11. Comen EA, Robson M. Inhibition of poly(ADP)-ribose polymerase as a therapeutic strategy for breast cancer. *Oncology (Williston Park).* 2010;24(1):55-62.

12. Bombard Y, Robson M, Offit K. Revealing the incidentalome when targeting the tumor genome. *JAMA.* (in press).

# 41 Central Nervous System Tumors

Kyle M. Walsh, Mitchel S. Berger, and Margaret R. Wrensch

## KEY POINTS

- *Disease summary:*
  - Primary central nervous system (CNS) tumors are a heterogeneous group of neoplasms arising from different cells of the CNS. CNS tumors may be associated with common genetic variation (sporadic tumors) and rare monogenic disorders (familial tumor syndromes).
  - Primary CNS tumors include both benign and malignant neoplasms, and in adults primarily consist of tumors of the neuroepithelial tissue and tumors of the meninges.
  - Tumors of neuroepithelial tissue account for approximately 34% of all primary brain and CNS tumors, and include in decreasing order of incidence: glioblastomas, lower-grade astrocytomas, oligodendrogliomas, ependymomas, and medulloblastomas. Neuroepithelial tumors are frequently malignant.
  - Tumors of the meninges account for approximately 36% of all primary brain and CNS tumors, and includes in decreasing order of incidence: meningiomas and hemangioblastomas. Tumors of the meninges are frequently benign.
- *Differential diagnosis:*
  - Symptoms of a primary CNS tumor can overlap with those of other neoplastic and non-neoplastic conditions, including metastatic brain tumors, peripheral nervous system tumors (eg, vestibular Schwannoma, chordoma), abscess or viral infection of the brain, cerebral infarct, cerebral hemorrhage, or encephalomyelitis (eg, multiple sclerosis, acute disseminated encephalomyelitis).
- *Monogenic forms:*
  - Numerous hereditary syndromes confer an increased risk for development of CNS tumors, including neurofibromatosis type 1, neurofibromatosis type 2, von Hippel-Lindau disease, tuberous sclerosis, Lynch syndrome, familial adenomatous polyposis, Li-Fraumeni syndrome, Cowden syndrome, melanoma-neural system tumor syndrome, and Gorlin syndrome (Table 41-1).
- *Family history:*
  - A family history of glioma confers approximately a twofold increased risk for development of glioma. Similarly, a family history of meningioma confers 3.5-fold increased risk for development of meningioma.
- *Twin studies:*
  - Twin or heritability studies have not been conducted for sporadic CNS tumors.
- *Environmental factors:*
  - Ionizing radiation increases CNS tumor risk. Personal history of allergies decreases meningioma and glioma risk. Men have a 20%-60% increased risk for glioblastoma compared to women, while women have a more than two-fold increased risk for meningioma compared to men.
- *Genome-wide associations:*
  - Genome-wide association studies (GWAS) have identified a single meningioma risk locus and eight independently significant glioma risk loci (Table 41-2).
- *Pharmacogenomics:*
  - In tumor genomes, *IDH1* or *IDH2* mutation, 1p or 19q codeletion, and *MGMT* promoter hypermethylation are all correlated with improved prognosis and an increased response to chemotherapy in patients with glioma.

## Diagnostic Criteria and Clinical Characteristics

***Diagnostic Criteria for CNS Tumors:*** While a comprehensive neurologic examination is needed, conclusive diagnosis of a CNS tumor requires some form of neuroradiologic imaging, most commonly gadolinium-enhanced magnetic resonance imaging (MRI). Determination of tumor type and histology can further be achieved:

- A full patient workup is necessary to diagnose a primary CNS tumor and exclude the possibility that the identified lesion is a metastasis from a primary tumor at another anatomic site.
- MRI may indicate the specific tumor type, especially in the case of meningiomas, and can further visualize the tumor and its relationship to the surrounding normal brain.

- Accurate diagnosis of a CNS tumor requires a tissue sample for histologic study, obtained either by biopsy or open surgery. Histopathologic diagnosis of low-grade glioma using only stereotactic biopsy comes with substantial risk of inaccuracy due to sampling error.
- A definitive diagnosis of tumor type or grade requires examination of tissue sections stained by hematoxylin and eosin.
- Important additional information may be obtained by a trained neuropathologist through immunohistochemical staining and cytogenetic testing of tissue sections.

***Clinical Characteristics:*** Local brain invasion, compression of adjacent regions and increased intracranial pressure in patients with a primary CNS tumor can manifest as a number of different symptoms, including:

*Table 41-1* **Mendelian Disorders With Increased CNS Tumor Susceptibility**

| Gene (Chromosome Location) | Disorder or Syndrome | Mode of Inheritance | Phenotypic Features | Associated CNS Tumors |
|---|---|---|---|---|
| *NF1* (17q11.2) | Neurofibromatosis type 1 | Dominant | Neurofibromas, schwannomas, café-au-lait macules | Astrocytoma, optic nerve glioma |
| *NF2* (22q12.2) | Neurofibromatosis type 2 | Dominant | Acoustic neuromas, meningiomas, neurofibromas, eye lesions | Meningioma, ependymoma |
| *VHL* (3p25.3) | von Hippel-Lindau disease | Dominant | Hemangioblastomas, renal cell carcinoma, pheochromocytoma, café-au-lait spots | Hemangioblastoma |
| *TSC1, TSC2* (9q34.14,16p13.3) | Tuberous sclerosis | Dominant | Development of multisystem nonmalignant tumors | Giant cell astrocytoma, cortical tubers |
| *MSH2, MLH1, MSH6, PMS2* | Lynch syndrome | Dominant | Predisposition to gastrointestinal, endometrial and other cancers | Glioblastoma, other gliomas |
| *APC* (5q22.2) | Familial adenomatous polyposis | Dominant | Predisposition to gastrointestinal, endometrial, and other cancers | Medulloblastoma |
| *TP53* (17p13.1) | Li-Fraumeni syndrome | Dominant | Predisposition to numerous cancers, especially breast, brain, and soft tissue sarcoma | Glioblastoma, other gliomas |
| *PTEN* (10q23.31) | Cowden syndrome | Dominant | Multiple hamartomas, increased cancer risk | Cerebellar gangliocytoma |
| *p16/CDKN2A* (9p21.3) | Melanoma-neural system tumor syndrome | Dominant | Predisposition to malignant melanoma and malignant brain tumors | Glioma, meningioma, ependymoma |
| *PTCH1* (9q22.32) | Gorlin-Goltz syndrome | Dominant | Predisposition to multiple basal cell carcinomas, odontogenic keratocysts, skeletal abnormalities | Medulloblastoma |
| *IDH1/IDH2* (2q33.3/15q26.1) | Ollier disease/ Maffucci syndrome | Acquired postzygotic mosaicism/ dominant with reduced penetrance | Development of intraosseous benign cartilaginous tumors, cancer predisposition | Glioma |

- Headache
- Nausea or vomiting
- Papilledema
- Generalized or focal seizures, especially in the case of gliomas
- Subtle cognitive dysfunction, including memory deficit and personality change
- Aphasia, apraxia, sensory loss, muscle weakness, and visual deficits may be observed and often reflect the function of the involved areas of brain

## Screening and Counseling

*Screening:* Increased risk of a CNS tumor is a characteristic symptom of numerous monogenic familial syndromes (Table 41-1). Relatives of an individual diagnosed with such a syndrome are themselves candidates for genetic testing to determine mutation status. Depending on the specific syndrome, such individuals may benefit from enhanced medical screening tailored to detect tumors associated with the particular syndrome.

*Table 41-2 CNS Tumor-Associated Susceptibility Variants*

| Candidate Gene (Chromosome Location) | Associated Variant | Relative Risk | Frequency of Risk Allele | Putative Functional Significance | Associated Disease Phenotype |
|---|---|---|---|---|---|
| MLLT10 (10p12.31) | rs11012732-A | 1.46 | 0.32 | Unknown | Meningioma |
| TERT (5p15.33) | rs2736100-G | 1.27 | 0.49 | Unknown | All glioma subtypes |
| EGFR (7p11.2) | rs2252586-T | 1.18 | 0.30 | Unknown | All glioma subtypes |
| EGFR (7p11.2) | rs11979158-A | 1.23 | 0.83 | Unknown | All glioma subtypes |
| CCDC26 (8q24.21) | rs55705857-G | 5.15 | 0.026 | Unknown | Oligodendroglial tumors/IDH mutated astrocytoma |
| CDKN2A, CDKN2B (9p21.3) | rs1412829-C | 1.42 | 0.61 | Unknown | Glioblastoma/ astrocytoma |
| PHLDB1 (11q23.3) | rs498872-T | 1.18 | 0.69 | Unknown | IDH mutated glioma |
| TP53 (17p13.1) | rs78378222-C | 2.35 | 0.0192 (Iceland) | Alteration of poly-adenylation signal impairs TP53 mRNA processing | All glioma subtypes |
| RTEL1 (20q13.33) | rs6010620-G | 1.52 | 0.23 | Unknown | All glioma subtypes |

While several genetic variants common in human populations confer moderately increased risk for CNS tumors (Table 41-2), genetic testing for disease-associated single-nucleotide polymorphisms (SNPs) has not been validated and is not currently available. **Counseling:** In a sample of individuals with no known history of a hereditary tumor syndrome, a family history of glioma conferred a statistically significant twofold increased risk for development of glioma. Similarly, a family history of meningioma conferred a statistically significant 3.5-fold increased risk for development of meningioma. A portion of this increased familial risk is due to common genetic variants, which in the case of glioma may show histology-specific associations (Table 41-2). In the case of CNS tumors, common genetic variants have not been incorporated into commercial genetic testing or risk prediction models and therefore are not yet part of genetic counseling practice.

Numerous familial syndromes confer an increased risk for development of CNS tumors. As outlined in Table 41-1, these disorders can all be inherited in an autosomal dominant manner, but have varied penetrance and expressivity. For more information on counseling individuals with respect to the disorders listed in Table 41-1, please refer to chapters on the specific monogenic disorder of interest.

## Management and Treatment

**Management:** In the case of low-grade or benign tumors, active surveillance is frequently undertaken to monitor tumor growth and progression. This is particularly true for patients with asymptomatic meningiomas, where treatment is initiated only if the tumor grows substantially or becomes symptomatic. Active surveillance may also be undertaken for patients with low-grade glioma, although many neurosurgeons opt for maximal safe resection as a first-line treatment.

**Therapeutics:** *Meningioma*: Symptomatic meningiomas and asymptomatic tumors that are growing or infiltrating should be surgically resected if feasible. Resection is often curative. For patients in whom incomplete resection was performed because the tumor was inaccessible, or in the case of atypical and malignant meningiomas, radiation therapy is also warranted and has been shown to prevent tumor recurrence and slow tumor progression.

*Glioma*: Malignant glioma is initially treated with maximal surgical resection that maintains neurologic and cognitive function, with use of intraoperative motor mapping being shown to minimize morbidity. Patients receiving total resection still have relatively high rates of tumor recurrence, but adjuvant radiotherapy can improve both progression-free and recurrence-free survival following resection. For patients with glioblastoma, adjuvant chemotherapy is also utilized. Temozolomide is currently the standard-of-care chemotherapy agent in the treatment of glioblastoma. Although the utility of postoperative chemotherapy for patients with oligodendroglial or low-grade astrocytic tumors has not been demonstrated in phase III trials, it is commonly employed and has shown benefit in retrospective studies.

**Tumor Markers, Prognosis, and Pharmacogenetics:** Inherited genetic variants are not currently utilized in determining the course of treatment for patients with CNS tumors, with the exception of the familial tumor syndromes (Table 41-1) which require different disease management strategies. Somatic alterations observed in CNS tumors (Table 41-3) do have value in predicting response to treatment and may be incorporated into treatment strategies. In the case of glioma, many of these somatic mutations are associated with particular tumor grades and histologies.

Oligodendrogliomas have a better prognosis than astrocytic tumors of similar grade, and are also more responsive to chemotherapeutic agents. As tumors with an oligodendroglial component frequently harbor mutations in *IDH1* or *IDH2*, show 1p/19q codeletion, and have *MGMT* hypermethylation, these mutations are associated with better prognoses in glioma patients (Table 41-4). In the case of the *IDH1* or *IDH2* mutation and 1p/19q codeletion, this survival advantage may reflect that the tumor (eg, glioblastoma) has an oligodendroglial component, itself a good prognostic

*Table 41-3 Molecular Alterations Frequently Observed in CNS Tumors*

| Gene/Chromosome | Molecular Alteration | Observed Frequency in CNS Tumors |
|---|---|---|
| 22q | Deletion | >50% of sporadic meningiomas |
| IDH1/IDH2 (2q33.3/15q26.1) | Missense mutation | 70%-80% of low-grade glioma (WHO II)<br>65%-70% of anaplastic glioma (WHO III)<br><10% of glioblastoma (WHO IV) |
| EGFR (7p11.2) | Amplification/hypermorphic mutation | <10% of low-grade and anaplastic glioma (WHO II and III)<br>>30% of glioblastoma (WHO IV) |
| 1p/19q | Codeletion | >80% of low-grade glioma (WHO II)<br>>60% of anaplastic glioma (WHO III)<br><25% of glioblastoma (WHO IV) |
| TP53 (17p13.1) | Loss-of-function mutations | ~30% of malignant glioma (WHO III and IV) |
| p16/CDKN2A, CDKN2B (9p21.3) | Deletion | ~50% of malignant glioma (WHO III and IV) |
| PTEN (10q23.31) | Loss-of-function mutations | ~25% of malignant glioma (WHO III and IV) |
| MGMT (10q26.3) | Promoter hypermethylation | >90% of low-grade glioma (WHO II)<br>>50% of anaplastic glioma (WHO III)<br><50% of glioblastoma (WHO IV) |
| FUBP1 (1p31.1) | Loss-of-function mutations | >10% of oligodendroglioma |
| CIC (19q13.2) | Loss-of-function mutations | >50% of oligodendroglioma |
| ATRX (Xq21.1) | Loss-of-function mutations | >10% of pediatric glioblastoma<br><10% of adult glioblastoma and oligodendroglioma |

factor. *MGMT* hypermethylation may confer a survival advantage independent of tumor histology, as *MGMT* is responsible for DNA repair following alkylating agent chemotherapy. Its silencing by hypermethylation may prevent repair of DNA damage and increase the efficacy of chemotherapeutic agents such as temozolomide. *IDH* mutation, 1p/19q codeletion, and *MGMT* hypermethylation frequently co-occur. Whether these alterations confer a survival advantage independent of tumor histology, or are simply molecular markers of less aggressive tumors remains to be determined.

## Molecular Genetics and Molecular Mechanism

Due to the high morbidity and mortality associated with CNS tumors, great efforts have been made to understand the etiology of these neoplasms. Heritable susceptibility to CNS tumors was originally suggested by the increased risk observed in patients with an affected first-degree relative, and also by the association of CNS tumors with numerous well-defined Mendelian disorders (Table 41-1). With the exception of linkage studies, genome-wide searches for heritable genetic causes of CNS tumors have thus far only been conducted in patients with glioma or patients with meningioma. In the case of meningioma, only a single GWAS has been published as of 2013. Further studies promise to expand meningioma SNP associations beyond the *MLLT10* locus.

GWAS of glioma patients have identified eight independently significant SNP associations, located in seven genes, that increase the risk for glioma development. Four of these genes appear to contribute to development of all glioma grades and histologies (*TERT*, *EGFR*, *TP53*, *RTEL1*), while the other three genes appear to contribute only to the development of certain histologic types (Table 41-2). SNPs near *CCDC26* appear to predispose primarily to oligodendroglial tumors and IDH-mutated astrocytomas, whereas SNPs in *PHLDB1* predispose to any IDH-mutated

*Table 41-4 Pharmacogenetic Considerations in CNS Tumors*

| Gene | Associated Medications | Goal of Testing | Variants | Effects |
|---|---|---|---|---|
| IDH1 (2q33.3) | Temozolomide | Prognosis | R132H | R132H—improved prognosis |
| Codeletion 1p/19q | Temozolomide | Prognosis | Codeletion | Deleted—improved prognosis |
| MGMT (10q26.3) | Temozolomide | Prognosis and efficacy | Promoter hypermethylation | Hypermethylated—increased chemosensitivity, improved prognosis |

glioma. SNPs near *CDKN2A* or *CDKN2B* confer increased risk for astrocytic tumors of all grades, including glioblastomas. The histologic specificity of these SNP associations is not yet definitive and remains an area of active research.

Whole-exome and whole-genome sequencing of glioma tumor tissue has identified a number of previously unrecognized genes that are involved in gliomagenesis. Most noteworthy has been the identification of *IDH1* and *IDH2* mutations in the majority of oligodendroglial tumors, more than half of the grade II and grade III astrocytomas, and approximately 10% of glioblastomas (grade IV). Sequencing oligodendrogliomas has also identified recurrent mutations in *FUBP1* and *CIC* on chromosomes 1p and 19q, respectively. As 1p/19q codeletion is also observed in greater than 80% of low-grade glioma (Table 41-3), this two-hit mechanism suggests that *FUBP1* and *CIC* act as tumor suppressors.

Tables 41-1 to 41-3 list genetic variants that increase the risk for development of CNS tumors, discovered either through GWAS, linkage studies, or tumor analyses, respectively. It has long been observed that mutations that cause Mendelian cancer syndromes occur in genes that also are frequently mutated in sporadic tumors. Thus, it is to be expected that loci in Table 41-1 largely overlap with those in Table 41-3. This is true for meningioma; constitutional *NF2* mutations cause neurofibromatosis type 2 and predispose individuals to the development of meningiomas, and somatic *NF2* mutations are identified in more than half of sporadic tumors.

An emerging theme in glioma research has been that the genes or pathways identified in linkage and tumor studies are also being identified in GWAS. This demonstrates that, in addition to the rare variation associated with Mendelian disorders, common genetic variation also contributes to gliomagenesis. While rare inherited loss-of-function mutations in *TP53* cause Li-Fraumeni syndrome, an inherited SNP found at a population frequency of approximately 2% also contributes to gliomagenesis. Additionally, 30% of sporadic gliomas show somatic loss of *TP53*. Because p53 is activated by DNA damage and oxidative stress, and responds by arresting cell division and promoting apoptosis, its role in tumor suppression is paramount. The *p16* or *CDKN2A* locus, which also appears in Tables 41-1 to 41-3, produces a protein that acts to stabilize p53. In this manner, the combination of linkage studies, GWAS and cytogenetics are beginning to shed light on the pathways involved in gliomagenesis.

Integrative genomics has recently shown promise in glioma research. SNPs associated with glioblastoma have been observed at the telomere-related genes *RTEL1* (regulator of telomere elongation helicase 1) and *TERT* (telomerase reverse transcriptase). Additionally, sequencing of glioblastoma tumors has identified recurrent mutations in *ATRX*, a gene that participates in chromatin remodeling at telomeres. A strong correlation has been observed between inactivation of *ATRX* and telomerase-independent telomere maintenance. As a result, a new model of gliomagenesis is being considered in which cancer cell immortalization is promoted by alternative lengthening of telomeres.

***Genetic Testing:*** For patients meeting screening criteria or belonging to an affected kindred, genetic testing is currently available for the dominantly inherited Mendelian disorders listed in Table 41-1. Prenatal testing is also available for a limited set of these disorders (eg, NF1). Please refer to chapters on the specific monogenic disorder of interest for additional information on the availability and appropriateness of genetic testing.

No role yet exists for genetic testing of patients with sporadic CNS tumors. However, genetic and cytogenetic testing of patients' tumors is routinely utilized to determine tumor histology and make better diagnoses. Genetic and cytogenetic testing of tumors also has a growing role in predicting patient survival and making treatment decisions, previously discussed and outlined in Table 41-4.

***Future Directions:*** Genome-wide studies of less common CNS neoplasms, such as ependymomas and hemangioblastomas, are on the horizon. Additional association studies of glioma and meningioma in non-Caucasian populations also appear warranted. As there is overlap between the genes identified from linkage studies of hereditary glioma tumor syndromes, glioma GWAS, and sequencing of glioma tumor genomes, approaches in integrative genomics promise to foster a better understanding of the complex processes underlying glioma and meningioma biology.

Genetic research on CNS tumors has, thus far, focused primarily on etiology. As the cost of genotyping and sequencing continues to decrease, pharmacogenomics will grow as a field. This is particularly important in the field of glioblastoma research, as median survival for glioblastoma patients remains around 15 months from diagnosis even for those receiving resection, radiation and temozolomide. Both constitutional polymorphisms and somatic mutations which correlate with better prognosis or response to treatment will be invaluable in increasing survival time and improving quality of life.

**BIBLIOGRAPHY:**

1. Central Brain Tumor Registry of the United States: http://www.cbtrus.org, Accessed July, 2012.

2. Hofer S, Lassman AB. Molecular markers in gliomas: impact for the clinician. *Target Oncol.* 2010;5(3):201-210.

3. Yano S, Kuratsu J, Kumamoto Brain Tumor Research Group. Indications for surgery in patients with asymptomatic meningiomas based on an extensive experience. *J Neurosurg.* 2006;105(4):538-543.

4. Weller M, Felsberg J, Hartmann C, et al. Molecular predictors of progression-free and overall survival in patients with newly diagnosed glioblastoma: a prospective translational study of the German Glioma Network. *J Clin Oncol.* 2009;27(34):5743-5750.

5. Sanai N, Chang S, Berger MS. Low-grade gliomas in adults. *J Neurosurg.* 2011;115(5):948-965.

6. Dobbins SE, Broderick P, Melin B, et al. Common variation at 10p12.31 near MLLT10 influences meningioma risk. *Nat Genet.* 2011;43(9):825-827.

7. Shete S, Hosking FJ, Robertson LB, et al. Genome-wide association study identifies five susceptibility loci for glioma. *Nat Genet.* 2009;41(8):899-904.

8. Wrensch M, Jenkins RB, Chang JS, et al. Variants in the CDKN2B and RTEL1 regions are associated with high-grade glioma susceptibility. *Nat Genet.* 2009;41(8):905-908.

9. Sanson M, Hosking FJ, Shete S, et al. Chromosome 7p11.2 (EGFR) variation influences glioma risk. *Hum Mol Genet.* 2011;20(14):2897-2904.

10. Stacey SN, Sulem P, Jonasdottir A, et al. A germline variant in the TP53 polyadenylation signal confers cancer susceptibility. *Nat Genet.* 2011;43(11):1098-1103.

11. Bettegowda C, Agrawal N, Jiao Y, et al. Mutations in CIC and FUBP1 contribute to human oligodendroglioma. *Science.* 2011;333(6048):1453-1455.

12. Heaphy CM, de Wilde RF, Jiao Y, et al. Altered telomeres in tumors with ATRX and DAXX mutations. *Science.* 2011; 333(6041):425.

## Supplementary Information

**OMIM References:**

[1] Tumor Protein p53; TP53 (#191170)

[2] Cyclin-Dependent Kinase Inhibitor 2A/p16(INK4A); CDKN2A (#600160)

**Alternative Name:**
• None.

*Key Words:* Glioma, glioblastoma, oligodendroglioma, astrocytoma, meningioma, ependymoma, hemangioblastoma, medulloblastoma

# 42 Esophageal Cancers

Nicholas B. Shannon and Rebecca C. Fitzgerald

## KEY POINTS

- *Disease summary:*
  - Esophageal cancers (ECs) are comprised of two main classes, esophageal adenocarcinoma (EAC) and esophageal squamous cell carcinoma (ESCC). Although globally ESCC is the more common of the two, in some western countries such as the United States of America and United Kingdom, EAC has become the dominant histology. Particularly high incidence rates of ESCC are observed in Iran, East Asia, and some African regions.
  - Rarely melanoma, sarcoma, small cell carcinoma, or lymphoma may arise.
  - More than 80% of the 481,000 yearly cases occur in developing countries; the disease is two to four times more common among males.
  - EAC is associated with Barrett esophagus (BE) as a consequence of gastroesophageal reflux disease (GERD) and obesity and usually occurs in the distal esophagus. ESCC is associated with smoking and alcohol and typically occurs in the mid and proximal esophagus.
  - The clinical presentation can usually be attributed to the direct local effects of the disease: dysphagia, sometimes accompanied by pain (odynophagia) and regurgitation of saliva or food. Weight loss is an early feature due to dysphagia and tumor-related cachexia in more advanced stages.

- *Differential diagnosis:*
  - It includes benign inflammatory esophageal stricture, esophagitis, gastric cancer, and achalasia or other motility disorders.

- *Monogenic forms:*
  - No single hereditary gene cause of EAC or ESCC is known to exist; however, tylosis is a Mendelian genetic syndrome, inherited in an autosomal dominant manner, and is associated with a high risk of developing ESCC (95% risk of developing ESCC by age of 65 years with type A). Linkage studies have suggested an association with the 17q25 locus tylosis esophageal cancer (TOC).

- *Family history:*
  - Increased risk of ESCC has been associated with a family history of upper gastrointestinal (GI) cancer probably due to inheritance of multiple low penetrance susceptibility genes. A first-degree relative is associated with one- to threefold increased risk and two or more affected first-degree relatives are associated with a 10-fold increased risk. Although several studies have shown familial aggregation of BE and EACC, linkage analysis in families has not been reported. Familial investigation of EC has primarily been performed in Asian populations; smaller Caucasian studies have shown a lack of evidence for familial susceptibility.

- *Twin studies:*
  - Although there have been no twin studies on EC, a genetic component to GERD has been demonstrated.

- *Environmental factors:*
  - The major risk factors for ESCC are tobacco smoking and alcohol consumption. ESCC is also associated with the consumption of burning-hot beverages and pickled foods. The main risk factor for EAC is reflux disease and obesity. There is a weaker risk association of EAC with tobacco smoking.

- *Genome-wide associations:*
  - Several associations have been identified by genome-wide association studies (GWAS) for ESCC; however, it is not known whether these are functionally important. Testing for single-nucleotide polymorphisms (SNPs) is not yet clinically validated.

- *Pharmacogenomics:*
  - The understanding and clinical application of genomics to therapy selection lags a long way behind other more common epithelial cancers.

## Diagnostic Criteria and Clinical Characteristics

Diagnostic evaluation should include

- A history to distinguish true esophageal dysphagia from oropharyngeal problems and likely dysmotility is critical. Clinical examination is mandatory but often noncontributory until in the advanced stages with palpable lymph nodes or liver enlargement. Nutritional status should be assessed.

- Blood count and serology, testing for nutritional status, inflammatory markers (eg, C-reactive protein [CRP], immunoglobulin G [IgG]), anemia, liver function.
- Endoscopic investigation is the investigation of choice. If there is no obvious lesion, chromoendoscopy utilizing Lugol iodine spray may be of benefit in high incidence areas for ESCC. Narrow band imaging and autofluorescence endoscopy may aid in the detection of early lesions in BE.
- Tissue sampling is mandatory to establish the diagnosis. Due to heterogeneity and tumor necrosis six biopsies are recommended.

If preinvasive lesions are identified, then multiple biopsy samples should be taken for the evaluation of dysplasia.

- Endoscopic ultrasound is useful to evaluate the depth of tumor invasion and lymph node involvement especially in the para-esophageal, gastric, and coeliac regions.
- Computed tomography (CT) is essential to provide information on local and systemic spread. Magnetic resonance imaging (MRI) is not currently part of the standard clinical staging algorithm. Positron emission tomography (PET) with fluorodeoxyglucose (FDG) should be used to help identify lymph node metastases and bone spread and may be useful to assess therapy response. CT and PET are increasingly performed as a combined modality.

- For tumors around the gastroesophageal junction with a gastric component laparoscopy is usually performed to assess the likely surgical approach (thoracotomy or laparotomy) and check for any peritoneal spread.

***Clinical Characteristics:*** Both ESCC and EAC have similar patterns of clinical presentation.

☞**PATTERNS OF DISEASE IN ESCC:** ESCC can present with dysphagia, weight loss, retrosternal or epigastric pain, and regurgitation caused by strictures. Superficial ESCC usually has no specific symptoms, but is sometimes associated with a tingling sensation, it is commonly observed as a slight elevation or shallow depression of the mucosal surface. Histopathologically ESCC

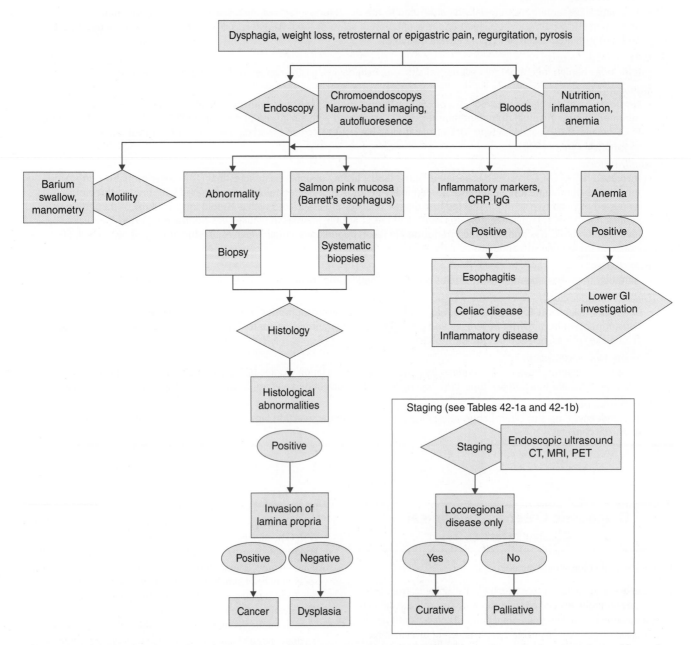

***Figure 42-1*** Algorithm for Diagnostic Evaluation of Patient With Upper Gastrointestinal (GI) Problems. Key evaluations in patients with esophageal cancer include endoscopy and histology for diagnosis followed by staging to inform on treatment decisions.

*Table 42-1a The Current (TMN7) Staging System for Esophageal Cancer*

| | |
|---|---|
| **T-stage** | |
| TX | Primary cannot be assessed |
| T0 | No evidence of primary |
| Tis | Tumour in situ/high-grade dysplasia |
| T1a | Tumour invades lamina propria or muscularis mucosae |
| T1b | Tumour invades submucosa |
| T2 | Tumour invades muscularis propria |
| T3 | Tumour invades adventitia |
| T4a | Tumour involves adjacent structures: pleura, pericardium, diaphragm, or adjacent peritoneum |
| T4b | Tumour involves other adjacent structures, eg, aorta, vertebral body, trachea |
| **N-stage** | |
| NX | Regional lymph nodes cannot be assessed |
| N0 | No regional lymph node metastasis |
| N1 | 1 to 2 regional lymph node metastases |
| N2 | 3 to 6 regional lymph node metastases |
| N3 | >6 regional lymph node metastases |
| **M-stage** | |
| MX | Distant metastasis cannot be assessed |
| M0 | No distant metastasis |
| M1a | Metastasis in celiac axis lymph nodes (station 9) |
| M1b | Other distant metastasis |
| **Grade** | |
| X | Grade cannot be assessed |
| 1 | Well differentiated |
| 2 | Moderately differentiated |
| 3 | Poorly differentiated |
| 4 | Anaplastic |

is defined as a squamous neoplasm that penetrates the epithelial basement membrane into the lamina propria or deeper tissue layers.

☞PATTERNS OF DISEASE IN BE: BE is the precursor lesion for EAC but is often clinically silent and may not be apparent in the presence of a large tumor mass. The symptomatology of BE when present is that of GERD usually manifesting as heartburn or acid regurgitation. Following repeated luminal injury the squamous esophageal epithelium is replaced by columnar epithelium.

The relative risk of EAC in patients with BE may be less than previously thought but is in the region of 0.33% per annum. In North America and some parts of Europe, the diagnosis of BE is restricted to columnar epithelium with goblet cells, elsewhere gastric metaplasia is also included in the definition.

☞PATTERNS OF DISEASE IN EAC: Symptoms of advanced EAC are similar to those of ESCC and principally include dysphagia and weight loss. Superficial EAC has no specific

*Table 42-1b Union Internationale Contre le Cancer/American Joint Cancer Committee (UICC/AJCC) Prognostic Groupings and Whether These Can Be Considered as Curative Disease Based on Survival Data*

| Prognostic Group | TNM Staging | Grade | Site | |
|---|---|---|---|---|
| Stage 0 | Tis N0 M0 | 1 | Any | Curative |
| Stage Ia | T1 N0 M0 | 1-2 | Any | Curative |
| Stage Ib | T1 N0 M0, T2 N0 M0 | 3, 1-2 | Lower | Curative |
| Stage IIa | T2 N0 M0 | 3 | Upper/middle | Curative |
| Stage IIb | T1-2 N1 M0, T3 N0 M0 | Any | Lower | Variable |
| Stage IIIa | T4a N0 M0, T3 N1 M0, T1-2 N2 M0 | Any | Upper/middle | Variable |
| Stage IIIb | T3 N2 M0 | Any | Any | Variable |
| Stage IIIc | T4a N1-2 M0, T4b any N M0, any T N3 M0 | Any | Any | Noncurative |
| Stage IV | Any T any N M1 | Any | Any | Noncurative |

symptoms. It can be discovered in patients presenting with symptoms of GERD, or during the surveillance of patients with BE. EAC is defined by the presence of invasion of the lamina propria.

☞**Extraesophageal Manifestations of EC:** Aside from lymph node involvement, typical sites of metastases include liver, lung, and adrenal glands. Compression of local structures in advanced disease may lead to airway obstruction and fistulas can occur into the bronchus and aorta.

## Screening and Counseling

**Screening:** Population screening for esophageal cancer has not been advocated despite its high mortality because of a lack of a suitable cost-effective, accurate method acceptable to patients. In high incidence areas for squamous cell cancer nonendoscopic cytologic devices have been trialed with limited success. Endoscopic screening with Lugol iodine spray is the gold standard to enable targeted biopsies to be performed; this is being used in high incidence areas such as China. Screening for BE relies on endoscopy and there has not been sufficient evidence to justify its use especially since endoscopic investigation is expensive, inconvenient, and uncomfortable, and carries a marginal risk of complications such as perforation and bleeding. Recent advances have been made with a nonendoscopic cell-sampling device coupled with a Barrett biomarker (TFF3) present in columnar epithelium.

There is some evidence for a role of serologic markers, including squamous cell carcinoma-related antigen (SCCA), carcinoembryonic antigen (CEA), and cytokeratin 19 fragment (CYFRA), although the data does not yet justify routine clinical use.

When preinvasive lesions are identified, endoscopic surveillance is generally recommended and intervention with endoscopic technologies such as endoscopic mucosal resection (EMR) and ablation techniques such as radiofrequency ablation (RFA) can be used for disease confined to mucosa.

**Counseling:** Although familial clustering is seen in esophageal cancer, it is unclear to what extent this is due to inherited or environmental factors. On the basis of current evidence it is not possible to give meaningful estimates of risk to family members unless tylosis is detected. It is reasonable in such families with affected first-degree relatives to perform a one-time screening endoscopy to look for preinvasive lesions. Individuals should be counseled on smoking cessation, alcohol moderation, and weight control.

## Management and Treatment for Invasive Cancer

**Management:** Following clinical staging, patients are usually divided into treatment groups based on whether the disease is locoregional and potentially curable or advanced with metastases for which palliative treatment is indicated.

☞**Local Palliation:** The main focus of care for incurable patients is palliation of dysphagia enabling them to eat. Esophageal obstruction can be treated by the use of expandable stents, which can be deployed endoscopically. Depending on the individual circumstances dilation, laser, or diathermy debulking of tumor may also be useful. For patients with a good performance status, palliative chemotherapy with or without radiotherapy may help to reduce

tumor burden, improve swallowing, and extend overall survival. The risks and benefits of these interventions need to be carefully weighed.

**Pain Control:** Pain may result from neural invasion of the tumor or metastases. In addition, pain may be experienced during EC treatment usually arising from esophageal tissue damage. Pain can be alleviated through standard pharmacologic analgesics. Nerve blocks may also be helpful in some cases.

**Chemotherapy and Chemoradiation:** For both ESCC and EAC chemotherapy is generally given in the neoadjuvant or preoperative setting. Increasingly triple modality therapy is given (chemoradiation followed by surgery) with clinical trial evidence for improved survival though at the expense of increased morbidity. In ESCC definitive chemoradiation may be considered and is particularly useful for those not fit for surgery. In the United Kingdom neoadjuvant chemotherapy is standard practice as established by the MRC OEO2 trial.

Molecular targeted therapies lag behind that for other epithelial cancers, but Her2 testing is increasingly being performed with the option to target the Her2 receptor in ongoing trials. If there is a significant gastric component Her2 targeted therapy may be given as standard on the basis of the TOGA trial data.

**Surgery:** The definitive treatment for patients with EC and submucosal invasion is esophagectomy with a gastric conduit to restore continuity, although this is only suitable for patients with localized disease (T1-3 disease without involvement of distant nodes or metastases). T4 disease can sometimes be resected depending on the adjacent structures involved; for example, it can be resected if invasion is into the pleura, but not if it is invading the aorta. Patients without submucosal invasion may instead be treated endoscopically (see below).

Surgery may be performed by a transthoracic (Ivor-Lewis) approach, permitting thorough lymphadenectomy, or a transhiatal approach, forming a high anastomosis with incomplete lymphadenectomy. Increasingly esophagectomy is performed laparoscopically; for patients with early disease a limited resection with regional lymphadectomy (Merendino procedure) may reduce postoperative morbidities. With improvements in technique and postoperative care, morbidity and mortality rates are now less than 5% in high-volume institutions.

**Endoscopic Therapy:** For patients with early-stage disease, endoscopic therapies offer a safer, less invasive option. Endoscopic mucosal resection (EMR or ER), and mucosal ablation using RFA are now becoming standard practice for EAC confined to the mucosa. In ESCC ablative therapy is also being performed successfully. Photodynamic therapy has largely been superseded by RFA in view of the phototoxicity. Argon plasma coagulation can be a useful adjunct for focal disease.

**Pharmacogenetics:** Testing for variants prior to assess potential chemotherapy efficacy is not clinically validated. In cisplatin-treated ESCC patients, variant alleles of *ERCC2* (D312N, K751Q) and *ERCC1* (8092C/A) which encode genes involved in nucleotide excision repair have been associated with improved survival; in contrast in patients who did not receive cisplatin, variant alleles had worse survival. Mutations in *MTHFR* are associated with decreased MTHFR activity, resulting in an increase in 5,10-methylenetetrahydrofolate ($CH_2FH_4$) concentration and fluorouracil (5-FU) activity. Thymidylate synthase (TS), a key enzyme in DNA synthesis is also involved in response to 5-FU, and a combination of *MTHFR* and *TS* variants has been associated with prolonged survival in ESCC patients (Table 42-2).

*Table 42-2 Pharmacogenetic Considerations in ESCC*

| Gene | Associated Medications | Goal of Testing | Variants | Effect |
|---|---|---|---|---|
| *MTHFR* (5, 10-methylenetetrahydrofolate reductase) | 5-FU | Efficacy | C677T, A1298C | Higher efficacy |
| *TS* (thymidylate synthase) | 5-FU | Efficacy | A277G | Higher efficacy |
| *ERCC2* (Excision repair cross-complementing 2) | Cisplatin | Efficacy | D312N, K751Q | Higher efficacy |
| *ERCC1* (Excision repair cross-complementing 1) | Cisplatin | Efficacy | 8092C/A | Higher efficacy |

## Molecular Genetics and Molecular Mechanism

Detailed study of familial predisposition to ESCC has focused on nonepidermolytic palmoplantar keratoderma (NEPPK or tylosis), which has been observed to segregate with ESCC in three pedigrees. The causative locus is known as the *TOC* gene and maps to 17q25 and is thought to be involved in the physical structure of stratified squamous epithelia. The genomic region containing the *TOC* gene is also associated with sporadic ESCC and EAC in loss of heterozygosity (LOH) studies.

Several polymorphisms have been associated with increased risk of developing ESCC (Table 42-3). In Asians, polymorphisms in *ALDH1B1* and *ALDH2*, the genes encoding aldehyde dehydrogenase, are associated with ESCC and are synergistic with alcohol use and smoking, leading to a 146-fold increased risk (OR = 146.4, 95% CI 50.5-424.5, n = 1071 cases, 2762 controls) in individuals with both genetic and environmental risk factors.

Somatic mutation of *TP53* (17p13) is an early event in ESCC, with some variation in frequency by geographic region. Amplification of cyclin D1 is another common event, and there is an association with accumulation of the Rb protein; both of these events are

associated with poorer survival. Amplification of proto-oncogenes has also been reported, including *EGFR* and *MYC*. Genes observed to be inactivated or lost include *CDKN2A*, *FHIT*, *TOC*, and the novel genes *DLEC1* and *DEC1*. Analyses of expression microarray profiles have identified a number of candidate oncogenes, tumor suppressors, and cancer-associated micro-RNAs with dysregulated expression. Many of these molecular features have also been linked to environmental exposures.

In EAC, the evidence for a familial association is more limited. Although association has been reported, population-based studies have suggested that the influence of genetic factors is limited, and is consistent with the rapid increase in incidence rates of EAC over the last 30 years. Although several associations have been identified for EAC in relatively small studies (*CCND1*, cyclin D1), these findings have not been replicated in larger case-control studies. Other relatively small studies have also identified associations in noncoding regions of genes (*MGMT*, *IGF1*), suggesting linkage disequilibrium with a functional variant or regulatory function.

Multiple somatic alterations have been observed in EAC (Table 42-4). *CDKN2A (p16)* is generally lost at an early stage in pathogenesis and *p53* mutation generally occurs by the time that invasive disease is established. Loss and gain of several chromosomal loci have been identified including gain of 8q (*MYC*) and

*Table 42-3 Disease-Associated Susceptibility Variants*

| Candidate Gene (Chromosome Location) | Associated Variant [effect on protein] | Relative Risk | Frequency of Risk Allele | Putative Functional Significance | Associated Disease Phenotype |
|---|---|---|---|---|---|
| *ADH1B* (4p15) | A227G [missense H48R] (rs1229984) | 1.85 | 0.23 (Japanese) 0.212 (1000 genomes) | Metabolism of alcohol | ESCC |
| *ALDH2* (12q24) | G1465* [missense stop-gain, E457*] (rs671) | 1.66 | 0.25 (Japanese) 0.057 (1000 genomes) | Metabolism of alcohol | ESCC |
| *PLCE1* (10q23) | A6414G [missense H1927R] (rs2274223) | 1.34 per allele | 0.209 (Chinese) 0.275 (1000 genomes) | GPCR pathways | ESCC |
| | C5964T [missense T1777I] (rs3765524) | 1.35 | 0.207 (Chinese) 0.281 (1000 genomes) | | ESCC |
| *MTHFR* (1p36) | C894T [missense A222V] (rs1801133) C677T | 1.57 | 0.325 (1000 genomes) | One-carbon metabolism pathway | ESCC |
| *ERCC2* (19q13) | T2245G [missense K751Q] (rs13181) | 1.25 | 0.235 (1000 genomes) | Nucleotide excision repair pathway | EAC |

*Table 42-4  Genetic Alterations in Esophageal Adenocarcinoma*

| Gene | Alteration | Frequency and Timing |
| --- | --- | --- |
| *TP53* | Mutation, LOH | 40%-88% increase from LGD, to HGD, and cancer |
| *SMAD4* | Loss, LOH | 40%-63% increase from LGD, to HGD, and cancer |
| *APC* | Promoter methylation, LOH | 50%-92% increase from LGD, to HGD, and cancer |
| *EGFR* | Overexpression | 31%-39% |
| *ErbB2* | Overexpression, amplification | 11%-43% late occurrence |
| *KRAS* | Mutation | 0%-36% |
| *CCND1* | Overexpression | 90% increase from BE |
| *CDKN2A (p16)* | Promoter methylation, LOH | 80% early occurrence |
| *AMACR* | Overexpression | 72%-96% increase from LGD, to HGD, and cancer |
| *CMYC* | Amplification | 83% |

LOH, loss of heterozygosity; LGD, low-grade dysplasia; HGD, high-grade dysplasia.

loss of 3p (*FHIT*), 5q (*APC*), and 18q (*SMAD4, DCC*). An increasing role for epigenetic alterations has been demonstrated by promoter methylation for E-cadherin, *APC*, *CDKN2A*, and *MGMT*. Early alterations in tumor suppressor genes, followed by loss of cell cycle checkpoints lead to ongoing genetic instability and EAC develops on this background of multiple clones of transformed cells. Despite considerable negative prognostic impact of many alterations, including ErbB2 amplification or overexpression, *TP53* mutations, and expression of *COX2*, *PRAP1* or *UPA*, and *MMP1*, there has been a difficulty in finding single molecular biomarkers of progression, which may be due to the heterogeneous nature of the disease. However advances are being made using *TP53*, p16, and DNA content, and future work may involve the development of panels of markers. In established, invasive EAC a panel of gene expression may predict outcome.

*Genetic Testing:* Currently no role exists for clinical genetic testing for susceptibility variants in the diagnosis or treatment of EC.

*Future Directions:* There is a requirement for large validated studies to determine the contribution of genetic susceptibility to ESCC and to EAC and to determine the potential of clinical testing for susceptibility alleles. Two GWAS studies including EAC are currently underway to identify susceptibility variants, Barrett's and Esophageal Adenocarcinoma Genetic Susceptibility Study (BEAGESS) and identification of inherited predispositions to BE and EAC (a Wellcome Trust Case Control Consortium 2, WTCCC2 study).

At the tissue level there is a requirement for biomarkers to predict the likelihood for progression from preinvasive disease, as well as to predict prognosis and response to therapy. In the future it may be possible to perform such tumor monitoring using blood-based assays.

Two large next-generation sequencing projects, the International Cancer Genome Consortium (ICGC) and The Cancer Genome Atlas (TCGA) are including cases of EA. It is hoped that the information from these studies will greatly expand current knowledge of the molecular pathology of this disease and may provide new options for prevention, treatment, or screening.

Overall the understanding and clinical application of genetics in EC lags being other more common epithelial cancers and chronic diseases. Further work is required to bring current knowledge through clinical use in aiding diagnosis and therapy selection. Increasing information on molecular pathology may allow the development of new therapeutic approaches in EC, for which the overall worldwide mortality rate remains above 84%.

**BIBLIOGRAPHY:**

1. Ferlay J, Shin HR, Bray F, Forman D, Mathers C, Parkin DM. GLOBOCAN 2008 v1.2, cancer incidence and mortality worldwide. *IARC CancerBase*. 2008;10. http://globocan.iarc.fr. Accessed November, 2011.

2. Bosman FT, Carneiro F, Hruban RH, Theise ND. WHO classification of tumours. *WHO Classification of Tumours of the Digestive System*. 4th ed. Vol 3. 2010;IARC.417.

3. Rice TW, Blackstone EH, Rusch VW. 7th edition of the AJCC Cancer Staging Manual: esophagus and esophagogastric junction. *Ann Surg Oncol*. 2010;17(7):1721-1724.

4. Desai TK, Krishnan K, Samala N, et al. The incidence of oesophageal adenocarcinoma in non-dysplastic Barrett's oesophagus: a meta-analysis. *Gut*. 2012;61(7):970-976.

5. Kadri SR, Lao-Sirieix P, O'Donovan M, et al. Acceptability and accuracy of a non-endoscopic screening test for Barrett's oesophagus in primary care: cohort study. *BMJ*. 2010;341:c4372.

6. Sakaeda T, Yamamori M, Kuwahara A, Nishiguchi K. Pharmacokinetics and pharmacogenomics in esophageal cancer chemoradiotherapy. *Adv Drug Deliv Rev*. 2009;61(5):388-401.

7. Toh Y, Oki E, Ohgaki K, et al. Alcohol drinking, cigarette smoking, and the development of squamous cell carcinoma of the esophagus: molecular mechanisms of carcinogenesis. *Int J Clin Oncol*. 2010;15(2):135-144.

8. Reid BJ. Cancer risk assessment and cancer prevention: promises and challenges. *Cancer Prev Res (Phila)*. 2008;1(4):229-232.

9. Lagergren J. Influence of obesity on the risk of esophageal disorders. *Nat Rev Gastroenterol Hepatol*. 2011;8(6):340-347.

10. Gao Y, Hu N, Han X, et al. Family history of cancer and risk for esophageal and gastric cancer in Shanxi, China. *BMC Cancer*. 2009;9:269.

11. Ong CA, Lao-Sirieix P, Fitzgerald RC. Biomarkers in Barrett's esophagus and esophageal adenocarcinoma: predictors of progression and prognosis. *World J Gastroenterol.* 2010;16(45):5669-5681.

12. Tanaka F, Yamamoto K, Suzuki S, et al. Strong interaction between the effects of alcohol consumption and smoking on oesophageal squamous cell carcinoma among individuals with ADH1B and/or ALDH2 risk alleles. Gut. 2010;59(11):1457-1464.

## Supplementary Information

### OMIM REFERENCES:

[1] Esophageal Cancer (#133239)

[2] Barrett Esophagus (#614266)

[3] Tylosis With Esophageal Cancer; TOC (#148500)

**Alternative Name:**

• None.

*Key Words:* Barrett esophagus, dysplasia, esophageal adenocarcinoma, esophageal squamous cell cancer, biomarkers

# 43 Lung Cancer

Rebecca S. Heist and Lecia V. Sequist

## KEY POINTS

- *Disease summary:*
  - Lung cancer is the leading cause of cancer mortality in the United States.
  - Approximately 85% of lung cancers are nonsmall cell lung cancer (NSCLC), and about 15% small cell lung cancer (SCLC). Among NSCLC, the incidence of adenocarcinoma is rising to surpass that of squamous cell carcinoma.
  - Presenting symptoms may include shortness of breath, cough, weight loss, or symptoms from a metastatic site such as headache or seizure from a brain metastasis or pain from a bony metastasis. Clinical symptoms typically present late in the course of disease and most patients are diagnosed with advanced lung cancer.
  - NSCLC staging uses the TNM system, in which T stage describes tumor size and location, N stage describes nodal status, and M stage describes metastases—the overall TNM defines if the cancer is stage I, II, III, or IV.
  - SCLC is staged as either limited stage or extensive stage, depending on the extent of the tumor and whether it can fit within a radiation port (limited) or not (extensive).

- *Differential diagnosis:*
  - It includes infection, metastatic cancer from another primary site, lymphoma, among others.

- *Monogenic forms:*
  - No single genetic cause of lung cancer is known to exist.

- *Family history:*
  - Some studies have suggested a slight increase in risk among first-degree relatives, but studies are confounded by smoking and exposure to secondhand smoke.

- *Environmental factors:*
  - Cigarette smoking is the leading cause of lung cancer and accounts for approximately 90% of all lung cancer cases in the United States. Both duration of smoking and number of cigarettes per day are directly correlated with lung cancer risk.
  - Environmental tobacco smoke, radon, occupational exposures to tar and soot, asbestos, and metals such as arsenic, chromium, and nickel, have also been associated with increased lung cancer risk.

- *Genome-wide associations:*
  - Recent genome-wide association studies (GWAS) have identified a region in the long arm of chromosome 15 (15q25) as being highly associated with lung cancer risks. This region on chromosome 15 contains several genes, including three that encode subunits of nicotinic acetylcholine receptor (nAChR): *CHRNA5*, *CHRNA3*, and *CHRNB4*, as well as other potential candidate genes including *IREB2* and *PSMA4*. It remains unclear whether the association is primarily related to the genetic variation in chromosome 15 affecting smoking behavior, or whether there is truly an independent association with lung cancer risk independent of the confounding effects of smoking behavior. Other potential lung cancer susceptibility loci identified by these GWAS studies mapped to 5q15.33 and 6p21.33.

## Diagnostic Criteria and Clinical Characteristics

### Diagnostic Criteria:

- Histologically or cytologically confirmed tissue biopsy showing lung cancer.
- Evaluation should include a full staging workup to assess for common sites of metastatic disease including chest computed tomography (CT) extending down through the liver and adrenals, positron emission tomography (PET) scan, and brain magnetic resonance imaging (MRI).

### Clinical Characteristics:

- Constitutional symptoms such as fatigue and weight loss are commonly seen.
- In general, symptoms are related to the growth of the primary tumor or metastatic disease.
- Symptoms related to primary tumor may vary based on location but could include locoregional symptoms such as cough, shortness of breath, and hemoptysis.
- Obstruction of central airways can lead to pneumonia, atelectasis, and worsening dyspnea.
- Chest wall involvement may cause pain.
- Superior vena cava (SVC) syndrome (tumor compressing or invading the SVC) manifests as dyspnea, facial swelling, venous distension in the neck and on chest wall, and occasionally headaches if cerebral edema is present.
- Apical tumors may impinge on the brachial plexus, causing pain, weakness or numbness of the upper extremity, or may lead to Horner syndrome (ipsilateral ptosis, miosis, anhidrosis).
- Symptoms related to metastases
  - Metastases to the bone may present with pain or pathologic fracture.
  - Central nervous system (CNS) metastases may manifest as headache, confusion, personality changes, or seizure. If there is leptomeningeal involvement, cranial nerve abnormalities may exist.
  - Pericardial effusion may cause tamponade. Pleural effusion will cause dyspnea.

## Screening and Counseling

*Screening:* Data regarding the efficacy of screening for lung cancer are evolving. Multiple studies in the past have shown no benefit in terms of overall mortality for lung cancer screening, but have largely been testing the value of chest x-rays (CXRs). The National Lung Screening Trial (NLST) is the first screening study in lung cancer to show a mortality benefit. The NLST enrolled more than 53,000 former and current smokers (at least 30 pack-years) ages 55 to 74 in a screening study comparing annual CXR × 3 to annual low-dose helical CT × 3. There was a relative reduction in mortality from lung cancer with low-dose CT screening of 20%.

*Counseling:* Smoking cessation is the most important counseling to provide.

## Management and Treatment

The treatment of lung cancer depends on histology and stage.

*Small Cell Lung Cancer:* Limited-stage SCLC is treated with a combination of chemotherapy and radiation. The addition of radiation during the first few cycles of platinum-based chemotherapy (usually cisplatin and etoposide) improves overall survival. Prophylactic cranial irradiation (PCI) also improves overall survival in limited-stage SCLC, because there is a high incidence of relapse in the brain and radiation can sterilize existing microscopic foci in the CNS.

For extensive-stage SCLC, chemotherapy alone is the standard. First-line therapy usually consists of platinum and etoposide. PCI can be considered in patients with good response.

*Nonsmall Cell Lung Cancer:* Stage I and II NSCLC (smaller tumors that have none or solely regional lymph node spread) is treated with upfront surgical resection when feasible. Multiple randomized control trials (RCTs) show a survival benefit from adjuvant chemotherapy in stage II disease. Data for adjuvant chemotherapy in stage I are mixed and suggest a benefit in stage IB cancers if the tumor size is greater than 4 cm, but not in stage IA or smaller IB tumors.

The standard of care for stage IIIA NSCLC (lymph node [LN] spread to the ipsilateral mediastinum) remains debatable. For patients in whom mediastinal LNs were not appreciated and underwent upfront surgery but were found incidentally to have IIIA disease on final pathologic analysis, adjuvant chemotherapy has demonstrated survival benefit in multiple RCTs. For patients in whom the mediastinal LNs were clinically enlarged from the time of diagnosis, a multimodality approach combining chemotherapy, radiation, and surgery is commonly used. In stage IIIB NSCLC (contralateral mediastinal lymph node involvement or direct invasion of the tumor into critical and unresectable structures) chemotherapy and radiation are combined and there is no role for surgery.

Stage IV NSCLC (metastases to the pleura, the other lung or distant organs) is treated with palliative chemotherapy. Platinum-based chemotherapy is the standard first-line regimen. For patients with adenocarcinoma, the addition of bevacizumab (vascular endothelial growth factor [VEGF] inhibitor) improves survival over platinum doublet alone. For patients with epidermal growth factor receptor (EGFR) mutations (see below), first-line therapy with an EGFR tyrosine-kinase inhibitor (TKI) improves progression-free survival (PFS) and quality of life (QOL).

## Molecular Genetics and Molecular Mechanism

*Genetic Testing:* The treatment of NSCLC has been revolutionized by the development of targeted agents against specific somatic genomic alterations that confer oncogene addiction. Genetic testing for these somatic alterations has become a part of routine clinical care in lung cancer. Testing can be performed on formalin-fixed paraffin-embedded tumor tissue for mutations such as *EGFR* and *KRAS*, among others, and fluorescence in situ hybridization (FISH) analysis for anaplastic lymphoma kinase (ALK) (Table 43-1). Multiple other somatic mutations are described in lung cancer, including *PIK3CA*, *BRAF*, and *Her2* mutations, among others. Identification of specific mutations is currently clinically important in making treatment decisions in cases of *EGFR*, *KRAS*, and *ALK*, and in other cases can direct patients and physicians to appropriate clinical trials of novel targeted agents.

*EGFR:* EGFR is a member of the ErbB receptor tyrosine kinase family, which also includes ErbB2 (Her2), ErbB3, and ErbB4. EGFR is a transmembrane protein consisting of an extracellular binding domain, a hydrophobic transmembrane segment, and a cytoplasmic tyrosine kinase domain. In response to ligand binding, EGFR is activated via dimerization and subsequent autophosphorylation of the tyrosine kinase domain. Phosphorylation activates downstream pathways including the MAPK, PI3K/AKT, and STAT signaling pathways and ultimately stimulates cell growth and proliferation.

Erlotinib and gefitinib are both small molecular TKIs of EGFR. Erlotinib is approved for the second- and third-line treatment of advanced NSCLC in the United States. Although approved for all NSCLC, a specific subset of patients has impressive regression of disease to EGFR TKI and derives more marked benefit. Retrospective analyses consistently demonstrated that Asian ethnicity, female gender, adenocarcinoma, and bronchioloalveolar histology, and nonsmoking history were clinical predictors of response to EGFR TKIs. However, the most powerful predictor of response is molecular, that is, the presence of sensitizing somatic mutations in the *EGFR* gene in the tumor. These activating *EGFR* mutations localize to a small region encoding the tyrosine kinase domain. In vitro studies showed that in the presence of EGF the mutated EGFR has significantly increased and prolonged activation as compared to wild type. The mutated receptors are also more sensitive to inhibition by EGFR TKI. The most common, "classical," mutations are an in-frame deletion in exon 19, and a missense mutation at codon 858 that leads to an arginine to leucine substitution (L858R). The presence of these mutations is closely correlated to the clinical and pathologic factors which were previously noted to be associated with response. Other "atypical" *EGFR* mutations, for example, exon 20 mutations, also are reported and have less sensitivity to EGFR TKI.

Genotype screening of EGFR is used to select patients with stage IV NSCLC who will receive EGFR TKIs in the first-line setting. Phase II studies of EGFR TKIs in patients with *EGFR* mutations show response rates of 55% to 90% with median PFS of approximately 9 months. Multiple studies have addressed the question of whether the sequence in which EGFR TKI and chemotherapy are given matters in the treatment algorithm. In general,

*Table 43-1 Somatic Molecular Genetic Testing*

| Gene | Testing Modality | Mutation Type | Detection Rate | Clinical Utility |
|------|-----------------|---------------|----------------|------------------|
| EGFR | Allele-specific PCR or direct sequencing | Exon 19 deletions L858R | 10% NSCLC but up to 50% of never-smokers with adenocarcinoma | EGFR TKI treatment with erlotinib or gefitinib in the first-line treatment of metastatic NSCLC improves PFS and QOL |
| ALK | "Break-apart" FISH assay | EML4-ALK translocation | 3%-5% NSCLC but may be up to 25% of never-smokers with adenocarcinoma | ALK inhibition with crizotinib in metastatic NSCLC has high response rate and long PFS |
| KRAS | Allele-specific PCR or direct sequencing | Missense mutations | 25% NSCLC | Less likely to respond to erlotinib |

these studies have consistently shown a PFS and QOL advantage to first-line EGFR TKI among patients who have *EGFR* mutations. However, there is not an overall survival difference seen, as these trials all allowed crossover, and patients with *EGFR* mutations appear to benefit from the EGFR TKI even when it is given in later lines of therapy.

Although response rates are high among patients with *EGFR* mutations, both de novo and acquired resistance remain issues. Numerous studies suggest that the atypical *EGFR* mutations are significantly less predictive of response as compared to the classical mutations. In addition, acquired resistance can develop via several mechanisms. The first described acquired resistance mechanism was a secondary *EGFR* mutation, *T790M*, which causes a threonine to methionine change at position 790 in the catalytic cleft of the EGFR tyrosine kinase domain, altering the relative affinity of adenosine triphosphate (ATP) versus EGFR TKI at the binding pocket (the drug competitively inhibits the ATP-binding site). MET amplification has also been identified as a mechanism of secondary resistance. Numerous clinical trials are ongoing that attempt to effectively target these mechanisms of drug resistance.

**ALK:** EML4-ALK translocations also confer an oncogene-addicted biology, are present in approximately 3% to 7% of NSCLC cases and are an important new molecular target in lung cancer. An inversion in chromosome 2 results in a fusion gene combining EML4 and ALK. EML4 is composed of an N terminal basic region, a hydrophobic echinoderm microtubule-associated protein like protein (HELP) domain, and WD repeats. The translocation results when the N terminal portion of EML4 is fused to the intracellular juxtamembrane region of ALK. The EML4-ALK fusion protein causes ligand-independent dimerization and constitutive activation of ALK. ALK signaling leads to activation of RAS-ERK, JAK3-STAT3, PI3K/AKT pathway signaling leading to cellular proliferation and growth.

ALK translocations in NSCLC are associated with younger age, nonsmoking history, adenocarcinoma histology, and signet-ring cell morphology. Patients with ALK translocations demonstrate impressive response to ALK inhibition. A large phase I study of the ALK inhibitor crizotinib demonstrated an overall response rate of 57% and disease control rate of 90% in patients with ALK translocation. The FDA has approved crizotinib for ALK translocated lung cancers. Resistance mutations within the kinase domain of EML4-ALK have already been described and newer agents are being developed to overcome these resistance mechanisms.

**KRAS:** *KRAS* mutations in lung cancer appear to be mutually exclusive to *EGFR* mutations and ALK translocations and are more often associated with smoking. The presence of a *KRAS* mutation has been associated with resistance to EGFR TKI therapy, and is considered a negative selection factor when considering the use of erlotinib.

**BIBLIOGRAPHY:**

1. Hung RJ, McKay JD, Gaborieau V, et al. A susceptibility locus for lung cancer maps to nicotinic acetylcholine receptor subunit genes on 15q25. *Nature.* 2008;452:633-637.

2. Amos CI, Wu X, Broderick P, et al. Genome-wide association scan of tag SNPs identifies a susceptibility locus for lung cancer at 15q25.1. *Nat Genet.* 2008;40(5):616-622.

3. Thorgeirsson TE, Geller F, Sulem P, et al. A variant associated with nicotine dependence, lung cancer and peripheral arterial disease. *Nature.* 2008;452:638-641.

4. McKay JD, Hung RJ, Gaborieau V, et al. Lung cancer susceptibility locus at 5p15.33. *Nat Genet.* 2008;40(12):1404-1406.

5. Wang Y, Broderick P, Webb E, et al. Common 5p15.33 and 6p21.33 variants influence lung cancer risk. *Nat Genet.* 2008;40(12):1407-1409.

6. Lynch TJ, Bell DW, Sordella R, et al. Activating mutations in the epidermal growth factor receptor underlying responsiveness of non-small cell lung cancer to gefitinib. *N Engl J Med.* 2004;350:2129-2139.

7. Paez JG, Janne PA, Lee JC, et al. EGFR mutations in lung cancer: correlation with clinical response to gefitinib therapy. *Science.* 2004;304:1497-1500.

8. Sequist LV, Bell DW, Lynch TJ, Haber DA. Molecular predictors of response to epidermal growth factor receptor antagonists in non-small cell lung cancer. *J Clin Oncol.* 2007;25(5):587-595.

9. Sequist LV, Martins RG, Spigel D, et al. First-line gefitinib in patients with advanced non-small cell lung cancer harboring somatic EGFR mutations. *J Clin Oncol.* 2008;26(15):2442-2449.

10. Mok TS, Wu YL, Thongprasert S, et al. Gefitinib or carboplatin-paclitaxel in pulmonary adenocarcinoma. *N Engl J Med.* 2009;361:947-957.

11. Maemondo M, Inoue A, Kobayashi K, et al. Gefinitib or chemotherapy for non-small cell lung cancer with mutated EGFR. *N Engl J Med.* 2010;362:2380-2388.

12. Mitsudomi T, Morita S, Negoro S, et al. Gefitinib versus cisplatin plus docetaxel in patients with non-small cell lung cancer harbouring mutations of the epidermal growth factor receptor (WJTOG3405): an open label, randomized phase3 trial. *Lancet Oncol.* 2010;11:121-128.

13. Rosell R, Moran T, Queralt C, et al. Screening for epidermal growth factor receptor mutations in lung cancer. *N Engl J Med.* 2009;361:958-967.

14. Kobayashi S, Boggon TJ, Dayaram T, et al. EGFR mutation and resistance of non-small cell lung cancer to gefitinib. *N Engl J Med.* 2005;352:786-792.

15. Engelman JA, Zejnullahu K, Mitsudomi T, et al. MET amplification leads to gefitinib resistance in lung cancer by activating ERBB3 signaling. *Science.* 2007;316:1039-1043.

16. Soda M, Choi YL, Enomoto M, et al. Identification of the transforming EML4-ALK fusion gene in non-small cell lung cancer. *Nature.* 2007;448:561-567.

17. Kwak EL, Bang YJ, Camidge DR, et al. Anaplastic lymphoma kinase inhibition in non-small-cell lung cancer. *N Engl J Med.* 2010;363(18):1693-1703.

18. Choi YL, Soda M, Yamashita Y, et al. EML4-ALK mutations in lung cancer that confer resistance to ALK inhibitors. *N Engl J Med.* 2010;363:1734-1739.

## Supplementary Information

**OMIM References:**

[1] Lung Cancer; (#211980)

[2] Cholinergic Receptor, Neuronal Nicotinic, Alpha Polypeptide 3; CHRNA3 (#118503)

[3] Cholinergic Receptor, Neuronal Nicotinic, Alpha Polypeptide 5; CHRNA5 (#118505)

[4] Smoking As a Quantitative Trait Locus 3; SQTL3 (#612052)

[5] Lung Cancer Susceptibility 1; LNCR1 (#608935)

[6] Lung Cancer Susceptibility 4; LNCR4 (#612593)

*Key Words:* Lung cancer, EGFR, ALK, KRAS, oncogene addiction

# 44 Cancers of the Small and Large Intestine

Manish Gala and Daniel C. Chung

## KEY POINTS

- *Disease summary:*
  - Colorectal cancer remains the second leading cause of cancer deaths in the United States, with an estimated 143,000 new diagnoses anticipated in 2012. The lifetime risk of any individual developing colon cancer is 5.1%. Often, the disease has no presenting symptoms, but can manifest through changes in bowel habits or appetite, vague abdominal pain, overt bleeding, occult blood loss, iron deficiency anemia, weight loss, or obstructive bowel symptoms. A significant number of afflicted individuals demonstrate a family history of colon cancer. Moreover, a small subset of these individuals will present with features of an established familial cancer syndrome. Careful integration of the family and personal history, physical examination findings, and endoscopic findings play a critical role in recognition and management of these high-risk individuals. Small bowel cancers remain rare, and account for less than 0.5% of all new cancers diagnosed. Malignancies of the small bowel include adenocarcinoma, lymphomas, carcinoids, and mesenchymal tumors. On occasion, cancers of the small bowel may also represent as a manifestation of a familial cancer syndrome.

- *Differential diagnosis:*
  - In the evaluation of an individual with a familial cancer syndrome, the first consideration should be an assessment of polyp burden. Lynch syndrome is the only defined nonpolyposis syndrome with colon and/or extracolonic cancers. Among those patients with polyposis, the main consideration is whether the polyps are adenomatous or hamartomatous. For those patients with large numbers of tubular adenomas, familial adenomatous polyposis (FAP) and *MUTYH*-associated polyposis (MAP) are in the differential diagnosis. Peutz-Jeghers syndrome (PJS), juvenile polyposis syndrome (JPS), and *PTEN* hamartomatous tumor syndromes (PHTS) are considered for those with hamartomatous polyposis.

- *Monogenic forms:*
  - Approximately 5% of colon cancer cases are linked to known familial colon cancer syndromes. Generally, these syndromes are broadly classified into polyposis or nonpolyposis syndromes. The most common nonpolyposis syndrome is Lynch syndrome (hereditary nonpolyposis colon cancer [HNPCC]), which accounts for 3% of all colon cancers. Polyposis syndromes include FAP, MAP, JPS, PJS, and PHTS. Of these polyposis syndromes, the first two are adenomatous polyposis syndromes and the latter three are rare hamartomatous polyposis syndromes. Many of these syndromes may also present with cancers outside of the colon including those of the small bowel, stomach, soft tissues, hepatobiliary system, uterus, ovary, urogenital tissues, skin, and central nervous system.

- *Family history:*
  - While only 5% of colon cancers are currently estimated to be linked to established colon cancer syndromes, over 25% of afflicted individuals may demonstrate a family history of colon cancer.

- *Twin studies:*
  - Analysis of Nordic twins demonstrates that the average genetic contribution to the risk of developing colon cancer is approximately one-third.

- *Environmental factors:*
  - Smoking, diet (red meat consumption), obesity (risk greater for men than women)

- *Genome-wide associations:*
  - While several loci have been identified, novel mechanisms and drug targets have yet to be elucidated from genome-wide association studies (GWAS).

- *Pharmacogenomics:*
  - Testing for specific, somatic mutations in colon cancers can assist in determining which chemotherapeutic agents to utilize. *KRAS* mutations in tumors have been associated with resistance to anti-EGFR agents. Individuals with stage II microsatellite instability (MSI)-high tumors may not benefit from chemotherapy.

## Diagnostic Criteria and Clinical Characteristics

### Small Bowel Cancers:

☞**DIAGNOSTIC CRITERIA:** Small bowel cancers include adenocarcinoma, lymphomas, carcinoids, and mesenchymal tumors (including gastrointestinal stromal tumors). Definitive diagnosis is often made by tissue analysis obtained via endoscopy, surgery, or interventional radiology. Carcinoid tumors and gastrointestinal stromal tumors (GISTs) may have suggestive radiographic appearances on computed tomographic (CT) scans, but tissue diagnosis should still be obtained if possible.

☞**CLINICAL CHARACTERISTICS:** Small bowel cancers remain rare, accounting for only 0.5% of new cancer cases each year. Clinical presentation may include vague, nonspecific abdominal pain, weight loss, obstructive symptoms, bleeding, or changes in bowel habits. Rarely, adenocarcinoma may be associated with a familial cancer syndrome (see later). Diseases of chronic inflammation such as Crohn disease may increase the risk of adenocarcinoma. Celiac disease has been associated with a risk of enteropathic T-cell lymphoma. Individuals with metastatic carcinoid tumors may present with carcinoid syndrome—a constellation of symptoms typically including flushing and diarrhea, but may also include palpitations, hypotension, and bronchoconstriction.

### Sporadic Colorectal Cancer:

☞**DIAGNOSTIC CRITERIA:** Diagnosis of colorectal cancer is often made by tissue obtained from endoscopy, surgery, or interventional radiology.

☞**CLINICAL CHARACTERISTICS:** Many individuals develop colon cancer without any symptoms. Indicative findings on laboratory studies include iron deficiency anemia. Symptoms range from vague abdominal pain, changes in bowel habits, anorexia, weight loss, occult or overt bleeding. A small percentage of individuals may present with synchronous colon cancers at the time of diagnosis, and complete examination of the colon should be performed if possible. Precursor lesions are thought to occur from adenomatous polyps or sessile serrated polyps, with the exception of inflammatory bowel disease in which dysplasia may be flat.

### Lynch Syndrome:

☞**DIAGNOSTIC CRITERIA:** Please see Table 44-1 for genetic differential diagnosis. Ultimately, diagnosis is established by genetic testing. The Amsterdam II criteria are used to make a clinical diagnosis of Lynch syndrome utilizing personal and family history of colon and extracolonic cancers. Individuals satisfying these criteria should proceed directly to germline testing of Lynch-associated genes. If genetic testing is negative and clinical suspicion remains high, such individuals should undergo similar clinical surveillance strategies as those with Lynch syndrome.

### Amsterdam II Criteria

Three relatives with a Lynch-associated cancer (colorectal, endometrial, small bowel, ureter, or renal pelvis) include all of the following:

1. One should be a first-degree relative of the two.
2. At least two successive generations should be involved.
3. Cancer in one of the affected individuals should be diagnosed before the age of 50 years.
4. FAP should be excluded in any cases of colorectal cancer.
5. Tumors should be verified by pathologic examination.

Individuals who do not satisfy Amsterdam II criteria may still have Lynch syndrome. The Revised Bethesda Guidelines were designed to identify those tumors that should undergo microsatellite instability testing and/or immunohistochemistry staining for loss of mismatch repair genes. If microsatellite instability or immunohistochemical loss is demonstrated, germline testing should be pursued to establish the diagnosis.

### Revised Bethesda Guidelines

1. Colorectal cancer diagnosed in a patient who is less than 50 years of age.
2. Synchronous or metachronous colorectal cancer or other Lynch-related cancer regardless of age.
3. Colorectal cancer with MSI-H histology (presence of tumor infiltrating lymphocytes, Crohn-like lymphocytic reaction, mucinous or signet-ring differentiation, or medullary growth pattern) diagnosed in a patient less than 60 years of age.
4. Colorectal cancer diagnosed in one or more first-degree relatives with a Lynch-related tumor, with one of the cancers being diagnosed under age 50 years.
5. Colorectal cancer diagnosed in two or more first- or second-degree relatives with Lynch-related tumors, regardless of age.

☞**CLINICAL CHARACTERISTICS:** Lynch syndrome may be responsible for 1% to 4% of all colon cancers. Patients develop few tubular adenomas that rapidly progress into colon cancer. Metachronous colon cancers can also be observed. The median age of presentation can range from 40 to 60 years depending on the particular Lynch-associated gene. In addition, other tumors such as endometrial, small bowel, ovarian, renal, and pancreatic cancers can be observed. Muir-Torre syndrome and Turcot syndrome are variants of Lynch syndrome in which sebaceous skin tumors and glioblastomas, respectively, are also observed.

### Familial Adenomatous Polyposis and MUTYH-Associated Polyposis:

☞**DIAGNOSTIC CRITERIA:** Individuals who present with 10 or more lifetime tubular adenomas, should be considered for genetic testing for these polyposis syndromes. First-degree relatives of individuals with FAP should also undergo testing. Diagnosis is made by direct germline testing for both disorders.

☞**CLINICAL CHARACTERISTICS:** FAP is the most common polyposis syndrome, with a prevalence of 1 in 5000 to 7000 persons. Affected individuals progressively develop hundreds to thousands of adenomatous colonic polyps beginning in the second decade of life and have an almost 100% risk of colorectal cancer typically by age 40 years, or 10 to 15 years after the initial development of polyposis. Attenuated forms (AFAP) also exist with fewer polyps and delayed presentation of colon cancer. About 90% of individuals may also develop duodenal, ampullary, or periampullary adenomas. Approximately 5% may develop ampullary cancers. Extracolonic cancers such as follicular and papillary thyroid cancers may be present in up to 12% of patients. Benign growths such as desmoids, osteomas, supernumerary teeth, epidermoid cysts, congenital hyperplasia of the retinal epithelium, or adrenal adenomas may also be present in FAP. This association between FAP and extracolonic benign growths has been designated as Gardner syndrome. Turcot syndrome is also observed with individuals with FAP. Individuals with *MUTYH*-associated polyposis can present with colonic and duodenal polyposis similar to those with FAP or AFAP.

### Juvenile Polyposis Syndrome

☞**DIAGNOSTIC CRITERIA:** Individuals must satisfy one of the three criteria: (1) more than three juvenile polyps in the colon, (2) any juvenile polyp outside of the colon, or (3) any juvenile polyp with a family history of JPS.

☞**CLINICAL CHARACTERISTICS:** Individuals with JPS present with multiple juvenile polyps throughout the entire gastrointestinal tract. Often individuals exhibit symptoms of bleeding, obstruction, and intussusception during childhood. JPS confers a 10% to 38% lifetime risk of colon cancer with an average age of diagnosis at 34 years, as well as a 15% to 21% lifetime risk of gastric and duodenal cancers.

### Peutz-Jeghers Syndrome:

☞**DIAGNOSTIC CRITERIA:** Clinical diagnosis of PJS include (1) two or more PJS polyps in the gastrointestinal tract, (2) one or more PJS polyps with characteristic mucocutaneous pigmentation, or (3) one or more PJS polyps with a family history of PJS.

☞**CLINICAL CHARACTERISTICS:** A rare diagnosis (1 in 150,000 persons), PJS is characterized by pigmented macules on lips, buccal mucosa, hands, and feet. These pigmented lesions may not be visible later in life. PJS results in the development of hamartomatous polyps characterized by a thick band of smooth muscle that may cause bleeding, intussusception, or obstruction. Polyps in the small bowel are more frequent than in the colon. The lifetime risk of colon cancer is 39%, and 93% for any malignancy. Other cancers include stomach, small bowel, pancreas, breast, sex cord, uterine, cervical, and melanoma.

### PTEN Hamartomatous Tumor Syndromes:

☞**Diagnostic Criteria:** PHTS consist of Cowden and Bannayan-Riley-Ruvalcaba syndromes (BRRS). Diagnostic criteria only exist for the Cowden syndrome. Pathognomonic criteria for Cowden syndrome include mucocutaneous lesions including six or more facial papules (of which three or more must be trichilemmomas), or cutaneous facial papules and oral mucosal papillomatosis, or oral mucosal papillomatosis and acral keratoses, or six or more palmoplantar keratoses. Major criteria include thyroid cancer, breast cancer, macrocephaly, Lhermitte-Duclos disease, and endometrial carcinoma. Minor criteria include noncancerous thyroid lesions, mental retardation, hamartomatous intestinal polyps, fibrocystic disease of the breast, lipomas, fibromas, genitourinary malformations, or tumors. To make a diagnosis in an individual, either one pathognomonic criterion or two major criteria (one must be macrocephaly or Lhermitte-Duclos disease), one major criterion and three minor criteria, or four minor criteria must be fulfilled. Diagnostic criteria for a relative of an individual with Cowden syndrome are less stringent; only one pathognomonic criterion, one major criterion, or two minor criteria are required.

☞**Clinical Characteristics:** Cowden syndrome is an autosomal dominant disorder with a prevalence of 1 in 200,000 persons. Individuals afflicted with Cowden syndrome may develop numerous intestinal hamartomatous polyps. The lifetime risk of colon cancer is estimated to range from 9% to 16%, with a median age of onset at 44 years. Individuals classically present with several mucocutaneous lesions (as described earlier). Thyroid disorders, breast disease, dysplastic gangliocytoma of the cerebellum, intracranial vascular malformations, macrocephaly, mental retardation, or genitourinary tumors and malformations may also be seen. Individuals with BRRS may present with similar findings of Cowden syndrome, but also with lipomas, penile lentigines, eye abnormalities, vascular anomalies, or myopathies.

## Screening and Counseling

**Screening:** Most sporadic colon cancers arise from adenomatous polyps or sessile serrated polyps over the period of several years in sporadic cases. Given the existence of a precursor lesion, several modalities have been employed to detect advanced adenomas or early cancers. These modalities include colonoscopy, flexible sigmoidoscopy, computed tomographic colonography (virtual colonoscopy), fecal DNA testing, fecal occult blood testing, double-contrast barium enemas, and fecal occult blood testing with sigmoidoscopy. Colonoscopy remains the preferred method by practitioners given complete, direct visualization of the entire colon and the ability to remove polyps at the time of the procedure. Colorectal cancer screening with colonoscopy is recommended for average-risk individuals starting at age 50 every 10 years. Shorter intervals are recommended for individuals who have polyps or a family history of colon cancer. Colonoscopy and flexible sigmoidoscopy have been demonstrated to reduce the number of colon cancer-associated deaths.

**Counseling:** On average, the risk of colon cancer in an individual with a first-degree family member is two times higher than the general population. If an individual has a first-degree relative who was diagnosed with colon cancer or advanced adenoma before the age of 60, or two or more first-degree relatives had colorectal cancer or advanced adenomas at any age, screening with colonoscopy is recommended at age 40 or 10 years before the youngest relative's diagnosis, whichever is the earlier date. Additional examinations should be repeated every 5 years. Individuals who demonstrate characteristics of a familial cancer syndrome, or are first-degree relatives of one, should be referred to a genetic specialist for further evaluation, testing, and more intensive screening.

## Management and Treatment

**Sporadic Colon Cancer:** After diagnosis, CTs of chest and abdomen or pelvis should be performed to stage the disease. For rectal cancers, a rectal magnetic resonance imaging (MRI) or transrectal ultrasound should also be performed. Carcinoembryonic antigen (CEA) levels should also be obtained. *KRAS* mutation status should be obtained for all cancers stage II and above. In addition, microsatellite instability (MSI) testing should be performed on all stage II cancers to determine the role for adjuvant chemotherapy. Supported by several cost-benefit analyses, some centers have initiated universal MSI testing of all colon cancers to identify Lynch syndrome in individuals who may not satisfy Amsterdam or Bethesda criteria.

**Lynch Syndrome:** Colonoscopy should be performed every 1 to 2 years beginning at age 20 to 25 years or 10 years earlier than the youngest colon cancer in the family. Annual colonoscopies should begin after age 40 years. Individuals with Lynch syndrome and colon cancer should have a subtotal colectomy with ileorectal anastomosis. Surveillance of the remaining rectum should be performed annually. Endometrial cancer screening is strongly recommended. Surveillance for other extracolonic tumors should be tailored to the family history. Aspirin (600 mg per day) may reduce the risk of developing both colonic and extracolonic tumors.

**Familial Adenomatous Polyposis:** Individuals with FAP should begin annual sigmoidoscopies at age 10 to 12 years. Once adenomas are detected, annual colonoscopies should be pursued. Prophylactic colectomy with ileorectal anastomosis, ileal pouch—anal anastomosis, or ileostomy remains the only definitive therapy. Timing of colectomy should take into account the number, size, and histology of polyps. Surgery is typically performed before the age of 25 years. Vigorous screening of any remaining rectum or the rectal cuff should be performed by sigmoidoscopy every 6 to 12 months. Patients with AFAP should undergo annual screening colonoscopies beginning at age 25 years, or younger depending on family history. The decision for endoscopic management versus colectomy in AFAP patients will depend on the severity of the phenotype. Given the high risk of duodenal or ampullary adenocarcinoma in FAP and AFAP patients, upper endoscopy with a forward and side-viewing endoscope should be performed prior to colectomy or by age 30. Repeat examination should be performed in 1- to 5-year intervals depending on endoscopic findings and histology. Annual thyroid ultrasounds and screening for childhood hepatoblastomas have been recommended by some groups.

**MUTYH-Associated Polyposis:** Colonoscopies should begin at age 18 to 20 years with repeat examinations performed every 1 to 2 years with great care to remove hyperplastic polyps and serrated adenomas, which can also occur in MAP. Colectomy can be considered in cases where the polyp burden mimics FAP. Guidelines for the screening of duodenal cancers in FAP or AFAP should be applied to MAP patients as well.

***Juvenile Polyposis Syndrome:*** Colonoscopy should be performed in those afflicted or at-risk family members, beginning at age 15 years every 1 to 2 years. Upper endoscopy should be performed every 1 to 2 years after the age of 25 years.

***Peutz-Jeghers Syndrome:*** Surveillance includes upper endoscopy and small bowel imaging every 2 to 3 years starting at 10 years of age, and colonoscopy every 2 to 3 years from the late teens. Magnetic resonance cholangiopancreatography (MRCP) or endoscopic ultrasound (EUS) with CA19-9 measurement should be performed every 1 to 2 years from age 30. Mammograms and breast MRI should be performed annually with breast examinations twice per year from age 25 years; testicular examinations for males should commence at age 10. Annual Pap smears should be performed in women from age 18.

***PTEN Hamartomatous Tumor Syndromes:*** Surveillance includes annual physical examination starting at age 18 or 5 years prior to the youngest cancer in the family. A baseline thyroid ultrasound should be performed at age 18, and consideration of annual examinations thereafter. An index colonoscopy should be performed at age 35 and repeat examinations within 5- to 10-year intervals. Annual dermatologic examinations should also be recommended. Given the higher rates of breast disease, women should undergo clinical breast examinations every 6 months starting at age 25 or 10 years prior to the youngest case. Annual mammography and breast MRI should begin at age 35 or 10 years prior to the youngest case. No firm recommendations exist for endometrial or urogential cancer screening, but patients should be educated about potential warning signs.

***Pharmacogenetics:*** See Table 44-2.

# Molecular Genetics and Molecular Mechanism

***Lynch Syndrome:*** Defects in the repair of short segments of nucleotide repeats called microsatellites underlie Lynch syndrome. *MLH1, MSH2, MSH6, and PMS2* are actively involved in DNA mismatch repair. 3' loss of *EpCAM* results in epigenetic silencing of *MSH2*. This mutator phenotype results in mutations in critical growth-regulatory genes with microsatellites in coding regions, such as *TGFβR2*.

***Familial Adenomatous Polyposis:*** Truncating mutations in *APC* result in accumulation of beta-catenin and activation of the Wnt pathway. As a result, beta-catenin can translocate into the nucleus, partner with the TCF4 transcription factor, and activate several growth-related genes.

***MUTYH-Associated Polyposis:*** *MUTYH* encodes a DNA glycosylase that excises adenine bases when they are inappropriately paired with guanine, cytosine, or 8-oxo-7,8-dihydroguanine. Biallelic mutations in *MUTYH* result in G:C to T:A transversions in coding regions of tumor suppressor genes, including *APC*, and oncogenes.

***Juvenile Polyposis Syndrome:*** Mutations in *MADH4, BMPR1A,* and *ENG* result in dysregulation of the transforming growth factor beta (TGFβ) signaling pathway, which controls a diverse set of processes including cell growth, differentiation, and apoptosis.

***Peutz-Jeghers Syndrome:*** *LKB1* or *STK11* encodes for a serine or threonine kinase that activates the adenosine monophosphate-activated protein kinase (AMPK) pathway which inhibits cell growth and proliferation. Mutations result in the inhibition of the AMPK system, and activation of mammalian target of rapamycin (mTOR)-related pathways.

**Table 44-1 Genetic Differential Diagnosis**

| Syndrome | Gene Symbol | Associated Findings |
|---|---|---|
| Lynch syndrome (hereditary non-polyposis colon cancer [HNPCC]) | *MLH1, MSH2, MSH6, PMS2, EpCAM* | Few polyps that rapidly progress to colon cancer with DNA microsatellite instability. Extracolonic cancers include endometrial, gastric, ovarian, urinary collecting system, skin, pancreatic, and bile duct cancers. |
| Familial adenomatous polyposis | *APC* | Hundreds to thousands of tubular adenomas in the colon, with development of colon cancer by the fourth decade of life. About 90% will also develop duodenal or periampullary adenomas. Attenuated forms of the disease also exist. |
| *MUTYH*-associated polyposis | *MUTYH* | Similar presentation to FAP, but autosomal recessive and greater variability in polyp number. |
| Juvenile polyposis syndrome | *MADH4, BMPR1A, ENG* | Juvenile polyps throughout upper and lower GI tract that may cause bleeding, obstruction, or intussusception. May develop gastric, duodenal, and colon cancer. |
| Peutz-Jeghers syndrome | *LKB1* | Pigmented macules on lips, buccal mucosa, hands, and feet. Hamartomatous polyps in the small bowel and colon that may cause bleeding, obstruction, or malignancy. |
| *PTEN* hamartomatous tumor syndromes | *PTEN* | GI hamartomatous polyps with features of Cowden syndrome and Bannayan-Riley-Ruvalcaba syndromes. |

Gene names: *MLH1*, MutL homolog 1; *MSH2, MSH6*, MutS homolog 2,6; *PMS2*, postmeiotic segregation increased 2; *EpCAM*, epithelial cell adhesion molecule; *APC*, adenomatous polyposis coli; *MUTYH*, MutY homolog; *MADH4*, mothers against decapentaplegic homolog 4; *BMPR1A*, bone morphogenetic protein receptor, type IA; *ENG*, endoglin; *LKB1*, liver kinase B1; *PTEN*, phosphatase and tensin homolog.

*Table 44–2* **Pharmacogenetic Considerations in the Treatments of Colon and Small Bowel Cancers**

| Gene | Associated Medications | Goal of Testing | Variants | Effect |
|------|------------------------|-----------------|----------|--------|
| KRAS | EGFR inhibitors (cetuximab or panitumumab) | Drug resistance | Hotspots at codon 12 and 13 | Resistance to anti-EGFR–based therapies |
| MSI status | Conventional chemotherapeutic regimen | Drug resistance | Panel of five markers employed. If two are positive, then tumor is deemed "MSI high" | No benefit of adjuvant chemotherapy in stage II MSI tumors versus surgery alone |
| KIT | Imatinib (Gleevec) | Dosing | Exon 9 mutations | Reduces efficacy of imatinib for GIST. Consider increasing dose from 400 mg per day to 800 mg |

MSI, microsatellite instability.

**PTEN Hamartomatous Syndromes:** *PTEN* negatively regulates AKT and mTOR-related growth pathways.

**Gastrointestinal Stromal Tumors:** A large fraction of GISTs demonstrate overexpression and activating mutations of the receptor tyrosine kinase, *KIT*. In a small subset of GISTs without *KIT* mutations, activating mutations of the platelet-derived growth factor alpha subunit *PDGFRA* or inactivating mutations of the subunits of succinate dehydrogenase (SDH).

**Genetic Testing:**

☞LYNCH SYNDROME: MSI testing and immunohistochemistry for loss of *MMR* genes can be performed on cancers and polyps. Direct gene sequencing and deletion analysis on germline DNA is commercially available. Nonsynonymous variants, missense variants, splice-site acceptor or donor mutations, insertions, and deletions can be found. Rare cases of germline epigenetic silencing have also been observed. Once an individual has been diagnosed, genetic testing of the specific mutation should be offered to first-degree relatives.

☞FAMILIAL ADENOMATOUS POLYPOSIS: Direct gene sequencing of *APC* is performed, typically revealing truncating mutations. Over 80% of patients demonstrating polyposis will have a mutation in this gene. More than 90% of pathogenic mutations are nonsense mutations which result in a truncated protein. Gene deletion is extremely rare. Classic FAP is associated with mutations between codons 169 and 1393. Severe phenotypes are seen with mutations between codons 1250 and 1464. AFAP typically correlates with mutations at the 5′ end, exon 9, and 3′ end of *APC*. Once an individual has been diagnosed, genetic testing of the specific mutation should be offered to first-degree relatives.

☞MUTYH-ASSOCIATED POLYPOSIS: Mutations in two hotspots, Y165C or G382D, account for 70% of all Caucasian mutations. Typically, these specific mutations are tested. Whole gene testing is also available. If a mutation is identified in the proband, siblings are at the highest risk given the autosomal recessive nature of the disorder. To clarify the risk in offspring, the spouse may be tested to assess for carrier status.

☞JUVENILE POLYPOSIS SYNDROME: Direct gene sequencing and deletion analysis of *MADH4*, *BMPR1A*, and *ENG* are available. Approximately 40% of cases demonstrate mutations in *MADH4* and *BMPR1A*. Should no mutation be found, careful periodic examination of first-degree relatives is warranted.

☞PEUTZ-JEGHERS SYNDROME: Direct gene sequencing and deletion analysis of *LKB1* is performed. Mutation or deletion of this gene accounts for only 50% to 60% of cases. If a mutation is found, first-degree relatives should be tested. Should no mutation be discovered in individuals that satisfy clinical criteria, careful physical examinations of first-degree relatives should be performed.

☞PTEN HAMARTOMATOUS SYNDROMES: Direct gene sequencing and deletion analysis of *PTEN* is performed. SDH subunit B, and SDH subunit D can be tested in individuals who present with features of Cowden syndrome and with no pathologic mutations in *PTEN*.

**Future Directions:** Clinical deployment of next-generation sequencing technologies offers the promise to discover novel germline variants associated with hereditary colon cancer. In addition, deep sequencing of tumors may also offer the promise of personalized treatment for gastrointestinal cancers.

**BIBLIOGRAPHY:**

1. Gala M, Chung DC. Hereditary colon cancer syndromes. *Semin Oncol.* Aug 2011;38(4):490-499.

2. Aaltonen LA, Salovaara R, Kristo P, et al. Incidence of hereditary nonpolyposis colorectal cancer and the feasibility of molecular screening for the disease. *N Eng J Med.* 1998;338:1481-1487.

3. Watson P, Lynch HT. The tumor spectrum in HNPCC. *Anticancer Res.* 1994;14:1635-1639.

4. Kinzler KW, Nilbert MC, Su LK, et al. Identification of FAP locus genes from chromosome 5q21. *Science.* 1991;253:661-665.

5. Nagase H, Miyoshi Y, Horii A, et al. Correlation between the location of germ-line mutations in the APC gene and the number of colorectal polyps in familial adenomatous polyposis patients. *Cancer Res.* 1992;52:4055-4057.

6. Sieber OM, Lipton L, Crabtree M, et al. Multiple colorectal adenomas, classic adenomatous polyposis, and germ-line mutations in MYH. *N Engl J Med.* 2003;348:791-799.

7. Howe JR, Roth S, Ringold JC, et al. Mutations in the SMAD4/DPC4 gene in juvenile polyposis. *Science.* 1998;280:1086-1088.

8. Su GH, Hruban RH, Bansal RK, et al. Germline and somatic mutations of the STK11/LKB1 Peutz-Jeghers gene in pancreatic and biliary cancers. *Am J Pathol.* 1999;154:1835-1840.

9. Hemminki A, Markie D, Tomlinson I, et al. A serine/threonine kinase gene defective in Peutz-Jeghers syndrome. *Nature.* 1998;391:184-187.

## Supplementary Information

**OMIM References:**

[1] Lynch Syndrome I; MSH2 (#120435)

[2] Colorectal Cancer, Hereditary Nonpolyposis, Type 2; HNPCC2, MLH1 (#609310)

[3] Colorectal Cancer, Hereditary Nonpolyposis, Type 4; HNPCC4, PMS2 (#614337)

[4] Colorectal Cancer, Hereditary Nonpolyposis, Type 5; HNPCC5, MSH6 (#614350)

[5] Colorectal Cancer, Hereditary Nonpolyposis, Type 8; HNPCC8, EPCAM (#613244)

[6] Familial Adenomatous Polyposis 1; FAP1, APC (#175100)

[7] Familial Adenomatous Polyposis 2; FAP2, MUTYH (#608456)

[8] Juvenile Polyposis Syndrome; JPS, MADH4, BMPR1A (OMIM# 174900)

[9] Peutz-Jeghers Syndrome; PJS, LKB1/STK11 (#175200)

[10] Cowden Syndrome; CD, PTEN, SDHB, SDHD (#158350)

[11] Bannayan-Riley-Ruvalcaba Syndrome; BRRS, PTEN (#153480)

**Alternative Names:**

- Lynch Syndrome: Hereditary Nonpolyposis Colorectal Cancer
- *MUTYH*-Associated Polyposis: Familial Adenomatous Polyposis Type 2
- Juvenile Polyposis Syndrome: Juvenile Intestinal Polyposis
- Peutz-Jeghers Syndrome: Hamartomatous Intestinal Polyposis, Polyps-and-Spots Syndrome
- Cowden Syndrome: Cowden Disease, Multiple Hamartoma Syndrome
- Bannayan-Riley-Ruvalcaba Syndrome: Bannayan-Zonana Syndrome, Riley-Smith Syndrome, Ruvalcaba-Myhre-Smith Syndrome

*Key Words:* Colon cancer, small bowel cancer, carcinoid, gastrointestinal stromal tumor, hereditary colon cancer, lynch syndrome, hereditary nonpolyposis colorectal cancer, familial adenomatous polyposis, *MUTYH*-associated polyposis, juvenile polyposis, Peutz-Jeghers syndrome, *PTEN* Hamartomatous tumor syndromes, Cowden syndrome, Bannayan-Riley-Ruvalcaba syndrome, Amsterdam criteria; Revised Bethesda Guidelines, adenomatous polyposis, hamartomatous polyposis

# 45 Pancreatic Cancer

Robert R. McWilliams

## KEY POINTS

- *Disease summary:*
  - Pancreatic cancer, like many adult-onset malignancies, is a complex genetic disorder, with the majority of cases apparently sporadic, with some identified environmental factors.
  - Pancreatic cancer often presents in the later stages of life, with a median age of approximately 70 years at diagnosis.
  - There is no commonly accepted screening test for pancreatic cancer.
  - Pancreatic cancer often presents at an advanced stage, with only 15% to 20% of patients surgically resectable at diagnosis.
- *Differential diagnosis:*
  - Cholelithiasis, peptic ulcer disease, poorly controlled type 2 diabetes, pancreatitis
- *Monogenic forms:*
  - Pancreatic cancer can arise in Peutz-Jeghers syndrome, Li-Fraumeni syndrome, hereditary pancreatitis, and individuals who harbor mutations in *BRCA1*, *BRCA2*, and *CDKN2A*.
- *Family history:*
  - 5% to 10% of pancreatic cancer patients report a family history of the disease.
- *Twin studies:* There is no reported increased incidence in twins of pancreatic cancer beyond that expected for first-degree relatives.
- *Environmental factors:*
  - Tobacco use, heavy alcohol use
- *Genome-wide associations:*
  - Several associations exist, with the non-O blood type in the *ABO* gene (rs505922) now being consistently replicated.
- *Pharmacogenomics:*
  - No pharmacogenetic or pharmacogenomic associations have been reported.

## Diagnostic Criteria and Clinical Characteristics

**Diagnostic evaluation should include both of the following:**

- Pancreas protocol computed tomography scan, which commonly shows a hypovascular mass in the pancreas
- Needle biopsy of primary tumor confirming adenocarcinoma or other histology (can be done on metastases if present at diagnosis)
- If pathologic confirmation is impractical, clinical diagnosis can be made in setting of pancreatic mass, elevated CA 19-9, and clinical syndrome including diabetes, weight loss, and epigastric pain.

**And the absence of**

1. Other tumor causing pancreatic mass such as, lymphoma, metastasis from lung, kidney, melanoma.

*Clinical Characteristics:*

☞ADENOCARCINOMA: The most common type of pancreatic cancer is adenocarcinoma, which comprises over 90% of pancreatic cancer. This type of malignancy has the poorest survival, and an expected prognosis of less than 6 months survival in advanced stages. For the minority of patients who present at a stage where surgical resection can be considered, full resection can offer a chance of cure. However, the vast majority of surgically resected patients will have a fatal recurrence of the disease. Adenocarcinoma is notoriously resistant to chemotherapy, though there have been recent studies suggesting higher responses to an aggressive combination regimen of irinotecan, oxaliplatin, 5-fluorouracil (5-FU), and leucovorin known as FOLFIRINOX.

☞ISLET CELL CARCINOMA: This less common malignancy of the pancreas is usually hormonally inactive. However, it is well known for its associated clinical hormonal syndromes such as insulinoma, gastrinoma, VIPoma, and glucagonoma. It may also be associated with the MEN1 syndrome, which often is associated with multiple pancreatic and duodenal tumors. Islet cell carcinoma appears more vascular on imaging studies than adenocarcinoma, and has a substantially better prognosis, often measured in years even for advanced disease.

☞ACINAR CELL CARCINOMA: This is a rare variant of pancreatic cancer emanating from the acinar cells, which produce the digestive enzymes released by the pancreas into the gut. This malignancy also has a good prognosis compared to adenocarcinoma.

## Screening and Counseling

*Screening:* There is no established, accepted screening for pancreatic cancer even in high-risk families. Endoscopic ultrasound studies are ongoing but not yet conclusive, and are limited by extensive abnormal imaging findings of the pancreas in such families. CA19-9 is not a useful screening mechanism to date.

*Counseling:* There are several genetic syndromes which have been determined to be genetically linked to pancreatic cancer risk. Among the most common are *BRCA1* and *BRCA2*, however penetrance is relatively low at approximately 5%. For affected families, breast and ovarian cancer generally represent greater threats to longevity. In *CDKN2A* (familial melanoma) families, penetrance is higher with reported frequencies of 20% to 50%. In either setting, maintenance of a healthy lifestyle including tobacco avoidance and avoidance of obesity are reasonable recommendations.

## Management and Treatment

### Management (Adenocarcinoma):

☞**SURGICALLY RESECTABLE DISEASE:** For tumors confined to the pancreas and not involving vital vascular structures such as the celiac trunk or superior mesenteric artery, surgical excision is generally performed. In some centers, neoadjuvant chemotherapy and radiation are given to patients prior to surgery. If surgery is performed primarily, adjuvant chemotherapy with gemcitabine, with or without radiation is generally performed, regardless of nodal involvement. Adjuvant therapy generally lasts 6 months in duration.

☞**LOCALLY ADVANCED CANCER:** For tumors generally limited to the pancreatic area but involving sufficient structures or tissue that precludes surgical resection, several therapies are employed. Radiation with chemotherapy sensitization such as 5-fluorouracil, capecitabine, or gemcitabine is often performed with a limited success in converting patients to resectability. Sometimes, systemic therapies such as FOLFIRINOX or gemcitabine-based therapy are given until progression of the malignancy.

☞**METASTATIC CANCER:** For metastatic pancreatic adenocarcinoma, therapeutic options range from FOLFIRINOX (most aggressive, but highest side effect profile) to gemcitabine (fewer side effects) with or without erlotinib, to palliative care alone. Participation in a clinical trial if available is strongly encouraged, as current options are limited.

### Therapeutics:

☞**CYTOTOXIC CHEMOTHERAPY:** Since its approval in 1997 gemcitabine has been the standard of care for advanced pancreatic adenocarcinoma. Gemcitabine is generally well tolerated with side effects primarily limited to cytopenias and fatigue; more substantial side effects are uncommon. However, multiple gemcitabine-based combinations have failed to show a substantial survival benefit over gemcitabine alone, which still remains the mainstay of therapy for many patients. In 2010, a phase III study performed in Europe showed a substantial survival benefit from the aggressive combination of FOLFIRINOX (oxaliplatin, irinotecan, 5-FU, and leucovorin) over gemcitabine therapy. However given the substantial toxicity of this combination, including neutropenia and gastrointestinal side effects, FOLFIRINOX is primarily used in patients with good performance scores and few comorbidities. Gemcitabine is still utilized in the second-line setting, either alone or in combination with other agents such as erlotinib. For patients receiving gemcitabine-based therapy in the first-line setting there is data showing a benefit to oxaliplatin, 5-FU, and leucovorin (OFF) over best supportive care. The majority of practitioners have used the FOLFOX schedule (which includes the same drugs as OFF, but in a slightly different schedule) in the second-line setting after gemcitabine failure. It is not known if FOLFIRINOX is more active than FOLFOX in any line of therapy.

☞**TARGETED THERAPY:** The only currently approved target therapy for pancreatic adenocarcinoma is erlotinib, a small molecule inhibitor of epidermal growth factor receptor (EGFR). The efficacy of this agent was demonstrated in a National Cancer Institute of Canada (NCIC) study in combination with gemcitabine, where the erlotinib arm had a longer survival than the gemcitabine alone arm. However this was a modest survival benefit, with a median difference in survival of less than 2 weeks, with the improvement in 1-year survival from 7% to 15%. Diarrhea and skin rash were prominent side effects in the combination arm; side effect profile

*Table 45-1 Disease-Associated Susceptibility Variants*

| Candidate Gene (Chromosome Location) | Associated Variant | Relative Risk | Frequency of Risk Allele | Putative Functional Significance | Associated Disease Phenotype |
|---|---|---|---|---|---|
| *BRCA1* | Truncating mutations/ deletions | Unknown | Rare | Homologous recombination defect | Associated with breast, ovarian, prostate cancer; pancreatic tumors may be more sensitive to platinum agents |
| *BRCA2* | Truncating mutations/ deletions | 4% | Rare | Homologous recombination defect | Associated with breast, ovarian, prostate cancer; pancreatic tumors may be more sensitive to platinum agents |
| *CDKN2A* | Missense mutations, deletions | 40% | Rare | Cell cycle defect | Associated with melanoma |
| *TP53* (17p13.1) | Missense mutations, deletions | Unknown | Rare | Complex | Li-Fraumeni syndrome |
| *ABO* | SNP rs505922 | 1.2 | 0.35 | Unknown | Non-O blood type |

along with the cost has limited the use of erlotinib in pancreatic cancer patients. Many other targeted agents are under investigation for therapy and pancreatic cancer but have not yet demonstrated survival benefit.

## Molecular Genetics and Molecular Mechanism

### *Genetic Testing:*

☞**CLINICAL AVAILABILITY OF TESTING:** Germline testing is available clinically for *BRCA1, BRCA2, CDKNA,* and *TP53.*

***Utility of Testing:*** Currently, testing can quantify risk to an individual, but does not carry any different screening recommendations if positive. Currently there are no known effective screening tools for persons at high genetic risk for pancreatic cancer outside of a clinical trial setting.

***Future Directions:*** Studies are in development for more effective screening mechanisms for early-stage pancreatic cancer. These include molecular profiling of blood samples, pancreatic use, and stool in addition to invasive and noninvasive imaging techniques. The challenge is identifying pancreatic cancer at a stage where it is not only surgically resectable, but when it has a low likelihood of metastasis. Smoking avoidance along with maintenance of a healthy body mass index are recommended for persons at risk.

### BIBLIOGRAPHY:

1. McWilliams RR, Rabe KG, Olswold C, De Andrade M, Petersen GM. Risk of malignancy in first-degree relatives of patients with pancreatic carcinoma. *Cancer.* 2005;104(2):388-394.

2. Amundadottir L, Kraft P, Stolzenberg-Solomon RZ, et al. Genome-wide association study identifies variants in the ABO locus associated with susceptibility to pancreatic cancer. *Nat Genet.* 2009;41(9):986-990.

3. Vaccaro V, Sperduti I, Milella M. FOLFIRINOX versus gemcitabine for metastatic pancreatic cancer. *N Engl J Med.* 2011;365(8):768-769.

4. Goggins M, Schutte M, Lu J, et al. Germline BRCA2 gene mutations in patients with apparently sporadic pancreatic carcinomas. *Cancer Res.* 1996;56(23):5360-5364.

5. Ghiorzo P, Gargiulo S, Nasti S, et al. Predicting the risk of pancreatic cancer: on CDKN2A mutations in the melanoma-pancreatic cancer syndrome in Italy. *J Clin Oncol.* 2007;25(33):5336-5337.

6. McWilliams RR, Wieben ED, Rabe KG, et al. Prevalence of CDKN2A mutations in pancreatic cancer patients: implications for genetic counseling. *Eur J Hum Genet.* 2011;19(4):472-478.

7. Burris HA, 3rd, Moore MJ, Andersen J, et al. Improvements in survival and clinical benefit with gemcitabine as first-line therapy for patients with advanced pancreas cancer: a randomized trial. *J Clin Oncol.* 1997;15(6):2403-2413.

8. Moore MJ, Goldstein D, Hamm J, et al. Erlotinib plus gemcitabine compared with gemcitabine alone in patients with advanced pancreatic cancer: a phase III trial of the National Cancer Institute of Canada Clinical Trials Group. *J Clin Oncol.* 2007;25(15):1960-1966.

9. Lal G, Liu G, Schmocker B, et al. Inherited predisposition to pancreatic adenocarcinoma: role of family history and germ-line p16, BRCA1, and BRCA2 mutations. *Cancer Res.* 2000;60(2):409-416.

10. Goldstein AM, Fraser MC, Struewing JP, et al. Increased risk of pancreatic cancer in melanoma-prone kindreds with p16INK4 mutations. *N Engl J Med.* 1995;333(15):970-974.

## Supplementary Information

### OMIM REFERENCES:

[1] Pancreatic Cancer (#260350)

[2] Familial Breast and Ovarian Cancer (#612555, #604370)

[3] Melanoma—Pancreatic Cancer Syndrome (#606719)

### Alternative Name:

- Pancreatic Adenocarcinoma

***Key Words:*** Pancreatic cancer

# 46 Pancreatic Neuroendocrine Tumors

Eugen Melcescu and Christian A. Koch

## KEY POINTS

- *Disease summary:*
  - Pancreatic neuroendocrine tumors (PNETs) are uncommon and represent only 1% to 2% of pancreatic neoplasms, about 85% of these tumors occur in the pancreas and 15% are extrapancreatic tumors.
  - Based on their clinical expression these tumors are categorized as either functional or nonfunctional.
  - Functional tumors (~50%) are characterized by abnormal secretion of (often) biologically active peptides mostly insulin, gastrin, glucagon, somatostatin, or vasoactive intestinal polypeptide (VIP).
  - Nonfunctional tumors are clinically silent although they can secrete neurotensin, pancreatic polypeptide or chromogranin A (CgA), but these peptide-like substances are not biologically active. Most nonfunctional PNETs have a malignant course. They are discovered usually when their size is large, have already invaded adjacent organs or metastasized.
  - Among functional tumors, insulinomas and gastrinomas account for 25% and 15% of the cases, respectively. The other functional PNETs are responsible for the remaining 15%.
  - Negative prognostic factors for PNETs are considered: metastasis, tumor diameter, angioinvasion, proliferative index Ki-67, lymph nodes, and mitoses. Localized disease has a 5-year survival rate of 60% to 100%, whereas regional and metastatic PNETs have a 40% and 29% survival rate, respectively.

- *Hereditary basis:*
  - Multiple endocrine neoplasia type 1 (MEN1): autosomal dominant trait with greater than 95% penetrance.
  - von Hippel-Lindau (VHL) syndrome: autosomal dominant pattern (80%); 20% due to a new mutation that occurred during the formation of reproductive cells or early in embryogenesis.
  - Neurofibromatosis type 1 (NF1): autosomal dominant (50%) or spontaneous mutations (50%).
  - Tuberous sclerosis: autosomal dominant pattern of inheritance; one-third of cases are inherited and two-thirds of people with tuberous sclerosis complex (TSC) are considered as sporadic; *TSC1* mutations–more frequent in familial cases while mutations in the *TSC2*–more often in sporadic cases.

- *Differential diagnosis:*
  - PNETs can be divided into functional and nonfunctional varieties. The functional PNETs lead to a recognizable clinical entity in which one or more hormones are secreted into the bloodstream. Nonfunctioning PNETs are initially asymptomatic and difficult to diagnose. Their diagnosis is more evident later in the disease course. Apart from that, a small number of PNETs are associated to four major genetic syndromes which can be recognized by their specific clinical features. Differential diagnosis has to take the family history (going back three generations) into consideration.

## Diagnostic Criteria and Clinical Characteristics

**Diagnostic Criteria:** WHO histologic classification of PNETs

- Well-differentiated endocrine tumors (benign or uncertain malignant potential)
- Well-differentiated endocrine carcinomas (low-grade malignancy)
- Poorly differentiated carcinomas (high-grade malignancy)
- Mixed endocrine-exocrine carcinomas

The European Neuroendocrine Tumor Society has adopted a staging system of PNETs considering cell characteristics or proliferation capacity of the tumor, and specific tumor node metastasis (TNM) staging system.

Three tumor grade categories were assigned to describe their proliferative behavior:

Grade I (Ki67 ≤2% or <2 mitoses per high-power field [HPF])—low proliferative index

Grade II (Ki67 3%-20% or 2-20 mitoses per HPF)—moderate proliferative index

Grade III (Ki67 <20% or <20 mitoses per HPF)—high proliferative index

The TNM staging system was subdivided into specific areas of the gastrointestinal (GI) system and takes into account tumor size, nodal and metastatic dissemination of these tumors. PNETs are frequently sporadic but they may be associated with genetic syndromes such as MEN1, VHL disease, NF1, or tuberous sclerosis. A recent study has shown that there is a different genetic expression between PNETs and pancreatic ductal adenocarcinomas. Genes most commonly affected by mutation in ductal adenocarcinomas are rarely affected in PNETs suggesting a different genetic mechanism involved in their pathogenesis.

PNETs are predominantly (50%) nonfunctional and have an indolent clinical course being diagnosed in an advanced stage.

An essential diagnostic approach of PNETs has to consider the specific clinical presentation of the disease (see the associated clinical findings in Table 46-1), personal medical and family history. The diagnosis of PNETs is complex and may include biochemical diagnosis, histopathology, and tumor imaging. PNETs can be identified using general and specific neuroendocrine markers. Common neuroendocrine markers in the diagnosis of PNETs and non-PNETs are:

- CgA (all different types of endocrine tumors)
- Neuron-specific enolase (NSE)
- Synaptophysin (P38)
- Protein gene product (PGP) 9.5

*Table 46-1  Genetic Differential Diagnosis*

| Syndrome | Gene Symbol | Associated Findings |
|---|---|---|
| Multiple endocrine neoplasia type 1 | MEN 1 | Hyperparathyroidism (≥90% of patients): asymptomatic hypercalcemia and/or nephrolithiasis<br>Pancreatic islet cell tumors (60%-70% of patients)<br>Pituitary tumors (15%-42% of patients) |
| von Hippel-Lindau syndrome | VHL<br>CCND1 | Hemangioblastomas (brain, spinal cord, retina), endolymphatic sac tumors, pheochromocytoma, renal cell carcinoma, pancreatic/renal/male genital tract cysts |
| Neurofibromatosis type 1 | NF1 | ≥6 café-au-lait macules >5 mm in diameter in prepubertal and >15 mm in diameter in adults, ≥2 neurofibromas, ≥2 Lisch nodules, axillary and inguinal freckling, optic gliomas, skeletal abnormalities, first-degree relative with NF1 |
| Tuberous sclerosis (*Roach et al., 1998) | TSC1<br>TSC2 | Major features: facial angiofibroma, periungual fibroma, hypomelanotic macules (more than 3), Shagreen patch, retinal nodular hamartomas, cardiac rhabdomyoma, subependymal giant cell astrocytoma<br>Minor features: pits in dental enamel, hamartomatous rectal polyps, bone or renal cysts, gingival fibromas |

*Possible Altered Genes in Pancreatic Neuroendocrine Tumors*

| Gene symbol | *DAXX*<br>*ATRX*<br>Genes in mTOR pathway (*TSC2, PTEN, PIK3CA*)<br>*TP53*<br>*PAX 8* |
|---|---|

*Reproduced with permission from Roach ES, Gomez MR, Northrup H. Tuberous sclerosis complex consensus conference: revised clinical diagnostic criteria. *J Child Neurol*. 1998;13:624-628.

Gene names: *MEN1*, multiple endocrine neoplasia 1; *VHL*, von Hippel-Lindau tumor suppressor; *CCND1*, cyclin D; *TSC 1*, hamartin or tuberous sclerosis 1; TSC 2, tuber in tuberous sclerosis 2; *NF1*, neurofibromin 1; *DAXX*, death-domain associated protein; *ATRX*, alpha thalassemia or mental retardation syndrome, X-linked; *mTOR*, mechanistic target of rapamycin (serine/threonine kinase); *TP53*, tumor protein p53; *PAX 8* (paired box 8).

- CD56
- MAP18
- CDX2 (intestinal NETs)
- Neuroendocrine secretory protein 55 (only in PNETs)

Determination of anterior pituitary hormones, ionized calcium, parathyroid hormone (PTH), and analyzing the menin gene are included in MEN1 screening. Symptoms arising from secreted hormones may lead to measurement of these hormones in the blood or tumor tissue for the initial diagnosis. Hormone-specific markers used in functioning PNETs are (see Table 46-2):

- Adrenocorticotropic hormone (ACTH)
- Calcitonin
- Insulin
- Growth hormone
- Growth hormone-releasing hormone (GHRH)
- Glucagon
- Gastrin
- Neurotensin
- Pancreatic polypeptide
- Somatostatin
- Serotonin
- VIP

The next step in diagnosing PNETs is represented by tumor imaging. Anatomic imaging of PNETs is essential for proper diagnosis and surgical management of the disease. Various imaging techniques have been employed in detection of PNETs. The most sensitive and specific imaging modalities considered are computed tomography (CT) and magnetic resonance imaging (MRI) followed by ultrasound.

**Transabdominal ultrasound** plays a limited role in evaluating these tumors because of difficulties related to imagining of the body and the tail region of the pancreas. Detection rates of ultrasound for pancreatic neuroendocrine tumor (NET) range from 0% to 66%.

**Transhepatic venous sampling** has a sensitivity of approximately 55%.

**Endoscopic ultrasound** has a sensitivity rate of 80% to 90%for PNETs.

**CT**—the use of multiphasic contrast-enhanced CT has improved its sensitivity up to 94.4%. A CT examination is recommended for detection of nodal and metastatic disease.

**MRI** is very useful for assessment of solid visceral organ lesions with a positive prediction value of 96%. The most typical MRI signs for these lesions are a T2 hyperintensity and T1 hypointensity. Gadolinium-enhanced MRI has a 40% sensitivity.

*Table 46-2 Laboratory Tests for Functioning PNETs*

| Functional PNETs | Diagnostic Tests |
|---|---|
| Insulinoma | Fasting serum glucose/proinsulin/insulin test<br>IGF-1, IGF-2<br>C-peptide suppression test<br>Angiography with percutaneous transhepatic pancreatic vein catheterization and calcium stimulation |
| Gastrinoma | Fasting serum gastrin (>1000 pg/mL)<br>Secretin stimulation test<br>Pentagastrin stimulated acid output<br>Basal acid output |
| Glucagonoma | Fasting serum glucagon test |
| VIPoma | Serum VIP (vasoactive intestinal peptide) test, $K^+$<br>Peptide histidine methionine plasma levels |
| Somatostatinoma | Fasting serum somatostatin test |
| PPoma | Preprandial PP concentration<br>Atropine suppression test, overstimulation test with secretin intravenously<br>Immunohistochemistry study |

- Functional imaging of PNETs is utilized for targeted detection of specific cell receptors leading to the localization of these tumors.
- The most common means of detection are somatostatin receptor scintigraphy, F18-fluorodeoxyglucose positron emission tomography (PET)/CT and F18-dihydroxyphenylalanine PET/CT.

**Somatostatin receptor scintigraphy (SRS)** is considered the gold standard for diagnosis, staging, and follow-up of these tumors.

An octreoscan has an overall sensitivity of approximately 80% to 90%, although it is lower for insulinomas (~40%). Ga-DOTA-TOC PET carries a sensitivity of 92% to 97%.

**Fluorodeoxyglucose (FDG) PET imaging** is a molecular imaging technique used for diagnosis of malignant tumors which are avid of glucose and necessitate higher levels of glucose to maintain their metabolism. FDG tumor uptake increases probably in relation to overexpression of glucose transporters GLUT-1, 3, and 5 and hexokinase. The sensitivities are around 50% for this imaging modality which may be more useful for prognostic purposes of PNETs.

**F18-dihydroxyphenylalanine PET/CT test** rests on the ability of neuroendocrine type cells to take up radiolabeled decarboxylate amino acid precursors and transport them into PNETs via the sodium independent system L. This test seems to be better in detection of PNET lesions compared with SRS. The overall sensitivities reported are in the range of 65% to 96% for the detection of individual lesions. Some authors have found better sensitivities rates for F18-dihydroxyphenylalanine PET/CT compared with conventional CT or SRS.

### Clinical Characteristics:

☞**Signs and Symptoms of a Functioning Islet Cell Tumor:** Nonfunctional PNETs (50%) are asymptomatic in early stages but, late in the course of the disease these tumors disseminate locoregionally or to a distant organ. MEN1 islet cell tumors are initially frequently nonfunctioning but may become active and secrete certain hormones in excess in middle-aged individuals. In VHL disease, endocrine pancreatic tumors are usually nonfunctioning. The symptoms of a functioning islet cell tumor depend on the type of hormone being produced and secreted. In Table 46-3 we describe the most common clinical presentations of islet cell tumors.

*Table 46-3 Clinical Presentation of Functional PNETs*

| Functioning PNETs | Symptoms |
|---|---|
| Insulinoma (17%) | Sweating, nausea, anxiety, tachycardia, palpitations, shaking, hunger, light-headedness, headache, visual disturbances, slurred speech, confusion, seizures |
| Gastrinoma (15%) | Recurrent stomach ulcers, abdominal pain, heart-burn, dysphagia, diarrhea |
| Glucagonoma (1%) | Skin rushes (necrolytic migratory erythema), decreased blood levels of amino acids, diarrhea, weight loss |
| Serotonin-secreting tumors (<1%) | Flushing, diarrhea, bronchoconstriction |
| Somatostatinoma (1%) | Diabetes mellitus symptoms, steatorrhoea, gall stones, hypochlorhydria, weight loss |
| VIPoma (2%) | Watery diarrhea, dehydration, hypokalemia, achlorhydria, abdominal pain or cramps, weight loss |

# Screening and Counseling

**Screening:** Mutations in the *MEN1* gene are localized in and around the open reading frame of the menin gene and are approximately 25% nonsense, 45% small deletions, 15% small insertions, less than 5% donor-splice mutations, and 10% missense mutations.

The genetic screening of familial MEN1 should sequence in and around the *MEN1* gene open reading frame. The detection of a known mutation in an individual will necessitate the testing of the other members of the family. The absence of *MEN1* germline mutations should be followed by the determination of MEN1-associated haplotype regarding the MEN1 locus (chromosome 11q13) and two or more other MEN1-affected family members will be required. If there is uncertainty that the trait in a family arises at the MEN1 locus, genetic linkage of the trait and the locus can be tested.

The screening of at-risk individuals for VHL syndrome should be started in childhood usually from the age of 5 years. Couples at risk for having a child with VHL can be sent to prenatal testing. Different screening modalities for specific tumors associated with the disease are recommended:

- Abdominal MRI (renal cell carcinomas)
- Head and spine MRI (hemangioblastoma) beginning in adolescence
- Plasma or urine fractionated metanephrines (pheochromocytoma)
- Ophthalmic examination (retinal angioma) in early childhood or infancy

Mutations in *NF1* lead to a truncated protein product. They are typically nonsense, frameshift, splice site mutations, or even missense mutations. An extended screening may increase the chance of detection to 95%. No efficient screening has been developed at this stage but regular dermatologic screening, blood pressure checks, and features related to pheochromocytoma (in <2% of patients with NF1) may be beneficial.

Surveillance screening in TSC is mandatory for people from a family affected by this condition. Most common surveillance means are fundoscopic examination, brain MRI, brain EEG, cardiac electrocardiography (ECG), echocardiography (ECHO), renal MRI, CT or ultrasound, dermatologic screening, neurodevelopmental testing, and pulmonary CT. The frequency of these tests varies for a child, adult, or relative affected by the disease.

Chorionic villus sampling (CVS) at about 10 to 12 weeks or amniocentesis at 16 to 18 weeks gestation can be recommended if a known disease-causing mutation is present in the family with TSC.

**Counseling:** Most cases of MEN1 are considered to have an autosomal dominant pattern of inheritance. However, MEN1 is a distinct autosomal disorder necessitating two altered copies of the *MEN1* gene to trigger tumor formation.

More than 1133 different germline (pathologic alleles variant) and 203 somatic mutations have been reported in MEN1 families and sporadic cases. In about 10% of MEN cases, mutations arise de novo and possibly will be passed down to subsequent generations. The majority of known studies have described a disease penetrance among *MEN1* germline mutation carriers of 82% to 99% by the age of 50 years.

Somatic *MEN1* mutations in sporadic tumors have been reported in 10% to 22% of parathyroid adenomas, 25% of gastrinomas, 10% to 22% of insulinomas, 50% of VIP-secreting tumors, and 25% to 35% of bronchial carcinoids.

VHL is an inherited autosomal dominant condition in which both alleles need to be mutated in order for the disorder to develop. Disease penetrance by the age of 60 years is more than 95%. The majority of VHL type 2 are caused by missense mutations that disrupt the VHL protein and are associated with pheochromocytoma. VHL type 1 is caused by large deletions and truncating mutations predisposing to hemangioblastomas or renal cell carcinomas and is rarely associated with pheochromocytoma.

NF1 is transmitted in an autosomal dominant (50%) or spontaneous mutation (50%). NF1 is inherited in an autosomal dominant manner. Two copies of the *NF1* gene must be altered to trigger tumor formation of NF1, compared with the classic form of autosomal dominant inheritance pattern where only one mutated copy is necessary. Half of affected individuals have NF1 as the result of a de novo *NF1* gene mutation. The sib of an affected individual has a 50% risk of inheriting the condition, but the disease manifestations are extremely variable.

The diversity of *NF1* mutations that occur in this disease makes genotype-phenotype correlation difficult. Large deletions have been linked to dysmorphic features and more mental retardation.

At present two clear correlations have been observed:

- **A whole *NF1* gene deletion:** early appearance of cutaneous neurofibromas, severe cognitive abnormalities and somatic overgrowth, large hands and feet, and dysmorphic facial features
- **A 3-bp in-frame deletion of exon 17 (c.2970-2972 delAAT):** typical pigmentary features of NF1, but no cutaneous or surface plexiform neurofibromas

TSC has an autosomal dominant pattern of inheritance, which means one copy of the altered gene in each cell will have the potential of triggering the disease. In about one-third of cases, an affected person inherits an altered *TSC1* or *TSC2* gene from a parent who has the disorder. Two-thirds of TSC cases result from sporadic genetic mutations, but their offspring may inherit it from them. *TSC1* mutations appear relatively frequent in familial cases of TSC, while mutations in the TSC2 gene are usually linked to sporadic cases (55%-90%). The most common missense mutations in TSC are at Arg611 (exon 16) and Pro1675Leu (exon 38), and 18 bp in-frame deletion in exon 40. Nonsense or frameshift mutations are also reported in TSC. About 15% to 20% of patients have no identifiable mutations. Tuberous sclerosis penetrance is now thought to be 100%. Genotype and phenotype correlation studies have shown a milder phenotype in patients with a *TSC1* mutation. Mental retardation and renal malignancy seem to be higher in individuals with *TSC2* mutations. *TSC1* mutations have been found less frequent in sporadic cases.

# Management and Treatment

The treatment of PNETs depends on several factors: symptoms, hormone secretion, tumor size, location, metastatic dissemination. The best therapeutic option in patients with localized or locoregional disease with minimal lymph node involvement is surgery.

**Surgical Treatment:** The initial presentation of the tumor indicates the surgical approach of the patient:

- Pancreaticoduodenal resection (Whipple operation)
- Distal pancreatic resection
- Tumor enucleation
- Lymph node dissection (malignancy)

Patients with limited liver metastases may benefit from surgical resection of the liver metastases. Resection of liver metastases may be beneficial for functioning and nonfunctioning tumors and may slow down the course of the disease.

Typical surgical procedures for liver metastases can be:

- Tumor enucleation
- Segmental resections
- Partial or extended hemihepatectomy

Advanced disease may be amenable to palliative surgical resection and tumor debulking. Individualized treatment in such cases is recommended. Selective embolization, transarterial chemoembolization, radiofrequency ablation, or liver transplantation may improve prognosis in such patients with metastatic liver disease.

**Medical Therapy:** Systemic chemotherapy is used in extended metastatic disease or when other palliative treatments have failed. *First-line treatment*: streptozotocin with 5-FU or doxorubicin. Most of the PNETs respond to this treatment and important tumor shrinkage is possible in 20% to 35% of the cases. Systemic therapy with somatostatin analogues (octreotide, lanreotide) may be considered in patients with unresectable or residual disease. *Interferon*: decreases circulating hormone levels in 30% to 60% of patients with endocrine gastrointestinal tumors producing symptomatic relief. Because PNETs have a generally indolent course even in operated metastatic disease, high survival rates have been reported.

**New Therapeutic Targets:**
- Multi-tyrosine kinase inhibitor—sunitinib, sorafenib, pazopanib
- Oral alkylating agents—temozolomide
- Inhibitors of mammalian target of rapamycin (mTOR)—everolimus, temsirolimus
- Antivascular endothelial growth factor (anti-VEGF) monoclonal antibody—bevacizumab
- Peptide receptor radionuclide therapy (PRRT)

## Molecular Genetics and Molecular Mechanism

**Syndrome/Gene/Locus:**

Multiple endocrine neoplasia type 1/*MEN1*/11q13
Von Hippel-Lindau syndrome/(*VHL, CCND1*)/3p25.3, 11q13
Neurofibromatosis type 1/*NF1*/17q11.2
Tuberous sclerosis/(*TSC1, TSC2*)/9q34,16p13.3

☞**MEN1:** It is a rare autosomal dominant hereditary cancer syndrome representing the development of a variety of tumors in diverse endocrine systems such as parathyroid glands, pancreatic islets, and pituitary gland, and even in nonendocrine tissues (>20 combinations of them). The *MEN1* gene is ubiquitously expressed and encodes a putative tumor suppressor protein called menin, which is involved in regulation of gene transcription, cell proliferation, apoptosis, and genome stability. Menin is primarily located in the nucleus where it exerts its aforementioned functions. The genetic screening of familial MEN1 should sequence in and around the menin protein's open reading frame. The histogenesis of PNETs is still unclear with some investigations regarding the ductal or acinar cell system as the origin.

☞**VHL SYNDROME:** Two distinct proteins are encoded by the *VHL* gene which is ubiquitously expressed: p30 and p19. These are involved in controlling oxygen-sensing pathways, microtubule stability and orientation, tumor suppression, cilia formation, regulation of senescence, cytokine signaling, collagen IV regulation, and formation of fibronectin matrix.

☞**NF1:** Various mutations could explain the extreme clinical variability of NF1. The mutated gene in NF1 encodes for a protein called neurofibromin. This protein plays a negative role in regulation of the Ras kinase pathway. Different types of mutations (deletions, missense, nonsense) of the *NF1* gene result in a dysfunctional suppressor protein and overgrowth of cells of various tissues (dermal, nervous system)

☞**TUBEROUS SCLEROSIS:** Two essential proteins for intracellular signaling pathways are coded by TSC1 and TSC2: hamartin and tuberin. As a result of their interaction a tuberin-hamartin complex is formed. This complex is considered essential for multiple intracellular signaling pathways controlling cell growth and proliferation.

**Genetic Testing:** DNA mutation analysis in well-differentiated pancreatic endocrine carcinomas should be sought for the following gene candidates:

- *MEN1, ATRX, DAXX, TSC2, PTEN, PIK3CA*
- mTOR pathway genes: *TSC2, PTEN, PIK3CA*
- Mutations affecting *ATRX* and *DAXX* genes (40% of PNETs)

The occurrence rates for PNETs in associated familial syndromes are as below:

- 85% to 100% of patients with MEN1
- 10% to 17%—VHL
- Less than or equal to 10% of patients—neurofibromatosis type 1
- Occasionally—in tuberous sclerosis

Specific genetic testing for these syndromes is recommended when family history and specific clinical and laboratory findings are suggesting either one of them. The genetic testing is available for the genes listed above. (see http://www.ncbi.nlm.nih.gov/sites/GeneTests/review?db=GeneTests).

**BIBLIOGRAPHY:**

1. Solcia E, Kloppel G, Sobin LH. Histological typing of endocrine tumors. *World Health Organization International Histological Classification of Tumors*. 2nd ed. Berlin, Germany:Springer; 2000.
2. Lubarsch O. Ueber denprimären Krebs des Ileum nebst Bemerkungenüber das gleichzeitige Vorkommen von Krebs und Tuberculose. *Virchows Arch Pathol Anat*. 1888;111:280-317.
3. Feyrter F. Über diffuse endokrine epitheliale Organe. *Zentralblatt-Innere Medizin*. 1938;59:546-556.
4. Langley K. The neuroendocrine concept today. *Ann N Y Acad Sci*. 1994;733:1-17.
5. Oberg K, Jelic S. Neuroendocrine gastroenteropancreatic tumors: ESMO clinical recommendation for diagnosis, treatment and follow-up. *Ann Oncol*. 2009;20(suppl 4):150-153.
6. Rindi G, Klöppel G, Alhman H, et al. TNM staging of foregut (neuro) endocrine tumors: a consensus proposal including a grading system. *Virchows Arch*. 2006;449:395-401.
7. Rindi G, Klöppel G, Couvelard A, et al. TNM staging of mid gut and hindgut (neuro) endocrine tumors: a consensus proposal including a grading system. *Virchows Arch*. 2007;451:757-762.
8. Jones S, Zhang X, Parsons DW, et al. Core signaling pathways in human pancreatic cancers revealed by global genomic analyses. *Science*. 2008;321:1801.
9. Evans DB, Skibber JM, Lee JE. Non-functioning islet cell carcinomas of the pancreas. *Surgery*. 1993;114:1175-1182.

10. Wilder RM, Allan FN, Power MH, Robertsson HE. Carcinoma of the islands of the pancreas. Hyperinsulinism and hypoglycemia. *J Am Med Assoc*. 1927;89:348-355.

11. Zollinger RM, Ellison EH. Primary peptic ulcerations of the jejunum associated with islet cell tumors of the pancreas. *Ann Surg*. 1955;142:709-728.

12. Verner JV, Morrison AB. Islet cell tumor and a syndrome of refractory watery diarrhea and hypokalemia. *Am J Med*. 1958;25:374-380.

13. Mallinson CN, Bloom SR, Warin AP, Salmon PR, Cox B. A glucagonoma syndrome. *Lancet*. 1974;ii:1-5.

14. Eriksson B, Arnberg H, Lindgren PG, et al. Neuroendocrine pancreatic tumours: clinical presentations, biochemical and histopathological findings in 84 patients. *J Intern Med*. 1990;228:103-113.

15. Modlin IM, Lye KD, Kidd M. A 5-decade analysis of 13,715 carcinoid tumors. *Cancer*. 2003;97:934-939.

16. Jiao Y, Shi C, Edil BH, et al. DAXX/ATRX, MEN1, and mTOR pathway genes are frequently altered in pancreatic neuroendocrine tumors. *Science*. 2011;331(6021):1199-1203.

17. Solcia E, Sessa F, Rindi R, Bonato M, Capella C. Pancreatic endocrine tumors. General concepts: non-functioning tumors and tumors with uncommon function. In: Dayal Y, ed. *Endocrine Pathology of the Gut and Pancreas*. Boca Raton: CRC Press; 1999:105-131.

18. Wilder RM, Allan FN, Power MH, Robertsson HE. Carcinoma of the islands of the pancreas. Hyperinsulinism and hypoglycemia. *J Am Med Assoc*. 1927;89:348-355.

19. Ramage JK, Davies AH, Ardill J, et al. Guidelines for the management of gastroenteropancreatic neuroendocrine (including carcinoid) tumours. *Gut*. Jun 2005;54(suppl 4):iv1-16.

20. Liu Y, Sturgis CD, Grzybicki DM, et al. Microtubule-associated protein-2: a new sensitive and specific marker for pulmonary carcinoid tumor and small cell carcinoma. *Mod Pathol*. Sep 2001;14(9):880-885.

21. McAuley G, Delaney H, Colville J, et al. Multimodality preoperative imaging of pancreatic insulinomas. *Clin Radiol*. 2005;60:1039-1050.

22. Rösch T, Lightdale CJ, Botet JF, et al. Localization of pancreatic endocrine tumors by endoscopic ultrasonography. *N Engl J Med*. 1992;326:1721-1726.

23. Gouya H, Vignaux O, Augui J, et al. CT, endoscopic sonography, and a combined protocol for preoperative evaluation of pancreatic insulinomas. *AJR Am J Roentgenol*. 2003;181:987-992.

24. Owen NJ, Sohaib SA, Peppercorn PD, et al. MRI of pancreatic neuroendocrine tumours. *Br J Radiol*. 2001;74:968-973.

25. Semelka RC, Custodio CM, CemBalci N, Woosley JT. Neuroendocrine tumors of the pancreas: spectrum of appearances on MRI. *J MagnReson Imaging*. 2000;11:141-148.

26. Carcinoid tumors, carcinoid syndrome, and related disorders. *Williams Textbook of Endocrinology*. 10th ed. Philadelphia, PA: Saunders; 2003:661-690.

27. Gabriel M, Decristoforo C, Kendler D, et al. 68Ga-DOTA-Tyr3-octreotide PET in neuroendocrine tumors: comparison with somatostatin receptor scintigraphy and CT. *J Nucl Med*. 2007;48:508-518.

28. Gambhir SS, Czernin J, Schwimmer J, Silverman DH, Coleman RE, Phelps ME. A tabulated summary of the FDG PET literature. *J Nucl Med*. 2001;42:S1-S93.

29. Zhao S, Kuge Y, Mochizuki T, et al. Biologic correlates of intratumoral heterogeneity in 18F-FDG distribution with regional expression of glucose transporters and hexokinase-II in experimental tumor. *J Nucl Med*. 2005;46:675-682.

30. Jager PL, Chirakal R, Marriott CJ, Brouwers AH, Koopmans KP, Gulenchyn KY. 6-L-18F-fluorodihydroxyphenylalanine PET in neuroendocrine tumors: basic aspects and emerging clinical applications. *J Nucl Med*. 2008;49:573-586.

31. Chandrasekharappa SC, Guru SC, Manickam P, et al. 1997 positional cloning of the gene for multiple endocrine neoplasia-type 1. *Science*. 276:404-407.

32. Lemos MC, Thakker RV. Multiple endocrine neoplasia type 1 (MEN1): analysis of 1336 mutations reported in the first decade following identification of the gene. *Hum Mutat*. 2008;29:22-32.

33. Brandi ML, Gagel RF, Angeli A, et al. Guidelines for diagnosis and therapy of MEN type 1 and type 2. *J Clin Endocrinol Metab*. 2001;86(12):5658-5671.

34. Maher ER, IseliusL, YatesJR, et al. Von Hippel-Lindau disease: a genetic study. *J Med Genet*. 1991;28:443-447.

35. Lemos MC, Thakker RV. Multiple endocrine neoplasia type 1 (MEN1): analysis of 1336 mutations reported in the first decade following identification of the gene. *Hum Mutat*. 2008;29:22-32.

36. Teh BT, Farnebo F, Phelan C, et al. Mutation analysis of the MEN1 gene in multiple endocrine neoplasia type 1, familial acromegaly, and familial isolated hyperparathyroidism. *J Clin Endocrinol Metab*. 1998;83:2621-2626.

37. Trump D, Farren B, Wooding C, et al. Clinical studies of multiple endocrine neoplasia type 1 (MEN1). *QJM*. 1996;89:653-669.

38. Carling T, Correa P, Hessman O, et al. Parathyroid *MEN1* gene mutations in relation to clinical characteristics of nonfamilial primary hyperparathyroidism. *J Clin Endocrinol. Metab*. 1998;83:2960-2963.

39. Goebel SU, Heppner C, Burns AL, et al. Genotype/phenotype correlation of *MEN1* gene mutations in sporadic gastrinomas. *J Clin Endocrinol Metab*. 2000;85:116-123.

40. Zhuang Z, Vortmeyer AO, Pack S, et al. Somatic mutations of the *MEN1* tumor suppressor gene in sporadic gastrinomas and insulinomas. *Cancer Res*. 1997;57:4682-4686.

41. Wang EH, Ebrahimi SA, Wu AY, Kashefi C, Passaro E Jr, Sawicki MP Mutation of the *MENIN* gene in sporadic pancreatic endocrine tumors. *Cancer Res*.1998;58:4417-4420.

42. Wu BL, Austin MA, Schneider GH, Boles RG, Korf BR. Deletion of the entire NF1 gene detected by the FISH: four deletion patients associated with severe manifestations. *Am J Med Genet*. 1995;59:528-535.

43. Upadhyaya M, Huson SM, Davies M, et al. An absence of cutaneous neurofibromas associated with a 3-bp inframe deletion in exon 17 of the NF1 gene (c.2970—2972delAAT): evidence of a clinically significant NF1 genotype-phenotype correlation. *Am J Hum Genet*. 2007;80:140-151.

44. Rendtorff ND, Bjerregaard B, Frödin M, et al. Analysis of 65 tuberous sclerosis complex (TSC) patients by TSC2 DGGE, TSC1/TSC2 MLPA, and TSC1 long-range PCR sequencing, and report of 28 novel mutations. *Hum Mutat*. 2005;26(4):374-383.

45. Sancak O, Nellist M, Goedbloed M, et al. Mutational analysis of the TSC1 and TSC2 genes in a diagnostic setting: genotype—phenotype correlations and comparison of diagnostic DNA techniques in tuberous sclerosis complex. *Eur J Hum Genet*. 2005;13: 731-741.

46. Akerstrom G. Management of carcinoid tumors of the stomach, duodenum and pancreas. *World J Surg*. 1996;20:173-182.

47. Norton JA, Warren RS, Kelly MG, Zuraek MB, Jensen RT. Aggressive surgery for metastatic liver neuroendocrine tumors. *Surgery*. 2003;134:1057-1065.

48. Moertel CG, Lefkopoulo M, Lipsitz S, Hahn RG, Klaassen D. Streptozotocin-doxorubicin, streptozotocin-fluorouracil or chlorozotocin in the treatment of advanced islet-cell carcinoma. *N Engl J Med*. 1992;326:519-523.

49. Aparicio T, Ducreux M, Baudin E, et al. Antitumour activity of somatostatin analogues in progressive metastatic neuroendocrine tumours. *Eur J Cancer*. 2001;37:1014-1019.

50. Öberg K, Lindstrom H, Alm G, Lundqvist G. Successful treatment of therapy-resistant pancreatic cholera with human leucocyte interferon. *Lancet*. 1985;i:725-727.

51. Rufini V, Calcagni ML, Baum RP. Imaging of neuroendocrine tumors. *Semin Nucl Med*. Jul 2006;36(3):228-247.

52. Everolimus approved for pancreatic neuroendocrine tumors. *The ASCO Post*. May 15 2011;2(8).

53. National Cancer Institute. Cancer Drug Information. FDA Approval for Sunitinib Malate. Pancreatic Neuroendocrine Tumors. http://www.cancer.gov/cancertopics/druginfo/fda-sunitinib-malate. Accessed August, 2013.

54. Duran I, Kortmansky J, Singh D, et al. A phase II clinical and pharmacodynamic study of temsirolimus in advanced neuroendocrine carcinomas. *Br J Cancer*. 2006;95(9):1148.

55. Hobday TJ, Rubin J, Holen K, et al. MC044h, a phase II trial of sorafenib in patients (pts) with metastatic neuroendocrine tumors (NET): a phase II consortium (P2C) study (abstract 4504). *J Clin Oncol*. 2007;25:199s.

56. Yao JC, Phan A, Hoff PM, et al. Targeting vascular endothelial growth factor in advanced carcinoid tumor: a random assignment phase II study of depot octreotide with bevacizumab and pegylated interferon alpha-2b. *J Clin Oncol*. 2008;26(8):1316.

57. Anlauf M, Schlenger R, Perren A, et al. Microadenomatosis of the endocrine pancreas in patients with and without the multiple endocrine neoplasia type 1 syndrome. *Am J Surg Pathol*. May 2006;30(5):560-574.

58. Vortmeyer AO, Huang S, Lubensky I, Zhuang Z. Non-islet origin of pancreatic islet cell tumors. *J Clin Endocrinol Metab*. Apr 2004;89(4):1934-1938.

59. Nordstrom-O'Brien M, van der Luijt RB, van Rooijen E, et al. Genetic analysis of von Hippel-Lindau disease. *Hum Mutat*. 2010;31:521-537.

## Supplementary Information

### OMIM REFERENCES:

[1] Multiple Endocrine Neoplasia Type 1; MEN1 (#131100)

[2] von Hippel-Lindau Syndrome; VHL, CCND1 (#608537, #168461)

[3] Neurofibromatosis 1; NF1 (#162200)

[4] Tuberous Sclerosis; TSC1, TSC2 (#605284, #191092)

### Alternative Names:

- Endocrine Adenomatosis, Multiple
- MEA1
- Wermer Syndrome
- von Recklinghausen Disease
- Tuberous Sclerosis Complex; TSC

*Key Words:* Pancreatic neuroendocrine tumors, well-differentiated endocrine tumors, poorly differentiated carcinomas, mixed endocrine-exocrine carcinomas, autosomal dominant pattern, multiple endocrine neoplasia 1, von Hippel-Lindau syndrome, neurofibromatosis type 1, tuberous sclerosis complex, germline mutations, chromogranin A, gastrin, neuron-specific enolase, synaptophysin, neuroendocrine secretory protein 55, ACTH, insulin, calcitonin, glucagon, VIP, somatostatin, serotonin, insulinomas, gastrinomas, F18-fluorodeoxyglucose PET/CT, F18-dihydroxyphenylalanine PET/CT, deletions, missense, nonsense mutationos

# 47 Hereditary Pheochromocytoma and Paraganglioma

Monica A. Giovanni and Justin P. Annes

## KEY POINTS

- *Disease summary:*
  - Paraganglia are clusters of neuroendocrine cells that comprise the sympathetic ganglia, the parasympathetic ganglia, and the adrenal medulla. A paraganglioma (PGL) is a tumor that derives from paraganglia.
  - The term pheochromocytoma (PHEO) is applied to catecholamine-secreting paragangliomas of the adrenal gland.
  - Extra-adrenal paragangliomas (ePGLs) may be categorized as either sympathetic (usually found in the abdomen) or parasympathetic (usually found in the head and neck; hnPGL) paragangliomas.
  - PHEOs and ePGLs most commonly present with hypertension, headache, anxiety, and/or palpitations.
  - hnPGLs usually present as an enlarging mass or with a mass effect such as a cranial nerve palsy (eg, Horner syndrome).
  - PGLs have an estimated prevalence of 1 in 5000 and an estimated incidence of 1 in 30,000.
- *Hereditary basis:*
  - Approximately 30% of PGLs are associated with an identifiable germline mutation; two-thirds of these cases are apparently sporadic.
    - The likelihood that a germline mutation is present is strongly influenced by the clinical presentation: presence of syndromic features, presence of a family history, tumor location, age of diagnosis, greater than one primary PGL or metastatic disease.
    - At least 10 PHEO- or PGL-predisposing genes have been identified.
  - PGLs show an autosomal dominant inheritance pattern with incomplete penetrance.
    - The tumor risk associated with several genes is influenced by the parent of origin (SDHD, SDHAF2, MAX) where tumor risk is associated with paternal inheritance.
- *Differential diagnosis:*
  - It is important to distinguish the multiorgan system syndromes that include PHEO or PGLs as a single feature (ie, von Hippel-Lindau [VHL], neurofibromatosis [NF], and multiple endocrine neoplasia [MEN]), from the familial tumor predispositions in which these tumors are the predominant feature (Table 47-1).

## Diagnostic Criteria and Clinical Characteristics

### Diagnostic Criteria for Familial Paraganglioma:

**At least one of the following**

- Single paraganglioma associated with an identified germline mutation
- Multiple paragangliomas in a single individual
- Paragangliomas in more than one generation
- Identification of a known paraganglioma causing germline mutation

**And the absence of**

- An alternative genetic syndrome such as NF1, VHL, or MEN2.

*Clinical Characteristics: Pheochromocytoma or ePGL:* Clinical features include intermittent hypertension, palpitations, and occasionally flushing. Familial paraganglioma is most often recognized in the setting of a single, apparently sporadic, pheochromocytoma.

*Glomus or carotid body tumors or hnPGL:* These tumors are primarily arise from the carotid body parasympathetic ganglia located at the bifurcation of the common carotid but may also arise from tympanic, vagal, jugular, or laryngeal ganglia. A female predominance is consistently observed. Most hnPGLs present as a painless neck mass. The metastatic potential of these tumors is relatively low but not absent.

## Screening and Counseling

*Screening:* In patients with an apparent sporadic pheochromocytoma or paraganglioma, up to 25% of these individuals will have an identifiable genetic (germline) mutation underlying that diagnosis with important implications for the patient and relatives. While NF1 can often be diagnosed on physical examination, the other entities require biochemical, radiographic, and/or genetic testing. Patients with MEN2A can exhibit elevated plasma calcitonin levels. Additionally, specific gene mutations in *VHL* have been recognized as the cause of familial pheochromocytoma in the absence of hemangioblastoma or renal cell carcinoma, termed VHL type 2C.

In an index case, the relative likelihood of these disorders can be predicted based on (a) age at diagnosis and (b) tumor characteristics. In general, germline mutation is more likely in younger patients and in the presence of multifocal disease with extra-adrenal location. While the mean age of diagnosis for familial paraganglioma is 28 to 34 years for PGLs, it should be noted that hereditary PGL has been diagnosed in very old age.

Although significant genetic heterogeneity exists, genetic testing strategies may be directed by a patient's clinical presentation, family history, and the relative frequency with which mutations in the specific gene is found.

*Table 47-1  Genetic Differential Diagnosis*

| Syndrome | Gene Symbol | Relative Frequency | Associated Findings |
|---|---|---|---|
| von Hippel-Lindau (see Chap. 129) | *VHL* | 20%-40% | Hemangioblastomas of the brain, spinal cord, and retina; renal cysts and clear cell renal cell carcinoma; and endolymphatic sac tumors. Risk of PHEO and other features are mutation specific. Mean age of PHEO is 29 years (PGL is rare). |
| Neurofibromatosis, type 1 (see Chap. 108) | *NF1* | 5%-15% | Cutaneous neurofibromas, plexiform neurofibromas, cafe-au-lait macules, axillary and inguinal freckling, Lisch nodules (iris hamartomas), optic glioma, sphenoid dysplasia, tibial pseudarthrosis, first-degree relative with NF1. Pheochromocytomas occur in approximately 1% of NF1 patients. |
| Multiple Endocrine Neoplasia, Type 2 (MEN2A) (see Chap. 81) | *RET* | 5%-15% | Medullary thyroid carcinoma (MTC), parathyroid adenoma/hyperplasia. PGLs typically present around age 40 years (decades after medullary thyroid tends to present), is confined to the adrenal gland, has low metastatic potential, and tends to secrete increased amounts of epinephrine. |
| PGL1 | *SDHD* | 20%-30% | PGLs are predominantly hnPGL (80%) but PHEOs (18%), ePGL (2%), and GIST (rare) also occur. The estimated penetrance of hnPGL is 80% and of PHEO is 30%. Parent of origin effect is observed. |
| PGL2 | *SDHAF2* | Rare | Primarily, if not exclusively hnPGLs. Parent of origin effect is observed. |
| PGL3 | *SDHC* | 3%-8% | PGLs primarily manifest as hnPGL (90%) though PHEO (5%) and ePGL (5%) do occur. Features such as renal cell carcinoma (7%) and gastrointestinal stromal tumors (GIST; 2%) are observed. |
| PGL4 | *SDHB* | 20%-30% | Variable PGLs are observed: ePGL (55%), PHEO (20%), and hnPGL (25%). SDHB-related PGLs are frequently malignant (20%-50%). Other features include renal cell carcinoma (3.5%) and gastrointestinal stromal tumors (GIST; 2%). |
| PGL5 | *SDHA* | Rare | PHEO and ePGL, GIST, Leigh syndrome (autosomal recessive) |
| PGLx | *TMEM127* | 1%-5% | PHEO, often bilateral with low malignant potential. hnPGL and ePGL have been observed. |
| PGLx | *MAX* | 1% | PHEO, often bilateral. Phenotype not fully delineated at present. Parent of origin effect is observed. |
| PGLx | *KIF1B* | Rare | PHEO. Not fully established as causative. |

Gene names: *VHL*, von Hippel-Lindau tumor suppressor; *NF1*, neurofibromin 1; *RET*, ret proto-oncogene; *SDHD*, succinate dehydrogenase complex, subunit D, integral membrane protein; *SDHAF2*, succinate dehydrogenase complex assembly factor 2; *SDHC*, succinate dehydrogenase complex, subunit C, integral membrane protein; *SDHB*, succinate dehydrogenase complex, subunit B iron sulfur; *SDHA*, succinate dehydrogenase complex, subunit A, flavoprotein; *TMEM127*, transmembrane protein 127; *MAX*, MYC-associated factor X; *KIF1B*, kinesin family member 1B.

☞**Presymptomatic Screening:**

• Annual symptom screening.
• Annual physical examination.
• Annual plasma or 24-hour urine metanephrine and normetanephrine measurement.
• Patients affected with an *SDHB* mutation should have annual MRI from skull base to the pelvis; patients harboring an *SDHA, C, D, TMEM127, SDHAF2*, or *MAX* mutation may not require imaging with the same frequency.
• Functional imaging may be used intermittently (every 5 years) and to determine if metastatic disease is present. The optimal nuclear study may depend on the tumor type.

*Glomus or carotid body tumors:* These tumors typically do not have endocrine properties. Surgical resection is the treatment of choice when limited neurologic and vascular risk is judged to be present. Permanent neurologic damage is described in 32% to 44% of patients who undergo surgical intervention. Patients should have metanephrine and normetanephrine levels measured prior to surgery to exclude an undetected ePGL or PHEO.

*Pheochromocytomas or ePGL:* Tumors located within the adrenal gland have a lower metastatic risk than ePGL which may be as high as 30%. Tumor resection is the treatment of choice for localized disease. Adrenal sparing surgical resection should be performed whenever possible. Adequate blood pressure control must be obtained prior to surgical intervention.

*GIST:* Tumors that are found in the stomach and lack somatic mutations in either KIT or PDGF-receptor alpha are likely to be associated with a germline mutation in a PGL-related gene. These patients should have a complete evaluation prior to surgical intervention.

**Counseling:** The PHEO or PGL syndrome is inherited in an autosomal dominant fashion. Each child of an affected parent has a 50% risk of inheriting the condition.

PGL1, PGL2, and MAX-related PGL are inherited as an autosomal dominant with *maternal imprinting*. In this case the disease phenotype is only transmitted via the father (50% risk) while carrier status without disease is inherited via the mother (50% risk). In the case of a documented maternally inherited pathogenic mutation of an imprinted gene, routine clinical and laboratory screening should continue but radiographic screening is not felt to be indicated.

Presymptomatic testing should be offered to all first-degree relatives of an affected individual. In situations of apparent de novo mutations, germline mosaicism in an unaffected parent and nonpaternity should be considered.

☞**AGE-ASSOCIATED PENETRANCE:** Accurate estimates of penetrance are not available at this time for PGL-associated genes. The numbers given below are likely biased in the upward direction.

- PGL1 (*SDHD* mutation) 48% by age 30 years and 73% by age 40 years
- PGL4 (*SDHB* mutation) 29% penetrance by age 30 years, and 45% by age 40 years
- TMEM127 presents at an older age (mean 41.5 years); unknown penetrance

☞**GENOTYPE-PHENOTYPE CORRELATION:** PGL4 is associated with abdominal disease that is frequently invasive and has a relatively high rate of metastasis (~40%). PGL1 may present with head and neck tumors in 89% of cases, may be multifocal and has a low rate of metastasis at first surgery. See Table 47-1 for additional details.

## Molecular Genetics and Molecular Mechanism

**Syndrome/Gene/Locus:**

PGL1/succinate dehydrogenase complex, subunit D (*SDHD*)/11q23.1

PGL2/succinate dehydrogenase complex assembly factor 2 (*SDHAF2*)/11q13.1

PGL3/succinate dehydrogenase complex, subunit C (*SDHC*)/1q23.3

PGL4/succinate dehydrogenase complex, subunit B (*SDHB*)/1p36.13

PGL5/succinate dehydrogenase complex, subunit A (*SDHA*)/5p15.33

PGLx/transmembrane protein 127 (*TMEM127*)/2q11.2

PGLx/MYC-associated factor X (*MAX*)/14q23.3

Succinate dehydrogenase (SDH) is a four subunit enzyme (SDH A, B, C, D) also known as mitochondrial complex II, which acts as a key component of the tricarboxylic acid cycle and oxidative phosphorylation respiratory chain. SDHAF2 is an assembly factor that facilitates complex formation. Disruption of the SDH complex function and loss of VHL result in elevated levels of transcription factor, hypoxia-induced factor 1α (HIF-1α) that is believed to drive tumorigenesis.

Pathogenic mutation of *TMEM127*, *MAX*, *NF*, and *RET* are believed to cause tumor formation by excessive activation of the mammalian target of rapamycin (mTOR) growth promoting signaling cascade.

**Genetic Testing:** DNA sequence and deletion analysis is clinically available for SDHAF2, SDHB, SDHC, and SDHD (see Gene Tests http://www.genetests.org/query?mim=168000). DNA sequence analysis is available for TMEM127 and Kif1B. The decision about which gene to test first is often based on the family history, the clinical presentation, and the overall incidence of mutations. The diagnostic value of performing immunohistochemical analysis of SDHA and SDHB on tumor tissue sections is still being evaluated. See the PGL testing strategy shown in Fig. 47-1.

**BIBLIOGRAPHY:**

1. Bayley JP, Kunst HP, Cascon A, et al. SDHAF2 mutations in familial and sporadic paraganglioma and phaeochromocytoma. *Lancet Oncol.* 2010;11:366-372.

2. Benn DE, Gimenez-Roqueplo AP, Reilly JR, et al. Clinical presentation and penetrance of pheochromocytoma/paraganglioma syndromes. *J Clin Endocrinol Metab.* 2006;91(3):827-836.

3. Burnichon N, Briere JJ, Libe R, et al. SDHA is a tumor suppressor gene causing paraganglioma. *Hum Mol Genet.* 2010;19:3011-3020.

4. Comino-Mendez I, Gracia-Aznarez FJ, Schiavi F, et al. Exome sequencing identifies MAX mutations as a cause of hereditary pheochromocytoma. *Nat Genet.* 2011;43:663-667.

5. Favier J, Brière JJ, Strompf L, et al. Hereditary paraganglioma/pheochromocytoma and inherited succinate dehydrogenase deficiency. *Horm Res.* 2005;63(4):171-179.

6. Gimenez-Roqueplo AP, Lehnert H, Mannelli M, et al. Phaeochromocytoma, new genes and screening strategies. *Clin Endocrinol (Oxf).* 2006;65:699-705.

7. Hao HX, Khalimonchuk O, Schraders M, et al. SDH5, a gene required for flavination of succinate dehydrogenase, is mutated in paraganglioma. *Science.* 2009;325:1139-1142.

8. Hoffman MA, Ohh M, Yang H, Klco JM, Ivan M, Kaelin WG Jr. von Hippel-Lindau protein mutants linked to type 2C VHL disease preserve the ability to downregulate HIF. *Hum Mol Genet.* 2001;10(10):1019-1027.

9. Jiménez C, Cote G, Arnold A, et al. Review: should patients with apparently sporadic pheochromocytomas or paragangliomas be screened for hereditary syndromes? *J Clin Endocrinol Metab.* 2006; 91(8):2851-2858.

10. Lips CJ, Landsvater RM, Höppener JW, et al. Clinical screening as compared with DNA analysis in families with multiple endocrine neoplasia type 2A. *N Engl J Med.* 1994;331:828-835.

11. Mariman EC, van Beersum SE, Cremers CW, et al. Fine mapping of a putatively imprinted gene for familial non-chromaffin paragangliomas to chromosome 11q13.1: evidence for genetic heterogeneity. *Hum Genet.* 1995;95:56-62.

12. Neumann HP, Bausch B, McWhinney SR, et al. Germ-line mutations in nonsyndromic pheochromocytoma. *N Engl J Med.* 2002;346:1459-1466.

13. Neumann HP, Eng C. The approach to the patient with paraganglioma. *J Clin Endocrinol Metab.* 2009;94:2677-2683.

14. Qin Y, Yao L, King EE, et al. Germline mutations in TMEM127 confer susceptibility to pheochromocytoma. *Nat Genet.* 2010;42: 229-233.

15. Rodríguez-Cuevas S, López-Garza J, Labastida-Almendaro S. Carotid body tumors in inhabitants of altitudes higher than 2000 meters above sea level. *Head Neck.* 1998;20(5):374-378.

16. Yeh IT, Lenci RE, Qin Y, et al. A germline mutation of the KIF1B beta gene on 1p36 in a family with neural and non-neural tumors. *Hum Genet.* 2008;124:279-285.

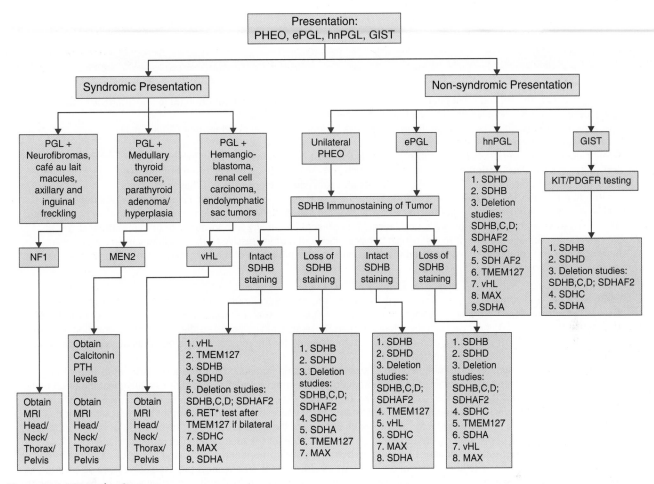

*Figure 47-1* PGL Testing Strategy.

17. van Naderveen FH, Gaal J, Favier J, et al. An immunohistochemical procedure to detect patients with paraganglioma and phaeochromocytoma with germline SDHB, SDHC, or SDHD gene mutations: a retrospective and prospective analysis. *Lancet Oncol.* 2008;10(8):764-771.

## Supplementary Information

### OMIM References:

[1] Paragangliomas 1; PGL1 (#168000)

[2] Paragangliomas 2; PGL2 (#601650)

[3] Paragangliomas 3; PGL3 (#605373)

[4] Paragangliomas 4; PGL4 (#115310)

[5] Paragangliomas 5; PGL5 (#614165)

[6] von Hippel-Lindau; VHL (#193300)

[7] Multiple Endocrine Neoplasia Type 2A; MEN2A (#171400)

[8] Neurofibromatosis Type 1; NF1 (#162200)

[9] MYC-Associated Factor X; MAX (#154950)

[10] Transmembrane Protein 127; TMEM127 (#613403)

[11] Kinesin Family Member 1B; KIF1B (#605995)

### Alternative Names:

- Familial Paraganglioma
- Paragangliomata
- Familial Glomus Tumor
- Chemodectomas
- Carotid Body Tumors
- Glomus Jugulare Tumors

*Key Words:* Pulsatile tinnitus, tympanic paraganglioma, palpitations, hypertension, diaphoresis, sweating, headache, cranial nerve palsy, anxiety, paraganglioma chemodectoma, carotid body tumor, glomus jugular tumor, pheochromocytoma, renal cell carcinoma, increased catecholamines, Horner syndrome, hearing loss

# 48 Prostate Cancer

Goutham Narla

## KEY POINTS

- *Disease summary:*
  - Prostate cancer is the second most fatal cancer for American men. It is the most common male noncutaneous cancer in developing countries, and a leading cause of death for men 60 years or older.
  - Age, African ancestry, and a positive family history are risk factors for disease development (Table 48-1).
  - Recent evidence suggests that approximately 10% of prostate cancers are hereditary.
  - Adenocarcinoma, cancer of glandular epithelial cells, is the most commonly diagnosed form.
  - Early diagnosis significantly improves treatment response and overall survival and is based on both biochemical studies using prostate-specific antigen (PSA) levels in patients and subsequent biopsies with Gleason scoring.
  - Treatment modalities for prostate cancer include hormone-based approaches, radiation, cytotoxic chemotherapy, and radical prostatectomy. Despite proper treatment many prostate cancer patients experience recurrence and will eventually develop aggressive metastatic prostate cancer, even when presenting initially with localized or indolent disease. No consistent biomarkers yet exist to distinguish between indolent and aggressive forms. Prostate cancer's genetic heterogeneity and complexity have hindered the elucidation and exploitation of the pathways driving pathogenesis and disease progression.

- *Hereditary basis:*
  - While age, race, and family history are known risk factors for prostate cancer, our understanding of the genetic basis of disease remains unclear. Germline mutations, often inherited in an autosomal dominant manner, may account for 9% of all prostate cancers and 45% of cases in men younger than 55 years. Linkage-based studies, positional gene cloning, and genome-wide association studies (GWAS) have been attempted and for the most part have been relatively unsuccessful in identifying the molecular basis for inherited risk.
  - Complex segregation analyses have modeled the effects of genetics on familial prostate cancer. Carter et al. imply that familial aggregation can be best explained by autosomal dominant inheritance of a rare, high-risk allele leading to an early onset of prostate cancer. The estimated cumulative risk of prostate cancer in this study was 88% for carriers and 5% for noncarriers by age 85 years. This inherited form of prostate cancer was estimated to account for a significant fraction of early-onset disease, and in total account for about 9% of all cases of the disease.
  - Men with a familial risk of prostate cancer represent an enriched pool for the identification of mutations and polymorphisms in tumor suppressor genes that lead to both the development and progression of the disease. This is based on the standard established methodologies and paradigms established for other cancer predisposition gene discoveries, in which the use of linkage analysis and positional gene cloning families is used to identify causative genes of interest. Genes identified in this manner can then be further examined and studied for their potential role in the progression of sporadic cancer. This approach has localized a number of prostate cancer-susceptibility loci and identified genes including *PTEN1*, *HPC1*, and *KLF6* (Table 48-2).
  - Race-associated differences in prostate cancer incidence and aggressiveness suggest an interaction between both hereditary and environmental factors. Epidemiologic studies have shown that the incidence of prostate cancer is highest in the Scandinavian countries while Asian countries have the lowest rates. African-American men have the highest risk for prostate cancer development, and in general are diagnosed with more advanced disease than Caucasians. African-American men also have higher mortality rates, even when diagnosed at the same clinical stage. The presence of significantly shorter CAG and GGC trinucleotide alleles of the androgen receptor gene in African Americans compared to non-African populations may represent a possible explanation for the increased risk, higher grade, and advanced stage of prostate cancer at diagnosis.

- *Twin studies:*
  - Retrospective, cohort, case-control, and twin studies, indicate family history to be a major risk factor for prostate cancer. These studies suggest that up to 10% of all prostate cancer cases may be a result of an inherited genetic predisposition to the disease. The number of affected family members and age at diagnosis accurately predict the risk of developing prostate cancer and its potential morbidity and mortality. Prostate cancer risk is increased among the first- and second-degree relatives of index patients with the risk of developing prostate cancer among the first- and second-degree relatives being directly proportional to the number of affected individuals in a given family and to earlier age at diagnosis of index cases (Table 48-3). In addition, the risk associated with having an affected brother is greater (relative risk [RR] = 3) than with having a father with prostate cancer (RR = 2.5). Currently, the only means the mortality associated with hereditary prostate cancer is early detection through screening to diagnose the disease while it is curable.

*Table 48-1  Risk Factors Associated With Prostate Cancer*

**Risk Factors**

| | |
|---|---|
| Age | Prostate cancer occurs more frequently in older men above the age of 50. The risk of developing prostate cancer increases with increasing age. |
| Family history | Family history is the strongest risk factor for prostate cancer. A man with one close relative (such as a father or brother) with prostate cancer has 2× the risk of developing prostate cancer than compared to man with no family history of the disease. If two close male relatives are affected, a man's lifetime risk of developing prostate cancer is increased fivefold. |
| Ethnicity | Prostate cancer risk is about 60% higher in African Americans than Caucasians. |
| Diet | A high-fat diet and low consumption of vegetables may be associated with an increased risk for prostate cancer. |
| Hereditary | Susceptibility to prostate cancer can be inherited. It is anticipated that 5%-10% of all prostate cancer cases are hereditary. In some families, a genetic predisposition to develop prostate cancer can be passed down from parent to child. |
| Prostate cancer screening | Screening tests include PSA and digital rectal examination (DRE). Currently there is no clinical testing for genes involved with prostate cancer.[a] |

[a]Men who are concerned about their hereditary risk because of family history should discuss their concerns with their physician and consider making an appointment with a trained genetic specialist.

*Table 48-2  Genetic Differential Diagnosis*

| Gene | Chromosome | Gene Function |
|---|---|---|
| PTEN1 (MMAC1/TEP1/MHAM) | 10q23.3 | Regulates the AKT signaling pathway; linked with cell regulation and apoptosis; loss of the PTEN1 protein correlates with loss of BCL2 in prostate tumors and contributes to chemoresistance. |
| HPC1 (PCS1) | 1q24-25 | Possible susceptibility locus for hereditary prostate cancer; mutation is seen in some with hereditary prostate cancer (families with multiple cases of early onset). |
| PCaP | 1q42-43 | Candidate for familial prostate cancer; linkage studies indicate it accounts for some cases. |
| HPCX | Xq27-28 | Accounts for approximately 16% of hereditary prostate cancers |
| CAPB | 1p36 | Evidence of linkage in those families with early onset (<66 years of age) |
| HPC20 | 20q13 | Evidence of linkage in families with less than five affected individuals and a later age at onset. No male-to-male transmission |
| KLF6 | 10p15 | Loss of heterozygosity analysis revealed that one KLF6 allele is deleted in some prostate cancer tumors downregulating p21 in a p53-independent manner to significantly increase prostate cell proliferation. Germline polymorphisms are associated with increased prostate cancer risk. |
| ELAC2 (HPC2) | 17p11.2-12 | Association between increased risk of developing prostate cancer and HPC2/ELAC missense mutations |
| RNASEL | 1q25.3 | Mutations have been associated with predisposition to prostate cancer and this gene is a candidate for the HPC1 allele. |
| BRCA1 | 17q21 | Evidence suggests that men with BRCA1 mutations may develop cancer at an earlier age (<65 years). Earlier age at diagnosis among carries of Ashkenazi founder mutations. Genetic testing is available for this gene. |
| BRCA2 | 13q12-13 | Evidence suggests that men with BRCA2 mutations may develop cancer at an earlier age (<65 years). A mutation in the central region of the BRCA2 gene may lower prostate cancer risk among men. Genetic testing for this gene is available. |
| MSR1 (SRA) | 8p22 | Important in susceptibility of prostate cancer for European and African-American men |

*Table 48-3 Family History Effect on Lifetime Risk of Clinical Prostate Cancer*[a]

| Family History | Relative Risk | % Absolute Risk |
|---|---|---|
| Negative | 1 | 8 |
| Father affected at 60 years or older | 1.5 | 12 |
| One Brother affected at age 60 years or older | 2 | 15 |
| Father affected before age 60 years. | 2.5 | 20 |
| One Brother affected before age 60 years. | 3 | 25 |
| Two affected male relatives[b] | 4 | 30 |
| Three or more affected male relatives[c] | 5 | 35-45 |

[a]Reproduced with permission from Bratt O. Hereditary prostate cancer: clinical aspects. *J Urol.* Sep 2002;168(3):9-0-913. Review.

[b]Father and brother, or two brothers, or a brother and a maternal grandfather or uncle, or a father and a paternal grandfather or uncle.

[c]The absolute lifetime risk for mutation carriers is probably 70% to 90% for high penetrance genes such as *HPC1*.

## Diagnostic Criteria and Clinical Characteristics

**Diagnostic Criteria:** The most commonly used diagnostic variables are serum PSA levels, DRE, and biopsy.

- DRE for growths in or enlargement of the prostate gland is used to identify potential cancer. A prostate tumor is often palpated as a hard lump.
- Serum PSA levels above 3 ng/mL may indicate prostate cancer.
- Biopsy of suspicious lesions on DRE or of the prostate in men with serum PSA levels above 3 ng/mL can provide histologic evidence in the prostate tissue of cancer.

**Prognostic Criteria:**

| Low risk | Gleason 2 to 6, and stage T1-T2a, PSA less than 10 ng/mL |
|---|---|
| Intermediate risk | Gleason 7, or stage T2b-T2c or PSA 10 ng/mL to 20 ng/mL |
| High risk | Gleason 8 to 10, or Stage T3-T4, PSA greater than 20 ng/mL |

A standard definition of hereditary prostate cancer is still lacking. One diagnostic schema is the Hopkins criteria for hereditary prostate cancer families. Families need to fulfill only one of these criteria to be considered to have hereditary prostate cancer:

1. Three successive generations of either the paternal or maternal lineages
2. Three or more affected first-degree relatives (son, brother, father)
3. A minimum of two relatives affected at 55 years of age or younger

**Clinical Characteristics:** Screening for prostate cancer using serum PSA levels is controversial. While used in the United States routinely, significant controversy exists about its utility in Europe and Great Britain where it is used far less, often if at all. In general, the majority of prostate cancers are still identified through symptomatic presentation of the disease to primary care providers when the disease is in advanced stage. Symptoms of prostate cancer include difficulty urinating, decreased force of urination, hematuria, blood in semen, swelling in legs, pelvic discomfort, and bone pain. To confirm the diagnosis of prostate cancer, PSA testing, DRE, ultrasound, and biopsy are routinely performed. Because a positive family history increases the positive predictive value of PSA testing, family history should always be assessed and a three-generation pedigree should be constructed for each patient in deciding whether to perform biopsies in a patient with a PSA level of 3 to 10 ng/mL.

## Screening and Counseling

Currently there is no genetic testing available for prostate cancer. Even without genetic testing, African-American men and men with a strong family history of prostate cancer should begin screening by PSA and DRE at age 40. All other men should seek routine screening for the disease starting at the age 50. Genetic counseling may be useful for screening high-risk populations to identify early-stage disease.

## Management and Treatment

**Screening:** PSA, DRE, and prostate biopsy to diagnose the disease.

**Watchful waiting:** Closely monitoring without treating until symptoms appear or change. This is usually used in older men with other medical problems or in early-stage disease (T1).

**Brachytherapy:** Radiation therapy where radioactive materials are placed into the tumor (usually used in T1-T3 disease).

**Chemotherapy:** Chemical treatment to eradicate or halt the replication or spread of cancerous cells. Chemotherapy drugs can be administered orally, through infusion or injection into vein, muscle, or cutaneous tissue. It is often used after surgery or radiation.

**Cryotherapy:** Removal of tumor by using subzero temperatures.

**Hormone therapy:** Blocking trophic or anabolic hormones like testosterone may cause tumor regression.

**Radiation therapy:** Radiation is used for local control of the cancer at the site of the tumor. It may be used before or after surgery and is sometimes used in combination with chemotherapy.

**Prostatectomy:** Surgical removal of part (cancerous) or all of the prostate gland.

**BIBLIOGRAPHY:**

1. Burmester JK, Suarez BK, Lin JH, et al. Analysis of candidate genes for prostate cancer. *Hum Hered.* 2004;57(4):172-178.

2. Ruijter E, van de Kaa C, Miller G, Ruiter D, Debruyne F, Schalken J. Molecular genetics and epidemiology of prostate carcinoma. *Endocr Rev.* 1999;20(1):22-45.

3. Keetch DW, Humphrey PA, Smith DS, Stahl D, Catalona WJ. Clinical and pathological features of hereditary prostate cancer. *J Urol.* 1996:155:1841-1843.

4. Carter BS, Beaty TH, Steinberg GD, Childs B, Walsh PC. Mendelian inheritance of familial prostate cancer. *Proc Natl Acad Sci USA*. 1992;89:3367-3371.

5. Easton DF, Schaid DJ, Whittemore AS, Isaacs WJ; International Consortium for Prostate Cancer Genetics. Where are the prostate cancer genes?—a summary of eight genome wide searches. *Prostate*. 2003;57:261-269.

6. Fearon E. Human cancer syndromes: clues to the origin and nature of cancer. *Science*. 1997;278:1043-1050.

7. Edwards BK, Howe HL, Ries LA, et al. Annual report to the nation on the status of cancer, 1973-1999, featuring implications of age and aging on U.S. cancer burden. *Cancer*. 2002;94: 2766-2792.

8. Kittles A, Young D, Weinrich S, et al. Extent of linkage disequilibrium between the androgen receptor gene CAG and GGC repeats in human populations: implications for prostate cancer risk. *Hum Genet*. 2001;109:253-261.

9. Giovannucci E, Stampfer MJ, Krithivas K, et al. The CAG repeat within the androgen receptor gene and its relationship to prostate cancer. *Proc Natl Acad Sci USA*. 1997;94:3320-3323.

10. Ostrander EA, Stanford JL. Genetics of prostate cancer: too many loci, too few genes. *Am J Hum Genet*. 2000;67:1367-1375.

11. Bratt O. Hereditary prostate cancer: clinical aspects. *J Urol*. Sep 2002;168(3):906-913. Review.

12. Walsh PC. Surgery and the reduction of mortality from prostate cancer. *N Engl J Med*. 2002;347:839-840.

13. Frankel S, Smith GD, Donovan J, Neal D. Screening for prostate cancer. *Lancet*. 2003;361:1122-1128.

## Supplementary Information

**OMIM REFERENCES:**

[1] Prostate Cancer; MIM (#176807)

[2] Gene Map Locus: 1q25, 17p11, etc

*Key Words:* Urology, prostate biopsy, digital rectal examination, prostate genetics, prostate, prostate gland, prostate cancer, PSA or prostate-specific antigen, hereditary prostate cancer

# 49 Testicular Germ Cell Tumors

Christian Kratz and Mark H. Greene

## KEY POINTS

- *Disease summary:*
  - Testicular germ cell tumor (TGCT) is the most common cancer diagnosed among young Caucasian men, and is relatively rare in African-American men. Most affected individuals are diagnosed with seminomas or nonseminomas; however, mixed germ cell tumors also occur. Intratubular germ cell neoplasia (carcinoma in situ) precedes most invasive cancers. Affected men have a good prognosis if managed according to modern treatment strategies.

- *Differential diagnosis:*
  - Gonadal stromal tumors, various other rare histologies such as hematopoietic tumors, tumors of ducts or the paratesticular structures, spermatocytic seminoma, and others.

- *Monogenic forms:*
  - Monogenic forms are not known. TGCT can occur in individuals with disorders of sex determination. Men with Klinefelter syndrome are at increased risk of mediastinal germ cell tumors.

- *Family history:*
  - 1% to 2% of all cases of TGCT have a positive family history (familial TGCT). Linkage analysis has failed to identify statistically significant genomic regions which might harbor a highly penetrant gene. Familial cases are significantly younger than sporadic cases, a difference which is not clinically useful. Otherwise, the clinical features of familial and sporadic TGCT are remarkably similar. The most common number of affected persons in multiple-case families is two, and families with greater than or equal to three affected individuals are quite rare. It has been suggested that the combined effect of multiple, common, low penetrance alleles is responsible for the familial aggregation of TGCT. Testicular microlithiasis has been implicated in the pathogenesis of familial TGCT.

- *Twin studies:*
  - The risk of TGCT has been reported to be higher among twins than nontwins. Moreover, a 37-fold or 76.5-fold elevated risk of TGCT in dizygotic or monozygotic twin brothers of men with TGCT has been reported.

- *Environmental factors:*
  - Epidemiologic data strongly support the notion that TGCT has a strong environmental component; however, specific exposures associated with an increased TGCT risk remain unknown.

- *Genome-wide associations:*
  - Multiple genomic loci in which TGCT risk-modifying variants might reside have been identified recently. Disease-associated genetic variants (single-nucleotide polymorphisms [SNPs]) provide insight into disease pathogenesis, in that most are part of biologic pathways involved in testicular development or fertility. Testing for SNPs is not yet clinically validated to diagnose or guide management of TGCT.

- *Pharmacogenomics:*
  - The homozygous variant G/G of the *BLMH* gene SNP A1450G has been associated with reduced survival and higher prevalence of early relapses in patients treated with the chemotherapeutic agent bleomycin, one of the cornerstones of modern multidrug therapy for TGCT.

## Diagnostic Criteria and Clinical Characteristics

Diagnostic evaluation often includes the following:

- Serum markers: alpha-fetoprotein (AFP); beta-human chorionic gonadotrophic ($\beta$-HCG); and lactate dehydrogenase (LDH).
- Imaging: testicular ultrasound, chest x-ray, computed tomographic (CT) scan or magnetic resonance imaging (MRI) of abdomen and pelvis, and chest CT scan.
- MRI or CT of central nervous system (CNS) in advanced disease or in the presence of symptoms.
- Radionuclide bone scan: only in the presence of symptoms.
- Total testosterone, luteinizing hormone (LH), follicle-stimulating hormone (FSH), semen analysis, sperm banking.
- Surgical exploration of the affected testicle (inguinal orchiectomy; trans-scrotal orchiectomy contraindicated)

*Clinical Characteristics:* Patients with TGCT classically present with a painless, palpable tumor in the testis. More typically, they present with symptoms suggestive of orchitis, or epididymitis. About 10% of germ cell tumors have an extragonadal origin. Occasionally, patients present with symptoms caused by metastatic disease. Seminomas arise later in life (mean age = 35 years) *versus* nonseminomas (mean age = 25 years). Well-established clinical risk factors include cryptorchidism and male infertility. Recent data suggest an increased risk of TGCT in men undergoing solid organ transplantation.

## Screening and Counseling

*Screening:* There is no proven screening modality for TGCT in either the familial or general population setting. Testicular self-examination is commonly recommended as part of routine health care, but it has never been proven to be effective. Genetic testing for disease-associated SNPs is not clinically validated.

**Counseling:** Approximately 1% to 2% of all cases of TGCT have an affected family member (familial TGCT). No monogenic forms have been identified. Brothers and fathers of TGCT patients have 8 to 10- and 4 to 6-fold increased risks of TGCT, respectively.

## Management and Treatment

**Management:** After radical orchiectomy through an inguinal incision, the individual management includes surveillance, chemotherapy, or radiotherapy. Treatment decisions take into account disease stage as well as treatment side effects. Treatment for metastatic tumors is guided by the International Germ Cell Cancer Collaborative Group (IGCCCG) classification and generally includes cisplatin-based combination chemotherapy. Such therapy produces 90% to 95% cure rates even in patients with metastatic disease at diagnosis. In recurrent disease, high-dose chemotherapy can lead to cure.

## Molecular Genetics and Molecular Mechanism

The recognition that most of the SNPs associated with TGCT risk are located in or near genes with similar biologic effects has focused ongoing etiologic research on those signaling pathways. Variants in the phosphodiesterase gene *PDE11A* have been implicated as possible TGCT risk modifiers. In parallel with the clinical similarity between sporadic and familial TGCT, the genetic associations identified to date are also similar in these two groups of subjects (Table 49-1).

**Genetic Testing or Risk Assessment:** No role yet exists for genetic testing in the diagnosis or, clinical etiologic elucidation of TGCT. However, TGCT presents a unique combination of both strongly associated or readily identifiable clinical risk factors and very strongly associated SNPs which, when combined, may permit the construction of risk stratification tools with unusual discriminatory ability.

**Future Directions:** Recent genome-wide association studies (GWAS) have identified pathways relevant for TGCT pathogenesis. Future research will further define the underlying biology that drives these associations. Moreover, clinical studies will need to determine whether the identified risk SNPs may be of any clinical value. Notably, TGCT risk SNPs—particularly those in or near the *KITLG* gene—are considerably more strongly associated with risk than risk SNPs identified in other cancers, suggesting that there may be a special research opportunity in this setting. Lastly, somatic changes in TGCT need to be further defined.

**BIBLIOGRAPHY:**

1. Kanetsky PA, Mitra N, Vardhanabhuti S, et al. A second independent locus within *DMRT1* is associated with testicular germ cell tumor susceptibility. *Hum Mol Genet.* 2011;20:3109-3117.

2. Gilbert D, Rapley E, Shipley J. Testicular germ cell tumours: predisposition genes and the male germ cell niche. *Nat Rev Cancer.* 2011;11:278-288.

3. Turnbull C, Rapley EA, Seal S, et al. Variants near *DMRT1, TERT* and *ATF7IP* are associated with testicular germ cell cancer. *Nat Genet.* 2010;42:604-607.

4. Mai PL, Friedlander M, Tucker K, et al.The International Testicular Cancer Linkage Consortium: a clinicopathologic descriptive analysis of 461 familial malignant testicular germ cell tumor kindred. *Urol Oncol.* 2010;28:492-499.

5. Greene MH, Kratz CP, Mai PL, et al. Familial testicular germ cell tumors in adults: 2010 summary of genetic risk factors and clinical phenotype. *Endocr Relat Cancer.* 2010;17:R109-R121.

**Table 49-1 TGCT Disease-Associated Susceptibility Variants**

| Candidate Gene (or Locus) (Chromosome Location) | Associated Variant | Relative Risk (per allele odds ratio) | Frequency of Risk Allele | Putative Functional Significance |
|---|---|---|---|---|
| 1q22 | rs2072499 | 1.19 | 0.35 | |
| 1q24.1 | rs3790672 | 1.20 | 0.28 | |
| *DAZL* (3p24.3) | rs10510452 | 1.24 | 0.69 | Primordial germ cell differentiation |
| 4q24 | rs2720460 | 1.24 | 0.61 | |
| *CATSPER3, PITX1* (5q31.1) | rs3805663 | 1.25 | 0.63 | *CATSPER3:* germ cells motility, *PITX1:* telomerase regulation |
| *PRDM14* (8q13.3) | rs7010162 | 1.22 | 0.61 | Controls expression of pluripotency genes |
| 16q12.1 | rs8046148 | 1.32 | 0.79 | |
| *TEX14* (17q22) | rs9905704 | 1.21 | 0.67 | Protein kinase highly expressed in male germ cells |
| 21q22.3 | rs2839186 | 1.26 | 0.46 | |
| *HPGDS* (4q22.2) | rs17021463 | 1.19 | 0.420 | |
| *MAD1L1* (7p22.3) | rs12699477 | 1.21 | 0.380 | |
| *RFWD3* (16q22.3) | rs4888262 | 1.26 | 0.458 | |
| *PPM1E* (17q22) | rs7221274 | 1.39 | 0.620 | |
| *UCK2* (1q23) | rs3790665 | 1.37 | | Pyrimidine ribonucleoside kinase |

6.  Rapley EA, Turnbull C, Al Olama AA, et al. A genome-wide association study of testicular germ cell tumor. *Nat Genet.* 2009; 41:807-810.

7.  Kanetsky PA, Mitra N, Vardhanabhuti S, et al. Common variation in *KITLG* and at 5q31.3 predisposes to testicular germ cell cancer. *Nat Genet.* 2009;41:811-815.

8.  Oosterhuis JW, Looijenga LH. Testicular germ-cell tumours in a broader perspective. *Nat Rev Cancer.* 2005;5:210-222.

9.  Nathanson KL, Kanetsky PA, Hawes R, et al. The Y deletion *gr/gr* and susceptibility to testicular germ cell tumor. *Am J Hum Genet.* 2005;77:1034-1043.

10. Winter C, Albers P. Testicular germ cell tumors: pathogenesis, diagnosis and treatment. *Nat Rev Endocrinol.* 2011;7:43-53.

11. Crockford GP, Linger R, Hockley S, et al. Genome-wide linkage screen for testicular germ cell tumour susceptibility loci. *Hum Mol Genetics.* 2006;15:443-451.

12. Korde LA, Premkumar A, Mueller C, et al. Increased prevalence of testicular microlithiasis in men with familial testicular cancer and their relatives. *Br J Cancer.* 2008;99:1748-1753.

13. Horvath A*, Korde L*, Greene MH, et al. Functional phospho-diesterase 11A mutations may modify the risk of familial and bilateral testicular germ cell tumors. *Cancer Res.* 2009;69: 5301-5306.

14. Mai PL, Chen BE, Tucker K, et al. Younger age-at-diagnosis for familial malignant testicular germ cell tumor. *Fam Cancer.* 2009;8:451-456.

15. Kratz CP, Greene MH, Bratslavsky G, Shi J. A stratified genetic risk assessment for testicular cancer. *Int J Andrology.* 2011;34(4 pt 2):e98-e102.

16. Kratz CP, Han SS, Rosenberg PS, et al. Variants in or near *KITLG, BAK1, DMRT1,* and *TERT-CLPTM1L* predispose to familial testicular germ cell tumor. *J Med Genet.* 2011;48:473-476.

## Supplementary Information

**Alternative Name:**
*   Testicular Cancer

*Key Words:* Germ cell, seminoma, nonseminoma, microlithiasis

# 50 Renal Cell Carcinoma

Anna Newlin and Peter Hulick

## KEY POINTS

- *Disease summary:*
  - Approximately 50,000 new cases of renal cell carcinoma (RCC) are diagnosed each year.
  - RCCs are adenocarcinomas derived from renal tubular epithelium. Renal carinoma is comprised of several different types of cancer, each with a different histologic type, with a different clinical course, responding differently to therapy, and caused by different genes.
  - Histologically, there are five subtypes:
    - Conventional (clear cell) (70%-80%)
    - Chromophile (papillary) (10%-15%). Papillary is further classified into type 1 (5%) and type 2 (10% of cases) based on further genetic alterations, histologic, and genetic criteria
    - Chromophobe (3%-5%)
    - Collecting duct (1%)
    - Unclassified (1%)
  - RCC can be hereditary as well as sporadic or nonhereditary. While sporadic RCC is often a solitary lesion and most commonly presents in individuals in their 60s, inherited forms tend to be multifocal, bilateral, and have an earlier onset.
- *Hereditary basis:*
  - Renal cancer is hereditary in up to 4% of cases, and follows an autosomal dominant inheritance pattern with incomplete penetrance. In the absence of a diagnosed syndrome, the risk for family members of patients with RCC may increase fivefold. The highest risk appears to be confined to siblings of renal cell cancer patients, arguing for the potential of low penetrance genes acting in concert to elevate the risk of disease.
- *Differential diagnosis:*
  - It is important to distinguish the multiorgan system syndromes that include renal cancer as a single feature (ie, von Hippel-Lindau [VHL], Birt-Hogg-Dubé [BHD], and hereditary leiomyomatosis renal cell cancer [HLRCC]) from the familial tumor predispositions (ie, hereditary papillary renal carcinoma [HPRC]), in which renal cancer is the only major finding. Thus, it is imperative to inquire about associated features if there is clinical suspicion for an inherited syndrome in order to establish a clinical diagnosis or indication for genetic (germline) testing (Table 50-1).

## Diagnostic Criteria and Clinical Characteristics

**Diagnostic Criteria for Hereditary Renal Cancer:** Inherited forms tend to be multifocal, bilateral, and have an early onset (<60 years of age). The histologic type of renal cancer can help delineate the associated syndrome(s) and guide further evaluation (Table 50-2).

**Diagnostic Evaluation:**

☞CLEAR CELL: If a patient presents with predominantly clear cell RCC and has features suggestive of an inherited predisposition (young age of onset, multiple lesions), it is important to investigate for signs and symptoms suggestive of VHL. To establish a clinical diagnosis of VHL in a patient, without a known family history, two or more characteristic lesions as noted above are required. The majority of individuals with VHL (70%) develop retinal hemangioblastomas (which can be asymptomatic) by their mid-twenties. These can be detected on routine ophthalmoscopic examination and are often the initial manifestation of VHL, thus providing an important clinical clue for targeting the evaluation. In the absence of retinal findings, further imaging can assist in arriving at a diagnosis of VHL or potentially point to other hereditary renal carcinoma syndromes.

- **Computed tomographic (CT) scan or magnetic resonance imaging (MRI)** to establish the presence of

- Central nervous system (CNS) hemangioblastomas (VHL)
- Pheochromocytomas that exhibit high signal intensity on T2-weighted MRI, which may help differentiate them from adrenal cortical nodules (VHL, SBHD)
- Paragangliomas particularly in the head and neck region (SBHD)
- Endolymphatic sac tumors identified with high signal intensity with T1 imaging on MRI as a mass on the posterior wall of the petrous part of the temporal bone (VHL)
- Multiple, bilateral lung cysts which can lead to unexplained spontaneous pneumothoraces (BHD)
- Subependymal glial nodules, cortical tubers, and subependymal giant cell astrocytomas (tuberous sclerosis complex [TSC])
- **Ultrasound examination** for evaluation of the epididymis and broad ligament, and for less expensive screening of the kidneys (VHL)
- **Measurement of urinary catecholamine metabolites** (VMA, metanephrine, and total catecholamine) to detect elevations that may suggest pheochromocytoma even in the absence of hypertension (VHL, SBHD)

☞PAPILLARY TYPE 1:
- **Germline MET mutation analysis** is recommended for patients with bilateral, multifocal papillary RCC as well as for those with a family history of type 1 papillary RCC.

*Table 50-1 Genetic Differential Diagnosis*

| Syndrome | Gene Symbol/Locus | Associated Findings |
|---|---|---|
| von Hippel-Lindau | *VHL/*3p25 | Hemangioblastomas of the cerebellum, brain stem, spinal cord, and retina; pancreatic and renal cysts, endolymphatic sac tumors, pheochromocytoma, and clear cell carcinoma |
| Hereditary papillary renal carcinoma | *MET/*7q31 | Bilateral multifocal type 1 papillary renal cancer, can be later onset (50-70 years) |
| Birt-Hogg-Dubé | *FLCN/*17p11.2 | Cutaneous fibrofolliculomas, pulmonary cysts, spontaneous pneumothoraces, multifocal oncocystosis |
| Hereditary leiomyomatosis renal cell cancer | *FH/*1q42.1 | Cutaneous and uterine leiomyomas |
| Tuberous sclerosis | *TSC1/*9q34 *TSC2/*16p13.3 | Seizures, mental retardation, angiomyolipoma, hamartomas in multiple organs, clear cell, papillary and chromophobe renal tumors |
| Succinate dehydrogenase, subunit B | *SDHB/*1p36.1-p35 | Pheochromocytoma and/or paraganglioma |

Gene names: *VHL*, von Hippel-Lindau tumor suppressor; *MET*, MET proto-oncogene; *FLCN*, folliculin; *FH*, fumarate hydratase; *TSC1* and *TSC2*, tuberous sclerosis complex 1 and 2; *SDHB*, succinate dehydrogenase complex, subunit B iron sulfur.

☞**Papillary Type 2:**
- **Pathologic confirmation of multiple cutaneous leiomyomas and uterine leiomyomata** (fibroids) in a simplex case or single leiomyoma in the presence of a positive family history of HLRCC.

☞**Chromophobe, Oncocytoma, Oncocytic Hybrid Renal Tumor:** BHD should be strongly considered when a patient presents with multiple foci of tumors with multiple histologic subtypes contained within the same kidney. This unique presentation of renal pathology is typical of BHD and should trigger an evaluation for associated findings (fibrofolliculomas, trichodiscomas or angiofibromas, acrochordons, and lung cysts) and consideration of genetic testing of the folliculin gene.

**Pathologic confirmation of**
- **Fibrofolliculoma** including five or more facial or truncal papules, with or without a family history of BHD.

*Table 50-2 Histologic Subtypes and Associated Syndromes*

| | |
|---|---|
| Clear cell | Von Hippel-Lindau, Birt-Hogg-Dubé, SDHB, TSC2, HLRCC |
| Papillary type 1 | Hereditary papillary renal carcinoma, TSC |
| Papillary type 2 | Hereditary leiomyomatosis renal cell cancer |
| Chromophobe, oncocytoma, ncocytic hybrid renal tumor | Birt-Hogg-Dubé (classically has several tumors with differing pathology in the same kidney), SDHB, tuberous sclerosis (angiomyolipoma more common) |
| Angiomyolipoma | Tuberous sclerosis |

- **Facial angiofibroma** in an individual who does not fit the clinical criteria of TSC or multiple endocrine neoplasia type 1 (MEN1).

*Clinical Characteristics:*
- Endolymphatic sac tumors: Hearing loss of varying severity.
- Fibrofolliculoma: Commonly found on the face and neck as a yellowish and dome-shaped papule.
- Hemangioblastomas of the brain, spinal cord, and retina: Clinical features include vision loss, headaches, gait disturbances.
- Paragangliomas: Generally slow growing and benign in nature. They commonly occur in the head and neck region.
- Pheochromocytoma: Clinical features include intermittent hypertension, palpitations, and occasionally flushing.

## Screening and Counseling

*Screening:* In an index case, the relative likelihood of these disorders can be predicted based on (a) age at diagnosis, (b) tumor characteristics, and (c) presence of associated features. In general, a germline mutation is more likely in younger patients and in the presence of multifocal disease. While HPRC can be diagnosed based on the presence of bilateral, multifocal, type 1 papillary RCC, the other entities require more targeted imaging, histopathologic confirmation of skin lesions, biochemical, and/or genetic testing.

Although HPRC is typically late onset (age of onset in the fifth, sixth, and seventh decades), an early-onset form recently has been described in which the disease appears in the second and third decades.

*Counseling:* VHL, HPRC, BHD, HLRCC, TSC1/TSC2, and SDHB (PGL4) are inherited in an autosomal dominant fashion with variable penetrance and expressivity. Each child of an affected parent has a 50% risk of inheriting the condition.

Molecular genetic testing for the family-specific mutation allows for early identification of at-risk family members, improves diagnostic certainty, and reduces costly screening procedures in at-risk relatives who have not inherited the family-specific disease-causing mutation. Presymptomatic testing should be offered to all first-degree relatives of an affected individual. In situations of apparent de novo mutations, germline mosaicism in an unaffected parent and nonpaternity should be considered.

☞PENETRANCE: Almost 100% in VHL and TSC. Based on their respective triad of clinical manifestations, penetrance of BHDS and HLRCC is considered to be very high. The occurrence of renal tumors among HLRCC patients has been estimated at 2% to 21%.

☞GENOTYPE-PHENOTYPE CORRELATION: Maranchie et al. identified a significantly higher incidence of RCC in patients with partial germline *VHL* mutations versus those with complete *VHL* gene mutations. In BHD, mutations can appear throughout the folliculin gene but there is a mononucleotide C tract located in exon 11 that accounts for a significant (44%) proportion of mutations identified. What remains to be seen is whether mutations in this region offer a significant difference in phenotype with regards to clinical management.

## Management and Treatment

*VHL:* Early surgery (nephron-sparing or partial nephrectomy when possible) for RCC; renal transplantation following bilateral nephrectomy. Surveillance for associated features, as well as RCC, is vital to minimize morbidity. Ophthalmologic examination and neurologic examination should be performed annually after diagnosis. At 5 years of age, catecholamine screening on an annual basis is to be performed. At 15 years of age a baseline audiology examination, MRI brain or CNS, and abdominal imaging should be performed. CNS imagining is generally repeated every 2 years and abdominal imagining annually.

*BHD:* When possible, nephron-sparing surgery is the treatment of choice for renal tumors, depending on their size and location. Total nephrectomy may be necessary in some cases, though tumors tend to be slow growing. There are no established surveillance guidelines but repeating abdominal imagining every 2 to 3 years appears reasonable if baseline scan is normal.

*HPRC:* Parenchymal-sparing surgery (partial nephrectomy) is recommended when the largest renal tumor approaches 3 cm in size. Patients who have tumors less than 3 cm generally are managed with observation.

*HLRC:* Kidney tumors associated with HLRCC have an aggressive disease course. Therefore, these tumors must be managed with caution until more is known about the natural history. Because of the aggressive nature of renal cancers associated with HLRCC, total nephrectomy should be strongly considered in individuals with a detectable renal mass.

*Tuberous Sclerosis:* Angiomyolipomas greater than 3.5 to 4 cm in diameter have the greatest risk of hemorrhage. It is recommended that those with symptomatic angiomyolipomas greater than 3.5 to 4 cm be considered for prophylactic renal arterial embolization or renal-sparing surgery.

*SDHB:* The clinical course, and thus management of RCC, is primarily guided by histologic subtype and extent of the underlying cancer. It is a common practice to have annual imaging screening for paragangliomas and pheochromocytomas, in addition to biochemical screening, for patients who are mutation positive. Evidence for RCC screening is less established, but extending the screening to include RCC seems reasonable especially given that some familial RCC families with *SDHB* mutations do harbor paragangliomas and pheochromocytomas in their family history.

*Therapeutics:*
- VHL—The VHL protein regulates hypoxia-inducible factor (HIF) and signals it for ubiquitin-mediated degradation. When VHL is mutated, HIF levels increase and downstream targets related to cell growth and angiogenesis remain activated including vascular endothelial growth factor (VEGF) and platelet-derived growth factor (PDGF). Tyrosine kinase inhibitors (TKIs), such as sunitinib, have been developed to target the receptors of these factors. In addition, inhibitors of HIF transcription, temsirolimus, have been developed to help target the entire pathway.

## Molecular Genetics and Molecular Mechanism

*Syndrome/Gene/Locus:*
  VHL/*VHL*/3p25
  Hereditary papillary renal carcinoma/*MET*/7q31
  Birt-Hogg-Dubé/*FLCN*/17p11.2
  Hereditary leiomyomatosis/*FH*/1q42.1
  Tuberous sclerosis/*TSC1* and *TSC2*/9q34 and 16p13.3
  PGL4/*SDHB*/1p36.1-p35

*Genetic Testing:* DNA sequence analysis is clinically available for VHL, FH, MET, TSC1 and TSC2, SDHB (see Gene Tests http://www.genetests.org)

☞SENSITIVITY OF TESTING:
- Approximately 100% of patients with VHL have mutations that are identifiable by bidirectional sequence analysis, +/− dosage studies.
- Of patients diagnosed with BHD on a clinical basis, mutation in *FLCN* is expected to be identified in approximately 80% of cases.
- *FH* mutations have been identified in 76% to 100% of clinically diagnosed individuals with HLRCC.
- Approximately 20% of individuals with TSC do not have an identifiable mutation.

*Future Directions:* Through understanding the primary events that underlie tumorigenesis in patients who have hereditary renal carcinoma and elucidating the downstream alterations resulting from these events, the mechanisms by which such processes can be blocked or reversed are slowly being revealed. The discovery of these same mutations and involved pathways in nonrenal tumors and sporadic forms of cancer has helped usher in the era of molecular therapeutics and alternative management strategies for the treatment of kidney cancer. For example, studies of the tricarboxylic acid cycle and the VHL-HIF pathways have provided the foundation for therapeutic approaches in patients with HLRCC-associated kidney cancer as well as other hereditary and sporadic forms of RCC.

**BIBLIOGRAPHY:**

1. Adley B, Smith N, Nayer R, Yang X. Birt-Hogg-Dubé syndrome, clinicopathologic findings and genetic alterations. *Arch Pathol Lab Med.* 2006;130:1865-1870.

2. Maranchie JK, Afonso A, Albert PS, et al. Solid renal tumor severity in von Hippel Lindau disease is related to germline deletion length and location. *Hum Mutat.* 2004;23:40-46.

3. Nickerson M, Warren MB, Toro JR, et al. Mutations in a novel gene lead to kidney tumors, lung wall defects, and benign tumors of the hair follicle in patients with the Birt-Hogg-Dubé syndrome. *Cancer Cell*. Aug 2002;2(2):157-164.

4. Poulsen MLM, Budtz-Jørgensen E, Bisgaard ML. Surveillance in von Hippel-Lindau disease (vHL). *Clin Genet*. Jan 2010;77(1):49-59.

5. Grubb RL, Corbin NS, Choyke P, et al. Analysis of 3-cm tumor size threshold for intervention in patients with Birt—Hogg—Dube and hereditary papillary renal cancer [abstract 980]. San Antonio, Texas: American Urological Association National Conference; 2005.

6. Grubb RL, 3rd, Franks ME, Toro J, et al. Hereditary leiomyomatosis and renal cell cancer: a syndrome associated with an aggressive form of inherited renal cancer. *J Urol*. 2007;177(6):2074-2079; discussion 2079-2080.

7. Pasini B, Stratakis, CA. SDH mutations in tumorigenesis and inherited endocrine tumours: lesson from the phaeochromocytoma—paraganglioma syndromes. *J Intern Med*. 2009;266:19-42.

8. Ricketts C, Woodward ER, Killick P, et al. Germline SDHB mutations and familial renal cell carcinoma. *J Natl Cancer Inst*. Sep 3 2008;100(17):1260-1262.

9. Linehan WM, Pinto PA, Bratslavsky G, et al. Hereditary kidney cancer—unique opportunity for disease-based therapy. *Cancer*. 2009;115(suppl 10):2252-2261.

10. Vanharanta S, Buchta M, McWhinney SR, et al. Early-onset renal cell carcinoma as a novel extraparaganglial component of SDHB associated heritable paraganglioma. *Am J Hum Genet*. 2004;74(1):153-159.

## Supplementary Information

**OMIM REFERENCES:**

[1] Birt-Hogg Dubé Syndrome; FLCN (#135150)

[2] Hereditary Leiomyomatosis and Renal Cell Cancer; FH (#605839)

[3] Papillary Renal Cell Carcinoma; MET (#605074)

[4] Succinate Dehydrogenase Complex, Subunit B, Iron Sulfur Protein; SDHB (*185470)

[5] Tuberous Sclerosis; TSC1 and TSC2 (#191100)

[6] von Hippel-Lindau Syndrome; VHL (#193300)

**Alternative Names:**

- Fibrofolliculomas With Trichodiscomas and Acrochordons
- Succinate Dehydrogenase 2 (SDH2)
- Tuberous Sclerosis Complex
- Adenoma Sebaceum

*Key Words:* Renal cell carinoma, kidney cancer, clear cell, oncocytoma, chromophobe, papillary fibrofolliculoma

# 51 *PTEN* Syndromes

Charis Eng

## KEY POINTS

- *Disease summary:*
  - The *PTEN* syndromes or *PTEN* hamartoma tumor syndromes (PHTS) include all disorders that have germline *PTEN* mutations.
  - PHTS includes Cowden syndrome (CS), Bannayan-Riley-Ruvalcaba syndrome (BRRS), Proteus syndrome (PS), and Proteus-like syndrome.
  - Typically, PHTS is characterized by hamartomas that can affect derivatives of all three germ layers and a high risk of breast and thyroid cancers.
    - CS is a multiple hamartoma syndrome with a high risk of benign and malignant tumors of the thyroid, breast, and endometrium.
    - BRRS is a congenital disorder characterized by macrocephaly, intestinal polyposis, lipomas, and pigmented macules of the glans penis.
    - PS is a complex, highly variable disorder involving congenital malformations and overgrowth of multiple tissues.
    - Proteus-like syndrome is undefined but refers to individuals with significant clinical features of PS who do not meet the diagnostic criteria for PS.

- *Hereditary basis:*
  - PHTS is an autosomal dominant condition with incomplete penetrance and variable expressivity.
  - PHTS can be seen in isolated individuals or in segregating families.
  - Germline *PTEN* mutations are found in approximately 85% of CS, approximately 65% of BRRS, 20% PS, 50% of PS-like, and 5% in individuals with CS-like features.
  - Germline *SDHB* and *SDHD* variants are found in approximately 10% of CS or CS-like individuals without germline *PTEN* mutations.
  - Germline epimutation (promoter hypermethylation) of *KLLN* are found in approximately 35% of CS or CS-like individuals without germline *PTEN* mutations.

- *Differential diagnosis:*
  - The primary differential diagnoses to consider are other hamartoma syndromes, including juvenile polyposis syndrome (JPS) and Peutz-Jeghers syndrome (PJS), both inherited in an autosomal dominant manner.
  - **JPS** is characterized by predisposition for hamartomatous polyps in the gastrointestinal tract, specifically in the stomach, small intestine, colon, and rectum. The term "juvenile" refers to the type of polyp, not the age of onset of polyps. Juvenile polyps are hamartomas that show a normal epithelium with a dense stroma, an inflammatory infiltrate, and a smooth surface with dilated, mucus-filled cystic glands in the lamina propria. Approximately 70% of JPS is caused by germline mutations and large deletions in *SMAD4* and *BMPR1A*. Germline deletions involving *BMPR1A* and *PTEN* (both on 10q) are particularly associated with juvenile polyposis of infancy.
  - **PJS** is characterized by the association of gastrointestinal polyposis and mucocutaneous pigmentation. PJS-type hamartomatous polyps are most prevalent in the small intestine, but also occur in the stomach and large bowel in the majority of affected individuals. The Peutz-Jeghers polyp has a diagnostic appearance and is quite different from the hamartomatous polyps seen in CS or JPS. Clinically, Peutz-Jeghers polyps are often symptomatic (intussusception, rectal bleeding), whereas CS polyps are rarely so.
    - Perioral region pigmented macules are pathognomonic, particularly if it crosses the vermilion border. Hyperpigmented macules on the fingers are also common.
    - Approximately 70% of PJS are accounted for by germline mutations in *STK11*.
  - Less likely genetic differential diagnoses include
  - **Birt-Hogg-Dubé syndrome (BHD)** is characterized by typical cutaneous findings including fibrofolliculomas, trichodiscomas, and acrochordons; pulmonary cysts or history of pneumothorax; and renal tumors usually renal oncocytoma, chromophobe renal cell carcinoma, or a mixture of oncocytoma and chromophobe histologic cell types. Skin lesions typically appear during the third or fourth decade of life and increase in size and number with age. Lung cysts are mostly bilateral and multifocal; most individuals are asymptomatic but have a high risk for spontaneous pneumothorax. Approximately 15% of individuals with BHD syndrome have renal tumors; median age of tumor diagnosis is 48 years. *FLCN* (*BHD*), the gene encoding folliculin, is the only gene known to be associated with BHD.
  - **Neurofibromatosis type 1 (NF1):** The only two features seen in both NF1 and CS or BRRS are café-au-lait macules and fibromatous tumors of the skin. The diagnosis of NF1 is sometimes mistakenly given to individuals with CS or BRRS because of the presence of ganglioneuromas in the gastrointestinal tract. Germline mutations and rearrangements in *NF1* are found in greater than 85% of NF1 patients.
  - **Nevoid basal cell carcinoma (Gorlin) syndrome:** This syndrome is characterized by basal cell nevi, basal cell carcinoma, and diverse developmental abnormalities. Affected individuals can also develop other tumors and cancers, such as fibromas, hamartomatous gastric polyps, and medulloblastomas. However, the dermatologic findings and developmental features in CS and nevoid basal cell carcinoma (Gorlin) syndrome are quite different. Germline *PTCH* mutations are found in 65% to 70% of Gorlin syndrome patients.

## Diagnostic Criteria and Clinical Characteristics

*Diagnostic Criteria:*

- A presumptive diagnosis of PHTS is based on clinical signs (Table 51-1); by definition, however, the diagnosis of PHTS is made only when a *PTEN* mutation is identified (Table 51-2).
- Consensus diagnostic criteria for CS have been developed and updated each year by the National Comprehensive Cancer Network (NCCN). Clinical criteria have been divided into three categories:

### Pathognomonic Criteria:

- Adult Lhermitte-Duclos disease (LDD), defined as the presence of a cerebellar dysplastic gangliocytoma.
  - Mucocutaneous lesions
    - Trichilemmomas (facial)
    - Acral keratoses
    - Papillomatous lesions
    - Mucosal lesions

### Major Criteria

- Breast cancer
- Epithelial thyroid cancer (nonmedullary), especially follicular thyroid cancer
- Macrocephaly (occipital frontal circumference ≥97th percentile)
- Endometrial carcinoma

### Minor Criteria

- Other thyroid lesions (eg, adenoma, multinodular goiter)
- Mental retardation (IQ ≤75)
- Hamartomatous intestinal polyps
- Fibrocystic disease of the breast

*Table 51-1  Main System Involvement in PTEN Syndrome*

| System | Manifestation | Frequency |
|--------|--------------|-----------|
| Skin | Trichilemmomas, papillomatous papules | >90% |
| Thyroid | Benign thyroid neoplasias and hamartomas | 67% |
| | Epithelial thyroid carcinoma (FTC/FvPTC>PTC) | 10% |
| Breast (female) | Fibrocystic disease, fibroadenomas, hamartomas, adenosis | >50% (?) |
| | Breast carcinoma | 25-50% |
| Uterus | Fibroids, endometrial carcinoma | ? |
| CNS | Macrocephaly (megencephaly) | >74% |
| | Lhermitte-Duclos disease | ? |
| GI | Hamartomatous and other polyps | >90% |
| Vessels | Vascular malformations | ? |

*Table 51-2  Molecular Genetic Testing*

| Gene | Testing Modality | Mutation Type | Mutation Frequency |
|------|-----------------|---------------|-------------------|
| *PTEN* | Sequencing | Intragenic mutations | 80% for PHTS meeting full criteria |
| | MLPA | Large deletions and rearrangements | 10% of *PTEN* mutation-negative CS/CSL |

- Lipomas
- Fibromas
- Genitourinary tumors (especially renal cell carcinoma)
- Genitourinary malformation
- Uterine fibroids

**An operational diagnosis of CS is made if an individual meets any one of the following criteria:**

- Pathognomonic mucocutaneous lesions alone if there are
  - Six or more facial papules, of which three or more must be trichilemmoma *or*
  - Cutaneous facial papules and oral mucosal papillomatosis *or*
  - Oral mucosal papillomatosis and acral keratoses *or*
  - Six or more palmoplantar keratoses *or*
- Two or more major criteria *or*
- One major and at least three minor criteria *or*
- At least four minor criteria

In a family in which one individual meets the diagnostic criteria for CS listed above, other relatives are considered to have a diagnosis of CS if they meet any of the following criteria:

- The pathognomonic criteria *or*
- Any one major criterion with or without minor criteria *or*
- Two minor criteria *or*
- History of BRRS

**PTEN Cleveland Clinic Score:** Based on a prospective series of 3042 individuals with CS or CS-like phenotype, a multiple logistic regression-based model for scoring by clinical features was derived, which outperformed the NCCN criteria. A score of 10 derives a prior probability of 3% of finding a germline *PTEN* mutation and so is the selected threshold for suggesting clinical PTEN testing. This score has not been derived for *SDH* or *KLLN* alterations.

## Screening and Counseling

*Screening:* See Table 51-2.

*Counseling:* PHTS are autosomal dominant disorders with variable and age-related penetrance. Over 90% of individuals with CS have some clinical manifestation of the disorder by the late 20s.

For purposes of genotype-phenotype analyses, a series of 37 unrelated probands with CS were ascertained by the operational diagnostic criteria of the International Cowden Consortium,

1995 version. Association analyses revealed that families with CS and germline *PTEN* mutations are more likely to develop malignant breast disease when compared to families that do not have a *PTEN* mutation. In addition, missense mutations and mutations 5' to or within the phosphatase core motif appeared to be associated with involvement of five or more organs, a surrogate phenotype for severity of disease. Large germline deletions spanning *PTEN* and *BMPR1A* are associated with juvenile polyposis of infancy.

## Management and Treatment

### Evaluations of following initial diagnosis

To establish the extent of disease in an individual diagnosed with PHTS, the following evaluations are recommended:

- Complete history, especially family history
- Physical examination with *particular* attention to
  - Skin
  - Mucous membranes
  - Thyroid
  - Breasts
- Urinalysis with cytospin
- Baseline thyroid ultrasound examination at age 18 years or 5 years younger than the earliest age at thyroid cancer diagnosis in the family

***Surveillance:*** The most serious consequences of PHTS relate to the increased risk of cancers including breast, thyroid, endometrial, and to a lesser extent, renal. In this regard, the most important aspect of management of any individual with a *PTEN* mutation is increased cancer surveillance.

☞**COWDEN SYNDROME:**

### General

Annual comprehensive physical examination starting at age 18 years (or 5 years before the youngest component cancer diagnosis in the family), with attention paid to skin changes and the neck region

- Consider annual dermatologic examination.
- **Annual urinalysis:** Consider annual cytology and renal ultrasound examination if the family history is positive for renal cell carcinoma.
- Baseline colonoscopy at age 50 years (unless symptoms arise earlier). If only hamartomas are found, the American Cancer Society guidelines for colon cancer screening (ie, annual fecal occult blood testing and sigmoidoscopy every 5 years or colonoscopy every 10 years) should be followed.

☞**BREAST CANCER:**

- **Women**
  - Monthly breast self-examination beginning at age 18 years
  - Annual clinical breast examinations beginning at age 25 years or 5 to 10 years earlier than earliest known breast cancer diagnosis in the family (whichever is earliest)
  - Annual mammography and breast magnetic resonance imaging (MRI) beginning at age 30 to 35 years or 5 to 10 years before the earliest known breast cancer diagnosis in the family (whichever is earliest)
- **Men** should perform monthly breast self-examination.

☞**THYROID CANCER:**

- Baseline thyroid ultrasound examination at age 18 years or 5 years younger than earliest age at thyroid cancer diagnosis in the family
- Consider annual thyroid ultrasound examination thereafter (although annual neck examination may be sufficient)

☞**ENDOMETRIAL CANCER:**

- **Premenopausal women:** Annual blind repel (suction) biopsies beginning at age 35 to 40 years (or 5 years before the youngest endometrial cancer diagnosis in the family)
- **Postmenopausal women:** Annual transvaginal ultrasound examination with biopsy of suspicious areas

Note: Although the NCCN guidelines removed endometrial surveillance after 2007 (without expert PHTS input), it is prudent to ensure the minimal surveillance for endometrial cancer as detailed above, if family history is positive for this.

## Molecular Genetics and Molecular Mechanism

### Syndrome/Gene/Locus:

PHTS/*PTEN*/10q23

☞**DESCRIPTION OF BASIC GENE FUNCTIONS:** Although extensive functional research has been accomplished, the complete function of PTEN is not yet fully understood. PTEN belongs to a subclass of phosphatases called dual-specificity phosphatases that remove phosphate groups from tyrosine as well as serine and threonine. In addition, PTEN is the major phosphatase for phosphoinositide 3,4,5-triphosphate, and thus downregulates the PI3K/AKT pathway. In vitro and human immunohistochemical data suggest that PTEN traffics in and out of the nucleus. When PTEN is in the nucleus, it predominantly signals down the protein phosphatase and MAPK pathway to elicit cell cycle arrest. One of the nuclear functions of PTEN is to stabilize the genome. When in the cytoplasm, its lipid phosphatase predominantly signals down the AKT pathway to illicit apoptosis. Absent or dysfunctional PTEN causes upregulation of the AKT pathway and increased mammalian target of rapamycin (mTOR) signaling. Recently, phase II trials of mTOR inhibitors for PHTS show promising preliminary results.

***Genetic Testing:*** Clinical testing for *PTEN* is widely available and should comprise polymerase chain reaction (PCR)-based sequencing and large deletion **or** rearrangement testing. *PTEN* mutation analysis has clinical utility, clinical validity, and actionability.

***Addendum:*** A recent study based on prospective accrual of Cowden and Cowden-like individuals revealed that individuals with germline *PTEN* mutations carried higher lifetime risks of a range of cancers than previously believed. Lifetime risks were estimated at 85% for female breast cancer, 35% for epithelial thyroid carcinoma, 28% endometrial carcinoma, 33% renal cell carcinoma, mainly of the papillary and oncocytoma type, and 9% colorectal carcinoma, as well as 6% melanoma. Based on these lifetime risk estimates, new draft recommendations for high risk surveillance are as shown in Table 51-3.

*Table 51-3  New Draft Recommendations for High Risk Surveillance*

| | Pediatric (<18 years) | Adult Male | Adult Female |
|---|---|---|---|
| Baseline workup | Targeted history and physical examination<br>Baseline thyroid Ultrasound<br>Dermatologic examination<br>Formal neurologic and psychological testing | Targeted history and physical examination<br>Baseline thyroid Ultrasound<br>Dermatologic examination | Targeted history and physical examination<br>Baseline thyroid Ultrasound<br>Dermatologic examination |
| **Cancer surveillance** | | | |
| From diagnosis | Annual thyroid Ultrasound and skin examination | Annual thyroid Ultrasound and skin examination | Annual thyroid Ultrasound and skin examination |
| From age 30[a] | As per adult recommendations | | Annual mammogram (for consideration of breast MRI instead of mammography if dense breasts)<br>Annual endometrial sampling or transvaginal ultrasound (or from 5 years before age of earliest endometrial cancer) |
| From age 40[a] | As per adult recommendations | Biannual colonoscopy[b]<br>Biannual renal ultrasound/MRI | Biannual (every other year) colonoscopy[b]<br>Biannual (every other year) renal ultrasound / MRI |
| Prophylactic surgery | Nil | Nil | Individual discussion of prophylactic mastectomy or hysterectomy |

[a]Surveillance may begin 5 years before the earliest onset of a specific cancer in the family, but not later than the recommended age cutoff.

[b]The presence of multiple non-malignant polyps in patients with *PTEN* mutations may complicate non-invasive methods of colon evaluation. More frequent colonoscopy should be considered for patients with a heavy polyp burden.

**BIBLIOGRAPHY:**

1. Eng C. *PTEN* Hamartoma Tumor Syndrome (PHTS). In: Gene Reviews at Gene Tests: Medical Genetics Information Resource [database online]. Copyright University of Washington, Seattle, 2001-2011. http://www.ncbi.nlm.nih.gov/books/NBK1488/. Accessed July, 2011.

2. Zhou XP, Waite KA, Pilarski R, et al. Germline *PTEN* promoter mutations and deletions in Cowden/Bannayan-Riley-Ruvalcaba syndrome result in aberrant PTEN protein and dysregulation of the phosphoinositol-3-kinase/Akt pathway. *Am J Hum Genet.* 2003;73:404-411.

3. Marsh DJ, Coulon V, Lunetta KL, et al. Mutation spectrum and genotype-phenotype analyses in Cowden disease and Bannayan-Zonana syndrome, two hamartoma syndromes with germline *PTEN* mutation. *Hum Mol Genet.* 1998;7:507-515.

4. Tan MH, Mester J, Peterson C, et al. A clinical scoring system for selection of patients for *PTEN* mutation testing is proposed on the basis of a prospective study of 3,042 probands. *Am J Hum Genet.* 2011;88:42-56.

5. Mester J, Tilot AK, Rybicki LA, Frazier TW, Eng C. Analysis of prevalence and degree of macrocephaly in patients with germline *PTEN* mutations and of brain weight in *Pten* knock-in murine model. *Eur J Hum Genet.* 2011;19:763-768.

6. Heald B, Mester M, Rybicki LA, Orloff MS, Burke CA, Eng C. Frequent gastrointestinal polyps and colorectal adenocarcinomas in a prospective series of *PTEN* mutation carriers. *Gastroenterology.* 2010;139:1927-1933.

7. Hobert J, Eng C. Featured collaborative review (with Gene Reviews): *PTEN* hamartoma tumor syndrome (PHTS)—an overview. *Genet Med.* 2009;11:687-694.

8. Zbuk KM, Eng C. Cancer phenomics: RET and PTEN as illustrative models. *Nature Rev Cancer.* 2007;7:35-45.

9. Ni Y, Zbuk KM, Sadler T, et al. Germline mutations and variants in the succinate dehydrogenase genes in Cowden and Cowden-like syndromes. *Am J Hum Genet.* 2008;83:261-268.

10. Eng C, Peacocke M. *PTEN* mutation analysis as a molecular diagnostic tool in the inherited hamartoma-cancer syndromes. *Nature Genet.* 1998;19:223.

11. Tan MH, Mester JL, Ngeow J, Rybicki LA, Orloff MS, Eng C. Lifetime cancer risks in individuals with germline *PTEN* mutations. *Clin Cancer Res.* 2012;18:400-407.

## Supplementary Information

**OMIM REFERENCES:**

OMIM Entries for PHTS:
[1] BRRS; (#153480)
[2] Cowden Syndrome; (#158350)
[3] Proteus Syndrome; (#176920)
[4] PTEN (#601728)

**Alternative Names:**
- Multiple Hamartoma Syndrome (CS)
- Bannayan-Zonana Syndrome, Riley-Ruvalcaba-Smith Syndrome (BRRS)
- *MMAC1/TEP1* (*PTEN*)

***Key Words:*** Cowden syndrome or disease, multiple hamartomas, breast cancer, thyroid cancer, multinodular goiter, endometrial cancer, fibroids, mucocutaneous hamartomas, hamartomatous polyps, ganglioneuromatous polyps, trichilemmoma, scrotal tongue, dolichocephaly, Lhermitte-Duclos disease, dysplastic gangliocytoma of the cerebellum

# 52 Hereditary Breast and Ovarian Cancer

Monica A. Giovanni, Michael F. Murray and Judy E. Garber

## KEY POINTS

- *Disease summary:*
  - Breast cancer is a common disease panethnically. Approximately 15% to 20% of breast cancer is thought to cluster in families while only 5% to 10% is caused by single gene defects.
  - Ovarian cancer is far less common; approximately 10% to 25% of ovarian cancer is caused by single gene defects.
  - The monogenic form of breast and ovarian cancer, hereditary breast and ovarian cancer (HBOC), caused by mutation in *BRCA1* and *BRCA2* predisposes individuals and families to a high lifetime risk of breast and ovarian cancers as well as other cancers including the prostate and pancreas. *BRCA1*-specific lifetime risk for female breast cancer is 55% to 65%, with a 39% risk for ovarian cancer. *BRCA2*-specific lifetime risk for female breast cancer is 47%, with a 11% to 17% risk for ovarian cancer. *BRCA*-related male breast cancer risk is 7% with a 20% risk for prostate cancer.
  - *CHEK2*-related breast cancer is a more recently described disease association. Mutations in *CHEK2* within the context of a strong family history of breast cancer pose an increased risk, though there is much controversy around actual risk assessments. Studies within a European population, where a single mutation is common (1100delC), report a baseline risk of 6%, with that risk increasing to 44% in families in which two other relatives have a breast cancer diagnosis.
  - Genome-wide association studies (GWAS) have identified 11 loci that have repeatedly been associated with breast cancer in at least two published studies, see Table 52-1. Interestingly a study by Bolton et al. found a risk association for ovarian cancer which overlaps the observed risk for breast cancer at 19q13.11. This may indicate a *BRCA1*- and/or *BRCA2*-associated pathway driving these risks. The other observed associations may ultimately reveal new cancer risk pathways or new insights into the one associated pathway.

- *Hereditary basis:*
  - HBOC is an autosomal dominant cancer predisposition syndrome; some individuals with a disease-causing mutation may not develop an associated cancer in their lifetime, giving the appearance that the disease may skip generations.
  - CHEK2 also exhibits an autosomal dominant pattern of inheritance, though with lower lifetime risk of disease, a family history may not be apparent.

- *Differential diagnosis:*
  - It is important to distinguish the multiorgan system syndromes that include breast or ovarian cancer as a single feature (ie, Cowden syndrome, Li-Fraumeni syndrome, hereditary diffuse gastric cancer, Lynch syndrome, Peutz-Jeghers syndrome), from the familial tumor predispositions in which these tumors are often the only major finding (Table 52-2).

## Diagnostic Criteria and Clinical Characteristics

*Diagnostic Criteria for Hereditary Breast and Ovarian Cancer Syndrome:*

**National Comprehensive Cancer Network Criteria (NCCN)— at least one or more of the following:**

- Early-onset cancer (age <50 years), typically premenopausal breast cancer including both invasive and ductal carcinoma in situ (DCIS) breast cancers
- Two primary tumors of the breast or breast and ovarian or fallopian tube or primary peritoneal cancer in a single individual
- Two or more primary tumors of the breast or breast and ovarian or fallopian tube or primary peritoneal cancers in first- second- and third-degree relatives from the same side of the family
- At-risk populations (eg, Ashkenazi Jewish, Icelandic)
- Member of a family with a known *BRCA1* or *BRCA2* mutation
- Any male breast cancer
- Ovarian or fallopian tube or primary peritoneal cancer at any age

## Screening and Counseling

*Screening:* Individuals meeting the above criteria established by NCCN should be referred for counseling and possible genetic testing.

☞**FEMALE CANCER RISK:** Women who are found to have a disease-associated mutation in *BRCA1* or *BRCA2* should initiate breast cancer surveillance.

Breast surveillance recommendations for female mutation carriers include

- Self-breast examination—though studies suggest limited efficacy
- Clinical breast examination beginning at age 25 and repeated at 6-month intervals
- Mammography beginning at age 25 and repeated annually
- Breast magnetic resonance imaging (MRI) beginning at age 25 and repeated annually

There are currently no effective ovarian cancer surveillance methods.

*Table 52-1 Eleven Loci Repeatedly Associated With Breast Cancer Risk in GWAS*

| Loci | Reported Genes | Mapped Genes | Number of Studies |
|------|---------------|-------------|-------------------|
| 16q12.1 | TOX3, TNRC9 | TOX3-CHD9 | 5 |
| 2q35 | Intergenic | TNP1-DIRC3 | 5 |
| 10q26.13 | FGFR2 | FGFR2, ATE1 | 9 |
| 5q11.2 | MAP3K1 | RPL26P19-MAP3K1 | 2 |
| 8q24.21 | Intergenic | SRRM1P-POU5F1B | 3 |
| 11p15.5 | LSP1 | LSP1 | 2 |
| 5p12 | Intergenic | FGF10-MRPS30-HCN1 | 3 |
| 6q25.1 | ESR1, C6orf97 | CCDC170-ESR1 | 4 |
| 10q21.2 | ZNF365 | ZNF365 | 2 |
| 3p24.1 | SLC4A7 | SLC4A7 | 2 |
| 19p13.11 | ABHD8, ANKLE1, C19orf62 | BABAM1 | 2 |

☞**MALE CANCER RISK:** Men who are found to have a disease-associated mutation in *BRCA1* or *BRCA2* should initiate breast and prostate screening.

Surveillance recommendations for male mutation carriers include

- Clinical breast examination repeated annually
- Prostate-specific antigen testing annually
- Digital rectal examination annually

Because melanoma is an established risk associated with *BRCA2* mutations, annual clinical skin examinations are recommended. While pancreatic cancer is seen at a higher frequency in families with *BRCA1* and *BRCA2* mutations, there is no proven clinical surveillance available, however screening is sometimes offered to families affected by pancreatic cancer.

***Counseling:*** *BRCA1* and *BRCA2* are inherited in an autosomal dominant fashion. Each child of an affected parent has a 50%

*Table 52-2 Genetic Differential Diagnosis*

| Syndrome | Gene Symbol | Associated Findings |
|----------|-------------|---------------------|
| Hereditary breast and ovarian cancer syndrome (HBOC) | BRCA1, BRCA2 | *BRCA1*: Breast cancer with medullary histopathology, often estrogen receptor, progesterone receptor, and Her2 neu negative; ovarian cancer is typically epithelial. Pancreatic cancer *BRCA2*: Breast cancer that cannot be distinguished from sporadic cancer; 70% estrogen receptor and progesterone receptor positive, Her2 negative; ovarian cancer is typically epithelial. Melanoma and pancreatic cancer |
| Cowden syndrome (*PTEN syndromes*) | PTEN | Benign and malignant breast, thyroid (typically follicular), and endometrial tumors. Additional features include macrocephaly, trichilemmomas, and papillomas |
| Li-Fraumeni syndrome | TP53 | Breast cancer, soft tissue sarcoma, leukemia, osteosarcoma, melanoma, as well as colon, pancreatic, adrenal cortical, and brain cancers |
| Hereditary diffuse gastric cancer | CDH1 | Lobular breast cancer and diffuse gastric cancer, typically signet-ring carcinoma or isolate cell-type carcinoma |
| Lynch syndrome | MLH1, MSH2, MSH6, PMS2, EPCAM | Colorectal, endometrial, and ovarian cancers |
| Peutz-Jeghers syndrome | STK11 | Gastrointestinal hamartomatous polyps with mucocutaneous pigmentation; breast cancer risk is increased though not a hallmark of the syndrome; Lifetime breast cancer risk 40% |

Gene names: *PTEN*, phosphatase and tensin homolog; *TP53*, tumor protein p53; *CDH1*, cadherin 1; *CHEK2*, checkpoint kinase 2; *MLH1*, homolog to *Escherichia coli* MutL 1; *MSH2*, homolog of *E. coli* MutS 2; *MSH6*, homolog of *E. coli* MutS 6; *PMS2*, postmeiotic segregation increased 2; *EPCAM*, epithelial cellular adhesion molecule; *STK11*, serine or threonine protein kinase 11.

*Table 52-3 Molecular Genetic Testing*

| Gene | Testing Modality | Mutation Type | Ethnicity-Based Common Mutations |
|------|------------------|---------------|----------------------------------|
| BRCA1 | Sanger sequence analysis with MLPA, targeted mutation analysis when familial mutation is known | Sequence variant, slice site mutations, and exonic or multiexonic deletions | Ashkenazi-Jewish: 185delAG, 5382insC |
| BRCA2 | Sanger sequence analysis with MLPA, targeted mutation analysis when familial mutation is known | Sequence variant, slice site mutations, and exonic or multiexonic deletions | Ashkenazi-Jewish: 6174delT Icelandic: 999del5 |

risk of inheriting the condition. Presymptomatic testing should be offered to all first-degree relatives of an affected individual.

☞**Penetrance:**
- *BRCA1*
  - Female breast cancer risk: 55% to 65% by age 70 years
  - Ovarian cancer risk: 39% by age 70 years
- *BRCA2*
  - Female breast cancer risk: 47% by age 70 years
  - Ovarian cancer risk: 11% to 17% by age 70 years
- *BRCA-associated male cancer risk*
  - Male breast cancer risk: 7% by age 70 years
  - Prostate cancer risk: 14% by age 70 years

☞**Genotype-Phenotype Correlation:** Cancer risks differ by gene and may also by location of a mutation within the gene. Studies have found that in families with mutations in the ovarian cancer cluster region (OCCR) of exon 11 of *BRCA2*, there is a higher ratio of ovarian to breast cancer than families with a mutation elsewhere in *BRCA2*.

## Management and Treatment

*Prevention:* In addition to the surveillance recommendations detailed earlier, prophylactic surgical interventions should be considered as a method to prevent primary disease manifestations. Women who are found to have a disease-associated mutation in *BRCA1* or *BRCA2* should consider prophylactic mastectomy in consultation with the care team. Prophylactic mastectomy provides greater than 90% breast cancer risk reduction in individuals with *BRCA* mutations.

Additionally, women who are found to have a disease-associated mutation in *BRCA1* or *BRCA2* should consider prophylactic bilateral salpingo-oophorectomy (BSO) after their childbearing is completed and when the woman is physically and emotionally prepared in consultation with the care team. BSO provides greater than 90% ovarian and fallopian tube cancer risk reduction in individuals with *BRCA* mutations. Premenopausal BSO also reduces breast cancer risk up to 50%.

Chemoprevention has been found to reduce the incidence of breast cancer in some *BRCA*+ women. Tamoxifen has been found to reduce the incidence of estrogen receptor-positive breast cancer, but not estrogen receptor-negative breast cancer, suggesting that tamoxifen may provide more benefit in women with *BRCA2* mutations. Studies have shown that tamoxifen reduced the risk for breast cancer by up to 62% among healthy women with

*BRCA2* mutations. Importantly, significant adverse consequences of tamoxifen treatment included higher rates of endometrial cancer and thromboembolic episodes in those individuals who took the medication.

*Treatment:* The treatment of both breast and ovarian cancer in individuals with *BRCA1* or *BRCA2* mutations is similar to the approach taken in the sporadic forms. There are data suggesting that BRCA-associated tumors are more sensitive to agents exploiting DNA repair, including platinums and investigational agents like PARP inhibitors.

## Molecular Genetics and Molecular Mechanism

*Syndrome/Gene/Locus:*
Familial susceptibility to breast cancer 1/*BRCA1*/17q21
Familial susceptibility to breast cancer 2/*BRCA2*/13q12-13

*BRCA1* and *BRCA2* are described as caretaker genes that play critical roles in DNA repair, cell cycle checkpoint control, and maintenance of genomic stability (Table 52-3). They are thought to directly regulate the growth of tumors by inhibiting growth or promoting death.

*Genetic Testing:* DNA sequence analysis is clinically available for *BRCA1*, and *BRCA2*.

(See Gene Tests http://www.genetests.org/query?mim=168000.)

**Bibliography:**

1. Antoniou A, Pharoah PDP, Narod S, et al. Average risks of breast and ovarian cancer associated with BRCA1 or BRCA2 mutations detected in case series unselected for family history: a combined analysis of 222 studies. *Am J Hum Genet*. 2003;72:1117-1130.

2. Bolton KL, Tyrer J, Song H, et al. Common variants at 19p13 are associated with susceptibility to ovarian cancer. *Nat Genet*. 2010;42(10):880-884.

3. Cybulski C, Gorski B, Huzarski T, et al. CHEK2 is a multiorgan cancer susceptibility gene. *Am J Hum Genet*. 2004;75:1131-1135.

4. Hindorff LA, MacArthur J, Morales J, et al. A Catalog of Published Genome-Wide Association Studies. http://www.genome.gov/gwastudies.

5. King MC, Wieand S, Hale K, et al. Tamoxifen and breast cancer incidence among women with inherited mutations in BRCA1 and BRCA2: National Surgical Adjuvant Breast and Bowel Project (NSABP-P1) Breast Cancer Prevention Trial. *JAMA*. 2001;286:2251-2256.

6. Liede A, Karlan BY, Narod SA. Cancer risks for male carriers of germline mutations in BRCA1 or BRCA2: a review of the literature. *J Clin Oncol.* 2004;22(4):735-742.

7. National Comprehensive Cancer Network. Clinical practice guidelines in oncology, genetic/familial high-risk assessment: breast and ovarian.http://www.nccn.org.

## Supplementary Information

**OMIM REFERENCES:**

[1] Familial Susceptibility to Breast Cancer 1; BRCA1 (#604370)

[2] Familial Susceptibility to Breast Cancer 2; BRCA2 (#612555)

[3] Susceptibility to Breast and Colorectal Cancer; CHEK2 (#604373)

**Alternative Names:**
- Familial Susceptibility to Breast Cancer 1
- Familial Susceptibility to Breast Cancer 2

*Key Words:* Breast cancer, ovarian cancer, hereditary cancer syndrome

# 53 Obesity

Haya Al-Saud, Sadia Saeed, Rajkumar Dorajoo, and Phillippe Froguel

## KEY POINTS

- *Disease summary:*
  - Common obesity has conventionally been viewed as a disease that is caused by substantial changes in the human environment, for example, the increase in consumption of calorie-rich food and decrease in physical activity. There is also strong evidence that genes are critically involved in the development of obesity.
    - Obesity is a major risk factor for cardiovascular diseases, pulmonary diseases (such as sleep apnea), metabolic diseases (eg, diabetes and dyslipidemia), osteoarticular diseases, for several of the commonest forms of cancer, and for serious psychiatric illness.

- *Differential diagnosis:*
  - It includes depression, diabetes mellitus, type 1, diabetes mellitus, type 2, fatty liver, growth hormone deficiency, hiatal hernia, hirsutism, polygenic hypercholesterolemia, hypertension, hypothyroidism, insulinoma, Kallmann syndrome, and idiopathic hypogonadotropic hypogonadism, generalized lipodystrophy, nephrotic syndrome, polycystic ovarian disease (Stein-Leventhal syndrome), pseudo-Cushing syndrome, adiposa dolorosa (Dercum disease), partial lipodystrophies associated with localized lipohypertrophy.

- *Monogenic forms:*
  - They explain at least 5% of obesity cases.

- *Family history:*
  - The risk of developing obesity has been shown to be doubled if a person has a first-degree relative who is overweight, tripled if your first-degree relative is moderately obese, and five times greater if first-degree relative is morbidly obese.

- *Twin studies:*
  - Twins studies of human obesity have shown that the heritability of body mass index (BMI) is between 0.5 and 0.8. It was also shown that the concordance rate between monozygotic twin pairs is more than twice that of dizygotic pairs (~0.68 vs ~0.28).

- *Environmental factors:*
  - Change in lifestyle, decline in physical activity, and abundance of fat-rich foods have been regarded as the three major components of the obesogenic environment. In addition, there are other risk factors for development of obesity that include age, gender, sleep duration, antidepression drug consumption, exposure to chemicals, and ethnicity.

- *Genome-wide associations:* A main role in genome-wide association studies (GWAS) is in hypothesis generations and the putative genes identified that have shed novel insights in disease etiology, although additional studies would be necessary to prove and determine mechanistic roles. Many associations exist with obesity and have provided a valuable contribution in the area of genetics of obesity by effectively identifying several putative genetic loci associated with the common polygenic form of obesity (Table 53-1).

- *Pharmacogenomics:*
  - Testing for leptin gene mutations that causes leptin deficiency (Table 53-2)

## Diagnostic Criteria and Clinical Characteristics

***Diagnostic Criteria for Obesity:*** Diagnostic evaluation should include the following:

- BMI is currently used as the most accurate and reliable way of measuring how overweight you are. To estimate BMI, multiply the individual's weight (in pounds) by 703, then divide by the height (in inches) squared. This approximates BMI in kilograms per meter squared ($kg/m^2$). Classifications for BMI: underweight BMI less than 18.5 $kg/m^2$, normal weight BMI 18.5 to 24.9 $kg/m^2$, overweight BMI 25 to 29.9 $kg/m^2$, obesity (class 1) BMI 30 to 34.9 $kg/m^2$, obesity (class 2) BMI 35 to 39.9 $kg/m^2$, and extreme obesity (class 3) BMI 40 $kg/m^2$.

- An adult with normal weight should have a BMI between 18.5 and 24.9. A BMI between 25 and 29.9 is considered overweight. A BMI over 30 is considered obese.

- As well as calculating your BMI, some further tests can be done that can help determine if you are at increased risk of any

*Table 53-1* **Obesity-Associated Susceptibility Variants**

| Implicated Genes and Position | Associated Variant | Per Allele Increase in BMI (kg/m²) or WHR | Risk Allele Frequency in Europeans (%) | Putative Function Related to Obesity |
|---|---|---|---|---|
| **Loci associated with BMI** | | | | |
| *FTO* (16q22.2) | rs1558902 | 0.39 | 42 | Neuronal function possibly associated with appetite control |
| Near *MC4R* (18q22) | rs571312 | 0.23 | 24 | Hypothalamic signaling, rare mutations cause monogenic obesity |
| Near *TMEM18* (2p25) | rs2867125 | 0.31 | 83 | Neural development, highly expressed at the hypothalamus |
| Near *GNPDA2* (4p13) | rs10938397 | 0.18 | 43 | Highly expressed at the hypothalamus |
| *SH2B18* (16q11.2) | rs7359397 | 0.15 | 40 | *SH2B1* involved in neuronal control of energy homeostasis, leptin release |
| Near *NEGR1* (1p31) | rs2815752 | 0.13 | 61 | Growth promoter involved with neuronal outgrowth |
| *MTCH2-NDUFS3-CUGBP1* (11p11.2) | rs3817334 | 0.06 | 41 | *MTCH2* involved in cellular apoptosis, highly expressed at the hypothalamus |
| Near *KCTD15* (19q13.11) | rs29941 | 0.06 | 67 | Highly expressed at the hypothalamus |
| *SEC16B* (1q25) | rs543874 | 0.22 | 19 | - |
| *BDNF* (11p14) | rs10767664 | 0.19 | 78 | Neuronal appetite control, *BDNF* deletions involved with WAGR syndrome characterized by hyperphagia and severe obesity |
| Near *ETV5* (3q27) | rs9816226 | 0.14 | 82 | Highly expressed at the hypothalamus |
| *SLC39A8* (4q24) | rs13107325 | 0.19 | 7 | - |
| Near *PRKD1* (14q12) | rs11847697 | 0.17 | 4 | - |
| Near *GPRC5B-IQCK* (16q12.3) | rs12444979 | 0.17 | 87 | - |
| *QPCTL-GIPR* (19q13.32) | rs2287019 | 0.15 | 80 | *GIPR* encodes incretin receptor |
| Near *RBJ-POMC-ADCY3* (2p23.3) | rs713586 | 0.14 | 47 | *POMC* involved in hypothalamic signaling; rare mutations cause monogenic obesity |
| *TFAP2B* (6p12) | rs987237 | 0.13 | 18 | - |
| *MAP2K5-SKOR1* (15q23) | rs2241423 | 0.13 | 78 | - |
| *NRXN3* (14q31) | rs10150332 | 0.13 | 21 | Possible neuronal reward system control |
| *FAIM2* (12q13) | rs7138803 | 0.12 | 38 | Adipocyte apoptosis, highly expressed at the hypothalamus |
| *LRRN6C* (9q21.3) | rs10968576 | 0.11 | 31 | - |
| Near *FLJ35779-HMGCR* (5q13.3) | rs2112347 | 0.1 | 63 | - |
| Near *FANCL* (2p16.1) | rs887912 | 0.1 | 29 | - |
| *CADM2* (3p21.1) | rs13078807 | 0.1 | 20 | - |
| Near *TMEM160-ZC3H4* (19q13.32) | rs3810291 | 0.09 | 67 | - |
| Near *LRP1B* (2q22.2) | rs2890652 | 0.09 | 18 | - |
| *MTIF3-GTF3A* (13q12.2) | rs4771122 | 0.09 | 24 | - |
| *TNNI3K* (1p31.1) | rs1514175 | 0.07 | 43 | - |
| Near *ZNF608* (5q23.2) | rs4836133 | 0.07 | 48 | - |

*(Continued)*

*Table 53-1 Obesity-Associated Susceptibility Variants (Continued)*

| Implicated Genes and Position | Associated Variant | Per Allele Increase in BMI (kg/m²) or WHR | Risk Allele Frequency in Europeans (%) | Putative Function Related to Obesity |
|---|---|---|---|---|
| Near *PTBP2* (1p21.3) | rs1555543 | 0.06 | 59 | - |
| Near *RPL27A-TUB* (11p15.4) | rs4929949 | 0.06 | 52 | *TUB* involved in sensorineural regulation |
| *NUDT3-HMGA1*(6p21.31) | rs206936 | 0.06 | 21 | |
| **Loci associated with WHR, independent of BMI** | | | | |
| *RSPO3* (6q22.33) | rs9491696 | 0.05 | 52 | Vascular development |
| Near *NFE2L3* (7p15.2) | rs1055144 | 0.04 | 21 | - |
| Near *VEGFA* (6p21.1) | rs6905288 | 0.04 | 56 | Vascular development, key mediator of adipogenesis |
| Near *GRB14* (2q24.3) | rs10195252 | 0.04 | 60 | Associated with insulin and triglyceride levels |
| *TBX15-WARS2* (1p12) | rs984222 | 0.03 | 37 | Transcription factor involved in adipocyte and specific adipose depot development |
| *NISCH-STAB1* (3p22.1) | rs6784615 | 0.03 | 94 | Interacts with insulin receptor substrate |
| Near *LYPLAL1* (1q41) | rs4846567 | 0.03 | 28 | Encodes protein believed to act as a triglyceride lipase and is upregulated in subcutaneous adipose tissue |
| Near *ITPR2-SSPN* (12p21.1) | rs718314 | 0.03 | 74 | - |
| Near *HOXC13* (12q13.13) | rs1443512 | 0.03 | 24 | Transcription factor involved in cell spatial distribution in embryonic development |
| Near *LY86* (6p25.1) | rs1294421 | 0.03 | 39 | Lipopolysaccharide recognition molecule |
| Near *ADAMTS9* (3p14.1) | rs6795735 | 0.03 | 41 | Involved in cell spatial distribution in embryonic development |
| *DNM3-PIGC* (1q24.3) | rs1011731 | 0.03 | 57 | Involved in glucose transporter expression in adipocytes |
| *ZNRF3-KREMEN1* (22q12.1) | rs4823006 | 0.02 | 57 | - |
| *CPEB4* (5q35.2) | rs6861681 | 0.02 | 34 | Involved in polyadenylation regulation |

health complications because of your obesity like measuring your blood pressure, waist circumference, and glucose and lipid levels.

**Clinical Characteristics:** Obesity is characterized by an excess of adiposity irrespectively where the excessive fat depots are. Obesity by itself is not a disease but a state and at least originally it is not always associated with metabolic and cardiovascular abnormalities.

## Screening and Counseling

**Screening:** Genetic screening could be done when monogenic forms of obesity, for example, leptin (*LEP*), leptin receptors (*LEPR*), prohormone convertase 1 (*PC1*), pro-opiomelanocortin (*POMC*), and melanocortin receptor (*MCR4*) genes are suspected, in particular in children with severe overweight and with appetite abnormalities. A chromosomal abnormality (eg, a deletion on

*Table 53-2 Pharmacogenetics in Obesity*

| Gene | Associated Medications | Goal of Testing | Variants | Effect |
|---|---|---|---|---|
| Leptin | Recombinant human leptin | Efficacy | ΔG133, Arg105Trp | High efficacy |

chromosome 16p) could be assessed in children with severe obesity and developmental delay.

*Counseling:* Many patients or families want to know their risk for developing obesity. Several monogenic forms of obesity result from the disruption of the leptin-melanocortin pathway. A lot of these mutations are found in consanguineous families. Families that have children with congenital leptin deficiency can benefit from genetic counseling, prognostication, and therapy by daily subcutaneous injections of leptin that dramatically reduced body weight (98% of which was fat mass). Although specific treatment for the other forms of monogenic obesity, for example, MC4R, POMC, and PC1 are not available yet, patients that carry these mutations are very likely to respond to pharmacotherapy.

## Management and Treatment

*Therapeutic Lifestyle Changes:* Most obese patients should adopt long-term nutritional adjustments to reduce caloric intake. Increase in physical activity is also important as it increases energy expenditure. Also, behavioral therapy should be pursued as it teaches self-monitoring, stress management, stimulus control, problem solving, cognitive restructuring, and social support.

*Pharmacotherapy:* Maybe helpful for high-risk patients with a BMI of greater than or equal to 30 kg/m$^2$. There are a number of antiobesity drugs available; however, a lot of them are not US Food and Drug Administration (FDA) approved. The only widely used drug is

*Orlistat:* Xenical (orlistat 120 mg), also known as tetrahydrolipstatin, was approved as a prescription product by FDA in 1999. Its primary function is preventing the absorption of fats from the human diet, thereby reducing caloric intake. This drug is used for obesity management accompanied with a reduced caloric diet, and it is also used to reduce the risk of regaining weight after prior weight loss. In 2007, Alli (orlistat 60 mg) was approved to be used for weight loss in overweight adults in conjunction with a low-calorie or fat diet.

*Surgery:* Bariatric surgery is actually the most effective weight loss option for patients who are morbidly obese, defined with a BMI greater than or equal to 40 kg/m$^2$ or a BMI of greater than or equal to 35 to 39.9 kg/m$^2$ and they have severe obesity-related medical complications, for example, hypertension, type 2 diabetes (T2D), or sleep apnea. Potential patients should also have tried to lose weight by diet therapy and have been unsuccessful in losing weight. A lot of cohort studies have shown that bariatric surgery decreases medical complications and mortality rates associated with obesity. The two most popular bariatric surgery procedures are the Roux-en-Y gastric bypass (RYPG) and laparoscopic adjustable gastric banding (LAGB). After RYPG and LAGB, patients lose 60% and 50% of their excess body weight, respectively.

*Pharmacogenetics:* Leptin is a gene that includes 167 amino acid peptides. Mutations in that gene cause congenital leptin deficiency. It is produced and secreted by adipocytes, and mediates adipose tissue mass by elevating thermogenesis and restricting food intake through both central and peripheral mechanisms. Recent studies have suggested that after intracerebroventricular administration of leptin in human and rats, adipose tissue showed a rapid decrease and features of apoptosis.

## Molecular Genetics and Molecular Mechanism

There is strong evidence that genes are critically involved in the development of obesity. Human single genetic defects were first described in mid 1990s and have led to severe obesity with the absence of developmental delays. These rare cases of monogenic obesity provided the first direct evidence that genetic factors play a considerable role in body weight regulation.

*LEP* and *LEPR* mutations were both first discovered in consanguineous families, which have led to a deeper understanding of appetite control. The hypothalamus in particular plays an important role in the regulation of appetite, body weight, and physical activity. It is now clear that obesity is a neuroendocrine disorder in which environmental factors and genetic predisposition both have an effect on the development of the disease.

Extensive studies have revealed mutations in other genes of the leptinergic-melanocortinergic pathway causing monogenic obesity. Examples are found in *PC1*, *POMC*, and melanocortin receptor (*MC4R*) genes. In the case of autosomal dominant mutations (*MC4R*), these mutations are found in total in about 2% in extremely obese adults and 3% to 6% of severely obese children. There remain, however, many obese individuals with apparently monogenic obesity (including individuals from consanguineous families) in whom mutations in the known obesity genes have been excluded.

GWAS is another approach used to investigate the association between common genetic variations and the disease in question. It has provided a valuable contribution in the area of genetics of obesity by effectively identifying several putative genetic loci associated with the common polygenic form of obesity.

*FTO* was the first locus incontrovertibly associated with obesity through an initial GWAS for T2D. In this study, variants at the intron 1 of the *FTO* gene lost their associations with T2D when study participants' BMI was taken into consideration, implying that the associations detected were mediated through obesity. The associations of *FTO* with BMI and risk for obesity have been independently identified by other large-scale studies.

A major finding from the discovery of *FTO* (even more for subsequent loci) was that the effect sizes of common variants associated with polygenic obesity would be modest. This has prompted collaborative efforts to increase sample sizes and power in studies through meta-analyses and these efforts have successfully identified as many as 32 loci for BMI associations and 14 others for central obesity measures that are independent of overall obesity. Genetic markers associated with obesity identified through GWAS are summarized in (Table 53-1).

A main role in GWAS is in hypothesis generations and putative genes identified have shed novel insights in disease etiology, although additional studies would be necessary to prove and determine mechanistic roles. Several of the loci detected for BMI or overall obesity indicate a prominent role at the hypothalamus. Furthermore, at least three loci detected (*MC4R*, *BDNF*, and *POMC*), well characterized functions at the hypothalamic control of energy homeostasis has been identified, and severe mutations result in monogenic forms of obesity. These findings highlight that obesity may also be a disorder of the central nervous system rather than a peripheral energy storage problem. Conversely, most loci detected for central obesity measures point to a more prominent role in distribution of fat in the body.

Not more than 5% of the heritability of the BMI is explained by the 40 single-nucleotide polymorphisms (SNPs) that are associated with obesity through GWAS. Therefore, there is a major gap in adiposity heritability which is unlikely to be totally explained by frequent SNPs. Copy number variations (CNVs) are DNA segments of 1 kb or larger whose copy number varies among different alleles. CNVs can also be termed as deletions, insertions, duplications, and complex multisite variants found in all humans.

The extent of which different CNVs may vary in their effects on phenotype is dependent on which genes they may overlap with and if they have any effect on gene function or not. Whole genes may vary in copy number and as a consequence may lead to a variation in gene expression, where gains and losses in copy number will increase and decrease gene expression levels. It has been estimated that CNVs account for 17.7% of heritable variation in gene expression and as a result may be phenotypically harmful. Some common gene CNVs have been found to increase susceptibility to certain complex diseases. A couple of studies have found disease association with variants. A substantial amount of these associations has been found to be involved with the immune system, cancer, brain development, and autism.

The investigation of rare great saphenous veins (GSVs) in children with "extreme" syndromic forms of obesity (eg, where obesity is seen with learning disability and other dysmorphic features) has also recently been very fruitful. Our group has also recently reported a highly penetrant form of obesity in subjects with a BMI of greater than 40 kg/m$^2$ that have been found to have rare deletions of at least 500 kb at 16p11.2, first identified in children with learning disability, which was present at appreciable frequencies in collections of obese adults and children in European populations.

***Genetic Testing:*** No genetic testing is available to diagnose the common form of obesity. If a monogenic form of obesity is suspected, the relevant gene may be sequenced. Molecular karyotyping may be indicated when obesity is associated with intellectual disability and/or dysmorphia.

***Future Directions:*** Apart from structural variants affecting genes involved in appetite it is also proposed that rare point mutations in genes coding for key proteins in the energy balance may also contribute to the genetics of obesity. With the development of next-generation sequencing it is now possible to identify rare mutations impairing genes involved in appetite regulation or in metabolism that can greatly contribute to obesity risk at the individual level. That may explain why some people are more vulnerable than others to the obesogenic current environment. It is likely that more progress will be made soon in the genetics of obesity opening avenues for better prevention and treatment of the disease.

## BIBLIOGRAPHY:

1. Blakemore AI, Froguel P. Is obesity our genetic legacy? *J Clin Endocrinol Metab.* 2008;93(11 suppl 1):S51-S56.
2. Froguel P, Blakemore AI. The power of the extreme in elucidating obesity. *N Engl J Med.* 2008;359(9):891-893.
3. Walley AJ, Asher JE, Froguel P. The genetic contribution to non-syndromic human obesity. *Nat Rev Genet.* 2009;10(7):431-442.
4. Montague CT, Farooqi IS, Whitehead JP, et al. Congenital leptin deficiency is associated with severe early-onset obesity in humans. *Nature.* 1997;387(6636):903-908.
5. Hinney A, Vogel CI, Hebebrand J. From monogenic to polygenic obesity: recent advances. *Eur Child Adolesc Psychiatry.* 2010;19(3):297-310.
6. Farooqi IS, O'Rahilly S. Monogenic human obesity syndromes. *Recent Prog Horm Res.* 2004;59:409-424.
7. Farooqi S, O'Rahilly S. Genetics of obesity in humans. *Endocr Rev.* 2006;27(7):710-718.
8. Frayling TM, Timpson NJ, Weedon MN, et al. A common variant in the FTO gene is associated with body mass index and predisposes to childhood and adult obesity. *Science.* 2007;316(5826):889-894.
9. Dina C, Meyre D, Samson C, et al. Comment on "A common genetic variant is associated with adult and childhood obesity." *Science.* 2007;315(5809):187; author reply 187.
10. Scuteri A, Sanna S, Chen WM, et al. Genome-wide association scan shows genetic variants in the FTO gene are associated with obesity-related traits. *PLoS Genet.* 2007;3(7):e115.
11. Heid IM, Jackson AU, Randall JC, et al. Meta-analysis identifies 13 new loci associated with waist-hip ratio and reveals sexual dimorphism in the genetic basis of fat distribution. *Nat Genet.* 2010;42(11):949-960.
12. Speliotes EK, Willer CJ, Berndt SI, et al. Association analyses of 249,796 individuals reveal 18 new loci associated with body mass index. *Nat Genet.* 2010;42(11):937-948.
13. de Smith AJ, Walters RG, Froguel P, Blakemore AI. Human genes involved in copy number variation: mechanisms of origin, functional effects and implications for disease. *Cytogenet Genome Res.* 2008;123(1-4):17-26.
14. Bochukova EG, Huang N, Keogh J, et al. Large, rare chromosomal deletions associated with severe early-onset obesity. *Nature.* 2010;463(7281):666-670.
15. Walters RG, Jacquemont S, Valsesia A, et al. A new highly penetrant form of obesity due to deletions on chromosome 16p11.2. *Nature.* 2010;463(7281):671-675.
16. Stranger BE, Forrest MS, Dunning M, et al. Relative impact of nucleotide and copy number variation on gene expression phenotypes. *Science.* 2007;315(5813):848-853.
17. Herrera BM, Lindgren CM. The genetics of obesity. *Curr Diab Rep.* 2010;10(6):498-505.

## Supplementary Information

**OMIM REFERENCES:**

[1] Leptin; LEP (#164160)

[2] Leptin Receptor; LEPR (#601007)

[3] Melanocortin 4 Receptor; MC4R (#155541)

[4] Pachyonychia Congenita, Type 1; PC1 (#167200)

[5] Pro-opiomelanocortin; POMC (#176830)

***Key Words:*** Obesity, bariatric surgery

# 54 Diabetes Mellitus Type 1

Adi Bar-Lev and Helen C. Looker

## KEY POINTS

- *Disease summary:*
  - Diabetes mellitus type 1 (T1DM) is a disorder of insulin secretion which can be subdivided into type 1A (immune mediated) and type 1B (nonimmune mediated).
  - The vast majority of T1DM is type 1A, characterized by both acute and chronic sequelae of hyperglycemia.
  - T1DM has a peak age of onset before the age of 20 years and is the commonest form of diabetes seen in children in the United States.
  - Because insulin production is impaired, T1DM is characterized by an absolute requirement for exogenous insulin and, unlike type 2 diabetes (T2DM), frequently presents as a medical emergency with hyperglycemia, dehydration, and ketoacidosis.
- *Differential diagnosis:*
  - Neonatal diabetes, T2DM, maturity-onset diabetes of the young (MODY)
- *Monogenic forms:*
  - While there is no monogenic form of DM type 1A, there is a monogenic autosomal recessive form of type 1B. This ketosis-prone DM (KPDM) is caused by mutations in the *PAX4* gene. Clinically distinct from type 1A, KPDM is characterized by an intermittent absolute requirement for insulin.
- *Family history:*
  - Risk of T1DM in the general population is 0.5%, while, the presence of an affected sibling is associated with a disease risk of 6% to 10%. The risk associated with an affected parent varies with gender. Offspring of an affected father have a risk of 6%, while offspring of an affected mother have a risk of only 2%.
- *Twin studies:*
  - Monozygotic twins have a concordance rate of 45%, compared with a 25% concordance rate for dizygotic twins.
- *Environmental factors:*
  - Unlike T2DM, lifestyle factors of diet and exercise are not implicated in the development of autoimmune T1DM; however, some associations have been noted between obesity and the development of T1DM. Past studies have suggested exposure to cow's milk, and certain viral illnesses (Coxsackie B, rubella, and mumps), may increase the risk of T1DM in some patients. Recent cohort analysis examining the effects of early exposure to cow's milk calls this long-standing theory into question.
- *Genome-wide associations:*
  - While much of the genetic susceptibility to T1DM is attributable to the human leukocyte antigen (HLA) region, many other associations exist. Please see Tables 54-1 and 54-2 for review of candidate genes and loci.
- *Pharmacogenomics:*
  - At this time, no pharmacogenetic testing has been established in guiding treatment of T1DM. Mechanisms elucidated by candidate genes and phenotype-modifying alleles may drive future research into possible pharmacogenomic applications.

## Diagnostic Criteria and Clinical Characteristics

### Diagnostic Criteria for Diabetes:

- Fasting plasma glucose greater than or equal to 126 mg/dL (6.7 mmol/L) *plus* symptoms *or* on greater than one occasion
- Random plasma glucose greater than or equal to 200 mg/dL (11.1 mmol/L) *plus* symptoms
- 75 g oral glucose tolerance test leading to 2-hour plasma glucose greater than or equal to 200 mg/dL

As of January 2010, the use of glycosylated hemoglobin ($HbA_{1c}$) criteria for the diagnosis of DM has been accepted by the American Diabetes Association. In addition to the established criteria earlier, these guidelines allow for $HbA_{1c}$ greater than or equal to 6.5% to be considered diagnostic of diabetes, with $HbA_{1c}$ 5.7% to 6.4% classified as prediabetes. In the case of T1DM, the International Expert Committee recommendations on which these guidelines were based specified that $HbA_{1c}$ should be used only in the absence of classic clinical symptoms.

Unlike T2DM, T1DM frequently presents with ketoacidosis. Therefore, a young lean patient presenting with clear ketoacidosis can receive a diagnosis of T1DM without further confirmatory testing. The overweight patient warrants further investigation given the increasing incidence of T2DM in childhood.

Diagnostic evaluation for T1DM should include

- Insulin or C-peptide less than 5 μU/mL, or 0.6 ng/mL is suggestive of T1DM. Note that a patient with T2DM in a high glucose state may temporarily have low C-peptide, but insulin secretion function should recover following the acute episode.
- Glutamic acid decarboxylase (GAD) antibodies—titers are high in T1DM.
- Islet cell antibodies—titers are high in T1DM.
- Thyroxine and thyroid antibodies may be checked to assess risk for thyroid dysfunction.

*Table 54-1  Type 1 Diabetes Association With HLA Typing*

| MHC Class (Chromosome Location) | HLA Type | Relative Risk or Odds Ratio | Frequency of Risk Allele | Putative Functional Significance | Associated Disease Phenotype |
|---|---|---|---|---|---|
| Class I (6p21.3) | HLA-A8 | RR 2.12 | | Interaction with TCR and KIR | |
| | HLA-A W15 | RR >1.5 | | Interaction with TCR and KIR | |
| | HLA-B*39 | RR>1.5 | | Interaction with TCR and KIR | |
| Class II (6p21.1) | HLA-DR3 (B8) | Risk increased (OR ~6.8) | 15% nondiabetic population | Presentation of antigens to CD4+ cells | Increased association with autoantibodies, especially GADA |
| | HLA-DR4 (B15) | Risk increased (OR ~6.8) Fathers with DR4 are more likely to transmit DR4 to their offspring than are mothers with DR4. Patients with both B8 and B15 antigens have greatly increased risk (synergistic effect on IDDM predisposition) | 22% nondiabetic population; 43% diabetic population; DR3/DR4 occurs in 35% diabetic population | Presentation of antigens to CD4+ cells. Associated with insulin-reactive clonally expanded T cells | Increased association with autoantibodies, especially GADA. Shows antibody response to exogenous insulin |
| | HLA-DRB1*04 | Risk increased | | Presentation of antigens to CD4+ cells | Associated with insulin and IA-2 autoantibodies |
| | HLA-DQA1*0301 | Risk increased | | Presentation of antigens to CD4+ cells | Associated with insulin and IA-2 autoantibodies |
| | HLA-DQB1*0302 | Risk increased (OR ~6.8) | | Presentation of antigens to CD4+ cells | Associated with insulin and IA-2 autoantibodies |
| | HLA-DQw8 | Risk increased | | Presentation of antigens to CD4+ cells | Associated with autoantibodies, especially GADA |
| | HLA-DQw1.2 | Risk decreased (RR is 0.37 for DQw1.2/DQw8, indicating dominant protective effect of DQw1.2) | 2.3% of diabetic population; 36.7% of nondiabetic population | Presentation of antigens to CD4+ cells | |
| | HLA-DQA1*0102-DQB1*0602 | Risk decreased | | Presentation of antigens to CD4+ cells | Protective effect may occur after disease process has started (association with + antibodies in absence of clinical disease) |

*(Continued)*

*Table 54-1* **Type 1 Diabetes Association With HLA Typing (Continued)**

| MHC Class (Chromosome Location) | HLA Type | Relative Risk or Odds Ratio | Frequency of Risk Allele | Putative Functional Significance | Associated Disease Phenotype |
|---|---|---|---|---|---|
| | HLA-DR2 | Risk decreased | | Presentation of antigens to CD4+ cells | |
| MICA: MHC class I chain-related gene A (6p21.3) | MICA5 | Increased risk for T1DM diagnosis age <25 | | Binds NKG2D and stimulates NK and T-cell effect or functions | Early age of onset. |
| | MICA5.1 | Increased risk for T1DM only for diagnosis at age >25, and in combination with high-risk MHC class II haplotypes | | Binds NKG2D and stimulates NK and T-cell effect or functions | Late age of onset (also confers risk for LADA) |

TCR, T-cell receptor; KIR, killer immunoglobulin-like receptor; NK, natural killer cells.

*Table 54-2* **Type 1 Diabetes-Associated Non-HLA Susceptibility Variants**

| Candidate Gene (Chromosome Location) | Associated Variant (DB SNP) | Odds Ratio | Putative Functional Significance |
|---|---|---|---|
| PTPN22 (1p13.2) | rs2476601 | OR 2.05 | Lymphoid protein tyrosine phosphatase, nonreceptor type 22. LYP downregulates signaling from T-cell receptor, the mutation enhances function leading to increased T-cell suppression. |
| BACH2 (6q15) | rs11755527 | OR 1.13 | Basic leucine zipper transcription factor 2 |
| TNFAIP3 (6q23.3) | rs6920220 | OR 1.09 | Tumor necrosis factor, alpha-induced protein 3 |
| | rs10499194 | OR 0.90 | |
| PTPN2 (18p11.21) | rs45450798 | OR 1.28 | Protein tyrosine phosphatase, nonreceptor type 2 |
| | rs478582 | OR 0.83 | |
| CD226 (18q22.2) | rs763361 | OR 1.16 | CD226 molecule |
| TAGAP (6q25.3) | rs1738074 | | T-cell activation GTPase-activating protein (coregulated with IL-2) |
| SH2B3 (12q24) | rs3184504 | | Lymphocyte adaptor protein |
| KIAA0350 (16p13) | rs2903692 | | Predicted to encode a sugar-binding C-type lectin |
| | rs725613 | | |
| | rs17673553 | | |
| ERBB3 (12q13.2) | rs2292239 | OR 1.31 | Tyrosine kinase type cell-surface receptor, HER3 |

*Clinical Characteristics:* T1DM is a disorder of insulin secretion. The resulting insulin deficit causes both acute symptoms, as well as long-term sequelae.

> **Effects of acute hyperglycemia:** polyuria, polydipsia, weight loss (with or without polyphagia), and blurred vision. Diabetic ketoacidosis is common with T1DM; the associated electrolyte derangements are life-threatening.
>
> **Effects of chronic hyperglycemia:** impaired growth, susceptibility to infections, retinopathy, nephropathy, as well as peripheral and autonomic neuropathy. In addition to microvascular complications, DM is associated with macrovascular atherosclerotic disease, ischemic heart disease, and cerebrovascular disease.

## Screening and Counseling

*Screening:* In contrast with T2DM, current guidelines do not recommend screening for T1DM in the general population. Risk assessment by HLA typing may be of some benefit to siblings of affected patients but is not a routine test. At this time, monitoring of at-risk patients is generally accomplished by screening for islet autoantibodies.

*Counseling:* Concordance for monozygotic twins is 45%, whereas dizygotic twin concordance is 25%. While the monozygotic concordance rate is significant, it is far from 100%, indicating a strong role for, as yet unidentified, environmental factors.

For siblings of patients with T1DM, the average reported risk is 6%, with an observed risk of DM by age 50 of 10%. In comparison with the 0.5% risk in the general population, the family history indicates a 20-fold increase in risk. That the risk of disease is higher for dizygotic twin siblings than for nontwin siblings may be explained by increased environmental similarity, including intrauterine exposures.

For offspring of a father with T1DM, the risk of disease is 6%; for those with a mother with T1DM, the risk of disease is 2%. The underlying mechanism for this gender-based difference has yet to be established but may be influenced by genetic factors (Tables 54-1 and 54-2).

Of note, regardless of gender, the risk to offspring has been shown to be twofold when a parent is diagnosed before age 11 years as compared with diagnosis after age 11 years.

## Management and Treatment

Because T1DM is a disorder of insulin secretion rather than insulin sensitivity, patients are critically dependent on exogenous insulin. The decision to initiate insulin versus oral hypoglycemic medicines is based on clinical differentiation between T1DM and T2DM, rather than genetic assessment.

*Pharmacogenetics:* Within T1DM, pharmacogenetic distinctions have not yet been established to guide treatment. Future directions may include genetic screening of patients with T1DM to help guide prevention of microvascular complications (see section on *MVCD* genes later).

Diabetes developing in the first 6 months of life (neonatal diabetes) is initially treated with insulin but is not necessarily a form of T1DM. Neonatal diabetes can be either permanent or transient (in which case the patient often goes on to develop T2DM later in childhood or early adulthood). Several causative mutations have now been identified for both types of neonatal diabetes, and genetic testing is now recommended for all neonatal diabetes patients. Older children and adults who were initially diagnosed with neonatal diabetes may also benefit from genetic testing if it was not undertaken at the time of diagnosis (see Genetic Testing section). This includes testing for known mutations in *KCNJ11* and *ABCC8*, as mutations in these genes are associated with diabetes that is often more easily controlled by high-dose sulfonylureas instead of insulin.

## Molecular Genetics and Molecular Mechanisms

Two subtypes of T1DM have been established: type 1A and type 1B. Type 1A is immune mediated, and accounts for the vast majority of T1DM. Type 1B, which includes rare nonimmune forms, is genetically distinct. We will focus on type 1A for the majority of this chapter, and discuss type 1B separately. (For all intents and purposes, T1DM refers to type 1A unless otherwise specified.)

*Molecular Genetics:* Genetic susceptibility to T1DM can best be described as complex. To comprehensively elucidate the currently known genetic associations, we will break these down into three categories: 1. HLA typing, 2. candidate gene findings, and 3. loci identified by linkage. We will also address additional associations found to modify not the risk for diabetes itself, but the severity of complications. As of October 2009, 43 separate loci have been identified.

☞**THE HLA REGIONS:** Approximately 50% of genetic susceptibility to T1DM can be accounted for by variations in the HLA regions on 6p21. While multiple loci within the HLA complex have associations with T1DM, genotyping for HLA-DR and HLA-DQ alone allows for identification of high-risk individuals with 90% of T1DM patients having at least one of the recognized high-risk haplotypes at these loci compared to 20% of the general population.

**A word on overlap with T2DM:** In individuals with HLA class II risk haplotypes (DR3[17]-DQA1*0501-DQB1*02 or DR4*0401/4-DQA1*0301-DQB1*0302), there was shown to be a higher risk of impaired glucose tolerance, both with and without GAD antibodies. It is possible that the known clustering of T1DM and T2DM in some families may be mediated in part by the HLA locus.

☞**NON-HLA CANDIDATE GENES:** Genome-wide association studies (GWAS) and candidate gene analyses have yielded evidence for the role of non-HLA genes in T1DM susceptibility. While the associated risks are generally smaller than with established high-risk HLA haplotypes, the elucidated pathways may present points for potential intervention.

☞**ADDITIONAL LOCI IDENTIFIED BY LINKAGE:** Extensive linkage analysis has yielded the identification of the so-called "IDDM loci" 1 to 18 (except 14 and 16). Many of these loci currently have only preliminary or minimal evidence for T1DM susceptibility. We include here only those with highly significant LOD scores, or a putative functional significance of interest (Table 54-3).

☞**VARIANTS AFFECTING PHENOTYPE:** The microvascular complications of diabetes (*MVCD*) genes have been associated with increased susceptibility to proliferative retinopathy,

*Table 54-3 Type 1 Diabetes-Linked Loci*

| IDDM Gene (Chromosome Location) | Associated Gene/Marker | LOD Score/Sibling Risk | Putative Functional Significance |
|---|---|---|---|
| *IDDM1* (6p21) | HLA region including *TNFA* | LOD 116.3, sibling risk 3.35 | |
| *IDDM2* (11p15.5) | VNTR polymorphism, in 5′ region flanking insulin gene (*INS*) *D11S922* | LOD 1.87 sibling risk 1.16 Increased risk conferred with paternal transmission, suggesting role of imprinting | Affects level of expression of insulin gene in thymus |
| *IDDM12* (2q33) | *CTLA4* gene | LOD 3.57 | CTLA4 (cytotoxic T-lymphocyte associated)-costimulatory molecule expressed by activated T cells |
| *IDDM15* (6q21) | *D6S283* (closest marker) | LOD 22.39 sibling risk 1.56 | |

nephropathy, and neuropathy. Variation in *MVCD1*, for example, leads to increased vascular endothelial growth factor (VEGF) activity, and thus to microvascular proliferation. At present seven *MVCD* genes have been identified (Table 54-4).

**A word on diabetes type 1B:** A minority of patients with T1DM have clear insulin deficiency and are susceptible to ketoacidosis, but show no evidence of autoimmunity, and variable HLA association. Type 1B diabetes does not appear to represent a single etiology but is characterized by episodic ketoacidosis, with varying degrees of insulin dependence between episodes, often with only an intermittent absolute requirement for insulin. The majority of these patients are of African or Asian ancestry, suggesting a genetically distinct disorder with clear phenotypic differences.

The prevalence of atypical diabetes is estimated to be 0.1% to 0.8% in Africa and 1.2% to 1.6% in the Caribbean. The prevalence may be higher in obese persons of African ancestry living in the United States and Europe. In a study of West Africans with KPDM, the most common atypical form, mutations in the *PAX4* gene (7q32) conferred blunted insulin secretion in response to glucose, with variable degrees of insulin resistance (higher in patients with obesity). Of KPDM patients of West African ancestry, 4% are homozygous *R113W*. The rarer *R37W* mutation confers a more severe phenotype. In contrast, a US study of KPDM found no evidence of mutation in *PAX4* or in several other candidate genes concluding that this form was not predominantly of a monogenic etiology.

*Table 54-4 Type 1 Genes With Variants Affecting Diabetes Phenotype*

| Gene | Also Known as | Location |
|---|---|---|
| *VEGF* | *MVCD1* | 6p12 |
| *EPO* | *MVCD2* | 7q21 |
| *ACE* | *MVCD3* | 17q23 |
| *IL1RN* | *MVCD4* | 2q14.2 |
| *PON1* | *MVCD5* | 7q21.3 |
| *SOD2* | *MVCD6* | 6p25.3 |
| *HFE* | *MVCD7* | 6p21.3 |

**Molecular Mechanisms:** The clear association of risk for T1DM (particularly the autoimmune subcategory of type 1A) with the HLA region is not surprising. MHC class I heavy chains are encoded within the HLA region on chromosome 6 (the light chain, B2-microglobulin, is encoded on chromosome 15). HLA-A, HLA-B, and HLA-C all interact with T-cell receptor (TCR) molecules as well as with the products of the killer immunoglobulin-like receptor (KIR) genes expressed on natural killer cells and some T cells.

For MHC class II (HLA-DR, HLA-DP, and HLA-DQ), both alpha and beta chains are encoded on 6p21.1. Variability exists in DP and DQ alpha and beta chains; the DR alpha chain is not polymorphic, with variability conferred by DR beta chain only. The precise mechanism whereby variability within HLA molecules causes T1DM remains uncertain. Failure of T cells to successfully present self-peptides to T cells in the thymus can lead to a failure of self-tolerance and thus the development of autoimmunity. It has also been postulated that there is also a failure in peripheral tolerance with the presentation of specific peptides to T cells. Different MHC class II antigens may be related to alterations in conformation which then alter the ability of certain peptides to be presented to T cells.

While the non-HLA associations tend to be less potent, their mechanisms contribute to our understanding of T1DM, as well as autoimmune disease in general. As examples, both *PTPN22* and *CTLA4* are associated with T1DM as well as other autoimmune conditions.

*PTPN22* codes for lymphoid protein tyrosine phosphatase (LYP) which interacts with C-terminal Src kinase (CSK) to downregulate T-cell receptor signaling. The rs2476601 single-nucleotide polymorphism (SNP) (C-T at 1858) causes an arginine to tryptophan substitution (R520W) that disrupts LYP complex formation with CSK. The mutation actually results in increased activity leading to reduced T-cell activation. This mechanism has also been reported to modify risk in other autoimmune conditions such as rheumatoid arthritis, systemic lupus erythematosus (SLE), and Graves disease.

Cytotoxic T-lymphocyte associated (*CTLA4*) is a member of the immunoglobulin superfamily. It is expressed by activated T cells and acts as a costimulatory molecule binding to B7-1 and B7-2 on antigen-presenting cells (APCs). *CTLA4* acts to override the TCR-induced stop signal necessary for T cell and APC conjugate formation. The resultant decrease in T-cell and APC conjugation leads to decreased cytokine production. T1DM has been associated with an increased transmission of the G allele of the 49A or G SNP in exon 1. This same polymorphism in *CTLA4* has also been shown with Graves disease, celiac disease, and SLE.

Other associated genes are related only to risk for T1DM rather than to autoimmunity in general—an example would be the variable number of tandem repeats (VNTR) associated with the insulin gene (*INS*). Three alleles are considered based on the VNTRs—the class I allele has the least VNTRs and the class III has the most. Homozygotes for class I alleles are at highest risk for T1DM while class III alleles are associated with increased expression of insulin in the thymus. It is thought that this could protect against T1DM by allowing greater exposure of T cells to insulin in the thymus allowing development of tolerance, or by allowing the development of insulin responsive T-regulatory cells.

***Genetic Testing:*** At this time, clinical genetic testing is available for forms of permanent neonatal diabetes mellitus (PNDM) and *KCNJ11*-related transient neonatal diabetes mellitus (see Gene Tests). Such testing is useful in predicting the course of disease, which varies with genotype (testing for PNDM includes all five known associated genes: *KCNJ11, ABCC8, INS, GCK,* and *PDX1*).

For T1DM, clinical genetic testing is not currently pursued. While HLA typing may be useful in risk assessment for siblings, such testing may become more routine if clinically beneficial prevention strategies are developed.

***Future Directions:*** Strategies for improved prediction of the development of T1DM are critical for studies of prevention or disease modification. In addition to predictive value, the candidate genes discussed offer potential targets for intervention (eg, selective inhibition of *PTPN22* may be useful in the subset of T1DM patients for whom this gene is implicated). The *MVCD* genes provide similar opportunities for disease modification. Would patients at increased risk of microvascular complications benefit from earlier initiation of an angiotensin-converting enzyme (ACE) inhibitor? For patients with excessive VEGF activity, could there be a role for bevacizumab? Certainly providing VEGF inhibition to patients with diabetes poses a risk for hypertension and proteinuria, but genetic testing may allow us to identify the subset of patients with diabetes and VEGF hyperactivity that may benefit from such treatment. In essence, the genetic variations discussed in this chapter serve as a basis for the development of personalized medicine in the treatment of diabetes.

## BIBLIOGRAPHY:

1. American Diabetes Association. Diagnosis and classification of diabetes mellitus. *Diabetes Care.* 2008;31(suppl 1):S55-S60.

2. Concannon P, Rich SS, Nepom GT. Genetics of type 1A diabetes. *N Engl J Med.* 2009;360:1646-1654.

3. Haaland WC, Scaduto DI, MaldonadoMR, et al. A-beta-subtype of ketosis-prone diabetes is not predominantly a monogenic diabetic syndrome. *Diabetes Care.* 2009;32:873-877.

4. International Expert Committee. International Expert Committee report on the role of the A1C assay in the diagnosis of diabetes. *Diabetes Care.* 2009;32(7):1327-1334.

5. Kent SC, Chen Y, Bregoli L, et al. Expanded T cells from pancreatic lymph nodes of type 1 diabetic subjects recognize an insulin epitope. *Nature.* 2005;435:224-228.

6. Li H, Lindholm E, Almgren P, et al. Possible human leukocyte antigen-mediated genetic interaction between type 1 and type 2 diabetes. *J Clin Endocr Metab.* 2001;86:574-582.

7. Redondo MJ, Eisenbarth GS. Genetic control of autoimmunity in type I diabetes and associated disorders. *Diabetologia.* 2002;45(5):605-622.

8. Savilahti E, Saarinen KM. Early infant feeding and type 1 diabetes. *Eur J Nutr.* 2009;48(4):243-249.

9. Schneider H, Downey J, Smith A, et al. Reversal of the TCR stop signal by CTLA-4. *Science.* 2006;313:1972-1975.

10. Shiina T, Hosomichi K, Inoko H, Kulski JK. The HLA genomic loci map: expression, interaction, diversity and disease. *J Hum Genet.* 2009;54:15-39.

11. Sobngwi E, Mauvais-Jarvis F, Vexiau P, Mbanya JC, Gautier JF. Diabetes in Africans. Part 2. Ketosis-prone atypical diabetes mellitus. *Diabetes Metab.* 2002;28:5-12.

12. Umpierrez GE, Smiley D, Kitabchi AE. Ketosis-prone type 2 diabetes mellitus. *Ann Intern Med.* 2006;144:350-357.

13. Vang T, Congia M, Macis MD, et al. Autoimmune-associated lymphoid tyrosine phosphatase is a gain-of-function variant. *Nat Genet.* 2005;37:1317-1319.

14. T1Dbase. http://www.T1dbase.org, Accessed October, 2009.

15. dbMHC. http://www.ncbi.nlm.nih.gov/projects/gv/mhc. Accessed November, 2009.

## Supplementary Information

### OMIM REFERENCES:

[1] Diabetes Mellitus, Insulin-Dependent; IDDM (*222100)

[2] Major Histocompatibility Complex, Class I, A; HLA-A (*142800)

[3] Major Histocompatibility Complex, Class II, DR-ALPHA; HLA-DRA (*142860)

[4] Major Histocompatibility Complex, Class I Chain-Related Gene A; MICA (*600169)

[5] Cytotoxic T-Lymphocyte Associated 4; CTLA4 (*123890)

[6] Protein Tyrosine Phosphatase, Nonreceptor Type 22; PTPN22 (*600716)

[7] Microvascular Complications of Diabetes, Susceptibility to 1; MVCD1 (#603933)

[8] Diabetes Mellitus, Ketosis-Prone; KPD, PAX4 (#612227)

***Key Words:*** Diabetes, diabetic retinopathy, major histocompatability complex, ketoacidosis

# 55 Diabetes Mellitus Type 2

Sruti Chandrasekaran and Braxton D. Mitchell

## KEY POINTS

- *Disease summary:*
  - Diabetes is a chronic metabolic disorder characterized by high levels of blood glucose that may lead to micro- and macrovascular complications if not controlled effectively. Type 2 diabetes mellitus (T2DM), which is characterized by defects in insulin secretion and insulin action, is the most common form of diabetes.

- *Differential diagnosis:*
  - Secondary causes of hyperglycemia should be considered. The classic differential diagnosis includes type 1 diabetes, maturity-onset diabetes of the young (MODY), pancreatic dysfunction, gestational diabetes, and other causes of obesity and insulin resistance, such as Cushing syndrome, acromegaly, polycystic ovarian disease, and drug-induced hyperglycemia (glucocorticoids).

- *Screening:*
  - Routine screening for T2DM should be performed in overweight patients, including children, possessing additional risk factors at least in every 3 years. In the absence of risk factors, testing for diabetes should begin at age 45.

- *Hereditary basis:*
  - T2DM is a polygenic disorder with 40% to 60% heritability. About 2% to 3% of diabetes is inherited as monogenic forms of diabetes; the most common monogenic forms are referred as MODY to distinguish them from type 1 and type 2 diabetes.

- *Family history and twin studies:*
  - The risk of developing T2DM in siblings of patients with T2DM is up to three times higher than that of the general population. Monozygotic twins have a 60% or higher long-term concordance rate for diabetes, much higher than the 25% concordance rate observed for T1DM in monozygotic twins.

- *Environmental factors:*
  - Obesity, sedentary lifestyle

- *Genome-wide associations:*
  - At least 37 variants have been associated with T2DM. All have small effect sizes and the known risk alleles, even collectively, do a poor job at predicting the future development of diabetes.

- *Pharmacogenetics:*
  - Identifying genetic variants that predict response to the blood glucose-lowering effects of antidiabetic medications is of great interest because of the high prevalence of diabetes and the large number of patients prescribed such medications. At present, there is insufficient basis for prescribing medication based on genotype.

## Diagnostic Criteria and Clinical Characteristics

**Diagnostic Criteria for Diabetes:**

**One of the following**

1. Fasting plasma glucose (FPG) greater than or equal to 126 mg/dL
2. Two-hour plasma glucose greater than or equal to 200 mg/dL during an oral glucose tolerance test (OGTT).
3. In a patient with classic symptoms of hyperglycemia or hyperglycemic crisis, a random plasma glucose greater than or equal to 200 mg/dL
4. Hemoglobin $A_{1c}$ greater than or equal to 6.5%

**Diagnostic Criteria for Prediabetes:**

**One of the following**

1. FPG between 100 to 125 mg/dL
2. Two-hour plasma glucose of 140 to 199 mg/dL during a 75-g OGTT
3. Hemoglobin $A_{1c}$ of 5.7% to 6.4%

**Clinical Characteristics:** Diabetes is characterized by high levels of plasma glucose. T2DM, which is due to defects in insulin sensitivity and/or insulin secretion, is the most common form of diabetes, affecting 8.3% of the US population with 18.8 million people

diagnosed and about 7 million undiagnosed. The clinical symptoms include weight loss, increased urination, increased thirst, hunger, blurred vision, asthenia, tiredness, irritability, and a characteristic darkening of skin in body folds and creases (acanthosis nigricans). Patients with T2DM can present with frequent and recurrent infections of the bladder, gums, skin, and vagina, ulcers that are difficult to heal, and numbness and tingling sensation of the hands and feet with or without other classic symptoms of diabetes. The discovery of abnormal blood glucose readings is frequently made during routine screening, emphasizing the importance of screening and counseling of these patients.

☞COMPLICATIONS OF DIABETES: The major T2DM-associated complications arise from micro- and macrovascular complications, and may include retinopathy, nephropathy, neuropathy, cardiovascular disease, cerebrovascular disease, and autonomic dysfunction in the form of erectile dysfunction, postural hypotension, and urinary incontinence.

## Screening and Counseling

**Screening for Type 2 Diabetes:** Screening for type 2 diabetes is noteworthy because the same test that is used for screening is also used for the diagnosis of the disease. Routine screening for diabetes should follow these guidelines:

1. Testing should be considered in all adults who are overweight (body mass index [BMI] $\geq25$ kg/m$^2$) and have additional risk factors:

   Physical inactivity; first-degree relative with diabetes; high-risk race or ethnicity (eg, African American, Latino, Native American, Asian American, Pacific Islander); women who delivered a baby weighing 9 lb or greater or previously diagnosed with gestational diabetes (GDM); hypertension (140/90 mm Hg or on therapy for hypertension); high-density lipoprotein (HDL) cholesterol level less than 35 mg/dL and/or a triglyceride level greater than 250 mg/dL; women with polycystic ovarian syndrome (PCOS); hemoglobin A$_{1c}$ greater than 5.7%, impaired glucose tolerance, or impaired fasting glucose on previous testing; other clinical conditions associated with insulin resistance (eg, severe obesity, acanthosis nigricans); or history of cardiovascular disease

2. In the absence of the above criteria, testing for diabetes should begin at age 45.

3. If screening results are normal, testing should be repeated at least at 3-year intervals, with consideration of more frequent testing depending on initial results and risk.

4. FPG, hemoglobin A$_{1c}$, or OGTT is appropriate to screen for diabetes and to assess the risk for future diabetes.

Obesity and T2DM are appearing at alarming rates in children. The recommended screening in children and youth according to American Diabetes Association (ADA) guidelines includes the following:

- Overweight (BMI >85th percentile for age and sex, weight for height >85th percentile, or weight >120% of ideal for height)

**Plus any of the two of the following four risk factors**

1. Family history of T2DM in a first- or second-degree relative
2. Race or ethnicity (Native American, African American, Latino, Asian American, Pacific Islander)
3. Signs of insulin resistance or conditions associated with insulin resistance (acanthosis nigricans, hypertension, dyslipidemia, PCOS, or small-for-gestational-age birth weight)
4. Maternal history of diabetes or GDM during the child's gestation

In these high-risk children, it is recommended that testing be initiated at age 10 years or at the time of puberty (whichever is earlier), and that testing be repeated in every 3 years.

*Counseling:* While the heritability of T2DM is 40% to 60%, consistent with a moderate tendency of the disease to cluster in families, there is not a strong genotype-phenotype correlation; that is, the known risk alleles for T2DM have a relatively low penetrance. If a patient has T2DM, the lifetime risk of his or her sibling becoming affected is up to three times higher than that of the general population. Monozygotic twins have a 60% or higher long-term concordance rate for diabetes, much higher than the 25% concordance rate observed for T1DM in monozygotic twins. Much of the familial clustering of T2DM is thought to be due to shared lifestyle risk factors among family members against the backdrop of an increased genetic susceptibility. Counseling to prevent T2DM thus chiefly involves promoting diabetes protective behaviors, such as physical activity and weight control.

## Management and Treatment

A primary goal of blood glucose screening is to detect prediabetes and prevent or delay the onset of diabetes through effective lifestyle intervention and counseling. The beneficial effects of lifestyle changes and weight management on reducing diabetes risk have been well established. In the Diabetes Prevention Program nondiabetic individuals with elevated fasting and postprandial glucose concentrations were randomized into placebo, metformin, and intensive lifestyle intervention arms. The goals of the intensive lifestyle intervention arm were a 7% decrease (or greater) in body weight and at least 150 min/wk of physical activity. After 3 years of follow-up, diabetes incidence was 58% lower in the lifestyle group (and 31% lower in the metformin group) compared to the placebo group. Based on these and other data, the American Diabetes Association (ADA) recommends lifestyle change as a cornerstone in the treatment of diabetes.

Management of established T2DM is typically based on intensive lifestyle changes coupled with pharmacotherapy with the goal of reducing the micro- and macrovascular complications that accompany the disease. A hemoglobin A$_{1c}$ goal of less than 7% has been recommended by ADA and less than 6.5% by the American Association of Clinical Endocrinologists. The Veterans Administration guidelines recommend individualizing glycemic targets for individuals based on the presence or absence of comorbidities.

*Nonpharmacologic Methods:* This includes medical nutrition therapy, diabetes self-management, and counseling that stress the importance of physical activity to effectively manage blood glucose control and improve insulin sensitivity.

*Pharmacologic Therapy:* This includes noninsulin and insulin-based therapies. Noninsulin-based therapies include biguanides, sulfonylureas, glinides, alpha-glucosidase inhibitors, thiazolidinediones (TZDs), DPP-4 inhibitors, GLP-1 agonists, amylin agonists, bile acid sequestrants, and dopamine agonists. Insulin-based therapies include long-, intermediate-, and short-acting insulin therapies and the use of insulin pumps.

☞**BIGUANIDES:** The major drug in this class is metformin. It works by decreasing hepatic glucose output, lowering fasting glycemia, increasing insulin-mediated glucose utilization in muscle or liver. Its antilipolytic effect reduces free fatty acids which in turn reduces substrate for gluconeogenesis. Metformin is weight neutral, has no risk of hypoglycemia, and on average results in a hemoglobin A$_{1c}$ reduction of 1.5% to 2%. The major side effects include a metallic taste in mouth, mild anorexia, nausea, diarrhea, and interference with B$_{12}$ absorption. Metformin is renally excreted and it has to be renally dosed and it is contraindicated in patients with a glomerular filtration rate (GFR) less than 30.

☞**SULFONYLUREA:** The major drugs in this class include glyburide, glimepiride, glipizide, gliclazide. These drugs enhance insulin secretion by binding to the K$_{ATP}$ channel (sulphfonylurea [SU] receptor) on beta cells, resulting in depolarization and opening of Ca$^{2+}$ channels, increasing insulin secretion. SUs result in a hemoglobin A$_{1c}$ reduction of about 1.5%. The disadvantage with this class of drug is weight gain and hypoglycemia. Side effects include nausea, skin reactions (photosensitivity), and abnormal liver function tests.

☞**GLINIDES:** This class includes repaglinide and nateglinide which work by stimulating insulin secretion by binding to a different site on the SU receptor. Since they are short acting they are usually given three times a day with meals. Though the risk of hypoglycemia is less than the SUs, this group of drugs also causes hypoglycemia and weight gain. A hemoglobin $A_{1c}$ reduction of about 1.5% is achieved with this group of medications.

☞**ALPHA-GLUCOSIDASE INHIBITORS:** The drug in this class is acarbose, which works by reducing the rate of polysaccharide absorption in the proximal small intestine thus lowering postprandial glucose levels. The average hemoglobin $A_{1c}$ reduction is about 0.5% to 0.9%. Acarbose is weight neutral but causes gastrointestinal discomfort and patient tolerability is low due to these side effects.

☞**TZDs:** Drugs include rosiglitazone and pioglitazone. These medications are peroxisome-proliferator-activated receptor gamma (PPARγ or PPARG) modulators and increase sensitivity of muscle, fat, and liver to insulin by increasing glucose transporter expression and by inhibiting hepatic gluconeogensis. The hemoglobin $A_{1c}$ reduction is about 1% to 1.4%; side effects include weight gain, fluid retention, and peripheral edema and are contraindicated in class III or IV heart failure. Rosiglitazone carries a black box warning about its increased risk of myocardial infarction and death from cardiovascular disease. In 2011 French and German medical agencies suspended the use of pioglitazone because of a potential increased risk of bladder cancer; the US FDA mandated a black box warning about bladder cancer and the use of pioglitazone.

☞**DPP-4 INHIBITORS:** The drugs in this class include sitagliptin, saxagliptin, and linagliptin. This class of drug works by inhibiting dipeptidyl peptidase-4, the enzyme which degrades glucagon-like peptide (GLP) and gastric inhibitory polypeptide (GIP) and increases glucose-mediated insulin secretion. DPP-4 inhibitors result in a hemoglobin $A_{1c}$ reduction of 0.6% to 0.9% and the side effects include increased risk of upper respiratory tract infection, urinary tract infection, C-cell hyperplasia, and pancreatitis. They are weight neutral and have decreased incidence of hypoglycemia. The FDA has approved them as monotherapy or in combination with TZD, SU, or metformin in the treatment of diabetes.

☞**GLUCAGON-LIKE PEPTIDE-1 AGONISTS:** The two drugs that are FDA approved in this class are exenatide and liraglutide. They potentiate glucose-stimulated insulin secretion by binding to the GLP-1 receptor on the beta cell and suppress glucagon secretion and slow gastric motility. They also work in the brain by decreasing appetite and food intake. This class of drug has an average hemoglobin $A_{1c}$ reduction of 0.5% to 1% and the major side effects include nausea, vomiting, diarrhea, and risk of pancreatitis. Liraglutide has been shown to cause C-cell hyperplasia. The advantage of this class is weight loss of about 2 to 3 kg in average. They do not cause hypoglycemia by themselves, although they can do so in combination with other insulin-secreting drugs, such as SU.

☞**AMYLIN AGONISTS:** Pramlinitide is a synthetic analogue of the beta-cell hormone amylin which acts by slowing gastric emptying and inhibiting glucagon production in glucose-dependent fashion. This class of drug predominantly decreases postprandial glucose excursions. It is approved for use as adjunctive therapy with regular insulin or rapid-acting insulin analogues and is associated with a hemoglobin $A_{1c}$ reduction of about 0.5% to 0.7% and a weight loss of about 1 to 1.5 kg over 6 months. The major side effect is nausea.

☞**BILE ACID SEQUESTRANTS:** This class of drugs has recently been approved for treatment of type 2 diabetes. The drug colesevelam, representative of this class, is believed to work by reducing endogenous glucose production, increasing incretin secretion, and reducing glucose absorption. Hemoglobin $A_{1c}$ reduction is

very modest at 0.3% to 0.4%. Major side effects include constipation, nausea, and dyspepsia. These drugs are weight neutral. They can reduce low-density lipoprotein (LDL) cholesterol and triglycerides, adding to their utility for patients with dyslipidemia.

☞**DOPAMINE AGONIST:** A timed-release bromocriptine (Cycloset) is FDA approved for type 2 diabetes, and its actions work centrally by modulating serotonin, noradrenaline, and dopamine in brain. These drugs are associated with a modest hemoglobin $A_{1c}$ reduction of 0.5% to 0.7% and they are weight neutral; they have not been shown to cause hypoglycemia. Nausea, vomiting, dizziness, and headache are side effects with this class of medication.

☞**INSULIN:** Insulin is effective in all patients, including those with long-standing diabetes who fail the earlier-mentioned therapies. Insulin is available as long-, intermediate-, and short-acting insulin. Long-acting insulin (glargine and detemir) is usually dosed once a day and its effects last for 24 hours. They are basal insulin. Insulin regular, aspart, lispro, glusiline are bolus insulin and they are given preprandially. NPH is an intermediate-acting insulin and NPH and is available as premixed insulin where it is mixed with short-acting insulin. Only short-acting insulin can be used in insulin pumps; this can be a convenient strategy for managing diabetes.

☞**NEWER DRUGS IN THE PIPELINE:** SGLT-2 inhibitors work by enhancing glucosuria and are currently waiting for FDA approval for diabetes management. Glucagon receptor antagonists work by reducing hepatic glucose overproduction. Glucokinase activators promote hepatic glucose uptake, and pancreatic insulin secretion and sirtuins (resveratrol) mimic the effects of dietary restriction with resulting enhanced glucose utilization, improved insulin sensitivity, and increases in exercise tolerance.

***Bariatric Surgery:*** Bariatric surgery in some patients has been shown to resolve diabetes and/or eliminate the need or pharmacologic therapy. In the hands of experienced surgeons the risk associated with surgery is minimal. Bariatric surgery is recommended for patients with BMI greater than 40 kg/m$^2$ and in those with BMI greater than or equal to 35 kg/m$^2$ with a life-threatening illness that can be improved by weight loss (eg, sleep apnea, type 2 diabetes, heart disease etc).

***Pancreas Transplant:*** While generally considered a treatment option for type 1 diabetes, pancreatic transplants may sometimes be performed in patients with type 2 diabetes, who comprise 6.6% of all transplant patients with diabetes. In patients with type 2 diabetes, indications for pancreatic transplant include age less than 50 to 55 years; BMI less than 30 to 32 kg/m$^2$; fasting C-peptide less than 10 ng/mL; total daily dose of insulin less than 1 U/kg/d; absence of smoking; absence of complications of diabetes including amputation, severe vascular and cardiac disease; and history of dietary and medication compliance.

***Pharmacogenomics of Antidiabetic Drugs:*** The recognition that there is interindividual variability in response to many blood glucose-lowering medications has stimulated interest in assessing whether polymorphisms in drug-metabolizing genes, drug target genes, and diabetes-risk genes influence the response to these drugs. Although some positive associations have been reported in the literature (eg, polymorphisms in *CYP2C9*, *ABCC8*, and *KCNJ11* associated with the blood glucose-lowering response to SU therapy and polymorphisms in organic cation transporter 1 [*SLC22A1*] associated with metformin response), most associations have yet to be replicated. The one exception is a polymorphism (rs11212617) in *ATM*, the ataxia telangiectasia mutated gene, which has recently been associated with variation in the glycemic response to metformin in a large genome-wide association study (GWAS) with replication. *ATM* is involved in DNA repair and cell cycle control, and plays a role in the effect of metformin upstream of AMP-activated protein kinase. However, the clinical significance of this specific association is probably low since the associated single-nucleotide polymorphism (SNP) explains only 2.5% of the variance in metformin response.

## Molecular Genetics and Molecular Mechanism

T2DM is a polygenic disorder for which defects in insulin secretion and insulin action are required. Glucose regulation is a tightly controlled process that involves glucose production from liver (gluconeogenesis), transport of glucose into target cells (insulin action), and secretion of insulin from the pancreas. Defects in any of these processes can disrupt glucose homeostasis and lead to hyperglycemia. The initial genetic studies were association studies involving

candidate genes from the insulin signaling system or were related to pancreatic beta-cell development and function. These studies led to the discovery of the Pro12Ala (rs1801282) variant in *PPARG* and the Glu23Lys (rs5210) variant in the potassium channel gene *KCNJ11*; both variants increase the risk for the development of T2DM. Recent genome-wide studies have implicated many previously unreported genes in type 2 diabetes susceptibility (Table 55-1). One surprise is that the large majority of all of the discovered genes seem to be related to pancreatic beta-cell dysfunction; very few are related to insulin action. Additionally, a T2DM-associated variant in the *FTO* gene appears to exert its effect primarily by increasing adiposity. To date, at least 37 variants have been associated with T2DM, many through GWAS and in genes not previously suspected as being involved in glucose metabolism (Table 55-1). The mechanisms by which most of the discovered genes influence diabetes susceptibility is unknown; of the genes with known connections to diabetes, some are related to pancreatic beta-cell dysfunction, and a few are related to insulin action.

*Table 55-1 Molecular Genetic Testing*

| Candidate Gene | Full Name | Associated Variant (s) | Relative Risk | Frequency of Risk Allele in Caucasians |
|---|---|---|---|---|
| PPARG | Peroxisome-proliferator-activated receptor gamma | rs1801282 | 1.14 | 0.92 |
| KCNJ11 | Potassium inwardly rectifying channel, subfamily J, member 11 | rs5219 | 1.15 | 0.50 |
| TCF7L2 | Transcription factor 7-like 2 | rs7903146 | 1.37 | 0.25 |
| FTO | Fat mass and obesity associated | rs8050136 | 1.15 | 0.45 |
| HHEX | Hematopoietically expressed homeobox | rs1111875 | 1.13 | 0.56 |
| SLC30A8 | Solute carrier family 30 (zinc transporter), member 8 | rs13266634 | 1.12 | 0.75 |
| CDKAL1 | CDK5 regulatory subunit-associated protein 1-like 1 | rs7754840 | 1.12 | 0.31 |
| CDKN2A/2B | Cyclin-dependent kinase inhibitor 2A (and 2B) | rs10811661 | 1.20 | 0.79 |
| IGF2BP2 | Insulin-like growth factor 2 mRNA binding protein 2 | rs4402960 | 1.17 | 0.29 |
| HNF1B | Hepatocyte nuclear factor 1 homeobox B | rs757210 | 1.12 | 0.43 |
| JAZF1 | Juxtaposed with another zinc finger gene 1 | rs864745 | 1.10 | 0.52 |
| CDC123/CAMK1D | Cell division cycle 123 homologue (Saccharomyces cerevisiae); Calcium/calmodulin-dependent protein kinase 1D | rs12779790 | 1.11 | 0.23 |
| TSPAN8/LGR5 | Tetraspanin 8; leucine-rich repeat-containing G-protein coupled | rs7961581 | 1.09 | 0.23 |
| THADA | Thyroid adenoma associated | rs7578597 | 1.15 | 0.92 |
| ADAMTS9 | ADAM metallopeptidase with thrombospondin type 1 motif, 9 | rs4607103 | 1.09 | 0.81 |
| NOTCH2 | Notch homologue 2 (Drosophila) | rs10923931 | 1.13 | 0.11 |
| KCNQ1 | Potassium voltage-gated channel, KQT-like subfamily, member 1 | rs2237892, rs231362 | 1.40, 1.08 | 0.61 (in Japan), 0.52 |

*(Continued)*

*Table 55-1  Molecular Genetic Testing (Continued)*

| Candidate Gene | Full Name | Associated Variant (s) | Relative Risk | Frequency of Risk Allele in Caucasians |
|---|---|---|---|---|
| IRS1 | Insulin receptor substrate 1 | rs2943641 | 1.19 | 0.61 |
| DUSP9 | Dual specificity phosphatase 9 | rs5945326 | 1.27 | 0.12 |
| PROX1 | Prospero homeobox 1 | rs340874 | 1.07 | 0.50 |
| BCL11A | B-cell CLL/lymphoma 11A (zinc finger protein) | rs243021 | 1.08 | 0.46 |
| GCKR | Glucokinase (hexokinase 4) regulator | rs780094 | 1.06 | 0.62 |
| ADCY5 | Adenylate cyclase 5 | rs11708067 | 1.12 | 0.78 |
| WFS1 | Wolfram syndrome 1 (wolframin) | rs1801214 | 1.13 | 0.27 |
| ZBED3 | Zinc finger, BED-type containing 3 | rs4457053 | 1.08 | 0.26 |
| DGKB/TMEM195 | Diacylglycerol kinase, beta 90kDa; alkylglycerol mono-oxygenase | rs2191349 | 1.06 | 0.47 |
| GCK | Glucokinase (hexokinase 4) | rs4607517 | 1.07 | 0.20 |
| KLF14 | Kruppel-like factor 14 | rs972283 | 1.07 | 0.55 |
| TP53INP1 | Tumor protein p53 inducible nuclear protein 1 | rs896854 | 1.06 | 0.48 |
| TLE4 | Transducin-like enhancer of split 4 E(sp1) homolog, Drosophila | rs13292136 | 1.11 | 0.93 |
| CENTD2 | ArfGAP with RhoGAP domain, ankyrin repeat and PH domain 1 | rs1552224 | 1.14 | 0.88 |
| MTNR1B | Melatonin receptor 1B | rs10830963 | 1.09 | 0.30 |
| HMGA2 | High mobility group AT-hook 2 | rs1531343 | 1.10 | 0.10 |
| HNF1A | HNF1 homeobox A | rs7957197 | 1.07 | 0.85 |
| PRC1 | Protein regulator of cytokinesis 1 | rs8042680 | 1.07 | 0.22 |
| ZFAND6 | Zinc finger, AN1-type domain 6 | rs11634397 | 1.06 | 0.56 |

Adapted from Prokopenko, et al., 2008 and Billings LK, Florez JC, 2010.

*Monogenic Forms of Diabetes:* In contrast to T2DM, which is characterized by a polygenic inheritance, a small number of monogenic forms of diabetes have been identified. These disorders tend to be related to an impairment of the body's ability to produce insulin and are inherited in autosomal dominant fashion. The two primary forms of monogenic diabetes are neonatal diabetes mellitus (NDM) and MODY. Collectively, these account for 2% to 3% of all cases of diabetes. MODY usually occurs in children or adolescents but may be mild and not detected until adulthood. MODY is much more common than NDM, which occurs in newborns and young infants. Mutations in nine different genes have been associated with MODY: hepatocyte nuclear factor 4-alpha (*HNF4A*), glucokinase (*GCK*), hepatocyte nuclear factor 1-alpha (*HNF1A*), insulin promoter factor-1 (*IPF-1*), hepatocyte nuclear factor 1-beta (*HNF1B*), and neurogenic differentiation 1 (*NEUROD1*), Kruppel-like factor 11 (*KLF11*), carboxyl ester lipase (*CEL*), and paired box gene 4 (*PAX4*). NDM has been associated with mutations in two different genes: *KCNJ11* and ATP-binding cassette transporter subfamily C member 8 (*ABCC8*).

*Genetic Testing:* To date, at least 37 variants have been associated with T2DM. The most common of these are shown in Table 55-1 below. The effect sizes of these variants are relatively small and even collectively, these variants account for less than 10% of disease susceptibility. Because of their small effect sizes and low penetrance, these variants even collectively are not yet useful for clinical prediction, particularly if one accounts for clinical variables such as BMI and family history of diabetes.

*Future Directions:* Although recent genome-wide associations have identified at least 20 different polymorphisms associated with T2DM, for nearly all loci we do not yet know how the variant affects gene function, nor in most cases how altered function of the associated gene affects T2DM. Whether any of these discoveries will lead to new therapies is not clear.

Because the known variants account for a relatively small part of the genetic susceptibility to diabetes, there remains a significant genetic component to T2DM that has yet to be identified. Current research includes sequencing known candidate genes to detect rare variants having potentially large effect size that might be important for a small number of people. An additional line of current research is to consider the joint effects of lifestyle variables such as body size and sedentary behavior, on genetic risk.

Research into the potential role of pharmacogenomics in T2DM management is just beginning. There is a need for more trials to identify variants associated with medication response. If successful, such research might reveal a benefit to tailoring glucose-lowering treatments to a patient's individual genetic constitution.

## BIBLIOGRAPHY:

1. American Diabetes Association. Standards of medical care in diabetes. *Diabetes Care.* Jan 2011;34(suppl 1):S11-S61.

2. International Expert Committee. International Expert Committee report on the role of the A1C assay in the diagnosis of diabetes. *Diabetes Care.* 2009; 32:1327-1334.

3. Centers for Disease Control and Prevention. National Diabetes Fact Sheet: national estimates and general information on diabetes and prediabetes in the United States. Atlanta, GA: U.S. Department of Health and Human Services, Centers for Disease Control and Prevention; 2011.

4. Kahn R, Alperin P, Eddy D, et al. Age at initiation and frequency of screening to detect type 2 diabetes: a cost-effectiveness analysis. *Lancet.* 2010;375:1365-1374.

5. Knowler WC, Barrett-Connor E, Fowler SE, et al. Reduction in the incidence of type 2 diabetes with lifestyle intervention or metformin. *N Engl J Med.* 2002;346:393-403.

6. Aguilar RB. Evaluating treatment algorithms for the management of patients with type 2 diabetes mellitus: a perspective on the definition of treatment success. *Clin Ther.* 2011;33(4):408-424.

7. Orlando G, Stratta RJ, Light J. Pancreas transplantation for type 2 diabetes mellitus. *Curr Opin Organ Transplant.* Feb 2011;16(1):110-115.

8. Holstein A, Seeringer A, Kovacs P. Therapy with oral antidiabetic drugs: applied pharmacogenetics. *Br J Diabetes Vasc Dis.* 2011;11:10-16.

9. The GoDARTS and UKPDS Diabetes Pharmacogenetics Study Group and The Wellcome Trust Case Control Consortium 2. Common variants near *ATM* are associated with glycemic response to metformin in type 2 diabetes. *Nat Genet.* 2011;43:117-120.

10. Pearson ER. Pharmacogenetics in diabetes. *Curr Diab Rep.* Apr 2009;9(2):172-181.

11. Altshuler D, Hirschhorn JN, Klannemark M, et al. The common PPARgamma Pro12Ala polymorphism is associated with decreased risk of type 2 diabetes. *Nat Genet.* Sep 2000; 26(1):76-80.

12. Gloyn AL, Weedon MN, Owen KR, et al. Large-scale association studies of variants in genes encoding the pancreatic beta-cell KATP channel subunits Kir6.2 (KCNJ11) and SUR1 (ABCC8)

confirm that the KCNJ11 E23K variant is associated with type 2 diabetes. *Diabetes.* Feb 2003;52(2):568-572.

13. Prokopenko I, McCarthy MI, Lindgren CM. Type 2 diabetes: new genes, new understanding. *Trends Genet.* 2008;24:613-621.

14. Billings LK, Florez JC. The genetics of type 2 diabetes: what have we learned from GWAS? *Ann N Y Acad Sci.* 2010;1212:59-77.

## Supplementary Information

### OMIM REFERENCES:

[1] MODY1—Maturity Onset Diabetes of the Young, Type 1; HNF4A (#125850)

[2] MODY2—Maturity Onset Diabetes of the Young, Type 2; GCK (#125851)

[3] MODY3—Maturity Onset Diabetes of the Young, Type 3; HNF1A (#600496)

[4] MODY4—Maturity Onset Diabetes of the Young, Type 4; PDX1 (#606392)

[5] MODY5—Maturity Onset Diabetes of the Young, Type 5; TCF2 (#137920)

[6] MODY6—Maturity Onset Diabetes of the Young, Type 6; NEUROD1 (#606394)

[7] MODY7—Maturity Onset Diabetes of the Young, Type 7; KLF11 (#610508)

[8] MODY8—Maturity Onset Diabetes of the Young, Type 8; CEL (#609812)

[9] MODY9—Maturity Onset Diabetes of the Young, Type 9; PAX4 (#612225)

[10] MODY10—Maturity Onset Diabetes of the Young, Type 10; INS (#613370)

[11] MODY11—Maturity Onset Diabetes of the Young, Type 11; BLK (#613375)

[12] Transient Neonatal Diabetes Mellitus; (#601410)

**Alternative Name:**

None

***Key Words:*** Maturity-onset diabetes of the young, transient neonatal diabetes mellitus, pharmacogenetics

# 56 Maturity-Onset Diabetes of the Young

Justin P. Annes

## KEY POINTS

- *Disease summary:*
  - MODY is estimated to explain 0.2% to 2% of adult diabetes diagnosed before 45 years of age, and is frequently misdiagnosed as either type 1 or type 2 diabetes.
  - The correct diagnosis of MODY is important to inform therapeutic interventions, disease prognosis, presymptomatic screening, and genetic counseling.
  - American Diabetes Association diagnostic categories of diabetes include type 1 diabetes, type 2 diabetes, gestational diabetes, and other specific types of diabetes. The various forms of maturity-onset diabetes of the young (MODY) are classified as "genetic defects of beta-cell function" within the "other specific types" category.

- *Hereditary basis:*
  - All forms of MODY are inherited in an autosomal dominant fashion.
  - Penetrance: Overall estimated at 80% to 95% lifetime; however, lower penetrance diabetes loci such as *HNF1B* (50%) contribute to MODY.
  - Prevalence of MODY is approximately 50 to 200 per million individuals.

- *Genetic differential diagnosis:*
  - It is important to distinguish MODY from mitochondrial diabetes and deafness (MIDD), neonatal diabetes mellitus (NDM), and syndrome-related diabetes.
  - MIDD represents up to 1% of diabetes and is characterized by maternal inheritance and deafness as the name suggests. The most common mitochondrial mutation (m.3243A>G) is also causative of several other mitochondrial syndromes including mitochondrial myopathy, encephalopathy, lactic acidosis and stroke-like episodes syndrome (MELAS) and therefore has phenotypic overlap.
  - NDM is diagnosed before 6 months and may be transient (TNDM) or permanent (PNDM) in nature. TNDM is caused by an imprinting defect in the 6q24 region that leads to excessive paternally derived expression of the *PLAGL1* and *HYMAJ* genes in approximately 70% of cases. PNDM, and less commonly TNDM, may be caused by a mutation in the constituents of the beta-cell K-ATP channel (*KCNJ11* or *ABCC8*). PNDM may also result from homozygous or compound heterozygous loss of function mutations in the *GCK* or *INS* genes. Mutations in the K-ATP channel are important to identify because they may be treated with high-dose sulfonylureas. Patients with TNDM are at increased risk for diabetes in adulthood.
  - Diabetes is associated with several genetic syndromes: Down syndrome, Klinefelter syndrome, Turner syndrome, Wolfram syndrome, Friedreich ataxia, Huntington disease, Laurence-Moon-Biedl syndrome, myotonic dystrophy, porphyria, Prader-Willi syndrome, lipodystrophy, and many others.

## Diagnostic Criteria and Clinical Characteristics

***Diagnostic Criteria for MODY:*** Historic diagnostic criteria for MODY are (1) hyperglycemia typically before age 25 years, (2) an autosomal dominant inheritance pattern affecting three generations, (3) absence of insulin therapy at least 5 years after diagnosis or significant C-peptide levels in a patient on insulin therapy indicating a beta-cell function defect, (4) absence of obesity or evidence of peripheral resistance. Families diagnosed with MODY frequently violate the historic diagnostic criteria: They may present at a later age, have fewer affected generations, progress rapidly, and have an elevated body mass index (BMI).

MODY is a clinically heterogeneous group of disorders consequent to genetic heterogeneity, allelic heterogeneity, variable expressivity, and incomplete penetrance.

**Clinical criteria is expected to have a high specificity but a relatively low sensitivity**
- Nonketotic hyperglycemia
- Age less than 25 in at least one affected member

- Autosomal dominant inheritance pattern affecting three generations
- Evidence of a beta-cell secretion defect, retained C-peptide production

**And the absence of**
- Maternal inheritance with deafness, autoantibodies characteristic of type 1 diabetes

Patients that fail to meet these diagnostic criteria in the context of high clinical suspicion may still be appropriate for genetic evaluation. The 2008 best practice guidelines recommended *HNF4A*, *GCK*, and *HNF1A* gene analysis in patients demonstrating diabetes before age 25 years, a strong family history, and evidence of insulin independence.

***Clinical Characteristics:*** The clinical phenotype of MODY is variable (Table 56-1). Even family members with the same mutation may display variable disease severity. MODY is characterized by a defect in insulin secretion capacity even in presymptomatic affected individuals. Presentation may be precipitated by factors that unmask an underlying beta-cell defect by reducing insulin sensitivity. Precipitants include infections, medications such as steroids, puberty, pregnancy, and obesity. However, the most common

*Table 56-1* **Genetic Differential Diagnosis**

| Syndrome | Gene Symbol | Alternative Gene Symbols | Relative Frequency, f | Associated Findings |
|---|---|---|---|---|
| MODY1 | HNF4A | TCF14 | 5% | Progressive diabetes with related sequelae. Sulfonylurea therapy generally effective, insulin may be required. Reduced serum levels of triglycerides, alpolipoproteins AII and CIII, and HDL. Mutation carriers have an elevated birth weight and are likely to experience hypoglycemia with hyperinsulinemia at birth. |
| MODY2 | GCK | GLK, HK4, LGLK | 22%-48% (higher with screening of asymptomatic individuals) | Mild lifelong asymptomatic hyperglycemia. Elevated glucose set-point (impaired fasting glucose and glucose tolerance test); diabetes-related complications not anticipated unless significant decompensation of glucose homeostasis occurs. Treatment with diet and exercise. |
| MODY3 | HNF1A | TCF1 | 30%-58% | Progressive beta-cell failure in the second to fifth decade. Insulin therapy may be required but sulfonylurea therapy should be trialed even if patient is using insulin. CAD risk may be increased despite elevated HDL and suppressed hsCRP. Glycosurea is present prior to the development of diabetes. |
| MODY4 | PDX1 | IPF1, STF1, IDX1 | Rare | Obesity and hyperinsulinemia with a relatively delayed age of onset (35 years) is characteristic. Families recognized by homozygous mutant phenotype of pancreatic agenesis. |
| MODY5 | HNF1B | TCF2 | 5% | Abnormal kidney or genital tract development, progressive renal insufficiency. Diabetes is secondary to pancreatic atrophy. LFT abnormalities. Hyperuricemia and gout. |
| MODY6 | NEUROD1 | | Rare | Familial, apparently typical type 2 diabetes. |
| MODY7 | KLF11 | TIEG2, FKLF | Rare | Familial, apparently typical type 2 diabetes that may be more common among French Moroccans. |
| MODY8 | CEL | BSSL, BSDL | Rare | Diabetes and exocrine insufficiency. Recurrent abdominal pain, steatorrhea, reduced fecal elastase, and reduced x-ray attenuation as a result of pancreatic atrophy and fat infiltration |
| MODY9 | PAX4 | | Rare | Mild progressive diabetes. Reduced insulin secretion in euglycemic mutation carriers. Increased prevalence in the Japanese population. |
| MODY10 | INS | | Rare | The less common delayed presentation may be misdiagnosed as either type 1 or type 2 diabetes. |
| MODY11 | BLK | | Rare | Familial, apparently typical type 2 diabetes. |

presentation is asymptomatic hyperglycemia. MODY should be suspected in young hyperglycemic patients who lack characteristic features of type 2 diabetes (obesity, acanthosis nigricans, polycystic ovarian syndrome) or type 1 diabetes.

☞**MODY1 (*HNF4A*):** This disorder is phenotypically similar to MODY3 but approximately five times less frequent. Progressive diabetes with vascular complications necessitates appropriate therapy. Patients are typically sensitive to sulfonylureas though insulin therapy may be required. Biochemical findings include reduced levels of lipoprotein A1, lipoprotein A2, and, in contrast to MODY3,

HDL. Mutation carriers have an elevated birth weight and are likely to experience hypoglycemia with hyperinsulinemia at birth.

☞**MODY2 (*GCK*):** This condition is a relatively common form of MODY that is found in all racial groups and characterized by nonprogressive hyperglycemia, usually asymptomatic. The diagnosis is commonly suspected based on an incidental elevated glucose reading in a young individual or during pregnancy. *GCK* mutations represent 2% to 5% of patients diagnosed with gestational diabetes. Because treatment with hypoglycemic agents does not appear to improve $HbA_{1c}$ and the diabetes-related complications are not observed, treatment is focused on diet and exercise. However, MODY2 patients are susceptible to developing superimposed type 2 diabetes and should be treated accordingly in such cases. Homozygous or compound heterozygous *GCK* mutations cause PNDM.

The ideal treatment of MODY2 mothers during pregnancy has not been established. Unaffected fetuses of affected mothers have an elevated birth weight whereas affected fetuses from unaffected mothers have low birth weight.

☞**Mody3 (*HNF1A*):** This disorder is the most common MODY, is found in all ethnicities, presents as autosomal dominant diabetes with normal glucose at birth (unlike MODY2) with progressive beta-cell failure in the second to fifth decade. The penetrance of diabetes is estimated to be 63% by age 25 and 96% by age 55. Patients born to an affected mother present approximately 12 years earlier than those born to an unaffected mother. Patients often display the diagnostic features of MODY and require insulin therapy in approximately 30% to 40% of cases. However, treatment with a sulfonylurea therapy is successful in many cases even after many years of insulin therapy and should be tried prior to initiating insulin therapy.

The risk of coronary artery disease may be elevated out of proportion to the degree of glycemic control. In contrast to typical type 2 diabetes, biochemical markers of an *HNF1A* mutation include elevated HDL levels and suppressed hsCRP (CRP is transcriptionally controlled by *HNF1A*). Glycosurea is observed even prior to the development of diabetes.

☞**Mody4 (*PDX1*):** This rare form of hereditary diabetes has been demonstrated in a limited number of families. Suspicion of an underlying *PDX1* mutation may be triggered by pancreatic agenesis which is seen in homozygous Pro63fsx60 mutation carriers. Unexpectedly, MODY4 patients, heterozygous individuals, demonstrate obesity and hyperinsulinemia with a relatively delayed age of onset (35 years).

☞**Mody5 (*HNF1B*):** These patients have a combination of renal abnormalities (80% penetrant and include renal cysts, familial hypoplastic glomerulocystic kidney disease, renal malformations, atypical hyperuricemic nephropathy, and renal dysplasia), uterine and genital tract abnormalities, abnormal liver function tests (60% penetrant), diabetes (50% penetrant) characterized by pancreatic atrophy and exocrine dysfunction, gout or hyperuricemia, and biliary abnormalities. De novo mutation may be as high as 50% leading most families not to meet MODY diagnostic criteria. Abnormalities may include almost any component of the genital, reproductive, and urinary tracts. With respect to both diabetes and renal disease, a broad range of penetrance and expressivity is observed even among patients with the same mutation. Insulin therapy is most commonly required. Patients who demonstrate hyperuricemia and treatment with allopurinol improve renal function.

☞**Mody6 (*NEUROD1*):** A rare form of autosomal dominant diabetes with phenotypic descriptions ranging from relatively delayed onset (40 years) and hyperinsulinemia to more severe phenotypes.

☞**Mody7 (*KLF11*):** It is a rare form of autosomal dominant early-onset diabetes. May be more common in French Moroccan families.

☞**Mody8 (*CEL*):** This rare MODY is characterized by beta-cell dysfunction and exocrine insufficiency. The typical age of presentation is 30 to 40 years. Nondiabetic affected individuals have a normal glucose tolerance. Mild recurrent abdominal pain starts in the second decade, steatorrhea, reduced fecal elastase, and reduced

x-ray attenuation (HU) of the pancreas as a result of pancreatic atrophy and fat infiltration.

☞**Mody9 (*PAX4*):** This a rare form of MODY that may have a relatively high pathogenic allele frequency (R121W) in the Japanese diabetic population (2%). The phenotype is variable but does not appear to be severe (insulin requiring) in most affected individuals. The penetrance of diabetes among individuals harboring a heterozygous PAX4 R121W allele is low; however, these patients do exhibit decreased insulin secretion capacity. Mutations (sequence variants) in *PX4* have been associated with diabetes risk.

☞**Mody10 (*INS*):** Mutation in the INS gene is a relatively common cause of PNDM. Pathogenic INS mutations are rarely observed in MODY families and highly penetrant type 1 diabetes families. Insulin therapy is frequently required.

☞**Mody11 (*BLK*):** Mutations in *BLK* are a rare cause of moderately penetrant (84%) autosomal dominant diabetes that appears to be influenced by BMI (insulin demand). Beta-cell function is preserved in affected individuals.

## Screening and Counseling

*Screening:*

**MODY 2:** Predictive testing in at-risk individuals should be considered if an elevated fasting glucose is present.

**MODY1, 3, 4, 5:** Predictive testing may be used to identify presymptomatic affected individuals and guide counseling and management.

*Counseling:* MODY is inherited in an autosomal dominant manner. All children and first-degree relatives carry a 50% risk of being affected.

☞**Genotype-Phenotype Correlation:**

*HNF1A:* In general, mutations affecting the 3' portion of the gene (exons 8-10) delay presentation by 8 years compared to mutations located more upstream (exons 1-6).

*GCK:* Mutations that increase enzyme activity cause hyperinsulinemic hypoglycemia whereas mutations that impair enzyme activity cause hypoinsulinemic hyperglycemia.

## Molecular Genetics and Molecular Mechanism

*Syndrome/Gene/Locus/Function:*

MODY1/hepatocyte nuclear factor 4-alpha (*HNF4A*)/20q13.12/ orphan nuclear receptor, transcription factor, expressed in the liver, pancreatic islets, kidneys, and genital tract, that participates in beta-cell maturation, expansion, and function.

MODY2/glucokinase (*GCK*)/7p13/catalyzes the phosphorylation of glucose (Glucose → Glucose-6-P), serves as the beta-cell glucose sensor. Mutations may result in decreased activity (decreased glucose sensitivity, hyperglycemia) or increased activity (increased glucose sensitivity, hypoglycemia).

MODY3/hepatocyte nuclear factor 1-alpha (*HNF1A2*)/12q24.2/ transcription factor expressed in the liver, pancreatic islets, kidneys, and genital tract, that participates in beta-cell maturation, expansion, and function. Activity is modulated by *HNF4A*. MODY4/pancreas/duodenum homeobox protein-1 (*PDX1*)/13q12.1/ is a relatively islet-specific transcription factor that enhances insulin and somatostatin expression. This gene participates in beta-cell maturation, expansion, and function. *PDX1* plays a broader role in endoderm development. *PDX1* haploinsufficiency leads to decreased beta-cell mass and increased susceptibility to endoplasmic reticulum stress and beta-cell failure. The Pro63fsx60 mutation disrupts the transcriptional transactivating domain and encodes a dominant negative protein product that disrupts function of the wild-type allele.

MODY5/hepatocyte nuclear factor 1-beta (*HNF1B*)/17cen-q21.3/a broadly expressed transcription factor that participates in the development of the kidney, pancreas, liver, and Mullerian duct.

MODY6/neuronal differentiation 1 (*NEUROD1*)/2q11.2/a helix-loop-helix transcription factor that is expressed in beta cells and regulates the expression of insulin.

MODY7/Kruppel-like factor 11 (*KLF11*)/2p25.1/glucose-induced regulator of insulin gene expression that acts by inducing *PDX1* gene expression and acting directly on the insulin gene promoter.

MODY8/carboxyl ester lipase (CEL)/9q34.2/this gene is a major constituent of the pancreatic digestive secretion and catalyzes the hydrolysis of cholesterol esters.

MODY9/paired domain gene 4 (*PAX4*)/7q32.1/this gene is a DNA-binding transcription factor that is required for beta-cell differentiation.

MODY10/insulin (*INS*)/11p15.5/insulin is a peptide secreted by islet beta cells in response to glucose elevation. Insulin promotes cellular glucose uptake and storage (hepatocytes, myocytes).

MODY11/tyrosine kinase, B-lymphocyte specific (*BLK*)/8p23.1/*BLK* is a member of the src family of proto-oncogenes and encodes a nonreceptor tyrosine kinase. *BLK* is expressed in beta cells and upregulates the expression of *PDX1* and *NKX6.1* which, in turn, drive the expression of insulin.

*Genetic Testing:* DNA sequence and deletion analysis is clinically available for several of the MODY genes (see Gene Tests http://www.ncbi.nlm.nih.gov/sites/GeneTests/lab?db=genetests).

## BIBLIOGRAPHY:

1. Froguel P, Vaxillaire M, Sun F, et al. Close linkage of glucokinase locus on chromosome 7p to early-onset non-insulin-dependent diabetes mellitus. *Nature*. 1992;356:162-164.

2. Hattersley AT, Beards F, Ballantyne E, Appleton M, Harvey R, Ellard S. Mutations in the glucokinase gene of the fetus result in reduced birth weight. *Nat Genet*. 1998;19:268-270.

3. Horikawa Y, Iwasaki N, Hara M, et al. Mutation in hepatocyte nuclear factor-1 beta gene (TCF2) associated with MODY. *Nat Genet*. 1997;17:384-385.

4. Moller AM, Dalgaard LT, Pociot F, Nerup J, Hansen T, Pedersen O. Mutations in the hepatocyte nuclear factor-1alpha gene in Caucasian families originally classified as having Type I diabetes. *Diabetologia*. 1998;41:1528-1531.

5. Pearson ER, Starkey BJ, Powell RJ, Gribble FM, Clark PM, Hattersley AT. Genetic cause of hyperglycaemia and response to treatment in diabetes. *Lancet*. 2003;362:1275-1281.

6. Tattersall RB, Fajans SS. A difference between the inheritance of classical juvenile-onset and maturity-onset type diabetes of young people. *Diabetes*. 1975;24;44-53.

7. Vionnet N, Stoffel M, Takeda J, et al. Nonsense mutation in the glucokinase gene causes early-onset non-insulin-dependent diabetes mellitus. *Nature*. 1992;356:721-722.

8. Yamagata K, Oda N, Kaisaki PJ, et al. Mutations in the hepatocyte nuclear factor-1alpha gene in maturity-onset diabetes of the young (MODY3). *Nature*. 1996b;384:455-458.

# Supplementary Information

## OMIM REFERENCES:

[1] Maturity-Onset Diabetes of the Young 1; MODY1 (#125850)

[2] Maturity-Onset Diabetes of the Young 2; MODY2 (#125851)

[3] Maturity-Onset Diabetes of the Young 3; MODY3 (#600496)

[4] Maturity-Onset Diabetes of the Young 4; MODY4(#606392)

[5] Maturity-Onset Diabetes of the Young 5; MODY5 (#137920)

[6] Maturity-Onset Diabetes of the Young 6; MODY6 (#606394)

[7] Maturity-Onset Diabetes of the Young 7; MODY7 (#610508)

[8] Maturity-Onset Diabetes of the Young 8; MODY8 (#609812)

[9] Maturity-Onset Diabetes of the Young 9; MODY9 (#612225)

[10] Maturity-Onset Diabetes of the Young 10; MODY10 (#613370)

[11] Maturity-Onset Diabetes of the Young 11; MODY11 (#613375)

## Alternative Names:

- Autosomal Dominant Diabetes.
- Mild Juvenile Diabetes Mellitus.
- Mason-Type Diabetes.
- MODY5 is also known as Atypical Familial Juvenile Hyperuricemic Nephropathy (FJHN), Glomerulocystic Kidney Disease, Hypopastic-Type FJHN, and Renal Cysts and Diabetes Syndrome (RCAD).
- MODY8 is also known as Diabetes-Pancreatic Exocrine Dysfunction Syndrome.
- MODY9 is also known as Ketosis-Prone Diabetes.

*Key Words:* Autosomal diabetes

# 57 Hypoglycemia

Eugen Melcescu and Christian A. Koch

## KEY POINTS

- *Disease summary:*
  - **Hypoglycemia** is defined as a decrease in the blood glucose level or its tissue utilization accompanied by typical signs and symptoms. Based on rate of decline (rapid or slow) in glucose blood levels, symptoms of hypoglycemia are classified mainly in two major categories: adrenergic and neuroglycopenic. Inadequate supply of glucose to the brain and other tissues may have a negative impact on their energy requirements and function.
  - **Whipple triad** defines a combination of three criteria used to diagnose hypoglycemia:
    - The presence of characteristic hypoglycemia symptoms
    - Low glucose levels and typical symptoms
    - The resolution of symptoms after the normalization of blood glucose
- *Hereditary basis:*
  - Hypoglycemia can be inherited as an isolated finding or as one component of a multisystem syndrome. Observed pattern of inheritance includes autosomal dominant, autosomal recessive, and X-linked recessive. See Genetic Differential Diagnosis.
- *Differential diagnosis:*
  - Various disorders of excessive or underproduction of glucose have a genetic component. The most common forms of genetic hyperinsulinemia are represented by familial hyperinsulinemia hypoglycemia (FHH) (Table 57-1). Autosomal dominant and recessive forms are identified based on SUR1/Kir6.2 receptor mutations in the different genes that encoded it: *ABCC8, KCNJ11*. Other rarer genetic causes of hyperinsulinism have been linked to mutations that coded for different enzymes or receptors identified with other subtypes of FHH: *GCK, HADH, INSR, GLUD1, SLC16A1*.
  - In 50% of patients with hyperinsulinism, there are no identifiable genetic markers but single-nucleotide polymorphisms (SNPs) were reported in some infants with hypoglycemia.
  - Beckwith-Wiedemann syndrome is an autosomal dominant condition with variable penetrance and genomic imprinting should be a part of the differential diagnosis of hyperinsulinemia.
  - Glucose-processing defects (glycogen synthase deficiency, glycogen-storage disease, respiratory chain defects) are mostly manifested during infancy and early childhood. Defects in alternative fuel production (carnitine acyl transferase deficiency, hepatic HMG CoA lyase deficiency, long-chain or medium-chain or variably short-chain acyl-coenzyme A dehydrogenase deficiency) can destabilize the energy balance in the body making it difficult to accommodate a prolonged starvation or acute stress period.
  - Disorders of glucose underproduction are caused by inadequate glucose stores (prematurity, small for gestational age), glycogen synthase deficiency, glycogen-storage disease, or hormonal abnormalities.
  - Glycogen synthase deficiency is manifested as fasting hypoglycemia because of the liver's inability to store glucose, whereas in glycogen-storage disease there are problems with glucose release and gluconeogenesis.
  - Hormonal deficiencies (partial or complete) are expressed as autosomal recessive or X-linked recessive condition. Some of these hormonal deficiencies may be associated with transient or persistent hypoglycemia.

## Diagnostic Criteria and Clinical Characteristics

An essential energetic source for central nervous system (CNS) function is represented by glucose. About 90% of cerebral metabolism is based on this substrate and a rapid or slow decline in availability of glucose in the body will produce associated signs and symptoms. The main clinical manifestations of hypoglycemia can be comprised in two major clinical pathways:

- Symptoms caused by activation of the autonomic nervous system (ANS) and its counter-regulatory hormones: sweating, nausea, anxiety, tachycardia, palpitations, shaking, hunger
- Neuroglycopenic symptoms due to deficiency of glucose: headache, visual disturbances, slurred speech, restlessness, bizarre behavior, somnolence, confusion, seizures, ataxia, coma

The symptoms related to activation of the ANS generally appear before neuroglycopenic symptoms which occur when glucose levels are below 40 to 50 mg/dL.

Neonatal hypoglycemic clinical presentation is sometimes difficult to diagnose. Diseases manifesting in the neonatal period have a more severe presentation. Some of the following symptoms may raise the suspicion of low blood glucose: cyanotic episodes, apnea, poor feeding, brief myoclonic jerks, lethargy, somnolence, and seizures.

In neonates, common causes of hypoglycemia are considered the following:

- Transient: prematurity, sepsis, perinatal asphyxia, uncontrolled diabetes (mother)
- Permanent
  - Hyperinsulinemic hypoglycemia of infancy (HHI)
  - Carbohydrate metabolism disorders
  - Disorders of fatty acid oxidation

*Table 57-1* **Genetic Differential Diagnosis**

| Syndrome | | Gene Symbol | Associated Findings |
|---|---|---|---|
| Hyperinsulinemia | Hyperinsulinemic hypoglycemia Familial (HHF) 1 | *ABCC8* | Hypoglycemia in the newborn or infant, elevated serum insulin, low serum ketone bodies, hypotonia, poor feeding, apnea, increased glucose response to glucagon administration |
| | HHF 2 | *KCNJ11* | |
| | HHF 3 | *GCK* | Children—hypoglycemia, diaphoresis, behavior changes |
| | HHF 4 | *HADH* | Adults—altered mental status, headaches, lethargy, loss of consciousness |
| | HHF 5 | *INSR* | |
| | HHF 6 | *GLUD1* | |
| | HHF 7 | *SLC16A1* | |
| | Beckwith-Wiedemann syndrome (BWS) | *CDKN1C* *H19* *IGF2* *KCNQ1* *KCNQ1OT1* | About 85% cases of BWS are sporadic but some (<15%) cases of BWS are familial Classic form: hemihypertrophy, macroglossia, ear creases, ear pits, hypoglycemia (50% of babies), visceromegaly (liver, spleen, kidneys, or adrenals) midline abdominal wall defects (omphalocele, umbilical hernia, diastasis recti), associated embryonal malignancies: Wilms tumor, hepatoblastoma |
| | Islet cell adenoma or tumor-associated with MEN1 | *MEN1* | Multiple endocrine neoplasia type 1 is caused by mutation in the *MEN1* gene while MEN2A or MEN2B, is caused by mutations in the *RET* gene and MEN4 by a mutation in the *CDKN1B* gene. MEN1 characteristics: <br>• Hyperparathyroidism (≥90% of patients), asymptomatic hypercalcemia and/or nephrolithiasis <br>• Pancreatic islet cell tumors (60%-70% of patients). Fasting hypoglycemia is caused by insulinoma <br>• Pituitary tumors in 15% to 42% of MEN1 patients |
| Defects in alternative fuel production | Carnitine acyltransferase deficiency | *CPT1A* *CPT2* | Neonatal form—respiratory failure, hypoglycemia, seizures, hepatomegaly, liver failure, cardiomegaly Infantile form—hypoketotic hypoglycemia, seizures Adult form—rhabdomyolysis, myoglobinuria, recurrent myalgia |
| | Hepatic hydroxymethylglutaryl coenzyme A [HMG CoA] lyase deficiency | *HMGCL* | Presenting in the first year of life with vomiting, seizures, metabolic acidosis, hypoketotic hypoglycemia |
| | Long-chain and medium-chain acyl-coenzyme A dehydrogenase deficiency | *ACADL* *ACADM* | Vomiting, feeding problems, lowered consciousness fatty acid accumulation, hyperammonemia Hypoglycemia, early-onset cardiomyopathy, neuropathy, pigmentary retinopathy, sudden death |
| | Variably in short-chain acyl-coenzyme A dehydrogenase deficiency | *ACADS* | Neonatal form—poor appetite, developmental delay, seizures, myopathy, and nonketotic hypoglycemia Infant form (generalized)—acute acidosis, low muscle tone Adult form (localized)—chronic myopathy |
| Disorders of glycogenolysis | Glycogen synthase deficiency | *GYS2* | Fasting hypoglycemia, increased ketones, free fatty acids, low levels of alanine and lactate, and in severe cases recurrent hypoglycemic seizures Decreased glycogen stores in the liver and inadequate gluconeogenesis Primarily manifested during infancy and early childhood |
| | Glycogen-storage disease type Ia/b | *G6PC* | Hypoglycemia, lactic acidosis, hypertriglyceridemia, hyperuricemia, doll-like faces with fat cheeks, growth failure, hepatomegaly |

*(Continued)*

*Table 57-1  Genetic Differential Diagnosis (Continued)*

| Syndrome | | Gene Symbol | Associated Findings |
|---|---|---|---|
| | Glycogen-storage disease type III | AGL | Hypoglycemia, growth retardation, hypotonia cardiomyopathy (later), hepatomegaly |
| | Glycogen-storage disease type VI | PYGL | Hypoglycemia, hyperlipidemia, hyperketosis, hepatomegaly, and growth retardation in early childhood |
| | Fructose 1,6 diphosphatase deficiency | FBP1 | Hypoglycemia, metabolic acidosis, seizures, hypertension, miosis, fatty liver, ketone bodies |
| | Phosphoenol pyruvate deficiency I,II | PCK1 PCK2 | Hypoglycemia, metabolic acidosis, cerebral atrophy, liver failure, generalised muscle weakness, early death |
| | Pyruvate carboxylase deficiency | PC | Type A (infantile form)—fatigue, abdominal pain, muscle hypotonia, lactic acidosis<br>Type B (severe neonatal form)—hyperammonemia, liver failure, abnormal movements, death within the first 3 months of life<br>Type C (intermittent or benign form)—mildly delayed neurologic development, transient metabolic acidosis |
| | Hereditary fructose intolerance | ALDOB | Vomiting, abdominal pain, enlarged liver, hypoglycemia, jaundice, hemorrhage, kidney failure, or seizures |
| | Galactosemia | GALT GALK1 GALE | Hepatomegaly, cirrhosis, renal failure, brain damage, ovarian failure |
| Hormonal disorders | X-linked panhypopituitarism | SOX3 | Neonatal hypoglycemia, growth hormone deficiency, variable deficiencies of other pituitary hormones, hypoplasia of the anterior pituitary with hypoplasia or absence of the lower half of the infundibulum, normal psychomotor development |
| | X-linked adrenal hypoplasia congenita | NR0B1 | Hypogonadotropic hypogonadism (males), skeletal immaturity, adrenal insufficiency (dehydration, shock, hypoglycemia) |
| | Combined pituitary hormone deficiency 1 | PROP1 | Growth failure, developmental deficiency starting early in life, mild hypothyroidism, deficient secondary sexual development, infertility, ACTH deficiency (late onset) |
| | Glucocorticoid deficiency-1 | MC2R | Cutaneous hyperpigmentation, tall stature, craniofacial abnormalities, hypoglycemia, muscles weakness |
| Disorders of amino acid metabolism | Maple syrup urine disease Ia, b, II | BCKDHA BCKDHB DBT DLD | Mental or physical retardation, feeding difficulties and a maple syrup odor to the urine. MSUD patients are included into five phenotypes: classic, intermediate, intermittent, thiamine-responsive, and dihydrolipoyl dehydrogenase (E3)-deficient |
| Other | Neurofibromatosis 1 | NF1 | Six or more café-au-lait macules >5 mm in diameter in prepubertal and >15 mm in diameter in adult individuals, two or more neurofibromas of any type, two or more Lisch nodules freckles of the axillae, optic gliomas |

Gene names: *ABCC8,* ATP-binding cassette, subfamily C (CFTR/MRP), member 8; *KCNJ11,* potassium inwardly rectifying channel, subfamily J, member 11; *GCK,* glucokinase hexokinase 4; *HADH,* hydroxyacyl-CoA dehydrogenase; *INSR,* insulin receptor; *GLUD1,* glutamate dehydrogenase 1; *SLC16A1,* solute carrier family 16, member 1 monocarboxylic acid transporter 1; *CDKN1C,* cyclin-dependent kinase inhibitor 1C (p57, Kip2); *H19,* H19, imprinted maternally expressed transcript (nonprotein coding); *IGF2,* insulin-like growth factor 2 (somatomedin A); *KCNQ1,* potassium voltage-gated channel, KQT-like subfamily, member 1; *KCNQ1OT1,* KCNQ1 overlapping transcript 1 (nonprotein coding); *MEN1,* multiple endocrine neoplasia type 1 gene; *CPT1A,* carnitine palmitoyltransferase 1A; *CPT2,* carnitine palmitoyltransferase 2; *HMGCL,* 3-hydroxymethyl-3-methylglutaryl-CoA lyase; *ACADL,* acyl-CoA dehydrogenase, long chain; *ACADM,* acyl-CoA dehydrogenase, C-4 to C-12 straight chain; *ACADS,* acyl-CoA dehydrogenase, C-2 to C-3 short chain; *GYS2,* glycogen synthase 2; *G6PC,* glucose-6-phosphatase, catalytic subunit; *AGL,* amylo-alpha-1, 6-glucosidase, 4-alpha-glucanotransferase; *PYGL,* phosphorylase, glycogen, liver; *FBP1,* fructose-1,6-bisphosphatase 1; *PCK1,* phosphoenolpyruvate carboxykinase 1, soluble; *PCK2,* phosphoenolpyruvate carboxykinase 2 (mitochondrial); *PC,* pyruvate carboxylase; *ALDOB,* aldolase B, fructose-bisphosphate; *GALT,* galactose-1-phosphate uridylyltransferase; *GALK1,* galactokinase 1; *GALE,* UDP-galactose-4-epimerase; *SOX3,* sex-determining region Y-box 3; *NR0B1,* nuclear receptor subfamily 0, group B, member 1; *PROP1,* PROP paired-like homeobox1; *MC2R,* melanocortin 2 receptor; *BCKDHA,* branched-chain keto acid dehydrogenase E1, alpha polypeptide; *BCKDHB,* branched-chain keto acid dehydrogenase E1, beta polypeptide; *DBT,* dihydrolipoamide branched-chain transacylase E2; *DLD,* dihydrolipoamide dehydrogenase; *NF1,* neurofibromin 1–(after http://www.genenames.org).

- Glycogen storage diseases
- Galactosemia
- Amino acid and acid organic disorders

Causes of hypoglycemia in older infants, children, and teenagers

- Overtreatment with insulin in type 1 diabetes, sepsis, glycogen storage disease (GSD) type I or III or VI, phosphoenolpyruvate carboxykinase deficiency, disorders of fatty acid oxidation, amino acid and acid organic disorders (maple syrup urine disease, propionic acidemia), poisoning (drugs)

In young and older adults, the most frequent forms of hypoglycemia are

- Overdosing of diabetes mellitus with insulin or oral hypoglycemic agents, Addison disease, alcohol-induced hypoglycemia, insulin-secreting pancreatic tumor, postgastric bypass surgery

**History:** A pertinent diagnosis of hypoglycemia has to be based on history, clinical examination, and various laboratory data.

It is important to know the age of debut of hypoglycemia, information about the birth history, previous seizures, food intolerance, behavioral changes, fasting hypoglycemia, visceromegaly, family history of diabetes, and if various medications with potential of inducing hypoglycemia have been administrated. Other information may be necessary based on individual approach of the patients with possible hypoglycemia.

**Physical Examination:** A thorough physical examination can help us to sort out various conditions related to hypoglycemia. Specific physical findings have been linked to certain conditions where the low blood sugar is a component of the diagnosis. Because of a great number of conditions what can be accompanied by hypoglycemia a systematic approach relying on major clinical syndromes involved is desirable.

The following clinical signs are most common in patients with hypoglycemia:

- Tachycardia, inappropriate mood, seizure, coma
- Diplopia, papilledema, visual field defects (bilateral hemianopsia)
- Large body size—hyperinsulinism
- Failure to thrive, dysmorphic features, skeleton malformation, organomegaly
- Midline facial, cranial abnormalities (cleft lip or palate), microphallus, growth failure with decreased growth rate for age, hypotension, hyperpigmentation
- Jaundice concomitant with an enlarged liver, eye changes (cataracts)

**Laboratory:** A major step toward a refined diagnosis and urgent treatment of hypoglycemia is represented by obtaining accurate laboratory data. It is important to measure serum glucose concentration with a laboratory-based glucose analyzer prior to the administration of glucose.

Most of the authors define hypoglycemia based on the following serum glucose levels:

- Less than 60 mg/dL in men
- Less than 50 mg/dL in women
- Less than 40 to 45 mg/dL in infants and children

However, these levels are still disputed among physicians particularly in neonates. Typically once hypoglycemia is confirmed (by serum glucose levels and/or adequate symptoms), it is important to obtain what was defined in the classical literature as, "critical sample" of blood. As a part of initial diagnosis an initial blood sample should measure various metabolic precursors and hormones involved in glucose counter-regulation helping us to have a more systematic approach of the metabolic and hormonal imbalances of the patient.

**Blood Sample**
- Serum—glucose, electrolytes, bicarbonate, anion gap, insulin, C-peptide, growth hormone, cortisol, lactate, ammonia, pyruvate, beta-hydroxybutyrate, free fatty acid (FFA), total and free carnitine, branched-chain amino acid, toxicology screen for adults (ethanol, salicylates, sulphonylureas)
- Urine—ketones, C-peptide

Any abnormal titers of FFA should hint to a defect in fatty acid metabolism, while high plasma lactate levels point to a defect in gluconeogenesis, glycolysis, or respiratory-chain defects. Low cortisol, growth hormone, sex hormone levels should guide us to a possible diagnosis of hypopituitarism or adrenal insufficiency.

**Other Studies**
- Glucagon challenge
- Intra-arterial calcium stimulation with hepatic venous sampling
- Liver function tests, thyroid tests
- Blood cultures, chest radiograph, urinalysis
- Genetic analysis for genetic disorders associated with hyperinsulinism (FHH, BWS, etc)
- Abdominal ultrasonography, computed tomography (CT) scanning, magnetic resonance imaging (MRI) (head, pancreas)
- [18F]-Dopa positron emission tomography (PET) to differentiate focal from diffuse pancreatic islet tumors

## Screening and Counseling

**Screening:** Considering the variety of diseases which can be linked to hypoglycemia a systematic approach to the screening of the patients is desirable. When the hypoglycemic hyperinsulinism hypothesis is supported by clinical presentation in neonates various factors should be evaluated:

- Maternal factors: mother diabetes, maternal pre-eclampsia, drugs (beta-blockers, beta-agonists, hypoglycemics salicylates, sulfonamides)
- Fetal related factors: moderate-severe hypoxia, intrauterine growth retardation, low Apgar score (<5)
- Some neonates are at high risk and their screening for hypoglycemia is mandatory in the first hour of life:

  - Prematurely born babies
  - Newborns with abnormal weight (>4 kg or >2 kg)
  - Neonatal sepsis
  - Suggestive hypoglycemic symptoms: tachypnea, tachycardia, apnea, somnolence, poor feeding, brief myoclonic jerks, seizures

After the initial screening of individuals with immediate risk, more laborious steps are necessary to sort out the multitudes of conditions with potential of developing neonatal, infantile, or childhood persistent hypoglycemia.

Clinical signs and symptoms, parental medical history could be helpful but most of the cases will necessitate a complex laboratory, imaging, and genetic evaluation to obtain a definitive diagnosis.

Most inherited disorders of metabolism associated with hypoglycemia are rare diseases and the recognition of their specific presentation is crucial for their management. A timely diagnosis will avert or reduce early or later complications associated with hypoglycemia. A possible list with the most typical clinical features accompanying these diseases is presented as follows:

- Isolated hepatomegaly—glycogen storage disease
- Macroglossia, hemihypertrophy—Beckwith-Wiedemann syndrome (BWS)
- Microcephaly; anterior midline defects—panhypopituitarism
- Neuromuscular symptoms—hypoglycemic seizures in GSD type I
- Rhabdomyolysis, myoglobinuria—long-chain hydroxyacyl dehydrogenase deficiency
- Enlarged liver, abdominal pain, seizures—hereditary fructose intolerance
- Eye changes (cataracts)—galactosemia

***Counseling:*** Hyperinsulinemia hypoglycemia familial (HHF) 1,2,4, carnitine acyltransferase deficiency, hepatic hydroxymethylglutaryl coenzyme A [HMG CoA] lyase deficiency, long-chain and medium-chain acyl-coenzyme A dehydrogenase deficiency, short-chain acyl-coenzyme A dehydrogenase deficiency, glycogen synthase deficiency, GSD type III, VI (25% of cases), fructose 1,6 diphosphatase deficiency, phosphoenol pyruvate deficiency I, II, pyruvate carboxylase deficiency, hereditary fructose intolerance, galactosemia, glucocorticoid deficiency-1 (same of the cases), and combined pituitary hormone deficiency 2 are inherited in an autosomal recessive pattern. The child of an affected individual has a 25% chance of being affected, a 50% chance of being an asymptomatic carrier, and a 25% chance of not being affected at all. Families who have had one affected child, have a 25% chance of having an affected child in each subsequent pregnancy. No significant genotype-phenotype correlations have been identified. However, in galactosemia the following mutations have a certain correlation with prognosis of the disease:

- Good prognosis: heterozygous p.Gln188Arg mutation, D/G or p.Asn314Asp/p.Asn314Asp, homo/heterozygous p.Ser135Leu allele mutations, heterozygous p.Gln188Arg/p.Arg333Gly
- Poor prognosis: hetero/homozygous p.Lys285Asn

HHF 3,6 are inherited in an autosomal dominant fashion. Each sib of an affected parent has a 50% chance of being affected or an asymptomatic carrier of these conditions. Islet cell adenoma associated with MEN1 is also inherited in an autosomal dominant mode with greater than 95% penetrance. No significant genotype-phenotype correlations have been observed in patients with germline mutation in the *MEN1* gene.

BWS inheritance is complex and not well understood. Some cases (10%-15%) are associated with an autosomal dominant mode of inheritance with incomplete penetrance and preferential maternal transmission. Most individuals with BWS have normal chromosomes (<1% have chromosomal abnormalities) and no family history of the disease (85%).

In BWS, the following genotype-phenotype correlations have been described:

- For *CDKN1C* mutations—positive family history, omphalocele, and/or cleft palate
- Paternal uniparental disomy (UPD) for 11p15: isolated hemihyperplasia and Wilms tumor
- H19 hypermethylation: Wilms tumor
- Loss of methylation at *KCNQ1OT1*: monozygotic twinning and embryonal tumors other than Wilms tumor

X-linked panhypopituitarism, X-linked adrenal hypoplasia congenita, and some individuals with glucocorticoid deficiency-1 have an X-linked recessive inheritance; these conditions affect males who have inherited a recessive X-linked mutation from their mother. The females are only affected when they have inherited mutations in the same gene X-linked from both parents. A boy of a woman who is a carrier has a 50% risk of inheriting the disorder. A female child of a woman who is a carrier has a 50% risk of inheriting the gene mutation. If a boy has the disease he will pass it on to all daughters who will become carriers. The boy of an affected male will not inherit the condition.

Neurofibromatosis type 1 (NF1) is transmitted in an autosomal dominant (50%) and spontaneous mutation (50%) fashion. Half of affected individuals have NF1 as the result of a de novo *NF1* gene mutations. The sib of an affected individual has a 50% risk of inheriting the condition, but the disease manifestations are extremely variable.

The diversity of *NF1* mutations that occur in this disease makes genotype-phenotype correlation difficult.

For the moment two clear correlations have been observed:

- A whole *NF1* gene deletion: early appearance of cutaneous neurofibromas, severe cognitive abnormalities and somatic overgrowth, large hands and feet, and dysmorphic facial features
- A 3-bp in-frame deletion of exon 17 (c.2970-2972 delAAT): typical pigmentary features of NF1, but no cutaneous or surface plexiform neurofibromas

## Management and Treatment

Initial therapeutic measures are based on the severity of presenting symptoms and glucose levels. A patient in critical condition needs an ABCs emergency response and stabilization. Particular attention should be paid in neonates who are at risk of developing hypoglycemia. Infants born prematurely or small for gestational age have a high risk of hypoglycemia immediately after birth and the need to be put on an oral or intravenous (IV) form of glucose.

High-risk infants should be screened regularly with the aim of normalization of blood glucose to levels above 45 to 50 mg/dL. When the infant or child is alert, oral or nasogastric administration of glucose may be attempted at about 20 mL/kg of oral glucose solution.

In older children and adults who are awake and alert, about 20 to 30 g by mouth initially are sufficient with the monitoring of glucose at 15 to 20 minutes after.

- Initial therapy: IV administration of D10W (bolus) at a rate of
  - 2 to 3 mL/kg for infants
  - 1 mL/kg of D25W for children
  - 50 mL of 50% glucose for adults
- The rates of continuous infusion of D10W for an infant are 4 to 6 mg/kg/min. The doses should be adjusted in increments of

2 mL/kg/min (up to 12 mL/kg/min) in relation to the patient's response to therapy. For children and adults the maintenance doses vary based on glucose solution concentrations utilized.

- D25W and D50W IV are not recommended for infants suspected to have FHH due to rebound effects. If solutions of greater than 12.5% dextrose are needed a central venous catheter is required.
- The maintenance rates of more than 10 mg/kg/min hint to hyperinsulinemia.
- The weaning of IV glucose solution may begin when stable levels of blood glucose above minimum target (usually >60 mg/dL) for age and gender have been achieved for more than 12 hours.

Glucagon may be used in certain situations as another treatment option and should be given as 0.5 mg intramuscular (IM) (age <5 years) or 1 mg IM (age >5 years). Infants with inborn errors of metabolism affecting gluconeogenesis or glycogenolysis may not respond completely to this treatment.

In children with a hyperinsulinism (FHH) diagnosis, the frequent feeding may not be sufficient and other therapeutic agents need to be administered: diazoxide, octreotide, or nifedipine.

Surgery is an option for documented focal or diffuse lesions. If this therapy is chosen, partial (often distal) pancreatectomy may be tried. In some cases, up to 95% of pancreas has been removed.

Hormone replacement therapy (cortisol, growth hormone) is appropriate for children with hypoglycemia and hypopituitarism. When a pituitary or hypothalamus tumor is diagnosed cranial surgery may be an option.

In conclusion, the management of hypoglycemia combines a series of dietary measures (glucose) and second-line agents with the purpose of bringing the blood sugar levels to normal and determining the cause of hypoglycemia to prevent future relapses.

## Molecular Genetics and Molecular Mechanism

### Syndrome/Gene/Locus:

Familial hyperinsulinemia hypoglycemia
- *ABCC8*/11p15.1
- *KCNJ11*/11p15.1
- *GCK*/7p15-p13
- *HADH*/4q22-q26
- *INSR*/19p13.2
- *GLUD1*/10q23.3
- *SLC16A1*/1p13.2-p12

Beckwith-Wiedemann syndrome/*CDKN1C*, *H19*, *IGF2*, *KCNQ1*, *KCNQ1OT1*/11p15.5

Islet cell adenoma/MEN1/11q13

Carnitine acyltransferase deficiency/*CPT1A* or *CPT2*/11q13,1p32

Hepatic hydroxymethylglutaryl coenzyme A [HMG CoA] lyase deficiency/*HMGCL*/1pter-p33

Long-chain and medium-chain acyl-coenzyme A dehydrogenase deficiency/*ACADL, ACADM*/2q34-q35, 1p31

Variably in short-chain acyl-coenzyme A dehydrogenase deficiency/*ACADS*/12q22-qter

Glycogen synthase deficiency/*GYS2*/12p12.2

Glycogen storage disease type Ia/b/*G6PC*/17q21

Glycogen storage disease type III/*AGL*/1p21

Glycogen storage disease type VI/*PYGL*/14q21-q22

Fructose 1,6 diphosphatase deficiency/*FBP1*/9q22.2-q22.3

Phosphoenol pyruvate deficiency I, II/*PCK1* or *PCK2*/20q13.3, 14q11.2-q12

Pyruvate carboxylase deficiency/*PC*/11q13.4-q13.5

Hereditary fructose intolerance/*ALDOB*/9q22.3

Galactosemia/*GALT*/9p13

X-linked panhypopituitarism/*PHPX*/Xq27.2-q27.3, Xq26.3

X-linked adrenal hypoplasia congenita/*NR0B1*/Xp21.3-p21.2

Combined pituitary hormone deficiency 2/*PROP1*/5q

Glucocorticoid deficiency-1/*MC2R*/18p11.2

Maple syrup urine disease Ia, b, II/*BCKDHA, BCKDHB, DBT*/19q13.1-q13.2, 6q14, 1p31

Neurofibromatosis type 1/*NF1*/17q11.2

☞**FAMILIAL HYPERINSULINEMIA HYPOGLYCEMIA:** *ABCC8* and *KCNJ11* genes code for the proteins SUR1 (sulfonylurea receptor 1) and $K_{IR}6.2$ (ATP-sensitive inward rectifier potassium channel 11), proteins that are important constituents of the beta-cell $K_{ATP}$ channel. Stimulation or inhibition of insulin secretion is dependent on the metabolic state and electrical activity of the membrane of $K_{ATP}$ channel from pancreatic beta cells. Mutations of the *ABCC8* or *KCNJ11* genes will derange the functionality of this receptor ($K_{ATP}$) and will maintain the cell membrane depolarized irrespective of ATP/ADP ratio. As a consequence, the voltage-gated calcium channels will be opened and hyperinsulinemia will follow.

Glutamate dehydrogenase activity is dependent on ADP ribosylation. An increased ATP:ADP ratio is necessary for insulin secretion in pancreatic beta cells. As glutamate dehydrogenase increases (through some *GLUD1* mutation) more amino acids are broken down into alpha-ketoglutarate, the ATP:ADP ratio rises, and more insulin is secreted.

*GCK* mutations enable glucokinase enzyme activity at lower glucose levels and cause insulin hypersecretion.

☞**BECKWITH-WIEDEMANN SYNDROME:** Most of the cases (85%) of BWS are sporadic. The other cases (<15%) are related to genes that are imprinted on the short arm of chromosome 11 referred to as 11p15. In imprinted genes, only one parental copy is active while the other copy is silent. BWS is caused by mutation or deletion of imprinted genes within the chromosome 11p15.5 region. The genes identified to play a role in BWS are the following: *CDKN1C*, *H19*, *IGF2*, *KCNQ1*, *KCNQ1OT1*. Some patients have abnormal DNA methylation in different areas of 11p15 with the alteration of normal epigenetic marks involved in the regulation of imprinted genes from this region. Even with the modern armamentarium of genetic testing many molecular defects cannot be fully elucidated.

☞**ISLET CELL ADENOMA (MEN1):** MEN1 is a rare autosomal dominant hereditary cancer or tumor syndrome representing the development of a variety of tumors in divers endocrine systems such as parathyroid glands, pancreatic islets, and pituitary gland, and even in nonendocrine tissues (>20 combinations of them). The *MEN1* gene encodes a putative tumor suppressor protein called menin, which is involved in regulation of gene transcription, cell proliferation, apoptosis, and genome stability. Menin is primarily located in the nucleus where it exerts its aforementioned functions. The genetic screening of familial MEN1 should sequence in and around the menin protein's open reading frame.

☞**CARNITINE ACYL TRANSFERASE DEFICIENCY:** Long-chain fatty acids (LCFAs) are transported from cytosol into mitochondria by carnitine shuttle for beta oxidation. The translocation of long-chain acyl-CoAs to inner mitochondrial membrane necessitates carnitine palmitoyltransferase 1 (CPT1) and carnitine acylcarnitine translocase. CPT2 is located on the inner mitochondrial membrane and its role is to reconvert acylcarnitine equivalents to the acyl-CoA species. CPT1 is regulated at cellular level by malonyl-CoA. Mutations of *CPT1A* may cause a reduction in activity of CPT1 with an impairment of utilization of fatty acids for beta oxidation and fasting intolerance. Deficiency of these enzyme leads to accumulation of LCFAs in tissues (liver, brain, etc) and the manifestation of the disease.

☞**HEPATIC HYDROXYMETHYLGLUTARYL COENZYME A:** This enzyme plays an important role in leucine catabolism and cleavage of HMG-CoA to acetoacetic acid and acetyl-CoA, the last step of ketogenesis. Mutations in the *HMGCL* gene decreases the activity of hydroxymethylglutaryl coenzyme A and subsequently affects leucine catabolism and production of the ketones bodies. A deficient ketogenesis results in hypoglycemia and metabolic acidosis.

☞**LONG-CHAIN ACYL-COENZYME A DEHYDROGENASE DEFICIENCY:** Mutations in the *HADHA* gene cause long-chain acyl-coenzyme A dehydrogenase (LCHAD) deficiency. The *HADHA* gene is important in the production of an enzyme complex called mitochondrial trifunctional protein. This mitochondrial trifunctional protein comprises three different enzymes important for metabolization of LCFAs. LCFAs are essential sources of energy for human bodies. Mutations in the *HADHA* gene make this enzymatic complex dysfunctional and difficult to store these LCFAs. As a result the affected patient experiences lethargy and hypoglycemia.

☞**MEDIUM-CHAIN ACYL-COENZYME A DEHYDROGENASE:** Mutations in the *ACADM* gene will impair ketogenesis and plasma and tissue levels of carnitine. People with these defects will have intolerance to prolonged fasting and recurrent hypoglycemia.

☞**VARIABLY IN SHORT-CHAIN ACYL-COENZYME A DEHYDROGENASE DEFICIENCY:** Mutations in the *ACADS* gene lead to decreased levels of an enzyme called short-chain acyl-CoA dehydrogenase. The catabolism of short-chain fatty acids will be perturbed and energy storage from these compounds will be limited.

☞**GLYCOGEN SYNTHASE DEFICIENCY:** A deficiency in glycogen synthase caused by mutations in the *GYS2* gene will reduce the amount of glycogen that the body can store in the liver. Low amounts of glycogen in the liver are associated with inability to prolonged fasting, hypoglycemia, and low normal blood levels of lactate and alanine.

☞**GLYCOGEN STORAGE DISEASE TYPE IA/B:** Represents the most common GSD. Mutations present in the *G6PC* gene result in deficiency of the glucose-6-phosphatase. This deficiency in reducing glycogen breakdown will lead to increased storage of glycogen in liver and kidneys and diminished capacity to produce glucose during periods of fasting. Impaired production of glucose from glycogen and gluconeogenesis will cause severe hypoglycemia and lactic acidosis.

☞**GLYCOGEN STORAGE DISEASE TYPE III:** It is caused by deficiency of the glycogen debrancher enzyme and is associated with an accumulation of abnormal glycogen. Some mutations have been linked to a deficient activity of the enzyme amylo-1,6 glucosidase. This causes an accumulation of an abnormal glycogen in the liver, muscles, and heart. The disease is present in early life and childhood with hepatomegaly, hypoglycemia, muscle weakness, and cardiomyopathy.

☞**GLYCOGEN STORAGE DISEASE TYPE VI:** It is a disorder of glycogenolysis caused by deficiency of hepatic glycogen phosphorylase. A deficient enzyme that is caused by a mutated gene and is characterized by hepatomegaly, growth retardation, and mild hypoglycemia after prolonged fasting.

☞**FRUCTOSE 1,6 DIPHOSPHATASE DEFICIENCY:** Fructose-1,6-bisphosphatase deficiency determines an impaired gluconeogenesis. Glycogenolysis is still intact. Because glycogenolysis is not impaired, hypoglycemia occurs only during caloric restriction.

☞**PHOSPHOENOL PYRUVATE DEFICIENCY I, II:** It is a metabolic disorder resulting from impaired gluconeogenesis. The disease is caused by a reduced activity of either cytosolic *PEPCK1* or mitochondrial *PEPCK2* and has an autosomal recessive transmission.

☞**PYRUVATE CARBOXYLASE DEFICIENCY:** It results in inefficiency of the citric acid cycle and gluconeogenesis to produce enough energy for body requirements.

☞**HEREDITARY FRUCTOSE INTOLERANCE:** Fructose-1,6-bisphosphate aldolase is a tetrameric protein catalyzing the reversible conversion of fructose-1,6-bisphosphate to dihydroxyacetone phosphate and glyceraldehyde 3-phosphate. Munnich et al. have found that the B isoform of aldolase in the liver is controlled by diet. A fructose diet induces ALDOB mRNA expression in the liver compared with fasting states.

☞**GALACTOSEMIA:** In individuals with galactosemia, the metabolism of galactose is deficient due to diminished activity of the enzyme and toxic levels of galactose-1-phosphate in various tissues are accumulated.

☞**CONGENITAL ADRENAL HYPOPLASIA (X-LINKED):** DAX1 protein is an orphan member of the nuclear receptor (NR) superfamily that negatively regulates the transcription through retinoic acid receptor and binds in the nucleus to retinoic acid (RA)-responsive element.

☞**PANHYPOPITUITARISM, PROP1:** Inactivating mutations in *PROP1* result in deficiencies of prolactin (PRL), luteinizing hormone (LH), follicle-stimulating hormone (FSH), growth hormone (GH), or thyroid-stimulating hormone (TSH).

☞**FAMILIAL GLUCOCORTICOID DEFICIENCY 1:** The adrenocorticotropin (ACTH) receptor is a member of the G protein-coupled receptor family. Mutations in this receptor result in high levels of serum ACTH and low levels of cortisol.

☞**NEUROFIBROMATOSIS TYPE 1:** Various mutations could explain the extreme clinical variability of NF1. The mutated gene in NF1 encodes for a protein called neurofibromin. This protein plays a negative role in regulation of the Ras kinase pathway (p21 oncoprotein). Different types of mutations (deletions, missense, nonsense) result in a dysfunctional suppressor protein and overgrowth of cells of various tissues (derm, nervous system).

*Genetic Testing:* Genetic testing is available for the genes listed earlier (see http://www.ncbi.nlm.nih.gov/sites/GeneTests/review?db=GeneTests).

About 45% of individuals with familial hyperinsulinemic hypoglycemia (FHH) have mutations in *ABCC8,* 5% have mutations in the coding region of *KCNJ11,* and other 5% have mutations in *GLUD1.* A very small percentage of FHI cases have activating mutations in *GCK* or inactivating mutations in *HADH.* About 50% of individuals with FHH have no mutations. The genetic testing has to be based on clinical suspicion and the incidence of these conditions. The most common causes of hypoglycemia considered besides FHH are BWS, organic acidemias, galactosemia, hereditary fructose intolerance, glycogen storage diseases, carbohydrate metabolism disorders, and fatty acid oxidation disorders. Very rare diseases associated with hypoglycemia are phosphoenol-pyruvate carboxykinase deficiency, congenital adrenal hypoplasia (X-linked), panhypopituitarism, or familial glucocorticoid deficiency. The commonality of these conditions is related to their general incidence in the general population.

**BIBLIOGRAPHY:**

1. Cryer PE, Axelrod L, Grossman AB, et al. Evaluation and management of adult hypoglycemic disorders: an Endocrine Society Clinical Practice Guideline. *J Clin Endocrinol Metab*. Mar 2009;94(3):709-728.

2. Chuang DT, Shih VE. Maple syrup urine disease (branched-chain ketoaciduria). In: Scriver CR, Beaudet AL, Sly WS, Valle D, eds. *The Metabolic and Molecular Bases of Inherited Disease*. 8th ed. Vol II. New York, NY: McGraw-Hill; 2001:1971-2005.

3. Weksberg R, Shuman C, Beckwith JB. Beckwith-Wiedemann syndrome. *Europ J Hum Genet*. 2010;18:8-14.

4. Sigauke E, Rakheja D, Kitson K, Bennett MJ. Carnitine palmitoyltransferase II deficiency: a clinical, biochemical, and molecular review. *Lab Invest*. 2003;83(11):1543-1554.

5. Bonnefont JP, Djouadi F, Prip-Buus C, Gobin S, Munnich A, Bastin J. Carnitine palmitoyltransferases 1 and 2: biochemical, molecular and medical aspects. *Mol Aspects Med*. 2004;25(5-6):495-520.

6. IJlst L, Ruiter JPN, Hoovers JMN, Jakobs ME, Wanders RJA. Common missense mutation G1528C in long-chain 3-hydroxy-acyl-CoA dehydrogenase deficiency: characterization and expression of the mutant protein, mutation analysis on genomic DNA and chromosomal localization of the mitochondrial trifunctional protein alpha subunit gene. *J Clin Invest*. 1996;98:1028-1033.

7. Roe CR, Ding J. Mitochondrial fatty acid oxidation disorders. In: Scriver CR, Beaudet AL, Sly WS, Valle D, eds. *The Metabolic and Molecular Bases of Inherited Disease*. 7th ed. Vol II. New York, NY: McGraw-Hill; 2001:2297-2326.

8. Shen J, Bao Y, Liu HM, Lee P, Leonard JV, Chen YT. Mutations in exon 3 of the glycogen debranching enzyme gene are associated with glycogen storage disease type III that is differentially expressed in liver and muscle. *J Clin Invest*. 1996;98:352-357.

9. Woods KS, Cundall M, Turton J, et al. Over- and underdosage of SOX3 is associated with infundibular hypoplasia and hypopituitarism. *Am J Hum Genet*. 2005;76:833-849.

10. Dekelbab BH, Sperling MA. Recent advances in hyperinsulinemic hypoglycemia of infancy. *Acta Paediatr*. 2006;95:1157-1164.

11. Langley SD, Lai K, Dembure PP, Hjelm LN, Elsas LJ. Molecular basis for Duarte and Los Angeles variant galactosemia. *Am J Hum Genet*. 1997;60:366-372.

12. Lai K, Langley SD, Singh RH, Dembure PP, Hjelm LN, Elsas LJ. A prevalent mutation for galactosemia among black Americans. *J Pediatr*. 1996;128:89-95.

13. Robertson A, Singh RH. Outcomes analysis of verbal dyspraxia in classic galactosemia. *Genet Med*. 2000;2:142-148.

14. Elsas LJ 2nd, Lai K. The molecular biology of galactosemia. *Genet Med*. 1998;1:40-48.

15. Hatada I, Nabetani A, Morisaki H, et al. New p57KIP2 mutations in Beckwith-Wiedemann syndrome. *Hum Genet*. 1997;100:681-683.

16. Enklaar T, Zabel BU, Prawitt D. Beckwith–Wiedemann syndrome: multiple molecular mechanisms. *Expert Rev Mol Med*. 2006;8:1-19.

17. Catchpoole D, Lam WWK, Valler D, et al. Epigenetic modification and uniparental inheritance of H19 in Beckwith-Wiedemann syndrome. *J Med Genet*. 1997;34:353-359.

18. Young LE, Fernandes K, McEvoy TG, et al. Epigenetic change in IGF2R is associated with fetal overgrowth after sheep embryo culture. *Nat Genet*. 2001;27:153-154.

19. Wu BL, Austin MA, Schneider GH, Boles RG, Korf BR. Deletion of the entire NF1 gene detected by the FISH: four deletion patients associated with severe manifestations. *Am J Med Genet*. 1995;59:528-535.

20. Upadhyaya M, Huson SM, Davies M, et al. An absence of cutaneous neurofibromas associated with a 3-bp inframe deletion in exon 17 of the NF1 gene (c.2970–2972 delAAT): evidence of a clinically significant NF1 genotype-phenotype correlation. *Am J Hum Genet*. 2007;80:140-151.

21. McGarry JD, Brown NF. The mitochondrial carnitine palmitoyltransferase system: From concept to molecular analysis. *Eur J Biochem*. 1997;244:1-14.

22. Wang S, Robert M, Gibson K, Wanders R, Mitchell GA. 3-Hydroxy-3-methylglutaryl-CoA lyase (HL): mouse and human HL gene (HMGCL) cloning and detection of large gene deletions in two unrelated HL-deficient patients. *Genomics*. 1996;33:99-104.

23. Matsubara Y, Kraus JP, Yang-Feng TL, Francke U, Rosenberg LE, Tanaka K. Molecular cloning of cDNAs encoding rat and human medium-chain acyl-CoA dehydrogenase and assignment of the gene to human chromosome 1. *Proc Natl Acad Sci USA*. 1986;83:6543-6547.

24. Shen J, Bao Y, Liu HM, Lee P, Leonard JV, Chen YT. Mutations in exon 3 of the glycogen debranching enzyme gene are associated with glycogen storage disease type III that is differentially expressed in liver and muscle. *J Clin Invest*. 1996;98:352-357.

25. Lteif AN, Schwenk WF. Hypoglycemia in infants and children. *Endocrinol Metab Clin North Am*. 1999;28:619.

26. Munnich A, Besmond C, Darquy S, et al. Dietary and hormonal regulation of aldolase B gene expression. *J Clin Invest*. Mar 1985;75(3):1045-1052.

27. Zanaria E, Muscatelli F, Bardoni B, et al. An unusual member of the nuclear hormone receptor superfamily responsible for X-linked adrenal hypoplasia congenita. *Nature*. 1994;372:635-641.

28. Raphael Rubin, David SS. *Rubin's Pathology: Clinicopathologic Foundation of Medicine*. 5th ed. Baltimore: Wolters Kluwer Health: Lippincot Williams & Wilkins; 2008:201-203.

29. Feldkamp MM, Angelov L, Guha A. Neurofibromatosis type 1 peripheral nerve tumors: aberrant activation of the Ras pathway. *Surg Neurol*. 1999;51(2):211-218.

30. Dynkevich Y, Rother KI, Whitford I, et al. Tumors, IGF-2 and Hypoglycemia: Insights from the clinic, the laboratory and the historical archive. *Endocr Rev*. 2013 May 13. [Epub ahead of print]

## Supplementary Information

**OMIM REFERENCES:** Condition; Gene Name (OMIM#)

[1] Familial Hyperinsulinemia Hypoglycemia
- ABCC8(#600509)
- KCNJ11(#600937)
- GCK(#138079)
- HADH(#601609)
- INSR(#147670)
- GLUD1(#138130)
- SLC16A1(#610021)

[2] Beckwith-Wiedemann Syndrome; CDKN1C, H19, IGF2, KCNQ1, KCNQ1OT1 (#130650)

[3] Islet Cell Adenoma; MEN1 (#131100)

[4] Carnitine Acyltransferase Deficiency; CPT1A, CPT2 (#600528/#600650)

[5] 3-Hydroxymethyl-3-methylglutaryl-CoA lyase Deficiency; HMGCL (#246450)

[6] Long-Chain and Medium-Chain Acyl-Coenzyme A Dehydroge-nase Deficiency; ACADLD, ACADMD (#609016/#201450)

[7] Variably in Short-Chain Acyl-Coenzyme A Dehydrogenase Deficiency; ACADSD (#201470)

[8] Glycogen Synthase Deficiency; GYS2 (#138571)

[9] Glycogen Storage Disease Type Ia/b; G6PC (#232200)

[10] Glycogen Storage Disease Type III; AGL (#232400)

[11] Glycogen Storage Disease Type VI; PYGL (#232700)

[12] Fructose 1,6 Diphosphatase Deficiency; FBP1 (#611570)

[13] Phosphoenol Pyruvate Deficiency I; PCK1 (#261650)

[14] Pyruvate Carboxylase Deficiency; PC (#266150)

[15] Hereditary Fructose Intolerance; ALDOB (#612724)

[16] Galactosemia; GALT (#230400)

[17] X-Linked Panhypopituitarism; PHPX (#312000)

[18] X-Linked Adrenal Hypoplasia Congenita; NR0B1 (#300200)

[19] Combined Pituitary Hormone Deficiency 1; PROP1 (#262600)

[20] Glucocorticoid Deficiency-1; MC2R (#202200)

[21] Maple Syrup Urine Disease Ia, b, II; BCKDHA, BCKDHB, DBT (#248600)

[22] Neurofibromatosis 1; NF1 (#162200)

**Alternative Names:**
- Persistent Hyperinsulinemic Hypoglycemia of Infancy
- Nesidioblastosis of Pancreas
- Hypoglycemia, Hyperinsulinemic, of Infancy
- Exomphalos-Macroglossia-Gigantism Syndrome
- Wermer Syndrome
- CPT IA
- Hydroxymethylglutaric Aciduria
- LCHAD Deficiency
- MCHAD Deficiency
- Lipid-Storage Myopathy Secondary to Short-Chain acyl-CoA
- SCADH Deficiency
- Liver Glycogen Synthase
- Glucose-6-Phosphatase Deficiency
- Forbes Disease
- Cori Disease
- Hers Disease
- Phosphorylase Deficiency Glycogen-Storage Disease of Liver
- Fructose-1,6-Bisphosphatase, Liver
- PEPCK1
- Leigh Syndrome due to Pyruvate Carboxylase Deficiency
- Fructose-1,6-Bisphosphate Aldolase B
- Galactose-1-Phosphate Uridylyltransferase Deficiency
- Pituitary Dwarfism
- Addison Disease, X-Linked; AHX AHC With HHG
- Adrenal Unresponsiveness to ACTH
- ACTH Resistance
- Branched-Chain Ketoaciduria
- Branched-Chain Alpha-Keto Acid Dehydrogenase Deficiency
- von Recklinghausen Disease
- Hanhart Dwarfism
- Pituitary Dwarfism III

# 58 Multiple Endocrine Neoplasia Type 1

Paraskevi Xekouki, Evgenia Gourgari, and Constantine A. Stratakis

## KEY POINTS

- *Disease summary:*
  - The term multiple endocrine neoplasia 1 (MEN1) refers to a familial tumor syndrome characterized by the combination of tumors of the parathyroid glands, pancreatic islet cells, and anterior pituitary gland.
  - Patients may also develop adrenal cortical tumors, carcinoid tumors, facial angiofibromas, collagenomas, and lipomas.
  - Parathyroid tumors are the first manifestation of MEN1 in more than 85% of patients. In less than 15% of patients, the first manifestation may be an insulinoma or prolactinoma.
  - The frequency of MEN1 is estimated to be 1 case in 30,000 persons with a female to male ratio of 1:1.
  - The age of onset of endocrine tumors is usually in the teenaged years; however, the diagnosis is frequently delayed until the fourth decade of life.

- *Hereditary basis:*
  - The gene for MEN1 has been localized to chromosome band 11q13 and codes for a 610-amino acid protein, referred to as menin.
  - Loss of heterozygosity (LOH) has been found in the region associated with MEN1, suggesting that the gene has tumor suppression function consistent with Knudson's two hit hypothesis. More than 90% of tumors from MEN1 patients have LOH.
  - *MEN1* germline mutations are identified in about 80% to 90% of probands with familial MEN1 syndrome and about 65% of individuals with sporadic MEN1 syndrome (ie, a single occurrence of MEN1 syndrome in a family)
  - 5-10% of patients with MEN1 may not harbor mutations in the coding region of the *MEN1* gene; these individuals may have whole gene deletions or mutations in the promoter or untranslated regions.
  - More than 10% of the *MEN1* mutations arise de novo.

- *Differential diagnosis:*
  - **MEN4 syndrome:** Germline mutations in *CDKN1B*/p27 gene, encoding the p27kip protein, have been reported in (a) a small family presented with characteristics of MEN1: somatotropinoma, parathyroid tumors, and renal angiomyolipoma, (b) in a Dutch patient diagnosed with three lesions compatible with a diagnosis of MEN1: small-cell neuroendocrine cervical carcinoma, adrenocorticotropic hormone (ACTH)-secreting pituitary adenoma and hyperparathyroidism.
  - **Sporadic primary hyperparathyroidism (PHPT)**
    - It presents as a single parathyroid adenoma, mostly in the sixth decade of life.
    - Symptoms are due to hypercalcemia, in contrast to individuals with MEN1 syndrome, who are often asymptomatic and identified during evaluation for manifestations of MEN1 syndrome.
  - **Familial isolated hyperparathyroidism due to mutations other than MEN1**
    - *CASR*, the gene encoding the calcium-sensing receptor, responsible for familial benign hypercalcemia (FBH), also called familial hypocalciuric hypercalcemia (FHH or FBHH) and neonatal severe primary hyperparathyroidism (NSHPT).
    - *HRPT2*, the gene encoding parafibromin, which is responsible for the hyperparathyroidism-jaw tumor (HPT-JT) syndrome
  - **MEN2 syndrome**, caused by mutations in *RET* characterized by medullary thyroid carcinoma, pheochromocytoma, and PHPT.
  - **Familial isolated pituitary adenoma (FIPA)**
    - Germline mutations in the *AIP* gene, encoding aryl hydrocarbon receptor-interacting protein, have been identified in 15% to 20% of FIPA cases.
    - The causative gene or genes in the majority (70%-80%) of FIPA families is currently unknown.
  - **Zollinger-Ellison Syndrome (ZES)**
    - Gastric acid hypersecretion and severe peptic ulceration due to tumor (gastrinoma) of the duodenum or pancreas producing the hormone gastrin
    - Symptoms generally occur one decade later than in MEN1
    - 25% of all ZES can be attributed to MEN1
  - **Insulinoma**
  - **Carcinoid tumors**
    - Carcinoid tumors not associated with MEN1 syndrome usually occur in derivatives of the midgut and hindgut, are argentaffin positive, and secrete serotonin (5-hydroxytryptamine).

## Diagnostic Criteria and Clinical Characteristics

***Diagnostic Criteria:*** Clinical diagnostic criteria for MEN1 syndrome include the presence of two of the following endocrine tumors, which may become evident either by overproduction of polypeptide hormones or by growth of the tumor itself (Table 58-1).

- **Parathyroid tumors**
  - PHPT is the main MEN1-associated endocrinopathy, and the first clinical expression of MEN1 syndrome in 90% of individuals.
  - MEN1-associated PHPT in contrast to sporadic are (a) younger age (20-25 years), (b) even gender distribution, (c) multiglandular disease, (d) more severe bone involvement, (e) lower parathyroid hormone (PTH) levels.

*Table 58-1  Tumor Types in MEN1*

| Tumor Type | Prevalence in MEN1 | Hormone Secretion | Characteristics |
|---|---|---|---|
| Parathyroid adenoma | 100% by age 50 years | PTH | Hyperplasia or adenoma<br>Onset: between ages 20 and 25 years |
| Pituitary adenoma | 20%-40%<br>First clinical manifestation in 10% of familial cases and 25% of sporadic cases | Prolactinoma: most common pituitary tumor subtype (60%)<br>Growth hormone (GH) secreting: 10%-20%<br>GH/PRL secreting: 5%<br>ACTH secreting: 5%<br>TSH secreting: rare<br>15–30%: nonfunctional | Most commonly macroadenomas<br>Rarely malignant<br>Poor response of prolactinomas to dopamine agonists (only 44% of patients being controlled) |
| Well-differentiated GEP-NETS | 25%-75%<br>Multicentric and may undergo malignant transformation | Gastrinoma (40%): Zollinger-Ellison syndrome (ZES)<br>Insulinoma (4%): fasting hypoglycemia<br>Glucagonoma (2%): silent or hyperglycemia<br>VIPoma (2%):Watery diarrhea<br>Nonfunctioning pancreatic endocrine tumors: the most frequent tumors in MEN1 syndrome (80%-100% of cases) | 25% of all ZES can be attributed to MEN1<br>25% of individuals with MEN1 syndrome/ZES have no family history of MEN1 syndrome<br>The age of onset of insulinoma associated with MEN1 is generally one decade earlier than the sporadic counterpart (before the age of 40 years) |
| Carcinoid | 10%<br>Thymic carcinoids more prevalent in males than in females<br>Bronchial carcinoids more prevalent in females than in males | Usually nonhormone secreting<br>Thymic, bronchial, and gastric carcinoids rarely oversecrete ACTH, calcitonin, or GHRH<br>Rarely oversecrete serotonin or histamine and rarely can cause carcinoid syndrome | Usually in the foregut (eg, thymus, lungs, stomach, duodenum)<br>Appears as a large mass after age 50 years<br>Thymic carcinoids of MEN1 syndrome tend to be aggressive<br>Bronchial carcinoids, often multicentric, may exhibit both synchronous and metasynchronous occurrence<br>In contrast to thymic carcinoids, most bronchial carcinoids usually behave indolently |
| Adrenocortical tumors | 20%-40% | Nonfunctional cortical adenomas or diffuse or nodular hyperplasia: most often benign<br>Cortisol secreting: rare<br>Aldosterone secreting: rare<br>Adrenal carcinomas: rare | |
| Thyroid lesions | 15%-27% | Euthyroid goitre, follicular adenomas, papillary, follicular carcinomas | Not clear causative relation to MEN1 |
| Nonendocrine tumors associated with MEN1 | Skin:<br>(1) Facial angiofibromas (40%-80%)<br>(2) Collagenomas (0%-72%)<br>(3) Lipomas (3%-34%)<br>(4) Confetti-like hypopigmented macules (6%)<br>(5) Multiple gingival papules (6%)<br>Central nervous system:<br>(1) Meningioma<br>(2) Ependymoma<br>(3) Leiomyomas | | Angiofibromas:<br>-Often multifocal<br>-Mostly located on the central part of the face |

*Table 58-2 Number and Type of Mutations Identified in MEN1*

| Type of Mutation | Prevalence | Hotspot Mutations |
|---|---|---|
| Nonsense | 23% | Codon 98: c.292C>T/p. Arg98X<br>Codon 145: c.1243C>T/P Arg415X<br>Codon 460: c.1378C>T/p. Arg460X |
| Frameshift deletions/insertions | 41% | Codons 83-83: c.249_252delGTCT<br>Codons 210-211: c.628_631delACAG<br>Codon 516: c.1546delC<br>Codon 516: c.1546_1547insC |
| In-frame deletions or insertions | 6% | Codon 120: c.358_360delAAG |
| Splice-site mutations | 9% | Intron 4: c.784-9G>A |
| Missense | 20% | |
| Large deletions | 1% | |
| Total number of identified mutations: 1133 | | |

- PTHP is more severe in the presence of ZES and biochemical parameters of ZES worsen in the presence of hypercalcemia.
- **Pituitary tumors**
  - The first clinical manifestation of MEN1 syndrome in 25% of simplex cases (ie, a single occurrence of MEN1 syndrome in a family) and in 10% of familial cases.
  - Symptoms are similar to sporadic pituitary tumors.
  - Multiple adenomas are significantly more frequent in MEN1, especially with prolactin-adrenocorticotropic hormone.
- **Well-differentiated endocrine tumors of the gastroenteropancreatic (GEP) tract**
  - **Gastrinoma**
    - 40% of individuals with MEN1 syndrome have gastrinoma, which manifests as ZES usually before the age of 40 years.
    - Common symptoms are upper abdominal pain, diarrhea, esophageal reflux, acid-peptic ulcers, heartburn, weight loss, vomiting, gastrointestinal (GI) bleeding (hematemesis or melena), and ulcer perforation even without prior symptoms.
    - Typically, they are multiple small (diameter <1 cm) gastrinomas in the duodenal submucosa. Half have already metastasized before diagnosis.
    - Pancreatic gastrinomas are rare in MEN1 but more aggressive than duodenal gastrinomas.
    - Sustained hypergastrinemia leads to hyperplasia of the enterochromaffin-like (ECL) cells which may ultimately progress through to malignant gastric carcinoid.
  - **Insulinoma**
    - Mostly presents as symptomatic fasting hypoglycemia
    - Usually multicentric (10%-20%); 25% metastasize either to regional lymph nodes or to the liver
  - **VIPoma**
    - **W**atery **d**iarrhea, **h**ypokalemia, and **a**chlorhydria (WDHA syndrome) resulting from a vasoactive intestinal peptide (VIP)
    - 17% of patients with MEN1 develop VIPomas at some stage of their disease. Approximately 10% of neuroendocrine tumors of the GI tract (except carcinoids) are VIPomas.

- **Glucagonoma**
  - Glucagonoma syndrome: necrolytic migratory erythema, diabetes mellitus, weight loss, anorexia, glossitis, anemia, diarrhea, venous thrombosis (the 4D syndrome: diabetes, dermatitis, deep vein thrombosis, and depression)

*Note: MEN1* germline mutations have been reported in 20% to 57% of families with familial isolated hyperparathyroidism (FIHP), which is characterized by parathyroid adenoma or hyperplasia without other associated endocrinopathies (Table 58-2).

## Screening and Counseling

*Screening: MEN* gene screening should only be performed in individual patients with suspected MEN1 syndrome. It is recommended that testing be done if a patient has

- One endocrine tumor or hormonal excess syndrome characteristic of MEN1 (eg, primary hyperparathyroidism, endocrine gastroenteropancreatic tumor, anterior pituitary adenoma, adrenal adenoma) plus age less than 40 years or positive family history or multifocal tumor.
- Two or more endocrine tumors characteristic of MEN1 syndrome.
- Recurrent endocrine tumor characteristic of MEN1 syndrome.

First-degree relatives should be screened for the mutation only if the patient has been found to have a germline mutation. Further screening of unaffected family members that do not carry the mutation is not necessary since their risk is the same as in the general population, that is, less than 0.1%. MEN1 is extremely rare before adolescent. More than 95% of MEN1 appear after the age of 12 and therefore it is advisable that genetic testing be done around that age, when the adolescent can also consent and participate to decision management.

For those asymptomatic individuals who are found to have the mutation it is recommended that they should undergo

- At least annually, fasting blood sample for ionized Ca and albumin corrected Ca, PTH, gastrin, glycoprotein alpha subunit, glucagon, VIP, polypeptide (PP), chromogranin A, prolactin, insulin-like growth factor 1 (IGF1), thyroid-stimulating hormone (TSH), FT4, glucose and insulin, cholesterol, triglycerides and high-density lipoprotein (HDL), urea and electrolytes, liver function tests.

- Periodic routine imaging screening for adults with proven MEN1: Annual abdominal ultrasonography-examining pancreas, liver, and adrenals. After 35 years old, annually CT or MRI of chest and abdomen for bronchopulmonary carcinoid, thymic carcinoid, adrenal and gastroenteropancreatic tumors. After third to fifth decade, yearly pituitary MRI. After fifth decade yearly dual-energy x-ray absorptiometry (DXA) bone mineral density (BMD).

*Counseling:* MEN1 syndrome is inherited in an autosomal dominant manner. That gives each child of an affected parent a 50% risk of inheriting the condition. Approximately 90% of individuals diagnosed with MEN1 syndrome have an affected parent and 10% have de novo mutations. Prenatal diagnosis is available by amniocentesis performed at 15 to 18 weeks' gestation or chorionic villus sampling (CVS) at 10 to 12 weeks' gestation.

## Management and Treatment

- **PHPT**
  - Early parathyroidectomy is suggested to control (a) even mild PHPT, uncontrolled disease is associated with progressive decline in bone mineral density and early onset of osteoporosis; (b) hypercalcemia, which is a secretagogue for gastrin and exacerbates hypergastrinemia in patients with concurrent enteropancreatic disease.
  - Consider the use of bone antiresorptive agents prior to surgery to reduce hypercalcemia, limit PTH-dependent bone resorption, and future risk of osteoporosis.
  - The optimal surgical approach is controversial; approaches include either subtotal parathyroidectomy (resection of 3-3$^{1/2}$ parathyroid glands) or total parathyroidectomy and autotransplantation of parathyroid tissue to the forearm musculature (reduces the potential for permanent postoperative hypoparathyroidism).
  - A transcervical thymectomy at the time of initial parathyroidectomy also facilitates removal of ectopic parathyroid tissue and may reduce the risk of malignant thymic carcinoid in later life.
  - Reoperation for recurrent hyperparathyroidism is often required within 10 years of an initially successful parathyroidectomy (recurrence rate up to 56%); surveillance with PTH and/or serum calcium to assess for hypoparathyroidism following subtotal or total parathyroidectomy and possible recurrence.
- **Intra-abdominal neoplasia**

Surgery is the only curative treatment option for MEN1-related pancreatic neuroendocrine tumors (PNETs).

- **Insulinomas**
  - In MEN1 should always be operated. Distal pancreatic resection (DPR) combined with enucleation of tumors from the head has shown higher cure rates compared to enucleation alone.
- **Gastrinomas**
  - Unlike sporadic gastrinoma, in MEN1 this disease is rarely cured by surgery. Surgical intervention mostly is ineffective due to the multicentric duodenal submucosal distribution of MEN1 gastrinoma.
  - Most experts prefer distal pancreatectomy to the level of the portal vein with enucleation of any tumors in the pancreatic head, a duodenotomy with excision of any tumors in the first to fourth portion of the duodenum and a peripancreatic lymph node dissection, whereas other groups prefer a pylorus-preserving pancreaticoduodenectomy (PPPD).
  - Reoperation is indicated if (a) there is biochemically established recurrence of ZES, (b) an unequivocal lesion in at least two imaging procedures, and (c) diffuse metastases have been excluded.
  - Control of hyperacidity with proton pump inhibitors or H$_2$-receptor blockers to reduce gastric acid output is strongly recommended, while surgical control of PHPT and somatostatin analogues may ameliorate hypergastrinemia.
  - Periodic gastroscopic surveillance is important for identification of both peptic ulcer disease and gastric carcinoid.
- **VIPOMAs:**
  - Treatment of a patient with a VIPoma begins with replacement of fluid losses and correction of electrolyte abnormalities; somatostatin analogues (octreotide) decrease VIP secretion and it is the treatment of choice to control diarrhea. Interferon-alpha (IFN-$\alpha$) in addition to octreotide may control symptoms in patients who are resistant or refractory to octreotide alone.
- **Carcinoid tumors**
  - Long-acting somatostatin analogs can control the secretory hyperfunction associated with carcinoid syndrome; however, the risk for malignant progression of the tumor remains unchanged.
- **Pituitary tumors**
  - Treatment of pituitary tumors in MEN1 is not different from that of sporadic pituitary tumors.
  - Treatment success seems to differ between sporadic and MEN1 pituitary tumors; normalization of pituitary hypersecretion occurred in 42% of the MEN1 patients after treatment, compared with 90% of the patients with sporadic tumors.
- **Prevention of primary manifestations**
  - The only prophylactic surgery possible in MEN1 syndrome is thymectomy to prevent thymic carcinoid and it should be considered at the time of neck surgery for primary hyperparathyroidism in males with MEN1 syndrome, particularly those who are smokers or have relatives with thymic carcinoid.

## Molecular Genetics and Molecular Mechanism

*Syndrome/Gene/Locus*
Gene symbol: *MEN1*
Chromosomal locus: 11q13
Protein name: Menin

Menin is mainly located in the nucleus. The C-terminal part of menin contains sequences that are essential for the regulation of gene expression as well as nuclear localization domains. Menin is widely expressed and may play different roles in different tissues. Menin potentially interacts with the promoter regions of thousands of genes and may be involved in the regulation of several cell functions, including DNA replication and repair, and in transcriptional machinery. It interacts with *JunD*, leading to the formation of a growth inhibiting complex as well as with nuclear factor kB, the Smad family, DNA, cell-cycle regulators and a variety of other transcription factors, cell structural elements, and regulators of apoptosis. It has been hypothesized that menin may mediate its tumor suppressor action by regulating histone methylation in promoters of *HOX* genes and/or p18, p27, and possibly other CDK inhibitors.

***Genetic Testing:*** Genetic testing should be offered to at-risk members of a family in which a germline *MEN1* mutation has been identified in an affected relative. In those patients in whom a *MEN1* mutation could not be detected, a search for a partial or whole deletion of an MEN allele could be undertaken, prior to searching for mutations in other genes, such as *CDNKIB*.

When molecular genetic testing for an *MEN1* mutation is not possible or is not informative, individuals at 50% risk (eg, first-degree relatives) should undergo routine evaluation.

For current information on availability of genetic testing see Gene Tests Laboratory Directory at http://www.genetests.org/query?mim=168000

**BIBLIOGRAPHY:**

1. Falchetti A, Marini F, Brandi ML. Multiple endocrine neoplasia type 1. In: Pagon RA, Bird TD, Dolan CR, Stephens K, eds. Gene Reviews [Internet]. Seattle, WA: University of Washington, Seattle; 1993-2005 [updated 2010 Mar 02].

2. Thakker RV. Multiple endocrine neoplasia type 1 (MEN1). *Best Pract Res Clin Endocrinol Metab.* 2010;24(3):355-370.

3. Karges W, Schaaf L, Dralle H, Boehm BO. Concepts for screening and diagnostic follow-up in multiple endocrine neoplasia type 1 (MEN1). *Exp Clin Endocrinol Diabetes.* 2000;108(5):334-340.

4. Burgess J. How should the patient with multiple endocrine neoplasia type 1 (MEN 1) be followed? *Clin Endocrinol (Oxf).* 2010;72(1):13-16.

5. Pieterman CR, Vriens MR, Dreijerink KM, van der Luijt RB, Valk GD. Care for patients with multiple endocrine neoplasia type 1: the current evidence base. *Fam Cancer.* 2011;10:157-171.

6. Fendrich V, Langer P, Waldmann J, Bartsch DK, Rothmund M. Management of sporadic and multiple endocrine neoplasia type 1 gastrinomas. *Br J Surg.* 2007;94:1331-1341.

7. Desai KK, Khan MS, Toumpanakis C, Caplin ME. Management of gastroentero-pancreatic neuroendocrine tumors (GEP-NETs). *Minerva Gastroenterol Dietol.* 2009;55:425-443.

## Supplementary Information

***Key Words:*** Multiple endocrine neoplasia, menin, pituitary, parathyroid, insulinoma, gastrinoma, glucagonoma

# 59 Multiple Endocrine Neoplasia Type 2

Steven G. Waguespack, Elizabeth G. Grubbs, and Mimi I. Hu

## KEY POINTS

- *Disease summary:*
  - Multiple endocrine neoplasia type 2 (MEN2) is caused by a dominantly inherited or de novo activating (gain of function) mutation in the *RET* proto-oncogene.
  - MEN2A (95% of MEN2 cases) is characterized by the development of medullary thyroid carcinoma (MTC) in greater than 90% of affected patients, pheochromocytoma (PHEO) in up to 50% of cases, and/or primary hyperparathyroidism (PHPT) in up to 20% of mutation carriers. Depending on the specific *RET* mutation, cutaneous lichen amyloidosis (CLA) and Hirschsprung disease can also occur.
  - MEN2B (5% of MEN2 cases) is characterized by the universal and early development of MTC, high risk of PHEO (up to 50% of cases) and a highly penetrant, distinctive physical appearance.
  - A strong genotype-phenotype correlation exists in MEN2 such that MTC disease severity, the likelihood of developing PHEO and PHPT, and the age of disease onset can be estimated based on genetic testing results.
  - In *RET* mutation carriers, C-cell hyperplasia is the initial stage of tumor development that leads to microscopic noninvasive MTC (usually bilateral) and ultimately to lymph node and distant metastases due to frankly invasive carcinoma.
  - Familial MTC (FMTC) is currently considered to be a phenotypic variant of MEN2A with a high risk for MTC but decreased penetrance and/or delayed onset of the other neoplastic manifestations. There is significant overlap between *RET* mutations associated with FMTC and those of MEN2A.
- *Hereditary basis:*
  - MEN2A and MEN2B have an autosomal dominant inheritance pattern with almost complete penetrance of the MTC phenotype.
- *Differential diagnosis:*
  - There is no other genetic syndrome associated with the development of MTC. Other multiorgan system syndromes that include PHEO as a feature include von Hippel-Lindau disease, the familial paraganglioma syndromes, and neurofibromatosis type 1. Familial PHPT is most commonly associated with MEN1 but the differential diagnosis also includes familial isolated primary hyperparathyroidism, familial hypocalciuric hypercalcemia, and hyperparathyroidism-jaw tumor syndrome. Hirschsprung disease can be sporadic or associated with underlying chromosomal abnormalities and gene mutations, including inactivating (loss of function) *RET* mutations that are distinct from the MEN2-causing mutations. The differential diagnosis for the skeletal phenotype of MEN2B includes Marfan syndrome and homocystinuria; intestinal ganglioneuromatosis may also be associated with Cowden syndrome and type 1 neurofibromatosis.

## Diagnostic Criteria and Clinical Characteristics

### Diagnostic Criteria:

#### At least one of the following

- One or more of the MEN2-associated endocrine tumors in a patient who has an identified germline mutation in the *RET* proto-oncogene
- Identification of a known MEN2-causing germline mutation in the *RET* proto-oncogene, particularly with a positive family history of any of the known MEN2-related endocrine tumors
- A diagnosis of MTC in a patient who has one or more close relatives with histologically confirmed MTC
- A clinical diagnosis of MEN2 (prior to confirmation via genetic testing) would be highly suspected in a given patient with two or more of the endocrine tumors associated with MEN2 or a diagnosis of MTC in a patient with the clinical features of MEN2B

#### And the absence of

- Another identifiable multiorgan system genetic syndrome that explains the development of PHPT, PHEO, and/or physical examination findings in the proband or family

### Clinical Characteristics: (Tables 59-1 and 59-2)

☞**MEDULLARY THYROID CARCINOMA:** Arising from the parafollicular C cells, MTC is usually the first MEN2 manifestation. Years before clinical disease becomes apparent, MTC begins as C-cell hyperplasia, a precancerous finding that ultimately develops into microscopic and then macroscopic cancer that is typically multifocal, bilateral, and located in the middle to upper regions of the thyroid lobes. Clinical presentations can include a palpable thyroid and/or neck mass, compressive symptoms, or diarrhea related to elevated calcitonin levels and other substances secreted by the tumor. Some patients may have microscopic MTC identified incidentally during thyroid surgery for another indication and, with the onset of genetic testing, more individuals are being identified to have lesser degrees of disease due to early surgical intervention at a presymptomatic stage. Lymph node and distant metastases typically occur years after the onset of tumorigenesis, and the most aggressive clinical presentation occurs with MEN2B, followed by codon 634 mutations in MEN2A, and finally by the other known disease-causing mutations in RET. Cervical and mediastinal lymph nodes are the most common sites of metastatic disease; typical distant sites for MTC spread include the lungs, liver, and bone or bone marrow. Calcitonin and carcinoembryonic antigen (CEA) are excellent tumor markers for MTC, with rapid doubling times associated with more aggressive disease and a worse prognosis.

*Table 59-1  MEN2A Phenotype*

| System | Manifestation | Comments |
|---|---|---|
| Thyroid C cells | Medullary thyroid carcinoma | >90% of MEN2A cases |
| Adrenal medulla | Pheochromocytoma | 0%-50% of MEN2A cases |
| Parathyroid glands | Primary hyperparathyroidism | 0%-20% of MEN2A cases |
| Skin | Cutaneous lichen amyloidosis | Rare |
| GI tract | Hirschsprung disease | Rare |

☞**PHEOCHROMOCYTOMA:** The classic triad of clinical features includes diaphoresis, headache, and palpitations in a patient with episodic or sustained hypertension, but patients with PHEO may not have these classic features and may even be entirely asymptomatic. PHEO in patients with MEN2 usually arise within a background of adrenal medullary hyperplasia and are associated with an adrenergic clinical phenotype (elevation of epinephrine ± norepinephrine, in addition to their metabolites, metanephrine and normetanephrine, respectively). Individuals with MEN2 are at an increased risk for bilateral PHEO and an earlier age of onset, and these tumors may present synchronously or even prior to an MTC diagnosis, especially in MEN2A. Paragangliomas (catecholamine-producing tumors located outside of the adrenal gland) and malignant tumors are exceedingly rare in MEN2.

☞**PRIMARY HYPERPARATHYROIDISM:** PHPT in patients with MEN2A may be due either to a single parathyroid adenoma or multigland hyperplasia. The disease is diagnosed and evaluated similarly to sporadic PHPT.

☞**CUTANEOUS LICHEN AMYLOIDOSIS:** CLA is skin disorder of intense pruritus and secondary skin changes typically located in interscapular region of the back that becomes clinically manifest in some MEN2A patients during late adolescence or young adult life.

☞**HIRSCHSPRUNG DISEASE:** This is a congenital disease characterized by the complete absence of neuronal ganglion cells (aganglionosis) from a portion of the intestinal tract, primarily the distal colon. It is usually diagnosed shortly after birth due to delayed passage of meconium, constipation, and in more severe cases, emesis associated with abdominal pain and distention. Milder cases may not be diagnosed until adulthood. The gold standard for diagnosis is a rectal biopsy.

☞**MEN2B PHENOTYPE:** While some aspect of the MEN2B clinical phenotype is present in all MEN2B patients, individual manifestations have a variable presentation and are age dependent. Because of this and general unfamiliarity with the syndrome, the MEN2B diagnosis is almost always delayed, even in the presence of typical clinical features.

## Screening and Counseling

**Screening:** Patients who have a clinical diagnosis of MEN2 (eg, MTC plus PHEO; MEN2B phenotype) or a suspicion of MEN2 based on the diagnosis of an associated endocrine tumor and a family history of MEN2-associated neoplasia should undergo testing for a germline *RET* mutation. Genetic counseling is an integral part of the care of the patient documented with or suspected to have MEN2. A genetic counselor can obtain a comprehensive family history, share and update patients on relevant information regarding MEN2, and facilitate genetic testing of the patient and at-risk family members as indicated. Presymptomatic genetic testing should be offered to all first-degree relatives of an individual with a known *RET* mutation. Preimplantation and prenatal genetic testing of the *RET* proto-oncogene is also possible.

*Table 59-2  MEN2B Phenotype*

| System | Manifestation | Comments |
|---|---|---|
| Thyroid C cells | Medullary thyroid carcinoma | 100% of MEN2B cases |
| Adrenal medulla | Pheochromocytoma | ~50% of MEN2B cases |
| GI tract | Oral mucosal (Fig. 59-1) and intestinal ganglioneuromatosis[a] | ~100% of MEN2B cases |
| Skeleton | Marfanoid body habitus, narrow long facies, pes-cavus, pectus excavatum, high-arched palate, scoliosis, and/or slipped capital femoral epiphysis | ~75% of MEN2B cases |
| Eyes | Inability to make tears in infancy, thickened and everted eyelids, mild ptosis, and prominent corneal nerves (medullated corneal nerve fibers) | Varies |
| Other | Joint laxity; hypotonia or proximal muscle weakness, thickened lips; pubertal delay | Varies |

[a]Mucosal neuromas can also occur on the conjunctiva and in the urinary system. Symptoms of intestinal ganglioneuromatosis include constipation and feeding problems in infancy and the development of megacolon in the most severe cases.

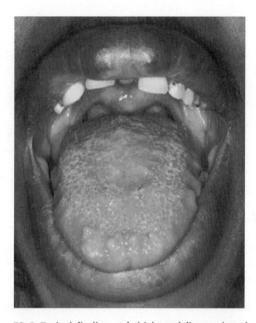

**Figure 59-1** Typical findings of thickened lips and oral mucosal neuromas are demonstrated in an adult with MEN2B. These oral manifestations of MEN2B are a highly penetrant component of the phenotype and can be an early clue to diagnosis in childhood.

Although most patients who present with apparently sporadic MTC are likely not to harbor a germline *RET* mutation, there is increased recognition that *RET* mutations, particularly those associated with less aggressive presentations of MTC, can be identified in such patients. This has led to the current recommendation for routine germline *RET* analysis in every patient diagnosed with MTC.

Patients with apparently sporadic PHEO would rarely harbor a germline *RET* mutation, but MEN2 should be considered in a young patient who presents with an adrenergic (elevated epinephrine ± norepinephrine) PHEO, especially if bilateral tumors are present. A patient would be unlikely to have PHPT as the initial manifestation of MEN2, so routine *RET* testing in a young patient with isolated PHPT is not routinely recommended unless there is a suggestive family history.

**Counseling:**

☞**INHERITANCE, PENETRANCE:** The MEN2 syndromes are highly penetrant disorders that are inherited in an autosomal dominant fashion. Each child of an affected parent has a 50% risk of inheriting the mutated *RET* gene. The probability of a de novo gene mutation is 5% or less in index cases with MEN2A and 50% or more in index cases with MEN2B. Nonpaternity and germline mosaicism in a clinically unaffected parent should be considered in situations of apparent de novo mutations.

☞**GENOTYPE-PHENOTYPE CORRELATION** (Fig. 59-2): After identification of *RET* as the causative gene in MEN2, it quickly became apparent that there were only a limited number of

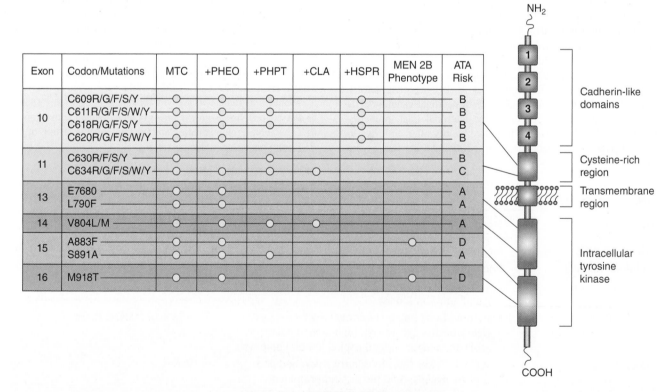

| Exon | Codon/Mutations | MTC | +PHEO | +PHPT | +CLA | +HSPR | MEN 2B Phenotype | ATA Risk |
|------|-----------------|-----|-------|-------|------|-------|------------------|----------|
| 10   | C609R/G/F/S/Y   | O   | O     | O     |      | O     |                  | B        |
|      | C611R/G/F/S/W/Y | O   | O     | O     |      | O     |                  | B        |
|      | C618R/G/F/S/Y   | O   | O     | O     |      | O     |                  | B        |
|      | C620R/G/F/S/W/Y | O   | O     |       |      | O     |                  | B        |
| 11   | C630R/F/S/Y     | O   | O     | O     |      |       |                  | B        |
|      | C634R/G/F/S/W/Y | O   | O     | O     | O    |       |                  | C        |
| 13   | E7680           | O   | O     |       |      |       |                  | A        |
|      | L790F           | O   |       |       |      |       |                  | A        |
| 14   | V804L/M         | O   | O     | O     | O    |       |                  | A        |
| 15   | A883F           | O   | O     |       |      |       | O                | D        |
|      | S891A           | O   | O     | O     |      |       |                  | A        |
| 16   | M918T           | O   | O     |       |      |       | O                | D        |

NH₂

1 2 3 4 — Cadherin-like domains

Cysteine-rich region

Transmembrane region

Intracellular tyrosine kinase

COOH

**Figure 59-2** The RET receptor and commonly mutated codons in MEN2A and MEN2B and their associated clinical phenotypes, including the recent risk stratification proposed by the American Thyroid Association to help determine the timing of early thyroidectomy. MTC, medullary thyroid carcinoma; PHEO, pheochromocytoma; PHPT, primary hyperparathyroidism; CLA, cutaneous lichen amyloidosis; HSCR, Hirschsprung disease. Adapted from Waguespack SG, Rich TA, Perrier ND, Jimenez C, Cote GJ. Management of medullary thyroid carcinoma and MEN2 syndromes in childhood. *Nat Rev Endocrinol.* 2011;7(10):596-607.

MEN2-causing mutations and that strong genotype-phenotype correlations were present.

MEN2A is most frequently due to mutations in *RET* exon 11 (codon 634 specifically) followed by mutations in exon 10 (codons 609, 611, 618, and 620 specifically). These mutations are located mostly in the extracellular cysteine-rich domain of the *RET* receptor. Other common mutations involve codons 630, 768, 790, 804, and 891. As molecular testing becomes widespread, more *RET* mutations and DNA variants (variants of unknown significance [VUS]) are being identified, which is contributing to an ever-changing spectrum of the MEN2A genotype and phenotype.

Patients with MEN2A and mutations in *RET* codon 634 have the highest risk of malignant C-cell disease followed by those with mutations in codons 609, 611, 618, 620, or 630, whereas mutations in codons 768, 790, 804, or 891 impart the lowest risk for clinically aggressive MTC.

In MEN2A, PHEO occurs most commonly in association with mutations in codon 634 and to a much lesser degree with mutations in codons 609, 611, 618, and 620. Primary hyperparathyroidism is chiefly associated with codon 634 mutations. Mutations in exon 10 (primarily codon 620, but also codons 609, 611, and 618) are associated with Hirschsprung disease. CLA has primarily been described in individuals with codon 634 mutations.

MEN2B is almost always due to the Met918Thr mutation (exon 16) located in the intracellular tyrosine kinase domain of the RET receptor. Rare cases can be attributed to a mutation caused by a two-base substitution in codon 883 (Ala883Phe, exon 15) or double *RET* mutations involving codon 804.

## Management and Treatment

See Table 59-3.

*Medullary Thyroid Carcinoma:* Cure rates are low when MEN2 patients have palpable MTC lesions. Consequently, surgical resection of the thyroid based on *RET* mutation prior to the development of clinically detectable disease offers the best chance for cure. The strong genotype-phenotype correlations that exist in MEN2 facilitate guidelines for treating presymptomatic patients with MEN2. Determining the appropriate age for thyroidectomy remains difficult, particularly in lower-risk *RET* mutations, and contemporary approaches to care incorporate knowledge regarding the genotype in addition to clinical data (ultrasound and calcitonin level).

For clinically apparent MTC, surgical resection consists of total thyroidectomy and central-compartment (level VI) lymph node dissection with the addition of compartment-focused lateral neck dissection for image- or biopsy-positive disease in those compartments. This treatment approach represents the most definitive curative modality available, with the adequacy of the initial operation being the most important determinant of outcome. Biochemical cure of MTC varies depending on the extent of lymph node involvement at the time of surgery (75%-90% in patients without lymph node involvement compared with 20%-30% in those with lymph node involvement).

For symptomatic or progressive metastatic MTC, vandetanib, an oral tyrosine kinase inhibitor, is approved in the United States based on the results of phases II and III studies that included MEN2 patients. Preliminary results from ongoing studies with other tyrosine kinase inhibitors also appear promising.

*Pheochromocytoma:* Medical therapy with a selective alpha-blocker, such as phenoxybenzamine, followed by a beta-blocker added a few days later is necessary to control hypertension and to optimize a patient for definitive therapy with surgical resection. Appropriate medical management and adequate hydration are essential to prevent a hypertensive crisis intraoperatively and postoperative hypotension.

Surgical resection is the treatment of choice for PHEO. As MEN2 patients are at high risk for bilateral disease, cortical-sparing adrenalectomy is considered to allow for exogenous steroid independence and to help reduce the risk of acute adrenal insufficiency.

☞PRIMARY HYPERPARATHYROIDISM: Surgical resection (parathyroidectomy for a single adenoma; subtotal parathyroidectomy

*Table 59-3 MEN2 Surveillance*

| Disease | Laboratory Testing | Radiologic Testing |
|---|---|---|
| Medullary thyroid carcinoma | • Calcitonin<br>• Carcinoembryonic antigen (CEA)<br>• Genetic testing (*RET* proto-oncogene)<br>• Fine-needle aspiration biopsy | • Ultrasound of thyroid/neck<br>• Cross-sectional imaging (CT/MRI) of the neck, chest, and abdomen (using a multiphase liver protocol) as clinically indicated |
| Primary hyperparathyroidism | • Calcium<br>• Intact parathyroid hormone<br>• 24-hour urine for calcium | • Ultrasound of thyroid/neck<br>• Tc99m sestamibi parathyroid scan<br>• 4D CT of the neck<br>• DXA scan, including distal forearm |
| Pheochromocytoma | • Plasma-free metanephrines/catecholamines<br>• 24-hour urine metanephrines/catecholamines | • CT/MRI of adrenals<br>• $^{123}$I/$^{131}$I -MIBG scintigraphy |
| Hirschsprung disease | • Rectal suction biopsy | • Abdominal x-ray<br>• Contrast enema<br>• Anorectal manometry |

CT, computed tomography; MRI, magnetic resonance imaging; 4D, four dimensional; $^{123}$I/$^{131}$I –MIBG, iodine-123 or iodine-131-meta-iodobenzylguanidine; DXA, dual-energy x-ray absorptiometry

in multigland disease) is indicated in patients with clinically relevant hypercalcemia. In a patient with mild PHPT, lifestyle and medical management strategies should be implemented, including maintenance of adequate oral hydration and avoidance of prolonged periods of immobilization. Antiresorptive therapies to treat osteoporosis can be utilized as clinically indicated, especially in those patients who may not be good surgical candidates. Cinacalcet (an oral calcimimetic that binds to the calcium-sensing receptor and can decrease parathyroid hormone levels and, in turn, serum calcium levels) can also be used to treat hypercalcemia as indicated. Patients who do not undergo surgery require routine monitoring of calcium levels, renal function, and bone densitometry.

☞**Cutaneous Lichen Amyloidosis:** CLA is the consequence of repeated scratching in response to intense pruritus. The use of topical capsaicin has been reported to have some efficacy in this setting.

*Hirschsprung Disease:* The goal of treatment is to resect the aganglionic segment of bowel while preserving sphincter function. The exact surgical approach is primarily based on surgeon preference.

# Molecular Genetics and Molecular Mechanism

*Syndrome/Gene/Locus:*

MEN2A (FMTC)/*RET* proto-oncogene/10q11.21
MEN2B/*RET* proto-oncogene/10q11.21

☞**Description of Basic Gene Functions:** *RET* is a member of the cadherin superfamily and it encodes a transmembrane receptor with intrinsic, ligand-stimulatable tyrosine kinase activity. The RET protein is a subunit of a multimolecular complex that binds growth factors of the glial-derived neurotropic factor (GDNF) family. It is crucial in neural crest development and subsequently has important roles in the development of the enteric nervous system, the kidney, and in spermatogenesis. MEN2 is caused by activating mutations that cause constitutive (ligand-independent) activation of the RET receptor. RET tyrosine kinase activity has become recognized as a "druggable" target in cancer therapeutics. The drug vandetanib, a potent inhibitor of the RET tyrosine kinase, in addition to vascular endothelial growth factor receptors 2 and 3, became the first agent approved by the FDA for the treatment of adults with symptomatic or progressive MTC, including patients with MEN2.

*Genetic Testing:* DNA sequence analysis of the *RET* proto-oncogene is widely available. As with any monogenic disorder, genetic testing should begin with the affected proband and be expanded to other family members only if a gene mutation is identified. Initial testing of *RET* includes sequencing of exons 10, 11, and 13-16, although directed testing (eg, exons 15 and 16 only in MEN2B; codon 634 only in a family with a known codon 634 mutation) is reasonable. In less than 2% of cases, individuals with hereditary MTC may have a *RET* mutation that cannot be detected in exons 10, 11, and 13-16; additional sequencing of exons 1-9, 12, and 17-21 should be considered in such cases, if the clinical suspicion for MEN2 is high. In cases where familial transmission is evident yet no mutation has been detected on exhaustive *RET* sequencing, at-risk individuals will need to be followed clinically.

**Bibliography:**

1. Moline J, Eng C. Multiple endocrine neoplasia type 2: an overview. *Genet Med.* Sep 2011;13(9):755-764.

2. Waguespack SG, Rich TA, Perrier ND, Jimenez C, Cote GJ. Management of medullary thyroid carcinoma and MEN2 syndromes in childhood. *Nat Rev Endocrinol.* 2011;7(10):596-607.

3. Kloos RT, Eng C, Evans DB, et al. Medullary thyroid cancer: management guidelines of the American Thyroid Association. *Thyroid.* 2009;19(6):565-612.

4. Cohen MS, Phay JE, Albinson C, et al. Gastrointestinal manifestations of multiple endocrine neoplasia type 2. *Ann Surg.* May 2002;235(5):648-654; discussion in 654-645.

5. Elisei R, Romei C, Cosci B, et al. RET genetic screening in patients with medullary thyroid cancer and their relatives: experience with 807 individuals at one center. *J Clin Endocrinol Metab.* Dec 2007;92(12):4725-4729.

6. Eng C, Clayton D, Schuffenecker I, et al. The relationship between specific RET proto-oncogene mutations and disease phenotype in multiple endocrine neoplasia type 2. International RET mutation consortium analysis. *JAMA.* Nov 20 1996;276(19):1575-1579.

7. Margraf RL, Crockett DK, Krautscheid PM, et al. Multiple endocrine neoplasia type 2 RET protooncogene database: repository of MEN2-associated RET sequence variation and reference for genotype/phenotype correlations. *Hum Mutat.* Apr 2009;30(4):548-556.

8. Frank-Raue K, Rondot S, Raue F. Molecular genetics and phenomics of RET mutations: impact on prognosis of MTC. *Mol Cell Endocrinol.* Jun 30 2010;322(1-2):2-7.

9. Moore SW, Zaahl MG. Multiple endocrine neoplasia syndromes, children, Hirschsprung's disease and RET. *Pediatr Surg Int.* May 2008;24(5):521-530.

10. Verga U, Fugazzola L, Cambiaghi S, et al. Frequent association between MEN 2A and cutaneous lichen amyloidosis. *Clin Endocrinol (Oxf).* Aug 2003;59(2):156-161.

11. Yen TW, Shapiro SE, Gagel RF, Sherman SI, Lee JE, Evans DB. Medullary thyroid carcinoma: results of a standardized surgical approach in a contemporary series of 80 consecutive patients. *Surgery.* Dec 2003;134(6):890-899; discussion 899-901.

12. Wells SA Jr., Gosnell JE, Gagel RF, et al. Vandetanib for the treatment of patients with locally advanced or metastatic hereditary medullary thyroid cancer. *J Clin Oncol.* Feb 10 2010; 28(5):767-772.

13. Wells SA Jr., Robinson BG, Gagel RF, et al. Vandetanib in patients with locally advanced or metastatic medullary thyroid cancer: a randomized, double-blind phase III trial. *J Clin Oncol.* Oct 24 2011.

14. Gild ML, Bullock M, Robinson BG, Clifton-Bligh R. Multikinase inhibitors: a new option for the treatment of thyroid cancer. *Nat Rev Endocrinol.* 2011;7(10):617-624.

15. Lee JE, Curley SA, Gagel RF, Evans DB, Hickey RC. Cortical-sparing adrenalectomy for patients with bilateral pheochromocytoma. *Surgery.* Dec 1996;120(6):1064-1070; discussion 1070-1071.

16. Santoro M, Melillo RM, Carlomagno F, Vecchio G, Fusco A. Minireview: RET: normal and abnormal functions. *Endocrinology.* Dec 2004;145(12):5448-5451.

17. Phay JE, Shah MH. Targeting RET receptor tyrosine kinase activation in cancer. *Clin Cancer Res.* Dec 15 2010;16(24):5936-5941.

**Acknowledgements:**

We are most grateful to Thereasa A Rich, MS, CGC for her thoughtful review of this chapter and to Gilbert J. Cote, Ph. D. for his contributions to Figure 59-1.

## Supplementary Information

**OMIM References:**

[1] Multiple Endocrine Neoplasia Type 2A; MEN2A (#171400)

[2] Familial Medullary Thyroid Carcinoma; FMTC (#155240)

[3] Multiple Endocrine Neoplasia Type 2B; MEN2B (#162300)

**Alternative Names:**

- Familial Medullary Thyroid Carcinoma
- Sipple Syndrome (MEN2A)
- Wagenmann-Froboese Syndrome (MEN2B)
- Mucosal Neuromal Syndrome (MEN2B)
- Multiple Endocrine Neoplasia, Type III; MEN3 (MEN2B)

**Key Words:** *RET* proto-oncogene, medullary thyroid carcinoma, calcitonin, carcinoembryonic antigen, C cell, hyperplasia, diarrhea, hypercalcemia, hyperparathyroidism, pheochromocytoma, paraganglioma, chromaffin cell, increased catecholamines, hypertension, cutaneous lichen amyloidosis, Hirschsprung disease, aganglionosis, constipation, megacolon, marfanoid, mucosal neuromas, ganglioneuromatosis, thickened lips, pescavus, high-arched feet, slipped capital femoral epiphysis.

# 60 Autoimmune Thyroid Diseases

Deirdre Cocks Eschler, Francesca Menconi, and Yaron Tomer

## KEY POINTS

- *Disease summary:*
  - Autoimmune thyroid disorders (AITDs) include Graves disease (GD) and Hashimoto thyroiditis (HT). Both are complex genetic diseases caused by the interplay of several genes with environmental triggers (eg, infection) resulting in disruption of normal thyroid function. AITDs are some of the most common autoimmune disorders and can be associated with other autoimmune diseases. Both are found in a higher prevalence among women with the age of onset most frequently between 30 and 50 years.
  - **Graves disease:** Production of thyrotropin (TSH) receptor stimulating antibodies (TRAb) results in overstimulation of the thyroid gland that causes an excessive production and inappropriate release of thyroid hormones resulting in clinical *hyperthyroidism*, as well as thyroid enlargement *(goiter)* due to hypertrophy and hyperplasia of thyroid follicles.
    - Symptoms are related to hyperthyroidism, as well as those that are specific to GD: Graves ophthalmopathy (GO) and Graves dermopathy.
  - **Hashimoto disease:** Also known as chronic lymphocytic thyroiditis, is the most common cause of hypothyroidism in the industrialized world with a higher prevalence in iodine sufficient areas and among smokers. It is characterized by lymphocytic infiltration of thyroid gland, causing thyroid cell death and resultant hypothyroidism.
    - Symptoms are related to the lack of thyroid hormones *(hypothyroidism)*.
- *Differential diagnosis:*
  - **GD:** Subacute thyroiditis, postpartum thyroiditis, silent thyroiditis, toxic multinodular goiter, toxic adenoma, surreptitious ingestion of thyroid hormones, drug-induced thyroiditis (eg, amiodarone, interferon)
  - **HT:** Primary myxedema, postpartum thyroiditis, drug-induced hypothyroidism (eg, amiodarone, interferon, lithium)
- *Family history:*
  - Familial predisposition to the development of AITD is very common. Several studies have reported a higher frequency of thyroid abnormalities in relatives of patients with AITD, most commonly the presence of thyroid antibodies.
- *Twin studies:*
  - It has been reported in several studies that the concordance rate in monozygotic twins is significantly higher than in dizygotic twins, both in GD and in HT. These findings support the notion that there is a clear inherited susceptibility in AITD.
- *Environmental factors:*
  - Iodine, infection, smoking, pregnancy, medications
- *Genome-wide associations:*
  - There are no genome-wide association studies (GWAS) reported to date. However, several genome-wide linkage and candidate gene studies have been reported. These studies identified several non-MHC susceptibility genes including *CTLA4*, *CD40*, *PTPN22*, thyroglobulin, and *TSHR*. In addition, the presence of arginine at position 74 of the HLA-DR beta chain was strongly associated with both GD and HT.

## Diagnostic Criteria and Clinical Characteristics

### Diagnostic Criteria for AITD:

☞**GRAVES DISEASE:** Diagnosis is based on the presence of primary hyperthyroidism plus at least one of the following: (1) clinically evident GO and/or dermopathy, (2) detectable serum TRAb, or (3) diffuse radioactive iodine uptake on thyroid scan.

Diagnostic evaluation should include

- The initial test to screen patients with symptoms of hyperthyroidism is a serum TSH. A low or undetectable level (normal levels 0.4-4 mU/L) should prompt testing of serum-free thyroxin (fT4) and total triiodothyronine (tT3). A suppressed TSH with a high serum fT4 and/or tT3 confirms primary hyperthyroidism. Note that it is important to test T3 since some patients develop T3 toxicosis and may have normal or low fT4 levels.

- **Serologic markers:** Though not necessary for the diagnosis, thyroid antibodies are present in most patients. While the TRAbs that cause GD are not easily measured, if high-sensitivity assays are used, they are detectable in over 95% of patients. TRAbs must be tested in pregnant women with a history of GD as high levels confer risk for neonatal Graves since TRAbs pass the placenta. In addition, thyroid peroxidase antibodies (TPOAbs) are positive in about three-quarters of patients and thyroglobulin antibodies (TgAbs) in about half of patients.
- **Thyroid examination:** A diffuse, firm enlargement of thyroid gland is present in most patients and is more common in patients younger than 50 years old. In some patients a bruit can be auscultated over the thyroid because of the increased blood flow to the gland.
- **Imaging studies:**
  - **Radioactive iodine uptake scan** can help distinguish GD from thyrotoxicosis caused by painless thyroiditis or postpartum thyroiditis, toxic multinodular goiter, toxic adenoma, and surreptitious ingestion of thyroid hormones.

In GD there is a homogenous increase in radioiodine uptake whereas in the other forms of thyrotoxicosis there is a low or focal radioiodine uptake.

- **Ultrasound with Doppler** may also help in the differential diagnosis with other causes of thyrotoxicosis; an increased blood flow to the gland is consistent with GD while low flow with destructive thyroiditis (painless or postpartum thyroiditis or some forms of drug-induced thyroiditis).
  - **CT scan of the neck:** In patients with symptoms of airway compromise, a computed tomographic (CT) scan of the neck should be done.

☞**HASHIMOTO THYROIDITIS:** Diagnosis is made in a patient with primary hypothyroidism plus evidence of autoimmunity. Diagnostic evaluation should include

- Screen patients with hypothyroid symptoms with serum TSH. High levels suggest hypothyroidism and require testing of serum fT4. High TSH and low fT4 confirm primary hypothyroidism (no need to test T3 which may be normal in early stages of hypothyroidism).
- **Serologic markers:** These are necessary for the diagnosis of HT (or autoimmune thyroiditis). Serum TPOAbs are positive in 90% to 95% of patients, and thyroglobulin antibodies in 60% to 80% HT. Antithyroid peroxidase antibodies are the more sensitive test; high levels correlate with thyroid dysfunction. Some patients have only positive antibodies with normal thyroid functions (subclinical disease). In these patients there is a 3% to 5% yearly risk of developing clinical disease.
- **Thyroid examination:** A goiter may be present and is most commonly firm, painless, and symmetric.
- **Imaging studies:** Imaging is not routinely indicated. Ultrasound would show a hypoechogenic thyroid, sometimes in a patchy pattern.
- Radioactive iodine uptake can be normal, increased, or decreased.
- **Thyroid biopsy:** While uncommon, patients with HT are at an increased risk of thyroid lymphoma and should have any dominant nodule biopsied by a fine-needle aspiration. The tissue of HT is characterized by lymphocytes (both B and T cells) infiltrating the thyroid gland. In addition, thyroid cells undergo changes and Hurthle cells are frequently identified.

*Clinical Characteristics:* Since thyroid hormones affect cellular functions in many tissues, symptoms of thyroid dysfunction are diverse and nonspecific. In GD there are also disease-specific symptoms thought to be related to autoantigen cross-reactivity with the skin and orbital tissues.

☞**GRAVES DISEASE:**
- Symptoms of hyperthyroidism
  - Most commonly weight loss despite increased appetite, palpitations, nervousness, fatigue, heat intolerance, tremor, insomnia.
  - Other symptoms are oligomenorrhea or amenorrhea, decreased libido, infertility, diarrhea, dyspnea, supraventricular tachycardias. Over time, increase in thyroid hormone can result in bone loss and osteoporosis, as well as glucose intolerance.
  - Elderly patients may not have classic symptoms (apathetic hyperthyroidism), or can develop atrial fibrillation which may be their presenting symptom.
  - Rarely, the disease may present with a thyroid storm: fever, altered mental status, psychosis, and tachycardia.

- Physical examination may reveal tachycardia, warm, moist skin, a tremor, hyperactive relaxation phase of deep tendon reflexes, a diffusely enlarged thyroid gland, and possibly a bruit heard over the gland.
- Symptoms specific to GD
  - **GO:** Most commonly manifests as burning sensation in the eyes, photophobia, and retro-ocular pressure. In severe cases, ocular pain, diplopia, and blurred vision may appear. Up to 50% of GD patients have clinical evidence of GO and it may develop within 1 year or before or after the diagnosis of hyperthyroidism. Smoking is a known risk factor.
  - **Graves dermopathy:** Lymphocytic infiltration of the skin ultimately causes a nonpitting edema, most frequently affecting the pretibial areas of the legs. It affects less than 1% of patients.
  - **Thyroid acropachy:** It is extremely rare. Results in swelling of the soft tissue and periosteal bone changes in the fingers or toes.

☞**HASHIMOTO THYROIDITIS:**
- Symptoms of hypothyroidism
  - Weight gain, cold intolerance, constipation, urinary retention (slowing of genitourinary [GU] and gastrointestinal [GI] tracts), menometrorrhagia, fatigue with slowed mentation, and occasionally heart failure.
  - **Physical examination** may reveal dry, cold, sometimes edematous skin, coarse hair, brittle nails, weight gain, delayed relaxation phase of deep tendon reflexes, bradycardia, and, in severe cases pleural or pericardial effusions.
  - **Laboratory:** If severe and not treated, patients can develop hypercholesterolemia, hyponatremia, and elevated homocysteine levels.

## Screening and Counseling

*Screening:* There is no current evidence for screening family members as currently there is no therapy for primary prophylaxis.
*Counseling:* While there is no need for genetic counseling, women with GD should be counseled about the risk of neonatal Graves and how to avoid it. Neonatal Graves is caused by TSH receptor stimulating antibodies crossing the placenta and stimulating the baby's thyroid. Therefore, women with Graves should be monitored carefully throughout pregnancy, by a thyroid specialist with experience in pregnancy, for TSH receptor stimulating antibodies and thyroid function. If the antibodies are positive, the baby should be monitored with fetal ultrasound for goiter. Immediately after delivery the baby should be observed, tested for thyrotoxicosis, and treated appropriately if neonatal Graves develops.

## Management and Treatment

*Graves Disease:* There are three treatment options for GD: antithyroid medications, radioactive iodine ablation, and surgery to remove the thyroid gland (total thyroidectomy).

☞**MEDICAL:**

- Commonly recommended for younger patients are antithyroid drugs—carbimazole and methimazole. Treatment is usually given for 6 to 18 months. The remission rate is 30% to 40% of those treated. Patients who are young, have large goiters, have eye involvement, or have high antibody titers at diagnosis are unlikely to achieve lasting remission with medical therapy alone. Rare but serious side effects include agranulocytosis and hepatic damage or failure. Propylthiouracil (PTU), formerly a common antithyroid medicine, is now rarely used because of its life-threatening hepatotoxicity. The only exception is during pregnancy where PTU is recommended over methimazole due to reports of aplasia cutis and choanal atresia in babies born to mothers taking methimazole.
- **Beta-blockers** can be used for symptomatic relief.
- If severe, for instance in thyroid storm, glucocorticoids can be used to decrease the conversion of T4 to T3, and iodine can be used (after starting antithyroid medications) to decrease the release of T4 and T3 from the thyroid.
- **Monitoring after treatment:** fT3 and fT4 will be the first markers to change, usually after about 4 weeks. Changes in TSH usually lag.

☞**RADIOACTIVE IODINE:** Radioactive iodine is effective in ablating the thyroid and inducing permanent hypothyroidism. It is particularly recommended for patients who are older or who fail to achieve permanent remission with medical management. Treatment involves oral ingestion of iodine-131. It is contraindicated in pregnant and breastfeeding women. Since radioactive iodine can accumulate in breast tissue it is recommended to delay radioactive iodine ablation up to a year after a woman stops breastfeeding. Iodine therapy can exacerbate GO, especially in smokers and those with severe GO, which may be in part prevented with concomitant glucocorticoid use. Treatment usually induces permanent hypothyroidism for which patients will need lifelong thyroid replacement therapy.

☞**SURGERY:** Total thyroidectomy is usually reserved for patients with large goiters, those with dominant, potentially malignant, nodules, or those who fail or refuse the above treatments. It is also used for pregnant women (during the second trimester) who fail medical management or require high doses of drugs.

☞**DISEASE-SPECIFIC TREATMENTS:**

- **Graves ophthalmopathy:** All patients with GO should be referred to an ophthalmologist. Most mild or even moderate cases of GO improve without drastic intervention. Treatment for GO involves treating the hyperthyroidism, smoking cessation, use of artificial tears, and, if severe, glucocorticoid therapy and/or orbital irradiation. If proptosis is severe after the acute phase of the disease it may require surgery with orbital decompression. Monoclonal antibodies against CD20 have also shown some promise in the treatment of GO.

**Hashimoto Thyroiditis:** Levothyroxine sodium (thyroxine), synthetic T4, is the treatment of choice once clinical hypothyroidism is present. It is indicated for most patients with TSH higher than the upper limit of normal, particularly in those with high-antibody levels. Treatment is lifelong and the starting dose is based on bodyweight and age; 1.6 to 1.8 µg/kg/d in adults, lower doses are given in elderly (about 0.5 µg /kg/d). After initiation of therapy, the T4 dose is adjusted based on the TSH levels. The goals of treatment are to normalize the TSH levels, and to correct the symptoms of hypothyroidism.

Absorption of thyroxine is affected by several drugs, including calcium, iron, and bile acid-binding resins. Therefore, thyroxine should be taken without other medications. Increased doses are required frequently in pregnancy and any patient planning to become pregnant should be monitored carefully before, during, and after pregnancy. In nonpregnancy patients serum thyrotropin should be measured 6 weeks after every dose adjustment and then annually in symptomatically stable patients. During pregnancy TSH should be measured more frequently.

## Molecular Genetics and Molecular Mechanisms

**Genetic Testing:** No need for genetic testing.
**Future Directions:** To date, six candidate genes have been identified in AITD (see Table 60-1). Future studies will try to correlate genotypes and phenotypes and identify subset of GD and HT patients who are affected by the different genetic variants.

**Table 60-1 Disease-Associated Susceptibility Variants**

| Candidate Gene (Chromosome Location) | Associated Variant | Putative Functional Significance |
|---|---|---|
| HLA-DR (6p21) | Arginine at position 74 of the HLA-DR beta chain | Pocket structure enables presentation of pathogenic peptides to T-cells |
| CTLA-4 (2q33) | Several: A/G49, CT60, 3'UTR (AT)n | Decreased CTLA-4 expression results in increased activation of T-cells |
| CD40 (20q13) | 5'UTR C/T SNP | Increased CD-40 expression results in increased activation of B-cells |
| PTPN22 (1p13) | Tryptophan/arginine substitution at codon 620 (R620W) | Mechanism unclear, possibly allowing escape of T-cells from tolerance |
| Thyroglobulin (8p24) | Several | Amino acid variants result in pathogenic peptides being presented to T-cells |
| TSHR (14q31) | Several in intron 1 | Mechanism unclear, possible changes in splicing |

Genetic predictors of development of agranulocytosis, or worsening of ophthalmopathy after radioactive iodine treatment would be very useful clinical tools.

## BIBLIOGRAPHY:

1. Pearce EN. Farwell, AP, Braverman, LE. Thyroiditis. *N Engl J Med.* 2003;348:2646-2655.

2. Tomer Y, Davies TF. Searching for the autoimmune thyroid disease susceptibility genes: from gene mapping to gene function. *Endocr Rev.* 2003;24:694-717.

3. Tomer Y, Huber A. The etiology of autoimmune thyroid disease: a story of genes and environment. *J Autoimmun.* 2009;32: 231-239.

4. Menconi F, Oppenheim YL, Tomer Y. Graves' disease. In: Shoenfeld Y, Cervera R, Gershwin ME, eds. *Diagnostic Criteria in Autoimmune Diseases.* Totowa, NJ: Humana Press; 2008:231-235.

5. Weetman AP. Graves' disease. *N Engl J Med.* 2000;343: 1236-1248.

6. Brent GA. Clinical practice. Graves' disease. *N Engl J Med.* 2008;358:2594-2605.

7. Rocchi R, Rose NR, Caturegli P. Hashimoto thyroiditis. *Diagnostic Criteria in Autoimmune Disease.* Totowa, NJ: Humana Press; 2010:217-220.

8. Vanderpump MPJ, Tunbridge WMG, French J M, et al. The incidence of thyroid disorders in the community: a twenty-year follow-up of the Whickham survey. *Clin Endocrinol (Oxf).* 1995; 43:55-68.

9. Cooper DS. Hyperthyroidism. *Lancet.* 2003;362:459-468.

10. Roberts CG Ladenson PW. Hypothyroidism. *Lancet.* 2004;363: 793-803.

## Supplementary information

**OMIM** REFERENCES:

[1] Graves disease: 275000

[2] Hasimoto disease: 140300

*Keywords:* Autoimmune thyroid disorders (AITD), Hashimotos thyroiditis (HT), Graves disease (GD)

# 61 Adrenal Insufficiency

Eugen Melcescu, Christian A. Koch

## KEY POINTS

- *Disease summary:*
  - Adrenal insufficiency is caused by a defective production of adrenal hormones due to a primary disorder of the adrenal gland or dysregulation of the hypothalamic-pituitary-adrenal axis.
  - Hereditary factors have been known to play a role in developing this condition.
  - Adrenal insufficiency is categorized as primary (failure of the adrenals to produce cortisol and/or aldosterone and/or androgens), secondary (deficient production of pituitary adrenocorticotropic hormone [ACTH]), or tertiary (impaired production of corticotropin-releasing hormone [CRH] by hypothalamus)
  - Primary adrenal insufficiency is classified as
    - Autoimmune—polyglandular syndromes type 1, 2, or other autoimmune conditions
    - Infectious—Waterhouse-Friderichsen syndrome (*Neisseria meningitidis, Mycobacterium tuberculosis, Streptococcus pneumoniae*, cytomegalovirus, histoplasmosis, etc)
    - Bilaterally metastatic disease: lung, breast, gastrointestinal carcinomas
    - Vascular-bilateral adrenal hemorrhage (hemorrhagic diathesis, trauma)
    - Genetic syndromes related to deficiency of enzymes in steroidogenesis and cholesterol metabolism, transcription factors, storage diseases, corticotropin receptor and signaling, sterol secretion, etc
    - Medications: mitotane, aminoglutethimide, ketoconazole, metyrapone, mifepristone RU486, megestrol, rifampicin, anticonvulsants (phenytoin), and others
  - Secondary adrenal insufficiency causes
    - Hypopituitarism (congenital, acquired, primary or metastatic tumor, radiation)
    - Iatrogenic (high-dose glucocorticoid therapy)

Clinical presentation of adrenal insufficiency is variable. Based on the causative factors various clinical expressions of the disease have been observed. The condition may have an abrupt or gradual onset or may appear in childhood or late in life.

- *Hereditary basis:*
  - Conditions inherited in an **autosomal recessive pattern**
    - 21-hydroxylase deficiency (the most common form of congenital adrenal hyperplasia (CAH))
    - 17-alpha-hydroxylase deficiency(<1% of all cases of CAH)
    - 11-beta-hydroxylase deficiency (represents 5%-8% of all cases)
    - 3-beta-hydroxysteroid dehydrogenase (HSD) type II deficiency
    - Lipoid congenital adrenal hyperplasia (the most severe form of CAH)
    - Smith-Lemli-Opitz (SLO) syndrome
    - Antley-Bixler syndrome with genital anomalies and disordered steroidogenesis
    - Wolman disease
    - Familial glucocorticoid deficiency 1 (>50% of patients do not have mutations in the *MC2R* gene)
    - Triple A syndrome
    - Polyglandular autoimmune syndrome type 1
    - Sitosterolemia
    - Zellweger syndrome
    - Panhypopituitarism: *HESX1, OTX2, LHX4, PROP1, TBX19*

Condition inherited in an **autosomal dominant inheritance**
  - Glucocorticoid receptor deficiency

Condition inherited in an **X-linked recessive pattern**
  - Congenital adrenal hypoplasia (X-linked)
  - Congenital adrenal hypoplasia (SF1 linked)
  - Adrenoleukodystrophy
  - Hyperglycerolemia
  - Panhypopituitarism: SOX3

## Diagnostic Criteria and Clinical Characteristics

As there are so many genetic etiologies without a uniform picture (ie, ambiguous genitalia for some, alacrima for others, mucocutaneous candidiasis in *AIRE* patients, etc), the biochemical screening and diagnosis prevails:

- Plasma cortisol at 8 AM less than 3 µg/dL
- Plasma cortisol less than 18 µg/dL (495 nmol/L) 30 to 60 minutes after 250 µg cosyntropin IV or IM
- Plasma aldosterone increment less than 5 ng/dL (150 pmol/L) after cosyntropin

*Clinical Characteristics:* The clinical presentation of adrenal insufficiency is directly correlated with the degree of loss of adrenal function.

**Table 61-1 Genes Associated With Different Presentations**

| Gene | CYP21A2 | CYP17A1 | CYP11B1 | HSD3B2 | CYP19A1 | POR | ABCD1 | SOX3 | HESX1 |
|------|---------|---------|---------|--------|---------|-----|-------|------|-------|
| **Presentation** | 21-OH | 17-alpha | 11-beta | 3-beta-HSD | P-450 | A-B | Adreno | Pan | Pan |
| **Ambiguous genitalia** | 1 | 3 | 2 | 4 | 3 | 3 | 4 | 4 | 4 |
| **Learning disability** | 4 | 4 | 4 | 4 | 4 | 2 | 1 | 1 | 1 |
| **Hypertension** | 3 | 2 | 1 | 4 | 4 | 4 | 4 | 4 | 4 |

Scale 1 to 4: 1 most likely and 4 least likely

21-OH, 21-hydroxylase deficiency; A-B, Antley-Bixler syndrome; Adreno, adrenoleukodystrophy; Pan, panhypopituitarism.

Individuals with chronic primary adrenal insufficiency may present with a variety of symptoms and clinical signs related to the extent of glucocorticoid, mineralocorticoid, and androgen deficiency. Patients with secondary adrenal insufficiency usually preserve their mineralocorticoid function for a while and consequently have no or less characteristic features of mineralocorticoid deficiency: dehydration, hyperkalemia, and hypotension.

Common clinical features for both primary and secondary (chronic) adrenal insufficiency are reduced strength, fatigue, anorexia, weight loss, hyperpigmentation (primary adrenal insufficiency), hypotension, dizziness, nausea, vomiting, tender abdomen, dehydration, confusion, diarrhea or constipation, myalgia, arthralgia hyponatremia, hyperkalemia, metabolic acidosis, loss of or decreased libido and of axillary and pubic hair (women only), amenorrhea, etc.

There are some clinical manifestations specific for primary adrenal insufficiency: postural hypotension (BP <110/70 mm Hg), salt-craving, tanning of the skin (hyperpigmentation)—patchy (palmar creases, mucous membranes, extensor surfaces, nipples) or generalized, vitiligo (if in the setting of polyglandular syndrome).

Adrenal crisis or acute adrenal insufficiency may be caused by a serious infection, acute stress, or hemorrhage of both adrenal glands precipitating the evolution of primary adrenal insufficiency. Adrenal crisis is not common in secondary adrenal insufficiency but can occur upon abrupt withdrawal of glucocorticoid, especially high-dose dexamethasone therapy. Symptoms and signs associated with adrenal crisis are the following: severe vomiting, diarrhea, dehydration, low BP, confusion, severe lethargy, fever, hyponatremia, hyperkalemia, shock, and coma.

For secondary adrenal insufficiency one should investigate for symptoms and signs of deficiency of other anterior pituitary hormones such as headache, diplopia, visual field defects. Their presence will suggest a pituitary or hypothalamic tumor.

## Screening and Counseling

*Screening:* Patients of certain ethnic groups such as Yupik Eskimos, Ashkenazi Jews, Slavics, Italians, and Hispanics are more commonly affected than Afrikaner and Asian people. Neonatal screening for 21-hydroxylase deficiency which accounts for greater than 90% of CAH cases, is performed routinely in many countries by measuring 17-hydroxyprogesterone. In addition, DNA analysis for *CYP21A2* mutations is helpful for determining carrier status and establishing the diagnosis prenatally. In infants and adolescents with hypertension, the more rare forms of CAH, 17-alpha-hydroxylase and 11-beta-hydroxylase deficiency should be considered. Anyone with ambiguous genitalia and/or virilization, precocious or delayed puberty, and/or unexplained sodium and potassium abnormalities should be checked for a defect in steroidogenesis as should be women with polycystic ovarian syndrome, evidence for estradiol deficit, and/or hirsutism (Table 61-1). Patients presenting with adrenal insufficiency and a personal or family history of such or other autoimmune disorders should be screened for polyglandular syndromes type 1 and 2 (Table 61-2).

*Counseling:* This is especially important for prenatal diagnosis to prevent virilization of a female fetus from an affected mother with 21-hydroxylase deficiency (21-OHD) CAH. One should distinguish between classic and nonclassic genotypes of 21-OHD CAH. In most patients with 21-OHD CAH, the genotype predicts disease severity, as the individual phenotype correlates with the greatest degree of residual enzyme activity from a mutant allele. In rare patients, this is not the case and may be related to additional alterations of the mutant allele, as shown in Argentinian 21-OHD CAH patients. In patients with salt-wasting 21-OHD CAH, homozygous deletions at the CYP21A2 locus are frequently identified. In classic 21-OHD CAH, a mutation on both *CYP21A2* alleles may lead to complete abortion of enzyme activity but genotype-phenotype discordance exists and may be explained by increased alternate splicing in cases where normal splicing is abolished. In nonclassic 21-OHD CAH, individuals may have a mixture between a mild and more severe mutation (ie, compound heterozygotes in ~ two-thirds of patients) at the CYP21A2 locus. However, there is also discordance between genotype and expected clinical phenotype.

Regarding germline mutations in the *PROP1* gene, there have thus far not been any cases with isolated gonadotropin (hypogonadotropic hypogonadism) deficiency. In individuals with *PROP1* mutations, often anterior pituitary hormones become deficient in the following order: growth hormone (GH), luteinizing hormone (LH) and follicle-stimulating hormone (FSH), thyroid-stimulating hormone (TSH), and adrenocorticotropic hormone (ACTH). However, the age of onset of the deficiency and its degree are variable even within the same family. As hypothyroidism usually is mild and occurring later in childhood, it usually is not combined with mental deficiency. No genotype-phenotype correlation exists in individuals with *PROP1* mutations.

## Management and Treatment

Acute manifestations of adrenal insufficiency may be life threatening.

*Treatment of Acute Adrenal Insufficiency:* Initial treatment should address correction of hypovolemia, electrolyte abnormalities, and steroid replacement: IV fluids (large quantities) and glucocorticoids should be given. Normal saline or 5% dextrose in 0.9% NaCl

*Table 61-2  Genetic Differential Diagnosis*

| Syndrome | Gene Symbol | Associated Findings |
|---|---|---|
| **Enzymes in steroidogenesis** | | |
| 21-hydroxylase deficiency | CYP21A2 | Four CAH forms: salt-wasting (SW), simple virilizing (SV), nonclassic (NC) late onset (attenuated), and cryptic<br>Babies (SW type): poor feeding, weight loss, dehydration<br>Other forms of CAH present with ambiguous genitalia, decreased fertility, hirsutism, short stature |
| 17-alpha-hydroxylase deficiency | CYP17A1 | Sexual infantilism, decreased/absent axillary and pubic hair, hypertension, hypokalemia |
| 11-beta-hydroxylase deficiency | CYP11B1 | Virilization, hypertension ($\uparrow$DOC), hypokalemia-classic form<br>Tall stature, advanced bone age, hirsutism, acne, infertility-nonclassic form |
| 3-beta-HSD type II deficiency | HSD3B2 | Pseudohermaphroditism presence or not of SW, hirsutism, accelerated growth, premature pubarche |
| Lipoid congenital adrenal hyperplasia | StAR | Severe defects in testicular and adrenocortical steroidogenesis, growth failure<br>Newborns: failure to thrive, $\downarrow$Na, $\uparrow$K, $\downarrow$s-cortisol |
| P-450-side-chain-cleavage deficiency | CYP19A1 | Clitoromegaly, polycystic ovaries, primary amenorrhea early/late-onset adrenal insufficiency |
| Smith-Lemli-Opitz syndrome | DHCR7 | Microcephaly, mental retardation, hypotonia, behavioral problems, malformations of the heart, lungs, kidneys, GI tract, and genitalia, syndactyly, polydactyly, hypospadias, photosensitivity |
| Antley-Bixler syndrome with genital anomalies and disordered steroidogenesis | POR | Ambiguous genitalia, midface hypoplasia, low-set ears choanal atresia, multiple joint contractures, infertility craniosynostosis, radiohumeral synostosis, visceral anomalies (genitourinary system) |
| **Storage disease** | | |
| Wolman disease | LIPA | Hepatosplenomegaly, poor weight gain, vomiting, diarrhea, developmental delay, anemia, calcification of the adrenal glands |
| **Pituitary insufficiency** | | |
| Panhypopituitarism | HESX1 | Septo-optic dysplasia, agenesis of the corpus callosum, panhypopituitarism, learning disabilities, delayed puberty |
| | OTX2 | Pituitary hypoplasia, neonatal hypoglycemia |
| | LHX4 | Hypoplastic anterior pituitary glands, deficiency of anterior pituitary hormones |
| | PROP1 | Deficiency of GH, TSH, PRL secretion, late-onset adrenal insufficiency |
| | TBX19 | Low ACTH and cortisol levels |
| | SOX3 | Hypopituitarism, mental and learning disabilities |
| **Transcription factors** | | |
| Congenital adrenal hypoplasia (X-linked) | NR0B1 | Hypogonadotropic hypogonadism (males), skeletal immaturity, adrenal insufficiency |
| Congenital adrenal hypoplasia (SF1 linked) | NR5A1 | Gonadal dysgenesis (small dysgenetic testes, absent uterus, clitoromegaly) |
| IMAGe syndrome | Unknown | IUGR, metaphysical, dysplasia, adrenal hypoplasia congenita, genital malformations |
| **Corticotropin receptor and signaling** | | |
| Familial glucocorticoid deficiency 1 | MC2R | Cutaneous hyperpigmentation, tall stature, craniofacial abnormalities, hypoglycemia, muscles weakness |

*(Continued)*

*Table 61-2* **Genetic Differential Diagnosis (Continued)**

| Syndrome | Gene Symbol | Associated Findings |
|---|---|---|
| Triple A syndrome | AAAS | Alacrima, achalasia, developmental delay, dysarthria, microcephaly, muscle weakness, peripheral neuropathy, hyperkeratosis, adrenal insufficiency |
| Glucocorticoid receptor deficiency | NR3C1 | Hirsutism, mild virilization, menstrual difficulties hypertension, hypokalemia, and metabolic alkalosis |
| **Autoimmune adrenalitis** | | |
| Polyglandular autoimmune syndrome type 1 | AIRE | Mucocutaneous candidiasis, hypoparathyroidism, Addison disease |
| Polyglandular autoimmune syndrome type 2 | | Addison disease, thyroid disease, type 1 diabetes mellitus |
| **Peroxisomal abnormalities** | | |
| Adrenoleukodystrophy | ABCD1 | Paraparesis, spasticity, weakness, learning and behavioral problems, aggressive behavior, adrenocortical insufficiency vision problems<br>Adrenomyeloneuropathy (slower progression) |
| **Sterol secretion** | | |
| Sitosterolemia | ABCG5 | Tendon and tuberous xanthomas, premature development of atherosclerosis, and abnormal hematologic and liver function tests, gonadal and adrenal failure |
| Sitosterolemia | ABCG8 | |
| **Glycerol kinase deficiency** | | |
| Hyperglycerolemia | GK | Three forms: infantile, juvenile, and adult<br>Infantile form: severe developmental delay<br>Adult form has no symptoms |
| **Disorders of peroxisome biogenesis** | | |
| Zellweger syndrome | PEX1,3,5,10,13,14,19,26 | Craniofacial abnormalities, polycystic kidneys, hepatomegaly hypospadias, agenesis of the corpus callosum |

Gene names: *CYP21A2*, cytochrome P450, family 21, subfamily A, polypeptide 2; *CYP17A1*, cytochrome P450, family 17, subfamily A, polypeptide 1; *CYP11B1*, cytochrome P450, family 11, subfamily B, polypeptide 1; *HSD3B2*, hydroxy-delta-5-steroid dehydrogenase, 3 beta- and steroid delta-isomerase 2; *StAR* (steroidogenic acute regulatory protein), *CYP19A1*, cytochrome P450, family 19, subfamily A, polypeptide 1; *DHCR7*,7-dehydrocholesterol reductase; *POR*, cytochrome P450 Oxidase; *LIPA*; lysosomal lipase acid; *HESX1*, HESX homeobox 1; *OTX2*, orthodenticle homeobox 2; *LHX4*, LIM homeobox 4; *PROP1*, PROP paired-like homeobox1; *TBX19*, T-box19; *SOX3*, sex-determining region Y-box 3; *NR0*, nuclear receptor subfamily 0, group B, member 1; *NR5A1*, nuclear receptor subfamily 5, group A, member 1; *MC2R*, melanocortin 2 receptor; AAAS, Allgrove, triple A; *NR3C1*, nuclear receptor subfamily 3, group C, member 1; AIRE, autoimmune regulator; ABCD1, ATP-binding cassette, subfamily D, member 1; *ABCG5*, ATP-binding cassette, subfamily G, member 5; *ABCG8*, ATP-binding cassette, subfamily G, member 8), *GK* glycerol kinase; *PEX*, peroxin.

IV in 500 to 1000 mL over 30 minutes should be administered initially followed by up to 3 to 4 L/24 h.

Hydrocortisone (or a different steroid) IV 2 mg/kg every 6 hours should be infused until resolution of acute symptoms occurs. Sometimes higher steroid doses are required to correct the electrolyte abnormalities. If the diagnosis of adrenal insufficiency is not clear-cut, hydrocortisone should be substituted with dexamethasone to eliminate the interferences with other subsequent investigations including the ACTH stimulation test.

Generally based on the evolution of the patient's condition, the hydrocortisone dose should be tapered in decrements of 20% to 30% over the next few days and converted to an oral substitution dose. For emergency situations in the future the patient should receive a 4-mg prefilled syringe with dexamethasone. This medication may be administered IM in such circumstances.

*Treatment of Chronic Adrenal Insufficiency:* Patients diagnosed with chronic adrenal insufficiency need to be educated about the necessity of lifelong replacement therapy and the dose adjustments required when a major stress or a surgical intervention survene.

If the patient has Addison disease, daily treatment with a glucocorticoid and a mineralocorticoid is advised. About 20 to 30 mg of hydrocortisone daily will suffice for most of the patients. Fludrocortisone may be used to replace the mineralocorticoid deficiency in doses of 0.05 to 0.15 mg po qd. Sufficient intake of sodium (3-4 g/d) should be assured.

Patients with Addison disease have to be instructed to wear a medical alert (Medic Alert) bracelet and an Emergency Medical Information Card which will alert the physician and help him to take the necessary emergency treatment measures.

During minor illnesses or surgeries the glucocorticoid dose should be increased two to three times for up to 3 days to provide the necessary adjustments. If major surgery is planned, higher doses are compulsory (up to 5-10 times the maintenance dose) to avert an adrenal crisis. The dose should then be tapered over the next few days to the maintenance daily dose.

## Molecular Genetics and Molecular Mechanisms

### Syndrome/Gene/Locus:

21-hydroxylase deficiency/*CYP21A2*/6p21.3

17-alpha-hydroxylase deficiency/*CYP17A1*/10q24.3

11-beta-hydroxylase deficiency/*CYP11B1*/8q21

3-beta-HSD type II deficiency/*HSD3B2*/1p13.1

Lipoid congenital adrenal hyperplasia/*StAR*/8p11.2

P-450-side-chain-cleavage deficiency/*CYP19A1*/15q23-q24

Smith-Lemli-Opitz syndrome/*DHCR7*/11q13.4

Antley-Bixler syndrome with genital anomalies and disordered steroidogenesis/*POR*/7q11.2

Wolman disease, LIPA/10q23.2-q23.3

Panhypopituitarism/*HESX1*/3p14.3

Panhypopituitarism/*LHX4*/1q25.2

Panhypopituitarism/*PROP1*/5q35.3

Panhypopituitarism/*TBX19*/1q24.2

Congenital adrenal hypoplasia (X-linked)/*NR0B1*/Xp21.3

Congenital adrenal hypoplasia (SF1 linked)/*NR5A1*/9q33

Familial glucocorticoid deficiency 1/*MC2R*/18p11.2

Glucocorticoid receptor deficiency/*NR3C1*/5q31

Triple A syndrome/*AAAS*/12q13

Polyglandular autoimmune syndrome type 1/*AIRE*/21q22.3

Adrenoleukodystrophy/*ABCD1*/Xq28

Sitosterolemia/*ABCG5*/8,2p21

Hyperglycerolemia/*GK*/Xp21.3

Zellweger syndrome/*PEX*/1p36.32, 1p36.22, 1q23.2, 2p16.1, 6q24.2, 7q21.2, 12p13.31, 22q11.21

**21-hydroxylase deficiency**, *CYP21A2*, 6p21.3: It is a structural gene for the adrenal microsomal cytochrome P450 specific for steroid 21-hydroxylation. The *CYP21A2* gene is responsible for making of 21-hydroxylase enzyme in the adrenal glands. Deficiency of this enzyme impairs the production of cortisol and aldosterone. Patients with the salt-wasting type have a completely nonfunctional enzyme.

**17-alpha-hydroxylase deficiency**, *CYP17A1*, 10q24.3: Mutations in the *CYP17A1* gene disrupt both 17 alpha-hydroxylase and 17,20-lyase activities in the steroidogenic pathway with deficiency in production of mineralocorticoids, steroids, androgens, and estrogens or progestins.

**11-beta-hydroxylase deficiency**, *CYP11B1*, 8q21: A mutated gene causes a deficient synthesis of cortisol and corticosterone of the adrenal gland with the accumulation of 11-deoxycortisol and 11-deoxycorticosterone and consequently high blood pressure.

**3-beta-HSD type II deficiency**, *HSD3B2*, 1p13.1: 3-beta-HSD II converts pregnenolone to progesterone, 17-hydroxypregnenolone to 17-hydroxyprogesterone and DHEA to androstenedione in the adrenals, and in the testes androstenediol to testosterone. This is a form of CAH that can produce ambiguous genitalia in both sexes.

**Lipoid congenital adrenal hyperplasia**, *StAR*, 8p11.2: A defect in the *StAR* gene will impact negatively adrenal or gonadal steroids. There is a StAR protein-dependent loss of steroidogenesis when the protein is mutated and a subsequent loss of steroidogenesis that is independent of StAR due to cellular damage from accumulated cholesterol esters. The individuals diagnosed with lipoid CAH are phenotypically females and need to be treated with mineralocorticoid and glucocorticoid to increase the chances of survival.

**P-450-side-chain-cleavage deficiency**, *CYP19A1*, 15q23-q24: Cholesterol side-chain cleavage enzyme is used in the debut of steroidogenesis to convert cholesterol to pregnenolone. Mutations in the *CYP11A1* gene lead to partial or complete 46, XY sex reversal.

**Smith-Lemli-Opitz syndrome**, *DHCR7*,11q13.4: Porter et al. (1996) offered the hypothesis of defective modification of the hedgehog proteins as a possible cause for SLO syndrome. 7-DHC reductase is involved in the final step of cholesterol synthesis and its mutated gene leads to various malformations in affected individuals.

**Antley-Bixler syndrome with genital anomalies and disordered steroidogenesis**, *POR*, 7q11.2: Cytochrome P450 oxidoreductase transfers electrons for the activation of both 17-alphahydroxylase and 21-hydroxylase.

Loss of POR protein affects steroidogenesis.

**Wolman disease**, *LIPA*, 10q23.2-q23.3: LIPA enzyme deficiency causes an accumulation of fat in the liver, gut, and other organs. This is believed to be the result of an impaired intracellular breakdown of various lipids.

**Panhypopituitarism**, *HESX1*, 3p14.3: A dysfunctional gene leads to abnormal development of the forebrain, eyes, pituitary gland, and other structures.

**Panhypopituitarism**, *LHX4*, 1q25.2: LHX3 and LHX4 are important factors in pituitary organogenesis having a pivotal role in proliferation and initial differentiation of pituitary-specific cell lineages.

**Panhypopituitarism**, *PROP1*, 5q35.3: Inactivating mutations in *PROP1* result in deficiencies of PRL, LH, FSH, GH, or TSH.

**Panhypopituitarism**, *TBX19*, 1q24.2: Mutations in *TBX19* gene affects the differentiation of the pituitary pro-opiomelanocortin (POMC) lineage.

**Congenital adrenal hypoplasia (X-linked)**, *NR0B1*, Xp21.3: DAX1 protein is orphan member of the nuclear receptor (NR) superfamily that negatively regulates the transcription through retinoic acid receptor and binds in the nucleus to RA-responsive element.

**Congenital adrenal hypoplasia (SF1 linked)**, *NR5A1*, 9q33: Steroidogenic factor-1 mutations may dysregulate the transcription of genes involved in reproduction, steroidogenesis, and male sexual differentiation.

**Familial glucocorticoid deficiency 1**, MC2R, 18p11.2: ACTH receptor is a member of the G protein-coupled receptor family. Mutations in this receptor result in high levels of serum ACTH and low levels of cortisol.

**Glucocorticoid receptor deficiency**, *NR3C1*, 5q31: Glucocorticoid receptors are bound to heat shock proteins in cytoplasm. Steroids are bound to this receptor and thereafter translocated to the nucleus and bound to specific sites on chromatin. Mutations in the *GCCR* gene affect glucocorticoid signal transduction and alter tissue sensitivity to glucocorticoids. An increase in the activity of the hypothalamic-pituitary-adrenal axis is needed to compensate for the lack of sensitivity to glucocorticoids of peripheral tissues.

**Triple A syndrome**, *AAAS*, 12q13: Mutations in the *AAAS* gene cause triple A syndrome. The gene is responsible for making of ALADIN protein found in the nuclear envelope and is considered essential for the movement of molecules into and out of the nucleus.

**Polyglandular autoimmune syndrome type 1**, *AIRE*, 21q22.3: A dysfunctional *AIRE* gene makes a mutated autoimmune regulator protein which can damage through autoimmunity various structures especially adrenal glands and parathyroid glands.

**Adrenoleukodystrophy**, *ABCD1*, Xq28: Mutations in the *ABCD1* gene impair peroxisomal beta oxidation and as a result the saturated very long-chain fatty acids (VLCFAs) are deposited in all tissues of the body. The most common targeted body structures are adrenal cortex and central nervous system. There are no clear relationships between genetic mutation and phenotypic presentation.

**Sitosterolemia**, *ABCG5*, 8,2p21: The genes involved in developing sitosterolemia synthesize two different protein members of the adenosine triphosphate (ATP)-binding cassette (ABC) transporter family which play a role in trafficking of sterols. The hyperabsorption of all sterols coupled with a deficient excretion of them are the culprit for developing premature coronary artery disease and gonadal and adrenal failure.

**Hyperglycerolemia**, *GK*, Xp21.3: Different mutations in the *GK* gene may cause primary adrenal hypoplasia. Seltzer et al. have found a restriction of glycerophospholipid synthesis and consequently a deficient activation of steroidogenesis.

**Zellweger syndrome**, *PEX*, 1p36.32, 1p36.22, 1q23.2, 2p16.1, 6q24.2, 7q21.2, 12p13.31, 22q11.21: Mutation in any of the genes involved in peroxisome biogenesis leads to the reduction or absence of functional peroxisomes in the cells of an individual protein required for the normal assembly of peroxisomes. The accumulation of VLCFAs and branched-chain fatty acids (BCFA) that are normally degraded in peroxisomes may affect the normal function of various tissues in human body.

*Genetic Testing:* Genetic testing is available for aforementioned genes.

(See http://www.ncbi.nlm.nih.gov/sites/GeneTests/review?db= GeneTests.)

A meticulous examination of the patient for clinical findings possibly associated with some genetic syndromes and a solid knowledge of the most common mutations for a certain genetic condition will help correctly diagnose these rare diseases and better prioritize the diagnostic testing. Among the conditions presented with deficiency of specific enzymes in steroidogenesis, 21-hydroxylase deficiency is the most common and lipoid congenital adrenal hyperplasia the most severe. When one clinically suspects panhypopituitarism, genetic testing should be considered especially for mutations in the *PROP1* gene, the most common known cause of this disorder (an estimated 12%-55% of cases). Mutations in other genes (*HEXS1*, *LHX3*, *TBX19*) are recommended to be tested after, because of the small number of patients affected. X-linked adrenal hypoplasia congenita is a disease which affects mostly males who present with signs of adrenal insufficiency either early or later in life. Autoimmune polyglandular syndrome type 1 is a rare condition

and some populations seem to be affected more frequently (Iranian Jews). Specific presentations of this condition include mucocutaneous candidiasis and later hypoparathyroidism and Addison disease which should lead to DNA sequencing of the *AIRE* gene. When a child has alacrima early in life (later achalasia and Addison disease), genetic testing for triple A syndrome should be performed. Adrenoleukodystrophy mainly affects the nervous system and the adrenal glands (mostly in males). Specific clinical findings may call for genetic testing of this condition. In Zellweger syndrome, both genetic tests involving the sequencing of *PEX* genes and biochemical testing may be helpful for diagnosis.

**BIBLIOGRAPHY:**

1. Bongiovanni AM, Root AW. The adrenogenital syndrome. *N Engl J Med.* 1963;268:1283-1289; 1342-1351; 1391-1399.

2. Oksana Lekarev, Alan Parsa, Saroj Nimkarn Karen Lin-Su, Maria I. New. Congenital adrenal hyperplasia. In: Leslie De Groot, ed. http://www.endotext.org/pediatrics/pediatrics8/pediatricsframe8. htm. Accessed June 2013.

3. Zanaria E, Muscatelli F, Bardoni B, et al. An unusual member of the nuclear hormone receptor superfamily responsible for X-linked adrenal hypoplasia congenita. *Nature.* 1994;372:635-641.

4. Tajima T, Fujieda K, Kouda N, Nakae J, Miller WL. Heterozygous mutation in the cholesterol side chain cleavage enzyme (p450scc) gene in a patient with 46,XY sex reversal and adrenal insufficiency. *J Clin Endocrinol Metab.* Aug 2001;86(8):3820-3825.

5. Smith DW, Lemli L, Opitz JM. A newly recognized syndrome of multiple congenital anomalies. *J Pediatr.* 1964;64:210-217.

6. McGlaughlin KL, Witherow H, Dunaway DJ, David DJ, Anderson PJ. Spectrum of Antley-Bixler syndrome. *J Craniofac Surg.* 2010;21:1560-1564.

7. Genin E, Huebner A, Jaillard C, et al. Linkage of one gene for familial glucocorticoid deficiency type 2 (FGD2) to chromosome 8q and further evidence of heterogeneity. *Hum Genet.* 2002;111:428-434.

8. Chrousos GP, Renquist D, Brandon D, et al. Glucocorticoid hormone resistance during primate evolution: receptor-mediated mechanisms. *Proc Natl Acad Sci.* 1982;79:2036-2040.

9. Charmandari E, Kino T, Ichijo T, Chrousos GP. Generalized glucocorticoid resistance: clinical aspects, molecular mechanisms, and implications of a rare genetic disorder. *J Clin Endocrinol Metab.* 2008;93:1563-1572.

10. Neufeld M, Maclaren NK, Blizzard RM. Two types of autoimmune Addison's disease associated with different polyglandular autoimmune (PGA) syndromes. *Medicine.* 1981;60:355-362.

11. Moser HW. Adrenoleukodystrophy: phenotype, genetics, pathogenesis and therapy. *Brain.* 1997;120:1485-1508.

12. Seltzer WK, Firminger H, Klein J, Pike A, Fennessey P, McCabe ERB. Adrenal dysfunction in glycerol kinase deficiency. *Biochem Med.* 1985;33:189-199.

13. Nicolas C. Nicolaides, Evangelia Charmandari, George P. Chrousos. Adrenal insufficiency. In: Leslie DG, ed. http://www.endotext. org/adrenal/adrenal13/adrenalframe13.htm. Accessed June 2013.

14. Verrijn Stuart AA, Ozisik G, de Vroede MA, et al. An amino-terminal DAX1 (NROB1) missense mutation associated with isolated mineralocorticoid deficiency. *J Clin Endocrinol Metab.* 2007;92:755-761.

15. Achermann JC, Meeks JJ, Jameson JL. Phenotypic spectrum of mutations in DAX-1 and SF1. *Mol Cell Endocrinol.* 2001;185: 17-25.

16. Melcescu E, Phillips J, Moll G, Subauste JS, Koch CA. 11Beta-hydroxylase deficiency and other syndromes of mineralocorticoid excess as a rare cause of endocrine hypertension. *Horm Metab Res.* 2012 Nov;44(12):867-78

## Supplementary Information

**OMIM References:**

Condition; Gene Name (OMIM#)

[1] 21-hydroxylase deficiency; CYP21A2 (#201910)

[2] 17-alpha-hydroxylase deficiency; CYP17A1 (#202110)

[3] 11-beta-hydroxylase deficiency; CYP11B1 (#202010)

[4] 3-Beta-HSD type II deficiency; HSD3B2 (# 201810)

[5] Lipoid congenital adrenal hyperplasia; StAR (# 201710)

[6] P-450-side-chain-cleavage deficiency; CYP19A1 (#118485)

[7] Smith-Lemli-Opitz syndrome; DHCR7 (#270400)

[8] Antley-Bixler syndrome with genital anomalies and disordered steroidogenesis; POR (#201750)

[9] Wolman disease; LIPA (#278000)

[10] Panhypopituitarism; HESX1 (#601802)

[11] Panhypopituitarism; OTX2 (#600037)

[12] Panhypopituitarism; LHX4 (#602146)

[13] Panhypopituitarism; PROP1 (#601538)

[14] Panhypopituitarism; TBX19 (#604614)

[15] Panhypopituitarism; SOX3 (#313430)

[16] Congenital adrenal hypoplasia (X-linked); NR0B1 (#300473)

[17] Congenital adrenal hypoplasia (SF1 linked); NR5A1 (#184757)

[18] Familial glucocorticoid deficiency 1; MC2R (#607397)

[19] Glucocorticoid receptor deficiency, NR3C1 (#138040)

[20] Triple A syndrome; AAAS (#605378)

[21] Polyglandular autoimmune syndrome type 1; AIRE (#607358)

[22] Adrenoleukodystrophy; ABCD1 (#300371)

[23] Sitosterolemia; ABCG5 (#605459)

[24] Sitosterolemia; ABCG8 (#605460)

[25] Hyperglycerolemia; GK (#300474)

[26] Zellweger syndrome; PEX 1, 3, 5, 10, 13, 14, 19, 26 (#214100)

**Alternative Names:**

- Addison Disease, X-Linked; AHX
- Congenital Adrenal Hyperplasia 1; CAH1
- Lipoid Hyperplasia, Congenital, of Adrenal Cortex With Male
- Steroidogenic Factor 1; SF1
- Dss-ahc Critical Region on the X Chromosome 1, Gene 1; DAX1
- Adrenal Unresponsiveness to ACTH
- Cytochrome p450 Side-Chain Cleavage Enzyme
- Adrenomyeloneuropathy; AMN
- Autoimmune Polyendocrinopathy-Candidiasis-Ectodermal Dystrophy; GCR; GRL
- Glycerol Kinase Deficiency
- SLO Syndrome
- Polydactyly, Sex Reversal, Renal Hypoplasia, and Unilobar Lung Lethal Acrodysgenital Syndrome
- Cerebrohepatorenal Syndrome

# 62 Pituitary Tumors and Syndromes

Eva Szarek, Paraskevi Xekouki, and Constantine A. Stratakis

## KEY POINTS

- *Disease summary:*
  - Pituitary tumors are typically of monoclonal origin (although not always); they are benign, often slow-growing, adenomas of the sella arising sporadically or rarely in the context of hereditary genetic syndromes accounting for 10% to 15% of all diagnosed intracranial neoplasms. Their true incidence is difficult to determine, as they are often asymptomatic. They can be effectively managed, as they are rarely malignant. Small pituitary tumors go largely undetected and are often only documented during postmortem studies; over 20% of the adult population may have a pituitary adenoma, identified incidentally by imaging studies (called "incidentalomas"). Significant morbidity occurs due to the pituitary tumor's effect on hormone secretion and compression of regional structures. Other symptoms include those from mass effects.

Pituitary tumors can be classified as follows:

1. Common tumors of the sella turcica
   a. Pituitary adenomas include nonfunctioning adenomas and tumors that hypersecrete hormones: growth hormone (GH)-omas (accounting for 20% of surgically treated lesions), prolactinomas (PRL; 50%), adrenocorticotropic hormone (ACTH)-producing adenomas (15%), and rarely thyroid-stimulating hormone (TSH)-omas, and gonadotropinomas (FSH-LH-omas).
   b. Craniopharyngiomas are epithelial tumors arising from remnants of Rathke pouch and account for 3% of all intracranial tumors.
   c. Supra- and parasellar meningiomas which account for 15% of all intracranial tumors.
   d. Miscellaneous benign cysts: Rathke cleft cysts, intrasellar colloid cysts, arachnoid cysts.
2. Rare tumors of the sella turcica: Optico-hypothalamic gliomas, metastases, chordomas, inflammatory lesions, germinomas, hypothalamic harmartomas, chondromas, epidermoids.
3. Miscellaneous pituitary tumors: Granular cell tumor, paragangliomas, pituitary carcinomas (~0.2% operated pituitary neoplasms), mucocele, chiasmatic cavernoma, hypothalamic lipoma, and sarcoidosis.

- *Pathogenesis:*
  - Pituitary tumors may be a manifestation of an underlying monogenic syndrome, such as McCune-Albright syndrome (MAS), multiple endocrine neoplasia type 1 (MEN1), Carney complex (CNC), multiple endocrine neoplasia type 4 (MEN4), and familial isolated pituitary adenomas (FIPA); alternatively, no single gene may be responsible. Some of these genes predispose to sporadic pituitary tumors, such as the aryl hydrocarbon receptor-interacting protein (*AIP*).

- *Twin studies:*
  - Pituitary tumors are rarely inherited, however, in the very small number of these patients there is usually a family history of other endocrine (parathyroid or pancreas) tumors.

- *Environmental factors:*
  - There are no known environmental causes.

- *Genome-wide associations:*
  - A suggestive linkage on chromosome 19q13.41 has been identified as a possible modifier for the severity of acromegalic features in patients with isolated familial somatotropinoma.

- *Pharmacogenomics:*
  - There are very few pharmacogenetic studies that assess the role of certain polymorphisms in the responsiveness to medications used in pituitary adenomas (eg, dopamine agonists and somatostatin analogues). *NcoI* T + genotype (homozygotes or heterozygotes for T allele), a D2 dopamine receptor (*DRD2*) polymorphism, has been associated with unresponsiveness to cabergoline treatment in patients affected with PRL-oma.

## Diagnostic Criteria and Clinical Characteristics

***Diagnostic Criteria for Pituitary Tumors:*** The investigation of a patient presenting with evidence of a pituitary tumor has three main objectives:

1. Investigation of any hormonal hypersecretion
2. Assessment of residual pituitary function
3. Examination of any mass effect of the tumor (including headaches, visual disturbances, and cranial nerve palsies)

Diagnostic evaluation should include (Fig. 62-1 algorithm)

- Visual fields and ophthalmologic evaluation in defining the presence of a chiasmal syndrome.
- Initial screening endocrine tests should include levels of prolactin, insulin-like growth factor 1 (IGF-1), LH, FSH, TSH, and alpha subunit, cortisol, and thyroxine (T4); men should have their testosterone level checked.
- Prolactin (PRL) levels
  - Serum PRL levels should be measured in any patient with a suspected sellar or suprasellar mass. If elevated, exclude

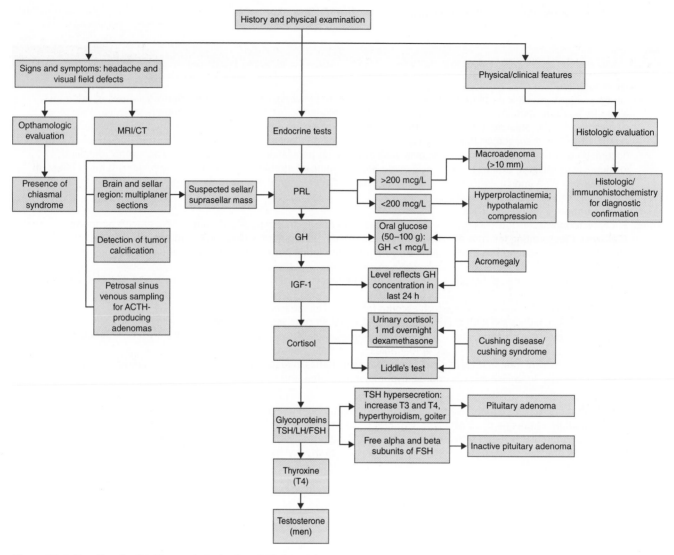

**Figure 62-1** Algorithm for the Diagnostic Evaluation of Pituitary Adenoma.

the possibility of pharmacologic and other factors (eg, pregnancy) prior to requesting extensive neuroimaging studies.

- Serum PRL level greater than 200 μg/L in a patient with an adenoma greater than 10 mm (macroadenoma) in size is diagnostic of a PRL-oma. Levels below this range in a macroadenoma suggest hyperprolactinemia secondary to hypothalamic compression.
- GH levels
  - GH levels are elevated in acromegaly but can fluctuate significantly.
  - Serum IGF-1 level is the best endocrinologic test for acromegaly. IGF-1 reflects GH concentration in the last 24 hours.
  - Oral glucose tolerance test is the definitive test for the diagnosis of acromegaly; a positive result is the failure of GH to decrease to less than 1 μg/L after ingesting 50 to 100 g of glucose.

- Cortisol levels—Cushing disease and Cushing syndrome
  - 24-hour urinary free cortisol, 1 mg overnight dexamethasone suppression test, and midnight cortisol have all been recommended as the screening tests.
  - For the confirmation and differential diagnosis of Cushing disease, several other diagnostic tests have been developed including corticotropin-releasing hormone (CRH) stimulation test, the high-dose dexamethasone suppression test, and Liddle test.
- Glycoprotein hormones—TSH, FSH, LH
  - Pituitary adenomas that are associated with TSH hypersecretion are uncommon. These patients have increased T3 and T4 levels, hyperthyroidism, and goiter with inappropriately high levels of TSH.
  - Free alpha and beta subunits of FSH are secreted by pituitary tumors thought to be inactive.
- Magnetic resonance imaging (MRI) of the brain and sellar region with multiplanar thin sections is of critical

importance. Pre- and postgadolinium images are recommended to ensure that primarily isointense lesions do not escape detection.

- Computed tomographic (CT) scan of the brain with sellar images may be sufficiently specific and can detect tumor calcifications (particularly useful for the differential diagnosis of other parasellar masses, eg, craniopharyngioma).
- Petrosal sinus venous sampling for ACTH-producing adenomas is performed in selective cases.
- Standard histologic examination and immunohistochemistry of these lesions confirm the diagnosis. The mutated form of *p53*, a tumor suppressor, can also be determined histologically. The presence of the mutated *p53* gene suggests a tumor with rapid, aggressive growth.

### Clinical Characteristics:

☞**GENERAL CHARACTERISTICS OF PITUITARY TUMORS:**

- Pituitary microadenomas: Intrasellar adenomas less than 1 cm in diameter that present with manifestations of hormonal excess without sellar enlargement or extension. Panhypopituitarism does not occur and usually can be treated successfully.
- Pituitary macroadenomas: Adenomas greater than 1 cm in diameter and cause sellar enlargement. Tumors 1 to 2 cm in diameter confined to the sella turcica can usually be treated successfully. Larger adenomas with suprasellar, sphenoid sinus, or lateral extension are more difficult to manage. Panhypopituitarism and visual loss are common findings.

☞**CLINICAL CHARACTERISTICS OF EACH PITUITARY TUMOR TYPE:**

- GH-omas (also known as somatotropinomas)
  - Children and adolescents present with gigantism.
  - Adults presenting with acromegaly manifest (1) changes in the size of the hands and feet, coarseness of the face, frontal bossing, and prognathism; (2) macroglossia; (3) hypertrichosis, hyperpigmentation, and hyperhidrosis; (4) respiratory difficulty and sleep apnea; (5) hypertension and diabetes mellitus; (6) cardiac complications resulting from acromegalic cardiomyopathy; (7) carpal tunnel syndrome; (8) colonic polyps (association with colon cancer).
- PRL-omas
  - Women: amenorrhea, galactorrhea, and infertility
  - Men: decreased libido, impotence, rarely galactorrhea
- ACTH-producing adenomas (Cushing disease)
  - Weight gain, centripetal obesity, "moon face," violet striae, easy bruisability, proximal myopathy, and psychiatric changes
  - Other possible effects including arterial hypertension, diabetes, cataracts, glaucoma, and osteoporosis
- TSH-omas
  - Hyperthyroidism with goiter (enlarged thyroid gland) in the presence of elevated TSH levels, the presence of headache as well as visual field defects are attributed to tumor expansion.
- Gonadotropinomas (FSH-LH-omas)
  - Usually large chromophobe adenomas presenting with visual impairment due to tumor mass effect. Rarely, these tumors are associated with precocious puberty or resumption of bleeding in postmenopausal women.
- Nonfunctioning adenomas
  - Headache and visual field disturbances are the usual presenting symptoms.

- Endocrine manifestations often precede the diagnosis for months or years, but the symptoms are subtle and maybe missed. The most common are hypogonadism, hypothyroidism, and hypoadrenalism.

☞**CLINICAL CHARACTERISTICS IN GENETIC SYNDROMES:**

- MEN1
  - Because of the low prevalence of the syndrome, MEN1 is responsible for only 2.7% of all pituitary adenomas.
  - About 40% of patients with MEN1 have pituitary adenoma.
  - Pituitary tumors in MEN1 appear to be larger and more aggressive than in patients without MEN1, with macroadenomas being present in 85% of the former, compared with only 42% of the sporadic cases.
  - PRL-omas predominate among both MEN1-associated adenomas and non-MEN1 pituitary adenomas. MEN1-related PRL-omas are usually macroadenomas (84%), and show higher rates of invasion than in non-MEN1 PRL-omas.
  - MEN1-associated pituitary tumors are significantly more likely to cause symptoms due to tumor size and have a significantly lower rate of hormonal normalization than non-MEN1.
- MAS arises from an activating *gsp* mutation in the *GNAS1* gene located on chromosome 20q13.2.
  - Pituitary lesions are usually hyperplastic and are less commonly adenomatous.
  - GH hypersecretion in MAS differs from the classical acromegaly; patients are generally young at the onset of the disease (<20 years) and diagnosis is usually based on growth acceleration rather than dysmorphic features, which are difficult to assess owing to fibrous dysplasia present in the syndrome.
- FIPA
  - This familial condition is characterized by pituitary tumors of all types in members of a single kindred in the absence of mutations in genes related to MEN1 or CNC.
  - In FIPA, tumors may be of homogeneous phenotype within a family or members of the same family may have different pituitary tumor types (heterogenous).
  - Pituitary tumors in patients with FIPA tend to present 4 years earlier than the sporadic ones, are significantly larger, and tend to have a higher rate of invasion in the cavernous sinus.
  - Mutations of the *AIP* gene (aryl hydrocarbon receptor-interacting protein) may account for 15% of FIPA families.
- CNC
  - The pituitary is one of multiple endocrine organs affected in CNC, and features hypersomatotropinemia and hyperprolactinemia, often beginning in adolescence. Clinically evident acromegaly due to a GH-producing tumor is a relatively infrequent manifestation of CNC. As with MAS, somatomammotrophic hyperplasia, a precursor of GH-producing adenoma, may precede clinically evident acromegaly in CNC patients.
- MEN4

Two families have been reported harboring a mutation in the *CDKN1B* gene:

- A German family exhibiting acromegaly, primary hyperparathyroidism, renal angiomyolipoma, and testicular cancer among various members
- A Dutch patient with a pituitary adenoma (Cushing disease), a cervical carcinoid tumor, and hyperparathyroidism

## Screening and Counseling

***Screening:*** Pituitary tumors are of endocrine origin and occur sporadically and for the most part remain unknown. The hereditary risk to relatives is not generally increased should a single family member present with a particular tumor (Fig. 62-1).

Screening for mutations in candidate genes related to familial syndromes involved in pituitary tumorigenesis (MEN1, MEN4, FIPA, CNC) should be offered to all patients presenting with a pituitary tumor in young age, other multiple tumors, a family history of endocrinopathy or an affected relative in whom a germline mutation of the genes involved has been identified. If molecular genetic testing is not possible or is not informative, individuals at risk (such as first-degree relatives of an individual with a familial syndrome) should undergo routine biochemical-clinical evaluation.

- Patients with a family history of pituitary tumors in the absence of MEN1 or CNC should be actively considered for *AIP* testing.
- Patients with sporadic pituitary tumors should also be considered for *AIP* screening, particularly if they are young and have aggressive tumors.
- The age in which screening should start differs for each familial disease; for MEN1 recommendations is as early as 10 years.

*Note:* MAS is not inherited because it is caused by a postzygotic mutation in the *GNAS1* gene that occurs very early in development. Therefore, genetic screening to the rest of the family members is not indicated.

***Counseling:*** Once a pathogenic mutation in one of the genes predisposing to familial syndromes has been identified in a proband, referral to a clinical geneticist is advised. Genetically predisposed subjects may benefit greatly from early identification by DNA analysis, especially at a presymptomatic stage.

- Genetic counseling of relatives of patients in FIPA families with *AIP* mutations is more difficult due to the uncertainty about the penetrance of disease. However, based on the reported data the penetrance of pituitary tumors in FIPA with *AIP* mutations is high, exceeding 50%.
- Approximately 90% of individuals diagnosed with MEN1 syndrome have an affected parent whereas approximately 10% have de novo mutations.
- If a parent of the proband is affected or harbors a mutation, the risk to the siblings is 50%; each child of an individual with MEN1 has a 50% chance of inheriting the mutation.
- When a *PRKAR1A* mutation is identified in individuals with CNC, genetic analysis should be proposed to first-degree relatives at the same time as the first cardiac ultrasound.

*Note:* At present, no recommendation has been made for prenatal diagnosis in the described familial syndromes.

## Management and Treatment

The treatment of pituitary tumors is dependent on tumor type, function, as well as size. Initial evaluation needs to determine the presence and type of hormone hypersecretion, any hormonal deficiencies, assessment of the need for replacement therapy, the presence of any visual disturbances, and the presence of extracellular extension. Therapeutic treatment may include one, or a combination of, transphenoidal or frontal surgery, radiotherapy and pharmacologic medicines. Since most pituitary tumors are benign, surgery improved long-term outcome in patients presenting with visual disturbances and suprasellar extensions.

***Transphenoidal Surgery:*** Surgical removal is generally performed on patients with secretory tumors, such as GH-, ACTH-, TSH-omas as well as nonfunctioning tumors. The exception to this is PRL-omas, in which the preferred treatment is medical with the use of dopamine agonists. These agents reliably result in tumor size and treat hyperprolactinemia. In the rare instances in which the tumor is excessively large, surgery would generally be the first-line of treatment. Success depends on tumor size, invasion of bone or dura, previous therapy, as well as surgeon experience.

For small, well-defined GH-microadenomas, cure rates reach up to 90%, whereas for patients with macroadenomas cure rates typically do not exceed 50%. Hemihypophysectomy may be curative in 80% of patients with clearly defined biochemical features of ACTH-dependent Cushing disease. If the immediate postoperative cortisol level is less than 3 μg/dL, a 95% 5-year remission rate can be expected. For clinically nonfunctioning tumors and the very rare TSH-omas (which present as macroadenomas), a relatively high incidence of postoperative tumor regrowth, even after apparently complete resection, has been reported.

### Pharmacologic Medicines:

☞**DOPAMINE AGONISTS:** Medical management of PRL-omas with dopamine agonists has been widely recommended as the treatment of choice. Dopamine agonists normalize PRL levels and reduce tumor size in about 60% to 70% of patients with macroadenomas and restore vision in those with optic chiasm suppression. Bromocriptine (2.5-15 mg/daily) and cabergoline (0.25-1 mg twice weekly) are widely used. Since its introduction, cabergoline has surpassed bromocriptine due to longer duration of action (twice a week vs daily dosing), higher clinical effectiveness in restoring ovulatory cycles and fertility, better tolerability and a fewer, but similar, side effects compared to bromocriptine. Dopamine agonists are also used in GH/PRL-cosecreting adenomas. Usual side effects include nausea, vomiting, constipation, headache, dizziness, and orthostatic hypotension. Valvulopathy has been reported following long-term administration of cabergoline.

☞**SOMATOSTATIN ANALOGUES:** Of the five somatostatin receptor (SSTR) subtypes, SSTR2 and SSTR5 are preferentially expressed on somatotroph and thyrotroph cell surfaces and mediate suppression of GH and TSH secretion. Due to antiproliferative and antitumorigenic effects somatostatin analogue therapy is associated with tumor shrinkage in a significant proportion of patients with acromegaly.

- Octreotide binds predominantly to SSTR2 and less avidly to SSTR5 and inhibits GH secretion with a 45 times greater potency than that of native somatostatin; single subcutaneous administration of octreotide (50 or 100 μg) suppresses GH secretion for up to 5 hours.
- Long-acting somatostatin analogues, octreotide-LAR, (20-30 mg intramuscularly), and lanreotide (60, 90, 120 mg) formulations are convenient (subcutaneously every 28 days), enhance compliance, and allow sustained biochemical control. Pasireotide (SOM230), a more recent SST analogue, has been found to have a 40-fold increased affinity to SST5 than other somatostatin analogues. Pasireotide is considered a very promising medication for ACTH-secreting adenomas, which frequently express SST5.

Usual side effects are gastrointestinal with up to half of patients initially experiencing diarrhea, nausea, or abdominal discomfort, but in most patients these are transient. New gallstones were reported to occur within the first year of therapy, in about 15% of patients. Additional patients may develop gallbladder sludge or microlithiasis. The routine use of surveillance gallbladder ultrasonograms in asymptomatic patients is not necessary, but symptomatic patients should be managed as clinically appropriate.

☞**GH-Receptor Antagonist (Pegvisomant):** A modified human GH which competes with endogenous GH for binding to the GH receptor (GHR) without activating it, thereby blocks the GH-initiated signaling and IGF-I production. In doses 10 to 20 mg/daily subcutaneously it was shown to normalize IGF-1 levels in up to 90% of patients. Generally it is well tolerated; redness or swelling at the injection site, pain, diarrhea, or nausea have been reported. Significant, but reversible, liver function abnormalities have been reported in a small number of patients (<1%).

*Radiotherapy:* Treatment with radiotherapy, in most cases, prevents further tumor growth and reduces hormone hypersecretion. Reduction in hypersecretion usually occurs within 6 months, yet the return to normal hormone levels may take up to 5 to 10 years. The procedure most often benefits patients with significant residual tumors and in whom the use of pharmacologic medicines have been unresponsive. It is important to note that the major risk of radiotherapy is the development of hypopituitarism (total or partial). Other risks include vascular damage causing cerebral ischemia, seizures, and the development of other brain and pituitary malignancies, as well as damage to the optic chiasm, optic nerves, and cranial nerves with subsequent development of ophthalmoplegia (vision loss). The incidence of risk increases with the length of treatment. Thus close follow-up and monitoring is strongly indicated.

1. Conventional external beam radiation therapy is delivered via high-energy sources in total doses of 4000 to 5000 cGy, given in daily doses of 180 to 200 cGy. Treatment is successful in 80% of patients with acromegaly but only 55% to 60% of patients with Cushing disease.

2. Intensity-modulated radiation therapy (IMRT) is an advanced form of three-dimensional radiation therapy which uses a computer-driven platform that moves the patient around as the radiation is delivered. IMRT allows the treating physician to shape the radiation beams and aim them at the tumor from several angles.

3. Stereotactic radiosurgery or stereotactic radiation therapy delivers a large, precise radiation dose to the tumor area in a single session or in a few sessions. This permits careful targeting of the tumor and thus less harm to the remaining normal pituitary gland; it also reduces radiation exposure to normal brain. A head frame is attached to the skull to help precisely aim the radiation beams. Once the exact location of the tumor is known from CT or MRI scans, radiation may be delivered. Several forms of stereotactic radiotherapy are used:

   A) Gamma Knife radiosurgery uses stereotactic CT-guided cobalt-60 gamma radiation. This technique has the ability to aim multiple beams of radiation of defined width at the desired intracranial target. Treatments are typically limited to one visit.

   B) Cyber Knife uses a small linear accelerator attached to a robotic arm which moves the beam to different positions during the course of treatment, all converging in the treatment area. Unlike the Gamma Knife, a head frame is not required for submillimeter accuracy. The robotic arm moves around the patient and applies real-time adjustments to treatment delivery based on variation in patient setup.

   C) Proton radiation (also known as proton beam therapy) is the most advanced radiation therapy technique available. The technique uses a particle accelerator to target the tumor with a beam of protons. Due to the physics of proton particles, protons enter the body and deposit most of their energy specifically to the final portion of their trajectory and stop; this is referred to as the Bragg peak. Thereby, these beams allow for more sparing of surrounding normal tissue from exposure to ionizing radiation compared with the other mentioned technologies. Due to these properties, a higher dose can be administered to the tumor. Briefly, a proton beam is generated through three steps: (1) hydrogen atoms (protons) are separated from water molecules by hydrolysis, (2) protons are injected into a cyclotron (large, 90-200 ton, electromagnetic device), and (3) protons are accelerated between two electrodes to nearly two-thirds the speed of light. Protons are guided into treatment rooms through a series of electromagnets. The radiotherapist can then customize the shape and focus of the beam to the target (ie, tumor). Given the equipment required for the generation of proton therapy, the centers are enormous, often three stories high, and extremely expensive. Currently, there are 10 operating beam centers in the United States.

## Molecular Genetics and Molecular Mechanism

The pathogenesis of pituitary adenomas has been attributed to diverse mechanisms involving cell cycle regulation, epigenetic silencing, and signaling pathways. This section outlines the important aspects of the molecular genetics and molecular mechanisms involved in pituitary tumorigenesis; further information can be found in the reviews by Xekouki et al. and Melmed.

Table 62-1 lists pituitary adenomas and their associated susceptibility variants.

1. **Cell cycle regulation** involves cyclins that stimulate cyclin-dependent kinases (CDKs). When activated, these kinases phosphorylate and inactivate a key negative regulator of the cell cycle—retinoblastoma-associated protein (Rb), a tumor suppressor protein. The active, hypophosphorylated form of Rb binds to E2F transcription factors, which restrains cell cycle progression through the G1 to S phase (the synthesis phase in which DNA is replicated). This function of Rb acts to prevent damaged DNA being replicated. By contrast, when phosphorylation is induced by complexes of cyclin and CDKs, Rb releases bound E2F transcription factors, which enables cell cycle progression.

   Cyclins D and E are found overexpressed in nonfunctioning pituitary adenomas, however, the mechanism for pituitary cell cycle dysregulation remains obscure. Cyclins A, B, E are more abundant in larger, high proliferative pituitary adenomas. *Rb1*-deficient mice develop pituitary intermediate-lobe tumors; nevertheless, somatic mutations of the *Rb1* gene do not appear to play a significant role in pituitary tumorigenesis. Interestingly, methylation of CpG islands in the Rb1 promoter and of other cell cycle regulatory genes of the Rb1 pathway (p16INK4a and p15INK4b) resulting in gene silencing are a frequent finding in sporadic pituitary tumors. In contrast, deregulation of

*Table 62-1 Pituitary Adenoma-Associated Susceptibility Variants*

| Candidate Gene (Chromosome Location) | Syndrome | Function (of gene product) | Associated Disease Phenotype | Nonendocrine Features |
|---|---|---|---|---|
| *PRKAR1A* (17q23-q24) | Carney complex | Tumor suppressor gene gatekeeper. Encodes regulatory subunit type 1α of cAMP-dependent PKA. PKA inhibits ERK1/2 cascade of MAPK pathway at c-Raf-1. | Pituitary adenoma | Myxoma: cardiac, breast, cutaneous, oropharynx, female genital tract Pigmented skin lesions: lentigines, blue nevi Other features: large-cell calcifying Sertoli cell tumor, schwannoma (psammomatous melanotic schwannoma), and breast ducal adenoma |
| *MEN1* (11q13) | MEN1 | Tumor suppressor gene gatekeeper Binds promoter of CDK inhibitors (p27$^{kip1}$ and p18$^{Ink4c}$) enabling transcriptional activation Interacts with the serine 5 phosphorylated C-terminal domain of RNA pol II and other transcription factors (eg, c-Jun and NF-kB) | Pituitary adenomas: PRL (most common), GH, TSH, ACTH, or nonsecretory | Occasionally lipoma, facial angiofibroma |
| *AIP* (11q13.2) | Pituitary adenoma predisposition | Tumor suppressor gene Binds and stabilizes aryl hydrocarbon receptor which is the main effector of cellular response to environmental toxins. Aryl hydrocarbon complex also binds to Hsp90 | Pituitary adenoma: GH-secreting, PRL-secreting, ACTH-secreting | No nonendocrine features have been reported |
| *GNAS1* (20q13.32) | McCune-Albright syndrome; polyostotic fibrous dysplasia | Oncogene | Acromegaly | Brachydactyly and mental retardation; prolonged bleeding time |
| | Cushing syndrome | | Pituitary adenoma, ACTH-secreting | |
| p27$^{kit1}$ *CDKN1B* (12p13) | MEN4 | Blocks the cell cycle in the G0/G1 phase upon differentiation signals or cellular insult; also regulates cell motility and apoptosis | Combinations of tumors of parathyroids, pancreatic islets, duodenal endocrine cells, and the anterior pituitary | Less common includes spinal cord ependymomas, angiofibromas, and lipomas |
| *SOX2* (3q26.33) | Pituitary adenoma predisposition | Proposed tumor suppressor gene | Hypopituitarism, deficiencies in GH, TSH, and ACTH | Microphthalmia, optic nerve hypoplasia, and abnormalities of the central nervous system |

E2F transcription factors leads to pituitary hyperplasia without progression to tumor formation, owing to premature cell senescence. Another important gene is *p53*, which inhibits cell cycle progression or induces apoptosis. Mutations in *p53* are found in many human cancers, but do not appear to play a major role in pituitary adenomas; abnormal expression has been reported in some pituitary carcinomas.

Two families of CDK inhibitors—the INK4a/ARF (p16, p15, p18) and cip/kip inhibitors (p21, p27, p57)—normally act as tumor suppressors by negatively regulating progression through the G1 and S phases of the cell cycle. These proteins inhibit CDK kinase activity preventing phosphorylation and inactivation of pRb. Knockout mice lacking p27 have been shown to develop multiorgan hyperplasia and intermediate-lobe pituitary tumors secreting ACTH. The expression of p27 is reduced in pituitary adenomas (including corticotroph, lactotroph, somatotroph, gonadotroph, and thyrotroph adenomas), compared with the normal cells from which they are derived, and completely lost in metastatic pituitary adenomas.

2. **Epigenetic silencing** has been identified in numerous tumor suppressor genes considered important in the pituitary. These genes include *p27^{kip1}*, the maternally expressed protein 3A (MEG3A; maps to 14q32.2), the *ZAC* tumor suppressor gene (also known as the pleomorphic adenoma gene-like 1, *PLAGL1*; maps to 6q24.2), the high mobility group A2 (*HMGA2*; maps to 12q14-15), the pituitary tumor transforming gene (*PTTG1*, maps to 5q35.1), and the potential tumor formation candidate Ikaros (Ik) (maps to 7p13-p11.1). The *PTTG1*, *MEG3A*, and *ZAC* genes have been implicated in pituitary tumorigenesis on the basis of their promoter methylation and are high expression in the normal pituitary, but have not been detected in pituitary adenomas.

*MEG3A* is a human homolog of the mouse maternally imprinted *Gtl2* gene. *Gtl2* has been suggested to be involved in fetal and postnatal development and to function as RNA. *MEG3A* is highly expressed in the normal human pituitary. In contrast, no MEG3A expression was detected in human clinically nonfunctioning pituitary tumors. These data indicate that this imprinted gene may be involved in pituitary tumorigenesis. Interestingly, MEG3A tumor-suppressive properties have been identified to be p53- and Rb-mediated, the two important tumor-suppressor pathways.

HMGA2, a member of the high mobility group A (HMGA) family, is a small, nonhistone, chromatin-associated protein binding DNA in AT-rich regions. HMGA family members are abundantly expressed during embryogenesis, but not in normal adult tissue. They have no intrinsic transcriptional activity; however, they regulate transcription by altering the architecture of chromatin and facilitating the assembly of multiprotein complexes of transcriptional factors. Mice overexpressing *HMGA2* develop mixed GH/PRL cell pituitary adenomas. In humans, rearrangement and amplification of the *HMGA2* gene expression seems to occur predominantly in PRL-omas, and HMGA2 mRNA abundance correlates with pituitary tumor size and proliferation.

*PTTG1* is an oncogene that serves as a marker of malignancy grades in several endocrine malignancies. Physiological PTTG1 properties include securin activity, DNA damage or repair regulation and involvement in organ development and metabolism. Overexpression of *PTTG1* causes cell transformation in vitro, and expression of this regulator is induced during initiation of

estrogen-induced pituitary tumor formation. Pituitary-directed *PTTG1* overexpression in transgenic mice results in focal pituitary hyperplasia and adenoma formation. Cloning of *PTTG1* in pituitary tumors has shown that approximately 90% of pituitary adenomas overexpress this gene compared with normal pituitary tissue, which expresses very little *PTTG1*.

Ik, an interesting transcription factor, is abundantly expressed during development in hormone-producing corticotroph cells. It binds to the pro-opiomelanocortin promoter to activate the endogenous gene. Altered expression of Ik isoforms have been implicated in human pituitary tumorigenesis through their actions on FGFR4 transcription. The dominant negative isoform of this protein, Ik6, is expressed in nearly half of all primary pituitary tumors, enhancing cell survival with antiapoptotic features. In these tumors, Ik is not expressed and its loss is associated with CpG island methylation and concomitant histone modification.

3. **Signaling pathways** involve the activation of a number of different pathways, such as those involving the protein serine—threonine kinases, tyrosine kinases, and others that ultimately affect the function of a variety of transcription factors and cell cycle genes. Errors in these processes have been implicated in the development of familial as well as sporadic pituitary tumors.

*Gsα/protein kinase A/cAMP pathway*

G-proteins (composed of three heterodimers: Gα, Gβ, and Gγ) belong to the family of proteins involved in regulating effector molecules such as adenylyl cyclase (AC) and ion channels. The major G-proteins involved in hormone action are Gs (stimulates AC), Gi (which inhibits AC, regulates $Ca^{2+}$ and $K^+$ channels), and Gq/11 (which acts through stimulation of phospholipase Cβ). Gs protein mutations have been reported in 30% to 40% of sporadic GH-omas; only GH-secreting tumors have been described in patients with MAS. MAS is a genetic syndrome caused by a postzygotic mutational event in the gene coding for Gsα (*GNAS*) and increased cAMP formation occurring in a mosaic fashion early in embryonic life. The *GNAS* locus maps on human chromosome 20q13. cAMP normally mediates growth hormone-releasing hormone (GHRH) signaling, the mutated somatotroph G-protein activation bypasses the requirement of GHRH-mediated activation, and persistent high levels of cAMP activate PKA signaling, leading to phosphorylation of CREB, leading to constitutive GH hypersecretion and proliferation of somatotroph cells. Compared with GNAS mutation-negative tumors, the former are smaller and believed to be slower proliferating, have increased intratumoral cAMP, do not respond vigorously to GHRH, and show better sensitivity to somatostatin analogs. However, no difference has been found in age, sex, and duration of the disease or cure rate between patients with and without the mutation. GNAS-activating mutations are rarely detected in nonfunctioning adenomas (<10%) or in ACTH-secreting adenomas (6%) and are absent from PRL- and TSH-omas. A sevenfold increase in phosphodiesterase (PDE) activity has been demonstrated in tumors harboring *GNAS* mutations that most probably counteract the activation of the cAMP pathway.

Inactivating mutations in the gene encoding for the regulatory subunit 1-α (R1a) of PKA (PRKAR1A) are responsible for more than 60% of patients presenting with CNC, a rare autosomal dominant condition described in approximately 500 individuals to date. *PRKAR1A* acts as a tumor-suppressor gene of the 17q22-24 PRKAR1A locus in CNC tumors. This gene is normally expressed and not mutated in all sporadic somatotroph tumors.

### MAPK & PI3K/Akt pathways

Six distinct groups of MAPKs have been characterized in mammals. Extracellular signal-regulated kinases (ERK1 and ERK2), also known as the classical MAPK signaling pathway, are preferentially activated in response to growth factors and regulate cell proliferation and cell differentiation. Signal transduction is often initiated by receptor tyrosine kinases, such as those of the Ret family, IGF-1 receptor, EGF, VEGF, and FGF receptor families. Ligand binding results in engagement and activation of the MAPK cascade comprised of the Ras/Raf (the product of the *BRAF* gene), MEK and ERK kinases. Sustained ERK signaling promotes the accumulation of genes required for the cell cycle, such as cyclin D1, and represses the expression of genes that inhibit proliferation. Of the members of the Ras-MAPK signaling pathway, Ras and Raf are proto-oncogenes. Gain-of-function mutations (activating mutations) of these genes drive a cell toward cancer. Common cancers with oncogenic Ras activation include pancreatic (90%), thyroid (60%), and colorectal (45%) cancers. Furthermore, 35% of cancers show increased MAPK activity. Experimental studies in animals have shown that in cultures of rat pituitary lactotrophs, IGF-1-induced proliferation, and this was abolished by the presence of a MAPK pathway inhibitor, whereas it inhibited apoptosis through activation of the PI3K/Akt. In GH4C1 somatolactotroph cell lines overexpressing wild-type $Gs\alpha$ protein and Gs protein (GSP) oncogene it was shown that cAMP levels were 10-fold lower in wild-type $Gs\alpha$-overexpressing cell lines compared with mutant cells. It is worth noting that sustained MAPK and ERK1/2 activation was observed in both cell lines through a PKA-dependent pathway. Additionally, forskolin—an agent that increases intracellular levels of cAMP, induced a large increase in ERK1/2 activity in GSP-negative tumors, suggesting that the ERK1/2 activity could be attributed to the cAMP/PKA pathway—an indication supporting the role of the ERK1/2 pathway in pituitary tumorigenesis. Nevertheless, in nonfunctioning pituitary adenomas, the increase of cAMP has resulted in a reduction in ERK1/2 pathways, indicating that cAMP (through activation of PKA) may induce cell growth or arrest depending on the cell type.

### Transcription factors

Expressions of transcription factors in pituitary adenomas are likely to reflect the origin of tumorigenic cells. However, their presence in pituitary adenoma development remains unclear. The most important transcription factors are listed here.

- PROP1

    Early development and differentiation of GH-, PRL-, TSH-, and the gonadotropin-secreting cells involve prophet of Pit-1 (*Prop-1;* MIM# 601538). *PROP1* has both DNA-binding and transcriptional activation ability. Elevated expression of Prop-1 may predispose pituitary tumor formation, as shown in mice overexpressing Prop-1. Overexposure, long-term, induces formation of Rathke cysts, pituitary hyperplasia, and nonfunctioning adenomas. Although PROP1 is widely expressed in pituitary adenoma subtypes in humans, its expression does not correlate with clinical behavior.

- PIT1

    Early differentiation of GH-, TSH-, and PRL-secreting pituitary cells is controlled by pituitary specific transcription factor-1 (*Pit-1;* MIM# 173110). PIT1 responsible for pituitary development and hormone expression in mammals and is a member of the POU family of transcription factors involved in the regulation of mammalian development. Its expression is identified in GH-, TSH-, and PRL-secreting pituitary adenomas. Nonfunctioning pituitary adenomas may also be PIT1 positive, suggesting that this subclass of adenomas may arise from an early cell precursor.

- DAX1

    DAX1 (*NR0B1*, MIM# 300473) is an orphan member of the nuclear receptor (NR) superfamily. Its main function is in the proper formation of the adult adrenal gland whereby its expression has been shown in all regions of the hypothalamo-pituitary-adrenal-gonadal axis during development as well as in adult tissues. Clinically, DAX1 is expressed in nonfunctioning pituitary adenomas of the gonadotroph lineage. PRL- and GH-omas are negative for DAX1.

- SOX2

    SOX2 (MIM# 184429), a member of the SOXB1 family of transcription factors, is a widely expressed progenitor and stem cell marker. SOX2 haploinsufficiency, in mice and humans, has been associated with variable hypopituitarism associated with anterior pituitary hypoplasia, suggesting an important role in anterior pituitary development. It has been recently reported, in two unrelated patients with *SOX2* haploinsufficiency, the development of nonprogressive pituitary tumors of early onset, suggesting SOX2 can act as a tumor suppressor. It is important to note that SOX2 may have an oncogenic potential, as has been demonstrated in breast cancer, squamous lung cancer, small cell lung carcinoma, meningiomas, glioblastomas as well as prostate cancer; all in which *SOX2* has been upregulated. The role of SOX2 in pituitary tumor formation may be linked to its role in the control of the cell cycle through its interaction with the canonical Wnt signaling pathway. Wnt signaling plays an essential role during pituitary development whereby it controls proliferation of Rathke pouch precursors and the differentiation of the PIT1 lineage

**Future Directions:** It is expected that in the next 5 years, many more defects will be identified; hopefully, these discoveries will also lead to new (and exciting) pharmacologic intervention strategies. Future work should focus on understanding the molecular mechanisms that control pituitary tumor transformation, where intracellular signaling molecules will constitute not only diagnostic or prognostic markers but also novel therapeutic targets.

**BIBLIOGRAPHY:**

1. Melmed S. Pathogenesis of pituitary tumors. *Nat Rev Endocrinol.* 2011;7(5):257-266.
2. Hemminki K, Forsti A, Ji J. Incidence and familial risks in pituitary adenoma and associated tumors. *Endocr Relat Cancer.* 2007;14(1):103-109.
3. DiGiovanni R, Serra S, Ezzat S, Asa SL. AIP mutations are not identified in patients with sporadic pituitary adenomas. *Endocr Pathol.* 2007;18(2):76-78.

4. Khoo SK, Pendek R, Nickolov R, et al. Genome-wide scan identifies novel modifier loci of acromegalic phenotypes for isolated familial somatotropinoma. *Endocr Relat Cancer.* 2009;16(3):1057-1063.

5. Filopanti M, Lania AG, Spada A. Pharmacogenetics of D2 dopamine receptor gene in prolactin-secreting pituitary adenomas. *Expert Opin Drug Metab Toxicol.* 2010;6(1):43-53.

6. The Endocrine Society Clinical Guidelines.

7. Batista DL, Riar J, Keil M, Stratakis CA. Diagnostic tests for children who are referred for the investigation of Cushing syndrome. *Pediatrics.* 2007;120(3):e575-e586.

8. Daly AF, Tichomirowa MA, Beckers A. The epidemiology and genetics of pituitary adenomas. *Best Pract Res Clin Endocrinol Metab.* 2009;23(5):543-554.

9. Pellegata NS, Quintanilla-Martinez L, Siggelkow H, et al. Germline mutations in p27Kip1 cause a multiple endocrine neoplasia syndrome in rats and humans. *Proc Natl Acad Sci USA.* 2006;103(42):15558-15563.

10. Georgitsi M, Raitila A, Karhu A, et al. Germline CDKN1B/ p27Kip1 mutation in multiple endocrine neoplasia. *J Clin Endocrinol Metab.* 2007;92(8):3321-3325.

11. The National Association for Proton Therapy. Proton Therapy Centers. http://www.proton-therapy.org/map.htm. Accessed 2012.

12. Xekouki P, Azevedo M, Stratakis CA. Anterior pituitary adenomas: inherited syndromes, novel genes and molecular pathways. *Expert Rev Endocrinol Metab.* 2010;5(5):697-709.

13. Melmed S. Mechanisms for pituitary tumorigenesis: the plastic pituitary. *J Clin Invest.* 2003;112(11):1603-1618.

14. Sandrini F, Kirschner LS, Bei T, et al. PRKAR1A, one of the Carney complex genes, and its locus (17q22-24) are rarely altered in pituitary tumours outside the Carney complex. *J Med Genet.* 2002;39(12):e78.

15. Alatzoglou KS, Andoniadou CL, Kelberman D, et al. SOX2 haploinsufficiency is associated with slow progressing hypothalamo-pituitary tumours. *Hum Mutat.* 2011;32(12):1376-1380.

## Supplementary Information

**OMIM REFERENCES:**

[1] Pituitary Adenoma, Prolactin-Secreting; AIP (#600634)

[2] Pituitary Adenoma, Growth Hormone-Secreting; AIP (#102200)

[3] Acromegaly; GNAS (#102200)

[4] Pituitary Adenoma, ACTH-Secreting; AIP (#219090)

**Alternative Names:**
- Incidentalomas
- Prolactinomas
- Growth Hormone-Producing Adenomas
- Adrenocorticotropic Hormone-Producing Adenomas
- Thyroid-Stimulating Hormone-Producing Adenomas
- Gonadotropinomas
- Craniopharyngiomas
- Optico-Hypothalamic Gliomas
- Pituitary Carcinoma
- Paraganglioma
- Hypothalamic Lipoma

***Key Words:*** Pituitary adenoma, McCune-Albright syndrome (MAS), multiple endocrine neoplasia type 1 (MEN1), Carney Complex (CNC), familial isolated pituitary adenomas (FIPA), acromegaly, Cushing disease

# 63 Disorders of Sexual Differentiation

Alan A. Parsa, Oksana Lekarev, Maria I. New, Mabel Yau, and Ahmed Khattab

## KEY POINTS

- *Disease summary:*
  - Genetic sex is determined by the paternally inherited X or Y chromosome. Once established sexual determination, the commitment of the primordial gonads to becoming testes or ovaries, will follow and lead to the final phase of sexual differentiation which is the subsequent development of the internal and external genitalia. Sexual differentiation under normal circumstances is under the control of a 35 kb region of the Y chromosome known as the *SRY* gene. A defect anywhere in this process can cause disorders of sexual differentiation and can be classified as one of the following:
  - 46,XY disorders of gonadal determination
  - 46,XX disorders of gonadal determination
  - 46,XY disorders of androgen biosynthesis and action
  - Luteinizing hormone (LH) receptor defects
  - Disorders of antimüllerian hormone (AMH) or antimüllerian hormone receptor
  - Androgen excess
- *Monogenic forms:*
  - All enzymatic defects associated with the adrenals are monogenic.
- *Family history:*
  - A pedigree of at least three generations should be obtained to evaluate consanguinity.
- *Environmental factors:*
  - Fetal exposure to compounds with estrogenic effects (xenoestrogens) such as herbicides, pesticides, polychlorinated biphenyls (PCBs), polystyrenes, as well as antiandrogens such as the polyaromatic hydrocarbons, linuron, vinclozolin. Androgen exposure includes inadvertent contact by the mother with testosterone creams used by a family member or the mother taking progestin-containing oral contraceptives.

## Diagnostic Criteria and Clinical Characteristics

***Diagnostic Criteria for Sexual Differentiation:*** Diagnostic criteria should include

All those being evaluated for a disorder of sexual differentiation will need a rapid and complete evaluation including

1. Serum hormone concentrations
2. Genotype
3. Extensive pedigree searching for abnormalities of sex development in family members including infertility

***Clinical Characteristics:***

☞CLINICAL AND GENETIC FEATURES OF SEXUAL DIFFERENTIATION: See Table 63-1.

*46,XY Disorders of Sexual Determination (DSD):* The *SRY* gene, a 35-kb region located on Yp11.3, is a key genetic component of sex determination. A mutation or deletion in this region will cause maldevelopment of testicular tissue which affects both internal and external genitalia. Approximately 1:20,000 live births are affected with one of the following conditions:

1. **Complete gonadal dysgenesis (CGD):** Also known as Swyer syndrome or 46,XY pure gonadal dysgenesis. Only 15% to 20% with CGD have been identified to have a defect in the *SRY* gene. Patients are born without normal testicular tissue (streak gonads) bilaterally and express phenotypic female external and internal genitalia. Subjects are assigned the female sex and go unrecognized at birth. Streak gonads may be inherited in an autosomal dominant, autosomal recessive, X-linked, or Y-linked manner depending on the gene involved.

Diagnosis is made during adolescence or adulthood due to pubertal delay, lack of secondary sexual characteristics, or primary amenorrhea. In CGD, if breast tissue develops or menstruation occurs, an estrogen-secreting tumor should be suspected and *must* be investigated. Stature is normal to tall with eunuchoid habitus. A pelvic ultrasound reveals a normal vagina, uterus, and fallopian tubes with the absence of Wolffian structures and ovaries. Serum markers showing hypergonadotropic hypogonadism along with a karyotype and ultrasound of the internal organs can help make the proper diagnosis. Diagnosis is based on the appearance and histologic features of both gonads. The risk of gonadal tumors is 30% if testicular tissue is identified.

2. **Mixed or partial gonadal dysgenesis (GD):** Mixed GD typically refers to a disorder in which one gonad is a streak while the other is normal or partially dysgenetic. The most common karyotype of mixed GD is mosaicism for 45,X or 46,XY. A few patients have 46,Xi(Yq) karyotype. Partial gonadal dysgenesis refers to a condition in which gonadal development is an intermediate between streak and normal bilaterally. 46,XY nonmosaic karyotype is common. The gonads can be found anywhere along the lines of testicular descent. Each gonad may possess a different degree of functional testicular tissue with each secreting different amounts of testosterone and AMH. This dictates the extent of Wolffian and müllerian duct proliferation and regression and may be asymmetrical correlating with the degree of ipsilateral gonadal development. The amount of testosterone produced will also affect the degree of genital ambiguity. An utriculovaginal pouch is a common feature. Patients with partial GD are born with female external genitalia, and the diagnosis is usually made during adolescence when the patient is evaluated for primary amenorrhea or lack of secondary

*Table 63-1 Hormonal and Genetic Aspects of Disorders of Sexual Differentiation*

**XY**

| 46,XY DSD | Inheritance | External Genitalia | Internal Genitalia | Presentation | Hormone profile | Risk of gonadal tumor | Treatment | Chromosome |
|---|---|---|---|---|---|---|---|---|
| Complete Gonadal Dysgenesis | AR, X-linked, Y-linked | Female | Female | Present with pubertal delay, no secondary sex characteristics, primary amenorrhea | ↑FSH, LH no ↑ in T with hCG. Compete GD: ↓↓ T, DHT, $E_2$ | Present | Estrogen replacement beginning at puberty Prophylactic/ therapeutic gonadectomy | Multiple: Yp11.3 9p24.3 9q33 12q13.1 |
| Mixed/Partial GD | AR, X-linked, Y-linked | variable | variable | Ambiguous genitalia, pubertal delay, amenorrhea (depends on the amount of functional testicular tissue) | Mixed/Partial GD: ↓ T, DHT, $E_2$, nml to ↓AMH | Present | Estrogen if reared as female, Testosterone if reared as a male. | Multiple: Yp11.3 9p24.3 9q33 12q13.1 |
| Testicular Regression Syndrome | AR limited to Males | variable | M | Lack of secondary male characteristics | ↑FSH, LH ↓↓ T, DHT, $E_2$ ↓↓ AMH No response to hCG | None | Testosterone if reared as a male | unknown |
| 5α-reductase type 2 deficiency | AR | Ambiguous or F | M | Virilization during puberty, | Nml FSH, LH Nml T,$E_2$, ↓DHT, ↑ Ratio T/DHT (>30) | ? | Depends on which gender role the patient decides during adolescence or puberty | 2p23 |
| P450 Oxoreductase deficiency | AR | variable | M | variable | ↑ 17-OHProg ↑ Prog ↓ F, DHEA ↓ $\Delta^4$ steroid, T | none | Ad hoc | 7q11.2 |
| 17β-hydroxysteroid dehydrogenase type 3 deficiency | AR | F | M | Virilization during puberty | Nml to ↑ $\Delta^4$ steroid ↑ratio $\Delta^4$/T (>15) ↓ T, DHT | none | Testosterone at puberty | 9q22 |
| Complete androgen insensitivity | X linked recessive | F | M or rudimentary mullerian | Infertile, amenorrhea + breast development | ↓ FSH, LH Nml to ↑AMH Nml $\Delta^4$ steroid Nml T, DHT ↑↑ hCG response | None | Estrogen if castrated | Xq11-q12 |

*(Continued)*

Table 63-1 Hormonal and Genetic Aspects of Disorders of Sexual Differentiation (Continued)

**XY**

| 46,XY DSD | Inheritance | External Genitalia | Internal Genitalia | Presentation | Hormone profile | Risk of gonadal tumor | Treatment | Chromosome |
|---|---|---|---|---|---|---|---|---|
| Partial Androgen insensitivity | X linked recessive | variable | M | variable | Nml FSH, LH; Nml to ↑ AMH; Nml $\Delta^4$ steroid; Nml T, DHT ↑↑ hCG response | None | Dependent on sex assignment | Xq11-q12 |
| Leydig cell hypoplasia | AR | Type I: F; Type II: ambiguous | M | variable | ↑ LH, nml FSH\↑ AMH; ↓ T, DHT, $E_2$; ↓hCG response; Nml ratio $\Delta^4$steroid/T | ? | Type I: Estrogen; Type II: Estrogen if raised as a female, T if raised as male | 2p21 |
| Persistent Müllerian duct syndrome | AR | M | M + F | Müllerian derivatives discovered incidentally | Nml hormonal profile | none | none | Type I: 19p13.3; Type II: 12q13 |

**XX**

| 46, XX DSD | Inheritance | External Genitalia | Internal Genitalia | Presentation | Hormone profile | Risk of gonadal tumor | Treatment | Chromosome |
|---|---|---|---|---|---|---|---|---|
| Ovotesticular DSD | Unknown | variable | M + F (variable) | variable | ↑ LH, FSH; ↓ T, DHT; No ↑ with hCG; Nml AMH | ? | Varies with the degree of ambiguity | X |
| Testicular DSD | Unknown | M | M | Small testicles (if descended), gynecomastia, azoospermia | ↑ LH, FSH; ↓ T, DHT; No ↑ with hCG; Nml AMH | none | Testosterone | SRY translocation to X |
| XX gonadal dysgenesis | Unknown | F | F | Amenorrhea, no secondary sexual characteristics (Turner's syndrome is most common) | ↑↑ LH, FSH ↓ $E_2$ | none | Estrogen | 2p16 |
| P450 aromatase deficiency | AD | Ambiguous/M | F | Virilization stops after delivery; Mother virilization during pregnancy | ↑ FSH, LH, $\Delta^4$steroid, T; ↓ $E_2$, Estrone; ↑ 16-OHAn (maternal) | none | Estrogen | 15q21.1 |

sexual characteristics. Once a presumptive diagnosis is made by karyotype of peripheral leukocytes in 46,XY patients, fluorescent in situ hybridization (FISH) for SRY or for Yp can be performed. There are only certain isolated and syndromic forms of 46,XY GD which can be diagnosed by molecular genetic techniques including comparative genomic hybridization or sequencing of known genes. The risk of gonadoblastoma is approximately 20% to 30% and can occur as early as 15 months of life. Precise diagnosis is made after prophylactic or therapeutic gonadectomy.

3. **Testicular regression syndrome (TRS):** Initial testicular development occurs in all cases. An unknown insult embryologically causes the degeneration of the testicular tissue either unilaterally or bilaterally. A vascular event has been postulated. Internal and external genital development will vary depending on when the complete loss of testicular tissue occurs. External genitalia can range from normal female, if regression occurs before 8 to 10 weeks gestation, to normal male genitalia, if occurring late in fetal development (after 12-14 weeks). If regression occurs during late fetal life it has also been termed "vanishing testes syndrome." Patients are typically found to have a primitive epididymis and spermatic cord ending blindly or to a fibrous nodule. Rarely do patients present as a female with primary amenorrhea. It is reported that TRS affects up to 5% of males born with cryptorchidism, and as high as 12% of cryptorchid patients older than 1 year. TRS caries an insignificant risk of malignancy and must thus be differentiated from gonadal dysgenesis, which carries a significant risk.

*46,XX Disorder of Sex Determination:*

1. **Ovotesticular DSD:** Previously known as true hermaphroditism. The subject will exhibit both testicular (seminiferous tubules) and ovarian (follicles) gonadal tissue within in the same gonad (ovotestes) or an ovary on one side and testicle on the other. Half of the time, the patient will have ovotestes on one side with a normal ovary or testes on the contralateral side. Bilateral ovotestes occurs in 20% of cases. The mixture of gonadal tissue causes a variance of internal and external genital development and will depend on the gonads hormonal status. A degree of müllerian duct regression is consistent in all forms and a unicornuate uterus is a common finding. Patients can be highly masculinized (predominantly testicular tissue) with bilateral palpable scrotal gonads with a prostatic vagina being the only müllerian remnant structure. They may also be phenotypically female (mostly ovarian tissue) with a fairly well-developed adnexa and vagina, and half of which will menstruate. About 10% of these patients are SRY-positive by FISH, and this aids in distinguishing ovotesticular DSD from 46,XX testicular DSD which is 90% SRY-positive. Levels of LH, follicle-stimulating hormone (FSH), estradiol, testosterone, and dihydrotestosterone (DHT) will be normal. AMH is a good marker to test for functioning testicular tissue. Diagnosis is confirmed when both gonads are examined histologically showing evidence of ovarian follicles and testicular tissue. There is approximately 5% risk of gonadal tumors, and this is more prevalent in those with abdominal gonads possessing testicular tissue.

2. **XX gonadal dysgenesis:** As phenotypic females, abnormal complement of the X chromosome is the most common cause of ovarian dysgenesis. Female genitalia are normal but due to early ovarian failure patients do not experience normal puberty. Amenorrhea is a common presenting complaint along with the lack of secondary sexual characteristics. The most common form

is Turner syndrome. Frequently females are diagnosed when presenting for a workup of short stature and a routine karyotype is performed. Müllerian structures are normal, and histologic studies of the gonads demonstrate bilateral streaks. Ovarian failure with hypergonadotropic hypogonadism is observed. The molecular basis of gonadal dysgenesis is unknown for the majority of cases though the FSH receptor (gene *FSHR*, 2p16) has been implicated.

3. **XX testicular DSD:** Caused by the translocation of the *SRY* gene to the X chromosome, approximately 85% of patients are born with normal male external genitalia with two testicles, no evidence of müllerian structures and azoospermia. In these patients 90% are SRY-positive by FISH in contrast to 10% being SRY-positive in 46,XX ovotesticular DSD. The majority of patients present during puberty with a normal size phallus and pubic hair along with gynecomastia, and small testes. It has been reported that gender identity and gender role is male for those with unambiguous genitalia.

*46,XY Androgen Biosynthesis or Action:*

1. **5-α reductase type 2 deficiency (SRD5A2):** Mapped to 2p23. 5-α reductase is responsible for the conversion of testosterone to dihydrotestosterone (DHT). Two forms of this enzyme exist: type 1, found in peripheral tissues including skin fibroblasts, becomes active around the time of puberty; type 2, expressed in genital skin tissue and male accessory sex organs, is the major active enzyme from fetal life until puberty.

   In utero, external genitalia development is under the control of DHT. DHT deficiency will therefore prevent masculinization of the male external genitalia. Physical findings may be minimal (ie, isolated micropenis or isolated hypospadias) to severe (ie, perineal hypospadias, bifid scrotum, or even normal female genitalia with a slightly enlarged clitoris). Commonly, patients present with female external genitalia and are raised as females during childhood. Testes are present and can be located intraabdominally or within the inguinal canal bilaterally. Müllerian regression and Wolffian duct preservation are unaffected due to the normal activity of Sertoli cells. Ejaculatory ducts typically end in a blind vaginal pouch or perineum close to the urethra.

   During puberty, possibly due to the activity of 5-α reductase type 1, spontaneous virilization occurs. The phallus enlarges and labioscrotal folds become rugated and pigmented. The testes enlarge and may descend into the labioscrotal folds. Acne, prostate enlargement, and fine facial hair ensue. Gynecomastia does not occur. Normal sperm production may occur in those with descended testes making fertility possible, though most are infertile. About half of patients will change sex from a female gender role to a male gender role during adolescence or early adulthood.

2. **Congenital lipoid hyperplasia:** (15q23-q24, 8p11.2) See section on Congenital Adrenal Hyperplasia.

3. **3-β hydroxysteroid dehydrogenase deficiency:** (1p13.1) See section on Congenital Adrenal Hyperplasia.

4. **17-α hydroxylase/17,20 lyase deficiency:** (10q24.3) See section on Congenital Adrenal Hyperplasia.

5. **P450 oxoreductase deficiency (POR):** (7q11.2) POR is a flavoprotein required for the proper action of all microsomal p450 enzymes including those involved in steroidogenesis. Unlike the earlier defects which involve only one enzyme, POR deficiency may cause partial enzymatic defects in multiple enzymes. Diagnosis becomes difficult since patients present with a wide

range of phenotypes from undervirilized males with partial 17-α-hydroxylase deficiency to overvirilized females with partial 21-hydroxylase deficiency. Levels of serum hormones are variable. This is a rare condition and children may present with ambiguous genitalia or as adolescents with amenorrhea and/or polycystic ovary syndrome (PCOS).

6. **17-β hydroxysteroid dehydrogenase type 3 deficiency:** A mutation in the gene *HSD17B3* affects the conversion of androstenedione to testosterone. The enzyme is expressed primarily in the gonads and maps to chromosome 9q22. The incidence is 1:147,000. Patients are commonly born with female external genitalia. At puberty patients may experience increased virilization with enlargement of the clitoris or phallus, muscle development, breast development, male pattern body hair, voice deepening, and descent of testes. Plasma levels of testosterone will normalize in the range of a pubertal male. XY patients are usually raised as females while half will adopt a male gender role in adolescence or early adulthood.

*Defects in Androgen Activity in the 46,XY:*

1. **Complete androgen insensitivity (CAIS):** The androgen receptor (AR) which is mapped to chromosome Xq11-q12, plays a key role in the differentiation of male internal and external genitalia, the maintenance of spermatogenesis as well as the regulation of hair growth and sex drive. The AR allows androgen sensitive cells to respond to androgens such as testosterone and DHT. If these hormones cannot bind to the androgen receptor, a 46,XY individual will be phenotypically female with infertility and amenorrhea. Physical examination will show a short, blind-ending vagina, with absent or rudimentary müllerian structures. Gonads may be intra-abdominal or inguinal. Subjects will have normal breast development, bone maturation, with none to sparse pubic and axillary hair. Stature is above the female average. Patient identity and behavior is feminine with no gender dysphoria. With over 300 mutations identified, the majority of cases show a single-amino acid substitution in the AR gene as the cause. A sequence analysis of all eight exons of the AR gene will detect 95% of the mutations. The incidence CAIS is between 2 and 5 per 100,000 genetically male births.

2. **Partial androgen insensitivity (PAIS):** (Xq11-q12) This is a heterogeneous condition due to the partial sensitivity of androgen receptors to androgens. Patients present with phenotypes varying from predominantly female external genitalia with clitoromegaly, labial fusion, and inguinal or labial testes to predominantly male external genitalia with simple (glandular or penile) or severe (perineal) hypospadias with a normal-sized penis and descended testes. The testes are functional and cause regression of the müllerian ducts and variable development of Wolffian ducts. At puberty, breast development and lack of penile enlargement with scant pubic hair are prominent features. Testes remain small and there is azoospermia. Only 50% of mutations will be detected upon sequencing the AR gene and thus may require a detailed family history showing the X-linked recessive inheritance of the disorder.

*Luteinizing Hormone Receptor Defects in the 46,XY:*

1. **Leydig cell hypoplasia:** In utero, Leydig cells, found in the testicles, promote testicular decent and produce testosterone which gets converted to DHT by 5-α-reductase type 2. DHT is the key component of in utero development of male external genitalia. In Leydig cell hypoplasia, Sertoli cells of the testes secrete AMH normally causing müllerian regression. Leydig cell hypoplasia is an autosomal recessive disorder involving an inactivating mutation in the luteinizing hormone or choriogonadotropin receptor gene (LHCGR) found on chromosome 2p21. Two forms exist: type 1 and type 2.

   a. Type 1, a severe form, involves the complete inactivation of the *LHCGR* gene and thus there is no Leydig cell function. With no testicular testosterone to be converted to DHT, external genitalia are normal female with undescended testes. There is full regression of müllerian structures due to normal Sertoli cell function and AMH release. At puberty the child will present with lack of female secondary sexual characteristics and primary amenorrhea.

   b. Type 2, mild form, is variable and depends on the degree of Leydig cell function and testosterone production. Phenotypes can include micropenis, cryptorchidism, severe hypospadias, and small testes. These patients will also have normal müllerian regression owing to normal Sertoli cell function. Spermatogenesis is incomplete due to hyalinization of the seminiferous tubules. In both cases laboratory studies will show low testosterone levels with elevated LH and normal FSH. There is no significant rise in testosterone levels when stimulated with human chorionic gonadotropin (hCG).

*Disorders of Antimüllerian Hormone or Antimüllerian Hormone Receptor in the 46,XY:*

1. **Persistent müllerian duct syndrome (PMDS):** AMH, a hormone released by testicular Sertoli cells, causes the regression of müllerian structures in utero. Two forms exist which produce the same phenotype: type I, a mutation in the gene producing AMH mapped to chromosome 19p13.3 and type II, a mutation in the AMH receptor mapped to 12q13. Both conditions do not allow full regression of the müllerian duct. The patient may have a uterus with fallopian tubes and no ovaries. Leydig cells function normally; therefore, male internal and external genitalia are unaffected with full fertility potential. Diagnosis is commonly incidental during unrelated abdominal surgery.

*Androgen Excess:*

1. **Maternal androgen intake:** Mothers who take progestin-containing oral contraceptives are at risk of causing 46,XX genital virilization, though it is very rare. The intake of androgens or androgen mimics will also place the 46,XX fetus at risk. Other causes of excess androgens can be tumors such as leuteomas or a cystic ovarian condition known as hyperreactio luteinalis.

2. **Congenital adrenal hyperplasia (CAH):** Please refer to Chap. 64.

3. **POR:** Please refer to earlier section on POR.

4. **P450 aromatase deficiency:** A mutation in the gene *CYP19A1* encoding P450 aromatase. This results in the inability to convert C19 steroids, including testosterone, to estrogens (C18 steroid). The initial manifestation of aromatase deficiency is placental with maternal virilization. An elevated level of androgen precursors in the maternal liver will cause maternal virilization as well as XX virilization. Low plasma concentrations of maternal estriol will also help with prenatal diagnosis.

Defective aromatization in the gonads will prevent the XX or XY child from having the normal growth spurt during puberty. Instead, these children experience a rapid linear growth and are typically tall owing to estrogen deficiency and failure of epiphyseal fusion. The delay in skeletal maturity leads to tall stature. Osteoporosis and bone pain are common. XX patients do not undergo spontaneous puberty and often have polycystic ovaries, increased virilization, and amenorrhea without breast development. The XY males experience normal puberty, since testosterone production is unaffected, though they will be infertile due to the lack of estrogen which is essential to spermatogenesis.

## Screening and Counseling

**Screening:** At the present time the only newborn screen that exists for steroid disorders is for 21-hydroxylase deficiency. Otherwise, genetic counseling for disorders of sexual differentiation occurs on a patient by patient basis. Since many of these disorders have an autosomal recessive mode of inheritance, family members of an affected person should be counseled to possible risks to having affected children. A careful pedigree is essential.

**Counseling:** An essential part of management for all those with DSD is the collaboration of an experienced multidisciplinary team including an endocrinologist, psychologist or psychiatrist, gynecologist, genetic counselor, and urologist or surgeon. Communication is essential between the family and patient. Support groups will also help the child or adult assimilate better with society and not regard his or her condition as a handicap.

## Management and Treatment

**Management:** When a child is born with ambiguous genitalia, great care must be made to assign the proper sex of the child. Parents are often greatly distressed and assume that the medical and nursing staff know what the gender assignment of the baby really is. Great care must be taken when discussing the baby with parents. Since it is unnatural to discuss a baby without using gender terms such as "he" or "she," it is easy to accidentally refer to the baby in a gender-oriented way. Great pressure is placed on the medical staff to make it better by prematurely assigning the child's gender. This can lead to more confusion and distress later if the suggested sex of rearing is at odds with the initial "off the cuff" decision. In the United States, there is a 60-day grace period in which the birth certificate must be completed. If the "wrong" sex is entered, it is very difficult to change and involves judicial intervention. The later the physician-imposed sex assignment is made, the more doubtful it is that a long-term gender identity will be stable.

**Therapeutics:**
1. Psychologic
   a. Gender assignment or reassignment as well as timing for surgery are very important. A psychologic evaluation should be thorough and conducted by an experienced team. Therapy should be directed at both the parents and child.
   b. Although there is no consensus as to the appropriate age to fully disclose a condition, it is recommended to proceed gradually with children and to adapt the disclosure to the child's cognitive and psychologic development. Tradition and family culture should be given great consideration in disclosure.
2. Hormone replacement
   a. Glucocorticoids are used most commonly in congenital adrenal hyperplasia to suppress the pituitary gland's oversecretion of adrenocorticotropic hormone (ACTH). This in turn will decrease elevated precursor hormones. Careful attention should be taken to avoid iatrogenic Cushing syndrome by administering too high a dose in an attempt to normalize all hormone levels (more information can be found in the CAH section).
   b. Testosterone is used in the treatment of those with testosterone deficiency (ie, 46,XX testicular DSD, 17-β-hydroxysteroid deficiency). Testosterone treatment by conversions to estrogens can compromise final adult height and should be avoided if possible until the patient has achieved appropriate height potential. If this is not possible, low doses should be used to maximize growth potential and may be used in conjunction with growth hormone if needed. Different forms of testosterone exist and treatment will vary depending on what is best for the patient. One therapy is the use of testosterone enanthate given intramuscularly every 3 to 4 weeks, starting at 100 mg and increasing by 50 mg every 6 months to 200 to 400 mg. High initial doses can cause priapism and should be avoided. Once normal levels of testosterone are achieved, maintenance dosage of 50 to 400 mg given every 2 to 4 weeks should be sufficed. Testosterone may also be given in the form of a patch or gel. For those with functioning Sertoli cells, hCG can be used to stimulate testicular testosterone production. This can help minimize adverse effects of exogenous testosterone administration.
   c. Estrogen can be given as an oral tablet or a patch with a goal of promoting secondary sexual characteristics in females with hypogonadism. It is also used to prevent osteoporosis. The patch is preferred since it delivers a more predictable dose by avoiding the first-pass through the liver as is seen in the oral form. The oral form should be used with caution in those with liver disease and estrogen-sensitive neoplasia. The initial dose should be the lowest possible dose and be slowly increased to a maximum of 0.625 mg/d of conjugated estrogens. During conditions such as 46,XX gonadal dysgenesis up to 1.25 mg/d may be used.

## Molecular Genetics and Molecular Mechanism

**Testicular Development** The genetic control of gonadal development is complex. As per the current understanding SF1, WNT4 and WT1 are the transcription factors and genes expressed in the common embryological urogenital ridge for development of gonads, kidneys and adrenal cortex. In the bipotential gonad several genes such as *WT1, SF1, LHX9, LIM1, GATA4, DHH, WNT4* and *FGF9* are expressed. SF1 and WT1 up-regulate SRY expression in pre-Sertoli cells and initiate the male gonad development. *SF1* is expressed in the hypothalamus, the pituitary, the gonads and the adrenal glands. *SF1* gene stabilizes the intermediate mesoderm which leads to formation of adrenal and gonadal primodial cells. SF1 also plays an important role in spermatogenesis, Leydig cell function in males; follicle development and ovulation in females. *WT1* is important for gonadal and renal development in urogenital ridges. During gonadal differentiation, WT1 is expressed in the coelomic epithelium and later in Sertoli and granulosa cells. *WT1* mutations lead to gonadal dysgenesis associated with Wilms tumor/or glomerular nephrotic syndrome with changes of diffuse mesangial sclerosis called Denys-Drash and Frasier syndrome.

SRY is sort of a master switch for testis determination. The gene lies on the short arm of the Y chromosome close to the pseudoautosomal region 1. Thus the susceptibility of SRY translocation onto the X chromosome results XX males (80% of cases); mutations and deletions of the SRY are responsible for 15% of XY females. SOX9 is a target gene of SRY and is strongly up-regulated in Sertoli cells. A double dose of SOX9 expression is required its action in XY males. A heterozygous mutations result in haploinsufficiency resulting in campomelic dysplasia, gonadal dysgenesis sex-reversal in 46,XY individuals. *SOX9* then up-regulates *FGF9* and has a role in inducing mesonephric cell migration into the developing fetal testis and Sertoli cell differentiation. If the expression of *FGF9* gene is favored over *WNT4/RSPO1*; the signals are shifted in favor establishing the male pathway. If *WNT4/RSPO1* is over expressed activating the β-catenin pathway favoring female development. SRY also directly inhibits β-catenin pathway mediated stimulation of *WNT4*. *ATRX* (X-encoded DNA-helicase) mutation results in mental retardation, α-thalassemia and gonadal dysgenesis in XY individuals. CBX2 is a transcriptional regulator whose disruption in mice causes several defects including retardation of embryonic gonadal formation and gonadal sex reversal in XY fetuses. The second step in male sex differentiation, is a more straightforward process. Anti Müllerian hormone (AMH) secreted by the testicular Sertoli cells acts on its receptor in the Müllerian ducts to cause their regression. Testosterone secreted by the testicular Leydig cells acts on the androgen receptor in the Wolffian ducts to induce the formation of epidydimis, deferent ducts and seminal vesicles. The second step thus requires the normal genetic expression of *AMH* gene and *AMH-R* gene, G-protien LHCG receptor gene, androgen receptor gene and several genes involved in the steroidogenic pathway such as StAR protein, *CYP11A1*, 3βHSD-2, 17 α-hydroxylase and 17,20 lyase enzyme, 17β-hydroxysteroid dehydrogenase type 3 (17βHSD-3).

***Ovarian Development*** During the bipotential stage, *WNT4*, *RSPO1*(R-spondinsare) and β-catenin seem to have both pro-ovarian and anti-testicular activities from early embryonic life, while *FOXL2* may also have similar actions postnatally. Ovarian differentiation also requires transcription factors such as LHX1, EMX2 and PAX2 necessary for intermediate mesoderm development. The differentiation of gonadal ridge is regulated by SF1, LHX9 and WT1. Genes such as *DAX1*, *MAGEB*, *WNT4* and FST should be expressed to antagonize testis. A duplication of *DAX1* results in sex-reversal in 46,XY patients Since the expression is dosage sensitive an altered number of DAX1 copies seems to result in abnormal gonadal differentiation. *WNT4* is a secreted protein that functions as a paracrine factor to regulate several developmental mechanisms. In humans, a duplication of *WNT4* expression causes ambiguous genitalia of 46,XY patients due to low androgen

production. *WNT4* is also involved in the internal genital tract differentiation. β-catenin and FOXL2 are both required to suppress *SOX9* expression during normal ovary development. Loss of function mutations in the human *RSPO1* gene is important for ovarian differentiation and a mutation can mutation result in the formation of ovotestes in the XX fetus FOXL2 is a transcription factor expressed in germ and somatic cells more strongly in the female than the male fetal gonad from the 8th fetal week. Mutations in the human *FOXL2* gene result in a variety of phenotypes in females with premature ovarian failure, streak gonads, eyelid abnormalities characterized by blepharophimosis, ptosis and epicantus inversus.

## BIBLIOGRAPHY:

1. Arboleda V, Vilain E. Disorders of sexual development. In: Yean and Jaffe's *Reproductive Endocrinology*, 6th ed. Philadelphia:Saunders Elsevier, 3013, pp. 2191–2228.

2. Rey RA, Josso N, Forest MG. Diagnosis and treatment of disorders of sexual development. In: Jamieson JL, DeGroot LJ. *Endocrinology*, 6th ed. Philadelphia:Saunders Elsevier, 2013, pp. 687-701.

3. Carillo AA, Danon M, Berkovitz GP. Disorders of sexual differentiation. In: Lifshitz F, ed. *Pediatric Endocrinology*, 4th ed, New York:Marcel Dekker, 2004, pp. 546-592.

4. De Santa Barbara P, Bonneaud N, Boizet B, Desclozeaux M, Moniot B, Sudbeck P, Scherer G, Poulat F, Berta P 1998 Direct interaction of SRY-related protein SOX9 and steroidogenic factor 1 regulates transcription of the human anti-Mullerian hormone gene. Mol Cell Biol 18:6653-6665

5. Giuili G, Shen WH, Ingraham HA 1997 The nuclear receptor SF-1 mediates sexually dimorphic expression of Mullerian Inhibiting Substance, in vivo. Development 124:1799-1807.

6. Vilain E, McElreavey K, Jaubert F, Raymond JP, Richaud F, Fellous M 1992 Familial case with sequence variant in the testis-determining region associated with two sex phenotypes. Am J Hum Genet 50:1008-1011

7. Pelletier J, Bruening W, Kashtan CE, Mauer SM, Manivel JC, Striegel JE, Houghton DC, Junien C, Habib R, Fouser L, et al. 1991 Germline mutations in the Wilms' tumor suppressor gene are associated with abnormal urogenital development in Denys-Drash syndrome. Cell 67:437-447.

8. Gwin K, Cajaiba MM, Caminoa-Lizarralde A, Picazo ML, Nistal M, Reyes-Mugica M 2008 Expanding the clinical spectrum of Frasier syndrome. Pediatr Dev Pathol 11:122-127

9. Correa RV DS, Bingham NC, Billerbeck AE, Rainey WE, Parker KL, Mendonca BB. 2004 A microdeletion in the ligand binding domain of human steroidogenic factor 1 causes XY sex reversal without adrenal insufficiency. J Clin Endocrinol Metab 89(4):1767-72

10. Kohler B, Lin L, Ferraz-de-Souza B, Wieacker P, Heidemann P, Schroder V, Biebermann H, Schnabel D, Gruters A, Achermann JC 2008 Five novel mutations in steroidogenic factor 1 (SF1, NR5A1) in 46,XY patients with severe underandrogenization but without adrenal insufficiency. Hum Mutat 29:59-64

# 64 Congenital Adrenal Hyperplasia

Alan A. Parsa, Oksana Lekarev, Maria I. New, Mabel Yau, and Ahmed Khattab

## KEY POINTS

- *Disease summary:*
  - Congenital adrenal hyperplasia (CAH) is a group of autosomal recessive inherited disorders of steroidal biosynthesis caused by a variety of enzymatic defects (Fig. 64-1).
  - Most cases of CAH can be accounted for by deficiencies in 21-hydroxylase (21-GHO): 90% to 95% of cases and 11β-hydroxylase (OHO): 3% to 8%.
  - Deficiencies in 21-hydroxylase and 11β-hydroxylase cause decreased cortisol production, that lead to a lack of negative inhibition of adrenocorticotropic hormone (ACTH) and oversecretion of ACTH. This increase in ACTH drives the adrenal glands to attempt to produce more cortisol but this increase is blocked by enzyme deficiencies. Adrenal precursors are thus shunted into the androgen pathway resulting in increased androgen synthesis, which does not require these enzymes.
  - Phenotypes can range widely depending on the degree of enzyme deficiency.
  - Hyperandrogenism is a key feature seen in 21-OHD and 11β-OHD.

- *Hereditary basis:*
  - These are autosomal recessive genetic disorders; thus both parents are typically carriers of *CYP21A2* or affected with 21-hydroxylase deficiency for the fetus to be affected.
  - Though less common, new mutations can arise in *CYP21A2*.

- *Differential diagnosis:*
  - In 46,XX, maternal androgen exposure, P450 oxoreductase deficiency (POR), ovotesticular disorder of sexual differentiation (DSD), mixed gonadal dysgenesis
  - In 46,XY, incomplete androgenization of genitals, 5α-reductase deficiency, nonclassic *StAR*

## Diagnostic Criteria and Clinical Characteristics

***Diagnostic Criteria for CAH:*** Diagnostic evaluation should include

- Newborn screen for 21-hydroxylase deficiency in all children born in the United States.
- All patients born with ambiguous genitalia must have a detailed hormonal and genetic evaluation.
- Genotyping is necessary as each mutation can cause a different phenotype.
- Hormonal determination
  - The gold standard for establishing hormonal diagnosis of 21-hydroxylase deficiency (21-OHD) is the corticotropin stimulation test (250 μg cosyntropin intravenously), measuring levels of 17-OHP at baseline and 60 minutes. These values can then be plotted on a nomogram to ascertain disease severity (Fig. 64-2). There is significant overlap between carriers and unaffected.
  - Assessment of fertility potential.
- Electrolytes should be monitored closely for hyponatremia and hyperkalemia and treated immediately; salt-wasting is present in 75% of patients with classic 21-OHD and can be life threatening. Plasma renin and aldosterone ratio is elevated.
- Extra doses of corticosteroids must be given during illness, trauma, and surgery to avoid crisis and death.

### Clinical Characteristics:

☞ CLINICAL FEATURES OF CAH:

Hyperandrogenism is a clinical feature consistent in both 21-OHD and 11β-OHD.

*46,XX females:* Genital virilization occurs only in the androgen-responsive external genitalia. Since females with CAH have normal ovaries and do not produce anti-Müllerian hormone (AMH), the internal genitalia (uterus and fallopian tubes) develop normally from the Müllerian anlage. Genital virilization can vary greatly depending on the amount of androgens exposed to in utero. The degree of virilization is classified into five Prader stages:

- Stage I: clitoromegaly without labial fusion
- Stage II: clitoromegaly and posterior labial fusion
- Stage III: greater degree of clitoromegaly, single perineal urogenital orifice, and almost complete labial fusion
- Stage IV: increasingly phallic clitoris, urethra-like urogenital sinus at base of clitoris, and complete labial fusion
- Stage V: penile clitoris, urethral meatus at tip of phallus, and scrotum-like labia (appear like males without palpable gonads)

*Childhood:* Depending on the amount of androgens exposed postnatally, an affected female may enter precocious pseudopuberty with early appearance of acne and axillary and pubic hair; rapid somatic growth with advanced epiphyseal maturation may lead to early epiphyseal closure and likely short stature.

*Adults:* Postpubertal females may develop progressive clitoral enlargement, deepening of the voice, increased muscle bulk, hirsutism, medication-resistant acne, and/or male pattern alopecia (temporal balding). Menstrual abnormalities, including oligomenorrhea or amenorrhea, and infertility may become evident.

*46,XY males:* In utero will not be affected by excess adrenal androgens and will thus be born with normal external genitalia which may be hyperpigmented.

*Childhood:* If left undetected males may also enter precocious pseudopuberty presenting similar to the females but with

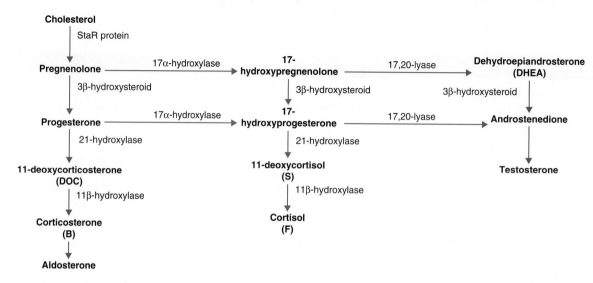

**Figure 64-1** Schematic of Steroid Synthesis in CAH.

progressive penile enlargement but small volume of testes. Signs of excess adrenal androgens in the adult male may be difficult to assess, but may notably lead to decreased testicular size and testicular testosterone production as well as impaired spermatogenesis. These abnormalities are due to the effects of excess adrenal androgens on gonadotropin secretion.

*Adult:* A complication of inadequate hormonal control of CAH is hyperplastic nodular testes. Many adult male patients are found to have adenomatous adrenal rests within the testicular tissue. These tumors have been reported to be ACTH dependent and to regress following adequate steroid therapy. For males, these testicular adrenal rests that can also occur in females with salt-wasting CAH and are associated with an increased risk of infertility.

21-OHD—The degree of deficiency in 21-hydroxylase can be phenotypically categorized into two distinct forms: classic, which encompasses two clinical syndromes: salt-wasting and nonsalt-wasting (simple virilizer); and nonclassic. Females with nonclassic 21-OHD possess the biochemical defect but do not have ambiguous genitalia.

**Salt-wasting 21-OHD:** Along with the signs of hyperandrogenism, the newborn will present with failure to thrive, hyponatremia, hyperkalemia, inappropriate natriuresis, and high plasma renin activity due to low aldosterone within the first few weeks of life. If severe and untreated, hypotension, cardiac arrhythmias, vascular collapse, shock, and death can occur. As an adult these patients are fragile to illnesses, stressful events, and accidents. High doses of steroids are needed to prevent serious complications, such as shock and death.

**Simple-virilizing 21-OHD:** Comprises approximately 25% of the classic type. The neonate will produce enough aldosterone to prevent salt loss and its complications. If not picked up during newborn screening, affected males, who are born with normal genitalia, may present with precocious pseudopuberty from the effects of hyperandrogenism as described above.

**Nonclassic 21-OHD:** It is the most common form of CAH and can present at any age after birth. There is typically no genital abnormality in these females. Diagnosis may be made when evaluated for symptoms of excess androgens including early puberty or later in life in females for causes of infertility, menstrual abnormalities, hirsutism, obesity, cystic acne.

Polycystic ovarian syndrome (PCOS) may also be seen as a secondary complication in these patients. Adult males may present with the signs of hyperandrogenism as described in the section earlier, but symptoms are often mild, and some patients may not present until being evaluated for infertility.

**11β-hydroxylase deficiency (11β-OHD):** Along with the clinical presentation of excess androgen as described earlier, the key feature of 11β-OHD is suppressed renin and hypertension. Despite failure of aldosterone production, overproduction of the precursor deoxycorticosterone (DOC), a less potent in vivo mineralocorticoid, causes salt retention and hypertension. Elevated blood pressure is usually not identified until later in childhood or in adolescence and is loosely correlated with the elevation in DOC. The degree of virilization does not strongly correlate to blood pressure, and fatal vascular accidents can occur in minimally virilized patients. Maintaining good blood pressure control is important since complications of long-standing uncontrolled hypertension, including left ventricular hypertrophy, retinal vein occlusion, and blindness have been reported in 11β-OHD patients. Potassium depletion develops concomitantly with sodium retention, but hypokalemia is variable. Renin production is suppressed secondary to mineralocorticoid-induced sodium retention and volume expansion. Aldosterone production is low secondary to low serum potassium and low plasma renin. Diagnosis is made by genetic testing (DNA analysis).

**Other forms of CAH:**

**3β-hydroxysteroid dehydrogenase (3β-HSD) deficiency:** There are two forms of 3β-HSD: type I and II. Type II is expressed in the adrenal cortex and gonads while type I, usually not affected in CAH, is found in the liver and other peripheral tissues. 3β-HSD deficiency in its classic form results in insufficient cortisol production. Females can be born with normal or virilized genitalia. The degree of virilization relates to the peripheral conversion of DHEA to testosterone by type I enzyme in the periphery. Males typically will have incomplete virilization of the external genitalia due to type II 3β-HSD deficiency in the gonads, characterized by micropenis, perineal hypospadias, bifid scrotum, and a blind vaginal pouch with or without salt-wasting due to the lack of mineralocorticoids. Gynecomastia is common at pubertal age.

**17α-hydroxylase deficiency (17α-OHD)/17, 20 lyase deficiency:** Affecting approximately 1% of patients with CAH,

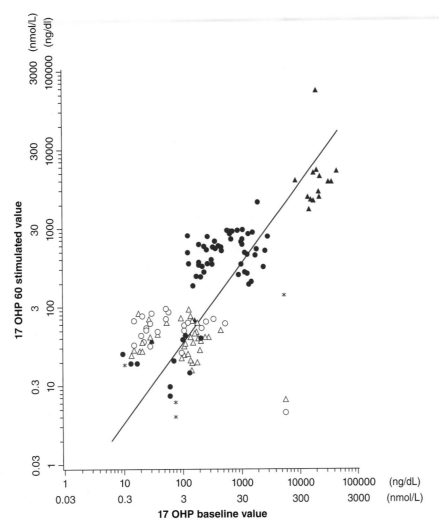

**Figure 64-2** Nomogram Relating Baseline to 60' ACTH-Stimulated Serum Concentrations of 17-Hydroxyprogesterone. The coordinates are logarithmic. A regression line for all data points is shown.

this enzyme deficiency blocks the production of sex steroids and glucocorticoids. The result is sexual infantilism in 46,XX females and undervirilized genitalia in 46,XY males. Increased levels of DOC and corticosterone will suppress renin activity leading to low renin-low aldosterone hypertension with metabolic alkalosis and hypokalemia. Diagnosis usually occurs in females with failure to develop secondary sexual characteristics and in males with undervirilization of genitals.

**Congenital adrenal lipoid hyperplasia (StAR protein deficiency):** Males with congenital adrenal lipoid hyperplasia are born with female-appearing external genitalia. Females have a normal genital phenotype at birth but remain sexually infantile without treatment. Salt-wasting occurs in both males and females. If not detected and treated, lipoid CAH may be fatal.

**P450 oxidoreductase (POR) Deficiency:** POR is a flavoprotein required for the proper action of all microsomal p450 enzymes including those involved in steroidogenesis. Unlike the earlier defects which involve only one enzyme, POR deficiency can cause partial enzymatic deficiencies in

multiple enzymes. This makes it difficult to diagnose since patients will present with a wide range of phenotypes ranging from undervirilized males with partial 17α-hydroxylase deficiency to overvirilized females with partial 21-hydroxylase deficiency. Levels of serum hormones are variable. This is a very rare condition and children may present with ambiguous genitalia or as adolescents with amenorrhea and/or PCOS.

## Screening and Counseling

**Screening:** When both parents are known to be carriers of a mutation for CAH or who have a child with known CAH, they are considered to be "at risk." These couples should be counseled about having future children. In planning for a future pregnancy, prenatal diagnosis and treatment with dexamethasone may be offered and discussed in detail. Since treatment must be initiated prior to 9 weeks gestation and the earliest screen is done at 10 to 12 weeks gestation (based in most cases on direct mutational analysis using allele-specific polymerase chain reaction [PCR] on DNA from

**Table 64-1** *Genes Associated With Congenital Adrenal Hyperplasia*

| Condition | Gene Symbol | Genital Ambiguity | Diagnostic Hormones | Androgens | Mineralocorticoid | Incidence |
|---|---|---|---|---|---|---|
| 21-hydroxylase deficiency | CYP21A2 | F | ↑17OHP before and after ACTH, ↑ACTH, ↑PRA | Excess | Deficiency | 90%-95% |
| 11β-hydroxylase deficiency | CYP11B1 | F | ↑DOC, ↑11-dexoxycortisol and DOC before and after ACTH, ↑serum androgens, ↑ACTH, ↓PRA, hypokalemia | Excess | ↑DOC ↓Aldo | 5% |
| Congenital lipoid adrenal hyperplasia | StAR | M | Low/absent levels of all steroid hormones Decreased/absent response to ACTH, ↑ACTH, ↑PRA | Deficiency | Deficiency | Rare |
| 3β-hydroxysteroid dehydrogenase deficiency | HSD3B2 | M (±F) | ↑17-OHPreg, ↑DHEA, ↓17OHP, ↓androstenedione ↑ACTH, ↑PRA ↑Δ⁵ steroids before and after ACTH, ↑Δ⁵/Δ⁴ serum steroids | Deficiency | Deficiency | Rare |
| 17α-hydroxylase/ 17,20-lyase deficiency | CYP17A1 | M | ↑DOC, ↑18-OHDOC, ↑corticosterone, ↑18-hydroxycorticosterone, ↓17α-hydroxylated steroids and poor response to ACTH, ↑ACTH, ↓PRA | Deficiency | Excess | Rare |
| Cytochrome P450 oxidoreductase deficiency | POR | Highly variable | ↑ACTH, ↑Prog, ↑17OHP, ↓DHEA, ↓Δ⁴, ↓T, normal electrolytes | Highly variable | Highly variable | Rare |

17OHP, 17-hydroxyprogesterone; ACTH, adrenocorticotropic hormone; PRA, plasma renin activity; 17OHPreg, 17-hydroxypregnenolone; DOC, deoxycorticosterone; Aldo, aldosterone; DHEA, dehydroepiandrosterone; Prog, progesterone; T, testosterone; Δ⁴, androstenedione.

chorionic villus samples) treatment must begin prior to knowing whether or not the fetus is affected. Parents must understand that prenatal treatment will prevent ambiguous external genitalia in an affected female, but will not eliminate the disorder.

As of July, 2008, newborn screening for 21-OHD became part of routine practice in all 50 states in the United States. Blood is taken from a heel stick and placed on a Guthrie card to be sent for analysis of 17-hydroxyprogesterone levels. By stratifying values to age and birth weight a fairly accurate diagnosis of the severity of the enzymatic defect can be made. Sensitivity of the test is lower in females than in males. A follow-up ACTH stimulation test may be needed for inconclusive results and should be done after 24 hours of life to prevent false positives. The nonclassic form is not picked up by new born hormonal screen.

*Counseling:* All those affected as well as carriers wanting to become pregnant should have a detailed discussion with their clinician and possibly a geneticist regarding issues such as pregnancy, fertility, growth, and surgery. Support groups should be introduced to help the child assimilate better. All those affected should be well aware that treatment is lifelong and not curative. A medical alert bracelet should be worn at all times indicating their risk of adrenal insufficiency.

The genes associated wit the enzyme deficiencies that cause CAH are listed in Table 64-1.

## Management and Treatment

The management and treatment of CAH require close monitoring. Laboratory findings alone do not suffice. Therapy is based on clinical judgment, side effects of the medications, laboratory results, as well as patient input. It is very important to have the patient involved in every step of the decision making to avoid issues such as noncompliance.

*Hydrocortisone:* Hydrocortisone (HC) requires multiple daily doses and is the drug of choice for children since growth is less impacted compared to dexamethasone or prednisone. The usual requirement dose is 10 to 15 mg/m²/d divided into two or three daily doses for classic and 5 to 10 mg/m²/d for nonclassic patients. Hydrocortisone does not suspend well in liquids, thus tablets should be used, and oral liquid suspensions should be avoided. For children, tablets can be embedded in marshmallows.

| 17-hydroxyprogesterone | Androstenedione | Testosterone |
|---|---|---|
| <1000 | <200 | Normal age appropriate range |

If the body becomes stressed (ie, fever, vomiting, accident), a stress dose of two to three times the daily dose divided to three times daily may be required. A patient undergoing surgery may need up to five times the daily dose and if unable to take oral medications an IM dose is recommended. The clinician should be very keen on avoiding overtreatment, which could lead to growth suppression and Cushing syndrome, as well as undertreatment, which could result in hirsutism, acne, weight gain, and poor growth. HC does not pass the placenta and is used in affected mothers whose fetus is considered unaffected.

***Dexamethasone:*** A long-acting steroid with a half-life of 36 to 50 hours, dexamethasone has been shown to stunt linear growth and should be avoided in children until after complete maturation of epiphyseal plates. The usual dose required is 0.25 to 0.5 mg nightly. Because it crosses the placenta, it is also the drug of choice in prenatal therapy for an affected female fetus. The optimal dosage is 20 µg/kg/d per maternal prepregnancy body weight in three divided doses with a maximum dose of 1.5 mg daily. If undertaken, this treatment should be initiated as soon as pregnancy is confirmed and no later than 9 weeks after the last menstrual period. The mother's blood pressure, weight, glycosuria, $HbA_{1c}$, symptoms of edema, striae, and other possible adverse effects of dexamethasone treatment should be carefully observed throughout pregnancy. Urinary estriol may be monitored in the mother after 15 to 20 weeks of gestation to indicate fetal adrenal suppression, and to assure compliance.

***Prednisone:*** An intermediate-acting steroid with a half-life of 18 to 30 hours, it is typically given twice daily at a dose of 5 to 10 mg/d. Prednisone itself is inactive until it passes through the liver to become its active metabolite, prednisolone. It should therefore be given cautiously in those with hepatic disorders. The goal is the same as hydrocortisone. Prednisone should not be used in pregnancy due to incomplete crossing of the placenta.

***9α-Fludrocortisone:*** A mineralocorticoid is used mostly in saltwasters to help maintain sodium and balance renin levels. The usual dose required is 0.1 mg daily with normal sodium and potassium levels being the goal. This dose may diminish with age and care should be taken not to oversuppress the renin-angiotensin axis to prevent complications of hypertension and mineralocorticoid activity.

***Sodium Chloride (Salt Tablets):*** Supplemental sodium chloride is given to infants with salt-wasting CAH in conjunction with 9α-fludrocortisone since breastmilk and formula contain very little sodium. Sodium chloride may also be given in older children and adults if there is difficulty maintaining normal sodium levels. A dose of 8 to 10 mEq/kg/d usually suffices.

***Surgery:*** The aim of surgical reconstruction in females with ambiguous genitalia caused by CAH is generally to remove the redundant erectile tissue, preserve the sexually sensitive glans clitoris, and provide a normal vaginal orifice that functions adequately for menstruation, intromission, and delivery. A medical indication for early surgery in females other than for sex assignment is recurrent urinary tract infections as a result of pooling of urine in the vagina or urogenital sinus.

## Molecular Genetics and Molecular Mechanism

*CYP21A2*, the gene encoding 21-hydroxylase enzyme (OMIM# 201910), is mapped to the short arm of chromosome 6 (6p21.3).

The inactive pseudogene for *CYP21A2*, denoted *CYP21A1P*, is 98% homologous to the active *CYP21A2* gene. The pseudogene is located 30 kb away from the active gene and contains deleterious mutations that render it nonfunctional. The majority of mutations found in *CYP21A2* derive from the pseudogene during either meiotic recombination or gene conversion. De novo mutations in the active gene can also occur but account for a small percentage of the transmission. To date, more than 100 mutations have been described, including point mutations, small deletions, small insertions, and complex rearrangements of the gene. Approximately 95% to 98% of the mutations causing 21-OHD have been identified through molecular genetic studies of gene rearrangement and point mutations arrays. Hormonally and clinically defined forms of 21-OHD CAH are associated with distinct genotypes characterized by varying enzyme activity demonstrated through in vitro expression studies. The classic phenotype is predicted when a patient carries two severe mutations. The nonclassic phenotype is caused by a mild/mild or severe/mild genotype, as is expected in an autosomal recessive disorder. Table 64-2 demonstrates the common mutations in *CYP21A2* and their related phenotypes. It is not always possible, however, to accurately predict the phenotype on the basis of the genotype—such predictions have been shown to be 90% to 95% accurate with some nonconcordance.

***Future Directions:*** Glucocorticoid replacement has been an effective treatment for CAH for the past 50 years and remains its primary therapy; however, the management of these patients presents a challenge because inadequate treatment as well as oversuppression can both cause complications. Adult short stature is frequently encountered in patients with CAH despite adequate glucocorticoid treatment. Data from our group and others have shown that patients with CAH are about 10 cm shorter than their parentally based target height. Our group was recently able to demonstrate that the combination of growth hormone and luteinizing hormone-releasing hormone (LHRH) analog improved final adult height by 8 cm when compared to CAH subjects treated only with glucocorticoid and mineralocorticoid therapy.

Some data show that children may be treated with lower doses of hydrocortisone if an androgen receptor antagonist (flutamide) and an aromatase inhibitor (testolactone) are utilized; however, the safety profile of the use of these medications in children has not been well studied. Antiandrogen treatment may also be useful as adjunctive therapy in adult women who continue to have hyperandrogenic signs despite good adrenal suppression.

Bilateral adrenalectomy is a radical but effective measure in some cases. A few patients who were extremely difficult to control with medical therapy alone showed improvement in their symptoms after bilateral adrenalectomy. Because this approach renders the patient completely adrenal insufficient, however, it should be reserved for extreme cases and is not a good treatment option for patients who have a history of poor compliance with medication.

Cell-free fetal DNA harvested from the mother's blood is a technique which is currently being developed to determine the sex of the fetus prior to the sixth week of gestation. If this technology becomes commercially available, it will decrease the amount of invasive procedures (chorionic villus sampling [CVS] and amniocentesis) as well as unnecessary prenatal therapy to male fetuses, which account for 50% of high-risk pregnancies.

Gene therapy, currently in development, is a promising future treatment strategy.

*Table 64-2* **Genetic Testing for 21-Hydroxylase Deficiency**

| Exon/Intron/Deletion | Mutation Type | Mutation | Phenotype | % Enzyme Activity | References |
|---|---|---|---|---|---|
| **Causative Mutations in Classic 21-OHD** | | | | | |
| Deletion | 30-kb deletion | - | SW | Severe (0%) | White et al. (1984) |
| Intron 2 | Aberrant splicing of intron 2 | 656 A/C-G | SW, SV | S (ND) | Higashi et al. (1988) |
| Exon 3 | 8-base deletion | G110 Δ8nt | SW | Severe (0%) | White et al. (1994) |
| Exon 4 | Missense mutation | I172N | SV | Severe (1%) | Amor et al. (1988) Tusie-Luna et al. (1990) |
| Exon 6 | Cluster | I236N V237E M239K | SW | Severe (0%) | Amor et al. (1988) Tusie-Luna et al. (1990) |
| Exon 8 | Nonsense mutation | Q318X | SW | Severe (0%) | Globerman et al. (1988) |
| Exon 8 | Missense mutation | R356W | SW, SV | Severe (0%) | Chiou et al. (1990) |
| Exon 10* | Missense mutation | R483P | SW | Severe (1%-2%) | Wedell and Luthman (1993) |
| **Causative Mutations in Nonclassic CAH** | | | | | |
| Exon 1 | Missense mutation | P30L | NC | Mild (30%-60%) | Tusie-Luna et al. (1991) |
| Exon 7 | Missense mutation | V281L | NC | Mild (20%-50%) | Speiser et al. (1988) |
| Exon 8* | Missense mutation | R339H | NC | Mild (20%-50%) | Helmberg et al. (1992) |
| Exon 10* | Missense mutation | P453S | NC | Mild (20%-50%) | Helmberg et al. (1992) Owerbach et al. (1992) |

NC, nonclassic; SW, salt-wasting; SV, simple virilizing; kb, kilobase; ND, not determined; *, not routinely assayed.

From New MI. Extensive clinical experience: nonclassical 21-hydroxylase deficiency. From Nonclassical 21-Hydroxylase Deficiency. *J Clin Endocrinol Metab*. 2006;91(11):4205-4214.

**BIBLIOGRAPHY:**

1. New MI, White PC. Genetic disorders of steroid metabolism. In: Thakker RV, ed. Genetic and molecular biological aspects of endocrine disease. London, UK: Bailliere Tindall; 1995:525-554.

2. New M, Lorenzen F, Lerner A, et al. Genotyping steroid 21-hydroxylase deficiency: hormonal reference data. *J Clin Endocrinol Metab*. 1983;57(2):320-326.

3. White PC, Speiser PW. Congenital adrenal hyperplasia due to 21-hydroxylase deficiency. *Endocr Rev*. 2000;21(3):245-291.

4. New MI. Extensive clinical experience: nonclassical 21-hydroxylase deficiency. *J Clin Endocrinol Metab*. 2006;91:4205-4214.

5. Lo J, Schwitzgebel V, Tyrrell J, et al. Normal female infants born of mothers with classic congenital adrenal hyperplasia due to 21-hydroxylase deficiency. *J Clin Endocrinol Metab*. 1999;84(3):930-936.

6. Morel Y, Murena M, Nicolino M, Carel JC, David M, Forest MG. Correlation between genetic lesions of the CYP21B gene and the clinical forms of congenital adrenal hyperplasia (CAH) due to 21-hydroxylase deficiency: report of a large study of 355 CAH chromosomes. *Hormone Res*. 1992;37:13.

7. Speiser PW, Dupont B, Rubinstein P, Piazza A, Kastelan A, New MI. High frequency of nonclassical steroid 21-hydroxylase deficiency. *Am J Hum Genet*.1985;37(4):650-667.

8. Lin-Su K, Vogiatzi MG, Marshall I, et al. Treatment with growth hormone and luteinizing hormone releasing hormone analog improves final adult height in children with congenital adrenal hyperplasia. *J Clin Endocrinol Metab*. 2005;90(6):3318-3325.

9. New M. et al. Extensive personal experience: prenatal diagnosis for congenital adrenal hyperplasia in 532 pregnancies. *J Clin Endocrinol Metab*. 2001;86:5651-5657.

## Supplementary Information

**OMIM REFERENCES:**

[1] *CYP21A2*; (#201910)

[2] *CYP11B1*; (#610613)

[3] *StAR*; (#600617)

[4] *HSC3B2*; (#201810)

[5] *CYP17A1*; (#609300)

[6] *POP*; (#124015)

# 65 Osteopenia and Osteoporosis

Mona Walimbe and Dolores Shoback

## KEY POINTS

- *Disease summary:*
  - Osteoporosis is a common disease characterized by low bone mass, microarchitectural disruption, and skeletal fragility resulting in an increased risk for fracture. Osteoporosis results from the interactions of multiple genetic loci, physiologic changes across the lifecycle, and disorders that secondarily influence bone mass and strength as well as environmental factors.
  - Primary osteoporosis includes juvenile osteoporosis (affects children or young adults with normal gonadal function), type 1 osteoporosis (postmenopausal women), or type 2 (age-associated or senile) osteoporosis.
  - Type 1 osteoporosis develops in postmenopausal women, typically aged 50 to 65 years, and is characterized by a phase of accelerated loss of bone mass especially from trabecular sites with an increased risk of fractures of the distal forearm and vertebral bodies.
  - Type 2 osteoporosis occurs in men and women older than 70 years and represents bone loss associated with aging and other factors such as nutritional deficiencies. Fractures usually occur in cortical and trabecular bone, including hip, wrist, and vertebral fractures.
  - Secondary osteoporosis refers to bone loss that occurs as a result of an underlying disease, hormone deficiency, or medication (Table 65-1). Many patients have overlap in these designations as well. For example, elderly postmenopausal women may have vitamin D deficiency in addition to chronic estrogen deficiency.
- *Differential diagnosis:*
  - This includes renal osteodystrophy, osteomalacia, and many secondary causes for loss of bone mass including those in Table 65-1.
- *Monogenic forms:*
  - There are several monogenic causes of osteoporosis as described in Table 65-2. There is no single genetic etiology for postmenopausal or for senile osteoporosis. Bone mineral density (BMD) is likely a complex polygenic trait.
- *Family history:*
  - Studies on the genetics of osteoporosis have shown that BMD and other skeletal characteristics such as the ultrasound properties of bone, skeletal geometry, and bone turnover have significant heritable components. Heredity and genetics may determine as much as 60% to 70% of an individual's peak bone mass. Affected first-degree relatives and a strong family history confer a higher risk for osteoporosis. It is not clear, however, to what extent the relative risk of osteoporosis is increased in an individual with an affected first-degree relative.
- *Twin studies:*
  - Twin studies have demonstrated that BMD is highly heritable with estimates from a cohort study in the United Kingdom demonstrating 50% to 80% heritability for BMD; another study showed heritability at the lumbar spine was 78% and at the femoral neck was 84%. These figures are consistent with other twin studies.
- *Environmental factors:*
  - Multiple lifestyle factors have been shown to contribute to the pathogenesis of osteoporosis (Tables 65-1 and 65-3).
- *Genome-wide associations:*
  - Although previous linkage and candidate gene studies have provided few replicated loci for osteoporosis, genome-wide association studies (GWAS) have produced multiple candidate genes. To date, several GWAS for osteoporosis and related traits have been conducted.
- *Pharmacogenetics:*
  - Genetic variants of osteoporosis that may be more or less responsive to certain forms of therapy have not been identified thus far. As a result, pharmacogenetics does not currently play a role in selecting the treatment of osteoporosis.

## Diagnostic Criteria and Clinical Characteristics

### Diagnostic Criteria for Osteoporosis and Osteopenia:

- The World Health Organization (WHO) has provided a densitometric definition of osteoporosis for postmenopausal women based on dual-energy x-ray absorptiometry (DXA) measurements of BMD.
- Normal BMD is characterized by a value above 1 standard deviation below the reference mean for young adult females (T-score ≥−1 SD).
- Low bone mass or **osteopenia** is characterized by a value greater than 1 but less than 2.5 standard deviations below the young adult female reference mean (T-score <−1 and >−2.5 SD).
- **Osteoporosis** is characterized by a value 2.5 standard deviations or more below the young adult female reference mean (T-score ≤−2.5).
- **Severe osteoporosis** is characterized by a value greater than 2.5 standard deviations below the young adult female reference mean in the presence of one or more fragility fractures.
- In premenopausal women, men less than 50 years of age and children, the WHO BMD diagnostic classification should not be applied.

*Table 65-1* Conditions, Diseases, and Medications That Are Associated with Bone Loss and Osteoporosis

| | |
|---|---|
| **Lifestyle factors** | Systemic mastocytosis |
| Alcohol abuse | Thalassemia |
| Chronic low calcium intake | **Rheumatologic and autoimmune diseases** |
| Inadequate physical activity and immobilization | Ankylosing spondylitis |
| Vitamin D insufficiency | Systemic lupus |
| Tobacco use | Rheumatoid arthritis |
| **Genetic disorders (discussed in this chapter)** | **Central nervous system disorders** |
| **Hypogonadism** | Parkinson disease |
| Androgen insensitivity | Stroke |
| Hyperprolactinemia | Multiple sclerosis |
| Premature ovarian failure and menopause | Spinal cord injury |
| Anorexia nervosa and bulimia | **Miscellaneous conditions and diseases** |
| Turner syndrome | Post-organ transplantation bone disease |
| Klinefelter syndrome | End stage renal disease |
| Hypopituitarism | Chronic metabolic acidosis |
| **Endocrine disorders** | Hypercalciuria |
| Hypercortisolism | Weight loss |
| Type 1 and 2 diabetes mellitus | Chronic obstructive lung disease |
| Primary hyperparathyroidism | **Medications** |
| Thyrotoxicosis | Aluminum (in antacids) |
| **Gastrointestinal disorders** | Cyclosporine A and tacrolimus |
| Celiac disease | Proton pump inhibitors |
| Inflammatory bowel disease | Heparin |
| Primary biliary cirrhosis | Depo-medroxyprogesterone |
| Malabsorption | Glucocorticoids ($\geq$ 5 mg/d prednisone or equivalent for $\geq$ 3 months) |
| Chronic pancreatic disease | Aromatase inhibitors |
| **Hematologic disorders** | Gonadotropin releasing hormone antagonists and agonists |
| Multiple myeloma | Thiazolidinediones |
| Monoclonal gammopathies | Thyroid hormones (in excess) |
| Sickle cell disease | |

Modified from The 2013 Clinician's Guide to Prevention and Treatment of Osteoporosis, National Osteoporosis Foundation.

In these groups, the diagnosis of osteoporosis should not be made on the basis of densitometric criteria alone. The International Society for Clinical Densitometry (ISCD) recommends that instead of T-scores, ethnic or race adjusted Z-scores should be used, with Z-scores of −2 or lower defined as either "low BMD for chronologic age" or "below the expected range for age."

- The relative risk of fracture increases as BMD decreases.
- Fragility fractures are defined as fractures that occur following a fall from standing height or less or with minimal to no trauma.

### Clinical Characteristics: General and Disease Specific:

☞**General:**
- Fragility fractures.
- Typical sites of fractures include spine, hip, femur, tibia, humerus, radius, ribs, and pelvis. Fractures of fingers, toes, face, and skull are typically not considered osteoporotic or fragility fractures.

- Height loss as an adult: historical greater than 4 cm or greater than 1.6 in; measured height loss greater than 2 cm or greater than 0.8 in; this may be seen with vertebral fractures and may lead to kyphosis.
- Many disorders that affect the acquisition of peak bone mass can also affect peak height attained in adolescence; growth retardation may be observed in childhood with such disorders.
- In the elderly, frailty and frequent falls are often clinical features of osteoporosis due to postmenopausal and senile bone loss.

☞**Disease Specific:**
- Cystic fibrosis
- Ehlers-Danlos syndrome
- Marfan syndrome
- Gaucher disease
- Hemochromatosis
- Homocystinuria

*Table 65-2  Genetic Differential Diagnosis for Osteoporosis/Osteopenia*

| Syndrome | Gene Name & Symbol | Associated Findings | Inheritance |
|---|---|---|---|
| **Cystic fibrosis** | Cystic fibrosis transmembrane conductance regulator (*CFTR*) | Multisystem disease affecting primarily the lungs but also the digestive, endocrine, reproductive systems. Osteoporosis is mainly secondary to pancreatic insufficiency leading to fat malabsorption and vitamin D deficiency | Autosomal recessive |
| **Ehlers-Danlos syndrome** | Many, but most commonly caused by defects in the fibrous proteins: *COL1A1*, *COL1A2*, *COL3A1*, *COL5A1*, *COL5A2*, *TNXB* or the enzymes: *ADAMTS2*, *PLOD1*[a] | Group of inherited connective tissue disorders caused by a defect in the synthesis of collagen type I or III | Various (see below) |
| *Types I and II (classical) | *COL5A1*, *COL5A2*, *COL1A1* | Affects type I and V collagen. Type 1 presents with severe skin involvement and type 2 presents with mild-moderate skin involvement | Autosomal dominant |
| *Type III and due to tenascin X deficiency (hypermobility) | *COL3A1*, *TNXB* | Characterized by extreme hypermobility | Autosomal recessive or autosomal dominant |
| *Type IV (vascular) | *COL3A1* | Defect in type III collagen synthesis. One of the more serious types of EDS as blood vessels and organs are more prone to tearing (rupture). Many patients have characteristic facial appearance (large eyes, small chin, thin nose & lips, lobeless ears), small stature with slim build with thin, pale, translucent skin | Autosomal dominant |
| *Type VI (kyphoscoliosis) | *PLOD1* | Deficiency of enzyme lysyl hydroxylase. Progressive curvature of the spine (scoliosis), fragile eyes, severe muscle weakness | Autosomal recessive |
| *Types VIIA & VIIB (arthrochalasis) | *COL1A1*, *COL1A2* | Affects type I collagen. Very loose joints, dislocations involving both hips. | Autosomal dominant |
| *Type VIIC (dermatosparaxis) | *ADAMTS2* | Extremely fragile and sagging skin | Autosomal recessive |
| **Marfan syndrome** | Fibrillin-1 gene (*FBN1*); a minority have mutations in the TGF-beta receptor 2 (*TGFBR2*) or TGF-beta receptor 1 (*TGFBR1*) gene | Characterized by aortic root dilatation, ectopia lentis, joint hypermobility, lumbosacral dural ectasia | Autosomal dominant |
| **Gaucher disease (type 1)** | Glucocerebrosidase gene (*GBA*) | Characterized by splenomegaly, hepatomegaly, anemia, thrombocytopenia, osteopenia and pathologic fractures, bone pain, growth retardation | Autosomal recessive |
| **Hemochromatosis** | Majority have *HFE* gene mutation. Other types include mutations in hemojuvelin, hepcidin, transferrin receptor 2, ferroportin 1, H-ferritin, L-ferritin | Mutations in the HFE gene cause increased intestinal iron absorption. The clinical manifestations are related to excess iron deposition in tissues such as the liver, heart, pancreas, pituitary (leading to hypogonadism which causes low bone mass). | Autosomal recessive |

*(Continued)*

*Table 65-2  Genetic Differential Diagnosis for Osteoporosis/Osteopenia (Continued)*

| Syndrome | Gene Name & Symbol | Associated Findings | Inheritance |
|---|---|---|---|
| **Homocystinuria** | Cystathionine beta synthase gene (CBS). May also involve the *MTHFR, MTR, MTRR, MMADHC* genes (play a role in converting homocysteine to methionine) | Increased risk of mental retardation, nearsightedness, scoliosis, megaloblastic anemia, osteoporosis. | Autosomal recessive |
| **Osteogenesis imperfecta** | Most have autosomal dominant mutation in *COL1A1* or *COL1A2*. In 10% of cases, patients have alternate mutations (usually autosomal recessive): FK506-binding protein 10 (*FKBP10* or *FKBP65* gene), *CRTAP, LEPRE1, PPIB, SERPINH1, SERPINF1, SP7/OSX* | 9 subtypes identified. Characterized by multiple fractures, short stature, occasionally blue sclerae and hearing loss.[2] | Mixed |
| **Osteoporosis-pseudoglioma syndrome** | Low-density lipoprotein receptor-related protein 5 gene (*LRP5*) | Characterized by congenital or infancy-onset visual loss and skeletal fragility recognized during childhood. | Autosomal Recessive |
| **Neurofibromatosis type 1** | Neurofibromin (*NF1*) | Café-au-lait macules, neurofibromas, freckling in the axillary or inguinal regions, optic glioma, Lisch nodules (iris hamartomas), bony lesions and osteoporosis | Autosomal Dominant |
| **Menkes steely hair syndrome** | ATPase, Cu++ transporting, alpha polypeptide gene (*ATP7A*) | Inability to regulate copper levels in the body. Mutations in ATP7A gene result in poor distribution of copper to the body's cells, causing accumulation in some tissues (small intestine & kidney) while other tissues (brain) have unusually low levels of copper. Those affected are characterized by sparse, kinky hair, failure to thrive and deterioration of the nervous system as well as osteoporosis. Children often do not live past age 3. | X-linked recessive |

[a]COL1A1, collagen, type 1, alpha-1; COL1A2, collagen, type 1, alpha-2;

COL3A1, collagen, type 3, alpha 1

COL5A1, collagen, type 5, alpha-1

COL5A2, collagen, type 5, alpha-2

TNXB, tenascin XB

ADAMTS2, a disintegrin-like and metalloproteinase with thrombospondin type 1 motif, 2

PLOD1, procollagen-lysine, 2 oxoglutarate 5-dioxygenase

[b]See dedicated chapter

**Table 65-3 *Common Risk Factors for Osteoporosis***

Age > 50 years

Female sex

Caucasian or Asian ethnicity

Family history of osteoporosis

Thin build or small stature (eg, body weight <58 kg or 127 lb)

Amenorrhea

Late menarche

Early menopause

Postmenopausal state

Physical inactivity or immobilization

Use of medications (such as anticonvulsants, corticosteroids, thyroid hormone supplementation, heparin, chemotherapeutic agents, androgen deprivation therapy)

Alcohol and tobacco use

Androgen or estrogen deficiency

Calcium or vitamin D deficiency

- Osteogenesis imperfecta
- Osteoporosis-pseudoglioma syndrome
- Neurofibromatosis type 1
- Menkes disease

## Screening and Counseling

**Screening:** In the United States and Canada, the majority of professional groups recommend BMD assessment in postmenopausal women 65 years or older regardless of risk factors. This recommendation is based on findings of greater fracture risk with advancing age beyond the seventh decade. Clinical trial data demonstrate reductions in fractures when postmenopausal women at highest fracture risk are treated. The BMD screening recommendations for men and for women younger than 65 years vary according to different groups of experts (Table 65-4).

Postmenopausal women and men older than 50 years should be clinically evaluated for osteoporosis risk in order to determine if there is a need for BMD testing. The greater the number of risk factors, the greater the risk of fracture. These include aging itself, hypogonadism and/or menopause, failure to have achieved peak bone mass in young adulthood (Table 65-5), and states of high bone turnover. The WHO fracture risk assessment tool (FRAX; found at http://www.shef.ac.uk/FRAX/) can be used for untreated patients between ages 40 and 90 to quantify the 10-year probability of a hip fracture or of the composite risk for four common osteoporotic fractures (clinical spine, forearm, hip, or proximal humerus).

Common risk factors for osteoporosis are listed in Table 65-3 as are the risk factors that, along with hip BMD by DXA, are used in the FRAX algorithm. Important secondary causes of osteoporosis are listed in Table 65-1. The potential skeletal complications of these disorders should be considered in the evaluation of patients with them.

**Table 65-4 *Bone Mineral Density Screening for Osteoporosis***

| Organization | Recommendations |
|---|---|
| **National Osteoporosis Foundation (NOF)[a] and International Society for Clinical Densitometry (ISCD)[b]** | |
| | *Women ≥65 years and men ≥70 years regardless of risk factors |
| | *Postmenopausal women <65 years and men 50-69 years when risk factors for bone loss or fractures are present |
| | *Adults with a fracture after age 50 |
| | *Adults with a condition or taking a medication associated with low bone mass or bone loss |
| | *Women during menopausal transition if there is a specific risk factor associated with increased fracture |
| | *Postmenopausal women discontinuing estrogen therapy |
| **American Association of Clinical Endocrinologists (AACE)[c]** | |
| | *All women ≥65 years |
| | *Any adult with a history of fracture not caused by severe trauma |
| | *Postmenopausal women <65 years with clinical risk factors for fracture |
| **United States Preventive Services Task Force (USPSTF)[d]** | |
| | *All women 65 years |
| | *Women <65 years whose fracture risk is equal to or greater than that of a 65 year old white woman with no additional risk factors |
| | *Current evidence is insufficient to assess the balance of benefits and harms of screening for osteoporosis in men |

[a]National Osteoporosis Foundation. Clinician's Guide to Prevention and Treatment of Osteoporosis. Washington, DC: National Osteoporosis Foundation; 2013.

[b]The International Society for Clinical Densitometry Official Positions. www.iscd.org/Visitors/positions/OfficialPositionsText.cfm

[c]American Association of Clinical Endocrinologists Medical Guidelines for Clinical Practice for the Diagnosis and Treatment of Postmenopausal Osteoporosis. http://www.aace.com/pub/pdf/guidelines/OsteoGuidelines2010.pdf

[d]U.S. Preventive Services Task Force. Screening for osteoporosis: U.S. preventive services task force recommendation statement. Ann Intern Med 2011;154:356.

The most common of the genetic disorders that cause osteoporosis are listed in Table 65-2. Screening is currently available for many of these conditions and screening and counseling of family members varies according to the individual disease. The reader is referred to the specific chapters dedicated to those diseases for more information.

**Table 65-5 *Examples of Disorders Associated With Reduced Peak Bone Mass***

| |
|---|
| Anorexia nervosa |
| Ankylosing spondylitis |
| Childhood immobilization (therapeutic bed rest) |
| Cystic fibrosis |
| Delayed puberty |
| Exercise-associated amenorrhea |
| Galactosemia |
| Intestinal or renal disease |
| Marfan syndrome |
| Osteogenesis imperfecta |
| Celiac disease |
| Male and female hypogonadism (eg, Turner or Klinefelter syndrome) |
| Juvenile arthritis |

**Counseling:** Counseling depends on the etiology of the osteoporosis. If related to specific Mendelian disease, risk for osteoporosis and transmission to the next generation can be significant.

## Management and Treatment

**Management:** Several interventions can be recommended universally to patients to reduce fracture risk. These include adequate daily calcium and vitamin D intake, regular weightbearing exercise, implementing strategies for fall prevention, and avoiding tobacco use and excessive alcohol intake.

Postmenopausal women and men aged 50 years or older should be considered for treatment if they have a hip or vertebral (clinical or morphometric) fracture, T-score less than or equal to −2.5 at the femoral neck, total hip or spine after appropriate evaluation excludes secondary causes, or osteopenia with a 10-year probability of hip fracture greater than or equal to 3% or a 10-year probability of major osteoporosis-related fracture greater than or equal to 20% based on the US-adapted FRAX algorithm. In addition, for cases of secondary osteoporosis, the underlying factor(s) that are causing or contributing to low bone mass should be addressed as well, as much as possible.

Drugs used for the prevention and treatment of osteoporosis usually act by one of two mechanisms: decreasing the rate of bone resorption or increasing the rate of bone formation. Increases in BMD are usually observed during the first 1 to 2 years of therapy, after which BMD may increase more slowly and/or reach a plateau. However, studies have indicated that patients on treatment with stable BMD still benefit from treatment through decreased fracture rates.

The antifracture benefits of FDA-approved drugs have mostly been observed in women with postmenopausal osteoporosis and prevalent fractures. FDA-approved osteoporosis treatments have been shown to decrease fracture risk in patients who have had fragility fractures or morphometric fractures by x-ray and/or have osteoporosis by DXA. These treatments may also reduce fractures in patients with osteopenia, but the evidence is not as strong.

**Therapeutics:**

☞**ANTIRESORPTIVE AGENTS:**

**Calcium:** The skeleton contains 99% of the body's calcium stores and when the exogenous supply is inadequate, bone tissue is resorbed from the skeleton to maintain serum calcium at a constant level. Therefore, adequate calcium and vitamin D intake are needed to maintain skeletal mass. Calcium and vitamin D supplements can suppress bone turnover, increase bone mass, and modestly decrease fracture incidence. Beneficial effects on fracture risk of these two agents are best demonstrated in elderly patients with relatively or frankly low calcium and vitamin D intake. The current recommended daily intake is 1300 mg/d for adolescents, 1000 mg/d for adults up to age 50, and 1200 mg/d for adults over 50 years. Increasing dietary intake is the recommended first-line approach; supplements should be used when adequate dietary intake cannot be achieved.

**Vitamin D:** Vitamin D and its metabolites play a major role in intestinal calcium absorption, bone health, muscle performance, and risk of falling. Current recommendations are for adults to maintain 800 to 1000 IU of vitamin D per day, with a desired 25-hydroxy vitamin D level of 30 ng/mL or higher. The exact level of 25-hydroxy vitamin D that constitutes sufficiency remains debated. Many patients are at risk for vitamin D deficiency, including those who are frail, homebound, hospitalized, and chronically ill. In addition, patients with malabsorption (eg, celiac disease), chronic kidney disease or limited sun exposure are also at risk.

**Estrogen:** Both estrogen and estrogen and progesterone therapy (hormone therapy) are approved by the FDA for the prevention of osteoporosis associated with menopause. Women who have not had a hysterectomy should receive progesterone as well (hormone therapy) to protect the uterine lining. The Women's Health Initiative (WHI) found that 5 years of hormone therapy reduced the risk of clinical vertebral fractures and hip fractures by 34% and other osteoporotic fractures by 23% but also reported increased risks of myocardial infarction, stroke, invasive breast cancer, pulmonary emboli, and deep vein phlebitis during 5 years of treatment with conjugated equine estrogen and medroxyprogesterone. Currently, estrogen or combined hormone therapies are recommended mainly for patients suffering from significant vasomotor effects of estrogen deficiency and early in menopause. In addition, they should be prescribed for the shortest duration possible. Nonestrogen treatments for osteoporosis are recommended before using estrogen or hormone therapy.

**Selective estrogen receptor modulators (SERMS):** These agents act as estrogens on some tissues and as antiestrogens on others. Raloxifene is the only FDA-approved SERM for both prevention and treatment of postmenopausal osteoporosis. It is an estrogen agonist at the bone and liver that promotes conservation of BMD. It is inert at the endometrium and a potent antiestrogen at the breast. Raloxifene decreases the risk of vertebral fractures and increases the risk of deep vein thrombosis to a degree similar to that observed with estrogen.

**Calcitonin:** The role of endogenous calcitonin in calcium metabolism is unclear but as a pharmacologic agent, it has been shown to inhibit osteoclastic bone resorption. Salmon calcitonin is FDA approved for the treatment of osteoporosis in women who are at least 5 years postmenopausal. It is available as an injection and also as a nasal spray. The side effects of the nasal spray include rhinitis and, rarely, epistaxis.

**Bisphosphonates:** Four bisphosphonates (alendronate, risedronate, ibandronate, and zoledronic acid) are FDA approved for the prevention and treatment of osteoporosis. Three bisphosphonates (alendronate, risedronate, and zoledronic acid) are approved for the treatment of glucocorticoid-induced osteoporosis in men and women and for the treatment of osteoporosis in men. Bisphosphonates inhibit osteoclast-mediated bone resorption. The approved bisphosphonates have been shown to reduce vertebral fractures and alendronate, risedronate, and zoledronic acid have been shown to reduce nonvertebral fractures, including hip fractures.

Side effects of oral bisphosphonate medications include gastrointestinal problems such as reflux, esophagitis, and gastric ulcers. There have been isolated and infrequent reports of osteonecrosis of the jaw in patients on oral bisphosphonates for treatment of osteoporosis and Paget disease. Osteonecrosis of the jaw is defined as the presence of exposed bone in the maxillofacial region that did not heal within 8 weeks after identification by a healthcare provider. The majority of cases of this jaw bone complication have occurred in patients with malignancies taking intravenous bisphosphonates at more frequent intervals and at much higher doses than the annual infusions of zoledronic acid used in patients with osteoporosis. Such complications often, but not invariably, follow dental procedures.

**Rank-L inhibition:** Denosumab, a human monoclonal IgG2 antibody to receptor activator of nuclear factor kappa B ligand or RANK-L has been approved by the FDA for the treatment of severe osteoporosis in patients with high risk for fracture. Studies have demonstrated significant reductions in spine, hip, and nonvertebral fractures in postmenopausal women with low BMD. This agent is also approved for the treatment of bone loss due to androgen deprivation therapy for prostate cancer and in women on adjuvant aromatase inhibitor therapy for breast cancer in both cases in patients at high risk for fracture.

☞**BONE-FORMING AGENTS:**

**Parathyroid hormone:** Although chronically elevated parathyroid hormone (PTH) levels can lead to bone pain, fractures and severe bone demineralization, intermittent and low-dose PTH can be a powerful bone-forming agent. Recombinant human PTH (amino acids 1-34) (teriparatide) is FDA approved for the treatment of osteoporosis in postmenopausal women and men at high risk for fracture. It is also approved for treatment of men and women at high risk for fracture from sustained systemic glucocorticoid therapy. It has been shown to reduce the incidence of both vertebral and nonvertebral fractures. Long-term carcinogenicity studies in rats demonstrated an increased risk for osteosarcoma. Thus far, it does not appear there is an elevated risk for osteosarcoma in humans. Individuals with an increased risk of osteosarcoma such as those with open epiphyses, prior radiation therapy to the skeleton, bone metastases, Paget disease, or a history of skeletal malignancy should not receive teriparatide therapy. The safety and efficacy of teriparatide have not been demonstrated beyond 2 years of treatment and so its treatment duration is limited to 2 years. Many clinicians follow teriparatide treatment with an antiresorptive treatment (eg, a bisphosphonate) to maintain or further increase BMD.

**Androgen:** Testosterone can increase bone mass in hypogonadal men and osteoporotic women but therapy of the latter group of patients is usually not well tolerated due to virilization. Fracture efficacy due to testosterone is unknown.

## Molecular Genetics and Molecular Mechanism

Table 65-6 lists genetic variants identified by a GWAS that are associated with osteoporosis, osteopenia, and/or BMD. Studies in which results were validated in a replication cohort are included.

*Future Directions:* Challenges in the field include identifying genetic determinants responsible for peak bone mass, fracture risk, and rates of bone loss and applying the information effectively in clinical management of the general population of patients without monogenic etiologies for skeletal fragility. Given the large number of genetic conditions in which skeletal fragility is an accompanying and often disabling feature of the disorder, the future anticipates the possibilities of gene therapy, enzyme or protein replacement, and/or stem cell therapy to address deficiencies in key skeletal factors to improve the clinical outlook for affected individuals.

**BIBLIOGRAPHY:**

1. American Association of Clinical Endocrinologists Guidelines for Clinical Practice for the Diagnosis and Treatment of Postmenopausal Osteoporosis. https://www.aace.com/sites/default/files/OsteoGuidelines2010.pdf. Accessed 2010.

2. Arden NK, Baker J, Hogg C, Baan K, Spector TD. The heritability of bone mineral density, ultrasound of the calcaneus and hip axis length: a study of postmenopausal twins. *J Bone Miner Res.* 1996;11:530-534.

3. Balemans W, Van Hul W. The genetics of low-density lipoprotein receptor-related protein 5 in bone: a story of extremes. *Endocrinology.* 2007;148:2622-2629.

4. Baim S, Binkley N, Bilezikian JP, et al. Official positions of the International Society for Clinical Densitometry and executive summary of the 2007 ISCD Position Development Conference. *J Clin Densitom.* 2008;11:75.

5. Compston J, Cooper A, Cooper C, et al. Guidelines for the diagnosis and management of osteoporosis in postmenopausal women and men from the age of 50 years in the UK. *Maturitas.* 2009;62:105.

6. Cummings SR, Bates D, Black DM. Clinical use of bone densitometry: scientific review. *JAMA.* 2002;288:1889.

7. Jacobs-Kosmin D, Shanmugam S. Osteoporosis. Medscape Reference. Herbert S. Diamond, ed. http://emedicine.medscape.com/article/330598-overview#aw2aab6b2b4aa. Accessed October 26, 2011.

8. Kanis JA, Johnell O. Requirements for DXA for the management of osteoporosis in Europe. *Osteoporos Int.* 2005;16:229.

9. Khosla S, Burr D, Cauley J, et al. Bisphosphonate-associated osteonecrosis of the jaw: report of a task force of the American Society for Bone and Mineral Research. *J Bone Miner Res.* 2007;22:1479-1491.

10. Leslie WD, Schousboe JT. A review of osteoporosis diagnosis and treatment options in new and recently updated guidelines on case finding around the world. *Curr Osteoporos Rep.* 2011;9:129.

11. Malfait F, Wenstrup RJ, De Paepe. Clinical and genetic aspects of Ehlers-Danlos syndrome, classic type. *Genet Med.* 2010;12:597-605.

*Table 65-6 Loci Revealed by Genome-Wide Association Studies (GWASs) for Osteoporosis and Related Traits*

**Candidate Loci Validated by GWAS**

| Gene | Gene Name | Gene Location | Associated SNPs | Putative Functional Significance |
|---|---|---|---|---|
| ESR1 | Estrogen receptor 1 | 6q25.1 | rs2504063, rs7751941 | Ligand-activated transcription factor important in hormone binding, DNA binding, and activation of transcription |
| PTH | Parathyroid hormone | 11p15.3-p15.1 | rs9630182, rs2036417, rs7125774 | Parathyroid hormone is involved in the regulation of calcium and bone metabolism |
| LRP5 | LDL receptor-related protein 5 | 11q13.4 | rs3781586, rs599083, rs4988321, rs3736228 | Regulator of osteoblast growth and differentiation, affecting peak bone mass in vertebrates. |
| FOXC2 | Forkhead box C2 | 16q24.3 | rs3751797 | Involved in Wnt/β-catenin signaling pathway, which has an essential role in the regulation of bone mass |
| SOST | Sclerostin | 17q11.2 | rs1877632, rs1534401, rs851084, rs851086 | Involved in Wnt/β-catenin signaling pathway, which has an essential role in the regulation of bone mass |
| SLC25A13 | Solute carrier family 25, member 13 | 7q21.3 | rs4729260, rs7781370 | Calcium-dependent mitochondrial solute transporter with a role in urea cycle function |
| MEPE | Matrix, extracellular, phosphoglycoprotein | 4q22.1 | rs727420 | Plays a role in the regulation of bone mineralization |
| TNFSF11 | Tumor necrosis factor ligand superfamily, member 11 (RANKL, receptor activator of nuclear factor kappa B ligand) | 13q14 | rs12585014, rs7988338, rs2148073, rs9594782, rs12721445m rs2277438 | Plays an important role in the regulation of bone remodeling and osteoclast development |
| TNFRSF11A | Tumor necrosis factor receptor superfamily, member 11a, NFκB activator (RANK, receptor activator of nuclear factor kappa B) | 18q22.1 | rs884205 | Plays an important role in the regulation of bone remodeling and osteoclast development |
| TNFRSF11B | Tumor necrosis factor receptor superfamily, member 11b (OPG, osteoprotegerin) | 8q24 | rs11995824, rs2062377 | Plays an important role in the regulation of bone remodeling and osteoclast development |

**New Loci For Other Osteoporosis Related Phenotypes**

| Gene | Gene Name | Gene Location | Associated SNPs | Putative Functional Significance |
|---|---|---|---|---|
| RAP1A | Ras-related protein | 1p13.2 | rs494453 | Important in adhesion and migration of lymphocytes |
| PLCL1 | Phospholipase C-like 1 | 2q33.1 | rs7595412, rs4850820, rs10180112, rs4850833 | Involved in inositol phospholipid-based intracellular signaling cascade |
| TBC1D8 | TBC1 domain family, member 8 | 2q11.2 | rs2278729 | May act as a GTPase-activating protein for Rab family protein(s) |

*(Continued)*

*Table 65-6  Loci Revealed by Genome-Wide Association Studies (GWASs) for Osteoporosis and Related Traits (Continued)*

**Novel Bone Mineral Density Loci**

| Gene | Gene Name | Gene Location | Associated SNPs | Putative Functional Significance |
|---|---|---|---|---|
| *GPR177* | G-protein coupled receptor 177 | 1p31.2 | rs1430742, rs2566755 | Involved in Wnt/β-catenin signaling pathway, which has an essential role in the regulation of bone mass |
| *TGFBR3* | Transforming growth factor, beta receptor III | 1p22.1 | rs1805113 | Multifunctional cytokine that modulates several tissue development and repair processes, including cell differentiation, cell cycle progression, cellular migration, adhesion, and extracellular matrix production |
| *FONG* | Formininotransferase N-terminal domain-containing gene | 2q33.1 | rs7605378 | Function of this gene as yet unknown |
| *GALNT3* | Polypeptide N-acetylgalactosaminyl-transferase 3 | 2q24.3 | rs1863196, rs6710518, rs4667492 | An enzyme that processes FGF23 into a glycosylated molecule which is biologically active |
| *CTNNB1* | Catenin beta 1 | 3p22.1 | rs87939, rs87938 | Involved in Wnt/β-catenin signaling pathway, which has an essential role in the regulation of bone mass. |
| *IBSP* | Integrin-binding sialoprotein | 4q22.1 | rs1054627 | Bone sialoprotein is an acidic glycoprotein that constitutes approximately 12% of the noncollagenous proteins in human bone and is synthesized by skeletal-associated cell types, including hypertrophic chondrocytes, osteoblasts, osteocytes, and osteoclasts |
| *ALDH7A1* | Aldehyde dehydrogenase seven family, member A1 | 5q31 | rs13182402 | Encodes an enzyme of the acetaldehyde dehydrogenase superfamily, which degrades & detoxifies acetaldehyde generated by alcohol metabolism. Acetaldehyde has been shown to inhibit osteoblast proliferation and decrease bone formation |
| *SOX4* | Sex-determining region Y-box 4 | 6p22.3 | rs9466056 | Lymphocyte-specific transcriptional activator |
| *MHC* | Major histocompatibility complex | 6p21 | rs3130340 | Associated with many immune-related diseases. The precise mechanism responsible for osteoporosis in this region is unknown |

*(Continued)*

**Table 65-6** *Loci Revealed by Genome-Wide Association Studies (GWASs) for Osteoporosis and Related Traits (Continued)*

| Gene | Gene Name | Gene Location | Associated SNPs | Putative Functional Significance |
|------|-----------|---------------|-----------------|-------------------------------|
| SFRP4 | Secreted frizzled-related protein 4 | 7p14 | rs1721400 | Member of SFRP family, which acts as soluble modulators of Wnt signaling. Overexpression of SFRP4 has been associated with reductions in bone mineral density |
| DCDC5 | Doublecortin domain-containing protein 5 | 11p14-p13 | rs16921914 | The protein encoded by this gene may bind tubulin and enhance microtubule polymerization |
| SOX6 | Sex-determining region Y-box 6 | 11p15.2-p15.1 | rs297325, rs4756846, rs7117858 | Member of the SOX gene family, thought to have a role in chondrogenesis and obesity-related insulin resistance |
| LRP4 | LDL receptor-related protein 4 | 11p11.2 | rs2306033, rs7935346 | Involved in Wnt/β-catenin signaling pathway, which has an essential role in the regulation of bone mass |
| SP7 | Transcription factor Sp7 | 12q13.13 | rs10876432, rs2016266 | Transcription factor that has an essential role in regulating osteoblast differentiation |
| IL21R | Interleukin 21 receptor | 16p12.1 | rs8057551, rs8061992, rs7199138 | Cytokine receptor that is important to bone biology and has been identified negatively to be correlated with the destruction of bone and cartilage |
| ADAMTS18 | ADAM metallopeptidase with thrombospondin type1 motif, 18 | 16q23.1 | rs16945612 | Allele change which leads to repression of two genes (BMP6 and RARa) which are involved in regulating osteoblast differentiation and bone remodelling |
| JAG1 | Jagged 1 | 20p12.2 | rs2273061 | Increase in bone mineral deposition |

12. Moller L, Mogensen M, Horn N. Molecular diagnosis of Menkes disease: genotype-phenotype correlation. *Biochimie*. 2009;91: 1273-1277.

13. National Osteoporosis Foundation. *Clinician's Guide to Prevention and Treatment of Osteoporosis*. Washington, DC: National Osteoporosis Foundation; 2013.

14. Papaioannou A, Morin S, Cheung AM, et al. 2010 clinical practice guidelines for the diagnosis and management of osteoporosis in Canada: summary. *CMAJ*. 2010;182:1864.

15. Qaseem A, Snow V, Shekelle P, et al. Screening for osteoporosis in men: a clinical practice guideline from the American College of Physicians. *Ann Intern Med*. 2008;148:680.

16. Richards JB, Kavvoura FK, Rivadeneira F, et al. Collaborative meta-analysis: associations of 150 candidate genes with osteoporosis and osteoporotic fracture. *Ann Intern Med*. 2009;151:528-537.

17. Rossouw JE, Anderson GL, Prentice RL, et al. Risks and benefits of estrogen plus progestin in healthy postmenopausal women: principal results from the Women's Health Initiative randomized controlled trial. *JAMA*. 2002;288:321.

18. Slemenda CW, Turner CH, Peacock M, et al. The genetics of proximal femur geometry, distribution of bone mass and bone mineral density. *Osteoporos Int*. 1996;6:178-182.

19. The International Society for Clinical Densitometry Official Positions. http://www.iscd.org/Visitors/positions/OfficialPositionsText .cfm

20. U.S. Preventive Services Task Force. Screening for osteoporosis: U.S. preventive services task force recommendation statement. *Ann Intern Med*. 2011;154:356.

21. Writing Group for the Women's Health Initiative Investigators. Risks and benefits of estrogen plus progestin in healthy postmenopausal women. *JAMA*. 2002;288:321-333.

22. Zheng HF, Spector TD, Richards JB. Insights into the genetics of osteoporosis from recent genome-wide association studies. *Expert Rev Mol Med*. 2011;13:e28.

23. Ng MY, Sham PC, Paterson AD, Chan V, Kung AW. Effect of environmental factors and gender on the heritability of bone mineral density and bone size. *Ann Hum Genet*. 2007;70:428-438.

## Supplementary Information

### OMIM REFERENCES:

[1] Cystic Fibrosis Transmembrane Conductance Regulator; CFTR (*602421)

[2] Ehlers-Danlos Syndrome Type I (#130000)

[3] Ehlers-Danlos Syndrome Type II (#130010)

[4] Ehlers-Danlos Syndrome Type III (#130020)

[5] Ehlers-Danlos Syndrome Type IV, Autosomal Dominant (#130050)

[6] Ehlers-Danlos Syndrome Type VI; EDS6 (#225400)

[7] Ehlers-Danlos Syndrome Type VII, Autosomal Dominant (#130060)

[8] Ehlers-Danlos Syndrome Type VII, Autosomal Recessive (#225410)

[9] Ehlers-Danlos Syndrome, Type VIII (%130080)

[10] Ehlers-Danlos Syndrome, Autosomal Dominant, Type Unspecified (130090)

[11] Marfan Syndrome: MFS (#154700)

[12] Gaucher Disease, Type 1 (#230800)

[13] Hemochromatosis; HFE (#235200)

[14] Homocystinuria due to Cystathionine Beta-Synthase Deficiency (#236200)

[15] Collagen, Type 1, Alpha-1; COL1A1 (+120150)

[16] Collagen, Type 1, Alpha-1; COL1A2 (*120160)

[17] Osteoporosis-Pseudoglioma Syndrome; OPPG (#259770)

[18] Neurofibromatosis, Type I; NF1 (#162200)

[19] Menkes Disease (#309400)

**Alternative Names:**

- Ehlers-Danlos Syndrome: Cutis Hyperelastica
- Osteoporosis-Pseudoglioma Syndrome: Osteogenesis Imperfecta, Ocular Form
- Menkes Disease: Copper Transport Disease; Hypocupremia, Congenital; Kinky Hair Syndrome; Menkes Syndrome; Steely Hair Syndrome; X-Linked Copper Deficiency

For other alternative names, please see chapters specific to those individual diseases.

***Key Words:*** Osteoporosis, osteopenia, bone mineral density, fractures

# 66 Albright Hereditary Osteodystrophy and Pseudohypoparathyroidism Type 1

Giovanna Mantovani and Francesca M. Elli

## KEY POINTS

- *Disease summary:*
  - Pseudohypoparathyroidism is a term applied to a heterogeneous group of disorders whose common feature is end-organ resistance to parathyroid hormone (PTH).
  - This spectrum of disorders includes pseudohypoparathyroidism type Ia (PHP-Ia), pseudopseudohypoparathyroidism (PPHP), pseudohypoparathyroidism type Ib (PHP-Ib), pseudohypoparathyroidism type Ic (PHP-Ic), and progressive osseous heteroplasia (POH).
  - The lack of responsiveness to parathyroid hormone results in low serum calcium, high serum phosphate, and inappropriately high serum parathyroid hormone.
  - PTH resistance, the most clinically evident abnormality, usually develops over the first years of life, with hyperphosphatemia and elevated PTH generally preceding hypocalcemia. Renal function is conserved through life and so seems to be bone mineral density (BMD).
  - Individuals with Albright hereditary osteodystrophy (AHO) have short stature, characteristically shortened fourth and fifth metacarpals, rounded face, ectopic ossifications, and often mild mental retardation.

- *Hereditary basis:*
  - PHP-Ia is caused by inactivating mutations in *Gs* gene and is inherited in an autosomal dominant manner. Patients inheriting the disease from the mother display all signs of AHO together with multihormone resistance, while patients inheriting the disease from the father have AHO with no evidence of resistance to hormone action (PPHP).
  - In PHP-Ib the defect is often sporadic but it may occasionally present as familial, with an autosomal dominant pattern of transmission (AD-PHP-Ib). Both sporadic and familial PHP-Ib are now known to be associated with disturbed imprinting at the *GNAS* locus.
  - POH is an autosomal dominant disorder caused by inactivating *GNAS* mutations of paternal inheritance.

- *Differential diagnosis:*
  - PHP type I is classically differentiated according to the presence (PHP-Ia and PHP-Ic) or absence (PHP-Ib) of AHO (Table 66-1).
  - In PHP-Ia and Ic patients resistance to hormones is not limited to PTH, but often includes thyroid-stimulating hormone (TSH), gonadotropins, and growth hormone-releasing hormone (GHRH), and patients may develop resistance to these different hormones with a variable severity and variable time course. Patients with PHP-Ia have been shown to have a partial deficiency (about 50%) of Gs activity due to a reduction in mRNA and protein, whereas this defect is absent in patients with PHP-Ic.
  - Patients showing the physical features of AHO without any evidence of PTH resistance are described as affected by PPHP. PPHP may be present either in kindreds in which PHP is present or as an isolated defect (AHO-like syndrome).
  - The molecular defect causing POH is the same as that causing PPHP. However, the observation that POH patients do not usually present with AHO, suggests that POH may be an extreme end of the spectrum of the AHO features seen in PPHP.

## Diagnostic Criteria and Clinical Characteristics

### Diagnostic Criteria for PHP:
- Elevated PTH levels
- Hypocalcemia
- Hyperphosphatemia
- Absence of hypercalciuria or impaired renal function
- Reduced calcemic and phosphaturic response to injected exogenous parathyroid hormone

### Clinical Characteristics:

**PHP-Ia:** In addition to PTH resistance, it is characterized by resistance to other hormones, including TSH, gonadotropins, and GHRH. It is associated with AHO, which includes short stature, obesity, round facies, subcutaneous ossifications, brachydactyly, and other skeletal anomalies. Some patients have mental retardation. Laboratory studies show a decreased cAMP response to infused PTH and defects in activity of the erythrocyte Gs protein.

**PPHP:** It is characterized by the physical findings of AHO without hormone resistance. Laboratory studies show a defect in Gs protein activity in erythrocytes.

**PHP-Ib:** It is characterized clinically by isolated renal PTH resistance. Patients usually lack the physical characteristics of AHO and typically show no other endocrine abnormalities, although resistance to TSH has been reported. However, patients may rarely show some features of AHO. Laboratory studies show a decreased cAMP response to infused PTH and, most recently reported, sometimes defects in Gs protein activity similarly to PHP-Ia patients.

**PHP-Ic:** It is clinically indistinguishable from PHP-Ia, therefore being characterized by the association of multihormone

*Table 66-1 Genetic Differential Diagnosis*

|  | AHO | Hormone Resistance | Heterotopic Ossification | PTH Infusion | Gsα Activity | GNAS Defect |
|---|---|---|---|---|---|---|
| PHP-Ia | Yes | Multiple: PTH, TSH, Gn, GHRH | Superficial | ↓cAMP ↓phosphaturia | ↓(50%) | Maternal inactivating mutations |
| PPHP | Yes | No | Superficial | Normal | ↓(50%) | Paternal inactivating mutations |
| PHP-Ib | No | PTH, TSH | No | ↓cAMP ↓phosphaturia | Normal/↓ | Imprinting dysregulation |
| PHP-Ic | Yes | Multiple: PTH, TSH, Gn | Superficial | ↓cAMP ↓phosphaturia | Normal | Few inactivating mutations reported |
| POH | No | No | Deep | NA | NA | Paternal inactivating mutations |

PHP, pseudohypoparathyroidism; PPHP, pseudopseudohyoparathyroidism; AHO, Albright hereditary osteodystrophy; POH, progressive osseous heteroplasia; Gn, gonadotropins; NA, not available.

resistance and AHO. Laboratory studies show a decreased cAMP response to infused PTH, but typically no defect in activity of the erythrocyte Gs protein.

**POH:** It is characterized by ectopic dermal ossification beginning in infancy, followed by increasing and extensive bone formation in deep muscle and fascia. These patients typically do not show any endocrine abnormality.

## Screening and Counseling

*Screening:* Most patients with PHP-Ia, PPHP, and POH carry an heterozygous inactivating mutation in Gsα-coding *GNAS* exons, and this diagnosis has important implications for the patient and/or close relatives. However, in about 20% to 30% patients no *GNAS* mutation is present. Recently, in a subset of patients with PHP and variable degrees of AHO, *GNAS* epigenetic defects similar to those classically found in PHP-Ib patients have been detected. This would propose that features of AHO may result from either mutations in Gs-coding exons or epigenetic defects, both defects resulting in silencing or reduction of Gs α transcription in selected tissues. Therefore, patients with AHO phenotype and abnormal Gs activity but absence of mutations in Gs-coding exons, should be tested for methylation defects at GNAS differentially methylated regions (DMRs).

Approximately 60% of PHP-Ib patients have imprinting defects at GNAS DMRs. PHP Ib is most often a sporadic disorder and displays *GNAS* imprinting abnormalities that involve multiple DMRs, but the genetic lesion underlying these epigenetic defects, if any, remains to be discovered: most of these cases could represent true stochastic errors in early embryonic maintenance of methylation. Paternal uniparental isodisomy (pUPD) of the long arm rather than of the entire chromosome 20 has been described as plausible cause of the disease in few sporadic PHP-Ib cases with broad *GNAS* methylation defects. Although rare, this should be taken into consideration for proper genetic counseling in these patients. On the other hand, sex-influenced autosomal dominant inheritance has been reported in familial cases, where PTH resistance develops only after maternal inheritance of the molecular defect. AD-PHP-Ib affected individuals and obligate carriers exhibit loss of methylation

only at GNAS exon A/B and a heterozygous microdeletion in the STX16 region, which host an imprinting control region (ICR) for GNAS A/B DMR. Recently, deletions removing the entire NESP55 DMR as well as part of *GNAS*-AS transcript have also been identified in some AD-PHP-Ib kindreds.

*Counseling:*

☞**INACTIVATING GNAS MUTATIONS:** Inactivating *GNAS* mutations are inherited in an autosomal dominant manner. Each child of an affected parent has a 50% risk of inheriting the condition. In particular, PHP-Ia is inherited as an autosomal dominant with *paternal imprinting*. In this case the disease phenotype is only transmitted via the mother (50% risk). PPHP and POH are inherited as an autosomal dominant trait with *maternal imprinting*. In this case the disease phenotype is only transmitted via the father (50% risk).

Presymptomatic testing should be offered to all relatives of an affected individual. In situations of apparent de novo mutations, germline mosaicism in an unaffected parent and nonpaternity should be considered.

**Genotype-phenotype correlation:** No correlations have been shown.

☞**IMPRINTING DEFECTS AT GNAS LOCUS:** Methylation defects involving multiple DMRs often underlie a sporadic disorder, but, for a correct counseling, it is important to exclude microdeletions involving the entire *GNAS* locus and UPD. In case of deletions, the disease phenotype is transmitted in an autosomal dominant fashion. Presymptomatic testing should be offered to all relatives of an affected individual. In situations of apparent de novo mutations, germline mosaicism in an unaffected parent and nonpaternity should be considered.

**Epigenotype-phenotype correlation:** No correlations have been shown.

## Management and Treatment

In general, PHP-I patients should be monitored annually for both blood biochemistries (PTH, calcium, phosphate, TSH) and urinary calcium excretion. Particular attention must be given in children to height, growth velocity, and pubertal development. Increasing

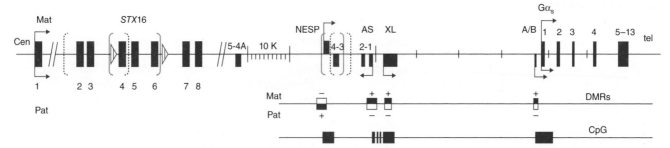

**Figure 66-1** Schematic graph of the *GNAS* locus and the *STX16* gene. Exons are indicated as black rectangles, STX16 and NESP-AS deletions as brackets, and allelic origin of transcription as broken arrows on the paternal (Pat) or maternal (Mat) allele. The four differentially methylated regions (DMRs) are represented below the genomic line by black boxes or + (methylated) or white boxes or − (unmethylated) on the Pat or Mat allele. The lower horizontal line shows the CpG islands identified by the Genome Browser software.

evidence suggests that, independently of growth curve, children should be screened with appropriate provocative tests for GH deficiency in order to eventually start treatment as soon as possible. Weight and body mass index (BMI) should be checked in order to start dietary or exercise intervention when appropriate. Careful physical examination and, when necessary, specific psychologic investigations should be performed annually in order to detect and follow the presence or evolution of specific AHO features (in particular heterotopic ossifications and mental retardation). Initial screening should include radiologic evaluation of brachydactyly.

The long-term therapy of hypocalcemia, in order to maintain normocalcemia, is with active vitamin D metabolites, preferentially calcitriol, with or without oral calcium supplementation. Patients should be also routinely screened and eventually treated for any associated endocrinopathy, in particular hypothyroidism and hypogonadism. Levothyroxine and sex hormones should be given following the same criteria, doses and follow-up as in any other form of hypothyroidism or hypogonadism.

There are no specific treatments for the various manifestations of AHO, even if subcutaneous ossifications may be surgically removed when particularly large or bothersome.

## Molecular Genetics and Molecular Mechanism

### Syndrome/Gene/Locus:

PHP-Ia/GNAS complex locus (*GNAS*)/20q13.32
PPHP/GNAS complex locus (*GNAS*)/20q13.32
PHP-Ib/GNAS complex locus (*GNAS*)/20q13.32
PHP-Ic/GNAS complex locus (*GNAS*)/20q13.32
POH/GNAS complex locus (*GNAS*)/20q13.32

*GNAS* is a complex imprinted locus and produces multiple transcripts: Gs-α, XLAS, NESP55, the A/B transcript, as well as an antisense *GNAS* transcript (GNASAS) (Fig. 66-1). The four main transcripts are produced through the use of alternative promoters and splicing of four unique first exons onto the shared exons 2 through 13. Gs-α is ubiquitously expressed and encodes a protein that stimulates adenylyl cyclase when activated by an agonist-occupied G protein-coupled receptor, thereby generating the second messenger cAMP. Gs-α is biallelically expressed with the exception of a small number of tissues, including renal proximal tubules, thyroid, gonads, and pituitary, where it is predominantly expressed from the maternal allele. XLAS is a large variant of Gs-α that is expressed exclusively from the paternal *GNAS* allele, primarily in neuroendocrine tissues and the nervous system. XLAS and Gs-α proteins are identical over their C-terminal portions, but they have distinct N-terminal domains. NESP55 is exclusively expressed from the maternal *GNAS* allele and encodes a chromogranin-like neuroendocrine secretory protein that, due to a stop codon in its unique first exon, shares no amino acid sequence with Gs-α. The A/B transcript, which uses the alternative first exon A/B (also referred to as exon 1A), and the antisense *GNAS* transcript, which consists of exons that do not overlap with any other *GNAS* exons, are ubiquitously expressed noncoding transcripts that are derived exclusively from the paternal *GNAS* allele. Consistent with their parent-specific expression, the promoters of the XLAS, NESP55, A/B, and antisense transcripts are within DMRs, and in each case the nonmethylated promoter drives the expression of the gene. In contrast, the promoter for Gs-α lacks methylation and is biallelically active in most tissues.

**Genetic Testing:** Clinically available analysis
- DNA direct sequencing for Gsα coding region
- COBRA (combined bisulfite restriction analysis) for *GNAS* DMRs methylation status
- Multiplex polymerase chain reaction (PCR) for STX16 3.3 and 4.4 Kb microdeletions

**BIBLIOGRAPHY:**

1. Mantovani G. Clinical review: pseudohypoparathyroidism: diagnosis and treatment. *J Clin Endocrinol Metab*. 2011; 96:3020-3030.

2. Kelsey G. Imprinting on chromosome 20: tissue-specific imprinting and imprinting mutations in the GNAS locus. *Am J Med Genet C*. 2010;154C:377-386.

3. Mantovani G, Spada A. Mutations in the Gs alpha gene causing hormone resistance. *Best Pract Res Clin Endocrinol Metab*. 2006;20:501-513.

4. Chase LR, Melson GL, Aurbach GD. Pseudohypoparathyroidism: defective excretion of 3', 5'-AMP in response to parathyroid hormone. *J Clin Invest*. 1969;48:1832-1844.

5. Farfel Z, Brickman AS, Kaslow HR, Brothers VM, Bourne HR. Defect of receptor-cyclase coupling protein in pseudohypoparathyroidism. *New Eng J Med*. 1980;303:237-242.

6. Levine MA, Downs RW Jr, Moses AM, et al. Resistance to multiple hormones in patients with pseudohypoparathyroidism: association with deficient activity of guanine nucleotide regulatory protein. *Am J Med*. 1983;74:545-556.

7. Faull CM, Welbury RR, Paul B, Kendall-Taylor P. Pseudohypoparathyroidism: its phenotypic variability and associated disorders in a large family. *Q J Med*. 1991;78:251-264.

8. Mantovani G, Ballare E, Giammona E, Beck-Peccoz P, Spada A. The Gs alpha gene: predominant maternal origin of transcription in human thyroid gland and gonads. *J Clin Endocrinol Metab*. 2002;87:4736-4740.

9. Mantovani G, Maghnie M, Weber G, et al. GHRH resistance in pseudohypoparathyroidism type Ia: new evidence for imprinting of the Gs alpha gene. *J Clin Endocrinol Metab*. 2003;88:4070-4074.

10. Juppner H, Schipani E, Bastepe M, et al. The gene responsible for pseudohypoparathyroidism type Ib is paternally imprinted and maps in four unrelated kindreds to chromosome 20q13.3. *Proc Nat Acad Sci USA*. 1998;95:11798-11803.

11. Liu J, Litman D, Rosenberg MJ, Yu S, Biesecker LG, Weinstein LS. A GNAS imprinting defect in pseudohypoparathyroidism type Ib. *J Clin Invest*. 2000;106:1167-1174.

12. Mantovani G, deSanctis L, Barbieri AM, et al. Pseudohypoparathyroidism and GNAS epigenetic defects: clinical evaluation of Albright hereditary osteodystrophy and molecular analysis in 40 patients. *J Clin Endocrinol Metab*. 2010;95:651-658.

ACKNOWLEDGEMENTS:

The work on Pseudohypoparathyroidism and GNAS is supported by a grant from the Italian Ministry of Health to G.M. (GR-2009-1608394).

## Supplementary Information

**OMIM REFERENCES:**

[1] Albright Hereditary Osteodystrophy; AHO (#168000)

[2] Pseudohypoparathyroidism Type Ia; PHP-Ia (#103580)

[3] Pseudohypoparathyroidism Type Ib; PHP-Ib (#603233)

[4] Pseudohypoparathyroidism Type Ic; PHP-Ic (#612462)

[5] Pseudopseudohypoparathyroidism; PPHP (#612463)

[6] Progressive Osseous Heteroplasia; POH (#166350)

[7] AHO-Like Syndrome (#600430)

***Key Words:*** Hormone resistance, *GNAS* gene, imprinting, methylation defects, brachydactyly, ectopic ossifications

# 67 Hypogonadotropic Hypogonadism

Ravikumar Balasubramanian and William F. Crowley, Jr.

## KEY POINTS

- *Disease summary:*
  - Kallmann syndrome (KS; hypogonadotropic hypogonadism and anosmia) and normosmic idiopathic hypogonadotropic hypogonadism (nIHH) represent the two major clinical presentations of humans with *isolated* deficiency of gonadotropin-releasing hormone (GnRH).
  - Both KS and nIHH are more common in males than females (~3:1) and affected patients present with either complete or partial absence of puberty.
  - During development, GnRH neurons arise from the embryonic olfactory placode and migrate *in utero* into the mediobasal hypothalamus where they secrete GnRH in a pulsatile manner. Combined developmental failure of both olfactory and GnRH neuronal migration result in KS, while isolated neuroendocrine failure of anatomically normal GnRH neurons results in nIHH.
- *Hereditary basis:*
  - 70% of KS or nIHH cases are apparently sporadic while the remainder is familial. However, on more detailed family expansion, a familial pattern can become evident. The inheritance pattern is heterogeneous. X-linked recessive, autosomal dominant, autosomal recessive, and oligogenic modes of inheritance are all documented.
- *Differential diagnosis:*
  - In adolescents presenting with delayed puberty, the main differential diagnosis is constitutional delay in puberty (CDP). Time is the major factor in distinguishing CDP and KS or nIHH as subjects with CDP eventually enter puberty spontaneously and achieve normal sexual maturation.
  - Other anatomic (CNS or pituitary tumors, head trauma, CNS irradiation, etc) or functional (chronic systemic illness, eating disorders, malnutrition) causes of hypogonadotropic hypogonadism must be excluded.

## Diagnostic Criteria and Clinical Characteristics

### Diagnostic Criteria for Isolated GnRH Deficiency:
**All of the following**
- Absent or incomplete puberty by age 18 years
- Serum testosterone less than or equal to 100 ng/dL in males or serum estradiol (E2) less than or equal to 20 pg/mL in females in the presence of inappropriately low or normal levels of pituitary gonadotropins (luteinizing hormone [LH] and follicle-stimulating hormone [FSH])
- All other anterior pituitary hormonal functions are normal and normal anatomy of the hypothalamus and pituitary fossa by magnetic resonance imaging (MRI)

**And the absence of**
- Functional etiology of hypogonadotropic hypogonadism (chronic systemic illness, eating disorders, malnutrition, chronic opiate ingestion, chronic glucocorticoid use, anabolic steroid use)
- Evidence of iron overload (hemochromatosis)

***Clinical Characteristics:*** Clinical manifestations vary with timing of onset of GnRH deficiency.

- Microphallus and cryptorchidism can be seen in infants with neonatal onset of GnRH deficiency and may prompt early diagnosis. Subjects with *TAC3/TACR3* signaling pathway mutations tend to exhibit a higher incidence of such neonatal defects.
- KS is characterized by the combination of complete anosmia or hyposmia occurring with isolated GnRH deficiency and

accounts for approximately 50% of subjects with isolated GnRH deficiency. Anosmia may also be recognized during early childhood prompting early assessment.
- The majority of KS and nIHH patients typically present in adolescence with completely absent or arrested early puberty. The remaining subjects present with incomplete puberty, including a characteristic "fertile eunuch" variant in male subjects wherein testicular development and spermatogenesis occur despite overt biochemical hypogonadism.
- An extremely rare presentation of isolated GnRH deficiency in males is the adult-onset variant, wherein patients who had otherwise completed normal puberty present with diagnostic criteria for GnRH deficiency later in adulthood.
- In approximately 10% KS or nIHH subjects, spontaneous reversal of GnRH deficiency may occur upon hormonal treatment. All KS or nIHH individuals should therefore be screened for spontaneous reversal by periodic withdrawal of hormonal therapy.

## Screening and Counseling

***Screening:*** At present, disease-causing mutations in 22 different causative genes have been identified in approximately 50% of subjects with isolated GnRH deficiency. A suggested algorithm for screening for mutations in the known genes using our current understanding of the phenotype-genotype correlations is shown in Fig. 67-1.

***Counseling:***

☞**INHERITANCE:** A detailed three-generation family history is a critical initial step for targeted genetic screening and predicting risk in family members. The evolving genetic

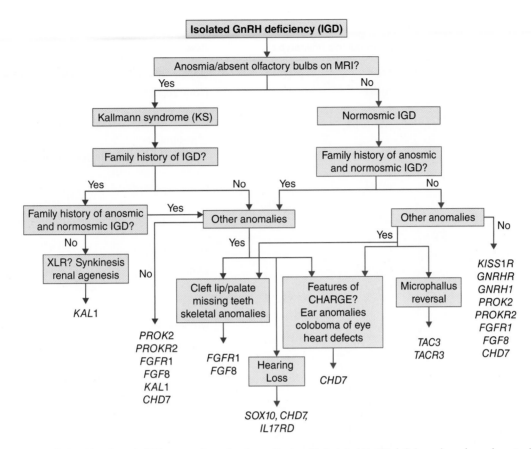

***Figure 67-1*** A proposed algorithm for prioritizing genetic testing for patients with isolated GnRH deficiency based on phenotypic information. Reproduced with permission from Au MG, Crowley WF Jr, Buck CL. Genetic counseling for isolated GnRH deficiency. Mol Cell Endocrinol. 2011;346:102-109.

architecture of human GnRH deficiency poses a significant genetic counseling challenge. Inheritance patterns vary depending on the causative gene and include X-linked recessive (*KAL1*), autosomal recessive (*GNRH1, GNRHR, KISS, KISS1R, TAC3, TACR3*), and autosomal dominant (*FGFR1, CHD7, SOX10*) patterns. Indeterminate inheritance patterns, overlap or mixed pedigrees (ie, KS and nIHH within a single pedigree), pedigrees with incomplete penetrance or variable expressivity warrant specific screening for the KS or nIHH overlap genes (*PROK2/PROKR2/FGF8/FGFR1/HS6ST1, FGF17, SPRY4, DUSP6*).

☞**GENOTYPE-PHENOTYPE CORRELATION:** The reproductive phenotype, while wide, is fairly similar across all genetic etiologies while the nonreproductive phenotypes offer valuable clues as to their genetic basis (Table 67-1). For example, nIHH subjects with microphallus or cryptorchidism at birth and "reversal" of GnRH deficiency in adulthood serve as phenotypic hallmarks of *TAC3* or *TACR3* pathway mutations. KS subjects with unilateral renal agenesis or synkinesis suggest *KAL1* gene mutations. Overlap or mixed pedigrees with presence of dental agenesis, cleft lip or palate and skeletal anomalies suggest *FGF8* or *FGFR1* pathway mutations. Presence of hearing loss has been strongly associated with *CHD7*, *SOX10* and *IL17RD* mutations. Presence of CHARGE syndrome features (**C**oloboma, **H**eart defects, **C**hoanal atresia, **R**etardation of growth and development, **G**enital abnormalities, and **E**xternal ear abnormalities) serve as pointers to *CHD7* mutations.

## Management and Treatment

Treatment options for hypogonadism in KS or nIHH subjects include sex steroids, gonadotropins, and pulsatile GnRH administration. Choice of therapy is determined by the particular life situation of the patient, that is, induction of secondary sexual maturation in pubertal patients versus the imminent need for fertility in other circumstances. When fertility is not desired in the near future, replacement with sex steroids is the most practical option in both sexes.

**KS or nIHH males:** In pubertal males, initial therapy with testosterone should be started at low doses and only gradually increased as secondary sexual characteristics are induced. Subsequently, adult doses can be maintained and further adjustments can be made based on serum testosterone levels. In neonatal male infants with microphallus, occasionally, low-dose testosterone can be given to promote penile growth.

**KS or nIHH females:** Initial treatment in adolescent females should consists of unopposed estrogen replacement to allow optimal breast development. When breast development has been optimized, a progestin should be added for endometrial protection and to regularize their menstrual cycles.

*Table 67-1  Genetic Differential Diagnosis and System Involvement*

| Gene Symbol | Reproductive Phenotype | Associated Findings |
| --- | --- | --- |
| *KAL1* | KS | Unilateral renal agenesis, bimanual synkinesis |
| *KISS1* | nIHH | None reported |
| *KISS1R* | | |
| *FGF8* | KS/nIHH | Cleft lip/palate; dental agenesis; skeletal anomalies |
| *FGFR1* | | |
| *PROK2* | KS/nIHH | ? Circadian/metabolic abnormalities |
| *PROKR2* | | |
| *GNRH1* | nIHH | None reported |
| *GNRHR* | | |
| *TAC3* | nIHH | Cryptorchidism; microphallus; reversibility |
| *TACR3* | | |
| *NELF* | KS | None reported |
| *CHD7* | KS/nIHH | Clinical overlap with CHARGE syndrome features |
| *HS6ST1* | KS/nIHH | None reported |
| *WDR11* | KS/nIHH | None reported |
| *SEMA3A* | KS | None reported |
| *IL17RD* | KS | Hearing loss |
| *SOX10* | KS | Hearing loss |
| *FGF17* | KS/nIHH | None reported |
| *DUSP6* | KS/nIHH | None reported |
| *SPRY4* | KS/nIHH | None reported |
| *FLRT3* | KS | None reported |

Gene names: *KAL1*, Kallmann syndrome 1 sequence; *KISS1*, kisspeptin; *KISS1R*, KISS1 receptor; *FGF8*, fibroblast growth factor 8; *FGFR1*, fibroblast growth factor receptor 1; *PROK2*, prokineticin 2; *PROKR2*, prokineticin receptor 2; *GNRH1*, gonadotropin-releasing hormone 1; *GNRHR*, gonadotropin-releasing hormone receptor; *TAC3*, tachykinin 3; *TACR3*, tachykinin receptor 3; *NELF*, nasal embryonic luteinizing hormone-releasing hormone (LHRH) factor; *CHD7*, chromodomain helicase DNA-binding protein 7; *HS6ST1*, heparan sulfate 6-O-sulfotransferase 1; *WDR11*, WD repeat domain 11 *DUSP6*, dual specificity phosphatase 6; *FGF17*, fibroblast growth factor 17; *FLRT3*, fibronectin leucine rich transmembrane protein 3; *IL17RD*, Interleukin 17 Receptor D; *SEMA3A*, semaphorin 3A; *SOX10*, SRY-box-10; *SPRY4*, sprouty homolog 4; (For a recent review of some of the genetics of each of the above genes see recent special edition of Molecular and Cellular Endocrinology, Genetics of GnRH deficiency (*Mol Cell Endocrinol*. Oct 22 2011;346[1-2]).

Many formulations of estrogens and progestins are available and these can be given in either cyclical or continuous fashion in accordance to individual patient preference.

**Fertility induction in KS or nIHH males:** Induction of fertility and gametogenesis requires special considerations therapeutically. Traditionally, exogenous gonadotropins are used to induce spermatogenesis in males. Treatment with human chorionic gonadotropin (hCG) is usually initiated at 1500 IU intramuscularly or subcutaneously every other day to normalize serum testosterone concentration as determined by trough testosterone levels drawn just prior to the next injection. Depending on the initial testicular volume, some males with KS/nIHH can produce sufficient sperm to achieve conception with hCG treatment alone. If testicular volume is prepubertal or if semen analysis reveals persistent azoospermia or marked oligospermia after 6 to 9 months of hCG therapy alone, FSH is usually added to the regimen at doses ranging from 37.5 to 150 IU, as either human menopausal gonadotropin (hMG) or recombinant formulation subcutaneously or intramuscularly.

Gynecomastia is a recognized side effect of hCG and can be minimized by gradually reducing the dose of hCG to the minimum required to sustain a serum testosterone concentration in the lower third of the normal range. An alternative method for induction of spermatogenesis is pulsatile GnRH but this therapy is not currently approved by the Food and Drug Administration for the treatment of infertility in men and thus is available for treatment of infertility in men only at specialized research centers. If infertility remains a problem despite successful spermatogenesis, in vitro fertilization is an option.

**Fertility induction in KS or nIHH females:** Pulsatile GnRH stimulation is an approved therapy for folliculogenesis in women with KS or nIHH. Intravenous administration of GnRH according to a physiologic regimen of administration fashioned to mimic that pattern of secretion of normal women across an ovulatory menstrual cycle recreates the hormonal dynamics of a normal cycle dynamics with the resulting ovulation of a single follicle. This therapy offers some advantages over the traditional treatment with exogenous gonadotropins in that it lacks the higher rates of both multiple gestation and ovarian hyperstimulation syndrome with their attendant morbidity and causes.

## Molecular Genetics and Molecular Mechanism

### Neurodevelopmental Genes Causing Only KS:

(i) *KAL1* or Kallmann syndrome 1 sequence: It encodes the extracellular matrix protein anosmin 1 which guides both olfactory axonal migration and GnRH neuronal migration.

(ii) *NELF* or nasal embryonic LHRH factor: Extracellular matrix molecule involved in guidance of olfactory axon projections and migration of GnRH neurons.

### Neuroendocrine Genes Causing Only nIHH:

(i) *GNRH1* or gonadotropin-releasing hormone 1 and *GNRHR* or gonadotropin-releasing hormone receptor: Hypothalamic decapeptide and its cognate pituitary receptor and pulsatile secretion result in pituitary secretion of LH and FSH.

(ii) *KISS1* or kisspeptin and *KISS1R* or *KISS1* receptor: Hypothalamic neuropeptide and its cognate receptor, essential for pulsatile GnRH secretion.

(iii) *TAC3* or tachykinin 3 and *TACR3* or tachykinin receptor 3: Hypothalamic neuropeptide crucial for GnRH secretion, primarily in the neonatal period and has key interaction with the KISS1 pathway in the hypothalamus.

### Overlap Genes Causing Both KS and nIHH:

*FGF8* or fibroblast growth factor 8 and *FGFR1* or fibroblast growth factor receptor 1: Growth factor pathway required for differentiation, migration, and function of GnRH neurons.

*PROK2* or prokineticin 2 and *PROKR2* or prokineticin receptor 2: Potential chemoattractant or guidance for olfactory axons and GnRH neuronal migration.

*CHD7*: Chromodomain helicase DNA-binding protein 7: Histone-binding and chromatin remodeling gene.

*HS6ST1*: Heparan sulfate 6-*O*-sulfotransferase 1: extracellular matrix component that functionally links *KAL1* with *FGFR1*.

*WDR11*: WD repeat protein that interacts with EMX1 homeodomain transcription factor, crucial to olfactory nerve development.

*SEMA3A*: Semaphorin 3A, an axonal pathfinding molecule with repulsive properties during embryonic development

*SOX10*: SRY-box 10, a transcription factor that is critical for neural crest development. Olfactory ensheathing cells, a SOX10 induced neural crest derivative is important for olfactory/GnRH axonal migration.

*IL17RD, SPRY4, FGF17, DUSP6 & FLRT3:* Members of the FGF syn-expression group that regulate the FGF signaling cascade in GnRH neuronal ontogeny.

**Genetic Testing:** At the time of this publication, CLIA-approved clinical laboratory genetic testing for KS or nIHH is only available for *KAL1*, *FGFR1*, and *CHD7*, though nearly 15 causative genes have been published in peer-reviewed scientific literature. A wider range of genetic testing for these genes is available on a research basis and the current list of available clinical and research-based testing, in addition to information about the laboratories conducting the testing, can be found on the National Center for Biotechnology Information's "GeneTests" website at http://www.ncbi.nlm.nih.gov/sites/GeneTests/.

## Bibliography:

1. Hoffman AR, Crowley WF Jr. Induction of puberty in men by long-term pulsatile administration of low-dose gonadotropin-releasing hormone. *N Engl J Med.* 1982;307(20):1237-1241.

2. Schwanzel-Fukuda M. Pfaff DW. Origin of luteinizing hormone-releasing hormone neurons. *Nature.* 1989;338(6211):161-164.

3. Balasubramanian R, Dwyer A, Seminara SB, Pitteloud N, Kaiser UB, Crowley WF Jr. Human GnRH deficiency: a unique disease model to unravel the ontogeny of GnRH neurons. *Neuroendocrinology.* 2010;92(2):81-99.

4. Hardelin JP, Dode C. The complex genetics of Kallmann syndrome: KAL1, FGFR1, FGF8, PROKR2, PROK2. Sexual development: genetics, molecular biology, evolution, endocrinology, embryology, and pathology of sex determination and differentiation. 2008;2(4-5):181-193.

5. Au MG, Crowley WF Jr., Buck CL. Genetic counseling for isolated GnRH deficiency. *Mol Cell Endocrinol.* 2011;346(1-2):102-109.

6. Sykiotis GP, Plummer L, Hughes VA, et al. Oligogenic basis of isolated gonadotropin-releasing hormone deficiency. *Proc Natl Acad Sci USA.* 2010;107(34):15140-15144.

7. Gianetti E, Tusset C, Noel SD, et al. TAC3/TACR3 mutations reveal preferential activation of gonadotropin-releasing hormone release by neurokinin B in neonatal life followed by reversal in adulthood. *J Clin Endocrinol Metabol.* 2010;95(6):2857-2867.

8. Nachtigall LB, Boepple PA, Pralong FP, Crowley WF Jr. Adult-onset idiopathic hypogonadotropic hypogonadism—a treatable form of male infertility. *N Engl J Med.* 1997;336(6):410-415.

9. Raivio T, Falardeau J, Dwyer A, et al. Reversal of idiopathic hypogonadotropic hypogonadism. *N Engl J Med.* 2007;357(9):863-873.

10. Balasubramanian R. Crowley WF Jr. Isolated GnRH deficiency: a disease model serving as a unique prism into the systems biology of the GnRH neuronal network. *Mol Cell Endocrinol.* 2011;346(1-2):4-12.

11. Kim HG, Kurth I, Lan F, et al. Mutations in CHD7, encoding a chromatin-remodeling protein, cause idiopathic hypogonadotropic hypogonadism and Kallmann syndrome. *Am J Hum Genet.* 2008;83(4):511-519.

12. Han TS, Bouloux PM. What is the optimal therapy for young males with hypogonadotropic hypogonadism? *Clin Endocrinol.* 2010;72(6):731-737.

13. Bouloux PM, Nieschlag E, Burger HG, et al. Induction of spermatogenesis by recombinant follicle-stimulating hormone (puregon) in hypogonadotropic azoospermic men who failed to respond to human chorionic gonadotropin alone. *J Androl.* 2003;24(4):604-611.

14. Martin KA, Hall JE, Adams JM, Crowley WF Jr. Comparison of exogenous gonadotropins and pulsatile gonadotropin-releasing hormone for induction of ovulation in hypogonadotropic amenorrhea. *J Clin Endocrinol Metabol.* 1993;77(1):125-129.

## Supplementary Information

### OMIM References:

[1] Kallmann Syndrome 1; KAL1 (#308700)

[2] Kallmann Syndrome 2; FGFR1 (#147950)

[3] Kallmann Syndrome 3; PROKR2 (#244200)

[4] Kallmann Syndrome 4; PROK2 (#610628)

[5] Kallmann Syndrome 5; CHD7 (#612370)

[6] Kallmann Syndrome 6; FGF8 (#612702)

[7] Hypogonadotropic Hypogonadism; PROK2, TACR3, FGFR1, CHD7, NELF, TAC3, KISS1R (#146110)

[8] Eunuchoidism, Familial Hypogonadotropic; GNRH1 (#227200)

**Alternative Names:**
- Idiopathic Hypogonadotropic Hypogonadism
- Hypothalamic Hypogonadism

***Key Words:*** Hypogonadotropic hypogonadism, Kallmann syndrome, idiopathic hypogonadotropic hypogonadism, delayed puberty, microphallus, micropenis, cryptorchidism, anosmia, hyposmia, fertile eunuch syndrome, hypogenitalia, GnRh deficiency, hypogonadotropism

# 68 **Celiac Disease**

Ryan Ungaro and Mark W. Babyatsky

## KEY POINTS

- *Disease summary:*
  - Celiac disease (CD) is a chronic inflammatory disease of the small intestine manifests as a dysregulated immune response to a known environmental trigger (gluten and its related proteins) in genetically susceptible individuals. The mainstay of treatment is a gluten-free diet.
  - CD is a common disease with a prevalence of up to 1% in Caucasian populations, but remains underdiagnosed. Classical presentation with malabsorption and gastrointestinal (GI) symptoms such as diarrhea or abdominal discomfort is relatively rare; more commonly, patients have vague symptoms or extraintestinal presentations including dermatitis herpetiformis, anemia, osteoporosis, short stature, infertility, fatigue, or transaminitis.
  - Serologic testing can aid in diagnosis of CD. The most sensitive and specific tests are antitissue transglutaminase (anti-tTG) or antiendomysial IgA antibodies. However, the gold standard of diagnosis is still demonstration of villous atrophy on duodenal biopsy and a clinical response to a gluten-free diet. Nearly all CD patients have HLA-DQ2 or HLA-DQ8 although a significant percentage of the normal population also carries these human leukocyte antigen (HLA) alleles; testing for HLA-DQ2 or DQ8 has excellent negative predictive value. A high prevalence of IgA deficiency mandates that when serology is negative but there is high clinical suspicion of CD, measurement of total IgA levels is indicated.
  - Patients with CD have an increased risk of malignancy (small intestinal adenocarcinoma and enteropathy-associated T-cell lymphoma). A subset of CD patients has refractory disease that will not respond to a gluten-free diet and is associated with a poorer prognosis.
  - CD is associated with other immune-mediated diseases, such as type 1 diabetes and inflammatory bowel disease, suggesting a common genetic background for these disorders.

- *Differential diagnosis:*
  - Collagenous sprue, Whipple disease, tropical sprue, Crohn disease, food intolerance (such as lactose), intestinal lymphoma, pancreatic insufficiency, bacterial overgrowth

- *Monogenic forms:*
  - No single gene is known to cause CD.

- *Family history:*
  - CD has a prevalence of 5% to 15% among first-degree relatives of affected patients.

- *Twin studies:*
  - Monozygotic twins have a 75% concordance rate in CD; dizygotic twins have an 11% concordance rate.

- *Environmental factors:*
  - The known triggering environmental antigen in CD is gluten, the protein found in wheat, and related proteins found in barley and rye. Gluten is composed of gliadin and glutenin proteins and has a high content of glutamine. tTG enhances the immunogenicity of gluten by deamidating glutamine, allowing gluten peptides to bind more strongly to HLA-DQ2 or DQ8 molecules on antigen-presenting cells (APCs) which then activate CD4+ T cells. A possible role for intestinal infections, such as rotavirus, in increasing the risk of CD has been implicated in the pathogenesis of CD.

- *Genome-wide associations:*
  - Genome-wide association study (GWAS) has confirmed the strong association of HLA-DQ2 and DQ8 with CD and uncovered many other susceptibility loci in CD, many of which encode genes involved in the immune response.

- *Pharmacogenomics:*
  - Pharmacogenetic testing currently does not have a role in CD.

## Diagnostic Criteria and Clinical Characteristics

### *Diagnostic Criteria for CD:*

☞DIAGNOSTIC EVALUATION FOR CD:

- Diagnostic testing for CD while the patient is on a gluten-containing diet.

- Serologic testing is often the first tests sent to diagnose CD. IgA antiendomysial antibodies and IgA antitissue tTG antibodies both have high sensitivity and specificity in screening for CD. Antiendomysial antibodies have a sensitivity of 90% to 97% and a specificity approaching 100%; anti-tTG antibodies have a sensitivity of 90% to 98% and specificity of 95% to 99%. Anti-tTG is preferred as testing for antiendomysial antibodies and is more operator dependent. Serum levels of these antibodies correlate with the degree of villous atrophy, and these tests may therefore have decreased sensitivity in milder disease. In contrast, IgA antigliadin antibodies have much lower sensitivity (no higher than 80%) and specificity (80%-90%).

- IgA deficiency is 10 to 15 times more common among patients with CD than in the general population with a prevalence of up to 3% and is important to consider in patients with negative IgA antiendomysial or anti-tTG antibodies with a high clinical suspicion for CD. If total IgA is low, serologic testing for CD can be performed using IgG antiendomysial or IgG anti-tTG antibodies. Some clinicians send total IgA levels with initial antiendomysial or anti-tTG antibody screening tests.

- The gold standard for diagnosing CD remains intestinal biopsy. Endoscopy should be performed even if serology is negative if there is high clinical suspicion. Biopsies should be obtained from the descending duodenum. Since the disease may be patchy, at least four biopsies should be taken. Endoscopy in patients with CD may demonstrate gross signs of villous atrophy including atrophic mucosa or scalloping of duodenal folds. However, these findings are neither sensitive nor specific for CD. Histology can range from partial to total villous atrophy. Other findings in CD include increased numbers of intraepithelial lymphocytes and hyperplastic, enlarged crypts, and increased numbers of inflammatory cells in the lamina propria.

- Genetic testing is helpful when other diagnostic tests are inconclusive. Nearly all patients with CD have HLA-DQ2 or HLA-DQ8 molecules (>99%). As the prevalence of these markers in the general population is high (30%-40%), HLA testing has poor specificity for CD and a high negative predictive value (near 100%). If these markers are absent, the diagnosis of CD is virtually excluded.

- Patients with positive histology must also demonstrate a clinical response to a gluten-free diet. If there is no response to treatment, other causes of villous atrophy should be considered. These include, but are not limited to, collagenous sprue, Whipple disease, tropical sprue, giardiasis, HIV enteropathy, eosinophilic gastroenteritis, Zollinger-Ellison syndrome, radiation- or chemotherapy-induced enteritis, Crohn disease, intestinal lymphoma, or food intolerance.

### *Clinical Characteristics of CD:*

☞PATTERNS OF DISEASE: The clinical presentation of CD in adults can vary greatly. It has been suggested that CD can be divided into several distinct phenotypes given the wide range of disease presentations. Patients with *classic* CD present with GI symptoms including diarrhea, steatorrhea, flatulence, and abdominal pain or flatulence. Classic CD presents similarly to irritable bowel syndrome (IBS); the diagnosis of CD should be considered in individuals meeting diagnostic criteria for IBS as the prevalence of CD in this population is increased more than fourfold compared to patients without IBS. In CD, these symptoms may be accompanied by other signs of malabsorption including weight loss, anemia, and vitamin deficiencies (eg, folate, vitamin D, calcium).

CD most commonly presents in an *atypical* form in which GI symptoms are mild or absent. Patients may present with extraintestinal findings such as iron deficiency, fatigue, osteoporosis, short stature, infertility, unexplained elevated liver enzymes, arthritis, dental enamel defects, aphthous ulcers, or neurologic symptoms such as ataxia, neuropathy, or migraine. Up to 14% of patients with iron deficiency anemia of unclear origin have CD.

*Silent* CD includes asymptomatic individuals found to have gluten-induced villous atrophy either after a positive serologic screening test or an incidental finding on endoscopy and biopsy. Lastly, patients with a previous diagnosis of CD that are now on a gluten-free diet without villous atrophy have *latent* disease.

☞ASSOCIATION WITH OTHER DISEASES: 6 is associated with a number of other disorders, many of which are autoimmune diseases. Dermatitis herpetiformis is another form of gluten sensitivity characterized by a pruritic, papulovesicular rash that affects up to 20% of CD patients and typically responds to a gluten-free diet. Other disorders associated with CD include type 1 diabetes, autoimmune thyroid disease, Addison disease, autoimmune hepatitis, primary biliary cirrhosis, autoimmune myocarditis, Sjögren syndrome, and inflammatory bowel disease. For example, the prevalence of CD in patients with type 1 diabetes ranges from 2% to 5%. Neurologic disorders such as peripheral neuropathy, headache, depression, ataxia, and epilepsy also appear to be associated with CD. Patients with osteoporosis have a significant prevalence of CD, ranging from 1% to 3.4%. CD also appears to be more common in patients with Down syndrome, Turner syndrome, and Williams syndrome.

☞COMPLICATIONS OF CD: CD is associated with a modest increase in all-cause mortality and may be increased in patients not adhering to a gluten-free diet. Some of the serious complications of CD include enteropathy-associated T-cell lymphoma, adenocarcinoma of the small intestine, and refractory CD. CD patients have an increased risk of both intestinal and extraintestinal non-Hodgkin lymphoma. Enteropathy-associated T-cell lymphoma is more common in older CD patients, develops in the proximal small intestine, and is associated with a poor prognosis. The diagnosis should be considered in patients with relapse of CD symptoms after response to a gluten-free diet. CD also increases the risk of proximal small bowel adenocarcinoma. About 5% of CD patients will develop refractory CD in which symptoms persist despite adherence to a gluten-free diet. Refractory CD can be characterized as type 1 or type 2. Type 1 is characterized by expansion of phenotypically normal intraepithelial lymphocytes. In contrast, intraepithelial lymphocytes in type 2 disease have an abnormal phenotype, lacking surface expression of CD3 and CD8. Patients with type 2 refractory CD have an increased risk of developing enteropathy-associated T-cell lymphoma or ulcerative jejunitis and have a high mortality rate (37%-60% within 5 years). A subset of patients with refractory CD responds to corticosteroid treatment.

## Screening and Counseling

*Screening:* Screening for CD in asymptomatic individuals in the general population is not currently recommended, but is for at-risk patients. This includes patients with possible atypical symptoms or diseases associated with CD (see earlier). Although many first- and second-degree relatives of patients with CD are screened, it is recommended that testing be conducted only if symptoms occur. It is recommended that patients with premature-onset osteoporosis or metabolic bone disease be screened for CD. It may be prudent to test at-risk patients more than once as up to 3.5% of first-degree relatives will seroconvert within an average of 2 years.

*Counseling:* CD has a prevalence ranging from 5% to 15% among first-degree relatives and a 75% concordance rate in monozygotic twins. In contrast, CD has an 11% concordance rate in dizygotic twins and a 30% concordance rate in HLA identical siblings. The odds ratio (OR) for developing CD is 1.7 in first-degree relatives and 2.5 for siblings. The prevalence can increase up to 20% for first- and second-degree relatives when a pair of siblings has the disease. CD is also increased in second-degree relatives with a prevalence ranging from 2.6% to 5.5%. For unclear reasons, two to three times as many women as men have the disease. Patients diagnosed with CD before the age of 36 or have a family history of autoimmunity also have an increased risk of developing other autoimmune diseases (HR = 2.65 and 2.36, respectively).

## Management and Treatment

The mainstay of treatment for CD is lifetime adherence to a gluten-free diet. Patients need to avoid all foods or products that contain wheat, rye, or barley. Safe substituted foods include rice, buckwheat, corn, quinoa, and sorghum. Although oats are tolerated by many CD patients, they may be contaminated with gluten. Adherence to a gluten-free diet can be very challenging and expensive. Contamination of food products with gluten is difficult to avoid. Patients with CD should therefore have consultation with an experienced dietitian and referral to an advocacy or support group. Most patients will experience symptomatic relief within a few weeks of starting a gluten-free diet. However, histologic improvement may lag, sometimes taking years, and often is incomplete. The gluten-free diet results in improved nutritional status and bone mass and is likely protective against non-Hodgkin lymphoma. Interestingly, adherence to a gluten-free diet appears to decrease the risk of developing other associated autoimmune diseases. Management of CD patients should also include careful evaluation for vitamin and mineral deficiencies. Patients may be deficient in folate, B vitamins, fat-soluble vitamins such as vitamin D, iron, and calcium. The American Gastroenterological Association also recommends obtaining a DEXA scan to evaluate for osteoporosis in adults diagnosed with CD 1 year after institution of a gluten-free diet in order to allow for stabilization of bone density. A third of patients with untreated CD exhibit splenic hypofunction and should be given pneumococcal vaccination.

Patients who are symptomatic on a gluten-free diet need thorough evaluation. Biopsy slides should be reviewed with an expert GI pathologist in adherence to a gluten-free diet through assessment by a dietician. Repeat small biopsy may be indicated and other diagnoses should be considered including other causes of villous atrophy (see earlier) as well as IBS, pancreatic insufficiency, bacterial overgrowth, or disaccharidase deficiency. The diagnosis of either enteropathy-associated T-cell lymphoma or refractory CD needs to be considered. Treatment of enteropathy-associated T-cell lymphoma involves chemotherapy with possible surgery for localized disease. Management of refractory CD involves aggressive nutritional support and vitamin repletion as well as continued adherence to a gluten-free diet. Treatment with immunosuppressive drugs can be considered but must be weighed against the chance of promoting progression to lymphoma. The expansion and proliferation of intraepithelial lymphocytes in refractory CD appears to be driven by interleukin 15 (IL-15) and therapies targeting this cytokine are currently under investigation.

*Pharmacogenetics:* Pharmacogenetic testing is currently not used in CD as the mainstay of therapy is diet modification. Pharmacogenetic considerations will likely become important if currently experimental biologic and immunomodulation therapies prove effective.

## Molecular Genetics and Molecular Mechanism

CD has long been understood to have a genetic basis as demonstrated through familial and twin studies. Linkage analysis, candidate gene association studies, and more recent GWAS have better defined specific genes associated with susceptibility to CD (Table 68-1). Uncovering genetic risk variants has allowed for the identification of potentially important underlying biologic and immunologic pathways in CD and may improve the ability to predict the disease risk.

The most important known genetic contributors to the pathogenesis of CD are the genes encoding the MHC class II molecules, HLA-DQ2 or HLA-DQ8. HLA-DQ molecules are heterodimers (composed of an α and β chain) expressed by APCs such as dendritic cells, macrophages, and B cells. HLA-DQ binds and presents foreign antigens to CD4+ T cells leading to subsequent activation of the adaptive immune system. Nearly all CD patients have either HLA-DQ2 or DQ8, while 30% to 40% of the general population expresses one of these HLA molecules. The vast majority of CD patients express HLA-DQ2 (up to 95%), which can be encoded by the DQA1*05 or DQB1*02 alleles in *cis* or less often in *trans* position with equal attributable risk. Most of the remaining CD patients have HLA-DQ8 (DQA1*03 and DQB1*0302). A small group of patients carry alleles that encode one chain of the DQ2 heterodimer molecule (DQA1*05 or DQB1*02 alleles). As mentioned above, testing for these genetic markers have high negative predictive value.

HLA-DQ2 and DQ8 molecules have pockets that preferentially bind negatively charged amino acids. When tTG encounters gluten in the intestinal mucosa, glutamine is converted to the negatively charged glutamate, increasing binding of gluten peptides to HLA-DQ2 and DQ8. In addition, HLA-DQ2 has a particular affinity for proline residues which are highly prevalent in gluten peptides. Patients who are homozygous for DQ2 have a four- to fivefold increased risk for developing CD compared to heterozygous patients. DQ2 homozygous patients also have enhanced T-cell proliferation and cytokine production in response to gluten as demonstrated by in vitro experiments. This may be due to the fact that homozygous patients, as compared to heterozygotes, are able to express greater numbers of DQ2 molecules that can bind gluten and subsequently activate CD4+ T cells.

*Table 68-1  Celiac Disease-Associated Susceptibility Variants*

| Candidate Gene (Chromosome Location) | Associated Variant | Odds Ratio | Frequency of Risk Allele | Putative Functional Significance | Other Diseases Associated With Gene |
|---|---|---|---|---|---|
| *HLA (6p21) | HLA-DQ2 HLA-DQ8 | OR = 7.04 (DQ2 cis) | 30%-40% general population | Antigen presentation to T cells | |
| *IL2 and IL21 (4q27) | rs13119723 | OR = 0.66 | | T-cell activation and proliferation, IFN-γ production | Type 1 diabetes, Graves disease, rheumatoid arthritis, psoriatic arthritis |
| *RGS1 (1q31) | rs2816216 | OR = 0.71 | | B-cell activation and chemokine signaling | |
| *IL18RAP (2q11-12) | rs917997 | OR = 1.27 | | IFN-γ production | Crohn disease, type 1 diabetes |
| *CCR3 (3p21) | rs6441961 | OR = 1.21 | | Leukocyte trafficking | |
| *IL12A (3q25-26) | rs17810546 | OR = 1.34 | | Induction of Th1 cells | Type 1 diabetes |
| *LPP (3q28) | rs1464510 | OR = 1.21 | | Unknown | |
| *TAGAP (6q25) | rs1738074 | OR = 1.21 | | T-cell cytoskeleton modulation | Type 1 diabetes |
| *SH2B3 (12q24) | rs653178 | OR = 1.19 | | T-cell receptor signaling | Type 1 diabetes |
| CTLA-4 (2q33) | AA polymorphism at exon 1 position 49 | OR = 2.36 | | Negative regulator of T-cell activation | Type 1 diabetes, systemic lupus erythematosus |
| ITGA4 (2q31) | rs6433894 | OR = 1.20 | | Immune cell adhesion and migration | |
| PBX3 (9q34.11) | rs7040561 | OR = 2.60 | | Immune cell maturation transcription factors | |
| PPP6C (9q34.11) | rs459311 rs458046 | OR = 1.70 | | Cell cycle transitions | |
| SERPINE2 (2q33) | rs6747096 | OR = 0.48 | | ECM production | |
| MYO9B (19p13.1) | rs2305764 | OR = 1.66 (heterozygous) OR = 2.27 (homozygous) | | Cytoskeleton and tight junction assembly | |
| PTPN22 (1p13.3) | rs2476601 | OR = 1.82 | | Negative regulator of T-cell receptor signaling | Type 1 diabetes |
| *TNFAIP3 (6q23.3) | rs2327832 | OR = 1.25 | | Negative regulator of NF-κB signaling | Systemic lupus erythematosus |
| *REL (2p16.1) | rs842647 | OR = 0.84 | | NF-κB transcription | Ulcerative colitis |
| Ubiquitin D | rs11724 | OR = 1.49 | | Negative regulator of NF-κB signaling | |

*Association found or confirmed in GWAS by van Heel et al, Hunt et al, or Trynka et al.

HLA-DQ2 and DQ8 are necessary but not sufficient to cause CD, in that 30% to 40% of the general population carries one of these risk variants yet only 2% to 5% of gene carriers actually develop the disease. The HLA contribution to the familial risk of CD is approximately 40%, signifying the importance of non-HLA genes and environmental factors in the determination of CD susceptibility. GWAS has identified non-HLA genes associated with

CD, similar to HLA genes, a majority of which are also involved in the immune response. These genes highlight the importance of immune pathways, in particular those that involve lymphocyte differentiation, activation, and signaling.

Immunologic studies have pointed to the importance of lymphocytes and adaptive immunity in the pathogenesis of CD. Both T cells and B cells appear to play a key role in the dysregulated immune response. Active CD is characterized by infiltration of the lamina propria by HLA-DQ2 or DQ8 restricted CD4+ T cells and an increase in the number of intraepithelial CD8+ cytotoxic T cells. In addition, autoantibodies directed against gliadin and tTG are also present. Gluten-specific CD4+ T cells have been identified in the lamina propria of patients with CD and secrete various proinflammatory cytokines. The predominant cytokine produced by activated CD4+ T cells in CD appears to be interferon-gamma (IFN-γ) which has many functions including stimulating fibroblasts and mononuclear cells to produce matrix metalloproteinases that can cause mucosal damage.

CD4+ T cells can also activate intraepithelial lymphocytes and induce B cells to secrete antigluten and anti-tTG antibodies. Cytotoxic intraepithelial lymphocytes are key effector cells in CD that can directly induce apoptosis in enterocytes resulting in villous atrophy. tTG does activate transforming growth factor-β, promoting differentiation of epithelial cells, a process that is disrupted in the mucosa of CD patients; anti-tTG autoantibodies may inhibit this action. Th17 T cells, which produce IL-17, have been shown to be key players in immune-mediated disease such as inflammatory bowel disease and rheumatoid arthritis. Recent studies have demonstrated that IL-17 expression is increased in the mucosa of patients with active CD and is enhanced by exposure to gliadin, although the functional role of IL-17 in CD is still under investigation.

Innate immune mechanisms also appear to play a role in the pathogenesis of CD. For example, the α-gliadin peptide p31-43 found in gluten may directly stimulate epithelial cells, macrophages, and dendritic cells to secrete IL-15 which promotes enterocyte apoptosis through upregulation of NKG2D receptors on intraepithelial lymphocytes and MICA ligands on intestinal epithelium.

Gene linkage analyses have found a susceptibility region on the long arm of chromosome 5 that contains a cytokine gene cluster although no specific risk variant or gene has been identified. Cytotoxic T lymphocyte antigen 4 (CTLA4) is an important negative regulator of T-cell activation and is associated with other autoimmune diseases including type 1 diabetes, Graves disease, and systemic lupus erythematosus. PTPN22 (protein tyrosine phosphatase nonreceptor 22) encodes a phosphatase that inhibits T-cell receptor signaling and has been associated with autoimmunity possibly because defects may allow survival of more autoreactive T cells during thymic development.

GWAS has uncovered multiple other potential susceptibility genes involved in T-cell activation and differentiation, including a region located on chromosome 4q27 that encodes the cytokines IL-2 and IL-21. IL-2 stimulates T-cell activation and proliferation and is important in maturation of regulatory T cells ($T_{reg}$) that help suppress immune responses. Of note, IL-2 knockout mice develop autoimmune disease. IL-21 expression is increased in the intestinal mucosa of CD patients and may cause T cells to be less responsive to $T_{reg}$ cells. IL-21 enhances both Th1 and Th17 immune responses. The association of IL-2 and IL-21 with CD highlights the potential importance of $T_{reg}$ cells and Th17 in CD. Interestingly, the region encoding the IL-23 receptor, which plays a key role in the Th17 pathway, was recently linked to CD; IL-23R mutations have also been associated with Crohn disease and ulcerative colitis. Other immune-related genes associated with CD include IL18RAP, IL12A, TAGAP, and SH2B3. IL12A encodes half of the cytokine IL-12 that can induce T cells that secrete IFN-γ. IL18RAP encodes part of the IL-18 receptor. IL-18 can induce T cells to secrete IFN-γ,

although the associated single-nucleotide polymorphism (SNP) appears to result in lower levels of IL18RAP mRNA. T-cell activation GTPase-activating protein (TAGAP) is expressed in activated T cells and may modulate cytoskeleton changes. SH2B3 is expressed in many immune cells, including dendritic cells and T cells, and appears to regulate T cell and cytokine receptor signaling. PBX3 (pre-B cell leukemia homeobox 3) has been associated with CD and encodes transcription factors that regulate immune cell maturation. Additionally, regulator of G-protein signaling 1 (RGS1) mutations have also been associated with CD, the protein is expressed in intraepithelial lymphocytes and regulates chemokine receptor signaling and B-cell activation. A SNP located near CCR3 and other genes encoding chemokine receptors was associated with CD, suggesting that chemokines that control immune cell recruitment have a role in the development of CD.

New gene associations in CD have identified a previously unidentified potential role for nuclear factor kappa B (NF-κB) signaling and may implicate innate immune pathways in the disease; implicated genes include TNFAIP3, REL, and Ubiquitin D. TNFAIP3 encodes for A20, which is required for terminating NF-κB signaling initiated by innate immune receptors such as toll-like receptors (TLRs). REL is a component of the NF-κB transcription complex. Ubiquitin D is strongly upregulated in the mucosa of CD patients and is involved in the degradation of molecules that inhibit NF-κB signaling and can also induce caspase-dependent apoptosis.

In terms of dysregulation of the immune response, there is overlap in the genetic background of CD and other autoimmune diseases with many shared risk-conferring genes (Table 68-1). This may help explain the epidemiologic associations of CD with such disorders and type 1 diabetes, autoimmune thyroid disease, and inflammatory bowel disease.

Independent of the immune response, patients with CD have increased permeability of the intestinal epithelium, suggesting that a defective epithelial barrier may contribute to disease pathogenesis perhaps by exposing lamina propria APCs and T cells to immunogenic gluten peptides. Several genes related to the intestinal barrier, including MYOB9, PARD3, and MAGI2, have been associated with CD. The MYOB9 (myosin IX B) gene encodes for a protein involved in epithelial cell cytoskeleton and tight junction formation. Mutations in MYOB9 have also been associated with increased risk of refractory CD type 2 as well as enteropathy-associated T-cell lymphoma. The PARD3 and MAGI2 genes, that encode tight junction scaffolding proteins, are also associated with ulcerative colitis, suggesting a common barrier defect.

The CD-associated gene alleles identified by GWAS and linkage or candidate gene analysis individually tend to have relatively modest effects on risk of developing the disease. A model incorporating both HLA and non-HLA genes to determine the risk of developing CD demonstrated that individuals carrying multiple non-HLA risk alleles had an increased risk of CD. Patients with greater than or equal to 13 risk alleles had an OR of 6.2. These findings support the idea that multiple genetic "hits" are necessary to develop CD, highlighting the complex genetic nature of the disease.

***Genetic Testing:*** Genetic testing for HLA-DQ2 or DQ8 has strong negative predictive value and can help to rule out CD when the diagnosis is uncertain. Recent studies have investigated the use of combined HLA and non-HLA genetic markers to predict the risk of developing CD although such testing currently has no clinical role. Resources for genetic counseling should be made available.

*Future Directions:* Although much progress has been made in the understanding of the genetics and pathogenesis of CD, many CD genetic risk factors remain to be elucidated as the HLA-DQ2 and DQ8 loci contribute up to 40% of the heritability while the currently known non-HLA genes associated with CD account for only 3% to 4% of the heritability. GWAS evaluates relatively common SNP variants (>5% minor allele frequency); rarer SNPs that may make a larger contribution to heritability can be missed. Increased understanding of known susceptibility genes and discovery of new risk variants will help elucidate the pathogenesis of CD and may provide future therapeutic targets.

## BIBLIOGRAPHY:

1. Dubois PC, Trynka G, Franke L, et al. Multiple common variants for celiac disease influencing immune gene expression. *Nat Genet.* 2010;4:295-302.

2. Trynka G, Hunt KA, Bockett NA, et al. Dense genotyping identifies and localizes multiple common and rare variant association signals in celiac disease. *Nat Genet.* Nov 6 2011;43(12):1193-1201.

3. Green PH, Jabri B. Coeliac disease. *Lancet.* 2003;362:383-391.

4. Green PH, Cellier C. Celiac disease. *N Engl J Med.* 2007;357:1731-1743.

5. Lincoln H, Green PH. Extraintestinal manifestations of celiac disease. *Curr Gastroenterol Rep.* 2006;8:383-389.

6. Cosnes J, Cellier C, Viola S, et al. Incidence of autoimmune diseases in celiac disease: protective effect of the gluten-free diet. *Clin Gastroenterol Hepatol.* Jul 2008;6(7):753-758.

7. Schuppan D, Junker Y, Barisani D. Celiac disease: from pathogenesis to novel therapies. *Gastroenterology.* 2009;137:1912-1933.

8. Jabri B, Sollid LM. Tissue-mediated control of immunopathology in coeliac disease. *Nat Rev Immunol.* 2009;9:858-870.

9. Romanos J, van Diemen CC, Nolte IM, et al. Analysis of HLA and non-HLA alleles can identify individuals at high risk for celiac disease. *Gastroenterology.* 2009;137:834-840.

10. Kupfer SS, Jabri B. Pathophysiology of celiac disease. *Gastrointest Endosc Clin N Am.* 2012;22:639-660.

11. Kumar V, Wijmenga C, Withoff S. From genome-wide association studies to disease mechanisms: celiac disease as a model for autoimmune diseases. *Semin Immunopathol.* Jul 2012;34(4):567-580.

## Supplementary Information

### OMIM REFERENCES:

[1] Celiac Disease; CD (#212750)

[2] Condition; Gene Name (OMIM#)

### Alternative Names:

- Celiac Sprue
- Gluten-Sensitive Enteropathy

*Key Words:* Celiac, sprue, enteropathy, gluten, gliadin, HLA, tissue transglutaminase

# 69 Acute and Chronic Pancreatitis

David Whitcomb

## KEY POINTS

- *Disease summary:*
  - Pancreatitis is a syndrome of multiple etiologies with strong genetic influences. Genetic variants and environmental factors affect susceptibility to injury and modify the inflammatory response.
  - **Acute pancreatitis (AP)** describes the clinical syndrome associated with sudden onset of pancreatic inflammation, usually associated with pancreatic injury. The majority of cases are caused by gallstones or alcohol withdrawal and multiple less-common etiologies. Approximately 20% of AP is idiopathic and/or genetic.
  - **Recurrent acute pancreatitis (RAP)** describes a condition in which AP occurs more than once. The etiology of RAP is similar to AP, except for a lower incidence of treatable causes (eg, gallstones), and higher incidence of idiopathic etiologies.
  - **Chronic pancreatitis (CP)** is a syndrome of pancreatic inflammation lasting over 6 months. Until recently, alcohol was considered to be the etiology in 70% to 90% of cases, but this has been disproven. There is no consensus on classification of subtypes, in part because of overlap of etiologies (eg, smoking and heavy chronic alcohol use). All of the known susceptibility genes for CP are linked to dysregulation of intrapancreatic trypsinogen. Unusual subsets of CP include autoimmune pancreatitis (~5%), and some rare congenital syndromes.
  - **Alcoholic pancreatitis (ACP)** is pancreatitis associated with excessive alcohol ingestion, usually greater than 60 g per day. Smoking is common in alcohol drinking patients, and the effects of the two are likely synergistic. Genetic factors increase the risk of alcoholic pancreatitis (unpublished).
  - **Hereditary pancreatitis (HP)** is an autosomal dominant disorder usually caused by mutations in the cationic trypsinogen gene (*PRSS1*) that begins with typical AP, RAP, and eventually CP. The high penetrance rate and early age of onset are useful in distinguishing HP from other forms of CP.
  - **CFTR-related pancreatitis** is used to describe patients with CP that is linked to variant mutations in the cystic fibrosis transmembrane conductance regulator gene (*CFTR*) but who do not meet diagnostic criteria for cystic fibrosis. Atypical CF (aCF) is a general term that covers the mild CF spectrum, including recurrent bronchitis, or lung infections with no pancreatic involvement. aCF includes late age of diagnosis and borderline or low sweat chloride levels (<60 mEq/L). Symptoms may be limited to the pancreas, but male infertility and chronic sinusitis are also common overlapping features. Complex genotypes with *CFTR* plus pancreatic secretory trypsin inhibitor gene (*SPINK1*) variants are common and associated with pancreatitis only.
  - **Autoimmune pancreatitis (AIP)** is inflammation of the pancreas driven by immune dysregulation rather than pancreatic injury. It is often associated with elevated IgG4 level and may have a dramatic response to steroid treatment.
- *Differential diagnosis:*
  - Acute pancreatitis is usually suspected with sudden, severe abdominal pain. Differential diagnosis includes myocardial infarction, dissecting aortic aneurysm, mesenteric thrombosis and/or ischemia, volvulus, intussusceptions, penetrating gastric or duodenal ulcer, biliary colic and acute cholecystitis. The correct diagnosis is usually made by abdominal imaging and/or marked elevation of digestive enzymes in the blood.

    Chronic pancreatitis is diagnosed with different criteria by different groups. In more advanced cases evidence of chronic pancreatitis include pancreatic atrophy, distortion, dilated pancreatic ductal systems, calcifications, and fibrosis. Other common features are diabetes mellitus and various patterns and severity of pain. The differential diagnosis includes pain from nonpancreatic sources, vascular calcifications, pancreatic duct dilatation from other causes (eg, intraductal papillary mucinous neoplasm [IPMN]) pancreatic insufficiency syndromes, and pancreatic cancer.
- *Monogenic forms:*
  - Three different genes that cause typical AP and CP: *PRSS1*, *CFTR*, and *SPINK1*. Additional genes cause syndromes that affect the pancreas to various degrees.
- *Family history:*
  - HP is an autosomal dominant form of recurrent acute pancreatitis with strong family histories. Phenotypic penetrance is between 60% and 80%, with median age of onset at 10 years. About half of the affected subjects will develop chronic pancreatitis with both pancreatic exocrine and pancreatic endocrine failure. There is an increased risk of pancreatic cancer, calculated to be a 70-fold increase in relative risk in some families.

    Familial pancreatitis is used to describe families in which pancreatitis occurs at greater frequency than would expected in the general population by chance alone. Many families have been found to have genetic variants that cluster in complex ways.
- *Twin studies:*
  - Monozygotic twins with disease-causing PRSS1 mutations appear to have similar disease penetrance of 80%, but the age of onset of symptoms and severity of disease appear to be highly similar in twins compared to the variance among unrelated subjects.
- *Environmental factors:*
  - Alcohol and smoking are the most common and well established.
- *Genome-wide associations:* First GWAS has been published. Whitcomb, D.C., et al. Common genetic variants in the CLDN2 and PRSS1-PRSS2 loci alter risk for alcohol-related and sporadic pancreatitis. *Nature genetics ePub.*(2012).
- *Pharmacogenomics:* None

## Diagnostic Criteria and Clinical Characteristics

### Diagnostic Criteria for Acute Pancreatitis:

**Diagnostic evaluation should include at least two of the following:**

- History consistent with acute pancreatitis, focused on the context, timing, character and location of pain, and the differential diagnosis.
- Serum amylase and lipase levels.
- Computed tomographic (CT) scan with or without contrast demonstrating pancreatic inflammation, peripancreatic fluid collections, or fat stranding. For acute pancreatitis, CT is a secondary test used to make the diagnosis if there is clinical suspicion but the patient does not have pain or elevated amylase or lipase or to rule our other causes for the clinical symptoms or to evaluate complications. It should only be done after fluid resuscitation and with consideration of renal function.

### Diagnostic Criteria for Chronic Pancreatitis:

**Diagnostic evaluation should include at least two of the following:**

- Symptoms lasting greater than 6 months.
- Histology demonstrating chronic inflammation and irregular fibrosis with destruction and loss of exocrine parenchyma with an irregular and patchy distribution in the interlobular spaces; intralobular fibrosis alone is not specific for chronic pancreatitis.
- CT scan demonstrating pancreatic structural abnormalities including any of the following: pancreatic ductal dilation, pancreatic parenchymal atrophy, pancreatic fibrosis, inflammatory mass, bile duct structure, pseudocysts, pancreatic calcifications, and absence of any evidence of pancreatic cancer or IPMN.
- Pancreatic function test that demonstrates exocrine insufficiency: Tests include human fecal elastase-1, fecal chymotrypsin levels, elevated fecal fat (steatorrhea), decreased pancreatic bicarbonate levels coming from the pancreatic duct (requiring intubation of the duodenum), decreased serum trypsinogen levels.
- Genetic testing includes the *PRSS1*, *CFTR* and the *SPINK1*, the chymotrypsin C gene (*CTRC*), and the calcium sensing receptor (*CASR*) with any of the above criteria. Genetic risk is not sufficient to make a diagnosis of chronic pancreatitis.

### Diagnostic Criteria for Autoimmune Pancreatitis:

**Diagnostic evaluation should include at least two of the following:**

- **Histology:** AIP is distinguished from other forms of pancreatitis by periductal lymphoplasmacytic infiltrate, inflamed cellular stroma with storiform fibrosis, obliterative phlebitis, and granulocytic epithelial lesions (GEL). Two types of AIP have been defined: type 1 typically has abundant (>10 cells/hpf) IgG4-positive cells (see below) and type 2 has GEL.
- **Serum IgG4 greater than 2 × upper limits of normal.** IgG4 levels may be normal or dramatically elevated. About 7% of pancreatic cancers have mildly elevated IgG4 levels.
- **Pancreatic imaging:** Features that are highly suggestive of AIP include a diffusely enlarged gland with featureless borders and delayed enhancement with or without a capsule-like rim. Focal areas of enlargement of pancreatic tissue without other features of pancreatic cancer are also common in AIP but are only considered consistent with AIP.
- **Other organ involvement:** AIP can be part of a systemic syndrome that includes involvement of the biliary tract, liver, salivary and lachrymal glands, kidneys, intestine or retroperitoneal fibrosis. There is also a common overlap with inflammatory bowel disease.
- **Response to corticosteroids:** AIP typically has a dramatic improvement in signs and symptoms with corticosteroid treatment. Extrapancreatic systems should also improve.

**Clinical Characteristics:** Both acute and chronic pancreatitis are inflammatory syndrome definitions largely by clinical criteria. Acute pancreatitis can be subclinical or mild, with vague abdominal pain and/or nausea. More severe disease is reflected by increasing pain and evidence of local inflammation with leukocyte elevation and elevation of digestive enzymes in the blood. Over the first 24 to 48 hours a subset of patients progress to systemic inflammation, manifest as the systemic inflammatory response syndrome (SIRS), defined as two or more features of (1) temperature greater than 38°C or less than 36°C, (2) HR greater than 90 BPM, (3) RR greater than 20/min or $PCO_2$ less than 32 mm Hg, (4) WBC less than 4000 or greater than 12,000 or 10% bands (immature neutrophils). About half of these patients will develop persistent SIRS (>24 hours), develop a vascular leak syndrome, pulmonary edema (from vascular leak, not from fluid overload), and multiorgan failure. Early goal-oriented fluid resuscitation and early enteral feeding are the only therapy known to shorten the duration of SIRS and reduce organ failure.

There is no consensus on the definition of early chronic pancreatitis. Indeed, the classic definitions are based on irreversible damage to pancreatic structure and function. Whatever the underlying etiology and mechanism of injury may be, the process of recurrent, severe, or persistent inflammation leads to complications of chronic inflammation in other organs. These include loss-of-organ function (ie, enzymes leading to nutrient maldigestion, islet cells leading to diabetes type 3c), fibrosis or sclerosis, a variety of pain syndromes, and increased risk of cancer (ie, pancreatic adenocarcinoma).

Autoimmune pancreatitis has an insiduous onset, often presenting with frequent presentation with obstructive jaundice with or without a pancreatic mass, histologically by a lymphoplasmacytic infiltrate and fibrosis and therapeutically by a dramatic response to steroids. Consensus diagnostic criteria have been published.

## Screening and Counseling

**Screening:** Screening for pancreatitis in the general population is not indicated. Presymptomatic genetic testing may be considered in families with hereditary pancreatitis (*PRSS1*) or familial pancreatitis (*SPINK1/CFTR/CFRC*) within the context of genetic counseling.

**Counseling:** Pancreatitis may be inherited in an autosomal dominant, autosomal recessive, multigene, or multifactorial manner. Patients who are candidates for genetic testing (or eligible family members) should receive appropriate genetic counseling prior to testing. The interpretation of the test depends on the results. A summary of the major disease-associated genes and common SNPs is given in Table 69-1.

**PRSS1 mutations:** Gain-of-function mutations in the *PRSS1* gene are associated with autosomal hereditary pancreatitis. Affected individuals typically inherit the disease gene, but de novo cases also occur, usually through conversion mutations between similar genes within the

**Table 69-1  *Disease-Associated Susceptibility Variants***

| Candidate Gene (Chromosome Location) | Associated Variant[a] [effect on protein] | Relative Risk | Frequency of Risk Allele | Putative Functional Significance | Associated Disease Phenotype |
|---|---|---|---|---|---|
| *PRSS1* 7q35 | *p.A16V, p.D22G, p.K23R, p.K231_I23INSIDK, p.N29I, N28T, Pv39A, p.R122H, pR122C* | >100 | Rare | Gain of function | Hereditary pancreatitis |
| *CFTR* 7q??? | Many (most are not functionally characterized) p.F508del is the most common severe mutation | ~3 | 2%-3% European ancestry | Protein misfolding, >95% loss of mutated CFTR function | F508del homozygote causes CF. Compound heterozygous genotypes result in severe to variable or atypical CF phenotypes depending on the less-severe variants. Pancreatitis may be the disease-defining phenotype. |
| *CFTR* 7q??? | p.R75Q | ~1.5 | ~7% healthy population | Reduction of bicarbonate conductance | As a compound heterozygous genotype (eg, with F508del), variable features of recurrent acute and chronic pancreatitis, chronic sinusitis, male infertility (CBAVD) |
| *SPINK1* | p.N34S | ~3 | 2%-3% healthy population | No known dysfunction | Modifies the severity of pancreatitis from multiple etiologies |
| *CTRC* | p.R254W, p.K247_R254del, and private mutations | Low | Rare | Rare | Contributes to a complex chronic pancreatitis trait |
| *CASR* | p.L173P, p.F391F, p.Q1011E *p.R896H, p.R990G* | Low | Low | Loss of function associated with SPINK1 mutations. Gain of function associated with alcohol etiology. | Contributes to chronic pancreatitis, usually as a complex genotype with SPINK1 p.N34S or heavy alcohol use. |
| *CTRC X* | rs12688220_C RR 1.39, MAF .26 | | | Altered CLDN2 localization | Increases risk of alcoholic pancreatitis, especially in men. |

[a]Italics indicate gain-of-function mutations.

CBAVD, congenital bilateral absence of the vas deferens.

trypsinogen gene cluster. The clinical phenotype has an 80% penetrance by age 20 years, with a median age of onset of 10 years. Patients with HP and no family history may have either a de novo mutation, have been adopted, are unfamiliar with the details of the family history, or have a paternity issue. A positive diagnosis therefore has implications for other family members and offspring. Patients with the mutation have a 50% chance that a child will have the disease gene, and 40% chance that the child will have symptoms. Genetic testing is used to confirm suspected diagnosis, which is important for limiting further evaluation into possible etiologies. In addition, the gene results are useful in guiding lifestyle choices, including strict avoidance of smoking and alcohol consumption, and healthy eating which may include vitamin and antioxidant supplements. A coexisting *SPINK1* mutation is a poor prognostic sign, and should prompt consideration

of total pancreatectomy with islet autotransplantation (TP/IAT) in symptomatic patients and a challenging clinical course.

A recent GWAS identified non-coding variants at the PRSS1-PRSS2 locus resulting in decreased expression of the trypsinogen genes (Whitcomb NG 2012). This locus was associated with a decreased risk of pancreatitis, further supporting the roll of trypsin in the etiology of various forms of recurrent acute and chronic pancreatitis.

***CFTR* mutations:** Loss-of-function mutations in *CFTR* are associated with sporadic and familial pancreatitis. If the patient has two *CFTR* gene mutations that are known to be functionally severe, then they likely have cystic fibrosis (CF). The classic form of CF is usually diagnosed at less than 5 years of age and is associated with an elevated sweat chloride test (>60 mEq/L) and pancreatic insufficiency. Occasionally, however, the symptomatic onset is acute pancreatitis. The diagnosis of cystic fibrosis is *not* based on genotype alone (ie, two severe mutations might be in *cis*), and the patient should be referred to a designated CF center for formal evaluation and testing. The diagnosis of CF is difficult to reverse if it is incorrect. The diagnosis of CF has tremendous implications for the patient and the family related to medical costs, complications, life expectancy, and social issues.

Patients with genotypes that include a functionally mild-variable *CFTR* mutation (eg, functional class IV) along with a second mild-variable or severe *CFTR* mutation have a CF. In these cases at least one of the CFTR molecules retains enough function to allow for normal organ function, unless there is a confounding genetic factor or strong environmental stressor. Thus, aCF can affect any of the organs also affected in classic CF. As with CF, a formal evaluation is warranted at a CF center prior to making a final diagnosis. If genetic testing is considered, complete *CFTR* sequencing is recommended. Full sequencing of *CFTR* is recommended when a patient has enough symptoms but only one identified *CFTR* mutation since there are hundreds of very rare or personal mutations. Over 1600 *CFTR* variants have been identified, but less than half have been proven to cause CF, and many are considered to be benign. The reason is that a variety of *CFTR* variants that were thought to be benign because they do not alter sweat chloride or cause dominant lung disease, are in fact associated with RAP and CP. These mutations (functional classification IVb) selectively disrupt bicarbonate conductance, but not chloride conductance. Since *CFTR* is critical in the pancreas, vas deferens, and sinuses for bicarbonate secretion, these organs are more sensitive to these mutations, resulting in pancreatitis, congenital bilateral absence of the vas deferens (CBAVD), and chronic sinusitis.

Patients with one *CFTR* severe (class I-III) or mild-variable (class IV or IVb) mutation plus a *SPINK1* mutation is at risk for RAP and CP. In this case the phenotype is limited to the pancreas. The patient does not need to be referred to a CF center because they are not at risk of life-threatening complications of lung disease. They are currently treated as typical RAP and CP.

*SPINK1* **mutations:** Pancreatic secretory trypsin inhibitor is an acute phase protein coded for by the *SPINK1* gene. SPINK1 is not expressed except in trace amounts under normal conditions. In the setting of inflammation the gene is markedly unregulated and serves as a feedback inhibitor of active trypsin. Loss-of-function mutations in *SPINK1* are common, with a prevalence of 1% to 3% in populations worldwide. They become important only when a condition coexists that results in recurrent trypsinogen activation to trypsin within the pancreas. Thus, *SPINK1* is a modifier gene.

*SPINK1* mutations are usually observed in familial pancreatitis (as an autosomal recessive trait), but also in sporadic cases. One common *SPINK1* mutation (p.N34S) appears to confer a very high risk of pancreatitis without concurrent major mutations or stressors. Penetrance is not known, but is thought to be above 60%. Age of symptom onset is also unclear, but is nearly always before age 20 years. A heterozygous *SPINK1* mutation confers a high risk of pancreatitis in complex genotypes including a mutation in *PRSS1*, *CFTR*, *CTRC*, or *CASR*. The age of onset of pancreatitis in patients with *SPINK1* complex genotypes is usually before age 20 years, although older ages of onset are being recognized. Patients with *SPINK1* mutations and pancreatitis generally have a more severe clinical course. In summary, *SPINK1* mutations can occur either as an autosomal recessive or a complex pattern.

*CTRC* **mutations:** The *CTRC* gene is a pancreatic digestive enzyme that is produced in small amounts in the pancreas. The function of CTRC appears to hydrolyze prematurely activated trypsin inside the pancreas in compartments with low calcium concentrations. *CTRC* mutations are uncommon, and the effect size appears to be much smaller than *PRSS1*, *CFTR*, or *SPINK1*. Recent studies suggest that mutations in *CTRC* are not sufficient to cause pancreatitis, but contribute to complex genotypes with *SPINK1*, *CFTR*, and *PRSS1* that further increase risk and severity of pancreatitis.

*CASR* **mutations:** The *CASR* is expressed in many cells, and genetic variants are involved in a variety of disorders and syndromes. There are both gain-of-function and loss-of-function mutations that have been characterized. Loss-of-function mutations are associated with pancreatic disease in a complex genotype with *SPINK1* mutations, and gain-of-function mutations are associated with pancreatitis in alcoholics. As with *CTRC* mutations the effects are thought to be milder than other pancreatitis-associated mutations.

*CLD2* **locus:** A recent GWAS identified a high-risk haplotype on the X chromosome encompassing the CLDN2 gene that increases risk of chronic pancreatitis, especially with alcohol consumption. The risk haplotype acts as a dominant factor in me (with only one X chromosome) but recessive in woman. Although the haplotype is common (minor allele frequency of 26%) it increases the risk of chronic pancreatitis by nearly 40%, and may partially explain why alcoholic chronic pancreatitis is much more common in men then women.

## Management and Treatment

*Management:* Pancreatitis describes the inflammatory response to a variety of factors that injure the pancreas. Therefore, the treatment is directed at identifying and eliminating or minimizing environmental stressors linked to etiology and progression, treating complications, and replacing lost function.

☞**LIFESTYLE:** The most important environmental factors associated with pancreatitis are cigarette smoking and alcohol consumption. Recent research demonstrates that alcohol alone confers a small susceptibility risk for pancreatitis (RR <2) and that a threshold of greater than 60 g of alcohol (> five standard drinks) per day must be exceeded. Furthermore, binge drinking is more risky than steady drinking. This is consistent with previous animal studies. The other recent finding was that cigarette smoking is an independent risk factor, that it is dose dependent, and confers an independent RR of greater than 2. Of equal importance is the suggestion that the effects of alcohol and smoking are multiplicative, with a RR of approximately 8. Continued drinking appears to accelerate the progression of RAP to CP, which may be irreversible. Therefore, patients with RAP and/or CP should avoid smoking and drinking alcohol.

*Therapeutics:*

☞**ANTIOXIDANTS:** The role of antioxidants is controversial. If they have a benefit, it appears to be limited to genetic and idiopathic forms of RAP and CP. This therapy does not appear to be beneficial in alcoholics.

☞**PAIN MANAGEMENT:** No single approach to pain management exists since pain occurs through multiple mechanisms including duct obstruction, acute inflammation, hyperstimulation, neural invasion with leukocytes, neuropathic pain, ischemia, etc. The pain syndrome is also aggravated by anxiety and depression. Most of the depression, disability, and poor quality of life are in the subset of patients with constant pain, rather than episodic pain. If the pain is believed to be related to duct obstruction or strictures, then endoscopic therapy should be considered. About 50% of patients will have significant and long-lasting relief from endoscopic therapy. Of those that fail, about 50% will respond to surgery. Medical therapies include over-the-counter pain medicine, narcotics, and pregabalin. Pregabalin was recently evaluated in a randomized, double-blind, placebo-controlled trial of patients with pain greater than 3 days per week. Significant pain relief was seen by week 3, and relief was twice that of placebo. In patients with intractable pain there is growing use of TP/IAT. This has been reported to be very effective in a subset of patients, but it is an irreversible procedure committing the patients to a lifetime of pancreatic enzyme replacement for pancreatic exocrine insufficiency. The long-term effects of islet cell autotransplantation in the liver continue to be evaluated. The possibility of TP/IAT should be considered early in patient management because many of the surgeries designed to improve pancreatic drainage reduce the number of islets and complicate this surgery.

☞**PANCREATIC ENZYME REPLACEMENT THERAPY:** Pancreatic enzyme replacement therapy (PERT) is indicated for patients with pancreatic exocrine insufficiency, including chronic pancreatitis. The enzymes are derived from porcine pancreas and are packaged in acid-resistant microspheres that mix with the meal, and are released when the pH is above levels that will destroy the enzymes. The medication is not targeted to the pancreas, but rather to the meal. Dosage depends on the amount of residual pancreas, the size and content of the meal, and biomarkers of effectiveness. Evidence of inadequate digestion includes fat in the stool (steatorrhea), bloating and diarrhea (possibly linked to bacteria fermenting undigested food), and markers of nutrition (serum prealbumin levels, fat-soluble vitamins, and vitamin $B_{12}$). Coordinating PERT with the meal and timing of digestion may be especially important in diabetics. Patients in whom treatment appears to be failing should be given acid suppression.

*Pharmacogenetics:* At this time there are no pharmacogenetic considerations in the treatment of pancreatitis.

# Molecular Genetics and Molecular Mechanism

*Genetic Testing:* *CFTR* gene panels are widely available, but only test for common severe mutations (eg, F508del), and miss the majority of pancreatitis-associated genotypes.

Currently, Ambry Genetics has exclusive license to test for *PRSS1* and hereditary pancreatitis mutations. They offer targeted testing as well as a pancreatitis panel with full *CFTR* and *SPINK1* screening.

*Future Directions:* The exocrine pancreas is a simple gland with two primary cell types, each with one primary function. Furthermore, the pancreas is protected from most environmental factors, with the exception of alcohol and smoking, which can be quantified using standardized techniques. The biology of these cells is well defined, allowing for the various genetic mutations to be localized and their effects modeled within the context of the exocrine gland. These features make the pancreatitis an optimal complex disease for modeling and simulation studies so that care of patients with early disease can be characterized and their care can be personalized.

**BIBLIOGRAPHY:**

1. Whitcomb DC. Genetic aspects of pancreatitis. *Annu Rev Med*. 2010;61:413-424.

2. Chen JM, Ferec C. Chronic pancreatitis: genetics and pathogenesis. *Annu Rev Genomics Hum Genet*. 2009;10:63-87.

3. Solomon S, Whitcomb DC, LaRusch J. PRSS1-related hereditary pancreatitis. In: Pagon RA, Bird TD, Dolan CR, Stephens K, eds. GeneReviews. Seattle, WA: University of Washington; 1993.

4. Rosendahl J, Landt O, Bernadova J, et al. CFTR, SPINK1, CTRC and PRSS1 variants in chronic pancreatitis: is the role of mutated CFTR overestimated? *Gut*. Apr 2013;62(4):582-592.

5. Ooi CY, Dorfman R, Cipolli M, et al. Type of CFTR mutation determines risk of pancreatitis in patients with cystic fibrosis. *Gastroenterology*. Jan 2011;140(1):153-161.

6. Schneider A, Larusch J, Sun X, et al. Combined bicarbonate conductance-impairing variants in CFTR and SPINK1 variants are associated with chronic pancreatitis in patients without cystic fibrosis. *Gastroenterology*. Jan 2011;140(1):162-171.

7. Rosendahl J, Witt H, Szmola R, et al. Chymotrypsin C (CTRC) variants that diminish activity or secretion are associated with chronic pancreatitis. *Nat Genet*. Jan 2008;40(1):78-82.

8. Larusch J, Whitcomb DC. Genetics of pancreatitis. *Curr Opin Gastroenterol*. Sep 2011;27(5):467-474.

9. Whitcomb, DC, Larusch J, Krasinskas AM, et al. Common genetic variants in the *CLDN2* and *PRSS1-PRSS2* loci alter risk for alcohol-related and sporadic pancreatitis. *Nature genetics*. 2012;44:1349-1354.

10. Shimosegawa T, Chari ST, Frulloni L, et al. International consensus diagnostic criteria for autoimmune pancreatitis: guidelines of the International Association of Pancreatology. *Pancreas*. 2011;40:352-358.

# Supplementary Information

**OMIM REFERENCES:**

[1] Hereditary Pancreatitis; PROTEASE, SERINE, 1; PRSS1 (#276000) (>90% of cases)

[2] Chronic Pancreatitis: Serine Protease Inhibitor, Kazal-Type 1; SPINK1 (#167790) (typically a complex genotype)

[3] Cystic Fibrosis, CF: Cystic Fibrosis Transmembrane Conductance Regulator; CFTR (#219700)

[4] Tropical Calcific Pancreatitis: Serine Protease Inhibitor, Kazal-Type 1; SPINK1 (#608189) (40% of cases)

*Key Words:* Trypsinogen/*PRSS1*, pancreatic secretory trypsin inhibitor/*SPINK1*, cystic fibrosis transmembrane conductance inhibitor/*CFTR*, pancreatitis, alcoholic pancreatitis, tropical pancreatitis, chronic pancreatitis, chronic calcific pancreatitis

# 70 Inflammatory Bowel Disease

Mark W. Babyatsky

## KEY POINTS

- *Disease summary:*
  - The inflammatory bowel diseases (IBDs) are prototypic complex genetic disorders, involving multiple interacting genetic loci and environmental factors that trigger disease.
  - IBD is comprised of two inter-related disorders, Crohn disease (CD), and ulcerative colitis (UC), as well as indeterminate colitis (IC). IC describes the 5% to 10% of IBD involving only the colon and is neither classic CD nor UC.
  - Clinical presentations of UC and CD overlap; both present with diarrhea, bloody diarrhea, abdominal pain, most extraintestinal manifestations, weight loss, and fever.
  - Anatomic involvement: *CD* can involve any portion of the gastrointestinal (GI) tract, most commonly the terminal ileum (5%-75%) and colon (20%-50%). CD causes transmural inflammation in all four layers of bowel wall; extension through the bowel wall can cause fistulae, abscesses, or perianal complications. Strictures secondary to fibrosis are relatively common. *UC* is localized to varying lengths of continuous inflammation proceeding proximally from the rectum; a discontinuous cecal patch may be present. UC is limited to mucosal and submucosal inflammation, and does not cause perianal or intra-abdominal disease; strictures are much less common than in CD.

- *Differential diagnosis:*
  - Infectious colitis (bacterial, viral, protozoal), pseudomembranous colitis (*Clostridium difficile* toxin), and ischemic colitis

- *Monogenic forms:*
  - No single gene cause of IBD is known to exist except perhaps for a rare form of CD (see IL-10 pathway later).

- *Family history:*
  - An affected first-degree relative confers a relative risk of 30 to 40 for CD and 10 to 20 for UC. Overlapping risk occurs since first-degree relatives of patients with CD have relative risk of 3.9 for developing UC.

- *Twin studies:*
  - Monozygotic twins have a 20% to 50% concordance rate in CD, much lower in UC.

- *Environmental factors:*
  - Luminal microbes or microbial products are implicated as "environmental" triggers for IBD.

- *Genome-wide associations:*
  - Many associations exist. Disease-associated genetic variants (single-nucleotide polymorphisms [SNPs]) provide insight into disease pathogenesis; testing for SNPs is not yet clinically validated to diagnose or guide management of IBD.

- *Pharmacogenomics:*
  - Testing for common thiopurine *S*-methyltransferase (TPMT) variants to guide management has proven validity in some clinical circumstances.

## Diagnostic Criteria and Clinical Characteristics

***Diagnostic Criteria for IBD:*** Diagnostic evaluation should include

- Stool studies including fecal leukocytes, culture for appropriate bacterial and parasitic cultures, assays for *C difficile* toxin, appropriate tests for possible viral etiologies (cytomegalovirus) and *Mycobacterium tuberculosis*.
- Colonoscopy with biopsy and ileum cannulation. *Granulomas* are present on endoscopic biopsies in approximately 10% of CD, crypt abscesses are indicative of UC.
- Serologic markers may be helpful; anti-*Saccharomyces cerevisiae* antibodies (*ASCA*) and antineutrophil cytoplasmic antibodies with perinuclear staining (*p-ANCA*) have high sensitivity for IBD in combination compared to other causes of intestinal inflammation, but sensitivity varies for different ethnic groups (much lower, eg, in regions endemic for tuberculosis). ASCA shows high specificity for CD, and p-ANCA for UC, although patients with CD limited to the colon may be positive for p-ANCA. Prognostic use of antibody concentrations in IBD remains under investigation.

- Upper GI imaging to assess for signs of ileal or other upper GI tract involvement.
- Workup for extraintestinal manifestations if clinically indicated.

***Clinical Characteristics:***

☞PATTERNS OF DISEASE IN CD:

**Fibrostenotic CD** can present with right lower quadrant pain as the most common symptom and can mimic acute appendicitis and present with pain, fever, and a palpable mass; alternatively, the pain may be colicky in nature, recurrent or progressive and associated with abdominal bloating, nausea, vomiting, and weight loss.

**Penetrating CD** can present with an intra-abdominal abscess with complications of fistulae to the perianal region, abdominal wall or bladder with associated drainage, urinary tract infections, pneumaturia or even fecaluria. Anal fissures are also specific for CD.

**Inflammatory colonic CD** can present identically to UC (see later).

☞**PATTERNS OF DISEASE IN UC:** UC presentation is less variable and is characterized by mucosal or submucosal inflammation of varying lengths of the colon but always involves the rectum. As such, clinical presentations include diarrhea that may be bloody, tenesmus, urgency, and crampy abdominal pain. Fever and weight loss may accompany severe disease.

**Extraintestinal manifestations of IBD:** Nonintestinal manifestations are similar for both CD and UC.

**Dermatologic manifestations** include the relatively common erythema nodosum that often correlate with acute flares. The more problematic pyoderma gangrenosum is much more common in UC than CD, and its course is independent of IBD activity.

**Joint manifestations** include peripheral arthritis that correlates with exacerbations of bowel disease, and central arthritis (ankylosing spondylitis or sacroiliitis) that does not correlate with bowel activity.

**Ocular complications** include conjunctivitis, episcleritis, and uveitis and may occur independent of bowel activity.

**Hepatobiliary complications** include nonalcoholic fatty liver disease, cholestasis, gallstones (CD>UC, particularly with ileal disease due to decreased bile acid reabsorption), and primary sclerosing cholangitis (UC>>CD), a fibrotic disorder of intra- and extrahepatic bile ducts that does not correlate with bowel disease activity.

**Renal complications** include kidney stones that are more common in CD than in UC. Oxalate absorption is increased in bowel inflammation leading to calcium oxalate stones. Uric acid stones also occur with increased frequency in CD.

## Screening and Counseling

**Screening:** No clear evidence for screening of family members exists. Genetic testing for disease-associated SNPs is not clinically validated. While suggestions of specific phenotypes related to specific SNPs exist such as stricturing ileal CD for the three most common *NOD2* SNPs, no current therapy for primary prophylaxis against IBD development is known, so these tests have no clinical utility at present.

**Counseling:** Familial clustering is common but not universal. Mendelian inheritance for a rare form of enterocolitis may exist but is exceedingly rare. Nevertheless, many patients want to know the risk for offspring during family planning and the risk for siblings of affected individuals. If a patient has IBD, the lifetime risk of a first-degree relative developing IBD is 10%; if two parents have IBD, the lifetime risk for each offspring may be as high as 36%. Genetic risk is much higher for CD than for UC with a relative risk of 3 to 40 for CD and 10 to 20 for UC. A first-degree relative of a proband with CD has a relative risk for developing UC of 3.9, while the relative risk of a UC proband developing CD is only 1.8.

## Management and Treatment

**Aminosalicylates:** For both forms of IBD, the aminosalicylates remain the most common first-line therapy in mild to moderate disease. Sulfasalazine, balsalazide, and olsalazine depend on colonic bacteria to release the active salicylate making them an effective treatment for UC and CD limited to the colon but much less effective in small intestinal involvement. Mesalamine is used preferentially in small intestinal CD. In addition to treating mild to moderate disease, salicylates reduce the incidence and severity of recurrence after surgical resection or medically induced remission. In UC, distal colonic inflammation can be treated with salicylate suppositories (proctitis) or enemas (proctosigmoiditis).

**Antibiotics and Probiotics:** Antibiotics have also shown to improve mild to moderate CD, particularly metronidazole and ciprofloxacin. Metronidazole also helps in the treatment of fistulous complications of CD but its use is limited by upper GI side effects and peripheral neuropathy. With recent understanding of the importance of the gut microflora, new strategies to eliminate or reduce proinflammatory bacteria or replace them with anti-inflammatory bacteria, also known as probiotics, should provide new treatment options. Clinical applications for using the microflora to treat IBD has not yet been optimized.

**Immune Modulating Agents:** Immunomodulatory medications are a mainstay of therapy. This should not be surprising, since genetic manipulation of many host immune factors in mice have demonstrated the importance of the mucosal response in the pathogenesis of IBD. In situations where IBD patients are refractory to steroids or develop flares on treatment with immunomodulators, consider superinfection with *C difficile* or opportunistic pathogens such as cytomegalovirus.

**Anti-TNF therapy:** Systemic antitumor necrosis factor (anti-TNF) therapy is the central treatment of moderate to severe CD, particularly in patients with fistulous disease but are also active in UC. Infection with *Mycobacterium tuberculosis* should be ruled out, since anti-TNF treatment can cause rapid and even fatal dissemination of tuberculosis. Anti-TNF therapy is also contraindicated in patients with abdominal abscesses or other bacterial infections.

**Azathioprine and 6-mercaptopurine:** Other immunomodulatory agents that are used frequently in the treatment of CD include azathioprine and its metabolite, 6-mercpatopurine, agents particularly effective in fistulous CD, prevention of relapses including those that occur postoperatively, and tapering patients off steroids. However, azathioprine and 6-mercaptopurine (6-MP) are limited by a slow onset of action (mean: 3 months) and side effects, most notably neutropenia. Genetic testing for TPMT, a key enzyme in the breakdown of azathioprine and 6-MP into nontoxic metabolites, is now widely available and has led to reduced toxicity (see later).

**Corticosteroids:** Glucocorticoids have long been used in acute flares and demonstrate more efficacy in UC than in CD. Importantly, steroid preparations are contraindicated in CD patients with fistulous disease or abscesses, and, in all IBD, can cause severe toxicity, including aseptic necrosis of susceptible bones, osteopenia, glucose intolerance, and cataracts. Budesonide, an oral steroid that is released in the ileum and undergoes rapid metabolism, is associated with fewer side effects but has no efficacy advantage over older steroid preparations. Of note, steroids have no role in prophylaxis against recurrence after surgery or medical remission. In distal UC, steroid enemas or foam are helpful in acute flares and show fewer side effects than other delivery methods.

**Cyclosporine:** A calcineurin inhibitor that inhibits T-cell activation, is effective, particularly when given at high doses intravenously, in patients with severe, refractory UC but its use is limited by side effects including renal failure and seizures and a lack of sustained remission in the absence of additional immunosuppressants.

**Methotrexate:** Another immunomodulator that has been shown to be effective in CD and usually has its onset of action with 8 weeks of starting therapy.

***Surgery:*** The major distinction in treatment of UC and CD is that surgery is curative for UC and should be avoided in CD due to the major risk of postoperative recurrence, particularly at the site of anastomosis. Even with recent advances in the medical treatment of IBD, surgery is still required in up to 50% of UC patients and up to 80% of CD patients with ileal involvement (50% with CD limited to the colon). In UC, indications for surgery include medical refractoriness, severe bleeding, and toxic megacolon; surgery is curative and most commonly involves a total colectomy and ileoanal anastomosis. The most common late surgical complication is inflammation of the pouch constructed as a J or S pouch using terminal ileum to avoid an ileostomy (pouchitis). This complication can be treated with antibiotics; probiotics may prevent recurrence. Surgery is often considered a last resort in CD, because, in contrast to UC, postoperative recurrence is very common. The most frequent indications for surgery in CD include refractoriness to medical treatment, steroid dependence, obstruction due to fibrotic stenosis of the terminal ileum, adhesions from prior CD surgery, massive bleeding, or abdominal fistulae or abscesses that do not respond to nonsurgical approaches. All patients should be started on either an aminosalicylate or immunomodulator such as azathioprine or 6-mercapotpurine postoperatively since these agents reduce postsurgical relapses.

***Pharmacogenetics:*** Pharmacogenetics is being incorporated rapidly into the treatment of patients with IBD (Table 70-1). TPMT, as noted earlier, is a key metabolic enzyme for azathioprine and 6-MP. Azathioprine is itself metabolized to 6-MP and eventually to active 6-thioguanine (6-TG). 6-MP can be inactivated by either TPMT or xanthine oxidase to nontoxic products. Mutations in the *TPMT* gene reduce TPMT activity, shunting metabolism to 6-TG and increasing toxicity, most importantly neutropenia; testing for TPMT enzyme activity in red blood cells or, preferably, genotype testing to detect the three major mutations that lower TPMT activity are both available and widely used before initiating therapy. Approved by the FDA, TPMT testing appears to be cost-effective. Methylenetetrahydrofolate reductase (*MTHFR*) mutations are associated with increased toxicity of methotrexate used to treat CD; testing is not yet widely available. Other mutations decrease

efficacy to infliximab, a TNF-α antibody, although clinical utility of these mutations have not been proven.

## Molecular Genetics and Molecular Mechanism

Many lines of evidence have long implicated a genetic predisposition for IBD including ethnic prevalence, associations with other genetic disorders, familial aggregation, and twin studies (monozygotic vs dizygotic concordance much higher in CD than in UC). Further, within families, the IBD phenotype is often strikingly similar. In the past 15 years, a multitude of mouse models bearing genetic modifications harbor IBD phenotypes; IBD in these models often vary in severity based on the background murine genetic strain, further suggesting important roles for genetic influences in the development of IBD. However, IBD is not a monogenic disorder, and is a model of a complex genetic disorder. The recognition of *NOD2* or *CARD15* as a CD susceptibility gene at the end of the 1990s was afforded by combination positional cloning strategies. More than 90% of the increased risk for CD in patients with results from three specific mutations of the *NOD2* or *CARD15* gene; homozygotes or compound heterozygotes for these mutations have a much higher prevalence of CD than heterozygotes or individuals not bearing any mutations. However, only a minority of patients with these variants develop actual CD, signifying that environmental factors are necessary for CD development in genetically susceptible hosts. The NOD2 or CARD15 protein recognizes bacterial peptidoglycans and regulates Paneth cell antimicrobial defensin expression, further defining the specific interactions between genes and environment in a human complex genetic disorder. Paneth cells are particularly abundant in the ileum and right colon, paralleling the location of CD in patients bearing *NOD2* or *CARD15* mutations.

Since the discovery of the role of *NOD2* or *CARD15*, more than 60 loci have been identified to confer IBD susceptibility (**replicated examples are noted in Table 70-2**), most commonly through large genome-wide association studies (GWASs), but occasionally through more traditional linkage analysis. Interestingly, these newer susceptibility genes help elucidate important pathways that are important in the pathogenesis of IBD, but that were poorly

***Table 70-1 Pharmacogenetics of Crohn Disease***

| Gene | Associated Medications | Goal of Testing | Variants | Effect |
|------|----------------------|-----------------|----------|--------|
| *TPMT* (thiopurine *S*-methyltransferase) | Azathioprine, 6-mercaptopurine | Safety and Efficacy | *2,*3A, *3C | Variants—lower dose WT—higher dose Less frequent WBC monitoring |
| *MTHFR* (5,10-methylene tetrahydrofolate reductase) | Methotrexate | Safety | *1298C | All side effects: nausea or vomiting, rash, abnormal LFTs |
| *FCGR3A* (Fc fragment of IgG, low affinity IIIa, receptor) | Infliximab | Efficacy | *G4985T | Lower efficacy |
| *FASLG* (FAS ligand) | Infliximab | Efficacy | *843TT | Lower efficacy; apoptotic pathway |
| *ABCB1* (ATP-binding cassette, subfamily B [MDR/TAP], member 1) | Glucocorticoids | Efficacy | *G2677TT *C3435T *843TT | Lower efficacy Steroid resistance Ethnic variation |

*Table 70-2  Crohn Disease-Associated Susceptibility Variants*

| Candidate Gene (Chromosome Location) | Associated Variant [effect on protein] (db SNP) | Relative Risk | Frequency of Risk Allele | Putative Functional Significance | Associated Disease Phenotype |
|---|---|---|---|---|---|
| *NOD2* (16q12.1) | C907T [nonsynonymous amino acid substitution P268S] (rs2066842) | | | Intracellular sensor of bacterial peptidoglycan | Ileal or ileoco-lonic CD |
| | C2209T [nonsynonymous amino acid substitution R702W] (rs2066844) | | | | |
| | G2827C [nonsynonymous amino acid substitution G908R] (rs2066845) | | | | |
| | 3121insC 1-BP INS, 3121C [frameshift/ premature stop codon] (rs2066847) | 1.5 heterozygous 3121insC  17.6 homozygous 3121insC | 8.4% among Jewish Caucasians and 8.1% among non-Jewish Caucasians | | |
| *IL23R* (1p31.3) | rs11209026 | | | IL23 receptor; innate and adaptive immune responses | CD, UC |
| *PTPN2* (18p11) | | | | IL23 pathway | CD |
| *IL12B* (5q33) | | | | IL23 pathway | CD |
| *IRGM* (5q33.1) | | | | Autophagy (mycobacteria) | CD |
| *ATG16Ll* (2q37.1) | | | | Autophagy (intracellular bacteria) | CD |
| *IBD5* (5q31) | | | | Specific genes unclear | CD, UC |
| *TNFSF15* (9q33.1) | | | | Tumor necrosis factor superfamily | C11 |
| HLA class II (6p[DRB1*0103]) | | | | Antigen presentation | Colonic CD, UC |
| *PTGER4* (5p13.1) | rs1373692 | | | Prostaglandin receptor E4 | CD |
| IL-10 ligand/ receptor | Multiple mutations | | | IL-10 anti-inflammatory pathway | CD |

*NOD2* formerly known as *CARD15*.

CD, Crohn disease; UC, ulcerative colitis

understood before these discoveries. Notably, the interleukin (IL)-23 receptor pathway (*IL23R, IL12b* [*p40 Ag*], *STAT3, JAK2*) confers risk for IBD, both for CD and UC. This immunoregulatory pathway is the key in the differentiation of Th17 cells, a recently described T-cell subset that secretes IL-17, an important mediator of antimicrobial defenses. IL-12 and IL-23 share a p40 subunit that binds to the IL-23 receptor, providing additional opportunities for

future therapeutic targets in IBD. Significantly, mutations of the IL-23 pathway are found in other autoimmune diseases, including psoriasis, Behcet disease, and ankylosing spondylitis (even patients without associated IBD). One intriguing gene family implicated in an enterocolitis resembling CD is the IL-10 or receptor pathway. Of note, IL-10 deficient mice have long been the standard murine model of enterocolitis most resembling CD. Recently, four patients, harboring mutations of either the *IL-10RA* or *B* subunit demonstrated an autosomal recessive pattern of CD-like enterocolitis, suggesting a possible rare monogenic disorder conferring CD risk. Other patients with CD-like disease and multiple fistulae demonstrated homozygous loss-of-function mutations in the *IL-10* gene itself. While more patients need to be studied for clinical validity, this ties the murine and human IL-10 correlation of genetic susceptibility to CD-like disease.

Autophagy, a catabolic process whereby cells utilize lysosomal machinery to degrade proteins including those made by intracellular pathogens, represents another essential pathway that has now been recognized through GWAS in IBD. Mutations in two genes, *ATG16L1* (autophagy of intracellular bacteria) and *IRGM* (mycobacterial autophagy) confer risk specifically for CD and again implicate genetic and environmental or bacterial interactions in the pathogenesis of IBD. Other candidate genes including *NCF4*, *PHOX2B*, and *FAM 92B* are also part of the autophagosomic pathway; mutations in these genes need to be independently reproduced but may further advance our understanding of CD pathogenesis and treatment targets in CD. Also associated by mutational analysis, the TNF family, known to be important by efficacious treatment of IBD with anti-TNF antibodies; mutations in *TNFSF15*, an inhibitor of angiogenesis, predispose to the development of CD. *HLA class II DRB1*0103* and perhaps other HLA mutations are part of antigen presentation to the mucosal immune system, and correlate with IBD, particularly with UC and CD limited to the colon.

In addition to these host genetic factors, bacterial genetics play an important role in the development and pathophysiology of IBD. As noted, many of the host genes implicated in CD pathogenesis are important in bacterial recognition (*NOD2* or *CARD15*), antigen presentation, native or adaptive immune responses or microbial autophagy. Recent metagenomic analysis of intestinal microbes demonstrates a restriction of bacterial lineages in patients with IBD. However, an expansion of the protobacterial lineages (adherent-invasive *Escherichia coli*, *Campylobacter concisus*, and enterohepatic *Helicobacter*) correlates most closely with the pathogenesis of IBD. Although specific pathogenic bacterial strains in IBD remain elusive, genetically modified mouse models demonstrate impressive phenotype specificity by distinct bacterial strains. Recently, distinct systems biology networks of genes examined in the microbiome of IBD patients compared to controls reveal some major variations that should shed light on additional candidate genes, many in metabolic pathways, that are associated with the development of IBD. Considering that the human intestine, particularly the colon, hosts sufficient numbers of bacteria to contain 100-fold more genes than the entire human genome, insights into the nature of bacterial genes and the proteins encode are likely to provide novel strategies for treating CD.

*Genetic Testing:* No role yet exists for genetic testing in the diagnosis of IBD. However, in treatment, genetic testing is indicated prior to the use of azathioprine or 6-MP for *TPMT* gene mutations.

*Future Directions:* The recent and current explosion in clinical genomics has already provided a wealth of new knowledge regarding the pathophysiology of CD and multiple opportunities for therapeutic interventions. Insights into autophagy, innate or adaptive immunity, and the human gut microbiome should provide new biologic targets for CD. While none of the genetic susceptibility gene variants have definitively provided genetic screening tools, larger-scale clinical studies correlating specific phenotypes or response to treatment with genotype may provide important new options for IBD prevention, treatment, or population screening. Genotype or phenotype correlations have been suggested and further research may confirm. For example, the HLA class II DRB1*0103 variant predicts either CD limited to the colon or UC.

Metagenomic and systems biology analysis of intestinal and colonic microflora should also yield new treatment or prevention options as we begin to understand the specific bacterial antigens that trigger disease in susceptible individuals. Finally, pharmacogenetics may soon predict individuals who may most benefit from certain medications as well as minimize drug toxicity, as we are already seeing with TMPT testing. While all of the outlined advances are new, IBD will continue to serve as a model for studying genetic or environmental interactions and for the realization of personalized medicine in the genomic era.

## BIBLIOGRAPHY:

1. Patel KK, Babyatsky MW. Medical education: a key partner in realizing personalized medicine. *Gastroenterology.* 2008;134:656-661.

2. Rioux JD, Xavier RJ, Taylor KD, et al. Genome-wide association study identifies new susceptibility loci for Crohn disease and implicates autophagy in disease pathogenesis. *Nat Genet.* 2007;39:596-604.

3. Limbergen JV, Russell RK, Nimmo ER, et al. The genetics of inflammatory bowel disease. *Am J Gastroenterol.* 2007;102:1-12.

4. Xavier RJ, Huett A, Rioux JD. Autophagy as an important process in gut homeostasis and Crohn's disease pathogenesis. *Gut.* 2008;57:717-720.

5. Goyette P, Labbe C, Trinh TT, et al. Molecular pathogenesis of inflammatory bowel disease: genotypes, phenotypes and personalized medicine. *Ann Med.* 2007;39:177-199.

6. Cho J, Weaver C. The genetics of inflammatory bowel disease. *Gastroenterology.* 2007;133:1327-1339.

7. Pena AS. Contribution of genetics to a new vision in the understanding of inflammatory bowel disease. *World Gastroenterol.* 2006;12:4784-4787.

8. Parkes M, Barrett PM, Prescott NJ, et al. Sequence variants in the autophagy gene IRGM and multiple other replicating loci contribute to Crohn's disease susceptibility. *Nat Genet.* 2007;39:830-832.

9. Xavier RJ, Podolsky DK. Unraveling the pathogenesis of inflammatory bowel disease. *Nature.* 2007;448:427-434.

10. Tysk C, Lindberg E, Jarnerot G, et al. Ulcerative colitis and Crohn's disease in an unselected population of monozygotic and dizygotic twins. A study of heritability and the influence of smoking. *Gut.* 1988;29:990-996.

11. Barrett JC, Hansoul S, Nicolae DL, et al. Genome-wide association defines more than 30 distinct loci for Crohn's disease. *Nat Genet.* 2008;40:955-962.

12. Pierik M, Rutgeerts P, Vlietnck R, Vermiere S. Pharmacogenetics in inflammatory bowel disease. *World J Gastroenterol.* 2006;12:3657-3667.

13. Glocker E-O, Kotlarz D, Klein C, Shah N, Grimbacher B. IL-10 and IL-10 receptor defects in humans. *Ann NY Acad Sci.* 2011;1246:102-107.

14. Glocker E, Grimbacher B. Inflammatory bowel disease: is it a primary immunodeficiency? *Cell Mol Life Sci.* 2012;69:41-48.

15. Greenblum S, Turnbaugh PJ, Borenstein E. Metagenomic systems biology of the human gut microbiome reveals topographical shifts associated with obesity and inflammatory bowel disease. *Proc Natl Acad Sci USA.* 2012;109:594-599.

16. Mukhopadhya I, Hansen R, El-Omar EM, Hold GL. IBD—what role do Protobacteria play? *Nat Rev Gastroenterol Hepatol.* 2012;19:219-230.

## Supplementary Information

**OMIM References:**

[1] Inflammatory Bowel Disease 1; IBD1 (#266600)

[2] Nucleotide-Binding Oligomerization Domain Protein 2; NOD2 (#605956)

[3] Blau Syndrome—Synovitis, Granulomatosis, With Uveitis and Cranial Neuropathies (#186580)

**Alternative Names:**

- Terminal Ileitis
- Regional Enteritis
- Granulomatous Enteritis
- Granulomatous Colitis
- Ileocolitis

***Key Words:*** colitis, ileitis, Crohn, IBD, microbiome, pharmacogenetics

# 71 Genetics of Constipation and Hirschsprung Disease

Melissa A. Parisi

## KEY POINTS

- *Disease summary:*
  - Constipation is defined as having a bowel movement less than three times per week. A newborn or infant that manifests severe congenital constipation may have a diagnosis of Hirschsprung disease (HSCR). HSCR, or congenital intestinal aganglionosis, is characterized by complete absence of neuronal ganglion cells in a portion of the intestinal tract resulting in complete or partial intestinal obstruction. Constipation is common, affecting at least 4 million Americans, and is associated with female gender, pregnancy, lower socioeconomic status, age over 65 years, and following childbirth or surgery. In contrast, HSCR is a relatively rare condition, affecting 1:5000 newborns with a male:female ratio of 4:1.
  - Constipation manifests with stools that are typically hard, dry, small in size, and difficult to pass.
  - Infants with HSCR frequently present in the first 2 months of life with symptoms of impaired intestinal motility such as failure to pass meconium within the first 48 hours of life, constipation, emesis, abdominal pain or distention, and occasionally diarrhea. HSCR should be considered in anyone with lifelong severe constipation, as the diagnosis may not be made until childhood or adulthood.
  - Suction biopsies of rectal mucosa or submucosa are the preferred diagnostic test for HSCR.
  - In 80% of individuals with HSCR, aganglionosis is restricted to the rectosigmoid colon (short-segment disease); in 15% to 20%, aganglionosis extends proximal to the sigmoid colon (long-segment disease); in about 5%, aganglionosis affects the entire large intestine (total colonic aganglionosis). Rarely, the aganglionosis extends into the small bowel or even more proximally to encompass the entire bowel (total intestinal aganglionosis).
  - HSCR may occur as an isolated finding or as part of a multisystem or chromosomal disorder. Syndromes associated with HSCR are diagnosed by clinical findings, cytogenetic analysis, or in some cases, by specific molecular or biochemical tests.

- *Differential diagnosis:*
  - Constipation is a symptom rather than a disease per se, and often occurs when there is inadequate fiber in the diet, lack of physical activity, or dehydration. Medications can cause constipation, as can irritable bowel syndrome, neurologic disorders (eg, stroke, Parkinson disease), metabolic or endocrine conditions (eg, diabetes, hypothyroidism), and systemic disorders (eg, lupus). The differential diagnosis for newborns with intestinal obstruction includes, in addition to HSCR, gastrointestinal malformations such as atresia or malrotation, meconium ileus due to cystic fibrosis, abnormalities of the enteric nervous system such as chronic intestinal pseudo-obstruction, and acquired factors such as maternal infection or intoxication or congenital hypothyroidism.

- *Monogenic forms:*
  - No single gene cause of constipation is known. There are six known genes that can cause nonsyndromic HSCR, and multiple causative genes implicated in syndromes associated with HSCR.

- *Family history:*
  - Constipation often runs in families, suggesting genetic predisposition or environmental factors such as diet. In individuals with nonsyndromic HSCR without a clear etiology, HSCR is considered to be a polygenic disorder with incomplete penetrance, variable expressivity, and a 4:1 predominance in males. The overall risk to siblings of an individual with HSCR is 4%. Syndromic forms of HSCR follow the Mendelian pattern of inheritance known for that condition.

- *Twin studies:*
  - Most case series of HSCR have inadequate sets of twins to draw conclusions.

- *Environmental factors:*
  - Diet, medications, and activity play a large role in gut motility, particularly constipation. Environmental factors also likely play a role in the penetrance of polymorphisms in genes such as *RET* to contribute to the development of HSCR.

- *Genome-wide associations:*
  - Genome-wide association studies (GWAS) have demonstrated the significant genetic contribution of the *RET* gene to HSCR, and have also implicated the *EDNRB* gene pathway and other genes as interacting with *RET*.

- *Pharmacogenomics:*
  - No specific pharmacogenomic associations are known, but there is promise that individualized treatments can be developed to treat various forms of constipation.

# Diagnostic Criteria and Clinical Characteristics

### Diagnostic Criteria for HSCR:

**Diagnostic evaluation should include at least one of the following:**

- Histopathologic demonstration of absence of enteric ganglion cells in the distal rectum. Suction biopsies of rectal mucosa and submucosa are the preferred diagnostic test because they can be performed safely without general anesthesia. Absence of ganglion cells in the submucosa of 50 to 75 sections examined from a biopsy establishes the diagnosis. Accessory findings include hypertrophic submucosal nerves and/or an abnormal acetylcholinesterase enzyme staining pattern.
- The diagnosis may be supported by anorectal manometry, abdominal radiographs that show a dilated proximal colon with empty rectum, or barium enema studies that demonstrate delayed emptying time and a funnel-like transition zone between proximal dilated and distal constricted bowel.
- Radiographic studies may be helpful in delineating the proximal extent of aganglionosis, but, intraoperative intestinal rectal biopsy is used to establish the precise boundary during surgical resection.

**And the absence of**

- Other known causes of intestinal obstruction

### Clinical Characteristics:

☞CONSTIPATION: Constipation is defined as having a bowel movement less than three times per week. Symptoms of constipation typically include stools that are hard, dry, small in size, and difficult to eliminate. Other symptoms can include pain with defecation and straining, bloating, and the sensation of a full bowel. Most individuals experience constipation at some time in their lives and it is typically self-limited and not serious. However, chronic constipation can ensue when the constipation is persistent and not responsive to standard measures. As defined by the American College of Gastroenterology Chronic Constipation Task Force, patients must report infrequent stools, difficult defecation or both for at least 3 of the previous 12 months. Constipation can occur when there is inadequate fiber in the diet, lack of physical activity, or dehydration. Chronic constipation can be categorized as functional or idiopathic, in which there is no identified underlying cause. Constipation can be secondary to another condition such as primary diseases of the colon (stricture, cancer, proctitis), metabolic disturbances or endocrine disorders (diabetes, hypothyroidism), neurologic disorders (stroke, Parkinson disease), systemic disease (lupus, multiple sclerosis), and use of medications such as narcotics. Constipation can be subtyped into dyssynergic defecation (pelvic floor dysfunction), pain-predominant constipation, irritable bowel syndrome (IBS)-related constipation, and slow-transit constipation; these are not mutually exclusive. Constipation is common, affecting at least 4 million Americans, and is associated with female gender, pregnancy, lower socioeconomic status, and age over 65 years, and can follow childbirth or surgery.

☞HSCR: Affected infants frequently present in the first 2 months of life with symptoms of impaired intestinal motility such as failure to pass meconium within the first 48 hours of life (50%-90% of newborns with HSCR), constipation, emesis, abdominal pain or distention, and occasionally diarrhea. Other symptoms of intestinal obstruction can include vomiting and neonatal enterocolitis and rarely, perforation of the gut. However, initial diagnosis of HSCR later in childhood or in adulthood occurs frequently enough that HSCR should be considered if an individual reports lifelong severe constipation. HSCR is due to absence of parasympathetic intrinsic ganglion cells in the submucosal and myenteric plexuses of the gut due to premature arrest of the migration of vagal neural crest cells in the hindgut during gestational development. Its classification is based on the extent of the aganglionic segment of bowel and includes the distal rectum and a variable length of contiguous proximal intestine.

Short-segment disease: Aganglionosis is restricted to the rectosigmoid colon (80% of cases)

Long-segment disease: Aganglionosis extends proximal to the sigmoid colon (15%-20% of cases)

Total colonic aganglionosis: Aganglionosis affects the entire large intestine (5% of cases)

Total intestinal aganglionosis: Aganglionosis extends into the small bowel or even more proximally to encompass the entire bowel (rare)

HSCR is a relatively rare condition, affecting 1:5000 newborns with a male:female ratio of 4:1. HSCR occurs as an isolated finding in 70% of affected individuals, but can be associated with a chromosomal abnormality in 12%. The most common chromosomal abnormality associated with HSCR is Down syndrome (trisomy 21), which occurs in 2% to 10% of all individuals with HSCR. The incidence of HSCR in individuals with Down syndrome is 2% to 15%. Although those with Down syndrome are at a 100-fold higher risk for HSCR than the general population, none of the established *HSCR* genes reside on chromosome 21; thus the association between trisomy 21 and HSCR remains unexplained, although rare HSCR-associated polymorphisms in *RET* and *EDNRB* have been identified in those with Down syndrome who have the condition. Other chromosomal aberrations associated with HSCR include deletions that encompass HSCR-associated genes: Deletion13q22 (*EDNRB*), Deletion10q11.2 (*RET*), and Deletion 2q22 (*ZEB2*). In these cases, associated features vary with the extent of deleted genetic material, but many manifest intellectual disability or developmental delay, distinctive facial features, growth retardation, hypotonia, and heart defects. HSCR is found in association with other congenital anomalies or birth defects in 18% of affected individuals in the absence of obvious chromosomal aberrations; malformations may affect the genitourinary, gastrointestinal, cardiac, and/or central nervous systems (including neuronal migration disorders). There are many syndromic forms of HSCR in which the HSCR is accompanied by other anomalies, and the inheritance pattern is dictated by the causative gene(s) (Table 71-1).

# Screening and Counseling

**Screening:** Screening is generally not indicated for HSCR, unless a first-degree relative of a proband with HSCR has symptoms of severe chronic constipation and has not been tested for HSCR. If a disease-associated mutation or polymorphism has been identified in a proband with HSCR, genetic testing of family members could be considered for prenatal risk counseling, although the low

*Table 71-1 Monogenic Syndromic Forms of HSCR*

| Syndrome | Associated Features | Mode of Inheritance | Chromosomal Locus/Gene Symbol | % With HSCR |
|---|---|---|---|---|
| Bardet-Biedl syndrome | Retinal dystrophy, obesity, ID, polydactyly, hypogenitalism, renal abnormalities | AR | At least 14 loci/genes | 2%-10% |
| Cartilage-hair hypoplasia | Short-limbed dwarfism, sparse hair, immune defects | AR | 9p21-p12/*RMRP* | 7%-9% |
| Congenital central hypoventilation syndrome (CCHS) | Hypoxia, reduced ventilatory drive, neuroblastoma | Variable | 4p12/*PHOX2B* 10q11.2/*RET* 5p13.1-p12/*GDNF* 20q13.2-q13.3/*EDN3* 11p13/*BDNF* 12q22-q23/*ASCL1* | 20% |
| Familial dysautonomia (Riley-Day syndrome) | Sensory and autonomic dysfunction (including abnormal sweat, tear, and saliva production) | AR | 9q31/*IKBKAP* | Unknown |
| Fryns syndrome | Distal digital hypoplasia, diaphragmatic hernia, CHD, craniofacial, ID | AR | Unknown | Unknown |
| Goldberg-Shprintzen megacolon syndrome | Craniofacial, microcephaly, ID, PMG | AR | 10q22.1/*KIAA1279* | Common[a] |
| L1 syndrome | ID, hydrocephalus, ACC, adducted thumbs | XLR | Xq28/*L1CAM* | Rare |
| Multiple endocrine neoplasia 2A (MEN 2A)/ FMTC | MTC, pheo, hyperparathyroidism[b] | AD | 10q11.2/*RET* | ≤1% |
| Multiple endocrine neoplasia 2B (MEN 2B) | MTC, pheo, mucosal and intestinal neuromas, skeletal abnormalities, corneal changes | AD | 10q11.2/*RET* | Rare |
| Mowat-Wilson syndrome | ID, microcephaly, craniofacial, CHD, ACC, epilepsy, short stature | AD | 2q22/*ZEB2* | 67% |
| Pitt-Hopkins syndrome | ID, microcephaly, hyperventilation, epilepsy, craniofacial | AD | 18q21.1/*TCF4* | Unknown |
| Smith-Lemli-Opitz syndrome | ID, hypospadias, 2/3 syndactyly, CHD, craniofacial | AR | 11q12-q13/*DHCR7* | Unknown |
| Waardenburg syndrome type 4 (Waardenburg-Shah syndrome) | Pigmentary abnormalities, deafness | AR (usually) AD | 13q22/*EDNRB* 20q13.2-q13.3/*EDN3* 22q13/*SOX10* | Common Almost 100% |

[a]Limited data are available.

[b]In FMTC, affected individuals do not have pheochromocytoma or hyperparathyroidism.

ACC, agenesis of the corpus callosum; AD, autosomal dominant; AR, autosomal recessive; ASCL1, achaete-scute complex, *Drosophila*, homolog of, 1; BDNF, brain-derived neurotrophic factor; CHD, congenital heart disease; DHCR7, 7-dehydrocholesterol reductase; FMTC, familial medullary thyroid carcinoma; ID, intellectual disability; IKBKAP, inhibitor of kappa light polypeptide gene enhancer in B cells, kinase complex-associated protein; L1CAM, neural cell adhesion molecule L1; MTC, medullary thyroid carcinoma; pheo, pheochromocytoma; PHOX2B, paired-like homeobox 2B; PMG, polymicrogyria; RMRP, RNAse mitochondrial RNA processing; TCF4, transcription factor 4; XLR, X-linked recessive; ZEB2, zinc finger E box-binding homeobox 2.

penetrance and high success rate of surgery typically do not necessitate such approaches.

**Counseling:** Workup for a child with HSCR should include a search for a chromosomal or syndromic cause utilizing a full physical examination, detailed family history (focusing on intestinal obstruction in infants and chronic constipation in adults), and genetic evaluation, typically including karyotype or chromosomal microarray analysis. HSCR is considered a neurocristopathy, and is often accompanied by other manifestations of disordered neural crest development and/or migration, such as pigmentary anomalies, hearing loss, cardiac conotruncal defects, craniofacial abnormalities, and central hypoventilation. If a proband has a chromosome abnormality related to HSCR (most likely accompanied by other congenital malformations and cognitive impairment), testing of parents is recommended to determine if it is de novo or the result of an inherited chromosomal rearrangement. Recurrence risks are based on the status of the parents. If the proband has a Mendelian form of HSCR associated with a syndrome (Table 71-1), testing for

the specific disorder should be considered with appropriate counseling depending on the mode of inheritance. Some individuals with nonsyndromic HSCR have a disease-causing mutation in the *RET* gene (Table 71-2) which can be inherited in an autosomal dominant manner with reduced penetrance of 50% to 70%. Several noncoding polymorphisms in RET also confer an increased or decreased risk of HSCR (Table 71-3), which in at least one case has a differential sex effect. In general, for probands with nonsyndromic HSCR without a clear etiology, HSCR is considered a polygenic disorder with incomplete penetrance, variable expressivity, and a 4:1 male predominance. The overall sibling recurrence risks is approximately 4%, and more precise empiric recurrence risks for HSCR in siblings are based on the length of aganglionic gut (Table 71-4).

☞**GENOTYPE-PHENOTYPE CORRELATIONS:** In general, identified mutations in *RET* and *EDNRB* have not predicted disease severity or extent. However, the presence of two mutations in any of the causative genes (Table 71-2), or the combination of heterozygous mutations in *RET* and *EDNRB* predicts higher penetrance and

---

**Table 71-2 Gene Mutations Associated With Isolated (Nonsyndromic) HSCR**

| Gene (Chromosome Location) | Inheritance | Frequency | Type of HSCR | Penetrance | Putative Mechanism | Mutations Associated With Syndromic Forms of HSCR? (Table 71-1) |
|---|---|---|---|---|---|---|
| *RET* (10q11.2) | AD | 17%-38% | Short segment | 50% for females 70% for males | Haploinsufficiency of tyrosine kinase receptor[a] | Yes |
| | | 70%-80% | Long segment | | | |
| | | 50% | Familial | | | |
| | | 15%-20% | Sporadic | | | |
| *GDNF* (5p13.1-p12) | AD[2] | <1% | Variable | Unknown | Haploinsufficiency of ligand for RET | Yes |
| *NRTN* (19p13.3) | AD[b] | <1% | Variable | Unknown | Haploinsufficiency of ligand for RET | Unknown |
| *EDNRB* (13q22) | AD/AR | 3%-7% | W276C | HSCR in 21% of heterozygotes; HSCR in 74% of homozygotes[c] | G-protein-coupled receptor function impaired | Yes[4] |
| | | | Variable | Unknown | | |
| *EDN3* (20q13.2-q13.3) | AD/AR | 5% | Variable | Unknown | Haploinsufficiency of ligand for EDNRB | Yes[d] |
| *ECE1* (1p36.1) | AD | <1% | Variable | Unknown | Defect in processing enzyme for EDN3 | Unknown |

[a]This does not completely explain the co-occurrence of an activating mutation in a conserved Cys residue that can cause both MEN 2A and HSCR.

[b]A mutation in this gene alone is insufficient to cause disease in most cases, but data are limited.

[c]This mutation is the cause of many but not all cases of HSCR and Waardenburg-Shah syndrome (especially in homozygotes) in the Mennonite population where incidence is 1:500.

[d]The syndromic form (Waardenburg syndrome type 4) is usually associated with homozygous mutations in this gene.

ECE1, endothelin-converting enzyme 1; EDN3, endothelin-3; EDNRB, endothelin B receptor; GDNF, glial cell line-derived neurotrophic factor; NRTN, neurturin; RET, REarranged during Transfection Proto-oncogene.

*Table 71-3 HSCR-Associated Susceptibility Variants*

| Candidate Gene (Chromosome Location) | Associated Variant(s) [effect on protein] (dbSNP) | Relative Risk | Frequency of Risk/Protective Allele | Putative Functional Significance | Associated Disease Phenotype |
|---|---|---|---|---|---|
| RET (10q11.2) | [SNP in −5 position relative to transcription] (rs10900296A>G) + RET +9.7 [intron 1 SNP in enhancer-like sequence] (rs2435357C>T)[a] + E2 [synonymous change p.A45A in exon 2] (rs1800858G>A) | 5.7-fold increase in HSCR susceptibility in males; 2.1-fold increase in susceptibility in females | <5% in Africans; 25% in Europeans; 40% in Chinese (risk allele) | The intron 1 SNP reduces the enhancer activity in vitro | HSCR |
| | E14 [synonymous change p.S836S in exon 14] (rs1800862C>T) + 3′utr [3′ UTR SNP (g.128496T>C)] (rs3026785)[a] | | 4%-8% in European Caucasians; 0% in Chinese (protective allele) | Increase expression of RET by stabilizing the mRNA transcript | Protective against HSCR (these 2 SNPs are in complete linkage disequilibrium) |
| NRG1 (8p12) | [intron 1 A>G of unknown significance] (rs16879552) | odds ratio of 1.68 | 32% in Chinese | NRG1 is expressed in neural crest cells of ENS and is a ligand for a receptor under SOX10 regulation | HSCR |
| | [intron 1 G>C of unknown significance] (rs7835688) | odds ratio of 1.98; increases to 19.53 in combination with RET rs2435357TT allele | 13% in Chinese | | |
| 9q31 | | | | Linked to disease in families with no or hypomorphic RET mutation | Long segment or short segment HSCR; strong family history |
| 3p21 | | | | Linked to increased susceptibility in families (in addition to RET and 19q12) | Short-segment HSCR |
| 19q12 | | | | Linked to increased susceptibility in families (in addition to RET and 3p21) | Short-segment HSCR |
| 16q23 | | | | Linked to increased susceptibility in Mennonite families (with RET and EDNRB) | HSCR |

[a]Predominant polymorphism believed to account for effect.
NRG, neuregulin.

**Table 71-4** *Recurrence Risks for Isolated HSCR Based on Length of Involved Gut*

| Proband | Sib | Risk to sib for HSCR when the proband has | |
|---|---|---|---|
| | | Long-Segment HSCR | Short-Segment HSCR |
| Male | Male | 17% | 5% |
| | Female | 13% | 1% |
| Female | Male | 33% | 5% |
| | Female | 9% | 3% |

more severe HSCR. In addition, two mutations in either *EDNRB* or *EDN3* predicts higher penetrance, more extensive intestinal aganglionosis, and the likelihood of manifestations of Waardenburg syndrome type 4 (WS4), a multisystem syndromic form of HSCR.

## Management and Treatment

***Management of HSCR:*** Surgical resection of the aganglionic segment of bowel and anastomosis of proximal bowel to the anus (transanal "pull-through") is the standard treatment for HSCR and can be performed as a single procedure or in stages. A variety of surgical anastomoses have been developed with the general goal of eliminating obstruction while preserving continence. A one-stage procedure is possible when the diagnosis is made before colonic dilatation occurs (typically, in short-segment disease); otherwise, a primary colostomy is usually necessary.

An effort is generally made to resect a variable length of gut just proximal to the aganglionic zone since this transitional area may have altered pathologic properties (eg, hypoganglionosis) and physiologic properties that are not conducive to normal intestinal motility. However, persistent intestinal dysmotility (usually constipation but sometimes diarrhea) after a pull-through procedure occurs in 10% to 15% of cases and may reflect an underlying abnormality of ganglionic gut that is not understood. Hirschsprung-associated enterocolitis can be a postsurgical complication with significant morbidity, and fistula or stenosis at the anastomosis site can also occur.

Individuals with extensive intestinal aganglionosis who develop irreversible intestinal failure may be candidates for intestinal transplantation.

***Management and Therapeutics of Constipation:*** The therapeutic interventions for chronic constipation depend in part in the suspected underlying etiology, the severity, and the duration. Some general interventions can help relieve symptoms and prevent recurrences.

**Diet:** Increasing fiber consumption to 20 to 35 g per day can help the intestinal tract form soft and bulky stools. Vegetables and fresh fruits, beans, whole grains, and bran cereals are typically high in fiber content. Limiting dietary intake of cheese, meat, ice cream, and processed foods can also be helpful.

**Lifestyle changes:** Increased physical activity, drinking adequate water and other liquids, and not ignoring the urge to have a bowel movement can all help improve symptoms of constipation.

**Laxatives:** Medications can help those individuals who still have constipation in spite of dietary and lifestyle interventions, particularly when used for a limited duration in combination with retraining to establish regular bowel habits. Types include bulk-forming laxatives (psyllium, methylcellulose, calcium polycarbophil), which must be taken with water and work by absorbing water in the intestine to make the stool softer; stool softeners and lubricants (docusate sodium and mineral oil), which moisten and/or grease the stool and prevent dehydration, particularly in the postoperative or postpartum periods; osmotic laxatives (magnesium, polyethylene glycol), which increase osmotic fluid flow through the colon; stimulants (senna, castor oil, bisacodyl), which cause rhythmic contractions of the intestinal musculature; saline laxatives (milk of magnesia), to draw water into the bowel when there is evidence of acute constipation without obstruction; chloride channel activators (lubiprostone), which stimulate intestinal fluid secretion by activating chloride channels, used especially for those with IBS and constipation symptoms. A gradual tapering off of laxatives may be necessary for those individuals who have used them chronically and whose bowels have developed dependence.

**Other agents:** One of the promising groups of therapies encompasses prokinetic agents to modulate the neural tone of the enteric nervous system and increase peristalsis. The best-known example was tegaserod (cisapride), a serotonin receptor agonist which was taken off the market due to concerns of induction of cardiac dysrhythmias. Other prokinetic agents such as combinations of specific serotonin receptor agonists with different serotonin receptor antagonists are under development. These agents could be particularly effective for individuals with slow transit constipation related to autonomic dysfunction involving the myenteric neurons and interstitial cells of Cajal. In some cases, surgery to correct an anorectal problem such as rectal prolapse, or an obstruction, such as in HSCR is warranted. If a medication such as a narcotic is to blame for symptoms of chronic constipation, discontinuing the medication may be effective; some specific opioid antagonists are being developed that target the peripheral receptors to avoid complications from central nervous system (CNS)-related side effects.

**Dyssynergic defecation or pelvic floor dysfunction (PFD):** For individuals with PFD, usually related to the inability to relax the anal sphincter and/or puborectalis muscles to defecate, and often associated with slow colonic transit, biofeedback has been shown to be effective in retraining the pelvic floor and abdominal muscles properly.

***Pharmacogenetics:*** No specific pharmacogenetic associations are known at this time for constipation or HSCR.

## Molecular Genetics and Molecular Mechanisms

The genes associated with isolated or nonsyndromic HSCR fall into two major groups: *RET* and related genes; and *EDNRB* and related genes. There is evidence that genes from these two pathways interact and that additive effects of mutations or variants in genes from both pathways contribute to the pathogenesis of HSCR.

**The RET Gene and Its Ligands:** The tyrosine kinase receptor RET (REarranged during Transfection Proto-oncogene) is expressed by enteric neural precursors after they leave the neural plate and throughout their colonization of the gut. Glial cell line-derived neurotrophic factor (GDNF) and NRTN (or NTN; neurturin) are two of the ligands for RET. Mutations in *GDNF* and *NRTN* have been identified in only a small minority of individuals with HSCR, and in almost all of those individuals, a mutation was also identified in *RET* or another *HSCR* gene, suggesting that mutation in one of the ligands is insufficient by itself to cause disease.

Mutations in *RET* appear to be dominant loss-of-function mutations with incomplete penetrance and variable expressivity. In fact, *RET* mutations alone are estimated to account for 7%-41% of all individuals with HSCR and 70%-80% of those with long-segment disease. Homozygous *RET* mutations have been associated with total colonic aganglionosis in some individuals. A *RET* mutation is identified in approximately 50% of all familial HSCR and 15% to 20% of sporadic HSCR. However almost all families with HSCR show linkage to the *RET* locus. The penetrance of RET mutations is approximately 50% in females and 70% in males. Several candidate loci that may be responsible for the incomplete penetrance and variable expressivity observed in individuals with *RET* mutations have already been identified.

Common polymorphisms in *RET* that do not cause amino acid changes are over-represented within a population of individuals with HSCR, adding further complexity to the task of determining if a sequence variant is a disease-causing mutation. In addition, specific *RET* haplotypes, including polymorphisms in promoter elements and 5′ introns, may also modify the risk of developing HSCR based on differences in RET protein expression, even in the absence of a pathogenic *RET* gene mutation. The most common *RET* polymorphism is found within the first intron in an enhancer region, has low penetrance, and confers differential effects in males and females, possibly explaining the increased incidence in males (Table 71-3). This polymorphism provides insights about a common multifactorial disorder: although it has low penetrance in comparison to *RET* mutations in the coding region, its higher prevalence in the population gives it relatively higher impact; it is likely to act synergistically with coding mutations to affect penetrance of HSCR; and an enhancer variant suggests that additional proteins might interact with this element to strengthen or weaken its effect on *RET* transcription, adding to the potential number of genetic, epigenetic, and/or environmental factors involved in disease causation.

**EDNRB and Related Genes:** The endothelin receptor type B (EDNRB) and its ligand, endothelin-3 (EDN3) are part of another cell signaling pathway that probably interacts with the RET pathway during enteric neural crest colonization. Synthesis of the mature active form of EDN3 requires post-translational modification by endothelin-converting enzyme 1 (encoded by *ECE1*, a gene rarely mutated in HSCR). *EDNRB* and *EDN3* mutations account for approximately 10% of individuals with HSCR. Within the Mennonite community, however, a significant proportion of affected individuals have a missense founder mutation in the *EDNRB* gene (Table 71-2), and some of these individuals have manifestations of WS4. In general, individuals with a heterozygous mutation in *EDNRB* or *EDN3* present with HSCR or occasionally features of WS4, while those with homozygous mutations in either gene are more likely to have more severe manifestations of WS4.

**Other Loci:** Additional genetic loci contributing to HSCR disease susceptibility have been mapped in several different studies, but the associated genes have not yet been identified with the exception of *NRG1* (Table 71-3).

**Recurrence Risks for HSCR:** See Table 71-4.

**Genetic Testing:** Clinical testing for many of the genes associated with syndromic forms of HSCR is available, and should be considered to confirm the diagnosis and inform recurrence risks, depending on the situation. Clinical testing is available for the entire coding region of the *RET* gene by sequence analysis, as well as duplication or deletion testing and prenatal testing in some laboratories. However, the clinical utility of *RET* gene testing is often limited to situations in which nonsyndromic monogenic HSCR is deemed likely and/or there is a strong family history and/or long-segment disease.

**Future Directions:** In the field of research on constipation, there is likely to be an emphasis on developing interventions that target the neurotransmitters and specific channels that govern gut motility. There is renewed interest in serotonergic receptor agonists and antagonists that will be highly specific, safe, and efficacious, without the side effects that caused cisapride to be taken off the market. Other therapies under development include promotility agents, chloride channel activators, guanylyl cyclase C receptor agonists, and opioid antagonists. And the promise of pharmacogenomic approaches lies in the ability to develop individualized therapeutic approaches for genetic differences that may underlie altered gut motility and predispose to chronic constipation.

With regard to future treatments for HSCR, one possibility includes cell therapies derived from neuronal precursor cells in the developing enteric nervous system that can be transplanted to the diseased gut. Equally important, HSCR remains the paradigm of a polygenic disorder with multiple genes and/or genetic pathways involved. Future studies are likely to uncover additional contributing genes, polymorphisms, and variants that allow for a complex but more robust understanding of the role of modifier genes and other factors that affect development of disease and risk assessment calculations. Ultimately, the field of HSCR genetics is likely to yield more insights into the complex migrations that neural crest derivatives make during embryonic gut development as well as the overall function of the enteric nervous system. This is an example where knowledge of a rare condition (HSCR) is likely to inform treatments of a quite common disorder (constipation).

**BIBLIOGRAPHY:**

1. Amiel J, Sproat-Emison E, Garcia-Barcelo M, et al. Hirschsprung disease, associated syndromes and genetics: a review. *J Med Genet.* 2008;45:1-14.

2. Attie T, Pelet A, Edery P, et al. Diversity of RET proto-oncogene mutations in familial and sporadic Hirschsprung disease. *Hum Mol Genet.* 1995;4:1381-1386.

3. Badner JA, Sieber WK, Garver KL, Chakravarti A. A genetic study of Hirschsprung disease. *Am J Hum Genet.* 1990;46:568-580.

4. Bolk S, Pelet A, Hofstra RM, et al. A human model for multigenic inheritance: phenotypic expression in Hirschsprung disease requires both the RET gene and a new 9q31 locus. *Proc Natl Acad Sci USA.* 2000;97:268-273.

5. Constipation. http://digestive.niddk.nih.gov/ddiseases/pubs/constipation/index.aspx. Accessed May 29, 2010.

6. Coran AG, Teitelbaum DH. Recent advances in the management of Hirschsprung's disease. *Am J Surg.* 2000;180:382-387.

7. Crowell MD, Harris LA, Lunsford TN, DiBaise JK. Emerging drugs for chronic constipation. *Expert Opin Emerg Drugs.* 2009;14:493-504.

8. Emison ES, McCallion AS, Kashuk CS, et al. A common sex-dependent mutation in a RET enhancer underlies Hirschsprung disease risk. *Nature*. 2005;434:857-863.

9. Garcia-Barcelo MM, Tang CS, Ngan ES, et al. Genome-wide association study identified NRG1 as a susceptibility locus for Hirschsprung's disease. *Proc Natl Acad Sci USA*. 2009;106:2694-2699.

10. Griseri P, Lantieri F, Puppo F, et al. A common variant located in the 3′UTR of the RET gene is associated with protection from Hirschsprung disease. *Hum Mutat*. 2007;28:168-176.

11. Kapur RP. Practical pathology and genetics of Hirschsprung's disease. *Semin Pediatr Surg*. 2009;18:212-223.

12. Lantieri F, Griseri P, Ceccherini I. Molecular mechanisms of RET-induced Hirschsprung pathogenesis. *Ann Med*. 2006;38:11-19.

13. Moore SW. Down syndrome and the enteric nervous system. *Pediatr Surg Int*. 2008;24:873-883.

14. Parisi MA. Hirschsprung disease overview. In: Pagon RA, Bird TC, Dolan CR, Stephens K, eds. *GeneReviews [Internet]*. Seattle, WA: University of Washington, Seattle; 1993-2010. 2002 Jul 12 [updated 2006 Dec 26].

15. Parisi MA, Kapur RP. Genetics of Hirschsprung disease. *Curr Opin Pediatr*. 2000;12:610-617.

16. Puffenberger EG, Hosoda K, Washington SS, et al. A missense mutation of the endothelin-B receptor gene in multigenic Hirschsprung's disease. *Cell*. 1994;79:1257-1266.

17. Ryan ET, Ecker JL, Christakis NA, Folkman J. Hirschsprung's disease: associated abnormalities and demography. *J Pediatr Surg*. 1992;27:76-81.

18. Sarioglu A, Tanyel FC, Buyukpamukcu N, Hicsonmez A. Hirschsprung-associated congenital anomalies. *Eur J Pediatr Surg*. 1997;7:331-337.

## Supplementary Information

**OMIM** REFERENCES:

[1] Hirschsprung Disease, Susceptibility to, 1; HSCR 1; RET (#142623)

[2] Hirschsprung Disease, Susceptibility to, 2; HSCR 2, EDNRB (#600155)

[3] Hirschsprung Disease, Susceptibility to, 3; HSCR 3, GDNF (#600837)

[4] Hirschsprung Disease, Susceptibility to, 4; HSCR 4, EDN3 (#131242)

**Alternative Names:**

- Hirschsprung Disease; HSCR
- Aganglionic Megacolon
- Megacolon, Aganglionic; MGC

*Key Words:* Constipation, Hirschsprung disease, RET gene, EDNRB gene, aganglionosis, motility

# 72 The Hereditary Hemochromatoses

David G. Brooks

## KEY POINTS

- *Disease summary:*
  - Iron is an essential dietary mineral that can become toxic when present in excess quantities or in a reactive state.
  - Hereditary hemochromatosis (HHC) is defined as a biochemical state of iron overload complicated by end-organ dysfunction such as diabetes, cirrhosis, or cardiomyopathy.
  - It is critical to recognize the general presenting symptoms or family history of HHC as this disease can be fatal if undiagnosed, but is the rare genetic disease that can be cured if detected and treated early.
  - The HHCs are a group of monogenic diseases with a common pathophysiology that features disruption of mechanisms regulating iron homeostasis resulting in excess iron accumulation.
  - The most common, classical form of the disease is type 1 or *HFE*-linked HHC which accounts for 80% of cases in Caucasian populations. The other types are rare and panethnic.
  - There are four other well-defined types of hereditary hemochromatosis caused by loss-of-function mutations in five genes.
  - The common pathophysiology underlying HHC is failure to prevent a rise in blood iron levels as evidenced by the fact that all five proteins either sense or control the level of iron.

- *Hereditary basis:*
  - Iron overload should only be attributed to hereditary causes after ruling out comorbid conditions such as other etiologies of liver disease or anemia that lead to secondary iron overload.
  - Types 1 to 3 HHC are autosomal recessive and result from loss-of-function mutations.
  - Type 4 is autosomal dominant due to heterozygous mutations of ferroportin with two distinct genotype-phenotype manifestations.

- *Differential diagnosis:*
  - The key is to distinguish uncomplicated iron overload from complicated iron overload that includes HHC.
  - It is imperative to differentiate other causes of liver disease where iron accumulation is secondary (eg, alcoholic or hepatitis virus cirrhosis) from HHC.
  - Other genetic disorders such as anemias and porphyria cutanea tarda are associated with secondary iron overload but have additional features that distinguish them from HHC.

## Diagnostic Criteria and Clinical Characteristics

### Diagnostic Criteria for HHC:

**All of the following**

- Primary iron overload usually evidenced as elevated plasma iron and transferrin saturation with hyperferritinemia without other identifiable cause of iron accumulation (Fig. 72-1).
- Evidence of organ dysfunction is highlighted earlier in Table 72-1. Most commonly this manifests as transaminitis, diabetes, impotence, arthritis, and arrhythmias.
- To prove hereditary etiology there must be evidence of two mutations in the same gene in types 1 to 3 or a single ferroportin mutation in type 4 disease (Table 72-2). In classical (type 1 disease), it is imperative that patients with two *HFE* mutations have *not* been misdiagnosed with HHC because the majority will not go on to develop disease due to reduced penetrance (see Counseling).

**And the absence of**

- Other comorbid conditions that could explain the iron overload.

**Clinical Characteristics:** There is no mechanism of active iron excretion, therefore regulating iron absorption from the intestine is the key in iron homeostasis; blood loss and pregnancy or lactation are the only proven mechanisms of iron loss and hence women are protected against HHC by menstrual bleeding until menopause.

The majority of daily iron needs are for erythropoiesis. Most iron to support RBC production is recycled from breakdown of old RBCs by the reticuloendothelial system with a minor component from dietary iron. The essential problem in type 1 HHC is slow, steady absorption of excess dietary iron such that by middle age (40s in men and 50s in women) there is not only iron overload but also end-organ damage. Thus, it is entry of iron into the blood that is in excess of that required to support erythropoiesis that is the initiating event in iron overload and hence HHC.

After transferrin is 100% saturated, nontransferrin-bound iron deposits quickly in the parenchyma of a characteristic set of organs as listed in Table 72-1. Iron accumulation in parenchymal cells triggers release of ferritin, resulting in hyperferritinemia, the degree of which is positively correlated with the degree of iron loading. The hallmarks of type 2 or juvenile hemochromatosis include early onset (<30 years of age) of massive iron overload causing cardiac and endocrine failure; there may not be sufficient time to result in liver failure.

## Screening and Counseling

**Screening:** The essential feature of all hemochromatoses is iron overload. For two reasons, screening for these disorders should be done with clinical chemistry tests for blood iron and not with genetic tests. First, there are widely available and affordable tests

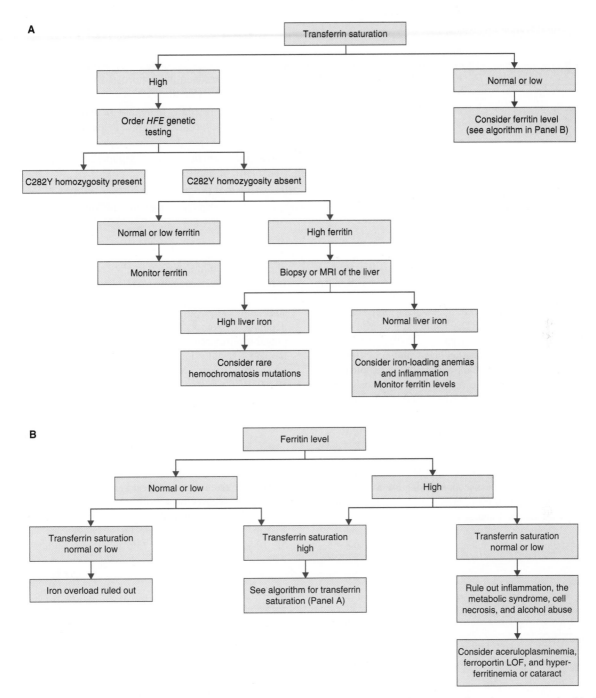

*Figure 72-1* Algorithm for Screening of Patients for Possible Iron Overload. (Adapted from Fleming R and Ponka P. Iron overload in human disease. *N Engl J Med* 2012; 366:348-59).

for serum iron that have excellent validity. Second, only the most common variety of hemochromatosis (type 1) is prevalent enough amongst Caucasians to merit consideration of screening by genetic testing. Furthermore, type 1 HHC features low penetrance (see Counseling), and thus *HFE* genetic testing does not warrant use as a screening test unless it is performed in an enriched population such as those with a very high local allele frequency as occur in some northwestern European populations.

Screening has an important role because of the general nonspecific presenting complaints of hemochromatosis and its curability

if detected early. The algorithm shown in Fig. 72-1 represents the best opportunity for screening by detecting signs of iron overload in the blood, followed by screening for other organs if evidence of abnormal blood iron parameters.

***Counseling:*** Type 1 HHC is almost always associated with homozygosity for the single founder *HFE* mutation *G845A*, encoding *C282Y* in the HFE protein. However, it is imperative *not* to diagnose patients harboring this genotype with hemochromatosis on the basis of genotype alone. They may have a predisposition to iron overload but without end-organ complications from iron,

*Table 72-1* **Organ System Involvement of HHC**

| System | Manifestation |
|---|---|
| Liver | Hepatocytic iron accumulation, hepatomegaly, transaminitis, fibrosis that can progress to cirrhosis, hepatocellular carcinoma, transplant, or death |
| Endocrine | Endocrine pancreatic islet cell iron accumulation resulting in insulin insufficiency and diabetes; anterior pituitary iron accumulation resulting in gonadotropin deficiency, impotence, and premature menopause |
| Heart | Iron accumulation triggering arrhythmia and restrictive cardiomyopathy and in juvenile hemochromatosis heart failure, transplant, or death |
| Joints | Synovial cell iron accumulation, arthropathy that progresses to chronic arthritis |
| Skin | Iron accumulation resulting in excess melanin production resulting in "bronze" appearance |

they do not meet criteria for HHC. This is because of incomplete penetrance. Evidence of increasing blood iron as "biochemical penetrance" of C282Y homozygosity is observed in 36% to 76% of homozygotes. However, evidence of end-organ complications is only observed in 2% to 38% of C282Y homozygous men and 1% to 10% of C282Y homozygous women.

When counseling patients and families with type 1 HHC it is critical to remember that it is iron overload that is important, not simply the inheritance of genetic variants that may or may not be penetrant. Hence, the counseling can be directive only in the setting of established iron overload with end-organ complications. It is prudent to counsel patients, especially males, with any *C282Y* alleles to avoid dietary iron supplements since they are protected against iron deficiency.

**Genotype-Phenotype Correlation:** Simple C282Y heterozygosity is common in Caucasians, approaching 6% to 10% allele frequency in some populations of northern European gene pools and cannot be considered causal of clinically significant body iron excess. Patients with this genotype may have a phenotype of relative resistance to iron deficiency anemia from a biochemical phenotype of mild increased iron absorption. Controversy exists regarding the very common *H63D* allele. In heterozygotes it confers no phenotype. In homozygotes the penetrance is so low that some authors have argued against attributing iron overload to this genotype without excluding all other possible causes. In compound heterozygotes (C282Y or H63D), the observed phenotype is one of steadily increasing transferrin saturation and ferritin levels rather than clinically significant iron overload (type 1 HHC).

## Management and Treatment

Management of HHCs is critical since symptomatic patients without treatment have a 5-year survival of 10%. The therapeutic strategy focuses on restoring iron homeostasis to the body through therapeutic bloodletting (phlebotomy), a highly efficient way to remove iron from the body. Phlebotomy can increase the 10-year survival rate to 75% in patients with cirrhosis and

*Table 72-2* **Molecular Genetic Testing**

| Gene | Class | Type and Inheritance | Mutation Type | Detection Rate |
|---|---|---|---|---|
| *HFE* | HFE linked | 1 = classical hemochromatosis, AR | *C282Y, H63D* plus rarer *S65C, R66C, I105T, R224G, V295A,* frameshift and deletions | C282Y & H63D common; other rare |
| *HFE2 (HJV)* | Hemojuvelin linked | 2A = juvenile hemochromatosis, AR | Typically homozygous private | Rare |
| *HAMP* | Hepcidin linked | 2B = juvenile hemochromatosis, AR | Private homozygous & compound heterozygous mutations | Rare |
| *TFR2* | Transferrin receptor 2 linked | 3 = juvenile hemochromatosis, AR | Private homozygous & compound heterozygous mutations | Very rare |
| *SLC40A1* (LOF) | Ferroportin linked | 4A = ferroportin disease, AD | *V162del, D157G, G80S, G490D* | Rare |
| *SLC40A1* (GOF) | Hepcidin-resistant ferroportin linked | 4B = hepcidin-resistant hemochromatosis, AD | *C326S/Y>N144D/T, Y64N* | Rare |

AR, autosomal recessive; AD, autosomal dominant; LOF, loss-of-function; GOF, gain-of-function.

normalize the life span in those without fibrosis. Iron chelator medications are available but are indicated in secondary iron overload (often due to recurrent transfusions for anemia), where phlebotomy is not appropriate. The efficacy, safety, and low cost of phlebotomy make it an appropriate modality for all primary iron overload disorders.

Iron is typically limiting for erythropoiesis thus phlebotomy can be performed at more frequent intervals on patients with hemochromatosis than from normal individuals. Patients with severe iron loading can tolerate weekly or biweekly phlebotomy without anemia for months to years. A running total of units of blood removed with corresponding hemoglobin level should be maintained. Each unit of blood removes 200 to 250 mg of iron, depending on the hemoglobin. Serum iron indices should be checked periodically during phlebotomy therapy. Goals include achieving a ferritin level below 50 ng/mL and transferrin saturation below 30%. After these goals have been reached, maintenance phlebotomy two to five times each year is typically required to prevent reaccumulation of iron.

Since the source of excess iron is dietary, removing iron supplements from the diet of a patient with hemochromatosis is imperative. Avoidance of vitamin C supplements is prudent since it aids absorption of iron. It is important for patients with evidence of liver disease to avoid other hepatotoxins such as alcohol. Iron is a growth-limiting nutrient in the pathogen *Vibrio*. Iron-loaded patients are advised to avoid raw seafood and shellfish from warm waters because of the increased risk for *Vibrio* infection and sepsis.

## Molecular Genetics and Molecular Mechanism

The underlying pathophysiology in HHC features disruption of the hepcidin-ferroportin axis. Most iron-overload disorders are associated with decreased hepcidin production; iron absorption and circulating hepcidin level are inversely correlated. This is because hepcidin, the "iron hormone," is produced in the liver and is sensitive to iron status within hepatocytes. Hepcidin controls the activity of ferroportin by attaching to it and targeting the protein for destruction in the lysosome. Since ferroportin is critical for exporting iron out of both the absorptive epithelium of the intestine and the reticuloendothelial cells, its downregulation by hepcidin decreases blood iron. Failure to downregulate ferroportin (eg, by abrogation of iron sensing) and hence hepcidin production leads to excess iron in blood which if left unchecked increases risk for hemochromatosis.

Type 4 HHC is also known as ferroportin disease and has two clinically and molecularly distinct subtypes. When mutations disrupt ferroportin-mediated iron export in subtype A, iron accumulates in reticuloendothelial macrophages and paradoxically is associated with low plasma iron. This manifests clinically as elevated splenic iron (compared to hepatic iron) by magnetic resonance imaging (MRI). This is a clinically mild form of iron overload with some patients having minimal symptoms despite extremely high (>2000 µg/L) ferritin values. Some experts have argued that type 4 HHC is an iron-overload disorder but not a hemochromatosis disorder because of the paucity of typical end-organ damage. In contrast, subtype B ferroportin mutations prevent hepcidin binding. Despite high serum hepcidin levels, patients develop iron overload and manifestations of HHC (Table 72-1).

***Genetic Testing:*** Genetic testing for *HFE*-linked hemochromatosis is widely available. Testing for the other, rarer types is available at specialty laboratories. Utility of testing is modest because biochemical measures of iron status can be used to diagnose and manage HHC.

## Bibliography:

1. Fleming R, Ponka P. Iron overload in human disease. *N Engl J Med.* 2012;366:348-359.

2. Brissot P, Bardou-Jacquet E, Troadec MB, et al. Molecular diagnosis of genetic iron-overload disorders. *Expert Rev Mol Diagn.* 2010;10(6):755-763.

3. Camaschella C, Poggiali E. Inherited disorders of iron metabolism. *Curr Opin Pediatr.* 2011;23:14-20.

4. Pietrangelo A. Hereditary hemochromatosis: pathogenesis, diagnosis and treatment. *Gastroenterology.* 2010;139:393-408.

5. Nadakkavukaran IM, Gan EK, Olynyk JK. Screening for hereditary haemochromatosis. *Pathology.* 2012;44:148-152.

6. Siddique A, Kowdley KV. Review article: the iron overload syndromes. *Aliment Pharmacol Ther.* 2012;35:876-893.

## Supplementary Information

### OMIM References:

[1] Condition; Gene Name (OMIM#)

[2] Type 1 Hereditary Hemochromatosis; HFE (#235200)

[3] Type 2A Juvenile Hemochromatosis; HJV (#602390)

[4] Type 2B Juvenile Hemochromatosis; HAMP (#613313)

[5] Type 3 Juvenile Hemochromatosis; TFR2 (#604250)

[6] Types 4A and B Hereditary Hemochromatosis; SLC40A1 (#606069)

### Alternative Name:
- Bronze Diabetes

***Key Words:*** Iron overload, transferrin saturation, ferritin, therapeutic phlebotomy

# 73 Wilson Disease

Eve A. Roberts

## KEY POINTS

- *Disease summary:*
  - Wilson disease (WD) is a disorder of hepatic copper disposition caused by mutations in the gene *ATP7B*, on chromosome 13, which encodes a metal-transporting $P_1$-type ATPase, known as the Wilson ATPase. In hepatocytes the Wilson ATPase assists in moving copper across intracellular membranes, which directly contributes to production of ceruloplasmin, a ferroxidase that is functional only when copper is incorporated. Additionally, the Wilson ATPase expedites excretion of copper into bile. Accordingly, in WD serum concentrations of ceruloplasmin are low and hepatic retention of copper develops, leading to liver injury. With progression of liver disease, copper spills out of the liver and accumulates in other organs, such as the brain, eyes, renal tubules, heart, and synovial membranes. Untreated WD is a progressive degenerative disease, nearly always associated with early death.
  - WD occurs worldwide, but it is rare. The average prevalence is 30 affected persons per million population, with a corresponding carrier frequency of approximately 1 in 90. More than 500 mutations have been identified, and 80% of affected individuals are compound heterozygotes. In some populations (including Iceland, Korea, Japan, Sardinia, and the Canary Islands) where the incidence in higher, there may also be a relatively circumscribed set of mutations. In northeastern Europe, the mutation *H1069Q* is found as at least one of the mutations in 35% to 75% of WD patients.
- *Hereditary basis:*
  - Autosomal recessive
- *Differential diagnosis (limited to principal disorders):*
  - **Hepatic**
    - Causes of elevated serum aminotransferases: chronic hepatitis B, chronic hepatitis C, nonalcoholic fatty liver disease (NAFLD), alcoholic hepatitis, alpha-1-antitrypsin deficiency, any drug-induced liver injury
    - Fatty liver: NAFLD, alcoholic liver disease, various rare metabolic disorders
    - Acute hepatitis: acute hepatitis A, B, C, E; cytomegalovirus (CMV), Epstein-Barr virus (EBV), human herpes virus 6 (HHV-6); unknown virus(es)
    - Autoimmune hepatitis-like: autoimmune hepatitis type 1 or 2, primary sclerosing cholangitis (with an autoimmune sclerosing cholangitis pattern)
    - Cirrhosis: principal causes of cirrhosis are covered already; other rare metabolic disorders (eg, citrullinemia type 2—mainly in East Asians)
    - Gallstones: cholesterol gallstones, typically idiopathic
    - Fulminant hepatic failure presentation: highly characteristic of WD but causes of acute liver failure require attention
  - **Neurologic**
    - Parkinson disease
    - Choreoathetosis—other causes
    - Pseudobulbar palsy—other causes
    - Tremors—other causes
    - Dysarthria—other causes
    - Familial dysautonomia
    - Epilepsy—other causes
  - **Psychiatric**
    - Organic brain syndromes
    - Primary causes of neuroses

## Diagnostic Criteria and Clinical Characteristics

### Diagnostic Criteria:

- **Genetic diagnosis:** identification of two disease-causing mutations in *ATP7B* (80% of patients are compound heterozygotes) or identification of homozygosity for one disease-causing mutation
- **Clinical diagnosis:** presence of hepatic or neurologic disorder consistent with WD + basal 24-hour urinary copper excretion greater than 0.6 μmol/d (>40 μg/d) + hepatic parenchymal copper concentration greater than 250 μg/g dry wgt

- Serum ceruloplasmin less than 50 mg/L is highly supportive of the diagnosis; serum ceruloplasmin less than 140 mg/L is highly consistent with the diagnosis; serum ceruloplasmin greater than 140 mg/L is still compatible with the diagnosis (serum ceruloplasmin may be normal).
- Employing greater than 0.6 μmol/d (>40 μg/d) as the threshold for diagnosing Wilson disease is more effective diagnostically than the previous customary value of 1.6 μmol/d (100 μg/d), which fails to identify 20% to 25% of patients. The diagnostic effectiveness of greater than 0.6 μmol/d (>40 μg/d) is particularly evident with pediatric patients.
- Hepatic parenchymal copper measurement greater than 100 μg/g dry wgt is consistent with the diagnosis; hepatic parenchymal

copper concentration greater than 70 μg/g dry wgt warrants further investigation; liver biopsy may be dangerous in patients with hepatic decompensation (coagulopathy and/or thrombocytopenia) and carries a 1/10,000 mortality rate overall; lack of facilities for performing the biopsy or for analyzing parenchymal copper content may also militate against obtaining this diagnostic information.

- Histologic findings on liver biopsy may also contribute to making the diagnosis of Wilson disease. These findings may include steatosis, glycogenated nuclei in hepatocytes, focal hepatocellular necrosis, fibrosis, or cirrhosis. Transmission electron microscopy may reveal changes in mitochondrial structure (variable shape and size, dilated tips of the mitochondrial cristae, dark bodies in the matrix) which are almost exclusively found with Wilson disease. Stainable copper is not a reliable diagnostic feature because it is a late finding and can also be found with severe cholestasis.
- Evidence of Kayser-Fleischer rings by slit-lamp examination by a competent specialist (present in ~60% of adults with hepatic Wilson disease and in ~90%-95% of adults with neurologic Wilson disease) is highly supportive of the diagnosis—note that Kayser-Fleischer rings may be present in various sorts of severe cholestatic liver disease.
- 24-hour urinary excretion after D-penicillamine challenge has been validated only in children. Contrary to the initial report, its diagnostic reliability is only moderate (not invariable).
- Head MR may reveal characteristic findings of WD, namely, the "face of the giant panda" in the midbrain on T2-weighted images. Basal ganglia abnormalities (high-signal intensity on T2, low-signal intensity on T1) may also be detected. Similar head MR findings may be found in other neurologic disorders including Leigh disease, hypoxic-ischemic encephalopathy, methanol poisoning, certain types of encephalitis, and extrapontine myelinolysis due to osmotic disequilibrium syndrome. MR is preferred to computerized tomography (CT).
- Incorporation of radioactive copper into ceruloplasmin is no longer utilized; incorporation of a nonradioactive isotope of copper into ceruloplasmin is unreliable as a diagnostic test.

**And the absence of**

- Definitive diagnosis of any hepatic, neurologic, or psychiatric disease in the extended differential diagnosis.

*Comment*: Note that the rare patient has been found who has both Wilson disease and autoimmune hepatitis, as well as a few patients with acute viral hepatitis superimposed on Wilson disease; also note that some patients with both nonalcoholic fatty liver disease and Wilson disease are bound to exist on a statistical basis; note that excluding all possible non-Wilsonian neurologic and psychiatric disorders may be extremely difficult.

*Clinical Characteristics:* WD is clinically pleiomorphic (Table 73-1). It can present principally as hepatic, neurologic, or psychiatric disease. The usual age range for clinical presentation is 5 to 45 years; younger individuals tend to have hepatic disease. WD mainly with a neurologic presentation has been newly diagnosed in older adults. Differentiation from other chronic liver disorders in young adults, such as autoimmune hepatitis, is important because treatment is different. Particularly in adults, differentiation from relatively benign neurologic problems, such as familial tremor, is critically important. Subtle presentations include episodes of self-limited jaundice due to transient hemolysis (not liver disease) and an obstetric history of repeated spontaneous abortions (Table 73-2).

With respect to hepatic disease, Wilson disease involves a spectrum severity from asymptomatic to acute liver failure. In some individuals, persistent asymptomatic hepatomegaly or nonspecific elevation of serum aminotransferases may be the earliest finding. Hepatic steatosis may occur, occasionally massive enough to resemble nonalcoholic fatty liver disease; this is diagnostically problematic if the individual is also overweight or obese. Some patients have acute hepatitis of only moderate severity, most often with features typical of autoimmune hepatitis (elevated serum IgG, positive nonspecific autoantibodies such as antismooth muscle antibody). Many patients still present with severe chronic liver disease: a small, shrunken cirrhotic liver, splenomegaly, and ascites. Wilsonian fulminant hepatic failure is a dramatic and distinctive clinical presentation. Widespread hepatocellular apoptosis releases copper into the bloodstream, where it destroys erythrocyte membranes and causes renal tubulopathy. Features are characteristic: severe Coombs-negative intravascular hemolysis, rapidly progressive renal dysfunction, comparatively low (200-1500 U/L) serum aminotransferases, and strikingly subnormal serum alkaline phosphatase. Serum copper is normal or elevated, and urinary copper is extremely elevated. Since the typical patient is unaware of having WD, the working diagnosis is acute viral or drug hepatitis. Delay in obtaining biochemical determinations relating to serum copper levels and 24-hour urinary copper excretion forces a clinical diagnosis so that appropriate treatment (liver transplantation) can be organized. Arithmetic formulations of routine laboratory data may help to point to the diagnosis of WD (Table 73-2).

Neurologic presentation of WD is usually with movement disorders (such as tremor) or with rigid dystonia resembling a Parkinsonian disorder (impassive facies, slowed ambulation, and drooling). Patients may have illegible, small, cramped handwriting. Unusual clumsiness for age may be identified by direct questioning. It is uncommon to have epilepsy as part of WD, but seizures may occur.

Psychiatric disorders may be the dominant clinical feature in approximately 20% of patients. Severe depression or various neurotic behavior patterns are typical. Frank psychosis is uncommon but a presentation resembling schizophrenia may occur. WD may be the cause of debilitating chronic psychiatric disease which has not been diagnosed definitively.

## Screening and Counseling

*Screening:* Screening is absolutely required for all sibs of a patient diagnosed with WD. The screening algorithm is somewhat different from algorithm for diagnosis, since its purpose is to identify individuals who may have WD and should therefore undergo more extensive clinical investigation.

Assessment of first-degree relatives should include medical history relating to jaundice, liver disease, and features of neurologic involvement; physical examination; serum copper, ceruloplasmin, liver function tests including aminotransferases, albumin, conjugated and unconjugated bilirubin; slit-lamp examination of the eyes for Kayser-Fleischer rings; basal 24-hour urinary copper. Anyone with abnormal findings requires further investigation, although the disorder may prove to be other than WD. Individuals without Kayser-Fleischer rings who have subnormal ceruloplasmin and abnormal liver tests may require liver biopsy to confirm the diagnosis. If available, molecular testing for *ATP7B* mutations or haplotype studies should be obtained and may be used as

*Table 73-1  System Involvement*

| System | Manifestation | Occurrence |
|---|---|---|
| Hepatic | • Asymptomatic hepatomegaly<br>• Isolated splenomegaly<br>• Persistently elevated serum aminotransferases<br>• Fatty liver<br>• Acute hepatitis of moderate severity<br>• Resembling autoimmune hepatitis<br>• Cirrhosis—compensated or decompensated<br>• Fulminant hepatic failure<br>• Gallstones (related to hemolysis) | Common (Wilsonian fulminant hepatic failure is uncommon, accounting for 5% of all acute liver failure) |
| Neurologic | • Movement disorders (tremor, involuntary movements)<br>• Drooling, dysarthria<br>• Rigid dystonia<br>• Pseudobulbar palsy<br>• Dysautonomia<br>• Migraine headaches<br>• Insomnia<br>• Seizures | Common |
| Psychiatric | • Depression<br>• Neurotic behavior patterns, including anxiety disorders<br>• Psychosis | Approximately 20% (psychosis less common) |
| Ocular | • Kayser-Fleischer (K-F) rings<br>• Sunflower cataracts | K-F rings: approximately 50% |
| Hematologic | Episodic hemolytic anemia, self-limited | Fairly common |
| Cutaneous | Lunulae ceruleae | Rare |
| Renal | • Aminoaciduria (renal Fanconi syndrome)<br>• Nephrolithiasis | Fairly common |
| Skeletal | • Premature osteoporosis<br>• Arthritis<br>• Rickets (related to renal disease) | Fairly common |
| Cardiac | • Cardiomyopathy<br>• Dysrhythmias | Uncommon |
| Pancreas | Pancreatitis | Rare |
| Endocrine | Hypoparathyroidism | Rare |
| OB-GYN | • Menstrual irregularities<br>• Infertility<br>• Repeated miscarriages | Not uncommon |

primary screening. Treatment should be initiated for all individuals over 3 years old identified as having Wilson disease by family screening. CT or MR imaging of the brain, not necessarily part of the screening process, should be obtained in those with presymptomatic WD as a baseline.

**Counseling:**

**Inheritance:** autosomal recessive with variable expression

☞GENOTYPE-PHENOTYPE CORRELATION: There is abundant evidence, from clinical experience and laboratory models, to show that mutations severely limiting the function of the Wilson ATPase are associated with early severe disease, which is usually hepatic.

## Management and Treatment

Availability of oral chelators from the mid-1950s onward dramatically improved the outlook for patients with WD, transforming it from a disease which was invariably fatal to one compatible with a productive life of normal or near-normal duration. The clinical outcome is best if treatment is started when the patient is still presymptomatic. Once started, treatment is lifelong (Table 73-3). Stopping treatment is associated with clinical deterioration, usually severe. The deterioration may not reverse on recommencing treatment. Treatment needs to be maintained during pregnancy; however, substituting trientine or zinc for D-penicillamine may be required. WD cannot be managed by diet alone. Copper-rich foods (organ meats, shellfish, nuts, chocolate, and mushrooms) should be avoided in the first year of treatment and taken sparingly thereafter. Vegetarians need supervision by a dietician since legumes, a mainstay of such diets, are high in copper. Patients with WD are best advised to abstain from alcohol. They should also maintain a healthy lifestyle: a well-balanced diet to keep body weight in a normal range and avoid abdominal obesity, and regular weightbearing exercise to ensure bone health. The benefit of antioxidants such as vitamin E has not been established through adequate clinical

**Table 73-2** *Algorithm for Diagnosis of an Adult Patient With Wilson Disease*

| Baseline Testing | Outcome | Further Action |
|---|---|---|
| **Adult with unexplained liver disease (liver enlargement, or abnormal liver biochemistries/synthetic function, or cirrhosis of undiagnosed etiology)—exclusive of apparent acute liver failure** | | |
| Serum copper, ceruloplasmin (CP); 24-h urine collection for basal 24-h urinary copper excretion; slit-lamp examination for Kayser-Fleischer (KF) rings | No abnormal findings<br>→ diagnosis of Wilson disease excluded════════════⟶ | Reassess at 6-month intervals if any doubts persist as to possibility of Wilson disease |
| | KF rings present; basal 24-h urinary Cu excretion >0.6 μmol (>40 μg/d); serum CP<140 mg/L<br>→ diagnosis very likely═══════⟶ | Commence treatment *or*[a] proceed to molecular testing and commence treatment, if confirmatory |
| | KF rings present; basal 24-h urinary Cu excretion >0.6 μmol; serum CP ≥140 mg/L (may be normal)<br>→ obtain molecular testing *or*[a] proceed to liver biopsy, if safe, for histology and hepatic copper quantification<br>• Hepatic copper >250 μg/g dry wgt → diagnosis confirmed=⟶<br>• Hepatic copper <250 μg/g dry wgt → diagnosis uncertain══⟶ | Commence treatment<br><br>Get molecular testing if not yet done *or*[a] reassess clinically |
| | KF rings absent; basal 24-h urinary Cu excretion >0.6 μmol; serum CP <140 mg/L<br>→ obtain molecular testing *or*[a] proceed to liver biopsy, if safe, for hepatic copper quantification<br>• Hepatic copper <50 μg/g dry wgt → Wilson disease excluded═══════════⟶<br>• Hepatic copper 51-250 μg/g dry wgt → Wilson disease possible═══════════⟶<br>• Hepatic copper >250 μg/g dry wgt → diagnosis confirmed=⟶ | Investigate alternative diagnoses<br>Get molecular testing, if not already obtained<br>Commence treatment |
| | KF rings absent; basal 24-h urinary Cu excretion <0.6 μmol; serum CP <140 mg/L<br>→ uncertain for Wilson disease: ascertain that urine collection was complete; if so, proceed to liver biopsy, if safe, for histology and hepatic copper quantification depending on histologic findings=⟶ | Evaluate hepatic copper quantification as above |
| **Adult with unexplained neurologic or psychiatric disease consistent with Wilson disease** | | |
| Image CNS by CT or MR (preferred); check liver biochemistries: AST, ALT, ALP, total and conjugated bilirubin, albumin, INR + CBC<br>Serum copper, ceruloplasmin (CP); 24-h urine collection for basal 24-h urinary copper excretion; slit-lamp examination for KF rings | • Head CT or MR may be normal or show characteristic features of Wilson disease═══════⟶<br>• Liver biochemistries may disclose unsuspected liver involvement═══════════⟶ | Retain as baseline or critical data<br>Liver sonography (ultrasound) and evaluate as above for hepatic presentation |
| **Adult sib of any adult newly diagnosed with Wilson disease** | | |
| Institute screening protocol without delay | (See text) | |

[a]Choice here depends on availability of timely, expert molecular testing.

The diagnostic algorithm for diagnosis of Wilsonian fulminant hepatic failure is entirely separate; special considerations apply; the diagnostic process is urgent and somewhat abbreviated; immediate consultation with a liver transplant team is absolutely required.

*Table 73-3 Drug Treatment of Adult Patient With Wilson Disease*

| Drug | Mode of Action; Dose | Neurologic Deterioration | Potential Side Effects | Other Issues |
|---|---|---|---|---|
| D-penicillamine | General chelator induces cupruria Typical adult dose: 500 mg bid or tid Maximum dose: 20 mg/kg/d; reduce by 25% when clinically stable | 10%-20% during initial phase of treatment | • *Initial hypersensitivity reaction*: fever, rash, proteinuria<br>• Lupus-like reaction<br>• Aplastic anemia<br>• Leukopenia<br>• Thrombocytopenia<br>• Nephrotic syndrome<br>• Degenerative changes in skin<br>• Elastosis perforans serpiginosa<br>• Serous retinitis<br>• Hepatotoxicity | Initial tolerability may be improved by starting with 250 mg daily and increasing dose by 250 mg every 3-4 days until target dose is reached. Should be stopped in any patient experiencing the *initial hypersensitivity reaction* and another drug substituted. Classified as a teratogen (actual risk in women with Wilson disease difficult to determine) Reduce dose slightly for surgery to promote wound healing and during pregnancy (if continued during pregnancy). Monitoring[a]: basal 24-h urinary Cu excretion (target is 200-500 μg/24 h [3-5 μmol/24-h]), complete blood count, urinalysis |
| Trientine | General chelator induces cupruria Typical adult dose: 500 mg or 600 mg bid Maximum dose: 20 mg/kg/d; reduce by 25% when clinically stable | 10%-15% during initial phase of treatment | • Gastritis<br>• Aplastic anemia rare<br>• Sideroblastic anemia | Reduce dose for surgery to promote wound healing and during pregnancy Safety in pregnancy has not been established. Monitoring[a]: basal 24-h urinary Cu excretion (target is 200-500 μg/24 h [3-5 μmol/24 h]), complete blood count, urinalysis |
| Zinc | Metallothionein inducer, blocks intestinal absorption of copper Usual adult dose: 50 mg elemental Zn three times daily *minimum* dose in adults: 50 mg elemental Zn twice daily | Can occur during initial phase of treatment, but uncommon | • Gastritis; biochemical pancreatitis<br>• Zinc accumulation<br>• Possible changes in immune function | No dosage reduction for surgery or pregnancy Less than the minimum daily dose is ineffective Adherence to the tid regimen (doses taken preferably away from meals) may be poor Safety in pregnancy has not actually been established. Overall effectiveness in hepatic Wilson disease long term seems to be imperfect. Monitoring[a]: basal 24-h urinary Cu excretion (target is <75 μg/24 h (1.2 μmol/24 h]), liver function tests, serum creatinine; serum or urinary zinc may be checked as measure of adherence |
| Tetrathiomolybdate | Chelator, blocks copper absorption | Reports of rare neurologic deterioration during initial treatment | • Anemia; neutropenia<br>• Hepatotoxicity | Experimental in the United States and Canada—not for routine administration Monitoring[a]: not yet established (short-term treatment only) |

[a]Monitoring protocol assumes assessment every 6 to 12 months and routinely includes review of the interval medical history and a pertinent physical examination.

research; however, vitamin E supplementation in pharmacologic diseases (400-800 IU/d by mouth) may be of value in some patients as adjunctive therapy.

## Molecular Genetics and Molecular Mechanism

*Syndrome/Gene/Locus: chromosome 13 (13q14.3):*

☞**DESCRIPTION OF CRITICAL GENE-PRODUCT FUNCTIONS:** The Wilson ATPase is required for incorporation of copper into nascent ceruloplasmin, which is produced in hepatocytes, and for biliary excretion of copper. The Wilson ATPase also participates in an intracellular mechanism for monitoring hepatocellular concentrations of copper.

*Genetic Testing:*

☞**CLINICAL AVAILABILITY OF TESTING:** Genetic testing is commercially available, but the quality and completeness of testing varies substantially from one facility to another. Complete characterization of the gene is available at some academic centers in the United States, Canada, and Europe. See database of Wilson disease mutations at http://www.wilsondisease.med.ualberta.ca/database.asp or EuroWilson data.

☞**UTILITY OF TESTING:** Genetic testing has proven benefit for detection of affected relatives, once the proband has been conclusively diagnosed clinically and characterized genetically. It is the investigation of choice for such diagnostic studies. It is also the investigation of choice for excluding the diagnosis of Wilson disease in a sib who might serve as a living-related donor for liver transplantation. It is a useful investigation for identifying atypically old patients. High-throughput analytical techniques for assessing the entire gene may enhance the role of genetic diagnosis as a routine investigation.

☞**MOLECULAR GENETIC TESTING**

- **High-throughput methods for mutation identification:** direct sequencing, denaturing high-performance liquid chromatography (DHPLC), and automated single-strand conformation polymorphism (SSCP) analysis. With all these methods the main challenge is to determine whether the identified gene alteration is actually causative of disease; mutation databases will be helpful here. This is an evolving area of current research.
- **In the absence of mutation identification:** haplotype analysis using close markers.

**BIBLIOGRAPHY:**

1. Thomas GR, Forbes JR, Roberts EA, Walshe JM, Cox DW. The Wilson disease gene: spectrum of mutations and their consequences. *Nat Genet.* 1995;9:210-217.

2. Medici V, Trevisan CP, D'Inca R, et al. Diagnosis and management of Wilson's disease: results of a single center experience. *J Clin Gastroenterol.* 2006;40:936-941.

3. Das SK, Ray K. Wilson's disease: an update. *Nat Clin Pract Neurol.* 2006;2:482-493.

4. Ala A, Walker AP, Ashkan K, Dooley JS, Schilsky ML. Wilson's disease. *Lancet.* 2007;369:397-408.

5. Merle U, Schaefer M, Ferenci P, Stremmel W. Clinical presentation, diagnosis and long-term outcome of Wilson's disease: a cohort study. *Gut.* 2007;56:115-120.

6. Roberts EA, Schilsky ML. Diagnosis and treatment of Wilson disease: an update. *Hepatology.* 2008;47:2089-2111.

7. Shanmugiah A, Sinha S, Taly AB, et al. Psychiatric manifestations in Wilson's disease: a cross-sectional analysis. *J Neuropsychiatry Clin Neurosci.* 2008;20:81-85.

8. Mak CM, Lam CW, Tam S. Diagnostic accuracy of serum ceruloplasmin in Wilson disease: determination of sensitivity and specificity by ROC curve analysis among ATP7B-genotyped subjects. *Clin Chem.* 2008; 54:1356-1362.

9. Wiggelinkhuizen M, Tilanus ME, Bollen CW, Houwen RH. Systematic review: clinical efficacy of chelator agents and zinc in the initial treatment of Wilson disease. *Aliment Pharmacol Ther.* 2009;29:947-958.

10. Prashanth LK, Sinha S, Taly AB, Vasudev MK. Do MRI features distinguish Wilson's disease from other early onset extrapyramidal disorders? An analysis of 100 cases. *Mov Disord.* 2010;25:672-678.

11. Weiss KH, Gotthardt DN, Klem D, et al. Zinc monotherapy is not as effective as chelating agents in treatment of Wilson disease. *Gastroenterology.* 2011;140:1189-1198.

12. Bennett J, Hahn SH. Clinical molecular diagnosis of Wilson disease. *Semin Liver Dis.* 2011;31:233-238.

## Supplementary Information

**OMIM REFERENCE:**

[1] Wilson Disease; *ATP7B* (#277900)

**Alternative Names:**
- Hepatolenticular Degeneration

*Key Words:* Liver, copper, Wilson ATPase, ATP7B, movement disorder, P1-type ATPases, metal-transporting, WD, WND

# 74 Gilbert Syndrome

Christopher DT. Corbett, Matthew J. Armstrong, and, Lee C. Claridge

## KEY POINTS

- *Disease syndrome:*
  - Gilbert syndrome (GS) is a hereditary defect in bilirubin metabolism.
  - It has a prevalence of 3% to 7% in the United States of America, but worldwide this varies immensely with levels approaching 10% in parts of Western Europe.
  - A 60% to 70% reduction in the liver's ability to conjugate bilirubin leads to unconjugated (indirect) hyperbilirubinemia which may intermittently manifest as clinical jaundice.
  - Jaundice due to GS does not indicate or result in liver damage.
  - GS itself has no long-term harmful effects and does not reduce life expectancy.
- *Hereditary basis:*
  - GS is an autosomal recessive inherited defect in the gene that codes for the enzyme uridine diphosphonate (UDP) glucuronyltransferase.
- *Differential diagnosis:*
  - Other genetic defects of bilirubin metabolism (Table 74-1)
  - Other causes of unconjugated hyperbilirubinemia such as hemolysis, drugs, and thyrotoxicosis
- *GS and Pharmacogenetics:*
  - Any drug which is metabolised via glucuronidation may have altered activity in patients with GS.
  - There is associated drug toxicity in GS with the chemotherapeutic agent, irinotecan. It is associated with an increased risk of neutropenia and diarrhoea.

## Diagnostic Criteria and Clinical Characteristics

GS can be confidently diagnosed with a thorough clinical history, examination, and routine biochemistry (Table 74-2 below).

Liver and/or biliary imaging and referral to a hepatologist are not needed. Histologically the liver is normal in GS and thus liver biopsy is not required. In cases where diagnostic doubt remains genetic testing can be performed, but this should rarely be necessary in clinical practice. In the age of genomics the provocation tests summarised below are of historic interest only. They are also impractical and nonspecific for GS.

1. **Fasting (Blood) test**: This involves a 48-hour fast from food. In GS, fasting precipitates a two- to threefold increase in unconjugated bilirubin, which then returns to normal within 24-hours of breaking the fast.
2. **Nicotinic acid and phenobarbital tests**: On injecting 50 mg of nicotinic acid intravenously a similar rise in bilirubin to the 48-hour fasting test would be expected, but within a shorter duration of 3 hours. Phenobarbital is an inducer of UDP glucuronyltransferase, and therefore administration can normalise bilirubin levels in patients with GS.

## Screening and Counseling

*Screening:* GS is an entirely benign condition; population screening and/or screening relatives of affected individuals is not necessary.
*Counseling:* GS is usually inherited in an autosomal recessive pattern. If both parents are unaffected carriers of the defective gene there is a 25% chance of offspring being affected. When only one parent is a carrier of the defective gene there is no chance of offspring being affected. Affected individuals will only pass on the condition to their offspring if their partner is also affected or an unaffected carrier.

GS is not a disease but simply an inborn variation in bilirubin metabolism resulting in a modest elevation of circulating unconjugated bilirubin. Jaundice may be precipitated by fasting, intercurrent illness, dehydration, surgery, physical exertion, and lack of sleep. Episodes of jaundice are not contagious, and will resolve spontaneously within a few days. There are no dietary restrictions and alcohol is safe within recommended limits.

GS can be associated with altered drug metabolism and this should be considered when prescribing (see Pharmacogenetic Considerations discussed later).

The condition does not reduce life expectancy or affect life insurance. Moreover, several epidemiologic studies have reported a lower incidence of cardiovascular disease in individuals with GS and this may be due to the antioxidant properties of bilirubin.

Patients should seek medical advice if an episode of jaundice is more severe or persistent than usual since this may indicate a separate condition.

## Management and Treatment

No treatment is required. The most important aspect of the management of this condition is to reassure patients and to avoid overinvestigation.

## Molecular Genetics and Molecular Mechanisms

UDP glucuronyltransferase is located in the endoplasmic reticulum of liver cells (hepatocytes) where it catalyses the conjugation of

*Table 74-1* **Genetic Differential Diagnosis**

| Syndrome | Gene Symbol | Metabolic Defect |
|---|---|---|
| Crigler-Najjar syndrome type I | *UGT1A* | Complete absence of bilirubin conjugation leading to severe jaundice in first few days of life. |
| Crigler-Najjar syndrome type II | *UGT1A* | Conjugating enzyme activity is less than 10%. It usually presents with persistent jaundice in childhood. |
| Dubin-Johnson Syndrome | *MRP2* | A defect in the bile canalicular multispecific organic anion transporter results in impaired excretion of anionic conjugates from hepatocytes into bile. Consequently there is a conjugated (direct) hyperbilirubinemia and a characteristic accumulation of pigments in the liver. There is also an abnormality of porphyrin metabolism in which >80% of urinary coproporphyrin is coproporphyrin I. |
| Rotor syndrome | Unknown gene | A disorder of hepatic storage which results in conjugated hyperbilirubinemia. |

Gene names: *UGT1A*, uridine diphosphonate glucuronyltransferase 1 family, polypeptide A cluster; *MRP2*, multidrug resistance protein 2.

bilirubin with glucuronic acid (glucuronidation) to form a water-soluble bilirubin diglucuronide which is excreted via the ATP-dependent transporter MRP2. There are several enzyme isoforms capable of conjugating a variety of substrates such as drugs and hormones. The gene expressing these enzymes has a complex structure and is located on chromosome 2 (2q37). There are five exons; exon 1 encodes for the region that confers the substrate specificity of each isoform, while exons 2 to 5 encode for the UDP-glucuronic acid binding site that is constant to all isoforms.

UDP glucuronyltransferase 1A1 (UGT1A1) is the isoform responsible for almost all bilirubin conjugation. Its expression depends on a promoter region containing a TATAA box. The most common polymorphism resulting in GS is due to the addition of an extra thymine (T) and adenine (A) dinucleotide to the TATAA box (UGT1A1*28). This impedes the binding of transcription factor IID leading to reduced expression of UGT1A1. However, additional heterozygous missense mutations in the coding region of UGT1A1 (Gly71Arg, Tyr486Asp, Pro364Leu) have also been identified and are particularly prevalent in Asian populations.

Studies have indicated that up to 16% of western populations may be homozygous for the UGT1A1*28 polymorphism, but only 3% to 10% of these populations have GS. This suggests that the genetic defect alone may not always be sufficient to completely manifest the syndrome. Furthermore, GS occurs more frequently in males than females and typically presents after puberty, this may be due to an inhibitory effect of androgens on UDP glucuronyltransferase.

***Pharmacogenetic Considerations:*** Drugs that inhibit UDP glucuronyltransferase activity such as gemfibrozil, and the protease inhibitors atazanavir and indinavir, can trigger episodes of jaundice. There is also a theoretical increase in the risk of myositis when statins are used in combination with gemfibrozil.

Although many drugs are partially metabolised by glucuronidation, reports of drug toxicity associated with GS are rare. The most documented example is of an increased risk of neutropenia and diarrhoea secondary to the chemotherapeutic agent irinotecan. The risk of irinotecan toxicity appears to be greatest when there is a combination of UGT1A1 and UGT1A7 polymorphisms. Altered

*Table 74-2* **Clinical Diagnostic Criteria**

| Diagnostic Clinical Features | Explanation |
|---|---|
| Unconjugated hyperbilirubinemia | Conjugated (direct) bilirubin is within the normal range and/or <20% of total bilirubin. |
| Normal liver enzymes and function tests | Normal alanine and/or aspartate transaminases, gamma-glutamyltransferase, alkaline phosphatase, and albumin indicate that liver pathology is unlikely to be present. |
| Absence of other causes of unconjugated hyperbilirubinemia<br>• Hemolysis<br>• Thyrotoxicosis<br>• Drugs (rifampicin, methyldopa, sulphasalazine, gemfibrozil) | <br><br>Normal reticulocyte count, lactate dehydrogenase and blood film<br>Normal thyroid function tests<br>Some drugs inhibit the activity of UDP glucuronyltransferase and can precipitate unconjugated hyperbilirubinemia. |
| No symptoms or signs that are suggestive of hepatobiliary disease | Absence of abdominal pain, pruritus, dark urine, and/or pale stools. There should be no bilirubinuria on urine dipstick because unconjugated bilirubin is not water soluble. |

metabolism of acetaminophen (paracetamol) has been demonstrated in a subgroup of patients with GS but recent studies suggest that acetaminophen is usually a substrate of a UDP glucuronyltransferase isoform other than UGT1A1.

Patients with GS should be told to inform medical staff of their condition if admitted to hospital and when prescribed new medication.

## BIBLIOGRAPHY:

1. Claridge LC, Armstrong MJ, Booth C, Gill PS. Gilbert's syndrome. *BMJ*. 2011;342:d2293.

2. Sieg A, Stiehl A, Raedsch R, Ullrich D, Messmer B, Kommerell B. Gilbert's syndrome: diagnosis by typical serum bilirubin pattern. *Clin Chim Acta*. 1986;54(1):41-47.

3. Schwertner HA, Vítek L. Gilbert syndrome, UGT1A1*28 allele, and cardiovascular disease risk: possible protective effects and therapeutic applications of bilirubin. *Atherosclerosis*. 2008;198(1):1-11.

4. Bosma PJ, Chowdhury JR, Bakker C, et al. The genetic basis of the reduced expression of bilirubin UDP-glucuronosyltransferase 1 in Gilbert's syndrome. *N Engl J Med*. 1995;333(18):1171-1175.

5. Hsieh TY, Shiu TY, Huang SM, et al. Molecular pathogenesis of Gilbert's syndrome: decreased TATA-binding protein binding affinity of UGT1A1 gene promoter. *Pharmacogenet Genomics*. 2007;17(4): 229-236.

6. Akaba K, Kimura T, Sasaki A, et al. Neonatal hyperbilirubinemia and mutation of the bilirubin uridine diphosphate-glucuronosyltransferase gene: a common missense mutation among Japanese, Koreans and Chinese. *Biochem Mol Biol Int*. 1998;46:21-26.

7. Owens D, Evans J. Population studies on Gilbert's syndrome. *J Med Genet*. 1975;12:152-156.

8. Rotger M, Taffe P, Bleiber G, et al. Gilbert syndrome and the development of antiretroviral therapy-associated hyperbilirubinemia. *J Infect Dis*. 2005;192(8):1381-1386.

9. Preuksaritanont T, Tang C, Qiu Y, Mu L, Subramanian R, Lin JH. Effects of fibrates on metabolism of statins in human hepatocytes. *Drug Metab Dispos*. 2002;30:1280-1287.

10. Lankisch TO, Schulz C, Zwingers T, et al. Gilbert's syndrome and irinotecan toxicity: combination with UDP-glucuronosyltransferase 1A7 variants increases risk. *Cancer Epidemiol Biomarkers Prev*. 2008;17(3):695-701.

11. Esteban A, Pérez-Mateo M. Heterogeneity of paracetamol metabolism in Gilbert's syndrome. *Eur J Drug Metab Pharmacokinet*. 1999;24(1):9-13.

12. Rauchschwalbe SK, Zühlsdorf MT, Wensing G, Kuhlmann J. Glucuronidation of acetaminophen is independent of UGT1A1 promotor genotype. *Int J Clin Pharmacol Ther*. 2004;42(2):73-77.

## Supplementary Information

### OMIM REFERENCE:

[1] Gilbert Syndrome (#143500)

### Alternative Names:

- Familial Benign Unconjugated Hyperbilirubinemia
- Constitutional Liver Dysfunction
- Familial Nonhemolytic Nonobstructive Jaundice
- Low-Grade Chronic Hyperbilirubinemia
- Unconjugated Benign Bilirubinemia

# 75 Nonalcoholic Fatty Liver Disease

Charissa Y. Chang and Scott Friedman

## KEY POINTS

- *Disease summary:*
  - Nonalcoholic fatty liver disease (NAFLD) refers to a spectrum of conditions involving excess fat accumulation in the liver. The term encompasses conditions ranging from simple steatosis to nonalcoholic steatohepatitis (NASH), which is defined by histologic findings of steatosis, inflammation, ballooned hepatocytes, Mallory-Denk bodies, and varying degrees of fibrosis. Simple steatosis is thought to have a benign prognosis, whereas a subset of individuals with NASH progress to end-stage complications of cirrhosis and hepatocellular carcinoma. The pathogenesis of NAFLD has not been clearly defined; however, there is a strong association with metabolic syndrome and insulin resistance.

- *Differential diagnosis:*
  - Alcoholic liver disease, viral hepatitis, autoimmune hepatitis, hemochromatosis, Wilson disease, medication-induced fatty liver disease (amiodarone, tamoxifen, valproic acid, TPN).

- *Monogenic forms:*
  - There is no single gene known to cause NAFLD. However, there are rare monogenic inherited disorders of lipid metabolism, insulin signaling, and mitochondrial function that result in hepatic steatosis. These disorders usually have other phenotypic manifestations which dominate over hepatic steatosis.

- *Family history:*
  - Small studies in kindreds demonstrate a higher prevalence of NAFLD among first-degree relatives of patients. One study demonstrated a 59% prevalence of fatty liver in siblings and a 78% prevalence of fatty liver in parents of children with NAFLD. About 18% of patients with NASH have an affected first-degree relative.

- *Twin studies:*
  - One study of monozygotic twins discordant for obesity demonstrated intrapair differences in liver fat that correlated with acquired obesity, suggesting the presence of strong nongenetic determinants of hepatic steatosis.

- *Environmental factors:*
  - Western diets containing increased amounts of high fructose corn syrup, saturated fats, and trans fats have been implicated in rising obesity trends and increasing incidence of NAFLD.

- *Genome-wide associations:*
  - The strongest association has been with a single-nucleotide polymorphism (SNP) variant in the *PNPLA3* gene (also called "adiponutrin"). Other SNPs have been described in patients with NAFLD (Table 75-1). Testing for gene variants is not yet clinically validated for diagnosis or management of NAFLD.

- *Pharmacogenomics:*
  - There are no known genetic predictors of response to pharmacotherapy.

## Diagnostic Criteria and Clinical Characteristics

### Diagnostic Criteria for Nonalcoholic Fatty Liver Disease:

**Diagnostic evaluation should include at least one of the following (Fig. 75-1 algorithm):**

- Exclusion of other causes of abnormal liver tests: hepatitis B, hepatitis C, autoimmune hepatitis, hemochromatosis, Wilson disease, drug- or alcohol-induced liver injury.
- Careful history taking to rule out alcoholic liver disease (guidelines suggest a threshold of <20 g/d in women and <40 g/d in men although these limits are not well established).
- Rule out other secondary causes of steatosis such as medications (valproic acid, amiodarone, tamoxifen, total parenteral nutrition).
- Anthropometric measurements (body mass index [BMI], waist circumference).
- Assessment for presence of metabolic syndrome (hypertension, increased waist circumference, dyslipidemia, diabetes).
- Testing for insulin resistance (homeostasis model assessment or HOMA index) if no overt diabetes present.
- Imaging to assess for steatosis (ultrasound, computed tomographic [CT] scan, magnetic resonance imaging [MRI]). Proton ($^1$H) magnetic resonance spectroscopy (MRS) can detect hepatic triglyceride content with high sensitivity. Its use has been limited to clinical trials and is not available for routine clinical use.
- Consider liver biopsy for definitive diagnosis and/or staging.

***Clinical Characteristics:*** Individuals with early stages of NAFLD are usually asymptomatic. The diagnosis is often made during evaluation of incidental liver test or imaging findings that suggest hepatic steatosis. There are currently no clinically available noninvasive tests to distinguish simple steatosis from NASH. Liver biopsy remains the gold standard for diagnosis of NASH, which carries a worse prognosis than simple steatosis. Pathologic findings on liver biopsy in patients with NASH include steatosis, inflammation, ballooned hepatocytes, Mallory-Denk bodies, and varying degrees of fibrosis. A subset of individuals with NASH develops fibrosis progression and eventual cirrhosis. Predictors of fibrosis progression have not been well defined. NASH is now recognized

*Table 75-1* **Nonalcoholic Fatty Liver Disease Associated Susceptibility Variants**

| Candidate Gene (Chromosome Location) | Associated Variant [effect on protein] (assayed by Affymetrix/ Illumina) | Relative Risk | Frequency of Risk Allele | Putative Functional Significance | Associated Disease Phenotype |
|---|---|---|---|---|---|
| *PNPLA3* Patatin-like phospholipase 3 (22q13.31) | Met148 [nonsynonymous amino acid substitution 1148M] rs738409 | Odds ratio 3.26 | 0.49 (Hispanics) 0.23 (European Americans) 0.17 (African Americans) | Loss-of-function mutation leading to impaired hydrolysis of triglycerides | Hepatic triglyceride accumulation (on ¹H MRS) Increased histologic severity (steatosis, inflammation, ballooning, and fibrosis) Increased histologic severity in pediatric NAFLD |
| *GCKR* (2p23.3-p23.2) | P-446L rs780094 | | 0.47 | Regulation of glucose storage/ disposal, provides substrates for de novo lipogenesis | Hepatic steatosis (on CT) Histologic NAFLD Increased LDL Increased triglycerides |
| *NCAN* (19p12) | P-91S rs2228603 | | 0.12 | Adhesion molecule | Hepatic steatosis (on CT) Histologic NAFLD Decreased LDL Decreased triglycerides |
| *LYPLAL1* (1) | rs12137855 | | 0.83 | Impaired triglyceride breakdown | Hepatic steatosis (on CT) Histologic NAFLD Decreased fasting glucose |
| *APOC3* Apolipoprotein C3 (11q23.1-q23.2) | rs2854116 (T-455C) rs2854117 (C-482T) | | | Increased apoli-poprotein C3 concentration, inhibition of lipoprotein lipase, impaired plasma triglyceride clearance | Hepatic steatosis, hypertriglyceridemia, insulin resistance |
| *ENPP1* Ectoenzyme nucleotide pyrophosphate phosphodiesterase 1/PC-1 (6q22-q23) | Lys121Gln | | | Modulation of insulin sensitivity | Fibrosis stage >1 in NAFLD |
| *IRS-1* Insulin receptor substrate-1 (2q36) | Gly972Arg | | | | Fibrosis stage >1 in NAFLD |
| *TNF-α* (6p21.3) | TNFA 238 | | | Inflammation, insulin resistance | Increased insulin resistance NASH |
| *MTTP* Microsomal triglyceride trans-fer protein (4q24) | −493G | | | Lipid metabolism | Hepatic steatosis |

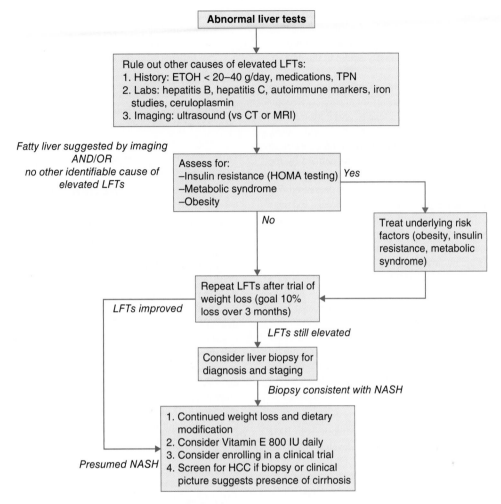

**Figure 75-1** Algorithm for Diagnostic Evaluation of Patient With NAFLD.

as an underlying cause of cases that might otherwise be diagnosed as cryptogenic cirrhosis. Clinical clues are a history of metabolic syndrome or obesity in a patient with cirrhosis and no other clear causes. Hepatocellular carcinoma can occur in patients with NASH, particularly in those who have progressed to cirrhosis.

Obesity and features of metabolic syndrome are common in individuals with NAFLD, highlighting the importance of screening for dyslipidemia, hypertension, and diabetes in those diagnosed with NAFLD. Cardiac comorbidities are common and are a significant cause of mortality in individuals with NASH. Other conditions associated with NAFLD include obstructive sleep apnea and polycystic ovary syndrome.

## Screening and Counseling

***Screening:*** There is not enough evidence to support genetic testing for disease-associated SNPs or screening of family members. The prevalence of NAFLD is higher in patients with metabolic syndrome and obesity compared to the general population. While there are no screening guidelines or cost-effective studies to support targeted screening, one approach is to screen patients with diabetes, hypertension, dyslipidemia, obesity, or a family history of metabolic

syndrome with alanine transaminase (ALT) testing. Liver tests can be normal in advanced stages of fibrosis, therefore a normal ALT does not rule out NAFLD and revised "normal" ALT thresholds (<19 U/mL for women, <30 U/mL for men) should be considered when interpreting ALT results.

***Counseling:*** Familial clustering has been described. Aside from rare inherited mitochondrial disorders and lipodystrophy syndromes, inheritance patterns have not been ascertained. Given the association between NAFLD and metabolic syndrome, patients and family members should seek routine medical care and age-appropriate screening for obesity, hypertension, and dyslipidemia.

## Management and Treatment

***Management:*** There are no proven pharmacologic treatment options. The mainstay of management involves lifestyle modification and treatment of underlying features of metabolic syndrome, including optimization of glycemic control in diabetics, treatment of hypercholesterolemia, and weight loss in those with obesity.

**Diet:** There are no large-scale clinical trials comparing different diets for treatment of NAFLD. However, a diet low in saturated fats, trans fats, and high-fructose corn syrup-containing products may help in reducing free fatty acids and reducing hepatic triglyceride accumulation. Ongoing studies are investigating the role of dietary supplementation with polyunsaturated fats (such as omega 3 fatty acids) in the amelioration of NASH.

**Exercise:** Exercise improves insulin resistance and has been shown to decrease hepatic steatosis in small studies. Recommendations for optimal exercise intensity or duration for the treatment or prevention of NASH have not been established. One case control study showed that only vigorous exercise (compared to moderate or total exercise), as defined by the US Department of Health and Human Services and the US Department of Agriculture, is associated with decreased risk for NASH and decreased risk for advanced fibrosis. Exercise should be recommended as part of an overall management plan to achieve weight loss and improve cofactors of metabolic syndrome; however, specific guidelines for the treatment of NASH are not available.

**Weight loss:** Weight loss in obese individuals with NASH has been shown to improve ALT and histology, particularly in morbidly obese individuals with NASH who have been observed to have regression of fibrosis and even cirrhosis following bariatric surgery. There are no large-scale controlled studies to support the use of pharmacologic weight loss agents in patients with NASH. Over-the-counter homeopathic weight loss agents have been implicated in drug-induced liver injury and should be discouraged due to uncertain benefit and potential harm.

It is important to note that there are ethnic differences in BMI thresholds for obesity; Asians and East Asians develop NASH at lower BMIs compared to non-Asians, possibly due to variations in visceral adipose distribution. As such, these differences should be taken into consideration when counseling patients on target BMI. Paradoxically, rapid weight loss exceeding 1.6 kg/wk has been associated with exacerbation of NASH, therefore, current guidelines recommend modest weight loss of 10% over 3 months in those who are overweight or obese.

*Therapeutics:* There are no proven pharmacologic agents which have been shown to clearly improve histologic findings in individuals with NASH. Potential therapeutic targets include insulin resistance, altered lipid metabolism, and hepatic inflammation associated with NASH.

**Vitamin E:** A recent multicenter placebo-controlled trial (PIVENS) demonstrated improvement in histologic findings in nondiabetic patients with NASH who were treated with vitamin E 800 IU/d for 96 weeks. Pioglitazone, a thiazolidinedione, did not provide significant improvement in histologic findings in the PIVENS trial compared to placebo, raising questions about the relative role of insulin resistance in the pathogenesis of NASH.

**Thiazolidinediones:** Thiazolidinediones (TZDs) improve hepatic insulin resistance and have therefore been studied in the treatment of NASH. Small pilot studies show improvement in ALT and some histologic features of NASH following treatment with TZDs; however, subsequent longer-term studies including the PIVENS trial have not shown significant improvement in fibrosis on paired biopsies. There is no proven role for TZDs in the treatment of NASH.

**Statins:** Small pilot studies show potential benefit from lipid-lowering agents in patients with NASH; however, no large-scale controlled trials exist. Statins have been shown to be safe in patients with chronic liver disease including NASH, therefore they should not be withheld in patients with NASH and dyslipidemia based on concern for potential hepatotoxicity.

*Pharmacogenetics:* There are no known genetic predictors of response to pharmacotherapy.

## Molecular Genetics and Molecular Mechanism

Ethnic differences in the prevalence of NAFLD and heritability studies provide evidence that genetic factors are involved in the propensity to develop NAFLD. The most convincing evidence for a gene variant associated with NAFLD comes from studies of PNPLA3. In 2008, a genome-wide association study (GWAS) of 9229 nonsynonymous sequence variants in subjects enrolled in the Dallas Heart Study revealed for the first time a single variant in PNPLA3 (I148M, rs738409), also known as adiponutrin, that is strongly associated with hepatic fat content as measured by $^1$H MR spectroscopy and hepatic inflammation as measured by aminotransferases. This association between the *PNPLA3* gene variant and NAFLD has been confirmed in two other GWAS studies and in other geographically diverse cohorts. The frequency of the variant rs738409 [G] allele is highest among Hispanics, intermediate in Caucasians, and lowest among African Americans, which is consistent with observed ethnic differences in prevalence of NAFLD. The rs738409 variant has been shown to correlate with measures of histologic severity in NASH (ballooning, fibrosis, inflammation, Mallory-Denk bodies). Interestingly, the association between *PNPLA3* variants and NAFLD appears to be independent of insulin resistance, BMI, or plasma triglycerides. This suggests that there are additional etiologic factors beyond insulin resistance that play a role in the development of NAFLD.

PNPLA3 encodes a protein expressed in liver and adipose tissue that belongs to the patatin-like phospholipase domain-containing family. While its function has not been fully elucidated, evidence suggests that it is a membrane-bound protein found in lipid droplets. The rs738409 variant of PNPLA3 encodes an isoleucine to methionine substitution at amino acid residue 148. Structural modeling suggests that this substitution leads to spatial hindrance of the catalytic domain of the protein, resulting in loss of function. PNPLA3 is thought to play a role in the hydrolysis of triglycerides. Loss of function associated with the rs738409 would therefore be predicted to result in accumulation of triglycerides in the liver. Interestingly, the PNPLA3 rs738409 [G] allele has also been found to correlate with disease severity in alcoholic liver disease.

A recent GWAS identified three additional variants in *NCAN*, *GCKR*, and *LYPLAL1* that correlate with steatosis on CT and histologic NAFLD. These variants have different effects on metabolic syndrome traits (Table 75-1) and highlight the possible presence of heterogenous pathways (insulin resistance, altered lipid metabolism) involved in the pathogenesis of NAFLD and a role for polygenic determinants of the NAFLD phenotype.

Other candidate genes that have been studied include those involved in lipid metabolism (*APOC3*), inflammation (*TNF*-α), insulin signaling (*ENPP1*), and insulin sensitivity (adiponectin) (Table 75-1). These gene variants have been less well studied than *PNPLA3*. A study in East Asian carriers of apolipoprotein C3 (*APOC3*) variant alleles C-482T, T-455C, or both showed an increase in plasma triglycerides and increased prevalence of NAFLD compared to wild-type homozygotes (38% vs 0%). When *APOC3* variants were compared to *PNPLA3* variants, *APOC3* accounted for 11%, *PNPLA3* accounted for 6.5%, and both accounted for 13.1% of variance, demonstrating a combined effect of having both gene variants and supporting a polygenic model of disease risk.

Monogenic inherited disorders that are associated with hepatic steatosis are rare and usually result in phenotypic extrahepatic manifestations that dominate over hepatic steatosis. However, they provide insight into pathogenesis of hepatic steatosis and can be considered in rare cases where the etiology of hepatic steatosis is unclear. These disorders include abetalipoproteinemia (MTTP), familial abetalipoproteinemia (APOB), citrullinemia type II (SLC25A13), familial partial lipodystrophy type 2 and type 3 (LMNA and PPARG, respectively), congenital generalized lipodystrophy (AGPAT2, BSCL2), neutral lipid storage disorder (PNPLA2, CGI-58), Wolman disease (LIPA), cholesterol ester storage disease (LIPA), medium-chain acyl coenzyme-A(CoA) dehydrogenase deficiency (ACADM), very long-chain acyl CoA dehydrogenase deficiency (ACADVL), and long-chain 3-hydroxy-acyl-CoA dehydrogenase deficiency (HADHA). Rare inherited mitochondrialopathies have also been associated with NASH and provide insight into the role of impaired fatty acid oxidation in the pathogenesis of NASH.

**Genetic Testing:** There are no clinically available tests for gene variants that predict NAFLD. Genetic testing may be useful in cases where a rare monogenic inherited disorder of lipid metabolism, lipodystrophy, or mitochondrial function is suspected.

**Future Directions:** The discovery of an association between the *PNPLA3* rs738409 (adiponutrin) gene variant and NAFLD, particularly with regard to its dissociation from insulin resistance, raises important questions about disease pathogenesis. Future studies will hopefully elucidate the functional role of adiponutrin and products of other gene variants in order to understand the various pathways involved in the pathogenesis of NASH. As more gene variants are discovered and existing variants are better described, it may be possible to guide therapeutic strategies based on genomic factors that predominate in individual cases of NASH (ie, increased insulin resistance versus abnormal lipid metabolism).

Other clinically relevant roles for gene studies are in the prediction of disease progression and in distinguishing between simple steatosis and NASH.

Finally, environmental factors related to diet and acquired obesity play a major role in the development of NAFLD. Further studies may help elucidate gene-environment interactions and guide preventive strategies in individuals who are at increased risk for NAFLD based on gene testing.

## Bibliography:

1. Hooper A, Adams L, Burnett J. Genetic determinants of hepatic steatosis in man. *J Lipid Res.* 2011;52:593-567.

2. Pietilainen K, Rissanen A, Kapril J, et al. Acquired obesity is associated with increased liver fat, intra-abdominal fat, and insulin resistance in young adult monozygotic twins. *Am J Physiol Endocrinol Metab.* 2005;288:E788-E774.

3. Das K, Das K, Mukherjee P, et al. Nonobese population in a developing country has a high prevalence of nonalcoholic fatty liver and significant liver disease. *Hepatology.* 2010;51:1593-1602.

4. Browning J, Szczepaniak L, Dobbins R, et al. Prevalence of hepatic steatosis in an urban population in the United States: impact of ethnicity. *Hepatology.* 2004;40(6):1387-1395.

5. Romeo S, Kozlitina J, Xing C, et al. Genetic variation in PNPLA3 confers susceptibility to nonalcoholic fatty liver disease. *Nat Genet.* 2008;1461-1465.

6. Yuan X, Waterworth D, Perry J, et al. Population-based genome-wide association studies reveal six loci influencing plasma levels of liver enzymes. *Am J Hum Genet.* 2008;83:520-528.

7. Speliotes E, Yerges-Armstrong L, Wu J, et al. Genome-wide association analysis identifies variants associated with nonalcoholic fatty liver disease that have distinct effects on metabolic traits. *PLoS Genet.* 2011;7(3):1-13.

8. Sookoian S, Castano G, Burgeno A, et al. A nonsynonymous gene variant in the adiponutrin gene is associated with nonalcoholic fatty liver disease severity. *J Lipid Res.* 2009;50:2111-2116.

9. Rotman V, Koh J, Zmuda D, et al. The association of genetic variability in patatin-like phospholipase domain-containing protein 3 (PNPLA3) with histological severity of nonalcoholic fatty liver disease. *Hepatology.* 2010;52:1274-1280.

10. Valenti L, Al-Serri A, Daly E, et al. Homozygosity for the patatin-like phospholipase-3/adiponutrin I148M polymorphism influences liver fibrosis in patients with nonalcoholic fatty liver disease. *Hepatology.* 2010;51:1209-1217.

11. Kantartzis K, Peter A, Machicao F, et al. Dissociation between fatty liver and insulin resistance in humans carrying a variant of the patatin-like phospholipase 3 gene. *Diabetes.* 2009:58:2616-2623.

12. He S, McPhaul C, Li J, et al. A sequence variation (I148M) in PNPLA3 associated with nonalcoholic fatty liver disease disrupts triglyceride hydrolysis. *J Biol Chem.* 2010;285(9):6706-6715.

13. Petersen KF, Dufour S, Harin A, et al. Apolipoprotein C3 gene variants in nonalcoholic fatty liver disease. *N Engl J Med.* 2010;362:1082-1089.

14. Dongiovanni P, Valenti L, Rametta R, et al. Genetic variants regulating insulin receptor signalling are associated with the severity of liver damage in patients with nonalcoholic fatty liver disease. *Gut.* 2010;59:267-27

## Supplementary Information

### OMIM References:

[1] Nonalcoholic Fatty Liver Disease, susceptibility to; NAFLD1 (#cu)

[2] Nonalcoholic Fatty Liver Disease, susceptibility to; NAFLD2 (#613387)

[3] Patatin-Like Phospholipase Domain-Containing Protein 3; PNPLA3 (#609567)

[4] Apolipoprotein C-III;APOC3 (#107720)

### Alternative Names:

- Nonalcoholic Fatty Liver Disease
- Nonalcoholic Steatohepatitis
- Fatty Liver

**Key Words:** Nonalcoholic steatohepatitis, NASH, nonalcoholic fatty liver disease, NAFLD, PNPLA3, adiponutrin, gene studies

# 76 Gallstone Disease

Marcin Krawczy and Frank Lammert

## KEY POINTS

- *Disease summary:*
  - Gallstone disease is a complex trait resulting from an interaction between genetic predisposition and environmental risk factors. In patients carrying rare monogenic mutations gallstones develop mostly due to genetic risk factors. On the other hand, in carriers of common risk variants, stones form predominantly due to environmental triggers interacting with these genetic variants.
  - Gallstone disease affects 10% to 50% of adults in developed countries; prevalence rates of gallstones in developing countries are rising constantly. The disease is rare in children.
  - Gallstones can be divided into three subtypes: cholesterol gallstones, which are most common (>95%) and compromise predominantly cholesterol, pigment gallstones that mainly consist of calcium bilirubinate, and mixed stones.
  - Nongenetic risk factors include age, parity, metabolic syndrome, obesity, and insulin resistance.
  - Most patients with gallstones remain asymptomatic throughout their lives; biliary colic represents the most common sign of symptomatic disease, which develops in 20% of patients.
  - In symptomatic patients early surgery is indicated due to recurrence of symptoms and high complication rates.
- *Differential diagnosis:*
  - Abdominal aneurysm, acute and chronic pancreatitis, biliary dyskinesia, diverticulitis, functional gastrointestinal disorders, peptic ulcer disease
- *Monogenic forms:*
  - Monogenic cholelithiasis is rare but the presence of predisposing variants substantially increases the risk of disease and the recurrence of stones after treatment. Bilirubin gallstones can be caused by single-gene mutations known to increase the risk of hemolytic anemias, in particular in children (hereditary spherocytosis: *ANK1, EPB42, SLC4A1, SPTA1, SPTB*; sickle cell disease: *HBB*; thalassemia major and intermedia: *HBB*; erythrocyte enzyme deficiencies: *AKI, G6PD, GPI, GSR, PGK1, PKLR, TPII*). Patients with risk variants of *ABCB4*, the gene encoding the hepatobiliary phosphatidylcholine floppase, develop the so-called low phospholipid-associated cholelithiasis (LPAC) syndrome.
- *Family history:*
  - Gallstone disease develops up to five times more frequently in family members of affected individuals.
- *Twin studies:*
  - Twin studies have demonstrated that in Europeans the genetic risk factors account for approximately 25% of total disease risk.
- *Environmental factors:*
  - Environmental effects account for 75% of gallstone risk.
- *Genome-wide association scans (GWASs):*
  - To date, one GWAS on gallstones has been published. The analysis of 280 cases and 360 controls in the screening panel, subsequently replicated in 1832 German and 167 Chilean patients, identified a common variant of the hepatobiliary cholesterol transporter (*ABCG8* p.D19H) as the first common genetic risk factor for gallstone formation in humans.

## Diagnostic Criteria and Clinical Characteristics

*Diagnostic criteria:*
- Presence of a colicky postprandial pain localized in epigastrium or in the right upper abdomen, in some patients accompanied by nausea or emesis.
- Detection of gallbladder or common bile duct stones by
  - Abdominal ultrasonography (US)
  - Magnetic resonance cholangiopancreatography (MRCP)
  - Endoscopic retrograde cholangiopancreatography (ERCP)
  - Endoscopic ultrasonography (EUS)

**Diagnostic evaluation should include at least one of the following (algorithm, Fig. 76-1):**

- Detection of gallstones in asymptomatic patients without signs of complications does not necessitate further evaluation.

- In symptomatic patients diagnostic evaluation should include
  - Blood tests including bilirubin, gamma-GT, alkaline phosphatase, alanine aminotransferase, lipase, and complete blood count.
  - Abdominal ultrasound to confirm or exclude presence of gallstones and their complications.
  - MRCP or EUS in patients with moderate probability of choledocholithiasis.
  - ERCP in case of common bile duct stones.
  - Abdominal CT scans in case of complications.

*Clinical Characteristics:*
- Individuals carrying gallstones can present with symptomatic and asymptomatic disease.
- Symptoms of gallstones can be nonspecific.
- Typical symptoms include colicky pain in the right upper quadrant, often radiating into upper back, lasting from at least 15 minutes to 5 hours.
- Acute cholecystitis should be suspected in case of colicky pain lasting for more than 5 hours, positive Murphy sign (ie,

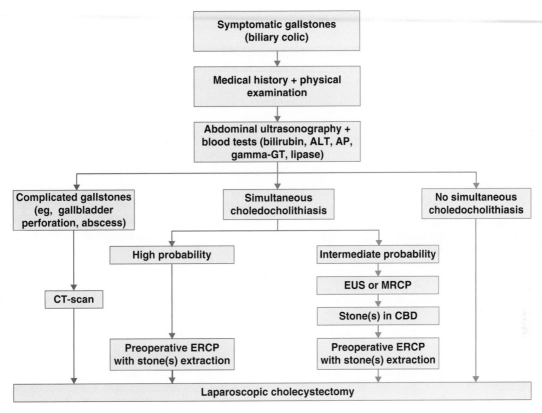

**Figure 76-1** Algorithm for Diagnostic Evaluation of a Patient With Biliary Colic.

tenderness above the gallbladder), fever, leukocytosis, and the following ultrasonographic features: thickening of the gallbladder wall (>3 mm), stratification of gallbladder wall into three layers, and fluid around gallbladder.

- Cholangitis should be diagnosed in case of jaundice, fever, and/or right upper quadrant abdominal pain (the so-called Charcot triad).

## Screening and Counseling

*Screening:* Genetic testing in gallstone patients and screening of family members should be considered in case of carriers of *ABCB4* mutations that substantially increase the risk of gallstone disease and recurrence after treatment (Table 76-1). Genetic testing for variants of *ABCB4* and *ABCB11*, encoding the hepatobiliary bile salt export pump, is also recommended for patients with biopsy findings compatible with chronic cholestatic liver disease of unknown etiology.

Gilbert syndrome is common, and the genetic testing is confirmatory for patients with isolated unconjugated hyperbilirubinemia. Nevertheless these patients, in particular men, carry at least twofold risk of cholesterol gallstones; apparently bilirubin precipitates may serve as nidus for cholesterol stone formation.

To date, the issue of screening common risk polymorphisms (*ABCG8*, *SLC10A2*, *UGT1A1*) has not been tested in large studies. No evidence-based strategy for preventing gallstones in individuals carrying common risk variants has been identified so far.

*Counseling:* Familial predisposition to gallstones is well documented. Nevertheless in patients carrying common variants predisposing to stone formation, environmental triggers (eg, diet, physical activity, multiparity, estrogens, octreotide, fibrates, and calcineurin inhibitors) seem to play key role in gallstone disease. Hence, counseling aimed at reducing the impact of these nongenetic risk factors is essential. On the other hand in case of monogenic cholelithiasis (eg, LPAC caused by *ABCB4* variants), lifestyle modification can only slightly reduce the risk of the disease. In these patients, prevention with ursodeoxycholic acid (UDCA) and testing of family members has been recommended.

## Management and Treatment

- In general, treatment of gallbladder stones in asymptomatic patients is not indicated. Nevertheless, prophylactic cholecystectomy has been recommended for the following conditions: gallbladder polyps greater than or equal to 1 cm, PSC patients with gallbladder polyps, porcelain gallbladder, stones greater than 3 cm. Prophylactic cholecystectomy is also considered in patients with sickle cell anemia (due to an increased risk of developing calcium bilirubinate stones as a result of chronic hemolysis) and in morbidly obese patients undergoing bariatric surgery.
- In symptomatic patients, analgesic therapy is required. Afterwards, surgical intervention is mandatory. To date, most patients with gallbladder stones undergo laparoscopic cholecystectomy.

*Table 76-1  Gallstone Disease-Associated Susceptibility Variants*

| Candidate Gene (Chromosome Location) | Associated Variant | Relative Risk | Frequency of Risk Variant | Putative Functional Significance | Associated Disease Phenotype |
|---|---|---|---|---|---|
| *ABCB4* (7q21) | Multiple variants | | | Decreased biliary phosphatidylcholine output | LPAC Chronic cholestasis |
| *ABCG8* (2p21) | c.55G>C (p.D19H) rs11887534 | OR = 2.2 | ~2% homozygous ~14% heterozygous | Increased biliary cholesterol output | Cholesterol stones |
| *ABCB11* (2q24) | Multiple variants | | | Decreased biliary bile salt output | Cholesterol stones Chronic cholestasis |
| *SLC10A2* (13q33) | c.378-105A>G rs9514089 | OR = 2.0 | ~11% homozygous | Decreased intestinal bile salt uptake | Cholesterol stones |
| *UGT1A1* (2q37) | Promoter variant A(TA)₇TAA UGT1A1*28 rs6742078 | OR = 2.3 | ~5% homozygous | Increased biliary bilirubin levels | Cholesterol stones Pigment stones |

*ABCB4*, hepatobiliary phosphatidylcholine floppase; *ABCB11*, hepatocanalicular bile salt export pump; *ABCG8*, hepatobiliary cholesterol transporter; LPAC, low phospholipid-associated cholelithiasis; OR, odds ratio; p, protein (amino acid number); *SLC10A2*, solute carrier 10A2; *UGT1A1*, UDP-glucuronosyl transferase 1.

- In case of acute cholecystitis, an early cholecystectomy (within 72 hours) is indicated.
- In patients with symptomatic bile duct stones, ERCP with stone removal, followed by early cholecystectomy in case of simultaneous gallbladder stones, is recommended.
- In patients with LPAC caused by *ABCB4* deficiency, long-term therapy with UDCA should be initiated to prevent occurrence or recurrence of the syndrome and its complications.

# Molecular Genetics and Molecular Mechanisms

Bile is composed of water, bile salts, phosphatidylcholine, cholesterol, and bilirubin. Adequate amounts of bile salts and phosphatidylcholine solubilize cholesterol and bilirubin in mixed micelles. The most common stones—cholesterol gallstones—precipitate in gallbladder from cholesterol supersaturated bile. Most gallstone patients display cholesterol bile supersaturation due to hypersecretion of cholesterols rather than hyposecretion of bile acids and phospholipids. According to twin studies as much as 25% of the gallstone risk in Europeans may be attributed to genetic predisposition. GWAS identified a common mutation of the hepatocanalicular cholesterol hemitransporter (*ABCG8* p.D19H) that promotes gallstone formation (Table 76-1). Based on serum lipid profiles, it has been hypothesized that individuals carrying the risk allele develop gallstones due to increased hepatic synthesis and secretion of cholesterol. Other defects observed in gallstone pathogenesis include increased synthesis of biliary mucin and gallbladder hypomotility. The latter factor leads to incomplete emptying of gallbladder content and to bile stasis. This in turn enhances formation of crystals, which grow into stones.

Black pigment gallstones are caused by augmented biliary secretion of bilirubin (eg, in the setting of hemolytic anemia), ineffective erythropoiesis (eg, in pernicious anemia), or spillage of excess bile salts into the large intestine, which promotes enterohepatic cycling of unconjugated bilirubin (in cystic fibrosis, extensive Crohn disease, or after ileocecal resection/bypass). The latter mechanism may also be caused by mutations of the *SLC10A2* (ileal sodium-dependent bile salt) transporter.

Carriers of the *UGT1A1* risk variant predisposing to the Gilbert syndrome are also at an increased risk of gallstone disease. In particular male carriers of the Gilbert syndrome *UGT1A1* promoter allele are prone to stone formation. In these individuals bilirubin crystals may serve as the primary nucleating factors on which cholesterol (and bilirubin) precipitates from supersaturated bile to grow gallstones.

*ABCB4* gene variants leading to deficiency of the hepatobiliary transporter for phosphatidylcholine, although less frequent, confer a higher risk for gallbladder (and intrahepatic) cholesterol stones as well as their recurrence after cholecystectomy. The LPAC syndrome often affects individuals of less than 40 years and is consistent with the spontaneous occurrence of cholelithiasis in mice lacking the *ABCB4* transporter.

***Genetic Testing:*** To date, genetic testing is not used in detecting or preventing gallstones. In patients with rare mutations that substantially increase the risk of developing gallstones, positive genetic test results might trigger primary prevention of symptomatic stones with UDCA.

***Future Directions:*** Quantification of individual gallstone risk based on multiple gene variants and environmental factors

- Identification of rare variants by targeted resequencing
- Identification of novel preventive strategies for individuals at highest stone risk
- Studies assessing the cost-effectiveness of pharmacologic interventions, for example, UDCA, statins and/or ezetimibe, in patients at risk of gallstone disease
- Development of new drugs that are tailored for carriers of genetic risk variants
- Evaluation of novel compounds such as modulators of the bile acid receptors FXR (nuclear receptor) and TGR5 (membrane receptor) in stone prevention and/or therapy

## Bibliography:

1. Buch S, Schafmayer C, Völzke H, et al. A genome-wide association scan identifies the hepatic cholesterol transporter ABCG8 as a susceptibility factor for human gallstone disease. *Nat Genet.* 2007;39:995-999.

2. Buch S, Schafmayer C, Völzke H, et al. Loci from a genome-wide analysis of bilirubin levels are associated with gallstone risk and composition. *Gastroenterology.* 2010;139:1942-1951.

3. Grünhage F, Acalovschi M, Tirziu S, et al. Increased gallstone risk in humans conferred by common variant of hepatic ATP-binding cassette transporter for cholesterol. *Hepatology.* 2007;46:793-801.

4. Katsika D, Grjibovski A, Einarsson C, Lammert F, Lichtenstein P, Marschall HU. Genetic and environmental influences on symptomatic gallstone disease: a Swedish study of 43,141 twin pairs. *Hepatology.* 2005;41:1138-1143.

5. Marschall HU, Krawczyk M, Grünhage F, et al. Gallstone disease in Swedish twins is associated with the Gilbert variant of UGT1A1. *Liver Int.* 2013;33:904-908.

6. Renner O, Harsch S, Schaeffeler E, et al. A variant of the SLC10A2 gene encoding the apical sodium-dependent bile acid transporter is a risk factor for gallstone disease. *PLoS One.* 2009;4:e7321.

7. Rosmorduc O, Poupon R. Low phospholipid associated cholelithiasis: association with mutation in the MDR3/ABCB4 gene. *Orphanet J Rare Dis.* 2007;2:29.

8. Stender S, Frikke-Schmidt R, Nordestgaard BG, et al. Sterol transporter adenosine triphosphate-binding cassette transporter G8, gallstones, and biliary cancer in 62,000 individuals from the general population. *Hepatology.* 2011;53:640-648.

9. Krawczyk M, Lütjohann D, Schirin-Sokhan R, et al. Phytosterol and cholesterol precursor levels indicate increased cholesterol excretion and biosynthesis in gallstone disease. *Hepatology.* 2012;55:1507-1517.

## Supplementary Information

### OMIM References:

[1] Gallbladder Disease 1; GBD1 (#600803)

[2] Gallbladder Disease 4; GBD4 (#611465)

[3] ATP-Binding Cassette, Subfamily G, Member 8; ABCG8 (#605460)

[4] UDP-Glucuronosyl Transferase (UGT)1A1; UGT1A1 (#191740)

### Alternative Names:

- Cholecystolithiasis
- Choledocholithasis

***Key Words:*** ABC transporter, cholecystectomy, cholelithiasis, cholesterol, ERCP, gallbladder, Gilbert syndrome, low phospholipid-associated cholelithiasis, solute carriers

# 77 Familial Autoinflammatory Diseases

Sylvie Grandemange, Isabelle Kone-Paut, and Isabelle Touitou

## KEY POINTS

- *Disease summary:*
  - Autoinflammatory diseases (AIDs) are illnesses of the innate immune system without high-titer autoantibodies or antigen-specific T cells in contrast to autoimmune diseases that relate to a deficit of acquired immunity. These diseases are characterized by recurrent fever and systemic inflammation, and the main complication is the risk of generalized or renal amyloidosis in untreated patients. Other sporadic, undefined, or complex disorders have been also linked to the AIDs group. This review will focus on hereditary recurrent fevers (HRFs).

- *Hereditary basis:*
  - Both dominant and recessive autosomal transmission, with incomplete penetrance

- *Differential diagnosis:*
  - Nonhereditary recurrent fevers, for example, PFAPA syndrome (Marshall syndrome)

## Diagnostic Criteria and Clinical Characteristics

### Diagnostic Criteria:

**Example: at least one of the following**

- Recurrent fever accompanied with various association of osteoarticular, cutaneous, and abdominal signs
- Biologic marker of inflammation (enhanced C-reactive protein [CRP]) during acute episodes
- Familial history

**And the absence of**

- Infection, antibodies

### Clinical Characteristics:

- Symptom-free periods, pediatric onset

## Screening and Counseling

**Screening:** See Fig. 77-1.

**Counseling:**

☞INHERITANCE, PENETRANCE: FMF and MKD are recessively inherited. TRAPS and CAPS are dominant diseases, but de novo mutations have been identified in rare cases of TRAPS and in all cases of severe forms of CAPS (also named, chronic infantile neurologic cutaneous and articular syndrome [CINCA]). Because of clinical similarities across AIDs, differential diagnosis is sometimes difficult. A decade ago, specific diagnosis has become possible after the discovery of the respective genes responsible for HRF (Table 77-1). The definitive genetic diagnosis of hereditary AIDs lies on the finding of unambiguous mutations in the causative genes, for example, *M694V* in the *FMF* gene, and *C30R* in the *TRAPS* gene. However, several variants are currently debated as to whether they are low-penetrance causing mutations or functional polymorphisms. Well-known examples are E148Q for *MEFV*, R121Q or P75L (old names R92Q and P46L) for *TNFRSF1A*, and V198M for *NLRP3*, respectively. A registry of mutations named infevers is available online at http://fmf.igh.cnrs.fr/ISSAID/infevers.

☞GENOTYPE-PHENOTYPE CORRELATION: The homozygote M694V genotype is associated with earlier onset and more frequent renal amyloidosis, but environmental factors may play a primary role overwhelming that of *MEFV* mutations. In TRAPS, mutations resulting in cysteine substitutions are associated with severe disease course and higher risk for secondary amyloidosis.

## Management and Treatment

The treatment depends on the HRF.

- In FMF, 1 mg daily colchicine therapy is effective in preventing acute episodes, as well as AA amyloidosis. A small proportion of patients with FMF respond poorly to colchicine, and it may be appropriate to increase the dose up to the maximum tolerated dose of approximately 3 mg/d under careful supervision (2 mg maximum in a child). The IL-1 RA agonist Anakinra has been reported effective in a few patients with FMF resistant or in case of intolerance to colchicine.

- The therapeutic options for MKD are still limited and most experiences rely on case reports. Some patients may respond to either nonsteroidal anti-inflammatory or high-dose steroids when given at crises onset. There are few reports of MKD patients who responded adequately to Anakinra and anti-TNF (Etanercept); however, data are too preliminary to confirm the advantage of IL-1 versus TNF blockade in this disease.

- Inflammatory episodes in TRAPS patients usually respond to nonsteroidal anti-inflammatory drugs or steroid treatment. However, long-term use of steroids may induce significant toxicity.

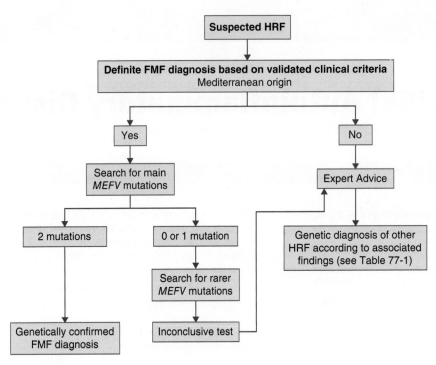

*Figure 77-1* Algorithm for Screening of Patient With Hereditary Recurrent Fever.

The first successful biotherapy administered in AIDs patient was the use of anti-TNF in a young TRAPS patient with renal amyloidosis. This therapeutic however later revealed not effective in all patients.

• First clinical experiences in small series of patients with CAPS features demonstrated the efficacy and safety of Anakinra, given daily subcutaneously at dosages ranging from 1 to 8 mg/kg. All patients responded to the drug at least partially. Alternatives to Anakinra are rilonacept (IL-1 trap) a fusion protein designed to attach to and neutralize IL-1 before it binds to the cell surface, and canakinumab, a potent anti-IL-1 monoclonal antibody. These two latter drugs are registered for use in United States and Europe for patients with CAPS.

The management of treated patients suffering from HRF includes clinical evaluation every 6 to 12 months depending on disease activity, as well as at least, in a stable patient, annual urinalysis, CRP and if possible serum amyloid A (SAA) dosage and white

*Table 77-1 Genetic Differential Diagnosis*

| Syndrome | Gene Symbol | Associated Findings |
|---|---|---|
| FMF: familial Mediterranean fever | *MEFV* (Mediterranean fever) | Recurrent fever lasting 1-3 days, almost exclusively patients of Mediterranean ancestry, peritonitis, monoarthralgia of the lower extremities, erysipelas-like erythema, splenomegaly |
| MKD: mevalonate kinase deficiency | *MVK* (mevalonate kinase) | Recurrent fever lasting 3-7 days, diarrhea, cervical adenopathies, acute abdomen bipolar aphtosis, arthralgia, maculopapular rash |
| TRAPS: TNF receptor-associated periodic syndrome | *TNFRSF1A* (tumor necrosis factor receptor superfamily 1A) | Recurrent fever lasting a few days to a few weeks, cervical stiffness, migratory erythema and myalgia, arthralgia |
| CAPS: cryopyrin-associated periodic syndrome | *NLRP3* (NLR family, pyrin domain containing 3) | Recurrent fever lasting a few hours to a few days, circadian profile, urticaria, arthralgia, and in severe cases, amyloidosis, deafness, blindness, bone deformation, meningitis |

Table 77-2 Syndrome/Gene/Locus/OMIM References/Alternative Names

| Acronym | Disease | | | | The Gene And Its Product | | | | |
|---|---|---|---|---|---|---|---|---|---|
| | Extended | Synonyme(s) | OMIM | Transmission | Locus Map | Acronyme | Extended | OMIM | Protein and synonyme(s) |
| FMF | Familial Mediterranean fever | Periodic fever, recurrent serositis | 249100 | Recessive | 16p13 | MEFV | MEditerranean FeVer | 608107 | Pyrin, Marenostrin |
| MKD | Mevalonate Kinase Deficiency | | | Recessive | | | | | |
| MA | Mevalonic Aciduria | | 610377 | | 12q24 | MVK | Mevalonate Kinase | 251170 | |
| HIDS | Hyper IgD Syndrome | | 260920 | | | | | | |
| TRAPS | TNF-Receptor Associated Periodic Syndrome | Familial Hibernian Fever; FHF | 142680 | Dominant | 12p13.2 | TNFRSF1A | Tumor Necrosis Factor Receptor Super Family 1A | 191190 | |
| CAPS | Cryopyrin Associated Periodic Syndrome | | | Dominant | 1q44 | NLRP3 | NLR pyrin domain containing protein 3 | 606416 | Cryopyrin, Cold Induced Autoinflammatory Domain-, Leucine-Rich Repeat and Pyd-Containing Protein 3; NALP3 Pyrin Domain-Containing Apaf1-Like Protein 1; PYPAF1, Caterpiller 1.1; CLR 1.1 |
| FCAS | Familial Cold Autoinflammatory Syndrome | Familial Cold Urticaria; FCU | 120100 | | | | | | |
| MWS | Muckle-Wells Syndrome | | 191900 | | | | | | |
| CINCA | Chronic Neurologic Cutaneous and Articular Syndrome | Neonatal-Onset Multisystem Inflammatory Disease; NOMID | 607115 | | | | | | |

*Table 77-3 Molecular Genetic Testing*

| Gene | Testing Modality | Mutation Type | Detection Rate |
|---|---|---|---|
| MEFV (Mediterranean fever) | Sequence analysis on genomic DNA from leucocytes | Almost exclusively substitutions | Up to 70% in patients from Mediterranean ancestry and clinical criteria. Less than 5% in other populations |
| MVK (mevalonate kinase) | | | >90% in patients with mevalonic aciduria and/or enzymatic defect |
| TNFRSF1A (tumor necrosis factor receptor superfamily 1A) | | | Less than 50% |
| NLRP3 (NLR family, pyrin domain containing 3) | | | |

blood cell count. Patients receiving colchicine must receive information on its potential toxicity in case of overdose, renal insufficiency, and in association to certain medications, for example, macrolids, statins, and cyclosporine. In patients receiving anti-IL-1 biologics, careful follow-up of leukocyte count, liver function, and cholesterol is needed every 3 to 4 months.

## Molecular Genetics and Molecular Mechanism

***Description of Basic Gene Functions:*** Innate immunity is our first line of defense against a wide range of exogenous and endogenous danger signal. Two main signaling pathways are defective in AIDs, those which lead to NF-κB activation, and those which allow the cleavage of pro-IL-1β via formation of a multiprotein platform named the inflammasome. Both enable the release of the active form of the proinflammatory pyrogenic interleukin-1β. HRFs are due to mutations in genes regulating either pathway. See Table 77-2.

- The exact function of the FMF protein named marenostrin or pyrin is not clear yet and probably complex. Contradictory studies show that it could both have an anti-inflammatory role through inhibition of IL-1β by sequestering an adapter protein (ASC) of the NLRP3 inflammasome, or act as a proinflammatory regulator through activation of IL-1β and by direct or indirect stimulation of the inflammasome, with rapid cell death and release of IL-1β.
- Mevalonate kinase (MK) is an essential enzyme in the isoprenoid and cholesterol synthesis. The MK enzyme catalyses the phosphorylation of mevalonic acid into 5-phosphomevalonate, which is the enzyme following the hydroxymethylglutaryl-coenzyme A reductase (HMGR) in the isoprenoid or cholesterol biosynthesis pathway. In case of cholesterol shortage, sterol regulatory element-binding proteins are synthesized to increase MK activity, and then cholesterol appears to be a main "sensor" of the pathway. MK enzyme deficiency results in mevalonic acid accumulation and end-product shortage. The role of this metabolic defect on inflammation is unclear but it has been demonstrated that the shortage of isoprenoid end products increases IL-1β secretion in MK-deficient peripheral blood mononuclear cells.

- TRAPS arises from mutations in TNFR1, a protein that mediates NF-κB signaling, and indirectly apoptosis and cytokine regulation. The impact of mutations in this receptor is probably multiple, on the receptor shedding, trafficking, or structure leading to cellular aggregates. In this disease, cells are more susceptible to inflammatory stimuli, and show sustained activation and decreased apoptosis.
- NLRP3 is a proinflammatory protein as it participates in the formation of inflammasome. In the absence of a trigger (bacteria, cell rupture, monosodium urate crystal), the leucine-rich repeat (LRR) domain of NLRP3 is thought to serve as an autoinhibitor by self-folding. Following the sensing of a proinflammatory component by the LRR domain, the molecule would spread out, dimerize, and associate through homotypic interaction with an adaptor protein to mediate the proteolytic processing of pro-IL-1β into its active form. Mutations cause constitutive activation of the inflammasome and enhance secretion of IL-1β.

### Genetic Testing (Table 77-3):

☞**Clinical Availability of Testing:** Genetic testing for FMF is available worldwide, and in United States of America and most European countries for the other HRF.

See Orphanet (http://www.orpha.net/consor/cgi-bin/index.php) and Genetest (http://www.ncbi.nlm.nih.gov/sites/GeneTests/?db=GeneTests)

☞**Utility of Testing:** A specific diagnosis is indispensable for a targeted treatment.

### Bibliography:

1. McDermott MF, Aksentijevich I. The autoinflammatory syndromes. *Curr Opin Allergy Clin Immunol.* 2002;2:511-516.
2. Touitou I, Kone-Paut I. Autoinflammatory diseases. *Best Pract Res Clin Rheumatol.* 2008;22:811-829.
3. The French FMF Consortium. A candidate gene for familial Mediterranean fever. *Nat Genet.* 1997;17:25-31.
4. The International FMF Consortium. Ancient missense mutations in a new member of the RoRet gene family are likely to cause familial Mediterranean fever. *Cell.* 1997;90:797-807.
5. Drenth JP, Cuisset L, Grateau G, et al. Mutations in the gene encoding mevalonate kinase cause hyper-IgD and periodic fever syndrome. International Hyper-IgD Study Group. *Nat Genet.* 1999;22:178-181.

6. McDermott MF, Aksentijevich I, Galon J, et al. Germline mutations in the extracellular domains of the 55 kDa TNF receptor, TNFR1, define a family of dominantly inherited autoinflammatory syndromes. *Cell.* 1999;97:133-144.

7. Hoffman HM, Mueller JL, Broide DH, et al. Mutation of a new gene encoding a putative pyrin-like protein causes familial cold autoinflammatory syndrome and Muckle-Wells syndrome. *Nat Genet.* 2001;29:301-305.

8. Feldmann J, Prieur AM, Quartier P, et al. Chronic infantile neurological cutaneous and articular syndrome is caused by mutations in CIAS1, a gene highly expressed in polymorphonuclear cells and chondrocytes. *Am J Hum Genet.* 2002;71:198-203.

9. Goldfinger SE. Colchicine for familial Mediterranean fever. *N Engl J Med.* 1972;287:1302.

10. Drewe E, McDermott EM, Powell RJ. Treatment of the nephrotic syndrome with etanercept in patients with the tumor necrosis factor receptor-associated periodic syndrome. *N Engl J Med.* 2000;343:1044-1045.

11. Hawkins PN, Lachmann HJ, McDermott MF. Interleukin-1-receptor antagonist in the Muckle-Wells syndrome. *N Engl J Med.* 2003;348:2583-2584.

12. Goldbach-Mansky R, Shroff SD, Wilson M, et al. A pilot study to evaluate the safety and efficacy of the long-acting interleukin-1 inhibitor rilonacept (interleukin-1 trap) in patients with familial cold autoinflammatory syndrome. *Arthritis Rheum.* 2008;58:2432-2442.

13. Lachmann HJ, Kone-Paut I, Kuemmerle-Deschner JB, et al. Use of canakinumab in the cryopyrin-associated periodic syndrome. *N Engl J Med.* 2009;360:2416-2425.

## Supplementary Information

**OMIM Reference:**

[1] Condition; Gene Name (OMIM#) See Table 77-2

**Alternative Name:** See Table 77-2.

*Key Words:* Recurrent fever, pediatric, systemic manifestations, inflammation

# 78 Common Variable Immune Deficiency

James M. Fernandez and Duane R. Wesemann

## KEY POINTS

- *Disease summary:*
  - Common variable immune deficiency (CVID) is a heterogeneous immunodeficiency disease characterized by low serum levels of the immunoglobulin isotypes IgG and IgA, impaired ability to produce specific antibodies after immunization and recurrent infections of the sinopulmonary or gastrointestinal tract.
  - First described in 1953 and later coined in 1973, CVID may present in childhood, adolescence, or adulthood and is the most common primary immunodeficiency syndrome that comes to medical attention.
  - In addition to being more susceptible to infections, CVID also can manifest aspects of immune dysregulation with noninfectious complications including autoimmunity (most typically autoimmune cytopenias), noninfectious gastrointestinal disease, granulomatous inflammation, lymphoid disease, and an increased risk of malignancy.
  - Although most cases of CVID are sporadic mutations, seven disease-causing or contributing genes have been identified that give rise to a CVID phenotype in the past 10 years.
- *Prevalence:*
  - The prevalence of CVID has been estimated at between 1:10000 and 1:100000 depending on geographic location.
- *Differential diagnosis:*
  - Because CVID is a diagnosis of exclusion, other causes of hypogammaglobulinemia must be ruled out. These include
  - X-linked agammaglobulinemia; X-linked lymphoproliferative disease; hyper-IgM syndromes; IgG subclass deficiency; selective antibody deficiency; secondary hypogammaglobulinemia; decreased production due to malignancy, drugs such as gold salts, penicillamine, antimalarial drugs, corticosteroids, phenytoin, carbamazapine, viral infections, and systemic illnesses causing bone marrow suppression are associated with the decreased production of immunoglobulins; increased loss due to protein-losing enteropathies, such as intestinal lymphangiectasia, nephrotic syndrome, burns, and other traumas leading to loss of fluids.

## Diagnostic Criteria and Clinical Characteristics

**Diagnostic Criteria for CVID:** CVID is defined as a diagnosis of exclusion.

The current PAGID diagnostic criteria state that CVID is probable in a male or female patient who has a marked decrease of IgG (at least 2 SD below the mean for age) and a marked decrease in at least one of the isotypes IgM or IgA, *and* fulfills *all* of the following criteria:

1. Onset of immunodeficiency at greater than 2 years of age.
2. Absent isohemagglutinins and/or poor response to vaccines.
3. Defined causes of hypogammaglobulinemia have been excluded.

**Clinical Characteristics:** Most patients with CVID are recognized to have a clinically significant immunodeficiency in the second, third, or fourth decades of life, after they have had several infections. Viral, fungal, and parasitic infections as well as bacterial infections may be causative.

The serum concentration of IgM is normal in about half of the patients. Abnormalities in T-cell numbers or function are common. The majority of patients have normal numbers of B cells; however, some have low or absent B cells with a unique subset being deficient in class switched memory B cells.

**Clinical Complications:**

☞**INFECTIONS:** Acute and chronic infections account for a large part of morbidity in patients with CVID. Recurrent respiratory tract infections are the most common feature, affecting up to 98% of patients, with the most common organisms isolated being *Streptococcus pneumoniae* and *Haemophilus influenzae*.

☞**BRONCHIECTASIS:** Recurrent respiratory tract infections can result in development of bronchiectasis, which is present in 4% to 76% of patients depending on the cohort.

☞**GASTROINTESTINAL COMPLICATIONS:** Approximately 20% to 60% of patients with CVID develop gastrointestinal disease. Diarrhea is the most frequently seen gastrointestinal manifestation in CVID with commonly identified pathogens including *Giardia*, *Campylobacter*, and *Salmonella* species. Infection with *Helicobacter pylori* infection is not uncommon and is associated with gastritis and an increased risk of development of malignancy.

Noninfectious pathologies have also been observed including pernicious anemia, inflammatory bowel disease, lymphocytic colitis, collagenous enterocolitis, and flattened villi. Abnormalities in liver function tests, autoimmune hepatitis, and primary biliary cirrhosis have been described in CVID.

☞**AUTOIMMUNITY:** Autoimmune disease is seen in 25% to 48% of CVID patients depending on the country. The most common diseases are autoimmune thrombocytopenia and autoimmune hemolytic anemia although multiple other immune diseases including vitiligo, psoriasis, pernicious anemia, rheumatoid arthritis, systemic lupus, Sjogren syndrome, primary biliary cirrhosis, hepatitis, and thyroiditis have all been described.

☞**GRANULOMATOUS DISEASE:** Granulomatous inflammation affects between 8% and 22% of patients with CVID and commonly affects the lungs, lymph nodes, and spleen but can be found in many other organs including liver, parotid glands, meninges, and bone marrow.

☞**MALIGNANCY:** The overall incidence of malignancy is increased in CVID with gastric carcinoma and non-Hodgkin lymphomas being the greatest risks with increased risks of 7 to 16 and 12 to 18 times higher, respectively. Multiple other malignancies have been observed to incur a greater risk with CVID including colorectal, breast, ovarian cancer, prostate, and multiple myeloma.

## Screening and Counseling

**Screening:** No single screening tool has been identified nor is required for the diagnosis of CVID. Genome-wide association study (GWAS) has identified many associations with CVID. When a primary humoral deficiency is suspected, serum levels of IgM, IgA, IgE, IgG, and IgG subclasses should be evaluated. Laboratory tests for antitetanus, H flu, and hepatitis B can be assessed for response to protein antigens if the patient has received these vaccines at least 1 month prior. Immune response to polysaccharide antigens can be assessed after receiving pneumovax by checking pneumococcal serotype antibodies at least 1 month prior to the vaccine.

Genetic testing for some of the more recognized mutations in CVID such as *TACI, ICOS, CD19, BAFF-R, MSH5* can be assessed for a molecular diagnosis and are available at specialized reference laboratories. Molecular testing is sometimes useful to exclude immunodeficiencies that arise from known genetic defects, such as some of the causes of hyper IgM syndrome.

Recently, a custom 300-kb resequencing array, the hyper-IgM/CVID chip, which interrogates 1576 coding regions from 148 genes implicated in B-cell development and immunoglobulin isotype switching has been developed.

**Counseling:** Approximately 10% of patients have at least one family member with either CVID or selective IgA deficiency.

Patients with known germline mutations in *CD19* or *ICOS* can expect autosomal recessive inheritance, whereas CVID due to germline inactivating mutation(s) in *TACI* can expect autosomal dominant inheritance. Carrier testing and prenatal diagnosis for pregnancies at increased risk for ICOS and TACI-associated CVID are available.

It is generally felt that family members and household contacts of patients with CVID may safely receive live vaccines without risk to the patient.

## Management and Treatment

**Management:**

☞REPLACEMENT IMMUNOGLOBULIN THERAPY: Replacement immunoglobulin therapy is the mainstay of treatment in CVID. Delivery of immunoglobulin through both the intravenous and subcutaneous routes appears to be safe and equally effective in preventing infections.

Current recommendations for immunoglobulin replacement involves starting a 400 mg/kg total monthly dose and then adjusting the dose to achieve a desired clinical effect. The ideal trough level to be achieved with immunoglobulin replacement therapy is debatable with suggestions ranging from levels greater than 800 mg/dL, greater than 700 mg/dL, and between 650 and 1000 mg/dL. Due to multiple factors such as IgG production rate, overall catabolism, metabolism, and comorbidities affecting clearance, each individual's pharmacokinetics change on a fairly routine basis. For these reasons, dose adjustment must be individualized and titrated to efficacy while being assisted by frequent trough levels. One needs to use caution when increasing the dose of infusion as the immunomodulatory mechanisms of high-dose IgG infusions may result

in altered expression and function of Fc receptors of IgG, impaired complement activation, altered cytokine profiles, and changes in cell proliferation, and therefore may have an immunosuppressive effect at high doses.

☞ANTIBIOTICS: Aggressive antibiotic regimens are usually given during acute respiratory infections to prevent long-term complications. If possible, specimen sampling and microbial susceptibility should be sent but should not delay starting empirical therapy. Typically an extended treatment course of 10 to 14 days is given per infectious episode.

Antibiotic prophylaxis should also be considered for frequent infections (> three per year) or severe infections or atypical sources of infection (eg, fungal). Clinical judgment on an individual patient basis must be used when designing overall patient treatment plans as some patients may benefit from both antibiotic prophylaxis as well as regular immunoglobulin therapy.

☞TRANSPLANT: Solid organ transplant: A few cases of lung and liver transplantation in CVID have been reported showing some short-term effect.

Stem cell transplantation: This represents a potential cure for the immunodeficiency but when and which subset of patients would benefit from transplant is still under much debate.

☞VACCINATIONS: There are no reports of CVID patients being affected adversely by vaccination with either live or other types of vaccines. CVID patients should receive the appropriate vaccines to prevent infectious diseases when travelling.

☞REFERRALS: If the patient's history, physical examination, and laboratory tests raise concern about a possible diagnosis of CVID, a referral to a clinical immunologist is indicated to assess vaccine responsiveness fully and to exclude other immune disorders. If CVID is confirmed, continued follow-up with a specialist at regular intervals is also advisable in order to follow immunoglobulin levels as well as participate in appropriate screening for further complications.

## Molecular Genetics or Molecular Mechanism

Most cases of CVID are sporadic in nature but approximately 10% of cases have been demonstrated to show familial clustering. Multiple genetic linkage studies in the 1980s showed an association on the human leukocyte antigen (HLA) region, but recently various gene mutations have been linked to the disease. A list of the most likely disease-causing mutations is listed below:

**TACI Mutations:** *TACI* is a receptor for the tumor necrosis factor (TNF)-related protein APRIL, which is needed for naïve B cells to obtain the ability to secrete IgA and IgG. B cells from *TACI* mutations are severely impaired in their ability. Mutations in *TACI* have been discovered in a significant proportion of patients with CVID, with 8.9% (50 out of 564) patients possessing at least one abnormal allele in the largest cohort of patients are analyzed.

**ICOS Mutations:** ICOS deficiency was the first genetic defect identified in patients with CVID. *ICOS* is a costimulatory molecule similar to CD28, which is expressed on activated T cells. Deficiency of ICOS is thought to inhibit the ability of T cells to provide cytokine "help" B cells need for antibody production. To date, 11 individuals from five different families have been identified, 9 of them with the same mutation.

***BAFF-R Mutation:*** A homozygous 24 bp in-frame deletion has been identified causing removal of an 8 hydrophobic amino acid sequence in the B-cell activating factor receptor (*BAFF-R*) transmembrane region resulting in undetectable BAFF-R protein expression on the B-cell surface. This is thought to cause reduced class-switched and nonclass-switched B cells. Mutations in *BAFF-R* have been identified in two individuals—a brother and sister pair born of a consanguineous marriage.

***CD19-Complex Mutations (CD19, CD21, CD81):*** *CD19* is expressed together with *CD21*, *CD81*, and *CD225* on the surface of mature B cells. *CD19* and *CD21* are B-cell specific antigens and are present on most other immune cells. Low or absent levels of CD19 protein on CD20+ B cells due to mutations appear to cause a decrease on class-switched memory B cells. These mutations are estimated to occur in about 1% of CVID patients and give an autosomal recessive inheritance.

***CD20 Mutations:*** *CD20* is a B-cell differentiation antigen widely expressed in B-cell development. Mutations in *CD20* may result in decreased B-cell proliferation and differentiation. This mechanism is used to the patient's advantage when treating certain autoimmune diseases with monoclonal antibodies targeting CD20. A homozygous mutation in *CD20* has been seen in one patient.

***MSH5 Mutations:*** *MSH5* is involved in DNA mismatch repair and meiotic homologous recombination and has been shown to play a role in CSR in mice and consequently a small cohort of American and Swedish patients with CVID were identified to have a *MSH5* mutation.

***GWAS:*** A total of 363 CVID patients and 3031 healthy controls were genotyped. Analysis of the data showed a significant association with the major histocompatibility complex (MHC) region and a suggestive association with a locus containing *ADAM28*, *ADAM7*, *ADAMDEC1*, and *STC1*. No association with the locus containing *TACI* was identified, nor were any patients with *TACI* mutations separately identified. This genome-wide analysis of SNP genotypes and CNVs uncovered multiple novel susceptibility loci for CVID, which the authors felt was consistent with idea that CVID is a heterogeneous disease. It is hopeful that the results will provide a new understanding of the immunopathogenesis of CVID.

## BIBLIOGRAPHY:

1. Janeway C, Apt L, Gitlin D. Agammaglobulinemia. *Trans Assoc Am Physicians*. 1953;66:200-202.

2. Cooper MD, Faulk WP, Fudenberg HH, et al. Classification of primary immunodeficie ncies. *N Engl J Med*. 1973;288(18):966-967.

3. Geha RS, Rosen F. *Case Studies in Immunology*. 5th ed. New York, NY: Garland Science, Taylor & Francis Group; 2008.

4. Yong PF, Thaventhiran JE, Grimbacher B. "A rose is a rose is a rose," but CVID is Not CVID common variable immune deficiency (CVID), what do we know in 2011. *Adv Immunol*. 2011;111:47-107.

5. Chapel H, Cunningham-Rundles C. Update in understanding common variable immunodeficiency disorders (CVIDs) and the management of patients with these conditions. *Br J Haematol*. 2009;145(6):709-727.

6. Cunningham-Rundles C, Bodian C. Common variable immunodeficiency: clinical and immunological features of 248 patients. *Clin Immunol*. 1999;92(1):34-48.

7. Chapel H, Lucas M, Lee M, et al. Common variable immunodeficiency disorders: division into distinct clinical phenotypes. *Blood*. 2008;112(2):277-286.

8. Ardeniz O, Cunningham-Rundles C. Granulomatous disease in common variable immunodeficiency. *Clin Immunol*. 2009;133(2):198-207.

9. Orange JS, Glessner JT, Resnick E, et al. Genome-wide association identifies diverse causes of common variable immunodeficiency. *J Allergy Clin Immunol*. 2011;127:1360.

10. Hare ND, Smith BJ, Ballas ZK. Antibody response to pneumococcal vaccination as a function of preimmunization titer. *J Allergy Clin Immunol*. 2009;123(1):195-200.

11. Blancas-Galicia L, Ramírez-Vargas NG, Espinosa-Rosales F. Common variable immunodeficiency. A clinical approach. *Rev Invest Clin*. 2010 Nov-Dec;62(6):577-582.

12. Wang HY, Gopalan V, Aksentijevich I, et al. A custom 148 gene-based resequencing chip and the SNP explorer software: new tools to study antibody deficiency. *Hum Mutat*. Sep 2010;31(9):1080-1088.

13. Hammarstrom L, Vorechovsky I, Webster D. Selective IgA deficiency (SIgAD) and common variable immunodeficiency (CVID). *Clin Exp Immunol*. 2000;120(2):225-231.

14. Bonilla FA. IgG replacement therapy, no size fits all. *Clin Immunol*. 2011 May;139(2):107-109.

15. Orange JS, Hossny EM, Weiler CR, et al. Use of intravenous immunoglobulin inhuman disease: a review of evidence by members of the Primary Immunodeficiency Committee of the American Academy of Allergy, Asthma and Immunology. *J Allergy Clin Immunol*. 2006;117(suppl 4), S525-S553.

16. Shehata N, Palda V, Bowen T, et al. The use of immunoglobulin therapy for patients with primary immune deficiency: an evidence-based practice guideline. *Transfus Med Rev*. 2010;24(suppl 1): S28-S50.

17. Roifman CM, Lederman HM, Lavi S, Stein LD, Levison H, Gelfand EW. Benefit of intravenous IgG replacement in hypogammaglobulinemic patients with chronic sinopulmonary disease. *Am J Med*. 1985;79(2):171-174.

18. Berger M, Rojavin M, Kiessling P, Zenker O. Pharmacokinetics of subcutaneous immunoglobulin and their use in dosing of replacement therapy in patients with primary immunodeficiency. *Clin Immunol*. 2011;139:133-141.

19. Jolles S. A review of high-dose intravenous immunoglobulin (hdIVIg) in the treatment of the autoimmune blistering disorders. *Clin Exp Dermatol*. Mar 2001;26(2):127-131.

20. Cunningham-Rundles C. How I treat common variable immune deficiency. *Blood*. 2010;116:7.

21. Salzer U, Warnatz K, Rizzi M, et al. B-cell activating factor receptor deficiency is associated with an adult-onset antibody deficiency syndrome in humans. *Proc Natl Acad Sci USA*. 2009;106(33):13945-13950.

22. Kopecky O, Lukesova S. Genetic defects in common variable immunodeficiency. *Int J Immunogenet*. 2007;34(4):225-229.

23. Takahashi N, Matsumoto K, Saito H, et al. Impaired CD4 and CD8 effector function and decreased memory T cell populations in ICOS-deficient patients. *J Immunol*. 2009;182(9):5515-5527.

24. Park MA, Li JT, Hagan JB, Maddox DE, Abraham RS. Common variable immunodeficiency: a new look at an old disease. *Lancet*. Aug 9 2008;372(9637):489-502.

25. Kuijpers TW, Bende RJ, Baars PA, et al. CD20 deficiency in humans results in impaired T cell-independent antibody responses. *J Clin Invest*. 2010;120(1):214-222.

26. Sekine H, Ferreira RC, Pan-Hammarstrom Q, et al. Role for Msh5 in the regulation of Ig class switch recombination. *Proc Natl Acad Sci USA*. 2007;104(17):7193-7198.

## Supplementary Information

**OMIM References:**

[1] Immunodeficiency, Common Variable, 1; Susceptibility to, 1; ICOS (#607594)

[2] Immunodeficiency, Common Variable, 2; Susceptibility to, 2; TACI (#604907)

[3] Immunodeficiency, Common Variable, 3; Susceptibility to, 3; CD19 (#107265)

[4] Immunodeficiency, Common Variable, 4; Susceptibility to, 4; BAFFR (#613494)

[5] Immunodeficiency, Common Variable, 5; Susceptibility to, 5; CD20 (#613495)

Gene/Locus:

| | |
|---|---|
| ICOS | 2q33 |
| TACI | 17p11 |
| CD19 | 16p11 |
| BAFFR | 22q13.2 |
| CD20 | 11q12.2 |

**Alternative Names:**
- Acquired Hypogammaglobulinemia
- Late-Onset Immunoglobulin Deficiency

*Key Words:* Common variable immune deficiency, immunodeficiency, hypogammaglobulinemia, IgA, IgG, IgE, IgM, recurrent infections, CD19, TACI, ICOS, late-onset hypogammaglobulinemia, acquired hypogammaglobulinemia, B cells

# 79 Hereditary Angioedema

Duane R. Wesemann and Rebecca Breslow

## KEY POINTS

- *Disease summary*
  - Hereditary angioedema (HAE) is a disorder characterized by episodic local subcutaneous and submucosal edema that typically involves the gastrointestinal and upper respiratory tracts.
  - There are three clinically indistinguishable types of the disorder. In HAE type I, serum levels of C1 esterase inhibitor (C1NH) are less than 35% of normal. In HAE type II, the levels are normal or elevated, but the protein is nonfunctional. HAE type III occurs exclusively in women. Both concentration and function of C1 inhibitor are normal and are precipitated or worsened by high estrogen levels.
  - The hereditary form accounts for approximately 2% of clinical angioedema cases and occurs in approximately 1 in 50,000 persons. It affects whites, African Americans, and all other ethnic groups.
- *Hereditary basis:*
  - Inheritance: autosomal dominant

## Diagnostic Criteria and Clinical Characteristics

***Diagnostic Criteria:*** The diagnosis is established in patients with one clinical criterion and one laboratory criterion. This is true for acquired disorders as well.

### Clinical Criteria:

- Self-limiting, noninflammatory subcutaneous angioedema without urticaria, recurrent, and lasting more than 12 hours.
- Self-remitting, recurrent abdominal pain lasting more than 6 hours without clear organic etiology.
- Recurrent laryngeal edema.
- A family history of recurrent angioedema and/or abdominal pain and/or laryngeal edema, if present, supports the diagnosis of HAE, although it is not required because the patient may have a new mutation or an acquired disorder.

### Laboratory Criteria:

- C1 inhibitor levels less than 50% of the lower limit of normal at two separate determinations (at least 1 month apart) with the patient in their basal condition and after the first year of life.
- C1 inhibitor function of less than 50% of normal at two separate determinations (at least 1 month apart) with the patient in their basal condition and after the first year of life.
- Mutation in C1 inhibitor gene altering protein synthesis and/or function. This is the only laboratory criterion that can be used to make the diagnosis in patients younger than 1 year of age.
- The criteria stipulate that C1 inhibitor antigenic levels and functional levels must be below 50%.

The following diagnostic algorithm (Fig. 79-1) was presented at an international consensus conference (Bowen et al, 2004).

Cutaneous eruptions are characterized by recurrent, nonpruritic angioedema in the absence of hives. Swelling can affect any area of the body, including the extremities, face, trunk, gastrointestinal tract, genitourinary regions, or upper airways. Abdominal symptoms include nausea, vomiting, abdominal pains, and diarrhea and may mimic infantile colic, acute appendicitis, or acute abdomen. Age of onset is variable, and the patient might present at less than 1 year of age with colic. Most patients experience their first attack by age 15, but the diagnosis may also be suspected in young adults, especially in retrospect of earlier symptoms. Although laryngeal symptoms may occur in early childhood, this tends to occur later. Attacks tend to last within 72 hours and usually are periodic, often followed by several weeks of remission.

Attack triggers are often unknown, but may include trauma, stress, menstruation, pregnancy, medicines (eg, oral contraceptives and angiotensin-converting enzyme [ACE] inhibitors), or infections.

## Screening and Counseling

***Screening:*** Screening for C1-INH deficiency is indicated when one or more of the following is present: recurrent angioedema without urticaria, unexplained recurrent episodes of self-limited, colicky, abdominal pain, a family history of angioedema, unexplained laryngeal edema, low C4 levels, especially in the setting of angioedema.

### Counseling:

Penetrance: Incomplete.

☞GENOTYPE-PHENOTYPE CORRELATION: Two genetic types of HAE result in indistinguishable phenotypic expression. Restriction endonuclease techniques demonstrate that multiple mutations can result in the affected phenotype. Those who inherit the abnormal gene can have a clinical spectrum ranging from asymptomatic to severely affected.

## Management and Treatment

***Acute Attacks:*** If laryngeal edema is present, airway assessment and management must always take precedence over any other treatments. If anaphylaxis is a diagnostic possibility, the patient should be given epinephrine (0.3 mg IM for adults, 0.01 mg/kg IM for children) without delay. Complement studies and/or serum tryptase levels should be obtained after the patient is stabilized. Any elevation in serum tryptase is consistent with anaphylaxis, although a normal level does not exclude it. The mainstay of therapy for acute HAE attacks is infusion of C1-INH replacement protein, the

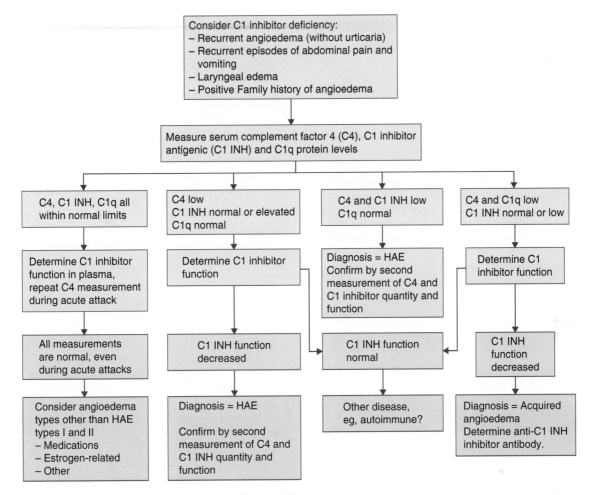

*Figure 79-1* Diagnostic Algorithm When Considering C1 Inhibitor Deficiency

two available products are Cinryze and Berinert. Use of C1-INH replacement protein results in rapid symptom reduction and reduced attack duration and is associated with a very low incidence of adverse effects. Cinryze, which originated in the Netherlands, is a purified human product which is dosed at 500 to 1500 U and infused intravenously. Berinert, the German product, is also derived from human plasma and administered intravenously. It is dosed at 20 U/kg body weight. A recombinant C1 inhibitor protein is currently in development but is not yet available for clinical use.

Fibrinolytics, such as epsilon-aminocaproic acid and tranexamic acid (not available in the United States) are older alternative agents and should be used according to established guidelines where available. In areas where these agents are not available, laryngeal attacks and severe abdominal attacks may be treated with repeated infusions of fresh frozen plasma (FFP), although there is a theoretical risk of exacerbating attacks with FFP and its use is controversial. The attenuated androgen danazol may also used for acute attacks by increasing levels of the C4 complement component. It may be given at 200 mg two to three times per day for acute attacks. After a favorable response, the dosage may be decreased by 50% or less at intervals of 1 to 3 months or longer as the frequency of attacks dictates. If an attack occurs, the dosage may be increased by up to 200 mg/d. Stanozolol, another attenuated androgen, is also an option and may be dosed up to 12 mg daily in the setting of an

acute attack. Mild-to-moderate abdominal attacks may be treated supportively with hydration and pain relief alone.

Two newer agents, ecallantide (Kalbitor) and icatibant (Firazyr), have recently been approved for the treatment of acute attacks. Ecallantide is a yeast-derived, reversible inhibitor of kallikrein which binds rapidly and with great avidity. It is approved for patients 16 years of age and older. A dose of 30 mg may be administered subcutaneously or intravenously, and its efficacy has been demonstrated in an extensive series of clinical trials. However, anaphylactic reactions to the product have been reported and, because of this, it must be administered by a healthcare professional. Icatibant is a bradykinin B2 receptor antagonist and is approved for treatment of acute attacks in adults. It is dosed at 30 mg SC, and has been shown to greatly reduce the median time to symptom relief without any significant drug-related adverse events. It may be self-administered at home, though patients are cautioned to seek emergency medical care following treatment of laryngeal attacks.

***Prevention or Prophylaxis:*** Cinryze is indicated for routine prophylaxis and is now considered as first-line therapy for prevention of HAE attacks. It is dosed at 500 to 1500 U administered IV every 3 to 4 days. It may be self-administered or given by a healthcare professional, depending on the individual situation. It may also be infused 1 hour prior to dental and surgical procedures as preprocedure prophylaxis. Attenuated androgens and fibrinolytics have also been used preprocedure for this purpose. Plasminogen activators are a theoretic risk, so use of these must be considered carefully. ACE inhibitors and estrogen-containing contraceptives should be avoided.

## Differential Diagnosis:

**Cutaneous or laryngeal swelling:** Allergic reactions and anaphylaxis, idiopathic angioedema, drug-induced angioedema (particularly ACE inhibitors or nonsteroidal anti-inflammatory drugs [NSAIDs]), allergic contact dermatitis, autoimmune conditions, thyroid disorders, superior vena cava syndrome, head and neck tumors, Cheilitis granulomatosa (Miescher cheilitis), Melkersson-Rosenthal syndrome, trichinellosis.

**Low C4 levels:** C4A deficiency (OMIM 120810), C4B (OMIM 120820)

**Low C1q levels:** C1q deficiency, hypocomplementemic urticarial vasculitis syndrome (HUVS), and SLE

## Molecular Genetics

The *C1-INH* gene encodes a soluble protease inhibitor that regulates the first component of the complement cascade (C1). Through inhibition of the C1 subcomponents (C1r and C1s) the activation of C4 and C2 is prevented. C1 inhibitor also inhibits several other serine proteinases including plasmin, kallikrein, and coagulation factors XIa and XIIa.

Patients with HAE type I (absent or low levels of an antigenically normal protein) appear to have a deletion of the C1 inhibitor gene or a truncated transcript because of a stop codon, whereas patients with HAE type II (elevated or normal levels of a dysfunctional protein) have a single base substitution. The two forms are clinically indistinguishable.

***Genetic Testing:*** Genetic testing is not required to confirm the diagnosis in adults, but is available. The diagnosis is made in infants occasionally by genetic typing.

**BIBLIOGRAPHY:**

1. Bowen T, Cicardi M, Farkas H, et al. Canadian 2003 International Consensus Algorithm For the Diagnosis, Therapy, and Management of Hereditary Angioedema. *J Allergy Clin Immunol.* 2004;114(3):629-637.

2. Schneider L, Lumry W, Vegh A, Williams AH, Schmalbach T. Critical role of kallikrein in hereditary angioedema pathogenesis: a clinical trial of ecallantide, a novel kallikrein inhibitor. *J Allergy Clin Immunol.* 2007;120:416-422.

3. Bork K, Frank J, Grundt B, Schlattmann P, Nussberger J, Kreuz W. Treatment of acute edema attacks in hereditary angioedema with a bradykinin receptor-2 antagonist (Icatibant). *J Allergy Clin Immunol.* 2007;119:1497-1503.

4. Agostoni A, Aygoren-Pursun E, Binkley KE, et al. Hereditary and acquired angioedema: problems and progress: proceedings of the third C1 esterase inhibitor deficiency workshop and beyond. *J Allergy Clin Immunol.* 2004;114(suppl 3):S51-S131.

## Supplementary Information

**Alternative Names:**
- Hereditary Angioedema, Type I
- Hereditary Angioedema, Type II
- Hereditary Angioneurotic Edema (HANE)
- Deficiency of C1 Esterase Inhibitor

***Key Words:*** Complement, angioedema, laryngeal swelling, wheezing, abdominal pain, stridor, swelling, C1 inhibitor

# 80 Deficiency of Components of the Complement System

Juan C. Cardet and Duane R. Wesemann

## KEY POINTS

- *Disease summary:*
  - Complement deficiencies are rare, and typically result in one or more of the following phenotypes: increased susceptibility to encapsulated bacteria (*Streptococcus pneumoniae*, *Haemophilus influenzae*, *Neisseria meningitidis*), and autoimmunity (systemic lupus erythematosus [SLE], atypical hemolytic uremic syndrome [HUS], and membranoproliferative glomerulonephritis [GN]).
  - This chapter does not address a single disease and its implicated genes, but rather a subdivision of the immune system. Deficiencies of the complement system (Table 80-1) will be discussed in clusters of similar phenotypic presentation. Given that the genetic basis for individual deficiencies of the complement components is sundry (and seldom clinically relevant), individual genes will be commented on only when germane to clinical management.

- *Overview of the complement system:*
  - Complement is a system composed of serum glycoproteins that coordinate cascades of events leading to clearance of foreign antigens and host-derived debris such as apoptotic cells. Complement is involved in recognition of micro-organisms, direct killing of micro-organisms, processing and clearance of immune complexes, as well as regulation of lymphocytes.
  - Three pathways of antigen recognition and activation converge in a common final pathway designed to permeabilize micro-organism invaders by way of a protein C5 to C9 protein complex that forms a pore in microbial lipid membranes. The pathways of activation are the classical, alternative, and mannose-binding lectin pathways (MBL). C1, C4, and C2 are early classical complement components. Factors D, B, are components of the alternative pathway. C3 and C5 to C9 are shared components. Complement regulatory proteins include factor I, factor H, C4-binding protein, and properdin. The proteins CD59 and DAF are also regulatory proteins whose deficiency is associated with paroxysmal nocturnal hematuria and are not described here. The C1 inhibitor protein (C1-INH) deficiency is associated with hereditary angioedema and is described in Chapter 79. There are multiple causes for secondary deficiencies of C3, for example, deficiency of factors H and I. Deficiency of some complement receptors are also implicated in leukocyte adhesion deficiency (LAD) and will not be discussed in this chapter.

- *Inheritance:*
  - Almost all complement components are inherited in an autosomal recessive fashion, except for properdin deficiency, which is X-linked recessive, and C1 esterase inhibitor deficiency, which is autosomal dominant. Heterozygously deficient individuals of components inherited in autosomal recessive fashion are typically asymptomatic.

- *Differential diagnosis:*
  - The differential diagnosis for adult-onset immune deficiency includes anatomic derangement (ie, fistula, cerebrospinal fluid [CSF] leak etc), common variable immune deficiency, specific antibody deficiency, antibody subclass deficiencies, congenital phagocyte dysfunctions, medication or toxin effects, hematologic cancers such as multiple myeloma or chronic lymphocytic leukemia, and HIV or AIDS.

- *Incidence:*
  - Complement deficiencies account for less than 1% of primary immunodeficiency states. Among C1 to C9 components, C2 deficiency is the most common in Western countries. Studies estimate 5/100,000 is completely deficient in C2.4 C9 deficiency is the most common in Japan. There are dozens of case reports of deficiencies in C1q, and C3. C4 protein is encoded in two genes, *C4A* and *C4B*, and a null mutation in at least one of the four gene products can be as high as 35% of the population.
  - Screening of 41,083 military recruits showed that 14 individuals (0.03%) had a deficiency of one of the classical complement components.
  - MBL deficiency is thought to be fairly common, with an 8% frequency in general population, making it the most common inherited immunodeficiency (arguably, given the absence of symptoms in many individuals) (see later).

## Diagnostic Criteria and Clinical Characteristics

**Diagnosis:** A diagnosis of a complement deficiency is made through clinical suspicion with confirmation with laboratory testing, as outlined later.

Measurement of CH50 is the best initial screening test for complement deficiencies. AH50 should be measured when deficits in the alternative pathway are suspected (this test is not available everywhere). The CH50 should be 0 for homozygous deficiencies of C1 to C8 components, and AH50 should be 0 for deficiencies in factor B, factor D, or properdin.

*Table 80-1 Genetic Differential Diagnosis of the Components of the Complement System*

| Genotype | Phenotypic Description | | |
| --- | --- | --- | --- |
| Deficiency | Infections | Autoimmunity | Other |
| Classical pathway: C1q, C1r, C1s, C4, C2 | Streptococcal and neisserial infections | SLE | • SLE onset usually in childhood, but adult cases reported<br>• Frequently antibody negative (ANA, DS-DNA) |
| Alternative pathway: Factor D, factor B, and properdin | Neisserial meningeal infections *frequently complicated by sepsis* | • One case report of a properdin-deficient patient with discoid lupus<br>• Autoimmunity found in mouse models not recapitulated in humans | • One case report of patient with dysfunctional factor B<br>• No homozygous factor B deficiency has yet been described<br>• Three families reported with factor D deficiency<br>• Properdin is the most common one of this group, and neisserial infections may be severe |
| Lectin pathway: MBL, MASP 1 and 2 | Severe infections only in early life or when comorbidities are present: cystic fibrosis or cancer patients | Rarely SLE | • Increased cardiovascular disease and atherosclerosis, gestational DM<br>• Typically asymptomatic in adulthood unless compounded with comorbidities |
| Convergence of the three pathways: C3 | Recurrent severe bacterial infections with encapsulated bacteria: neisserial, *S pneumoniae, H influenzae*: OM, PNA, meningitis | Rarely SLE | • +/– signs and symptoms of immune complex deposition |
| Terminal complement components final common pathway): C5-C9 | Severe recurrent infection by *Neisseria gonorrhea* or *N meningitidis* | Rarely SLE | • C9 deficiency associated with less severe symptoms<br>• Heterozygosity is *not* associated with disease.<br>• In the absence of C9, C5-C8 alone can create a permeability defect sufficient to lyse cells.<br>• Rare neisserial strains are usually isolated |
| Regulatory proteins (factor H, factor I, C4BP, MCP) | Severe pyogenic bacterial infections in factor I deficiency, less so in factor H and MCP, unknown in C4BP | GN, Atypical HUS in factor H deficiency and MCP, less so in factor I, unknown in C4BP | • Atypical HUS is verotoxin/diarrhea negative.<br>• Deficiencies of factors H, I, and MCP will lead to a consumptive, secondary deficiency of C3.<br>• Only one case report of a patient with C4BP deficiency, who presented with a Behcet-like illness<br>• Factor I deficiency clinically indistinguishable from primary C3 deficiency<br>• Factor H implicated in AMD |

SLE, systemic lupus erythematosus; GN, membranoproliferative glomerulonephritis; OM, otitis media; PNA, pneumonia; ANA: antinuclear antibodies; DS-DNA, double-stranded DNA; AMD: age-related macular degeneration.

- A CH50 that is 0 or very low along with a normal AH50 is suggestive of deficits in the early classical components (C1q, r, s, C2, or C4).
- An AH50 that is 0 or very low along with a normal CH50 is suggestive of deficits in the alternative pathway (factors B, D, or properdin).
- If both CH50 and AH50 are low then there are deficits in either C3 or terminal complement components (C5-C9).
- The CH50 for C9 deficiency is approximately half of normal levels but not 0, as some degree of cell lysis can be achieved by C5 to C8 even in the absence of C9.
- If CH50 and AH50 are normal, then homozygous deficiency of either classical or alternative pathway can be ruled out.

Low levels should be investigated, as a low CH50, C4, C2, and C3 can be low or undetectable due to a consumptive process such as infection or sepsis. Active connective tissue disease or vasculitis also can be associated with hypocomplementemia, as can autoantibodies such as C3 nephritic factor.

Importantly, a C3 hypocomplementemia will result in a propensity to infection regardless of its cause.

- Obtaining complement activation products such as C4d, C3-5a, Bb, or SC5b-9 might be necessary to differentiate an inherited complement deficiency from a consumptive process.
- A + family history, a deficit restricted to one complement component (as opposed to several), and a CH50 or AH50 equaling 0 (as opposed to being "low") all point toward an inherited deficiency and not a secondary deficiency.
- Specific deficiencies can be measured directly via ELISA. Serum levels of MBL, factor H, factor I, and properdin can be measured immunochemically, and some commercial laboratories offer such measurement techniques.
- If a C3 deficiency is suspected but a quantitative test is normal, then a C3 functional assay should be obtained.
- Some terminal complement deficiencies tend to occur more frequently in some ethnic groups than others, and C5 and C8 are more commonly deficient in Caucasians, C6 in African American, and C9 in Japanese.
- If recurrent infections are not limited to *Neisseria* species and are particularly severe, then checking for regulatory complement proteins and C3 is indicated.
- If recurrent infections are accompanied by a HUS or GN, then factors H and I, MCP, C3, C3 nephritic factor, and antifactor H antibodies should be checked. (C3 nephritic factor is an autoantibody against the C3 convertase that leads to C3 depletion, but its clinical presentation includes lipodystrophy in addition to infections and GN.)

*Clinical Characteristics:* Autoimmunity, especially SLE, is the most common presentation in patients with deficiency C1, C4, or C2. Incidence rates of SLE in patients with C1q and C4 deficiency are reported to be over 90% and 75%, respectively. Incidence rates of SLE in C2 deficiency are less (10%-15%). C4A deficiency (with normal C4B) is associated with SLE in 15% of patients. SLE associated with C1 and C4 (and their subcomponents) is associated with an equal male:female ratio, onset earlier in life, a 30% risk of GN, and multiorgan involvement, whereas SLE associated with C2 deficiency tends to behave more like common SLE.

Infections typically first occur in the first 2 years of life in early classical, C3, and regulatory protein-deficient patients, whereas they first occur in the teenage years in the alternate pathway and terminal complement-deficient patients. The risk of systemic infections is 20% in patients with early classical complement deficiencies (encapsulated bacteria), close to 75% of patients with deficiencies in the alternate pathway (meningococcal infections), close to 70% in C3-deficient patients (encapsulated bacteria, recurrent), close to 60% in patients with terminal complement deficiencies (neisserial infections, recurrent), 40% in patients deficient in factor H (encapsulated bacteria, recurrent), and 100% of patients deficient in factor I (encapsulated bacteria, recurrent).The relative risk of meningococcal disease in patients with deficiencies of the terminal complement components is 5000 in comparison with patients without these deficiencies.

MBL deficiency is common and leads to increased susceptibility to infection in patients who may be otherwise immunocompromised such as patients with cystic fibrosis, recipients of chemotherapy or newborns.

## Screening and Counseling

Screening is indicated in individuals suspected of having complement defects. Given that most complement components are inherited in an autosomal recessive fashion, and that heterozygotes are asymptomatic, screening of asymptomatic family members is not typically indicated. The exception is properdin, which is X-linked recessive and all reported cases are males. Genetic testing of family members is indicated.

## Management and Treatment

Neither purified nor recombinant isolated complement proteins are currently clinically available for the treatment of inherited complement deficiencies. Only supportive therapy is available, and consists of vaccination and prophylactic antibiotics. There are few randomized clinical trials addressing management or treatment guidelines. There are case reports of fresh frozen plasma (FFP) given emergently for the treatment of infections, with mixed results. Replacement of deficient proteins with FFP transfusion is not done due to a risk of infections, as well as by the potential production of autoantibodies to the deficient protein.

All routine vaccines are recommended and safe in complement deficiencies. Vaccines against, pneumococcus, meningococcus, and *H influenzae* are recommended for all complement-deficient patients, but patients with only terminal complement deficiencies may be treated only with tetravalent meningococcal vaccine. This vaccine given once every 3 years was found to maintain normal titers of anticapsular antibodies in patients with terminal complement deficiencies. The same cannot be said of early complement deficiencies, where antibody titers may not reach protective levels after vaccination.

Referral to an immunologist is indicated upon diagnosis of a complement deficiency.

Of the complement deficits leading to GN, only MCP deficiency is thought to be amenable to cure through renal transplantation, because while factors H and I are *soluble* proteins, MCP is a *transmembrane protein*, correctable with kidney.

## Molecular Genetics or Molecular Mechanism

The association with complement deficiencies with susceptibility to infection is because of impaired microbe killing. The paradoxical association with autoimmune disease, such as SLE and GN is thought to be secondary to impaired clearance of immune complexes and apoptotic cells (leading to an abundance of autoantigens and subsequent autoimmunization), in addition to altered cytokine regulation.Dysregulation of B-cell tolerance is also cited as a possible explanation since complement plays a role in physiologic B-cell tolerance.

***Genetic Testing:*** Currently, the demonstration of decreased levels of complement proteins as described earlier is the extent of the clinically relevant workup of complement deficiencies. While numerous genetic mutations have been found for most of the more than 30 proteins of the complement system, testing for these is not widely available. Because a genotype-phenotype correlation has not been delineated for the different mutations, discerning between them does not currently change clinical management.

### BIBLIOGRAPHY:

1. Walport MJ. Complement: parts 1 and 2. *N Engl J Med.* 2001; 344(14):1058-1144.

2. Botto M, Kirschfink M, Macor P, Pickering MC, Würzner R, Tedesco F. Complement in human diseases: lessons from complement deficiencies. *Mol Immunol.* 2009;46:2774-2783.

3. Colten HR. Navigating the maze of complement genetics: a guide for clinicians. *Curr Allergy Asthma Rep.* 2002;2(5):379-384.

4. Sjoholm AG, Jonsson G, Braconier JH, Sturfelt G, Truedsson L. Complement deficiency and disease: an update. *Mol Immunol.* 2006;43(1-2):78-85.

5. Ross SC, Densen P. Complement deficiency states and infection: epidemiology, pathogenesis and consequences of Neisserial and other infections in an immune deficiency. *Medicine.* 1984;63(5):243-273.

6. Worthley DL, Bardy PG, Mullighan CG. Mannose-binding lectin: biology and clinical implications. *Intern Med J.* 2005;35(9):548-555.

7. Wen 2004. Clinical and laboratory evaluation of complement deficiency. *J Allergy Clin Immunol.* 2004;113(4):585-593.

8. Palarasah Y, Nielsen C, Sprogøe U, et al. Novel assays to assess the functional capacity of the classical, the alternative and the lectin pathways of the complement system. *Clin Exp Immunol.* 2011;164:388-395.

9. Truedsson L, Bengtsson AA, Sturfelt G. Complement deficiencies and systemic lupus erythematosus. *Autoimmunity.* 2007;40(8):560-566.

10. Figueroa J, Densen P. Infectious diseases associated with complement deficiencies. *Clin Microbiol Rev.* 1991;4(3):359-395.

11. Platonov AE, Vershinina IV, Kuijper EJ, Borrow R, Käyhty H. Long term effects of vaccination of patients deficient in a late complement component with a tetravalent meningococcal polysaccharide vaccine. *Vaccine.* 2003;21:4437-4447.

12. Caprioli J, Noris M, Brioschi S. Genetics of HUS: the impact of *MCP*, *CFH*, and *IF* mutations on clinical presentation, response to treatment, and outcome. *Blood.* 2006;108:1267-1279.

## Supplementary Information

### OMIM REFERENCES:

Online Mendelian Inheritance in Man, OMIM®. McKusick-Nathans Institute of Genetic Medicine, Johns Hopkins University (Baltimore, MD), Jan 2012. http://omim.org/

[1] Complement component 1, q subcomponent, A chain;*C1qA* 1p36;120550

[2] Complement component 1, q subcomponent, B chain; *C1qB* 1p36;120570

[3] Complement component 1, q subcomponent, C chain;*C1qC* 1p36;120575

[4] Complement component 1, r subcomponent;*C1r* 12p13;216950

[5] Complement component 1, s subcomponent;*C1s* 12p13;120580

[6] *C2* 6p21;217000

[7] Complement component 4A;*C4A* 6p21;120810

[8] Complement component 4B;*C4B* 6p21;120820

[9] *C3* 19p21;120700

[10] *C5* 9q32;120900

[11] *C6* 5q13;217050

[12] *C7* 5q13;217070;

[13] Complement component 8, alpha subunit;*C8A* 1p32;120950

[14] Complement component 8, beta subunit;*C8B* 1p32;120960

[15] Complement component 8, gamma subunit;*C8G* 9q34;120930

[16] *C9* 5p13;120940

[17] *Factor B* 6p21;138470

[18] *Factor D* 19p13;134350

[19] *Factor H* 1q31;134370

[20] *Factor I* 4q25;217030

[21] *Properdin* Xp11;312060

[22] Mannose-binding lectin;*MBL* 10q11;154545

[23] Membrane cofactor protein;*MCP* 1q32;120920

[24] Mannan-binding lectin serine protease 1;*MASP 1* 3q27;600521

[25] Mannan-binding lectin serine protease 2;*MASP 2* 1p36;605102

[26] C4-binding protein alpha subunit;*C4BPA* 1q32;120830

[27] C4-binding protein beta subunit;*C4BPB 1*q32;120831

***Key Words:*** Complement, recurrent infections, systemic lupus erythematosus, SLE, autoimmunity, paroxysmal nocturnal hemoglobinuria, *Neisseria*, immune deficiency, properdin, factor B, factor D, factor I, MBL

# 81 Hemolytic Uremic Syndrome

Federica Mescla, Giuseppe Remuzzi, and Maina Noris

## KEY POINTS

- *Disease summary:*
  - Hemolytic uremic syndrome (HUS) is a rare disease (1-2 cases per 100,000) characterized by the triad of thrombocytopenia, nonimmune hemolytic anemia, and acute renal impairment, due to a microangiopathic lesion affecting especially the glomerular endothelium.
  - Around 90% of HUS cases, referred to as typical or diarrhea-associated HUS, are traceable to gastrointestinal infection with Shiga toxin (Stx)-producing bacteria such as *Escherichia coli* serotype 0157:H7, are usually heralded by bloody diarrhea and mostly affect children under 5 years. Causes of other distinct forms of HUS include infection by neuramidase-producing *Streptococcus pneumoniae*, a rare inborn error in cobalamin metabolism and quinine-induced antibodies.
  - The remaining 10% of cases are classified as atypical HUS (aHUS) and can be further distinguished into familial (<20%) and sporadic cases. aHUS occurs at any age and often carries a poor prognosis.

- *Hereditary basis:*
  - Genetic abnormalities have been identified in 50% to 60% of aHUS cases, both in familial and sporadic forms. Both autosomal recessive and dominant inheritance are possible; penetrance is incomplete and clinical expression variable.
  - All the genetic defects identified so far result in susceptibility to uncontrolled activation of the alternative pathway of the complement system on the surface of self cells.

- *Differential diagnosis:*
  - HUS-like presentations can occur in other forms of thrombotic microangiopathy, including thrombotic thrombocytopenic purpura (usually with predominant neurologic manifestations; very low levels of von Willebrand factor cleaving protease ADAMTS-13), disseminated intravascular coagulation (relevant prolongation of coagulation tests and fibrinogen consumption), scleroderma renal crisis, and malignant hypertension.
  - The diagnosis of aHUS is made by exclusion, in particular typical HUS must be ruled out on the basis of microbiologic findings (serologic or culture evidence of infection by bacteria-producing Stx, toxin assays), since up to 25% of Stx-associated HUS cases may not manifest diarrhea.
  - Among aHUS cases, genetic testing can distinguish between the seven main categories of genetic defects identified so far (Table 81-1); no genetic alteration is found in 30% to 40% of patients.

## Diagnostic Criteria and Clinical Characteristics

***Diagnostic Criteria for Genetic aHUS:*** aHUS is considered to have a genetic basis when at least one of the following conditions is present:

- Two or more members of the same family are affected by the disease at least 6 months apart and exposure to a common triggering infectious agent has been excluded.
- A disease-causing mutation is identified in one of the genes in which mutations are known to be associated with aHUS, irrespective of familial history.

Nonetheless, it is possible that at least a subset of the cases not fulfilling the above criteria carry yet to be identified genetic defects. ***Clinical Characteristics:*** About 60% to 70% of patients with genetic aHUS have childhood onset. A variety of triggering conditions have been described, including infections, pregnancy (10%-15% of aHUS cases in females manifest in pregnancy or postpartum), malignancies, transplantation, antiphospholipid syndrome, and use of drugs (calcineurin inhibitors, chemotherapy agents, oral contraceptives, interferon). No triggers are identifiable in about 50% of cases (idiopathic aHUS).

During acute episodes, key clinical findings are thrombocytopenia (often severe, below 60,000/mm³), microangiopathic hemolytic anemia with fragmented red blood cells—schistocytes—in peripheral blood smears, and acute kidney dysfunction (rise in serum creatinine, hypertension, oligoanuria, urinalysis abnormalities). Involvement of other organs, such as brain, heart, pancreas, and gastrointestinal tract, occurs in 20% of cases.

Typical renal histology findings affecting glomeruli and, in most severe cases, arterioles as well, comprise platelet-fibrin thrombi, narrowing of the capillary lumen and endothelial swelling, with detachment of endothelial cells from basal membrane and subendothelial deposition of electron-lucent fluffy material and cell debris.

Overall, renal prognosis is poor in most cases, with frequent relapses even after full recovery and progression to end-stage renal disease in 60% of patients.

## Screening and Counseling

***Screening:*** At present, a genetic mutation can be identified in 50% to 60% of aHUS cases, with important implications for the patient and close relatives. All patients presenting with clinical features compatible with aHUS should be screened for genetic alterations, including cases of pregnancy-associated HUS, in whom complement abnormalities have been reported in as much as 86% cases.

No clinical feature can reliably distinguish between different genetic defects. Determination of plasma levels of complement components C3, factor H (FH), and factor I (FI), search for autoantibodies against FH and analysis of surface expression of MCP on peripheral leukocytes by flow cytometry, if altered, can provide hints of the genetic defect most likely involved and therefore guide genetic testing strategy. If no information emerges following this first survey,

**Table 81-1 Genetic Abnormalities and Clinical Outcome in Patients With aHUS**

| Gene | Protein Affected | % aHUS | % Short-Term Remission With Plasma Therapy[a] | Rate of ESRD/Death[b] | Outcome of Kidney Transplantation |
|---|---|---|---|---|---|
| CFH (aHUS1) | Factor H | 25%-30% | 50%-60% (plasma exchange superior to plasma infusion) | 70%-80% | 80%-90% recurrence |
| MCP (aHUS2) | Membrane cofactor protein (CD46) | 10%-15% | No definitive indication for therapy; 80%-90% complete remission independently on plasma therapy | <20% | 15%-20% recurrence, long-term graft survival similar to graft recipients with other causes of ESRD |
| CFHR1, CFHR3, CFHR4 | Deletion of factor H-related 1, 3, 4; formation of autoantibodies antifactor H | 6%-10% | 70%-80% (plasma exchange combined with immunosuppression) | 30%-40% | 20% recurrence |
| CFI (aHUS3) | Factor I | 4%-10% | 25%-40% (larger quantities of plasma needed to achieve remission) | 60%-70% | 70%-80% recurrence |
| C3 (aHUS5) | Complement C3 | 4%-10% | 50%-60% | 60%-70% | 40%-50% recurrence |
| THBD (aHUS6) | Thrombomodulin | 5% | 50%-80% | 60% | 1 report of post-transplant recurrence |
| CFB (aHUS4) | Factor B | 1%-2% | 30%-40% (few data available) | 70% | Few data available (recurrence in one case), likely high risk |

[a]Remission includes both complete remission and partial remission (ie, hematologic remission with renal sequelae).
[b]ESRD denotes end-stage renal disease; rates refer to 5 to 10 years after disease onset.

genetic testing can be undertaken in a stepwise fashion, starting from more prevalent mutations and proceeding to less frequent ones, as resumed in the diagnostic algorithm presented in Fig. 81-1.

It is likely that "third generation" DNA sequencing systems, conjugating high throughput technology and accessible costs, will soon become widely available in clinical practice. In such setting,

screening for all known disease-associated genes with short turn-around times could become cost-effective, enabling recognition of concomitant genetic alterations in a single patient and laying the basis for a personalized pharmacogenomic-oriented approach.

***Genetic Counseling:*** Predisposition to aHUS is inherited in an autosomal dominant or autosomal recessive manner with

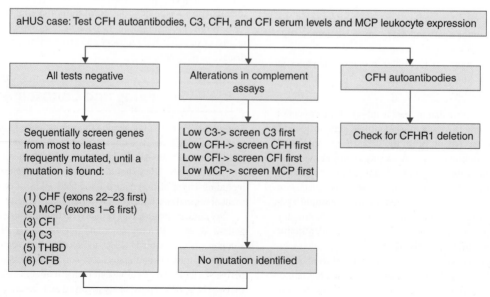

**Figure 81-1** Algorithm for Mutation Screening in New-Onset aHUS.

incomplete penetrance. Other rare reported possibilities are digenic inheritance (in 5% of cases, most commonly MCP with either complement facto I (CFI) or complement factor H (CFH) and uniparental isodisomy.

In cases with autosomal recessive inheritance, parents of affected individuals are obligate heterozygotes (carriers) and normally are asymptomatic, even if there are reports of rare adult-onset aHUS in carriers. Each sibling of a patient has a 25% chance of inheriting two disease-associated mutations, a 50% chance of being a carrier, and a 25% chance of inheriting no mutation; offsprings of affected individuals are obligate carriers.

Patients with autosomal dominant aHUS may have an affected parent or close relative, but in most cases family history is negative. The most frequent reason for this is incomplete penetrance; early death of relatives, late onset of disease in relatives, or de novo mutation in the proband are other possibilities. If a parent carries the mutation, the risk to the siblings of inheriting the mutation is 50%; if the mutation found in the proband cannot be identified in the parents—and paternity in ensured—the risk to the sibs is lower, but nonetheless greater than the general population, due to the possibility of germline mosaicism. Each child of an individual with autosomal dominant aHUS has a 50% chance of inheriting the mutation.

In autosomal dominant forms, penetrance is incomplete, around 50%. Known factors affecting penetrance include both concomitant genetic factors (eg, polymorphisms in the regulator of complement activator (RCA) cluster) and the earlier-cited recognized environmental triggers, likely acting as complement activators.

Presymptomatic genetic testing should be offered to first-degree relatives of aHUS patients carrying an identified genetic mutation. Prenatal diagnosis for pregnancies at increased risk is possible if the disease-associated mutation has been identified in the family.

☞GENOTYPE-PHENOTYPE CORRELATION: Clinical severity, age of onset, and disease progression often differ among individuals carrying the same mutations, making prediction of disease outcome for the individual based on single genetic mutations impossible. Greater insight into concomitant genetic risk factors for aHUS and their interplay with disease-associated mutations will likely enable to draw more precise genotype-phenotype correlations.

Nonetheless, identification of the genetic defect carries important prognostic information, mainly regarding overall renal survival, rates of response to plasma therapy, and post-transplantation recurrence, as recapitulated in Table 81-1. In general, FH mutations appear to be associated with the most severe disease phenotype, while most patients with MCP mutations remain dialysis independent, in spite of frequent recurrences; prognosis of patients with other genetic defects lies in the middle between these two extremes. Patients with antifactor H antibodies, often with deletions of *CFHR1* gene, have been reported to present a high frequency of gastrointestinal symptoms and extrarenal complications.

## Management and Treatment

Plasma exchange or infusion is the most well-established treatment approach in aHUS and should be started urgently. The rationale is to provide normal complement regulators and at the same time, in the case of plasma exchange procedures, remove dysfunctional factors or autoantibodies and avoid the risk of fluid overload. An overall 25% to 50% decrease in mortality with plasma therapy has been reported; different response rates to plasma manipulation have been reported on the basis of genetic defect (Table 81-1).

Plasma resistance or plasma dependence is possible and plasma unresponsiveness may develop after long-term therapy.

Immunomodulatory drugs (eg, corticosteroids, azathioprine, mycophenolate mofetil, rituximab) can be a useful adjunct to reduce the production of pathogenetic antibodies and risk of relapse in patients with anti-CHF autoantibodies.

Bilateral nephrectomy may be necessary in cases with severe manifestations (refractory hypertension, hypertensive encephalopathy, thrombocytopenia, and anemia) that are not responsive to conventional therapy.

Therapeutic agents targeting the complement system are very promising in the setting of aHUS. In particular eculizumab, a humanized monoclonal antibody that inhibits complement component C5, has recently received FDA approval for aHUS on the basis of excellent results in 37 patients with plasma resistant and dependent forms (http://www.fda.gov/AboutFDA/CentersOffices/CDER/ucm273089.htm).

Outcome of kidney transplantation in aHUS is highly variable on the basis of mutation type, as recapitulated in Table 81-1. Transplantation results are good in patients with MCP mutations and antifactor H antibodies, in whom normal MPC protein in the graft and immunosuppression, respectively, are beneficial. In the remaining cases, transplantation carries an elevated risk of recurrence with subsequent graft loss and is therefore relatively contraindicated. Pre-emptive plasma therapy and use of eculizumab have been shown to be promising strategies to ameliorate graft survival in such patients.

Given the predominantly hepatic synthesis of CFH and CFI, simultaneous liver-kidney transplantation represents an additional option for patients carrying such mutations. Experience in this field has been limited, and combined liver-kidney transplant remains a highly complex and risky procedure that needs to be reserved to very selected cases.

Following treatment of acute episodes, patients, particularly those maintaining residual kidney function, are at risk of relapse and thus need to be closely followed up.

## Molecular Genetics and Molecular Mechanism

*Gene/Protein/Locus:*
   CFH/complement factor H/1q32
   CD46/membrane cofactor protein/1q32
   CFI/complement factor I/4q25
   CFB/complement factor B/6p21.3 app
   C3/complement C3/19p 13.3-p13.2
   THBD/thrombomodulin/20p11.2
   CFHR3/complement factor H-related protein 3/1q31-q32.1
   CFHR1/complement factor H-related protein 1/1q31-q32.1
   CFHR4/complement factor H-related protein 4/1q31-q32.1

Up to now more than 200 aHUS-associated abnormalities affecting nine different genes have been characterized, and new mutations and novel candidate genes are being discovered. All the genetic defects identified so far are traceable to proteins taking part in the alternative pathway of complement activation. As shown in Fig. 81-2, the complement system is a set of plasma proteins that is activated on the surfaces of foreign organisms, amplifying inflammatory responses and contributing to the clearance

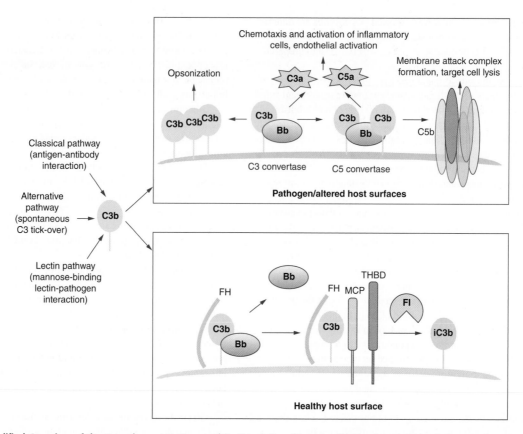

***Figure 81-2*** Simplified Overview of the Complement System and its Regulation. The complement is a system of plasma components that is activated through a proteolytic cascade on the surface of pathogens and altered cells, contributing to their clearance and reestablishment of homeostasis. All the characterized pathways of complement activation converge on cleavage of the central component C3 into C3a and C3b. C3b deposits on surfaces and associates with factor-D activated factor B –Bb-, forming the alternative pathway C3 convertase C3bBb. Further C3a and C3b are thus formed. Anaphylatoxin C3a is a potent inflammatory mediator, while C3b opsonizes cell surfaces and takes part in the assembly of C5 convertase C3bBb3b, with subsequent cleavage of C5 into anaphylatoxin C5a and C5b. The latter deposits on surfaces together with late complement components C6-C9, leading to cell lysis through the membrane attack complex.

On normal host surfaces, complement activity is inhibited by an array of physiological regulators. Among them, serine protease factor I –FI- cleaves C3b, giving inactive iC3b, in the presence of soluble cofactors (like factor H –FH-, a plasma protein that interacts with poly-anions on host surfaces), and membrane-bound complement regulators (like membrane cofactor protein -MCP- and thrombomodulin -THBD-). Moreover, factor H directly accelerates the decay of C3 convertase C3bBb and thrombomodulin is involved in the generation of thrombin-activatable-fibrinolysis inhibitor (TAFIa), a plasma carboxypeptidase B that cleaves C3a and C5a. Mutations in all these complement regulators have been detected in aHUS, predisposing to uncontrolled, destructive activation of complement alternative pathways on host cells.

of pathogens through a variety of mechanisms. Deposition of complement on healthy self-cells and host surfaces is prevented through a series of regulatory mechanisms, comprising both membrane-bound and soluble regulators. Defects in such mechanisms are found in aHUS, making patients more susceptible to inappropriate activation of complement on cell surfaces, especially at the level of glomerular endothelium and basal membrane, which leads to the endothelial injury and platelet activation typical of thrombotic microangiopathy.

Predisposition to excessive alternative pathway activation in aHUS occurs through three fundamental mechanisms:

- Loss-of-function mutations in negative regulators of the alternative complement pathway (serine protease factor I and its cofactors factor H, CD46, thrombomodulin)

- Gain-of-function mutations in C3 convertase components C3 and factor B, rendering them more resistant to regulatory mechanisms
- Genetic predisposition to formation of antifactor H antibodies, determining functional FH deficiency, as likely occurs in deletions involving *CFHR1* gene

***Genetic Testing:*** Mutation analysis of aHUS-related genes is currently time consuming, costly, and available only in reference laboratories. At present clinical testing is available for all identified aHUS-associated genetic defects, except CFHR1-CFHR4 deletion and *CFHR1* point mutations; more detailed and updated information on testing modalities and reference laboratories can be found on http://www.genetests.org. Turnaround time is usually in the order of weeks or months, so, at present, genetic information are usually not available during management of disease at its onset. Nonetheless, genetic testing plays an important role in the management of affected patients, providing prognostic information and guiding choices in the field of kidney transplantation (Table 81-1). Identification of unaffected carriers in the family is fundamental when considering the option of living related kidney donation, since nephrectomy for donation purposes could precipitate aHUS in asymptomatic, genetically predisposed individuals. Moreover, knowledge of carrier status makes it possible to avoid known HUS triggers and, if this is not possible, undergo adequate monitoring following exposure.

## BIBLIOGRAPHY:

1. Tarr P, Gordon CA, Chandler WL. Shiga-toxin-producing Escherichia coli and haemolytic uraemic syndrome. *Lancet.* 2005;365(9464):1073-1086.

2. Besbas N, Karpman D, Landau D, et al. A classification of hemolytic uremic syndrome and thrombotic thrombocytopenic purpura and related disorders. *Kidney Int.* 2006;70(3):423-431.

3. Noris M, Remuzzi G. Atypical hemolytic-uremic syndrome. *N Engl J Med.* 2009;361(17):1676-1687.

4. Kavanagh D, Goodship T. Genetics and complement in atypical HUS. *Pediatr Nephrol.* 2010;25(12):2431-2442.

5. Remuzzi G. von Willebrand factor cleaving protease (ADAMTS13) is deficient in recurrent and familial thrombotic thrombocytopenic purpura and hemolytic uremic syndrome. *Blood.* 2002;100(3):778-785.

6. Ruggenenti P, Noris M, Remuzzi G. Thrombotic microangiopathy, hemolytic uremic syndrome, and thrombotic thrombocytopenic purpura. *Kidney Int.* 2001;60(3):831-846.

7. Fakhouri F, Roumenina L, Provot F, et al. Pregnancy-associated hemolytic uremic syndrome revisited in the era of complement gene mutations. *J Am Soc Nephrol.* 2010;21(5):859-867.

8. Noris M, Bresin E, Mele C, Remuzzi G, Caprioli J. Atypical Hemolytic-Uremic Syndrome. Gene Reviews—NCBI Bookshelf. http://www.ncbi.nlm.nih.gov/books/NBK1367/?report=printable. Accessed on October, 2011.

9. Dragon-Durey MA, Sethi SK, Bagga A, et al. Clinical features of anti-factor H autoantibody-associated hemolytic uremic syndrome. *J Am Soc Nephrol.* 2010;21(12):2180-2187.

10. Ariceta G, Besbas N, Johnson S, et al. Guideline for the investigation and initial therapy of diarrhea-negative hemolytic uremic syndrome. *Pediatr Nephrol.* 2009;24(4):687-696.

11. Zuber J, Le Quintrec M, Sberro-Soussan R, Loirat C, Frémeaux-Bacchi V, Legendre C. New insights into postrenal transplant hemolytic uremic syndrome. *Nat Rev Nephrol.* 2011;7(1):23-35.

12. Saland JM, Ruggenenti P, Remuzzi G. Liver-kidney transplantation to cure atypical hemolytic uremic syndrome. *J Am Soc Nephrol.* 2009;20(5):940-949.

13. Legendre CM, Licht C, Muus P et al. Terminal complement inhibitor eculuzumab in atypical hemolytic-uremic syndrome. *N Engl J Med.* 2013; 368(23):2169-2181

## Supplementary Information

### OMIM REFERENCES:

[1] Complement Factor H-Related 4; CFHR4 (#605337)

[2] Complement Factor H-Related 3; CFHR3 (#605336)

[3] Thrombomodulin; THBD (#188040)

[4] Hemolytic Uremic Syndrome, Atypical, Susceptibility to, 1; AHUS1 (#235400)

[5] Complement Component 3; C3 (#120700)

[6] Complement Factor B; CFB (#138470)

[7] Complement Factor H-Related 1; CFHR1 (#134371)

[8] Complement Factor H; CFH (#134370)

[9] Membrane Cofactor Protein; MCP (#120920)

[10] Hemolytic Uremic Syndrome, Atypical, Susceptibility to, 2; AHUS2 (#612922)

[11] Hemolytic Uremic Syndrome, Atypical, Susceptibility to, 3; AHUS3 (#612923)

[12] Hemolytic Uremic Syndrome, Atypical, Susceptibility to, 4; AHUS4 (#612924)

[13] Hemolytic Uremic Syndrome, Atypical, Susceptibility to, 5; AHUS5 (#612925)

[14] Hemolytic Uremic Syndrome, Atypical, Susceptibility to, 6; AHUS 6 (#612926)

[15] Complement Factor I; CFI (#217030)

*Key Words:* Thrombotic microangiopathy, hemolytic anemia, thrombocytopenia, renal failure, hemolytic uremic syndrome, atypical hemolytic uremic syndrome, alternative pathway of the complement system, complement factor H, complement factor I, complement C3, complement factor B, membrane cofactor protein MCP, antifactor H antibodies

## 82 **Tuberculosis**

Tom H. M. Ottenhoff and Esther van de Vosse

- *Disease summary:*
  - Tuberculosis (TB) is an infectious disease that is caused by *Mycobacterium tuberculosis* (*Mtb*). Most individuals are able to control infection in an asymptomatic or latent stage (>90%), while only 3% to 10% of those infected will progress to develop active TB disease during their lifetime. Host susceptibility is dependent on multiple interacting genetic loci and environmental factors, such as coinfections (HIV), malnutrition, and immunosuppressive medication. Around 1.7 million people die from TB, and 9 million develop active TB disease each year.
  - TB most often presents as pulmonary TB (75%). Extrapulmonary TB can present as meningeal TB, TB lymphadenopathy, bone TB, spinal TB, skin TB, disseminated (miliary) TB, and in principle can affect any organ or tissue. Extrapulmonary TB is more commonly found in individuals with an acquired (HIV, tumor necrosis factor [TNF]-blocking medication) or primary immunodeficiency (PID).
  - Clinical systemic features of TB are mostly nonspecific, and include fever, night sweats, weight loss or cachexia, anemia, tachycardia, and fatigue. Local clinical features depend on the specific site of disease: persistent and productive cough and possibly hemoptysis in pulmonary TB, enlarged lymph nodes in TB lymphadenopathy, headache, and nuchal rigidity in meningeal TB, etc.
- *Differential diagnosis:*
  - For pulmonary TB bronchitis, bacterial pneumonia including pneumonia caused by nontuberculous mycobacteria (NTM) such as *Mycobacterium kansasii*, chronic obstructive pulmonary disease, sarcoidosis, lung cancer. For extrapulmonary TB disseminated infection with nontuberculous mycobacteria related to HIV or Mendelian susceptibility to mycobacterial disease, other disseminated granulomatous infections.
- *Monogenic forms:*
  - No single genetic cause of TB has been identified. TB is however occasionally found in patients with certain primary immunodeficiencies, such as genetic deficiencies in the interleukin-12 or -23/interferon-gamma axis or chronic granulomatous disease.
- *Family history:*
  - An affected first-degree relative confers a relative risk of 2.1 for TB.
- *Twin studies:*
  - Monozygotic twins have a 32% concordance rate, dizygotic twins have a 14% concordance rate for clinical TB, although environmental factors play a large role in these concordance rates.
- *Environmental factors:*
  - *Mycobacterium tuberculosis, Mycobacterium bovis* (the cause of bovine TB but also pathogenic in humans), or, less commonly and mostly in West Africa, *Mycobacterium africanum* infection is causative.
- *Genome-wide associations:*
  - TB susceptibility-associated genetic variants (Table 82-1) have been identified mainly through candidate gene studies. Most variants confer only a small additional risk for TB, and testing for genetic variants is therefore of no diagnostic value in TB. Genetic variants have provided insight into disease pathogenesis.
- *Pharmacogenomics:*
  - Testing for genetic variants to guide treatment of TB (Table 82-2) is not yet clinically validated.

## Diagnostic Criteria and Clinical Characteristics

**Diagnostic Criteria for TB:** Diagnostic evaluation should include the following:

- The gold standard for TB diagnosis is bacteriologic confirmation of samples from clinically suspected cases. Diagnosis of pulmonary TB should include repeated (minimum 2×), confirmed sputum microscopy; identification of acid-fast bacilli in a sample provides immediate diagnosis with high but not complete specificity. For smear-negative pulmonary TB and for extrapulmonary TB, more invasive diagnostic procedures

Table 82-1 Tuberculosis Disease-Associated Susceptibility Variants

| Candidate Gene (Chromosome Location) | Associated Variant [effect on protein] (SNP database ID) | Relative Risk | Frequency of Risk Allele[b] | Putative Functional Significance | Associated Disease Phenotype |
|---|---|---|---|---|---|
| P2RX7 (12q24) | **1513A>C** [nonsynonymous amino acid substitution E496A] (rs3751143) | 1.4 Allele 1513C | 13% in Russians, 15% in Turkish, 15% in Punjabi Indians, 25% in Vietnamese, 19% in Mexican mestizo, 17% in Tunisians | Ligand-gated cation channel responsible for ATP-mediated bacterial killing | Extrapulmonary TB susceptibility |
| SLC11A1[a] (2q35) | **1729 + 55del4** [TGTG deletion in 3'UTR] (rs17235416) | 1.4 Allele 55del4 | 16% in Gambians, 2% in Danish, 10% in Chinese, 8% in Koreans | Transporter involved in iron metabolism | TB susceptibility |
| | **1627G>A** [nonsynonymous amino acid substitution D543N] (rs17235409) | 1.3 Allele 1627A | 13% in Iranians, 12% in Chinese, 15% in Peruvians | | TB susceptibility |
| | **469 + 14G>C** [variation in intron 4] rs3731865 | 1.2 Allele 469+14C | 7% in Gambians, 9% in Chinese, 1% in Taiwanese, 34% in Peruvians | | TB susceptibility |
| | **5' (GT)n** [5' promoter GT repeat variation] (rs34448891) | Risk allele varies per population | 14% in Gambians, 16% in Tanzanians, 2% in Japanese, 4% in Taiwanese | | TB susceptibility |
| VDR (12q13.11) | **2T>A** [non-synonymous amino acid substitution M1K] (rs10735810) | 2.0 Allele 2T | 38% in Chinese, 28% in Tibetans | Vitamin D receptor pathway | TB susceptibility |
| TLR1 (4p14) | **743G>A** [non-synonymous amino acid substitution S248N] (rs4833095) | Risk allele varies per population | 71% in Germans, 25% in African-Americans | Receptor for recognition of mycobacterial lipoprotein | TB susceptibility |
| | **1805G>T** [non-synonymous amino acid substitution S602I] (rs5743618) | Risk allele varies per population | 32% in Germans, 90% in African Americans | | TB susceptibility |

| Gene (locus) | Variant | Risk allele odds ratio | Frequency[b] | Function | Association |
|---|---|---|---|---|---|
| *IL12B* (5q31.1-q33.1) | **1188T>G** [3'UTR variation] (rs3212227) | Risk allele varies per population | 69% in Guinea-Bissauans, 67% in African Americans, 17% in Russians | Subunit of IL-12 and IL-23, key cytokines in cell-mediated immunity | Pulmonary TB susceptibility |
| | **GC>TTAGAG** [promoter variation] (rs17860508) | 1.2-1.5 short allele | 48% Indians, 48% Chinese | | TB susceptibility |
| *TLR8* (Xp22) | **1A>G** [nonsynonymous amino acid substitution M1V] rs3764880 | 1.2-2.9 allele 1G | 24% in Indonesians, 76% in Russians, 50% in Turkish | Receptor for recognition of a mycobacterial molecule | Pulmonary TB susceptibility in males |
| *IFNG* (12q14) | **874T>A** [variation in intron 1] (rs2430561) | 0.7 allele 874T | 31% in Chinese, 44% in Spanish, 43% in Brazilians, 43% in Tunisians, 32% in South Africans, 36% in Pakistani | Dimerizes to form IFN-γ, a key cytokine in cell-mediated immunity | TB susceptibility |

Variants that were found in meta-analyses not to be associated with TB, and variants reported once to be associated with TB but have not been replicated in other populations are not included.

[a]*SLC11A1* is also known as *NRAMP1*.

[b]Frequencies of populations in which the allele was found associated with TB.

*Table 82-2 Pharmacogenetics in Tuberculosis*

| Gene | Associated Medications | Goal of Testing | Variants | Effect |
|------|------------------------|-----------------|----------|--------|
| NAT2 (N-acetyltransferase 2) | Isoniazid | Efficacy and safety | *5, *6, *7 *12, *13, *14 | Slow elimination, higher risk |
| CYP2E1 (cytochrome P450 2E1) | Isoniazid | Safety | *1B, *5A, *5B | Lower risk |
| GSTM1 (glutathione S-transferase mu 1) | Isoniazid | Safety | Null | Higher risk |

such as bronchoalveolar lavage or biopsy for acid-fast staining, polymerase chain reaction (PCR), culture and histopathologic examination may be required. For all types of TB, confirmation by culture is preferred, since this will allow drug susceptibility testing of the clinical *Mtb* strain, *Mtb* strain genotyping to evaluate transmission patterns and subtyping (assessment of virulence [eg, *Mtb* W/Beijing clades]) and differentiation from NTM or *M. bovis*.

- Chest radiography is a fairly sensitive method to identify pulmonary TB. Imaging techniques are important for the detection of extrapulmonary TB, to guide targeted specimen collection.
- A recently developed new DNA-based amplification test, GeneXpert MTB/RIF, can diagnose TB (and rifampicin resistance), but has been validated only in active pulmonary TB cases. The test lacks sensitivity in extrapulmonary TB, particularly meningeal TB, and in smear-negative pulmonary TB in HIV-infected individuals.
- Tuberculin skin testing (TST) is a helpful diagnostic tool in individuals in low-prevalence settings and in the absence of Bacillus Calmette-Guérin (BCG) vaccination. In high-prevalence areas the predictive value of the tuberculin skin test is low, due to high level of exposure to *Mtb*, concurrent BCG vaccination and likely NTM exposure. The sensitivity of the test is decreased in immunocompromised individuals.
- Interferon-gamma release assays (IGRA) based on stimulating blood cells with *Mtb*-specific antigens (ESAT6, CFP10, TB7.7) can detect infection but cannot distinguish between latent and active TB. These tests are therefore mainly useful in low incidence settings. IGRA remain more sensitive in the immunocompromised, compared to TST.
- HIV testing of all new cases of TB is generally recommended, as timely treatment of HIV infection improves prognosis. Combined treatment is complicated by interactions between multi-drug therapy (MDT) and many drugs used in antiretroviral therapy.
- In resource-poor settings there is often no access to mycobacterial culture such that the diagnosis remains based on clinical and radiologic criteria. WHO guidelines regarding the diagnosis of smear-negative and extrapulmonary TB, in the context of HIV, exist.

### Clinical Characteristics:

☞**GENERAL TB CHARACTERISTICS:** Many clinical features of TB are nonspecific, and are related to systemic inflammation, including prolonged fever, night sweating, weight loss, tachycardia, fatigue, and loss of appetite.

☞**PULMONARY TB:** Pulmonary TB can present with a persistent, productive cough, hemoptysis, shortness of breath, and pleural pain.

☞**EXTRAPULMONARY TB:** Patients with extrapulmonary TB can, but do not necessarily, present with systemic TB symptoms. However, they can present with a wide variety of symptoms, depending on the site of infection.

*Meningeal TB*: fever, headache or neck stiffness, vomiting, seizures, neurologic deficits, and decreased consciousness

*Spinal TB*: chronic back pain, accompanied by restriction of movement, paresis, spasticity

*TB lymphadenopathy*: enlarged peripheral lymph nodes, fistulae, enlarged intrathoracic or intra-abdominal lymph nodes that rarely can cause obstruction of blood vessels or the common bile duct

*Joint TB*: chronic and arthritic joint pain, swelling, and restriction of movement

*Disseminated or miliary TB:* any number of symptoms since nearly every organ can be affected. Symptoms can include abdominal pain, multiple erythematous papules in the skin, dyspnea. Signs include hepatosplenomegaly, enlarged lymph nodes, septic shock, acute respiratory distress syndrome, and even multiorgan failure.

## Screening and Counseling

**Screening:** No genetic screening of family members exists or is needed for TB. Genetic testing for disease-associated single-nucleotide polymorphisms (SNPs) is not clinically recommended nor validated.

TB is diagnosed in patients with a PID, such as Mendelian susceptibility to mycobacterial disease (MSMD, mutations in *IL12RB1, IL12B, IFNGR1, IFNGR2, STAT1*), or X-linked chronic granulomatous disease (mutations in *CYBB*). Genetic screening is relevant only for TB patients suspected of a PID in whom HIV has been excluded.

**Counseling:** Counseling is not required for most TB patients. Counseling for PID-associated TB is focused on the PID. Depending on the involved gene, the PID inheritance can be autosomal recessive, autosomal dominant, or X-linked and the defects can be partial or complete.

## Management and Treatment

### Management:

☞**THERAPEUTICS:** For adults with pulmonary TB, the most frequently used treatment is a combination of the first-line anti-TB drugs isoniazid, rifampicin, ethambutol, and pyrazinamide for 2 months, followed by isoniazid, rifampicin for 4 months. For adults with TB meningitis isoniazid, rifampin, ethambutol, and streptomycin may be used, for 12 months. All drugs are to be administered in a directly observed treatment program (DOTS) to increase compliance and reduce development of secondary antibiotic resistance. An increasing number of *Mtb* strains are resistant to first-line antibiotics and need to be treated with second-line (MDR-TB) or third-line (XDR-TB) regimens, which tend to have limited efficacy and more serious side effects. Ideally, empirical regimens are adjusted according to drug-susceptibility of *Mtb* strains, but culture and susceptibility testing are not widely available in many endemic regions.

☞**PREVENTION:** Infants or young children in high TB prevalence areas are routinely vaccinated with the attenuated *M. bovis* BCG vaccine. Although BCG is effective against meningeal TB and miliary TB in children, it has shown limited and inconsistent efficacy against pulmonary TB, which is the most frequent manifestation and only contagious form of the disease. BCG efficacy varies widely in human populations, and is least effective in areas with a high rate of infection with NTM. NTM may cause an immune response comparable to BCG, thereby masking or blocking the effect of the vaccine.

Isoniazid treatment of TST-positive and/or IGRA-positive TB-exposed individuals for 6 to 9 months affords 70 to 80 protective efficacy against developing active TB, but may have side effects. This approach is therefore generally limited to persons in whom the infection is acquired recently. In individuals that need anti-TNF treatment (rheumatoid arthritis, Crohn disease), or that are in need of immunosuppression for other reasons, latent TB infection has a very high risk of reactivation often with a severe course and should be screened for and, if present, treated before starting such therapy.

☞**PHARMACOGENETICS:** Pharmacogenetics is not yet incorporated widely in the treatment of patients with TB, although some limited pharmacogenetic information is available (Table 82-2).

Isoniazid can be inactivated by two different pathways: the first pathway involves *N*-acetyltransferase 2 (NAT2)-mediated acetylation, resulting in acetylisoniazid which is hydrolyzed to acetylhydrazine. Acetylhydrazine is oxidized by cytochrome P450 2E1 (CYP2E1) to form hydroxylamines, which are intermediates in the formation of established hepatotoxic metabolites. Some of these hepatotoxic metabolites can be detoxified by glutathione-*S*-transferase (GST). The second pathway involves direct hydrolysis of isoniazid to hydrazine, a potent hepatotoxin.

## Molecular Genetics and Molecular Mechanism

About one-third of the world population is infected with *Mtb*, of which only 3% to 10% develop TB disease. Genetic predisposition can explain part of this selective susceptibility. Studies of heritability using twins and other familial designs have convincingly implicated a genetic component contributing to outcomes of TB infection although to date the specific genes or genetic variation involved have remained elusive. Despite many genetic associations reported in particular populations, very few polymorphisms in candidate genes have been consistently replicated and validated as

being associated with TB. These discrepancies are, among others, due to population differences and differences between *Mtb* strains worldwide.

Animal models of TB infection have implicated a number of possible candidate genes, but with the exception of MSMD PID these often have ambiguous or disappointing patterns of replication in humans (eg, human *SP110* variation does not replicate the strong impact of its homologue *Ipr1* in in-bred mice). A number of host genetic factors have however been directly implicated in tuberculosis susceptibility in humans (Table 82-1), but strong genetic effects on tuberculosis risk have been difficult to detect both by candidate gene and genome-wide association studies (GWASs).

*Genetic Testing:* Except in the case of PID-associated TB, genetic testing does not have a role yet in identifying people at risk for TB. Each genetic variant only confers a small additional risk for developing TB, while environmental factors play the major role.

*Future Directions:* Due to the large number of environmental factors involved in development of TB, it will continue to be a challenge to identify genetic variants that influence risk of disease. Genetic screens will however likely to be used in the future to identify people at risk (eg, from PID) and selectively guide prevention interventions, such as (postinfection) vaccination or treatment of latent TB (pharmacogenetics). Next-generation deep sequencing will be helpful in identifying additional genetic factors.

**BIBLIOGRAPHY:**

1. Aissa K, Madhi F, Ronsin N, et al. Evaluation of a model for efficient screening of Tuberculosis contact subjects. *Am J Respir Crit Care Med.* 2008;177(9):1041-1047.

2. Simonds B. *Tuberculosis in Twins.* London, UK: Pitman Medical Punlishing Company; 1963.

3. van de Vosse E, Hoeve MA, Ottenhoff TH. Human genetics of intracellular infectious diseases: molecular and cellular immunity against mycobacteria and salmonellae. *Lancet Infect Dis.* 2004;4(12):739-749.

4. World Health Organization. *Treatment of Tuberculosis: Guidelines.* 4th ed. World Health Organization; Geneva, Switzerland; 2010.

5. Andersen P, Doherty TM. The success and failure of BCG—implications for a novel tuberculosis vaccine. *Nat Rev Microbiol.* Aug 2005;3(8):656-662.

6. Vynnycky E, Fine PEM. Lifetime risks, incubation period, and serial interval of tuberculosis. *Am J Epidemiol.* 2000; 152(3):247-263.

7. Kallmann FJ, Reisner D. Twin studies on the significance of genetic factors in tuberculosis. *Am Rev Tuberc.* 1942;47:549-574.

8. Bellamy R, Beyers N, McAdam KP, et al. Genetic susceptibility to tuberculosis in Africans: a genome-wide scan. *Proc Natl Acad Sci USA.* 2000;97(14):8005-8009.

9. Jepson A, Fowler A, Banya W, et al. Genetic regulation of acquired immune responses to antigens of Mycobacterium tuberculosis: a study of twins in West Africa. *Infect Immun.* 2001; 69(6):3989-3994.

10. Baghdadi JE, Orlova M, Alter A, et al. An autosomal dominant major gene confers predisposition to pulmonary tuberculosis in adults. *J Exp Med.* 2006;203(7):1679-1684.

11. van Crevel R, Parwati I, Sahiratmadja E, et al. Infection with *Mycobacterium tuberculosis* Beijing genotype is associated with polymorphisms in SLC11A1/NRAMP1 in Indonesian tuberculosis patients. *J Infect Dis.* 2010;200:1671-1674.

## Supplementary Information

**OMIM References:**

[1] Susceptibility to Mycobacterium tuberculosis (#607948)

[2] Mendelian Susceptibility to Mycobacterial Disease; IL12B, IL12RB1, IFNGR1, IFNGR2, STAT1 (#209950)

[3] Chronic Granulomatous Disease; CYBB (#306400)

**Alternative Names:**
- Consumption
- White Plague
- Phthisis

*Key Words:* Tuberculosis, diagnosis, treatment, genetic and environmental factors

# 83 Malaria

Susanna Campino, Grant Hill-Cawthorne, and Arnab Pain

## KEY POINTS

- *Disease summary:*
  - Malaria is a major parasitic infection in humans with significant global health impact. The pathogen *Plasmodium* completes its sexual maturation in mosquitoes, which in turn transmit sporozoites to humans while feeding on their blood. In humans, the liver incubates sporozoites allowing for their asexual reproduction before their release into the blood stream where they continue their reproduction in red blood cells (RBCs), altering their properties, and causing the various symptoms of malaria.

- *Differential diagnosis:*
  - Consider viral infections such as HIV seroconversion, dengue fever, hepatitis A, B, and E, influenza and viral hemorrhagic fevers. Bacterial infections with a similar presentation include typhoid, pneumonias, and leptospirosis.

- *Monogenic forms:*
  - Genetic host and pathogen factors are known to influence the disease risk. The best known host genetic factor is sickle cell hemoglobinopathy where carriers of this disease have an approximately 10-fold increase in protection against severe and complicated malaria.

- *Genome-wide associations:*
  - A number of genetic variants in the pathogen genome have been identified, some of which may serve as candidates for the development of more effective antimalarial therapies and vaccines.

- *Pharmacogenomics:*
  - Some antimalarial drugs can cause hemolysis in patients with glucose-6-phosphate dehydrogenase (G6PD) deficiency so measurement of G6PD activity is indicated.

## Diagnostic Criteria and Clinical Characteristics

**Clinical Characteristics:** Malaria should be suspected in anyone who has previously visited a malaria-endemic area, including those that took prophylaxis. Human malaria can be caused by five species of *Plasmodium* (*Plasmodium falciparum, Plasmodium vivax, Plasmodium ovale, Plasmodium malariae*, and the simian parasite *Plasmodium knowlesi*) out of which infections by *P falciparum* and *P vivax* are most common. Human infection with *P knowlesi* is thought to be a zoonosis and has only been reported in Southeast Asia.

☞**SIGNS AND SYMPTOMS:**

*Incubation period* can be as short as 6 days for naturally acquired infection. Most patients who have a *P falciparum* infection will present within 6 months of exposure. *P vivax* and *P ovale* may enter a hypnozoite stage in the liver with infections usually presenting more than 6 months, and occasionally years, after exposure. There is a risk of relapse if only the blood phase of the disease is treated and the hypnozoites are not cleared.

*Symptoms* are nonspecific and there are no pathognomonic features. Most patients complain of fever or sweats or rigors, myalgia, headache, and general malaise. Malaria may be misdiagnosed as influenza or another respiratory viral infection, or as gastroenteritis due to gastrointestinal symptoms and jaundice. The fever typically does not follow the classically described quotidian, tertian, or quartan patterns.

*Signs* are also nonspecific and reminiscent of many other conditions. A fever is not invariably present and hepatomegaly is uncommon in acute malaria. Children are more likely to have hepatosplenomegaly than adults.

*Severe or complicated falciparum malaria* may present with

- Metabolic acidosis (pH <7.35)
- Hypoglycemia (blood glucose <2.2 mmol/L)
- Shock
- Anemia (Hb <8 g/dL)
- Disseminated intravascular coagulopathy
- Pulmonary edema leading to acute respiratory distress syndrome
- Renal impairment or failure
- Impaired consciousness and/or seizures
- Jaundice

☞**HISTORY TAKING:** *A detailed exposure history* is essential. Obtain details of countries visited and regions within each country, including stopovers. Ask about accommodation, use of bed nets, mosquito repellent chemicals, and chemoprophylaxis. Ask about prophylactic drug combination, duration, side effects, adherence, and premature cessation.

**Differential Diagnosis:** Consider viral infections such as HIV seroconversion, dengue fever, hepatitis A, B, and E, influenza, and viral hemorrhagic fevers. Bacterial infections with a similar presentation include typhoid, pneumonias, and leptospirosis.

**Diagnosis:**

☞**DIAGNOSTIC INVESTIGATIONS FOR MALARIA:**

*Timing* of investigations is important. In suspected malaria cases blood should be taken for testing immediately. All tests should be communicated back to the clinician as positive or negative for malaria within 1 to 2 hours. Speciation should then be available within 12 hours, if not possible at the time of initial diagnosis. Ensure to stop chemoprophylaxis upon admission to hospital as this may interfere with parasite detection in the blood.

*Thick and thin blood films* are sensitive and specific for all *Plasmodium* species in the hands of an experienced light microscopist. A thin smear should be examined under oil emersion for 15 to 20 minutes and a thick smear for 5 to 10 minutes before being declared negative. If there is clinical suspicion of malaria but initial films are negative, then repeat films should be carried out after 12 to 24 hours and again after a further 24 hours. In pregnancy thick films can still be negative in severe infections due to the sequestration of parasites in the placenta.

*Percentage of infected RBCs* should be estimated if falciparum malaria is diagnosed as this has implications for the choice of treatment to be used.

*Rapid diagnostic tests (RDTs)* are not as sensitive or specific for the detection of nonfalciparum infections. However, due to the lack of expertise in many Western laboratories they are particularly useful for suspected cases of malaria presenting out of hours. These tests require small volumes of blood (2-50 µL) and therefore can be done on finger-prick samples. Targets vary but include histidine-rich protein-2 of *P falciparum* (PfHRP-2), parasite-specific (*P falciparum, P vivax*, or both) lactate dehydrogenase, or the pan-malarial *Plasmodium* aldolase. However, there are currently no specific tests available for *P malariae, P ovale*, or *P knowlesi*. They require higher parasite densities than a good light microscopist for detection and cannot be used for assessing response to therapy. Autoantibodies such as rheumatoid factor or heterophile antibodies may lead to false-positive results and false-negative results have been reported in high-grade parasitemias due to the prozone phenomenon.

*Polymerase chain reaction* is emerging but still of limited availability. It should be considered as the new gold standard as it is highly sensitive and specific and allows for speciation.

*Additional blood tests*

**Routine**
- Full blood count (anemia and thrombocytopenia)
- Urea and electrolytes (renal failure and metabolic disturbance)
- Liver function tests (hepatitis)
- Blood glucose (hypoglycemia due to disease, or baseline before treatment)

**Sick patients**
- Blood gases (metabolic acidosis)
- Blood culture (superinfections)
- Lactate (hyperlactatemia)
- Clotting studies (disseminated intravascular coagulopathy)

**Consider for differential diagnosis**
- Chest x-ray
- Computed tomography (CT) head and lumbar puncture
- Other infection screening samples, for example, urine, stool

*Notification of cases:* Your health authority is likely to require you to refer all cases of malaria to a central public health notification unit.

## Management and Treatment

### General Management:

☞**Nonfalciparum Malaria:**
- Malaria caused by *P ovale, P vivax*, or *P malariae* are rarely life threatening but severe or complicated cases (as defined in Signs and Symptoms) should be treated the same as falciparum malaria. *P knowlesi* can be confused by microscopists as *P malariae* but usually has high parasitemias (>1%) and should be treated as falciparum malaria.
- Can usually be managed on an outpatient basis.
- G6PD activity will need to be measured before discharge.

☞**Falciparum Malaria:**
- Admit to hospital.
- Certain categories of patients may deteriorate quickly: pregnant women, children, and the elderly.
- Mixed infections that include falciparum parasites should be treated as falciparum malaria.
- Measure initial parasite count—more than 2% parasitized red cells increase the chance of serious disease.

### Current Drugs Available:

*Artemisinin (and derivatives):* Natural antimalarials sourced from the sweet wormwood (*Artemisia annua*). All derivatives are metabolized to the active metabolite dihydroartemisinin, which acts on young ring-forming parasites. They produce rapid clearance of parasitemia and rapid resolution of symptoms. They do act against drug-resistant *P falciparum* strains but recrudescence is seen with short-duration monotherapies. Therefore, extended-duration combinations with mefloquine, lumefantrine, or tetracycline/doxycycline are recommended. Artemisinin-based combination therapies (ACTs) are the WHO recommended treatments for uncomplicated *P falciparum* malaria and in chloroquine-resistant uncomplicated *P vivax* infections. Parenteral artesunate is the WHO recommended treatment for severe malaria. Use of coartemether (artemether and lumefantrine) may be associated with hearing loss and is currently not recommended in the first trimester of pregnancy.

*Atovaquone/proguanil:* Fixed drug combination that is synergistic: inhibits electron transport and reduces the potential across the mitochondrial membrane. Usually used as malaria chemoprophylaxis where it acts at both the liver and the blood stage; effective in areas of Thailand where chloroquine and mefloquine resistance has been documented; can also be used for the treatment of noncomplicated *P falciparum* infection, including multidrug-resistant strains. Oral aphthous ulcers may occur and warfarin anticoagulation may be potentiated. Pregnancy, severe renal insufficiency, and hypersensitivity are contraindications.

*Chloroquine:* Still drug of choice for chemoprophylaxis in travelers going to chloroquine-sensitive areas. WHO second-line treatment (in combination with tetracycline or doxycycline or clindamycin) is the choice for uncomplicated *P falciparum* malaria. Chloroquine-primaquine is the treatment of choice for chloroquine-sensitive *P vivax* infections. Well tolerated except for its bitter taste. Black people may experience generalized pruritus. Retinal toxic effects are very unlikely to occur at the total dosage used for treating malaria. Contraindications include a history of epilepsy or generalized psoriasis.

_Mefloquine:_ Acts on the intraerythrocytic asexual stages by inhibiting heme polymerization within the food vacuole. It remains an effective chemoprophylaxis agent against malaria in chloroquine-resistant areas but adverse effects at high doses preclude extensive use as a treatment agent. Increasing mefloquine resistance is being seen in the border areas between Cambodia, Burma, and Thailand. Side effects are common (25%-50% of travelers using mefloquine for chemoprophylaxis). The most frequent side effects are vivid dreams, nausea, mood changes, insomnia, and gastrointestinal upset. Severe reactions such as seizure and psychosis are rare and reported in 1 in 6000 to 1 in 13,000 users. Mefloquine is therefore contraindicated in those with a known hypersensitivity reaction, history of serious psychiatric disease, or seizure disorder (but not childhood febrile seizures).

_Primaquine:_ Is the only agent in common use that is effective against the liver stage of _P ovale_ and _P vivax_ infections. It is also active against the blood stages and against gametocytes and therefore is used both for chemoprophylaxis and terminal treatment. Resistance is increasing so the recommended dose for radical cure has been increased for malaria acquired in Oceania and Southeast Asia. As the main contraindication is G6PD deficiency, all individuals should have their G6PD activity levels measured prior to treatment. Primaquine use is also contraindicated in pregnancy as the drug crosses the placenta and the infant's G6PD status cannot be determined in utero.

_Quinine:_ Oral therapy with quinine (with a second agent) is indicated for the treatment of uncomplicated falciparum malaria and as a step-down therapy after parenteral treatment of complicated malaria. As WHO has designated parenteral artesunate as the drug of choice for treating severe or complicated malaria, parenteral quinine is an alternative drug when artesunate is not available (such as in the United Kingdom where artesunate is available on a named-patient basis only).

_Other drugs:_

_Pyrimethamine-sulfadoxine_ is a fixed drug combination that inhibits folate synthesis in the parasite. However, it is of little use for the treatment of _P falciparum_ due to drug resistance in the Amazon basin, Southeast Asia, and Africa.

_Clindamycin_ inhibits the parasite apicoplast but is less effective than doxycycline or atovaquone/proguanil. It is therefore reserved for those cases where first-line drugs cannot be used (eg, pregnant women and young children).

_Doxycycline_ inhibits parasite protein synthesis. It is effective as chemoprophylaxis and treatment of chloroquine-resistant _P falciparum_ and can be used as prophylaxis against mefloquine-resistant isolates but has to be taken daily, increasing noncompliance. Side effects include photosensitivity, gastrointestinal upset, and rarely, esophageal ulceration. Doxycycline is contraindicated in pregnancy, breast-feeding women, and children less than 8 years of age.

**Pharmacogenetics:** It has been incorporated in malaria treatment for a long time. To achieve radical cure (elimination of the liver stage) of _P vivax_ and _P ovale_ an 8-aminoquinoline antimalarial needs to be used. As these can cause hemolysis in patients with G6PD deficiency, routine measurement of G6PD activity has been carried out for a number of years whenever a patient presents with nonfalciparum malaria.

# Molecular Genetics and Molecular Mechanisms

**Host Genetics: Genetic Predisposition to Malaria:** Genetic epidemiologic studies have demonstrated that host genetic factors influence the response to malaria significantly. It is likely that many different genes are involved, that interact with several other factors, such as environmental, parasite genetics, and complex life cycle, and host age and immunity. Several studies have identified candidate genes that can affect the response to malaria, mostly genes associated with RBC and the immune system. Table 83-1 summarizes some of the most convincing associations described over the past years. The classical example is the protective effect of certain RBC polymorphisms caused by abnormalities of hemoglobin structure and synthesis. In the late 1940s, Haldane pointed out that the high frequency of thalassemia in the Mediterranean was the result of selective pressure by malaria. One of the best examples is the hemoglobin S (HbS) or sickle cell hemoglobin. African children who are heterozygous for HbS appear to have approximately 10-fold increase in protection against severe and complicated malaria in a number of populations. The precise mechanism of resistance is yet to be established. It may involve reduction of parasite growth inside the RBC, increased splenic clearance or reduced cytoadherence of the infected RBC. On the other hand, the Duffy blood group antigen is expressed in the RBC of most people, except in populations from sub-Saharan Africa who are Duffy blood group-negative. _Plasmodium vivax_ needs the Duffy antigen to invade RBC and discovery has led to the development of a candidate vaccine against _P vivax_ that is under clinical trials.

Genetic interactions that determine protective immunity have also been implicated in protection against malaria but the evidence is less strong than the results for erythrocyte-related genes (Table 83-1) (reviewed in). Some genomic regions were identified which showed evidence for linkage to the parasitological and clinical phenotypes studied. A genome-wide association study (GWAS) of severe malaria in the Gambia used an assay consisting of approximately 500,000 single-nucleotide polymorphisms (SNPs) identified 19 hits including the sickle cell substitution. Further GWAS are being performed in Ghanaian, Kenyan, Malawian, and Vietnamese populations with larger sample sizes and using both case-control and affected-offspring parental trio designs using larger SNP arrays (www.malariagen.net).

**Plasmodium Genetics and Drug Resistance:** Historically, antimalarial drugs and mosquito control programs have significantly reduced malaria worldwide. However, the appearance and spread of drug-resistant parasites and insecticide-resistant mosquitoes has contributed to a substantial increase in malaria cases. In numerous parts of the world _P falciparum_ has become resistant to chloroquine (CQ) and to Fansidar (sulfadoxine-pyrimethamine [SP]), the two most common treatments in most endemic areas. Although other antimalarial drugs have been introduced, resistance to all antimalarial drug classes has been reported, including artemisinin (ART) derivatives. The development and spread of resistance could be the result of the overuse of antimalarial drugs, incomplete treatment courses, and the extensive genetic variability and high proliferation rate that permits resistant parasite populations to appear rapidly. A barrier to successful malaria vaccine and drug development has been our limited understanding of the genetic variability among _P falciparum_ parasites. Traditional genetic methods, which are

*Table 83-1  Host Genetics in Malaria*

| Gene/Locus | Protein | Observed Genetic Association with Malaria |
| --- | --- | --- |
| **Red blood cells related** | | |
| *HBB* | Beta-globin | HbS protects against severe malaria. HbC association is variable |
| *HBA* | Alpha-globin | Thalassemia protects against severe malaria |
| *FY* | Duffy antigen | duffy negative have complete protection against P vivax |
| *ABO* | Histo-blood group ABO system transferase | Blood group 'O' is associated with reduced risk of severe malaria |
| *GYPA* | Glycophorin A | Deficiency in RBC reduces P falciparum infection |
| *GYPB* | Glycophorin B | Deficiency in RBC reduces P falciparum infection |
| *GYPC* | Glycophorin C | Deficiency in RBC reduces P falciparum infection |
| *G6PD* | Glucose-6-phosphate dehydogenase | G6PD deficiency protects against severe malaria. |
| **Immune system related** | | |
| *HLA* (class I and class II) | | HLA-B53 and HLA-DRB1 associated with protection against severe malaria |
| *TNF* | tumor necrosis factor | Associated with severe malaria and re-infection risk |
| *IFNG* | interferon gamma | Associated with severe malaria and reduce risk of cerebral malaria |
| *IL10* | interleukin-10 | Variable association with severe malaria |
| *IL4* | interleukin-4 | Associated with antimalaria antibodies levels in the Fulani ethnic group |
| *TLR4* | Toll like receptor 4 | Variable association with severe malaria |
| **Parasite sequestration related** | | |
| *CD36* | thrombospondin receptor | Variable association with severe malaria |
| *ICAM1* | intercellular adhesion molecule-1 | Variable association with severe malaria |

For detailed associations see review of Kwiatkowski DP, 2005

experimentally difficult to apply in *P falciparum*, have been used to find mutations that contribute to resistance to certain antimalarials. *P falciparum* CQ resistance has been shown to be associated with mutations in the transporter gene *pfcrt* and genes encoding *P falciparum* dihydrofolate reductase (pfdhfr) and dihydrofolate reductase (pfdhps) have been shown to confer resistance to SP (reviewed in Table 83-2). Copy number and/or point mutations at the *P falciparum* multidrug-resistance (pfmdr1) gene have been associated with parasite response to mefloquine, quinine, ART, and other antimalarial drugs. However, the effect of these genes alone does not explain completely the drug resistance and unknown genes need to be discovered. Advances in genomic technologies, including whole-genome sequencing using next-generation technologies, are facilitating the mapping of hundreds of parasite genomes. These data are already contributing to understanding the parasite global diversity and biology, and will assist future GWAS to understand the molecular mechanisms of parasite-specific phenotypes, such as

resistance and invasion traits. Further advances in whole-genome sequencing technologies will assist with similar studies in the larger host and vector genomes.

***Plasmodium Genomics: Drug and Vaccine Development:*** Complete genome sequences of three out of five human-infecting malaria species (*P falciparum*, *P vivax*, and *P knowlesi*) are publicly available for exploitation as new drug targets and vaccine candidates. There are over 5300 malaria genes in each of the three primate malaria species sequenced. As malaria has become more tractable over the last decade, it has attracted more funding toward drug and vaccine development with establishment of public-private partnerships. The predicted malaria antigens are constantly being evaluated as possible vaccine candidates and some have entered clinical trials. The success of large-scale functional genomics studies to evaluate new drug or vaccine candidates requires the creation of appropriate molecular tools and reagents to support such experiments. Using the annotated genome-sequence information,

**Table 83-2 Genes Involved with Drug Resistance in Malaria**

| P. falciparum Gene | Protein | Observed Genetic Association with Malaria |
|---|---|---|
| PfCRT | digestive vacuole transmembrane protein | point mutations associated with resistance to chloroquine |
| Pfmdr1 | multidrug resistance protein | point mutations and copy number associated with resistance to chloroquine, mefloquine, halofantrine and other antimalarials |
| Pfdhfr | dihydrofolate reductase enzyme | point mutations associated with resistance to pyrimethamine |
| Pfdhps | dihydropteroate synthase enzyme | point mutations associated with resistance to sulfadoxin |

For detailed associations see review of Hayton K, 2008

a high-throughput recombinational cloning approach was used to generate a large number of expression clones in *P falciparum* for their subsequent evaluation as possible vaccine targets. Large-scale gene inactivation and other functional genomics studies in rodent malaria models and in *P falciparum* are providing new insights into biochemical and invasion pathways that may be targeted for drug discovery or for vaccine evaluation. The drug development efforts in malaria have shifted to modern cell-based assays providing drug efficacy information on greater than 1000s of chemical compounds at a relatively short period of time. Recently, an imaging-based high-content screening technique was used to evaluate over 4000 commercially available antimalarial compounds with previous antierythrocytic stage activity. This screening has resulted in identification of imidazolopiperazine compounds as effective inhibitors for both erythrocytic and exoerythrocytic (ie, hepatic stages) stages of the parasite. However, one of the challenges ahead is to understand the precise biochemical mechanism of action of the newly identified compounds to facilitate further improvement in efficacy through chemical modifications.

An effective vaccine is expected to provide the ideal and most cost-effective solution for preventing millions of cases on malaria in endemic regions. Currently, there is no commercially available and licensed vaccine available for malaria. Several lines of published evidence suggest that a prophylactic malaria vaccine is possible. Traditional approaches of malaria vaccine development primarily focused on targeting one of the parasite stages of development either within the human or in the mosquito vector. Vaccines against the pre-erythrocytic stages have produced the most promising results. Initial successes of inducing a malaria-protective response came over three decades ago with the use of irradiated live sporozoites in human. The result of a clinical trial of an injectable preparation of live attenuated sporozoites has just been reported to the scientific community. The first clinical trial using a purified malaria protein began two decades ago but so far only the circumsporozoite protein (CSP, the major surface protein of the malaria sporozoites) has produced reproducible protective results in human volunteers. The CS protein is indeed the immuno-dominant protective antigen in irradiated sporozoites and is responsible for 90% of the protection in a *Plasmodium yoelii*-infected PyCSP-tolerant mouse malaria model.

The most effective recombinant malaria vaccine tested to date is called RTS, S. RTS, S is a hybrid protein component composed of hepatitis B surface protein and the recombinant CS protein formulated in a multicomponent adjuvant known as AS01. The RTS, S clinical trials partnership has just published the interim result of a large multicenter phase III clinical trial, which is broadly in line with results (55% protection against all malaria episodes and 35% efficacy against severe malaria) obtained in phase II trial. The RTS, S has been in development over 25 years and is currently being developed by a public-private partnership between Glaxo-SmithKline (GSK) and the PATH Malaria Vaccine Initiative (MVI) with additional financial support from the Bill & Melinda Gates Foundation. Many other malaria vaccines are in various stages of development but the RTS, S/AS01 formulation is considerably more advanced toward registration and deployment. WHO has indicated that subject to satisfactory phase III trial results, it could recommend RTS, S as the first malaria vaccine for use in selected African countries in just over 3 years. The full results of the phase III trial on RTS, S/AS01 will be available in 2014. For details on a list of malaria vaccine candidates and major advances in malaria vaccine development, please see in.

***Future Directions:*** The recent explosion of large genomic datasets has already provided a wealth of new knowledge on pathophysiology, genetics of host resistance, natural diversity of malarial antigens, and aided in discovery of biochemical pathways that may pave ways for new therapeutic inventions in future. Large-scale genome variation studies of the parasite will allow us to understand the true population level diversity of all malarial antigens and drug-resistance markers and may provide vital clues to the development and spread of antimalarial drug resistance in the field across continents. Although there have been several recent advances in malaria vaccine development and testing, we still have some way to go before any of these vaccine candidates will reach the clinics in sub-Saharan Africa and in other malaria-endemic regions. Future studies may combine large number of host and parasite genotypes with clinical data in order to gain vital insights in genotype-phenotype correlations in malaria. Scientific discoveries made in these studies may eventually have a significant effect on the clinical management of malaria.

**BIBLIOGRAPHY:**

1. Moody A. Rapid diagnostic tests for malaria parasites. *Clin Microbiol* Rev. Jan 2002;15:66.
2. Marx A, Pewsner D, Egger M, et al. Meta-analysis: accuracy of rapid tests for malaria in travelers returning from endemic areas. *Ann Intern Med.* May 17 2005;142:836.

3. Jelinek T, Grobusch MP, Schwenke S, et al. Sensitivity and specificity of dipstick tests for rapid diagnosis of malaria in nonimmune travelers. *J Clin Microbiol*. Mar 1999;37:721.

4. Mackinnon MJ, Gunawardena DM, Rajakaruna J, Weerasingha S, Mendis KN, Carter R. Quantifying genetic and nongenetic contributions to malarial infection in a Sri Lankan population. *Proc Natl Acad Sci USA*. Nov 7 2000;97:12661.

5. Haldane J. Disease and evolution. *Ricerca Sci*. 1949;19:3.

6. Kwiatkowski DP. How malaria has affected the human genome and what human genetics can teach us about malaria. *Am J Hum Genet*. Aug 2005;77:171.

7. Campino S, Kwiatkowski D, Dessein A. Mendelian and complex genetics of susceptibility and resistance to parasitic infections. *Semin Immunol*. Dec 2006;18:411.

8. Jallow M, Teo YY, Small KS, et al. Genome-wide and fine-resolution association analysis of malaria in West Africa. *Nat Genet*. Jun 2009;41:657.

9. White NJ. Drug resistance in malaria. *Br Med Bull*. 1998;54:703.

10. Wongsrichanalai C, Meshnick SR. Declining artesunate-mefloquine efficacy against falciparum malaria on the Cambodia-Thailand border. *Emerg Infect Dis*. May 2008;14:716.

11. Hayton K, Su XZ. Drug resistance and genetic mapping in Plasmodium falciparum. *Curr Genet*. Nov 2008;54:223.

12. Meister S, Plouffe DM, Kuhen KL, et al. Imaging of Plasmodium liver stages to drive next-generation antimalarial drug discovery. *Science*. Dec 9, 2011;334:1372.

13. Epstein JE, Tewari K, Lyke KE, et al. Live attenuated malaria vaccine designed to protect through hepatic CD8 T cell immunity. *Science*. Oct 28 2011;334:475.

14. Kumar KA, Sano G, Boscardin S, et al. The circumsporozoite protein is an immunodominant protective antigen in irradiated sporozoites. *Nature*. Dec 14 2006;444:937.

15. Agnandji ST, Lell B, Soulanoudjingar, et al. First results of phase 3 trial of RTS,S/AS01 malaria vaccine in African children. *N Engl J Med*. Nov 17 2011;365:1863.

16. Hill AV. Vaccines against malaria. *Philos Trans R Soc Lond B Biol Sci*. Oct 12 2011;366:2806.

## Supplementary Information

*Key Words:* Malaria, host genetics, drug resistance, malaria vaccine

# 84 Genetics of HIV

Talia H. Swartz, Shirish Huprikar, and Benjamin K. Chen

## KEY POINTS

- *Disease summary:*
  - HIV is a blood-borne, sexually transmissible virus that causes immunodeficiency by infecting CD4+ helper T cells. The infection causes an inversion of the normal CD4/CD8 T-cell ratio, dysregulation of B-cell antibody production, and enhances susceptibility to opportunistic infections at advanced disease stages.
  - HIV is a lentivirus, part of the Retroviridae family, which is an enveloped, positive-sense RNA virus that replicates with a DNA intermediate called a provirus. The provirus integrates into the host-cell DNA and persists for the lifetime of the cell.
  - The disease is marked by three phases—acute HIV seroconversion, asymptomatic chronic HIV infection, and acquired immune deficiency syndrome (AIDS). Depending on the host genetics, the duration of each phase can vary. Acute seroconversion is marked by nonspecific symptoms including fever, flu-like illness, lymphadenopathy, and rash which may occur in half of all people infected with HIV. The asymptomatic infection may last for 5 to 10 years on average until the development of AIDS, which occurs when the CD4+ count falls below 200 cells/mm³. At this stage, individuals are at risk for opportunistic infections such as *Pneumocystis* pneumonia, esophageal candidiasis, mycobacterial disease, cryptococcal meningitis, cytomegalovirus (CMV) retinitis, and toxoplasmosis as well as malignancies such as lymphoma and Kaposi sarcoma.
  - For purposes of studying the susceptibility to HIV or AIDS, researchers have classified patients with atypical outcomes into four major categories: 1. exposed uninfected (EU) individuals who remain uninfected after repeated exposure to HIV; 2. rapid progressors (RP) with uncontrolled viremia who progress to a CD4 count below 350 within 3 years; 3. long-term nonprogressors (LTNP) who are infected, yet maintain stable CD4 count and low level viremia for more than a decade; and 4. elite controllers or suppressors (EC/ES) who can suppress viremia for a decade or longer. These classifications have provided some insights into how viral and host genetics contribute to variations in outcome.

- *Differential diagnosis of symptomatic HIV:*
  - Influenza, Epstein-Barr virus (EBV), and other viral syndromes, immunodeficiency such as severe combined immune deficiency (SCID), B-cell and T-cell deficiency

- *Monogenic forms:*
  - *CCR5Δ32* was a mutation identified in 1996 that protected against HIV infection in homozygotes. The mechanism of action is that HIV gp120 binds to CD4 to gain entry into the cell using CCR5 as the chemokine receptor to which HIV binds. Strong evidence for this mutation in homozygotes and partially in heterozygotes has demonstrated delayed HIV disease progression.

- *Family history:*
  - Not available

- *Twin studies:*
  - In HIV-discordant monozygotic twins, a reduction of naïve T cells with skewing of T-cell repertoire has been noted in the HIV-infected cohort.

- *Environmental factors:*
  - A few small studies have demonstrated environmental factors potentiating HIV progression and its sequelae. While tobacco abuse has not been shown to accelerate HIV progression, it has been shown to worsen opportunistic infections, particularly pulmonary infections. Stress and depression have additionally been shown to be associated with faster rates of progression. Additionally certain viral infections such as herpes simplex virus (HSV) increase risk for HIV transmission.

- *Genome-wide associations:*
  - Genetic associations with disease outcome are numerous. Disease-associated genetic variants (single-nucleotide polymorphisms [SNPs]) provide insight into disease pathogenesis. The first genome-wide association study (GWAS) in HIV-1 disease identified several variants and the most clinically relevant variant is the *HCP5* locus that tracks to the HLAB*5701 allele that is clinically validated in the management of HIV (Table 84-1). Subsequent studies have confirmed the KLA mapping as well as the chemokine co-receptor/ligand CCR5 loci.

- *Pharmacogenomics:*
  - Screening for HLA B*5701 is utilized for screening for abacavir hypersensitivity when abacavir is being considered as a component of the antiretroviral regimen.

*Table 84-1 Pharmacogenetic Considerations in HIV*

| Gene | Associated Medications | Goal of Testing | Variants | Effect |
|------|------------------------|-----------------|----------|--------|
| *HLA-B\*5701* (HLA marker) | Abacavir | Safety | *5701 | Hypersensitivity monitoring |

## Diagnostic Criteria and Clinical Characteristics

*Diagnostic Criteria for HIV:* **Diagnostic evaluation includes the following tests (Fig. 84-1 algorithm):**

- Positive (rapid) enzyme immunoassay
- Positive confirmatory western blot

    *or*

- HIV RNA (viral load)

    Once the diagnosis is made, further testing is recommended

- CD4 cell count and percentage
- HIV resistance testing (genotype)
- Coreceptor tropism assays (when considering maraviroc)
- HLA B\*5701 testing (when considering abacavir)
- CMV and *Toxoplasma* IgG testing
- Sexually transmitted disease (STD) screening (eg, syphilis)
- Cervical and anal cancer screening
- Screening for latent tuberculosis
- Viral hepatitis screening

An individual is tested either for general screening or for those who are at high risk. The enzyme immunoassay (EIA) is performed that is a rapid or point-of-care test with various forms (oral, blood). If the result is positive, a confirmatory western blot (WB) is performed. If the western blot is positive, the diagnosis is confirmed

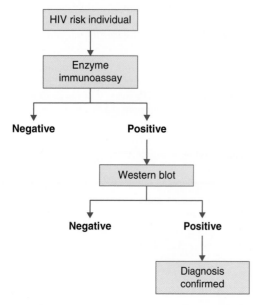

*Figure 84-1* Algorithm for Diagnostic Evaluation of Patient with HIV.

and the standard workup is recommended. The exception to this algorithm is that in the event of acute HIV, there is a seroconversion or "window" period in which antibodies to HIV are not yet detectable in the blood and therefore EIA and WB would be negative. In this situation, an HIV polymerase chain reaction (PCR) would be performed.

*Clinical Characteristics:*

**HIV disease is marked by three distinct stages, described below:**

1. *Acute seroconversion* is observed symptomatically in half of new patients infected with HIV. It is associated with fever, flu-like illness, lymphadenopathy, and rash and may be confused with numerous other viral and nonviral syndromes such as secondary syphilis or acute toxoplasmosis. During this time, the viral load rapidly rises but a rapid immunoassay enzyme test may not detect the HIV surface protein before several weeks have passed, causing a falsely negative result. For this reason, the HIV PCR assay is more sensitive during this period from 2 weeks to 6 months and if suspicion exists for acute HIV, an HIV PCR should be performed concomitantly with serologic testing (Fig. 84-1).

2. *Asymptomatic infection* may last for 5 to 10 years on average until the development of AIDS. This may vary by individual and treatment guidelines discussed later. For treated patients, adverse effects include side effects, drug interactions, and increased risk for cardiac and other metabolic complications. These individuals require assessment of cardiac risk factors and age-appropriate cancer screening, as this group is at higher risk than the general population. As the CD4+ count drops below 500 cells/mm³, individuals are at increased risk for infections including esophageal candidiasis and HSV; hematologic effects such as anemia and thrombocytopenia; and malignancies including Kaposi sarcoma and lymphoma.

3. AIDS occurs when the CD4+ count falls below 200 cells/mm³ or when an AIDS-defining condition develops irrespective of CD4 count. At this stage, individuals are at risk for opportunistic infections and malignancies as previously described. Individuals whose CD4 count is below 200 should receive prophylaxis against *Pneumocystis* and those whose CD4 count is below 75 should receive prophylaxis against *Mycobacterium avium* complex (MAC).

The graph (Fig. 84-2) depicts the time course of CD4+ cells and HIV viral load through the natural history of HIV infection. The initial infection is marked by an acute rise in viral load that reaches a peak with weeks of initial infection. During acute infection before the viral load peaks, rapid enzyme immunoassay may not detect virus, giving a false-negative result. After the acute infection, the viral load gradually decreases down to the individual's set point where the counts may remain stable for years. The CD4 count drops initially and then follows a more gradual progression and the individual may remain in this clinical latency or asymptomatic period for years until becoming symptomatic. Once the CD4 count falls below 200, the disease is classified as AIDS, which is an

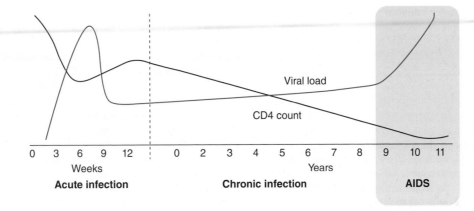

**Figure 84-2** Clinical Course of HIV Infection.
Modified with permission from HIV&AIDS Media Project, Epidemic Demystified; Journal Aids. N.p.,n.d. Web 12 Aug 2013.

absolute indication for antiretroviral therapy and puts the patient at risk for development of multiple infectious complications.

## Screening and Counseling

**Screening:** All individuals between 13 and 64 years of age should be screened for HIV regardless of recognized risk factors. Annual screening is recommended in high-risk individuals. HIV screening is recommended for all pregnant women and repeat screening in the third trimester is recommended in individuals with higher risk.
**Counseling:** Familial clustering is not characterized. No Mendelian forms exist. Counseling relates to risk of exposure and is important in partner identification and risk of infection based on specific contact.

## Management and Treatment

**Management:** Highly active antiretroviral therapy is indicated based on laboratory or clinical measures. Current guidelines suggest initiation of therapy in all individuals. In the past, the following populations were recommended for earlier initiation of therapy regardless of CD4 cell count:

- Symptomatic HIV disease
- Pregnant women
- HIV-1 RNA greater than 100,000 copies/mL
- Rapid decline in CD4 cell count, greater than 100 cells/mm$^3$
- Active hepatitis B or C virus coinfection
- Active or high risk for cardiovascular disease
- HIV-associated nephropathy (HIVAN)
- Symptomatic primary HIV infection
- High risk for secondary HIV transmission, that is, serodiscordant couples

Antiretroviral therapy was previously recommended on the basis of CD4 cell count in all patients with a history of an AIDS-defining illness or with a CD4 count less than 500 cells/mm$^3$ (a shift from prior paradigm of initiation <350 cells/mm$^3$). Therapy is now universally recommended for all infected invidiuals regardless of CD4 cell count.

**Therapeutics:** Several classes of antiretroviral drugs are in use. The preferred regimen for patients who are naïve to antiretroviral therapy should include a dual nucleoside or nucleotide reverse transcriptase inhibitor backbone in combination with a non-nucleoside reverse transcriptase inhibitor, a boosted protease inhibitor, or an integrase strand transfer inhibitor.

**Nucleoside reverse transcriptase inhibitors** (NRTI) are nucleos(t)ide analogs that are competitive inhibitors at the catalytic site of the reverse transcriptase and inhibit replication of virus. Major drugs in this class include abacavir (ABC), lamivudine (3TC), emtricitabine (FTC), tenofovir (TDF), and zidovudine (ZDV). The combination of tenofovir and emtricitabine (TDF/FTC) has been shown to be superior to other combinations in terms of virologic response and is favored as backbone for initial therapy. The renal toxicity is the major side effect associated with tenofovir. ABC has been associated with increased cardiovascular events and can cause a hypersensitivity reaction in patients with HLA-B*5701. This remains the paradigm of pharmacogenomics in the management of HIV.

**Non-nucleoside reverse transcriptase inhibitors** (NNRTI) are non-nucleoside analogs that bind reverse transcriptase and inhibit replication of virus. They act through allosteric inhibition of the reverse transcriptase causing a conformational change in the active site of the enzyme, decreasing affinity for nucleoside binding. These drugs are effective with excellent virologic response, low pill burden, and convenient dosing. They have long half-lives and a low genetic barrier to resistance. It takes a single mutation to confer resistance to the main drugs in this class, efavirenz (EFV) and nevirapine (NVP). Major adverse effects of efavirenz include skin rash and neuropsychiatric effects as well as teratogenicity. Nevirapine is associated with hypersensitivity and hepatotoxicity.

**Protease inhibitors** (PI) target the viral protease which is responsible for maturation of the virus particle. This class of inhibitors revolutionized the treatment of HIV as they have excellent virologic suppression and a significantly higher genetic barrier to resistance. They are most effective when boosted by ritonavir (RTV) which is a potent cytochrome p450-3A4 inhibitor. The main adverse effects of this class are dyslipidemia, insulin resistance, hepatotoxicity, and gastrointestinal (GI) upset. Drugs in this class include atazanavir (ATZ), darunavir (DRV), fosamprenavir (FPV), and lopinavir (LPV).

**Integrase strand transfer inhibitor** (INSTI) has recently been added to the first-line treatment guidelines. The first member was raltegravir (RAL) which has been shown to have a non-inferior response to efavirenz with fewer adverse events. It also has fewer drug interactions than the PI- or NNRTI-based regimens, but has a lower genetic barrier to resistance than with the boosted PI-based regimen.

**Entry inhibitors** are an emerging class of antiretroviral drugs that target surface proteins on either the HIV virus surface or on the surface of the CD4 cell. Examples of the first type include enfuvirtide (T-20) which is a gp41 inhibitor which blocks viral membrane fusion and maraviroc (MVC) which is a CCR5 coreceptor inhibitor that blocks fusion at the level of coreceptor engagement. Enfuvirtide is rarely used because it is only available in an injectable formulation and exhibits injection-related complications. Maraviroc has been shown to be effective in treatment-experienced patients and may be useful in early infection when the likelihood of having R5-tropic viral variants is greater than in late diseases. Because it is only effective against CCR5-tropic viral strains, the CCR5-tropism assay should be performed prior to initiation.

**Pharmacogenetics** has guided HIV treatment for more than a decade with HIV genotyping for resistance mutations. Viral genotyping is routinely performed on patients who are failing therapy and is useful in guiding therapeutic options. With the improvement in sequencing technology and the emerging recommendations, new guidelines recommend genotype testing on all newly diagnosed patients. With respect to host genomic sequencing, the field remains more in its infancy. A small number of host genes have an impact on pharmacotherapy. The most important example of this is abacavir hypersensitivity. About 5% to 8% of HIV patients who initiated antiretroviral therapy with abacavir developed a significant multiorgan hypersensitivity response. When initially identified, three markers together (HLA-B*5701, HLA-DR7, and HLA-DQ3) were shown to have a positive predictive value of 100% and negative predictive value of 97% for abacavir hypersensitivity. Since that time, HLA-B*5701 has been shown to be an excellent independent predictor. The incidence of abacavir hypersensitivity varies with group, found in 6% to 8% in Caucasians, 2% to 3% in African Americans; however, screening has been shown to be beneficial in both populations.

# Molecular Genetics and Molecular Mechanism

The interplay between host and pathogen genomics is an active area of study. Many genes are thought to influence the course of HIV infection and treatment. The genetic variants that affect drug metabolism and transport can modulate treatment response, adverse reactions, or the appearance of resistance mutations. The genetic variants that impact the natural history of HIV disease are generally related to HIV viral entry and immune response to viral infection. Information has been gained through observing individuals who have atypical patterns of HIV progression. Some individuals have varied patterns on the basis of their genetics that either accelerate or delay the natural history of the disease. These variants are described below and the important HIV disease-associated susceptibility variants are listed in Table 84-2.

### Genetics of Four Main HIV Progression Variant Categories:

☞**EXPOSED UNINFECTED:** EU individuals remain uninfected after large HIV inoculation. No specific genetic predisposition has been identified, however, these individuals have been shown to have robust noncytotoxic CD8+-cell anti-HIV responses in vivo and there has been evidence to suggest that high-risk individuals may have higher levels of CCL2, CCL4, CCL5, and CCL11 and HIV-specific IgA has also been implicated.

☞**RAPID PROGRESSORS:** RPs develop AIDS within less than 3 years with uncontrolled viremia. Some have been reported to progress within 1 year. The prognostic factors are multifactorial but characteristics common to this group are the detection of highly replicative dual tropic X4/R5 viruses. Dendritic cell-specific intracellular adhesion molecule-3-grabbing nonintegrin (DC-SIGN) is a well-characterized antiviral response in which mutations have also been noted in individuals will accelerated progression of disease.

☞**LONG-TERM NONPROGRESSORS:** LTNPs maintain stable CD4 count and low-level viremia for more than a decade. A significant number of studies have evaluated this population and among this group, the CCR5 mutations are most well characterized in terms of their ability to prevent HIV acquisition and delay AIDS progression through impaired HIV entry into cells. The Δ32 variant is the most prevalent mutation in this population and has been demonstrated to have prevalence in these individuals of 30%. It is on the basis of this understanding that the entry inhibitor class of antiretrovirals has been developed. By contrast, some mutations that interact or inhibit or downregulate CCR5 are associated with accelerated progression to AIDS. HLA typing subsets have also been implicated in this group, specifically related to individuals with the HLA-B*5705 and HLA-B*2705 who demonstrate substantially longer HIV course before progression to AIDS. In small sample sizes greater than 80% of LTNPs posses these alleles compared with approximately 10% of chronic progressors. An additional class of LTNPs has been identified who suppress viral progression on the basis of antibodies to HIV surface proteins including gp120 and gp41.

☞**ELITE CONTROLLERS OR SUPPRESSORS:** EC or ES can suppress viremia for a decade or longer to a level that is undetectable. The APOBEC group of genes is important in the study of long-term nonprogressors and elite controllers, as mutations in *APOBEC3G* have been shown to relate to delayed AIDS progression. This group of proteins is made up of cytidine deaminases that catalyze the deamination of cytosine to uracil in the nascent viral DNA causing mutations that are lethal for the virus. HLA complex P5 (*HCP5*) has been implicated as associated with 1% of HIV patients who demonstrate slowed progression of disease. The *HCP5* gene is located on chromosome 6, and the associated variant is known to be in high linkage disequilibrium with the *HLA* allele *B*5701*. HLA-B*57 and B*58 are associated with low viral load that is thought to boost cytotoxic T-lymphocyte activity. *KIR3DS1* or *KIR3DL1* allele and HLA class I alleles that encode an isoleucine at position 80 (HLA-Bw480I) had the slowest rates of progression to AIDS.

### Genetic Testing:
According to current guidelines, HIV genotypes are recommended in all newly diagnosed patients. The only host genetic testing done is for HLA B*5701 in the event that abacavir will be added to the backbone.

*Table 84-2* **HIV Disease-Associated Susceptibility Variants**

| Candidate Gene (Chromosome Location) | Associated Variant [effect on protein] | Relative Risk | Frequency of Risk Allele | Putative Functional Significance | Associated Disease Phenotype |
|---|---|---|---|---|---|
| ABCB1/MDR1 (7q21.1) | rs2032582 | | | MDR resistance pump | Reduced risk of NVP hypersensitivity |
| ABCC2 (10q24) | rs2273697 | | | Multidrug resistance-associated protein | TDF proximal renal tubulopathy |
| ABCC4 (13q32) | rs899494 | | | Multidrug resistance-associated protein | Higher levels of 3TC and ZDV |
| APOBEC3B (22q13.1) | n/a | | | Deletion of APOBEC3B | Accelerated AIDS progression |
| APOBEC3G (22q13.1) | rs35228531 | | | Activation-induced cytidine deaminases | Accelerated AIDS progression |
| ApoE (19q13.2) | rs429358 | | | Apolipoprotein E | RTV-associated dyslip-idemia/accelerated HIV progression |
| CCL5/RANTES (17q11.2) | rs2107538 | | | Downregulates CCR5 | Accelerated AIDS progression |
| CCR2 (3p21) | rs1799864 | | | Chemokine receptor | Delayed AIDS progression |
| CCR5Δ32 (3p21) | rs333 | 0.70 | 10% in individuals of European descent, 31% in LTNP | Truncated HIV coreceptor | Prevents HIV acquisition/delayed AIDS progression |
| CUL5 (11q22) | n/a | | | Ub-ligase cofactor | Accelerated AIDS progression |
| CXCR1 (2q35) | rs916093 | | | Modulation of CD4 and CXCR4 expression | Delayed AIDS progression |
| CYP2B6*6 (19q13.2) | rs2279343 | | | Cytochrome P450 | High EFV/NVP levels EFV neurotoxicity |
| DC-SIGN/CD209 (19p13) | rs1801157 | | | Receptor for viral infection | Accelerated AIDS progression |
| IFNG (12q15) | n/a | | | Aberrant IFN-γgamma regulation | Accelerated AIDS progression |
| IL-10 (1q32.1) | rs1800872 | | | Th2 cytokine downregulated | Accelerated AIDS progression |
| HLA-B (6p23) | rs2523619 | | | Blocks HIV escape | Delayed AIDS progression |
| HLA-B*27 (5p21.3) | n/a | | | Blocks HIV escape | Delayed AIDS progression |
| HLA-C*35 (6p21.3) | rs9264942 | | | Restricted CD8 response | Accelerated AIDS progress |
| HLA-B*57 (6p21.3) | rs2395029 | | | Blocks HIV escape | Delayed AIDS progression |
| HLA B*5701 (6p21.3) | rs10937275 | 6.9 | 6%-8% in Caucasians, 2%-3% in African Americans | Major histocompat-ibility complex | ABC hypersensitivity |
| HLA-DRB1 (6p21.3) | NG 002432 NM 002124 | | | Major histocompat-ibility complex | NVP hypersensitivity/rash |

*(Continued)*

*Table 84-2* **HIV Disease-Associated Susceptibility Variants (Continued)**

| Candidate Gene (Chromosome Location) | Associated Variant [effect on protein] | Relative Risk | Frequency of Risk Allele | Putative Functional Significance | Associated Disease Phenotype |
|---|---|---|---|---|---|
| *KIR* (19q13.4) | n/a | | | Antiviral NK cell activity | Delayed AIDS progression |
| *TNF-α* (6p21.3) | rs361525 | | | Cytokine signaling | ? accelerated lipoatrophy |
| *UGT1A* (2q37) | rs4233633 | | | UDP-glucuronosyl-transferase | ATZ-associated hyperbilirubinemia |

*Future Directions:* As viral genotyping and host genotyping become more cost-effective, antiretroviral therapy is likely to become even more genotype-driven. Low-cost deep sequencing may help to identify resistance mutations that are present at low frequency and may play a role in preventing the rapid evolution of resistance by tailoring drug regimens to a more detailed knowledge of pre-existing viral genotypes. With host genotyping, in addition to avoidance of adverse effects such as with abacavir and its associated hypersensitivity, future studies may identify genetic associations that may help to determine predisposition to resistance or treatment failure. In both cases, the genotyping information will likely be essential in the development of long-term antiretroviral therapy which minimizes the evolution of resistance or adverse complications.

Additionally, a better characterization of host factors impacting of HIV disease progression may help to identify which individuals would most benefit from early initiation of antiretroviral therapy. Lastly, greater knowledge of polymorphisms in host immune genes may also guide the most elusive intervention for HIV disease, preventive or therapeutic vaccines.

## BIBLIOGRAPHY:

1. An P, Winkler C. Host genes associated with HIV/AIDS: advances in gene discovery. *Trends Genet.* 2010;26(3):119-131.

2. Mothe B, Ibarrondo J, Llano A, Brander C. Virological, immune and host genetics markers in the control of HIV infection. *Dis Markers.* 2009;27:105-120.

3. Casado C, Colombo S, Rauch A, et al. Host and viral genetic correlates of clinical definitions of HIV-1 disease progression. *PLoS One.* 2010;5(6):e11079.

4. Chatterjee K. Host genetic factors in susceptibility to HIV-1 infection and progression to AIDS. *J Genet.* 2010;89:109-116.

5. Fellay J, Marzolini C, Meaden ER, et al. Response to antiretroviral treatment in HIV-1-infected individuals with allelic variants of the multidrug resistance transporter 1: a pharmacogenetics study. *Lancet.* 2002;359(9300):30-36.

6. Limou S, Zagury JF. Immunogenetics: Genome-Wide Association of Non-Progressive HIV and Viral Load Control: HLA Genes and Beyond. *Front Immunol.* 2013:4:118.

7. Kaur G, Mehra N. Genetic determinants of HIV-1 infection and progression to AIDS: susceptibility to HIV infection. *Tissue Antigens* 2009;73(4):289-301.

8. Mahungu TW, Johnson MA, Owen A, Back DJ. The impact of pharmacogenetics on HIV therapy. *Int J STD AIDS.* 2009;20(3):145-151.

9. Mallal S, Phillips E, Carosi G, et al. HLA-B*5701 screening for hypersensitivity to abacavir. *N Engl J Med.* 2008;358(6):568-579.

10. Thompson MA, Aberg JA, Cahn P, et al. Antiretroviral treatment of adult HIV infection: 2010 recommendations of the International AIDS Society—USA panel. *JAMA.* 2010;3:321-333.

## Supplementary Information

**OMIM REFERENCE:**

[1] Human Immunodeficiency Virus Type 1, Susceptibility to; HIV1 (#609423)

**Alternative Names:**

- Human Immunodeficiency Virus (HIV)
- Acquired Immunodeficiency Syndrome (AIDS)
- Highly Active Antiretroviral Therapy (HAART)
- Antiretroviral Therapies (ARVs)

*Key Words:* HIV, AIDS, highly active antiretroviral therapy (HAART), antiretroviral therapies (ARVs)

# 85 Hepatitis B and Hepatitis C Infection

Fuat Kurbanov and Chloe L. Thio

## HEPATITIS B INFECTION

### KEY POINTS

- *Disease summary:*
  - Hepatitis B infection is caused by the hepatitis B virus (HBV), which is transmitted through percutaneous and sexual routes. With an estimated 400 million people with chronic hepatitis B worldwide, HBV infection is currently one of the most prevalent infections. In the United States, there are an estimated 1.25 million people with chronic hepatitis B. A hepatitis B infection acquired in adulthood results in development of protective antibodies approximately 95% of the time. In the remaining approximately 5%, a chronic hepatitis B infection is established, which can lead to end-stage liver disease in 2% to 10% per year and in some infection progresses to liver failure and hepatocellular carcinoma. In HBV acquired in infancy or childhood, the majority of people become chronically infected. Several drugs are available for treatment of chronic hepatitis B, but in the majority of patients, treatment is long term (lifelong in some) since HBV is difficult to eradicate.

- *Major clinical forms of infection include*
  - Chronic hepatitis B—Chronic hepatitis B is defined as persistence of the hepatitis B surface antigen (HBsAg) for more than 6 months. It can be divided into active and inactive disease based on detection of HBV DNA and degree of necroinflammatory disease in the liver. It can be subdivided into HBeAg positive (usually active disease) and HBeAg negative (can be active or inactive) chronic hepatitis B.
  - Resolved hepatitis B—Previous HBV infection without further virologic, biochemical, or histologic evidence of active virus infection or disease. Serologically this is distinguished by absence of HBsAg but presence of antibodies to the hepatitis B core antigen (anti-HBc) and surface antigen (anti-HBs)

- *Differential diagnosis:*
  - Autoimmune hepatitis, viral hepatitis A, C, and E, HDV coinfection or superinfection, alcoholic hepatitis, nonalcoholic steatohepatitis (fatty liver), sclerosing cholangitis, Wilson disease, alpha-1-antitrypsin-deficiency-related liver disease, drug-induced liver disease

- *Monogenic forms:*
  - Not available

- *Family history:*
  - Not available

- *Twin studies:*
  - One study showed that monozygotic twins, who were infected with HBV, were more likely to become chronically infected compared to dizygotic twins or siblings.

- *Environmental factors:*
  - Hepatitis B is an infectious virus so exposure to virus via percutaneous or sexual contact is necessary to acquire the infection.

- *Genome-wide associations:*
  - Strong association established between genetic variation around HLA-DPA1 and HLA-DPB1 genomic region and chronic outcome of acute infection in Asian populations.

- Single-nucleotide polymorphism (SNP) in *KIF1B* on chromosome 1p36.22 is associated with hepatocellular carcinoma (HCC) development in Asian chronic HBV carriers.

- *Pharmacogenomics:*
  - Not available

## Diagnostic Criteria and Clinical Characteristics

### Diagnostic Criteria for Hepatitis B:

☞DIAGNOSTIC EVALUATION:
- Initial testing: HBsAg. Two positive tests separated by 6 months are required for the diagnosis of chronic hepatitis B.

- If chronic hepatitis B is diagnosed, then additional testing includes HBV DNA, hepatitis B e antigen, hepatitis B e antibody, liver function tests, liver imaging, and in some cases, a liver biopsy.

### Clinical Characteristics:

☞SYMPTOMS OF ACUTE HBV INFECTION: Acute infection symptoms and their severity can vary. The symptoms may include fever, fatigue, abdominal pain, jaundice, dark urine, light- or clay-colored stools, scleral icterus, nausea, vomiting, and anorexia. However, the infection can be asymptomatic.

☞**DISEASE PATTERNS IN CHRONIC HEPATITIS B:** Chronic hepatitis B is usually asymptomatic. Chronic liver disease develops slowly over decades and when symptoms occur can include abdominal pain, ascites, jaundice, easy bruising, decreased appetite, or encephalopathy. Laboratory manifestations include thrombocytopenia, coagulopathy, low albumin, and elevated transaminases. Hepatocellular carcinoma is usually asymptomatic until lesions become large. Diagnosis of hepatocellular carcinoma is with either liver ultrasound, computed tomography (CT) scan, or magnetic resonance imaging (MRI). The diagnosis is confirmed with a biopsy of the hepatic lesions.

☞**EXTRAHEPATIC MANIFESTATIONS OF CHRONIC HBV:** Many extrahepatic syndromes are immune mediated and are a consequence of deposition of circulating immune complexes, local immune complex formation induced by viral antigens, viral-induced autoantibodies, or a direct viral reaction to extrahepatic tissue sites. Examples include

- Polyarteritis nodosa—affects small- and medium-sized vessels, more common in Caucasian patients than in Asian patients.
- Glomerulonephritis—mainly seen in children but can occur in adults.
- A serum-sickness like "arthritis-dermatitis" prodrome—occurs with HBV acquisition and has variable joint and skin manifestations. Occasionally, the arthritis following the acute prodromal infection may persist; however, joint destruction is rare.
- Skin manifestations—usually palpable purpura.

## Screening and Counseling

*Screening:*
- Routine screening of family members for HBV is recommended if unvaccinated.

*Counseling:*
- Counseling of family members includes vaccination against HBV. Counseling does not involve human genetic information.

## Management and Treatment

Since adult-acquired acute hepatitis B usually results in the development of protective antibodies without treatment, most cases of acute hepatitis B do not need treatment. The exception to this is cases of acute infection with fulminant liver failure where treatment may be beneficial. In chronic hepatitis B, the HBV DNA level correlates with the risk for developing end-stage liver disease and hepatocellular carcinoma. Thus, patients with higher HBV DNA levels and evidence of inflammation are treated. Guidelines from the American Association of Liver Disease and the Infectious Diseases Society of America exist regarding who should be treated.

*Therapeutics Currently Approved by the FDA:*

☞**NUCLEOSIDE OR NUCLEOTIDE ANALOGUES:** These are oral agents, which inhibit the HBV polymerase. The major problem is emergence of drug-resistant variants, which occur most frequently with lamivudine. The most potent agents are tenofovir and entecavir and they have the highest genetic barrier to resistance, so development of drug resistance is uncommon in treatment-naïve patients. For that reason, these two agents are recommended first-line agents to treat chronic hepatitis B in treatment-naïve patients.

- Lamivudine (Epivir)
- Adefovir (Hepsera)
- Tenofovir (Viread)
- Telbivudine (Tyzeka)
- Entecavir (Baraclude)

☞**OTHER TREATMENTS:**
- Interferon alpha-2a—no longer used since pegylated interferon is available
- Pegylated interferon alpha-2a (Pegasys)
- Pegylated interferon alpha-2b (Intron A)

Patient's age, HBeAg status, ALT levels, liver disease stage, coinfection with HIV and/or hepatitis D virus (HDV) and/or hepatitis C virus (HCV), HBV DNA level, HBV genotype, previous treatment history, or presence of drug-resistant mutations are factors considered in treatment of hepatitis B.

Liver transplantation: Transplantation is reserved for people with advanced liver disease as measured by the model for end-stage liver disease (MELD) score, which estimates survival rates. Reinfection of the transplanted organ occurs universally without treatment, so prevention of reinfection with hepatitis B immune globulin and oral anti-HBV agents is recommended.

**Pharmacogenetics** has not yet been incorporated routinely in HBV treatment.

## Molecular Genetics and Molecular Mechanism

A recent genome-wide association study (GWAS) revealed a strong association of *HLA-DP* polymorphisms and HBV recovery in Asian populations (Japanese and Thai) (Table 85-1). The mechanism for this association has not been discovered.

Another GWAS carried on Chinese population revealed association between polymorphism in *KIF1B* on chromosome 1p36.22 and development of HCC. They suggested that carcinogenesis may be associated with decreased expression of KIF1B that might play a tumor-suppressor function.

*Genetic Testing:* The clinical role of genetic testing in diagnostics and treatment response is not yet established.

*Future Directions:* A study in European and Blacks found that a HLA-DP variant is also associated with HBV outcome although a different SNP was responsible for the association. The functional significance of these associations needs to be determined. Studies to determine genetic associations with treatment outcomes need to be performed.

*Table 85-1 Hepatitis B Virus Associated Variants*

| Candidate Gene (Chromosome Location) | Associated Variant [effect on protein] | Relative Risk | Putative Functional Significance | Associated Disease Phenotype |
|---|---|---|---|---|
| HLA chr6 (p21.3) | HLA-DPA1*0202-DPB1*0501 | 1.45 | Unknown | Chronic infection |
| | HLA-DPA1*0202-DPB1*030 | 2.31 | | |
| HLA chr6 (p21.3) | HLA-DPA1*0103-DPB1*0402 | 0.52 | Unknown | Protection from chronic infection |
| | HLA-DPA1*0103-DPB1*0401 | 0.57 | | |
| HLA chr6 (p21.3) | HLA-DRB1*1302 | 0.24 | Unknown | Protection from chronic infection |
| HLA chr6 (p21.3) | HLA A*0301 | 0.47 | | Protection from chronic infection |
| HLA chr6 (p21.3) | HLA B*08 | 1.59 | | Chronic infection |
| IFN-AR2 (Chr 21q22) | F8S | 2.8 | Surface expression | Chronic infection |
| CCR5del32 chr 3 (p21) | 32 base pair deletion | 0.53 | Non-functional protein | Protection from chronic infection |
| IL10RB chr 21 (q22) | K47E | 2.1 | RNA and surface expression | Chronic infection |
| mbl2 chr 10 (q11.2-q21) | Combination of promoter and exon 1 SNPs | Variable | Amount of mannose binding lectin (MBL) produced | Low MBL-chronic infection; High MBL-protection from chronic infection |
| TNF-alpha chr 6 (p21.3) | -308A or -863 C/C | 0.56 | Plasma TNF levels | Protection from chronic infection |
| IFNGR1 chr 6 (q23.3) | -56C/C | 0.71 | Higher transcription | Protection from chronic infection |

**BIBLIOGRAPHY:**

1. Frodsham AJ, Zhang L, Dumpis U, et al. Class II cytokine receptor gene cluster is a major locus for hepatitis B persistence. *Proc Natl Acad Sci USA*. 2006;103:9148-9153.

2. Gong QM, Kong XF, Yang ZT, et al. Association study of IFNAR2 and IL10RB genes with the susceptibility and interferon response in HBV infection. *J Viral Hepat*. 2009;16:674-680.

3. Kamatani Y, Wattanapokayakit S, Ochi H, et al. A genome-wide association study identifies variants in the HLA-DP locus associated with chronic hepatitis B in Asians. *Nat Genet*. 2009;41:591-595.

4. Lin TM, Chen CJ, Wu MM, et al. Hepatitis B virus markers in Chinese twins. *Anticancer Res*. 1989;9:737-741.

5. Lok AS, McMahon BJ. Chronic hepatitis B: update 2009. *Hepatology*. 2009;50:661-662.

6. Thio CL, Astemborski J, Thomas R, et al. Interaction between RANTES promoter variant and CCR5Delta32 favors recovery from hepatitis B. *J Immunol*. 2008;181:7944-7947.

7. Thio CL, Thomas DL, Karacki P, et al. Comprehensive analysis of class I and class II HLA antigens and chronic hepatitis B virus infection. *J Virol*. 2003;77:12083-12087.

8. Thursz MR, Kwiatkowski D, Allsopp CE, Greenwood BM, Thomas HC, Hill AV. Association between an MHC class II allele and clearance of hepatitis B virus in the Gambia. *N Engl J Med*. 1995;332:1065-1069.

9. Zeng Z, Guan L, An P, Sun S, O'Brien SJ, Winkler CA. A population-based study to investigate host genetic factors associated with hepatitis B infection and pathogenesis in the Chinese population. *BMC Infect Dis*. 2008;8:1.

10. Zhang H, Zhai Y, Hu Z, et al. Genome-wide association study identifies 1p36.22 as a new susceptibility locus for hepatocellular carcinoma in chronic hepatitis B virus carriers. *Nat Genet*. 2010;42(9):755-758.

## Supplementary Information

**OMIM REFERENCE:**

[1] Hepatitis B Virus, Susceptibility to; #610424

**Alternative Name:**

• HBV, susceptibility to Hepatitis B virus, resistance to

*Key Words:* HLA, MHC, MBL, CCR5

# HEPATITIS C INFECTION

## KEY POINTS

- *Disease summary:*
  - Hepatitis C infection is caused by the hepatitis C virus (HCV), which is primarily transmitted percutaneously but can also be transmitted through sexual contact. Acute HCV infection can either be spontaneously cleared (~30%) or lead to chronic hepatitis C, which predisposes to end-stage liver disease (ESLD) (liver cirrhosis and hepatocellular carcinoma). Chronic hepatitis C can be cleared by treatment in about 50% to 90% of patients with the newest drugs, but treatment success varies depending on several host and viral factors.
  - *Acute hepatitis C* refers to a short-term illness that occurs during the first 6 months after infection with HCV. Up to 80% of acute infections are asymptomatic. In the minority of patients who experience acute-phase symptoms, they vary from mild and nonspecific, to a disabling illness lasting several months. Fulminant hepatitis is rare, but can be fatal. Onset of symptoms is usually insidious, with fever, flu-like symptoms, malaise, anorexia, nausea, and abdominal discomfort, followed by jaundice (for most of symptomatic patients). Urine may become unusually dark, and stools quite pale. Liver enzyme levels are usually mildly elevated. Antibodies develop on average about 8 weeks after infection, but are not protective for reinfection.
  - Chronic hepatitis C is defined as persistence of HCV for more than 6 months, which is identified by HCV RNA in blood. Clinically, it is often asymptomatic but most have very mild elevations in liver enzyme levels. In 15% to 20% of cases, long-term carriage of the virus leads to ESLD.
- *Differential diagnosis:*
  - Autoimmune hepatitis, viral hepatitis A, B, and E, alcoholic hepatitis, nonalcoholic steatohepatitis (fatty liver), sclerosing cholangitis, Wilson disease, alpha-1-antitrypsin-deficiency-related liver disease, drug-induced liver disease
- *Environmental factors:*
  - Hepatitis C is an infectious virus, so exposure to virus via percutaneous or sexual contact is necessary to acquire the infection.
- *Genome-wide associations:*
  - Strong association exists between genetic variation around *IL28B* of chromosome 19 and natural or treatment-induced HCV clearance. A deletion polymorphism in a newly-identified gene, interferon lambda 4 (IFNL4), is in linkage disequilibrium with polymorphisms in IL28B (IFNL3), and is also associated with natural or treatment-induced clearance. Genetic variation in *ITPA* on chromosome 20 (20p13) has been shown to be predictive for ribavirin-induced anemia, which is one of the most common side effects of the current standard treatment for hepatitis C (combination of pegylated interferon-alpha and ribavirin) (Table 85-2).
- *Pharmacogenomics:*
  - Testing for *IFNL3* genotype to guide management may be useful but has not been studied. With the newer oral direct antiviral agents, the role of *IL28B* or *IFNL4* genotype in management is not clear. The utility of testing *ITPA* variants in clinical management has not been studied.

## Diagnostic Criteria and Clinical Characteristics

### Diagnostic Criteria for Hepatitis C:

**☞DIAGNOSTIC EVALUATION:**

- Initial testing: HCV antibody
- If HCV antibody is negative and suspect acute hepatitis C can test for HCV RNA in blood since antibodies take approximately 8 weeks to develop.
- If HCV antibody is positive, then test for HCV RNA to determine if infection is chronic. Two positive HCV RNA tests separated by 6 months define chronic hepatitis C. Two negative HCV RNA tests separated by 6 months define clearance of HCV.
- If chronic hepatitis C is diagnosed, then additional testing includes liver function tests, liver imaging, HCV genotype, and in some cases, a liver biopsy.

- *IFNL3B* genotype, *ITPA* genotype may be helpful prior to initiating therapy but further studies are needed.

### Clinical Characteristics:

**☞SYMPTOMS OF ACUTE HCV INFECTION:** Acute infection is usually asymptomatic. When symptoms occur they can include fever, fatigue, abdominal pain, jaundice, dark urine, light- or clay-colored stools, scleral icterus, nausea, vomiting, and anorexia.

**☞DISEASE PATTERNS IN CHRONIC HEPATITIS C:** Chronic hepatitis C is usually asymptomatic until end stage liver disease occurs. Chronic liver disease develops slowly over decades and when symptoms occur can include abdominal pain, ascites, jaundice, easy bruising, decreased appetite, and encephalopathy. Laboratory manifestations include thrombocytopenia, coagulopathy, low albumin, and elevated transaminases. Hepatocellular carcinoma is usually asymptomatic until lesions become large. Diagnosis of hepatocellular carcinoma is with alpha-fetoprotein and either liver ultrasound, computed tomography (CT) scan, or magnetic resonance imaging (MRI). In some cases, a biopsy of the hepatic lesions is also required.

**Table 85-2 Pharmacogenetic Considerations in Hepatitis C Treatment**

| Gene | Associated Medications | Goal of Testing | Variants | Effect |
|---|---|---|---|---|
| ITPA (inosine triphosphatase) | Ribavirin (RBV) | Safety | P32T (rs1127354) | Variant—protective against RBV-induced anemia<br>WT—predisposes to RBV-induced anemia |
| ITPA (inosine triphosphatase) | Ribavirin (RBV) | Safety | Splicing altered (rs7270101) | Variant—protective against RBV-induced anemia<br>WT—predisposes to RBV-induced anemia |
| IFNL3 | Pegylated interferon and ribavirin | Treatment response prediction | rs8099917 | Variant—nonsustained virologic response (SVR)<br>WT—SVR |
| IFNL3 | Pegylated interferon and ribavirin | Treatment response prediction | rs12979860 | Variant—non-SVR<br>WT—SVR |
| IFNL3 | Pegylated interferon and ribavirin | Treatment response prediction | rs8103142 | Variant—non-SVR<br>WT—SVR |
| IFNL3 | Pegylated interferon and ribavirin | Treatment response prediction | rs28416813 | Variant—non-SVR<br>WT—SVR |
| IFNL3 | Pegylated interferon and ribavirin | Treatment response prediction | rs4803219 | Variant—non-SVR<br>WT—SVR |
| IFNL3 | Pegylated interferon and ribavirin | Treatment response prediction | rs12980275 | Variant—non-SVR<br>WT—SVR |
| IFNL3 | Pegylated interferon and ribavirin | Treatment response prediction | rs8109886 | Variant—non-SVR<br>WT—SVR |
| IFNL3 | Pegylated interferon and ribavirin | Treatment response prediction | rs8105790 | Variant—non-SVR<br>WT—SVR |
| IFNL3 | Pegylated interferon and ribavirin | Treatment response prediction | rs10853727 | Variant—non-SVR<br>WT—SVR |
| IFNL3 | Pegylated interferon and ribavirin | Treatment response prediction | rs7248668 | Variant—non-SVR<br>WT—SVR |
| IFNL3 | Pegylated interferon and ribavirin | Treatment response prediction | rs10853728 | Variant—non-SVR<br>WT—SVR |
| IFNL3 | Pegylated interferon and ribavirin | Treatment response prediction | rs11881222 | Variant—non-SVR<br>WT—SVR |
| IFNL3 | Pegylated interferon and ribavirin | Treatment response prediction | rs581930 | Variant—non-SVR<br>WT—SVR |
| KIR | Pegylated interferon and ribavirin | Treatment response prediction | KIR2DL2 | NR |
| KIR | Pegylated interferon and ribavirin | Treatment response prediction | KIR2DL3 | SVR |
| IFNL4 | Pegylated interferon and ribavirin | Treatment response prediction | rs368234815 | TT/TT-SVR<br>ΔG/ΔG-non-SVR |

☞**EXTRAHEPATIC MANIFESTATIONS OF CHRONIC HCV:**
- Cryoglobulinemia which can lead to skin blotching, joint pain, vasculitis, peripheral neuropathy.
- Non-Hodgkin lymphoma is more common in people with chronic hepatitis C.
- Endocrine manifestations include diabetes mellitus, which is more common in people with chronic hepatitis C than in

the general population but a direct causal link has not been established.
- Renal complications include membranoproliferative glomerulonephritis, which is usually related to cryoglobulinemia. Can also get membranous nephropathy.
- Dermatologic manifestations with the most common being lichen planus.

## Screening and Counseling

*Screening:* Routine screening of family members is not recommended.

*Counseling:* Counseling of family members is to avoid practices associated with HCV transmission.

## Management and Treatment

Since not all patients progress to ESLD and since treatment, which has severe side effects, is successful in only approximately 50-90% of patients, not all patients are treated. Guidelines from the American Association of Liver Disease and the Infectious Diseases Society of America exist regarding treatment criteria, which differs based on the genotype (1-11) of the virus. The most common genotypes are 1-3.

*Therapeutics Currently Approved by the FDA:*
- Peginterferon alpha-2a *or*
- Peginterferon alpha-2b
  *with*
- Ribavirin

The dose and duration of pegylated interferon alpha and ribavirin are dependent on the HCV genotype, patient's weight,

*Table 85-3 Hepatitis C Virus Spontaneous Clearance Associated Variants*

| Candidate Gene (Chromosome Location) | Associated Variant [effect on protein] (assayed by affymetrix/illumina) | Relative Risk | Frequency of Risk Allele | Putative Functional Significance | Associated Disease Phenotype |
|---|---|---|---|---|---|
| *IL28B* chr19 (q13.2) | rs12979860 [unknown] | 5.6-7.3 | White: 0.14-0.47 Black: 0.45-0.77 Asian: 0-0.34 | IL28B regulatory region? | (T) viral persistence/ nonresponse |
| *IL28B* chr19 (q13.2) | rs8099917 [unknown] | 1.98-12.1 | White: 0.15-0.19 Black: 0.02-0.06 Asian: 0.08 | IL28B/A regulatory region? | (G) viral persistence/ nonresponse |
| *IL28B* chr19 (q13.2) | Lys70Arg [nonsynonymous IL28B 3d exon] (rs8103142) | 19.8 | Not available in HapMap | Cytokine properties? | (C) viral persistence/ nonresponse |
| *IL28B* chr19 (q13.2) | rs12980275 [unknown] | 14.9 | White: 0.34-0.43 Black: 0.53 Asian: 0.08 | Cytokine properties? | (G) viral persistence/ nonresponse |
| *IL28B* chr19 (q13.2) | rs11881222 [unknown] | 19.8 | White: 0.31 Black: 0.33 Asian: 0.07 | Cytokine properties? | (G) viral persistence/ nonresponse |
| *IL28B* chr19 (q13.2) | rs8105790 [unknown] | 19.8 | White: 0.22 Black: 0.28 Asian: 0.11 | Cytokine properties? | (C) viral persistence/ nonresponse |
| *KIR* chr19 (q13.4) *HLA* chr6 (p21.3) | KIR2DL3-HLA-C1 [weaker inhibition of NK] | 3.05 | White: 0.75-0.8 Black: 0.6 | Effect on NK suppression | Homozygosity for KIR2DL3-HLA-C1 associated with spontaneous clearance |
| *HLA* chr6 (p21.3) | HLA B*57 A*03 Cw*01 Cw*05 DRBI*01 DRBI*11 DQBI*03 DQBI*05 | 0.62 2.43 0.43-7.1 0.12 0.37 7.0 2.7 0.3 | N/A | Optimal pathogenic antigen presentation | Clearance |
| *HLA* chr6 (p21.3) | Cw4 DRBI*03 DRBI*07 DQBI*02 | 1.78 0.39 2.42 2.98 | | Suboptimal pathogenic antigen presentation | Persistence |
| IFNL4 | rs368234815 | 3.51-4.68 in African-Americans | White: 32.2 Black: 78.3 Asian: 6.7 | TT-no IFNL4 is transcribed | TT-viral clearance ΔG-viral persistence |

*Table 85-4* **Hepatitis C Liver Fibrosis**

| Candidate Gene (Chromosome Location) | Associated Variant [effect on protein] (assayed by affymetrix/illumina) | Relative Risk | Frequency of Risk Allele | Putative Functional Significance | Associated Disease Phenotype |
|---|---|---|---|---|---|
| *IFNGR2* | rs9976971 [unknown] | 2.95 | (A): White: 0.41 Black: 0.07 Asian: 0.45 | Interferon-gamma receptor 2 | In European patients |

and response to the first several weeks of therapy. The response to the therapy depends on several factors including HCV RNA level, ethnicity, HIV status, duration of HCV infection, body mass index, HCV genotype, and *IFNL3* genotype (Table 85-2). Patients with acute HCV infection have a much better response to therapy.

**Other Therapies:**

*Interferon-λ1:* This is a type III interferon that has been tested in phase 1b trials and is associated with antiviral activity. There is intense interest in this molecule because of the strong genetic association of IL28B (interferon-λ3) with HCV treatment response.

There are several direct-acting antivirals in phase II and III clinical trials.

*Liver transplantation:* Transplantation is reserved for people with advanced liver disease as measured by the model for end-stage liver disease (MELD) score, which estimates survival rates. Infection of the transplanted organ occurs universally so treatment may be needed.

Pharmacogenetics has not yet been incorporated routinely in HCV treatment since the *IFNL3* and *IFNL4* association are recent findings. However, it may prove to be useful to determine who should receive treatment, the duration of treatment, and whether a lead-in phase prior to giving direct-acting antiviral agents will improve response. Variation in the *ITPA* gene, which is associated with ribavirin-induced anemia, also has not been incorporated into clinical practice (Table 85-2).

## Molecular Genetics and Molecular Mechanism

The recent discovery of the association of *IFNL3* and *IFN-L4* with treatment response is a major breakthrough in the understanding of the role of host genomics in hepatitis C. Several single-nucleotide polymorphisms (SNPs) in *IFNL3* have been associated with HCV outcomes (Table 85-3) but whether any of them are causal is unknown. The *IFN-L4* association is newly discovered and the SNP leads to the production of *IFN-L4* whereas the wild type is a null allele. The highly associated SNPs are located several kilobases upstream of the *IFNL3* gene and thus may be in linkage disequilibrium with the causal SNP. Further studies are being undertaken to determine the causal SNP and then functional studies of this SNP will be needed. One study identified a polymorphism in *IFNGR2* to be associated with cirrhosis (Table 85-4).

**Genetic Testing:** The role of *IFNL3* genetic testing in treatment response is not yet clear.

**Future Directions:** The recent finding of strong associations of *IFNL3* variants and spontaneous and treatment-induced clearance of HCV has provided a key to further understand the immune response to HCV infection. Studies to determine the functional consequences of the implicated SNPs should offer insights into potential biologic targets for therapy.

Studies are now being done to determine how to use the knowledge of a patient's *IFNL3* genotype to maximize the therapeutic response and to minimize side effects and risk for developing drug-resistant HCV variants.

**Bibliography:**

1. Fellay J, Thompson AJ, Ge D, et al. ITPA gene variants protect against anaemia in patients treated for chronic hepatitis C. Nature. 2010;464: 405-408.

2. Ge D, Fellay J, Thompson AJ, et al. Genetic variation in IL28B predicts hepatitis C treatment-induced viral clearance. *Nature.* 2009;461:399-401.

3. Ghany MG, Strader DB, Thomas DL, Seeff LB. Diagnosis, management, and treatment of hepatitis C: an update. *Hepatology.* 2009;49:1335-1374.

4. Khakoo SI, Thio CL, Martin MP, et al. HLA and NK cell inhibitory receptor genes in resolving hepatitis C virus infection. *Science.* 2004;305:872-874.

5. Nalpas B, Lavialle-Meziani R, Plancoulaine S, et al. Interferon gamma receptor 2 gene variants are associated with liver fibrosis in patients with chronic hepatitis C infection. *Gut.* 2010;59:1120-1126.

6. Ochi H, Maekawa T, Abe H, et al. ITPA polymorphism affects ribavirin-induced anemia and outcome of therapy—a genome-wide study of Japanese HCV patients. *Gastroenterology.* 2010;139(4):1190-1197.

7. Rauch A, Kutalik Z, Descombes P, et al. Genetic variation in IL28B is associated with chronic hepatitis C and treatment failure: a genome-wide association study. *Gastroenterology.* 2010;138:1338-1345, 1345.e1-e7.

8. Suppiah V, Moldovan M, Ahlenstiel G, et al. IL28B is associated with response to chronic hepatitis C interferon-alpha and ribavirin therapy. *Nat Genet.* 2009;41:1100-1104.

9. Tanaka Y, Nishida N, Sugiyama M, et al. Genome-wide association of IL28B with response to pegylated interferon-alpha and ribavirin therapy for chronic hepatitis C. *Nat Genet.* 2009;41: 1105-1109.

10. Thio CL, Gao X, Goedert JJ, et al. HLA-Cw*04 and hepatitis C virus persistence. *J Virol.* 2002;76:4792-4797.

11. Thomas DL, Thio CL, Martin MP, et al. Genetic variation in IL28B and spontaneous clearance of hepatitis C virus. *Nature.* 2009;461:798-801.

12. Vidal-Castineira JR, Lopez-Vazquez A, Diaz-Pena R, et al. Effect of killer immunoglobulin-like receptors in the response to combined treatment in patients with chronic hepatitis C virus infection. *J Virol.* 2010;84:475-481.

13. Wang JH, Zheng X, Ke X, et al. Ethnic and geographical differences in HLA associations with the outcome of hepatitis C virus infection. *Virol J.* 2009;6:46.

14. Prokunina-Olsson L, Muchmore B, Tang W, et al. A variant upstream of IFNL3 (IL28B) creating a new interferon gene IFNL4 is associated with impaired clearance of hepatitis C virus. *Nat Genet.* 2013;45:164-171.

## Supplementary Information

**OMIM REFERENCES:**

[1] Hepatitis C Virus Susceptibility to; IL28B (#609352)

[2] Hepatitis C virus, resistance to

[3] Hepatitis C virus infection, response to therapy of

**Alternative Name:**

- HCV, susceptibility to

*Key Words:* IFNL3, IFNL4, HLA , KIR

# 86 Bronchitis and Pneumonia

Marcos I. Restrepo, Oriol S. Vidal, and Grant W. Waterer

## KEY POINTS

- *Disease summary:*
  - **Bronchitis** is the inflammation of the bronchial airway. Bronchitis can be divided into two categories, acute and chronic, each of which has different etiologies, pathologies, and therapies.
    - Acute bronchitis is often caused by infection. Viruses cause about 90% of cases of acute bronchitis, whereas bacteria account for fewer than 10%.
    - Chronic bronchitis is characterized by the presence of a productive cough that lasts for 3 months or more per year for at least 2 years. Chronic bronchitis most often develops due to recurrent injury to the airways caused by inhaled irritants. Cigarette smoking is the most common cause, followed by air pollution and occupational exposure to irritants. Acute exacerbations of chronic bronchitis are frequently caused by an infection.
  - **Pneumonia** is an inflammatory condition of the lung associated with fever, chest symptoms, and a lack of air space (consolidation) on a chest x-ray. Pneumonia is typically caused by bacteria but there are a number of other causes. Infectious agents include bacteria, viruses, fungi, and parasites.
    - Clinical presentations of bronchitis and pneumonia overlap; the two may have fever, cough, dyspnea, or extrapulmonary symptoms.
    - A diagnosis of pneumonia requires a chest radiograph showing consolidation in the lung parenchyma.
    - Anatomic involvement: bronchitis involves bronchial airway, between trachea and lung parenchyma. Pneumonia involves lung parenchyma, especially alveoli, distal airway, and interstitium.
    - This chapter is focused on acute respiratory infections, including acute bronchitis and pneumonia, and excludes acute exacerbations of chronic bronchitis which is recognized as a different condition by itself.

- *Hereditary basis:*
  - Susceptibility to pulmonary infectious diseases and its adverse outcomes has a strong genetic influence.
  - Although there are numerous reports of positive associations between gene polymorphisms and clinical outcomes, most of these are probably spurious or at best in linkage disequilibrium with the key genetic markers rather than being the "true" sites of polymorphic interest.
  - Genetic variation in mannose-binding lectin (*MBL2*), the IgG2A receptor (*FCGR2A*), and *CD14* are the best-validated markers of susceptibility to adverse outcomes from acute respiratory infections.
  - Rather than a few key polymorphisms determining risk, it appears that dozens, if not hundreds, of polymorphisms interact and contribute to total risk.

- *Differential diagnosis:*
  - Chronic obstructive pulmonary disease
  - Congestive heart failure
  - Lung cancer
  - Diffuse interstitial lung diseases
  - Pulmonary embolus
  - Pulmonary vasculitis

## Diagnostic Criteria and Clinical Characteristics

***Diagnostic Criteria:*** Acute respiratory infection is a clinical diagnosis defined by the presence of at least two of the following clinical signs:

- Cough
- Fever
- Shortness of breath
- Tachypnea
- Phlegm production of yellow, green, or bloodstained color

A chest radiograph is necessary to differentiate between bronchitis and pneumonia:

- The absence of a consolidation supports the diagnosis of bronchitis.

- The presence of a consolidation in lung parenchyma suggests the diagnosis of pneumonia.

***Clinical Characteristics:*** The most common symptoms of acute respiratory infections are fever, nonproductive or productive of purulent cough, dyspnea, pleuritic chest pain, chills, and mental status changes.

Patients present less commonly with diarrhea, new-onset or worsening confusion in elderly patients, and headache.

Clinical signs include fever or hypothermia, dullness to percussion, increased tactile and vocal fremitus, egophony, crackles, whispered pectoriloquy, and pleural friction rub.

## Screening and Counseling

***Screening:*** No clear evidence for screening of family members exists. Genetic testing for disease-associated single-nucleotide

*Table 86-1* **Impact of Genetic Polymorphisms on Clinical Outcomes in Acute Pulmonary Infection**

| Gene | SNP | Impact on Clinical Outcomes |
|---|---|---|
| Mannose-binding lectin (*MBL2*) | Gly54Asp (G/A) (rs1800450) | Increased risk of invasive pneumococcal disease |
| | Arg52Cys (C/T) (rs5030737) | Associated with higher severity and mortality |
| Immunoglobulin G receptor (*FCGR2A*) | Arg13His (C/T) (rs1801274) | Increased risk for bacteremic pneumococcal pneumonia and higher severity |
| *CD14* | CD14 -159C>T | Increased risk of septic shock and death from septic shock |

polymorphisms (SNPs) is not clinically validated. Apart from polymorphisms in *MBL2*, *FCGR2A*, and *CD14* there is no consensus on which polymorphisms are truly important.

*Counseling:* Few studies have evaluated the penetrance of different polymorphisms. In one study, homozygotes for certain "codon variants" in mannose-binding lectin (Table 86-1) of patients were observed to be at increased risk of developing invasive pneumococcal disease (IPD). However, this association was not found in smaller studies. A meta-analysis which combined all studies showed a significant association of homozygosity for variant alleles and IPD (Odds ratio [OR] 2.58, 95% confidence interval [CI] 1.38-4.80). These results were driven by the strong weight found on the large sample size study ($n = 337$).

No clear genotype-phenotype correlation has been found. The influence of many genetic polymorphisms is highly dependent on the infecting pathogen, so grouping all cases of bronchitis or pneumonia as one cohort greatly diminishes the ability to identify key associations.

## Management and Treatment

*Antimicrobial Therapies:* A major goal for therapy is eradication of the infecting organism, with resultant resolution of clinical disease. As such, antimicrobials are a mainstay of treatment.

Antimicrobials have been recognized by clinical guidelines as an important component in the management of acute bronchitis and pneumonia with a bacterial etiology. The challenge of identifying patients most likely to benefit from antimicrobial therapy is difficult in the clinical setting. However, appropriate risk stratification of patients, and the use of antimicrobials within the correct spectrum and for a suitable duration, can improve clinical outcomes while minimizing induction of antimicrobial resistance. Factors to be considered in antimicrobial agent selection include local tissue penetration, effects on bacteriologic eradication, duration of therapy, speed of resolution, and prevention or delay of recurrences.

The most common antibiotics used in acute bronchitis are amoxicillin and tetracycline, and alternative options include amoxicillin-clavulanate, macrolides, levofloxacin, and moxifloxacin. In pneumonia there is a need to cover atypical pathogens, particularly *Legionella*, whereas in bronchitis these pathogens are not a major clinical concern. The most common antimicrobials recommended by clinical practice guidelines for patients with pneumonia differ on the severity of the disease and if the patient requires hospitalization. The most commonly prescribed antimicrobials to treat hospitalized patients with pneumonia include monotherapy with fluoroquinolones or a combination of beta-lactams with fluoroquinolones or macrolides. In addition, for patients with severe pneumonia the recommendation is to stratify according to the risk of *Pseudomonas* infection (eg, chronic structural lung diseases, etc). For patients with severe pneumonia it is recommended to use a combination of beta-lactams plus a macrolide or a respiratory fluoroquinolone. Patients with bacteremic pneumococcal pneumonia should be started on a combination of antimicrobials which include a beta-lactam plus a macrolide.

*Non-Antimicrobial Therapies:* Short-acting inhaled beta-2-agonists (with or without a short-acting anticholinergic) are the preferred bronchodilators for treatment of an acute exacerbation of chronic bronchitis. Systemic corticosteroids can also improve lung function, arterial hypoxemia, and reduce the risk of early relapse in severe acute exacerbations.

Patients with severe pneumonia who require ICU care may benefit from low-dose systemic corticosteroids as an adjunct therapy in order to improve the elevated associated inflammatory cytokine response. However, further studies are needed to confirm the efficacy of systemic corticosteroids in patients with severe pneumonia.

## Molecular Genetics and Molecular Mechanism

To investigate genetic variability in susceptibility to acute pulmonary infection, a large number of polymorphisms in a diverse set of candidate genes have been studied. Polymorphisms in mannose-binding lectin, the IgG2A receptor, and CD14 are the best-recognized genetic markers associated with important clinical consequences (Table 86-1).

*MBL2*, formerly *MBL* is a soluble pattern-recognition molecule that binds micro-organisms and has an independent ability to activate the complement system. Several polymorphisms in the gene itself or in the promoter region can lead to variation in mannose-binding lectin serum concentration, influencing susceptibility to and the course of different types of infections. *MBL2* promoter region polymorphisms were found to be a risk factor for severe sepsis in earlier studies, but these results are not confirmed in other studies in pneumonia, *Legionella*, and sepsis. Some of the conflicting reports may be due to the variable number of polymorphisms studied or because of the significant variability in frequency of the variant alleles in different racial or ethnic groups.

There are three major classes of immunoglobulin G receptors expressed on human leukocytes: FcgRI (CD64); FcγRII (CD32), and FcγRIII (CD16). Human FcγRIIa (gene name *FCGR2A*) has two codominantly expressed allotypes arginine (Arg) or histamine (His) at position 131, of which Arg is associated with decreased binding of the IgG2 subclass. Different studies suggest that homozygosity for *FCGR2A* Asp/Asp is a risk factor for bacteremic pneumococcal pneumonia, although these results have not been replicated in another study. Complicating the assessment of the *FCGR2A* polymorphism is linkage disequilibrium with polymorphisms in interleukin-10 which is in the same region of chromosome 1. No published study to date has performed a full haplotype mapping across the entire *FCGR2A* and *IL10* region in patients with acute respiratory infection. Therefore, the most significant polymorphic area(s) remains unclear.

Studies of *CD14* polymorphisms have produced relatively consistent findings. A relatively common polymorphism (*CD14* -159C>T) is associated with an increased risk of septic shock and death from septic shock. However, since CD14 is not involved in signaling for most gram-positive pathogens, the effects that have been observed are likely more pronounced in gram-negative sepsis, which may explain in part the studies with negative findings.

Other putative genetic markers of susceptibility to infection have been studied, as polymorphisms in toll-like receptor genes, lipopolysaccharide-binding protein genes, or myeloid differentiation protein-2 genes. However, the results of these studies are not conclusive.

**Genetic Testing:** No role yet exists for genetic testing in the diagnosis of bronchitis and pneumonia.

**Future Directions:** The future in genetics in pulmonary infectious diseases is in large collaborative efforts creating exquisitely detailed (both clinically and microbiologically) cohorts allowing the use of state-of-the-art genetic techniques such as hypothesis-generating genome-wide association studies (GWAS) and haplotype mapping across entire chromosomes.

The bias of publishing only positive simple association studies in small cohorts has greatly hindered the progress in understanding the genetic influence on pneumonia and sepsis.

More detailed microbiologic data incorporated into the analysis are also needed in future studies.

The ultimate proof of a genetic marker's importance will be the successful development of a pharmacologic agent that improves outcome in those carrying the deleterious genotype, or the successful incorporation of genetic markers into clinical algorithms for the prognosis, diagnosis, prevention, or treatment of patients with acute respiratory infections.

## BIBLIOGRAPHY:

1. Burgner D, Jamieson SE, Blackwell JM. Genetic susceptibility to infectious diseases: big is beautiful, but will bigger be even better? *Lancet Infect Dis.* 2006;6(10):653-663.

2. Waterer GW. Polymorphism studies in critical illness—we have to raise the bar. *Crit Care Med.* 2007;35(5):1424-1425.

3. Endeman H, Herpers BL, de Jong BA, et al. Mannose-binding lectin genotypes in susceptibility to community-acquired pneumonia. *Chest.* 2008;134(6):1135-1140.

4. Roy S, Knox K, Segal S, et al. MBL genotype and risk of invasive pneumococcal disease: a case-control study. *Lancet.* 2002; 359(9317):1569-1573.

5. Brouwer MC, de Gans J, Heckenberg SG, Zwinderman AH, van der Poll T, van de Beek D. Host genetic susceptibility to pneumococcal and meningococcal disease: a systematic review and meta-analysis. *Lancet Infect Dis.* 2009;9(1):31-44.

6. Garcia-Laorden MI, Sole-Violan J, Rodriguez de Castro F, et al. Mannose-binding lectin and mannose-binding lectin-associate serine protease 2 in susceptibility, severity, and outcome of pneumonia in adults. *J Allergy Clin Immunol.* 2008;122:368-374.

7. Sutherland AM, Walley KR, Russell JA. Polymorphisms in CD14, mannose-binding lectin, and Toll-like receptor-2 are associated with increased prevalence of infection in critically ill adults. *Crit Care Med.* 2005;33(3):638-644.

8. Yuan FF, Wong M, Pererva N, et al. FcgammaRIIA polymorphisms in Streptococcus pneumoniae infection. *Immunol Cell Biol.* 2003;81(3):192-195.

9. Gibot S, Cariou A, Drouet L, Rossignol M, Ripoll L. Association between a genomic polymorphism within the CD14 locus and septic shock susceptibility and mortality rate. *Crit Care Med.* 2002;30(5):969-973.

## Supplementary Information

### OMIM Reference:

[1] No online Mendelian inheritance in man (OMIM#) references for bronchitis and pneumonia.

*Key Words:* Acute respiratory infections, bacterial bronchitis, bacterial pneumonia, sepsis

# 87 Gaucher Disease

Manisha Balwani and Robert J. Desnick

## KEY POINTS

- *Disease summary:*
  - Gaucher disease is a lysosomal storage disease (LSD) which results from the deficient activity of the degradative enzyme, acid β-glucosidase, and the lysosomal accumulation of its glycosphingolipid substrate, glucosylceramide (GL-1), primarily in the monocyte-macrophage system.
  - Three major clinical subtypes of Gaucher disease have been described. Type 1 is the most common, and is differentiated from type 2 and type 3 by a lack of primary central nervous system involvement.
  - Type 1 Gaucher disease is most common in the Ashkenazi Jewish population (~1 in 1000 affected; 1 in 15 is a carrier) and is characterized by hepatosplenomegaly, pancytopenia, and bone disease.
  - Type 2 Gaucher disease is characterized by onset in infancy and progressive psychomotor retardation with death by age 2. Individuals with type 3 diseases may have onset in infancy with a slowly progressive neurologic course and may survive into the third or fourth decade of life.

- *Hereditary basis:*
  - Gaucher disease (all subtypes) is inherited as an autosomal recessive trait. Heterozygous carriers are asymptomatic, and when both parents are carriers there is a 25% risk for an affected child with each pregnancy.

- *Differential diagnosis (Table 87-1):*
  - LSDs and mucopolysaccharidosis: Hepatosplenomegaly, which is seen in Gaucher disease, is present in other lysosomal storage diseases including types A and B Niemann-Pick disease and the mucopolysaccharidoses types I, II, III, VI, and VII. The presence of other clinical features as well as biochemical testing distinguishes these.
  - Saposin C deficiency: Patients with saposin C deficiency can present with symptoms similar to severe neuronopathic Gaucher disease. However, they have normal acid β-glucosidase activity.

## Diagnostic Criteria and Clinical Characteristics

*Diagnostic Criteria:* Diagnosis is established by

- Determining the acid β-glucosidase enzyme activity in peripheral blood leucocytes is diagnostic for all subtypes. Affected individuals will have activity which is markedly decreased to less than 10% of normal mean activity. Enzyme activity does not differentiate the subtypes or predict disease severity.
- Mutation analysis of the five most common mutations (N370S, L444P, 84GG, IVS2+1, and R496H) in the acid β-glucosidase gene will detect over 95% of mutations in Ashkenazi Jewish patients and around 50% to 60% in non-Jewish patients. DNA sequencing of the acid β-glucosidase gene will identify other mutations, and mutation analysis can predict disease subtype and prognosis.
- Bone marrow examination may show the presence of "Gaucher cells" which have a characteristic morphologic appearance. However, similar cells are seen in hematologic malignancies called "pseudo-Gaucher" cells. The bone marrow biopsy is not diagnostic, and determining the acid β-glucosidase enzymatic activity or acid β-glucosidase-specific mutations is required for the diagnosis.

*Clinical Characteristics:* Type 1 Gaucher disease patients have significant phenotypic heterogeneity. Patients may present with early-onset symptomatic disease in childhood or remain asymptomatic through life. Clinical characteristics of type 1 Gaucher disease include anemia, thrombocytopenia, hepatosplenomegaly, clinical or radiographic evidence of bone disease, and rarely, lung involvement. It is distinguished from types 2 or 3 disease by the absence of primary neurologic involvement. Commonly reported symptoms include easy bruising, bleeding, fatigue, bone or joint pain, abdominal pain, and fullness. More recently, Type 1 Gaucher disease has been associated with an increased risk for Parkinson. Types 2 and 3 disease have primary neurologic involvement, and can present with psychomotor retardation, oculomotor apraxia, and hypertonia.

## Screening and Counseling

*Screening:* Family screening: After molecular genetic testing has confirmed the presence of two disease-causing mutations in the proband, family members can be tested by targeted mutation analysis. Biochemical testing with acid β-glucosidase assay is not reliable for the identification of carriers.

Prenatal carrier screening: Prepregnancy carrier screening for Gaucher disease with targeted mutation analysis is offered to all

**Table 87-1 System Involvement**

| System | Manifestation |
|---|---|
| Skeletal | Marrow infiltration, Erlenmeyer flask deformity, lytic lesions, bone infarcts, avascular necrosis, and low bone density |
| Visceral | Hepatosplenomegaly |
| Hematologic | Cytopenias and acquired coagulation factor abnormalities |
| Pulmonary | Pulmonary hypertension |
| Immunologic | Polyclonal or monoclonal gammopathy |
| Metabolic | Low total and HDL cholesterol, high ferritin, elevated chitotriosidase, and angiotensin-converting enzyme levels[a] |
| Neurologic | Types 2 and 3 disease: psychomotor retardation, opisthotonus, oculomotor apraxia, retroflexion, spasticity |
| Cardiovascular | Homozygosity for the *D409H* mutation confers an atypical phenotype with valvular calcification |

[a]Biomarkers of Gaucher disease.

individuals of Ashkenazi Jewish ancestry. Prenatal testing as well as preimplantation genetic diagnosis is available to at-risk couples.

***Counseling:*** Gaucher disease is inherited as an autosomal recessive trait and affected individuals carry two disease-causing mutations. Parents of the proband are heterozygous and carry one mutant acid β-glucosidase allele. Siblings of the proband have a 25% risk of being affected, and if not affected, a 67% risk of being carriers. All offspring of an affected individual are obligate carriers. As the carrier frequency of Gaucher disease is high in the Ashkenazi Jewish population (~1:15), it is not uncommon to see affected parents and offspring.

Genotype-phenotype correlations in type 1 Gaucher disease are somewhat useful. In general, the presence of at least one *N370S* mutation precludes primary neurologic involvement. Individuals with two copies of the *N370S* mutation tend to have a milder disease as compared to those who are compound heterozygotes with one *N370S* allele in combination with a more severe mutation (*84GG, IVS2+1, L444P*, etc). However, there is significant variability even within the same genotype, highlighting the role of genetic modifiers.

## Management and Treatment

A comprehensive baseline examination to establish disease severity followed by annual follow-up to monitor disease progression and/or response to treatment is recommended for all types 1 and 3 patients regardless of symptoms. Type 2 patients are seen on a monthly basis or as needed. The baseline examination includes a detailed medical history including family history and physical examination. Laboratory studies include measurement of hematologic indices, liver function

tests, iron indices, cholesterol profile, and biomarkers of Gaucher disease activity including chitotriosidase, angiotensin-converting enzyme, and tartrate-resistant acid phosphatase. Radiologic studies include magnetic resonance imaging (MRI) or computed tomography (CT) scan of the abdomen for assessment of liver and spleen volumes, MRI of the femurs to assess marrow infiltration and infarcts, x-rays to assess bone age in children as well as infarcts, lytic lesions, and failure of bone remodeling (Erlenmeyer flask deformity), dual-energy x-ray absorptiometry (DEXA) for assessment of bone mineral density. In patients with types 2 and 3 Gaucher disease a detailed neurologic evaluation including MRI of the brain, electroencephalogram, and neuropsychometric testing are recommended.

Management of patients requires a multidisciplinary approach. Supportive care includes use of analgesics for pain management, joint replacement for chronic pain and limited range of motion, and/or transfusion of blood products for severe anemia or thrombocytopenia. Supplemental calcium, vitamin D, and bisphosphonates are used for patients with osteopenia or osteoporosis. Partial or total splenectomy has been used in the past for severe thrombocytopenia and severe pancytopenia which has a high risk of bleeding complications and/or infection. However, splenectomy is rarely used with the currently available therapeutic options.

Treatment options include

1. Enzyme replacement therapy: Administration of exogenous recombinant enzyme provides safe and effective therapy. The enzyme decreases the accumulated substrate, GL-1. Currently, there are three FDA approved enzyme replacements for treatment of Gaucher disease in the United States.

   Imiglucerase has been available since 1994 and has been shown to reverse hematologic and visceral involvement, improve quality of life, decrease frequency of bone pain and crises as well as improve bone density of Type 1 patients. More recently, Velaglucerase and Taliglucerase have received FDA approval for treatment of Type 1 Gaucher disease.

2. Substrate reduction therapy: The principle of substrate reduction is to reduce the rate of GL-1 synthesis to offset the catabolic defect and to restore the metabolic balance. This involves the oral administration of small molecules which can partially inhibit GL-1 biosynthesis. Miglustat is FDA-approved for those with mild-to-moderate type 1 Gaucher disease in whom enzyme replacement is not an option. Eliglustat, a specific inhibitor of the enzyme glucosylceramide synthase is in Phase 3 clinical trials for Type 1 Gaucher disease.

3. Bone marrow transplantation: This approach is limited by significant morbidity and mortality and not commonly used.

## Molecular Genetics and Molecular Mechanism

***Syndrome/Gene/Locus:***
Gaucher disease/acid β-glucosidase/1q21 (GBA)

Acid β-glucosidase is a glycoprotein composed of 497 amino acids. The enzyme functions in the lysosomes of all tissues and is responsible for hydrolyzing GL-1 to glucose and ceramide.

***Genetic Testing:*** Targeted mutation analysis of the common mutations causing type 1 Gaucher disease is especially useful for individuals of Ashkenazi Jewish descent (Table 87-2). Testing is available at academic medical centers and commercial testing laboratories.

*Table 87-2 Molecular Genetic Testing*

| Gene | Testing Modality | Mutation Type | Detection Rate |
|---|---|---|---|
| Acid β-glucosidase | Targeted mutation analysis | Five common mutations (*N370S, L444P, 84GG, IVS2+1, R496H*) | ~95% in Ashkenazi Jewish ~50%-60 % in other populations |
| Acid β-glucosidase | Sequencing | | ~98% |

Complete gene sequencing is also available and is recommended for those with enzyme levels in the affected range where targeted mutation analysis did not identify two disease-causing mutations. DNA analyses provide useful diagnostic confirmation as well as genotype-phenotype correlations. GBA is the only gene associated with Gaucher disease.

### BIBLIOGRAPHY:

1. Grabowski GA, Beutler E. Gaucher disease. In: Scriver C, Beaudet A, Sly W, Valle D, eds. The Metabolic and Molecular Bases of Inherited Diseases. 8th ed. New York, NY: McGraw-Hill; 2001:3635-3668.

2. Grabowski, GA. Gaucher disease: gene frequencies and genotype/phenotype correlations. *Genet Test.* 1997;1(1):5-12.

3. Charrow J, Andersson HC, Kaplan P, et al. The Gaucher Registry: demographics and disease characteristics of 1698 patients with Gaucher disease. *Arch Intern Med.* 2000;160:2835-2843.

4. Weinreb NJ, Aggio MC, Andersson HC, et al. Gaucher disease type 1: revised recommendations on evaluations and monitoring for adult patients. *Semin Hematol.* 2004;41(4 suppl 5):15-22.

5. Vellodi A, Tylki-Szymanska A, Davies EH, et al. Management of neuronopathic Gaucher disease: revised recommendations. *J Inherit Metab Dis.* 2009;32(5):660-664.

6. Weinreb NJ, Charrow J, Andersson HC, et al. Effectiveness of enzyme replacement therapy in 1028 patients with type 1 Gaucher disease after 2 to 5 years of treatment: a report from the Gaucher Registry. *Am J Med.* 2002;113(2):112-119.

7. Platt FM, Jeyakumar M. Substrate reduction therapy. *Acta Paediatr Suppl.* 2008;97(457):88-93.

8. Grabowski G, Horowitz M. Gaucher's disease: molecular, genetic and enzymological aspects. *Baillieres Clin Haematol.* Dec 1997;10(4):635-656.

9. www.genetests.org

10. Rosenbloom B, Balwani M, Bronstein JM, et al. The incidence of Parkinsonism in patients with type 1 Gaucher disease: data from the ICGG Gaucher Registry. *Blood Cells Mol Dis.* 2011;46:95-102.

## Supplementary Information

### OMIM REFERENCES:

[1] Gaucher Disease; Acid β-Glucosidase (606463), Gene locus 1q21 Acid β-Glucosidase

### Alternative Names:

- Acid β-Glucosidase
- β-Glucosidase, Acid
- Glucocerebrosidase
- Glucosylceramidase

*Key Words:* Lysosomal storage disease, splenomegaly, hepatomegaly, anemia, thrombocytopenia, bone disease

# 88 Fabry Disease

Robert J. Desnick

## KEY POINTS

- *Disease summary:*
  - Fabry disease is an X-linked lysosomal storage disease (LSD), which results from the deficient activity of the enzyme, α-galactosidase A (α-Gal A), and the lysosomal accumulation of glycosphingolipids with α-terminal galactosyl moieties, primarily globotriaosylceramide (GL-3).
  - Two major clinical subtypes have been described. The classic phenotype due to mutations that express little, if any, α-Gal A activity (<1% of mean normal) and present in childhood or adolescence, and a later-onset phenotype due to mutations that express residual enzyme activity (>1% of mean normal levels).
  - Newborn screening studies indicate the incidence in males of the classic phenotype to be about 1 in 25,000 to 40,000, while the later-onset phenotype is about 10 times more frequent in Europe and Taiwan.
  - Clinical manifestations of the classic phenotype include angiokeratoma, acroparesthesias, hypohidrosis, gastrointestinal symptoms, and a characteristic corneal keratopathy. With advancing age, the classic patients develop renal failure, cardiac disease, cerebrovascular disease, and premature demise.
  - Patients with the later-onset phenotype do not have endothelial glycosphingolipid deposition and lack the early manifestations of the classic phenotype. They develop renal failure, cardiac disease, or strokes later in life, typically between the third and fifth decades of life.
  - Enzyme replacement therapy (ERT) with recombinant α-Gal A has proven safe and effective in clinical trials.

- *Hereditary basis:*
  - Fabry disease (both subtypes) is inherited as an X-linked trait. Manifestations in heterozygous females can range from as severely affected as males to asymptomatic, primarily due to random X-chromosomal inactivation. All daughters of an affected male are heterozygous, while all sons will not inherit the Fabry gene. On average, 50% of sons of a heterozygous mother will be affected and 50% of daughters will be heterozygotes.

- *Differential diagnosis:*
  - **Acroparesthesias:**
    - Many of the symptoms in Fabry disease can be similar to those of other disorders, including rheumatoid or juvenile arthritis, rheumatic fever, erythromelalgia, lupus erythematosus, Raynaud syndrome, fibromyalgia, and multiple sclerosis. In children with acroparesthesias without any other major finding, "growing pains" may be attributed to their complaints.
  - **Angiokeratoma:**
    - Angiokeratomas, that are similar to or indistinguishable from the clinical appearance and distribution of the cutaneous lesions in Fabry disease, have been described in other lysosomal storage diseases, including fucosidosis (OMIM #230000), galactosialidosis (OMIM #256540), GM1-gangliosidosis (OMIM #230500), aspartylglucosaminuria (OMIM #208400), β-mannosidosis (OMIM #248510), and Kanzaki disease (OMIM #609242).
    - Angiokeratoma of Fordyce, angiokeratoma of Mibelli, and angiokeratoma circumscriptum are a few cutaneous disorders that have similar cutaneous lesions to those seen in Fabry disease. None have the typical histologic or ultrastructural lysosomal pathology of the Fabry lesion.
    - The angiokeratoma of Fordyce is similar in appearance to that of Fabry disease, but is limited to the scrotum, and usually appears after age 30.
    - The angiokeratomas of Mibelli includes warty lesions on the extensor surfaces of extremities in young adults and is associated with chilblains.
    - Angiokeratoma circumscriptum or naeviformus can occur anywhere on the body, is clinically and histologically similar to that of Fordyce, and is not associated with chilblains.
  - In adults, presence of arrhythmias, left ventricular hypertrophy (LVH), short PR interval, hypertrophic cardiomyopathy, proteinuria, renal insufficiency, transient ischemic attacks (TIAs), and strokes can all be consistent with Fabry disease. One should be on alert especially if there is a family history of these, and an X-linked inheritance pattern.
  - Male patients in hemodialysis or renal transplantation clinics, as well as in cardiac clinics and in stroke clinics, should be evaluated for unrecognized Fabry disease by demonstrating deficient α-Gal A activity in plasma or leukocytes. These results are diagnostic in males, but α-Gal A mutation analysis should be performed to identify the family mutation and for the diagnosis of heterozygotes for which the enzyme assay is unreliable due to random X-chromosomal inactivation.

## Diagnostic Criteria and Clinical Characteristics

### Clinical Characteristics (Table 88-1)

- The major early manifestations in classically affected males and some heterozygous females include acroparesthesias, angiokeratoma, hypohidrosis, and a characteristic corneal keratopathy. With advancing age, the glycosphingolipid (GL-3) deposition in the microvascular endothelial cells throughout the body leads to renal insufficiency and failure, cardiac and cerebrovascular events, and premature demise.

- Classically affected patients typically present with neuropathic pain in childhood or adolescence, which also

*Table 88-1 System Involvement*

| System | Manifestation |
|---|---|
| Skeletal | Mild, if any, skeletal involvement. Mild osteopenia in older patients |
| Visceral | Hypohidrosis in classically affected males from early childhood |
| Hematologic | Mild anemia in some patients |
| Pulmonary | Glycolipid storage in lungs can cause lung disease. Patients should not smoke |
| Immunologic | N/A |
| Metabolic | The deficient activity of $\alpha$-galactosidase A results in the systemic accumulation of the glycosphingolipid, globotriaosylceramide (GL-3), and related glycolipids, particularly in the microvascular endothelium |
| Neurologic | In childhood, burning, tingling pain in the extremities. In adults, TIAs and strokes can occur |
| Cardiovascular | Cardiovascular dysfunction may include left ventricular hypertrophy leading to hypertrophic cardiomyopathy, valvular abnormalities, and arrhythmias |
| Ophthalmologic | Characteristic corneal dystrophy on slit-lamp microscopy. Vision is not impaired. Tortuous conjunctival and retinal vessels, characteristic anterior and posterior cataracts |
| Renal | Glomerular involvement leads to renal insufficiency and failure |
| Dermatologic | Classically affected patients have diffuse angiokeratoma (telangiectasias) and hypohidrosis |
| Gastrointestinal | Classically affected males may have chronic postprandial pain and diarrhea |

can be misdiagnosed as erythromelalgia or fibromyalgia. Episodes of burning or tingling pain in the hands and feet (acroparesthesias) in children or adolescents are brought on by exercise, fever, stress, or changes in weather conditions. The pain may be chronic, or can be severe and last for days or even weeks.

- The presence of cutaneous lesions, termed angiokeratomas, which are actually telangiectasias, in affected males, sparse lesions appear in childhood or adolescence in the "swimsuit" region, especially in the umbilicus and on the scrotum. Heterozygous females from families with the classic phenotype may have sparse angiokeratomas on the breasts, flanks, and/or genital region.
- Decreased or absent ability to sweat, hypohidrosis or anhidrosis, is characteristic in classically affected males and many heterozygotes.
- The bilateral corneal dystrophy can be mimicked by use of certain drugs including amiodarone and chloroquine.
- With advancing age, classically affected males will develop renal insufficiency leading to dialysis and/or transplantation, cardiac disease including left ventricular hypertrophy leading to hypertrophic cardiomyopathy, arrhythmias, and cerebrovascular disease including TIAs and strokes.
- Prior to ERT, the average age of death prior to dialysis and renal transplant was about 40 years, with renal treatment, about 50 years in classically affected males.
- Males with the later-onset phenotype have residual $\alpha$-Gal A activity and lack the early manifestations in classically affected males, including the acroparesthesias, angiokeratoma, hypohidrosis, and the corneal keratopathy. They present later in life (third-eighth decades), with renal, cardiac, and/or cerebrovascular disease.

**Diagnostic Criteria (Fig. 88-1):**
- Suspect clinical manifestations include the following in classically affected males: childhood or adolescent onset of

acroparesthesias: pain in the fingers and toes, particularly during a fever, exercise, or stress. Typically these males also will have hypohidrosis, angiokeratomas in the swimsuit region, gastrointestinal manifestations (postprandial pain and diarrhea), and a characteristic corneal dystrophy only visible by slit-lamp microscopy. Later-onset patients present in the third to eight decade with renal insufficiency and failure, left ventricular hypertrophy, hypertrophic cardiomyopathy, and/or transient ischemic attacks or cryptogenic strokes.
- Demonstration of deficient plasma or leukocyte $\alpha$-Gal A activity in affected males. Confirm $\alpha$-Gal A enzyme deficiency by $\alpha$-Gal A mutation analysis to determine family mutations. Mutation analysis also provides genotype or phenotype correlation for classic and later-onset disease.
- For heterozygous females, the $\alpha$-Gal A activity can range from low to normal and therefore, all suspect heterozygotes are diagnosed by demonstration of the family mutation, which also provides genotype or phenotype information.
- Over 670 $\alpha$-Gal A mutations are known as of August, 2013.

**Clinical Characteristics:**

☞**PHENOTYPIC SPECTRUM:** There are two major subtypes of Fabry disease, the classic and later-onset phenotypes. Affected males with the classic phenotype have little, if any, $\alpha$-Gal A enzyme activity (<1% of mean normal), whereas males with the later-onset phenotype have residual enzymatic activity, typically greater than 1% of normal. In classically affected males, the progressive microvascular endothelial glycosphingolipid accumulation leads to the clinical manifestations including angiokeratomas, acroparesthesias, hypohidrosis, and gastrointestinal abnormalities. They also have a characteristic corneal opacity detectable early in childhood or adolescence. With advancing age, manifestations include renal insufficiency and failure, cardiac involvement, and cerebrovascular disease. Heterozygous females from Fabry families with the classic phenotype have a wide range of clinical manifestations that vary from asymptomatic to severely affected.

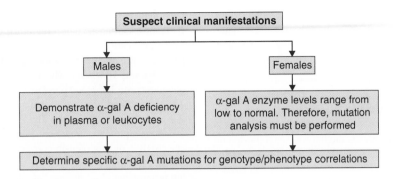

**Figure 88-1** Algorithm for Diagnostic Evaluation of Patient With Fabry Disease.

Affected males with the later-onset phenotype present in adulthood, usually lack the classical early manifestations (angiokeratomas, acroparesthesias, hypohidrosis, and corneal opacities), and develop renal and/or cardiac disease in the third to fifth decades of life. Heterozygous females from later-onset families may be asymptomatic or develop symptoms later in life, including cardiac and renal manifestations.

☞**THE CLASSIC PHENOTYPE:** The symptoms of the classic subtype of Fabry disease usually begin in childhood or adolescence. Early symptoms include the onset of acroparesthesias and the appearance of angiokeratomas. Pain is an early symptom of the classic phenotype. Affected individuals may experience episodes of severe burning pain in the hands and the feet (acroparesthesia) and sometimes in the arms and legs. Severe episodes of pain (Fabry crises) may last for hours to days and are frequently associated with exercise, fatigue, and/or fever. Classically affected individuals have decreased or absent sweat production (hypohidrosis or anhidrosis) and discomfort in warm temperatures (heat intolerance). The angiokeratomas are cutaneous macular-papular lesions that are reddish to dark-blue and are typically found in the area between the hips and the knees.

Classically affected males and about 90% of heterozygotes from classically affected families have a characteristic corneal opacity seen by slit-lamp microscopy that does not affect vision. Conjunctival and retinal vessels are tortuous and may appear cork screw like and/or dilated due to the glycosphingolipid accumulation in the vessel walls. Additional symptoms associated with Fabry disease may include dizziness, headache, generalized weakness, and fatigue.

Gastrointestinal symptoms are seen in at least 20% of classically affected Fabry patients. These include postprandial abdominal cramping, bloating, diarrhea, vomiting, and nausea. Patients may report alternating constipation and diarrhea. Progressive glycosphingolipid deposition in the kidney interferes with renal function; microvascular involvement of the kidney begins in childhood, progresses to isosthenuria, proteinuria, and tubular dysfunction, then with advancing age results in progressive renal disease and failure typically by age 35 to 45 years. Dialysis or renal transplantation is effective in correcting the renal disease, and renal transplants are not affected by the disease. All potential family donors should be evaluated to ensure that they are not affected or heterozygotes.

With maturity, most classically affected males experience cardiovascular and/or cerebrovascular disease. Cardiovascular dysfunction may include myocardial infarction, cardiac hypertrophy, valvular abnormalities, and arrhythmias, while cerebrovascular complications include risk of early stroke, hemiplegia, hemianesthesia, and TIAs. Most adult males have sinus bradycardia; atrioventricular (AV) conduction accelerations (short PR intervals) are more commonly seen in young patients without left ventricular hypertrophy. In older patients, bundle-branch-blocks and AV abnormalities are more commonly seen. GL-3 accumulation in heart valve tissue with secondary fibrosis and calcification can lead to valvular dysfunction rarely of hemodynamic significance. The progressive vascular involvement is a major cause of morbidity and mortality, particularly after treatment of the renal insufficiency by chronic dialysis or transplantation.

Other manifestations include lower extremity edema in the absence of significant renal disease, hypoalbuminemia, or varices. This lymphedema is due to the accumulation of GL-3 in the lymphatic vessels and nodes. Progressive high-frequency hearing loss occurs in classically affected males in the third to fifth decades of life. Tinnitus, and/or vertigo may also appear. The most likely cause of the acute hearing loss is microvascular events. Chronic hearing loss, however, is usually the result of GL-3 accumulation in the audiovestibular ganglia and vessels of the cochlea and is therefore termed sensorineural. Pulmonary involvement manifests as dyspnea, shortness of breath, intolerance to exercise, and wheezing. Pulmonary function tests may reveal an obstructive pattern. These pulmonary findings are seen especially in smokers. Depression, anxiety, and fatigue are also seen in affected individuals and will negatively impact quality of life.

Symptoms may increase with age due to the progressive involvement of the microvascular system leading to kidney failure, heart disease, and/or strokes. Kidney function decreases progressing to failure and the need for dialysis or transplantation typically by 35 to 45 years of age in affected males. Kidney involvement in female heterozygotes is more variable. Only about 10% to 15% of heterozygotes develop kidney failure. Heart disease includes heart enlargement (typically left ventricular hypertrophy, leading to hypertrophic cardiomyopathy), rhythm abnormalities, and heart failure. Involvement of very well blood vessels in the brain leads to strokes.

Additional symptoms sometimes associated with Fabry disease include delayed puberty, lack of or sparse hair growth, and malformation of the joints of the fingers. In some cases, affected individuals have abnormal accumulation of lymph in the feet and legs-associated swelling (lymphedema), which may result from disruption of lymph's normal drainage due to the glycosphingolipid accumulation in the lymphatic vessels and lymph nodes.

☞**THE LATER-ONSET PHENOTYPE:** Patients with the later-onset subtype typically do not have the angiokeratoma; they usually sweat normally, do not experience the Fabry pain or crises, and do not have heat intolerance or the corneal keratopathy. These individuals develop cardiac, renal, or cerebrovascular disease later in adult life, and have been identified by screening cardiac and hemodialysis clinics for unrecognized patients with Fabry disease.

## Screening and Counseling

*Screening:* Screening of patients in hemodialysis, renal transplantation, cardiac (especially patients with left ventricular hypertrophy and hypertrophic cardiomyopathy), and stroke clinics has identified previously unrecognized patients with classic and later-onset Fabry disease. The identification of an affected older patient leads to screening the family for other affected, especially younger males and symptomatic females who can benefit from earlier treatment.

Newborn screening for Fabry disease has been undertaken in Europe (Italy and Austria) and Taiwan. Pilot screening programs have been undertaken in Illinois and Washington, and newborn screening for Fabry disease has been legislatively mandated in several states in the United States.

*Counseling:*

☞X-LINKED INHERITANCE: Fabry disease is inherited as an X-linked trait. The gene that causes this disease is located on the long arm of the X chromosome (Xq22.1). There are over 660 mutations in the α-Gal A gene that cause Fabry disease. Once the diagnosis is made in an affected patient, the entire family should be screened by enzyme or mutation assays to identify all affected males and heterozygotes. Efforts should be directed to determine if the family has a classic or later-onset mutation. In general, absent enzyme activity results in the classic subtype, while patients with the later-onset subtype have residual enzyme activity. All affected individuals should be evaluated by a physician who has expertise in Fabry disease and by geneticists or genetic counselors who can inform family members on their risk of affected offspring and the availability of prenatal diagnosis. The severity and range of symptoms may vary among affected males, and especially heterozygotes in the same family. Not all males with Fabry disease have all of the symptoms of the disease.

☞GENOTYPE-PHENOTYPE CORRELATIONS: Certain mutations predict the early-onset classic phenotype including nonsense, and frameshift mutations, small out-of-frame deletions and insertions, whole exon deletions, and certain splice-site consensus sequence mutations, as well as missense mutations that are located in or near the enzyme's active site, or that render the enzyme unstable.

Mutations that predict the later-onset phenotype, include missense mutations that encode residual α-Gal A activity of which most are buried, or mostly buried in the enzyme structure; splicing mutations that retain a small percentage of normal transcripts (that encode the normal enzyme), and in-frame, small deletions, or duplications that encode residual enzymatic activity.

## Management and Treatment

*Management:* Consensus recommendations and guidelines for evaluation and management are available.

☞PAIN: The episodes of pain generally have precipitating causes such as physical exertion, fever and illness, changes in temperature, stress, etc. Patients should make every effort to avoid these precipitating factors, if possible. Patients with frequent severe pain may benefit from medications such as diphenylhydantoin (Dilantin), carbamazepine (Tegretol), or gabapentin (Neurontin). These medications must be taken every day to prevent the onset of pain and/or to reduce the frequency and severity of painful attacks.

☞RENAL DISEASE: Management of the Fabry nephropathy includes control of blood pressure, proteinuria, and hyperlipidemia. The target blood pressure in patients with chronic kidney disease (CKD) is below 130/80 mm Hg. A low sodium, low protein diet and presymptomatic treatment with angiotensin receptor blockers (ARBs) or angiotensin-converting enzyme (ACE) inhibitors should be administered. They are important in the management of the progressive renal disease, in addition to ERT in patients with proteinuria. For those patients with severely compromised kidney function, dialysis and kidney transplantation are available. The success of kidney transplantation offers the ability to restore kidney function in Fabry patients and has improved the overall prognosis for this disease. The disease does not recur in the kidney, because the normal enzyme in the graft prevents accumulation of GL-3.

☞CARDIOVASCULAR INVOLVEMENT: ACE inhibitors and ARBs also are mainstay treatment for left ventricular systolic dysfunction; diuretics can help relieve dyspnea. Pacemakers may be required. Internal cardioverter-defibrillators (ICDs) are used for patients who are considered to be at high risk of sudden cardiac death, due to ventricular tachycardia.

☞NEUROLOGIC DISEASE: Prophylaxis with antiplatelet or anticoagulant medication such as aspirin (81 mg/d) should be administered as TIAs or strokes are common in the older patients. Hearing loss can be treated with hearing aids, and noise trauma should be avoided to preserve hearing.

*Therapeutics:* ERT with human recombinant α-Gal A has been available since 2001 in Europe and 2003 in the United States. Treatment should begin early, at least as soon as clinical symptoms or signs are observed, particularly in affected males with the classic disease. Two preparations of the enzyme are available: agalsidase-alfa (Replagal; Shire Pharmaceuticals) and agalsidase-beta (Fabrazyme; Genzyme Corp). Only agalsidase-beta is FDA approved and commercially available in the United States. Although the two recombinant enzymes are kinetically and structurally similar, they are approved at different doses. Agalsidase-beta and -alfa are prescribed at 1 and 0.2 mg/kg every 2 weeks by intravenous infusion, respectively. Fabrazyme has been shown in randomized, double-blind, placebo-controlled clinical trials to clear the accumulated GL-3 from interstitial capillary endothelial cells of the kidney, and to stabilize the eGFR. ERT with agalsidase-beta also cleared the GL-3 from the vascular endothelial cells in the heart and skin. A Phase IV randomized, double-blind, placebo-controlled study in older Fabry patients with mild-to-moderate renal insufficiency demonstrated that agalsidase-beta slowed the progression of renal dysfunction. Subsequent studies have shown that the addition of ACE inhibitors or angiotensin II receptor blockers may augment the renal protective effects of enzyme replacement. Clinical trials of agalsidase-alfa have been reported including a phase 1 open-label trial evaluating a single dose from 0.007 to 0.1 mg/kg, a phase 2 single-site, double-blind, placebo-controlled trial, and a second phase 2 trial evaluating GL-3 clearance in the heart biopsies, which did not reach clinical significance.

Other therapies are in development including oral pharmacologic chaperone therapy using a small molecule monotherapy, migalastat (Amigal), to enhance the residual α-Gal A activity, and a adjunctive therapy administering both the pharmacologic chaperone and recombinant enzyme to patients with either subtype. Efforts to develop gene therapy remain preclinical at present.

*Table 88-2 Molecular Genetic Testing*

| Gene | Testing Modality | Mutation Type | Detection Rate |
|------|------------------|---------------|----------------|
| *GLA* | Gene sequencing<br>Gene dosage | All types<br>Large deletions | All affected males with α-Gal A enzyme deficiency have *GLA* mutations. Accurate for heterozygotes. |

## Molecular Genetics and Molecular Mechanism

**Syndrome/Gene/Locus:** Fabry disease is caused by mutations in the gene encoding the lysosomal hydrolase, a-Gal A. The *GLA* gene is located on the long arm of the X-chromosome (Xq22.1). As of August 2013, over 670 disease-causing mutations in the *GLA* gene have been reported. There are no common mutations and most mutations are family-specific or present in a few families (ie, "private mutations"). De novo mutations are rare. Genotype-phenotype correlations are predictable.

**Genetic Testing:** Confirmation of the clinical diagnosis in males is made by demonstration of deficient α-Gal A activity in plasma and/or leukocytes. Heterozygous females may have low to normal levels of enzymatic activity due to random X-chromosomal inactivation. Suspected heterozygotes require molecular α-Gal A gene analyses to identify the family mutation (Table 88-2).

- Determination of the α-Gal A activity and confirmation by α-Gal A mutation detection are available (see GeneTests, http://www.ncbi.nlm.nih.gov/sites/GeneTests/lab/clinical_disease_id/2775?db=genetests). The CLIA- and NYS-approved Mount Sinai Genetic Testing Laboratory routinely provides these services.
- Prenatal diagnosis of Fabry disease can be made by measuring α-Gal A activity and demonstrating the family-specific *GLA* mutation in amniotic cells at about 15 weeks of pregnancy or at about 10 weeks of pregnancy in chorionic villi.
- Pilot studies of newborn screening have been undertaken in Italy, Austria, USA, and Taiwan.
- By genotype analysis, the incidence of the classic phenotype was between 1 in approximately 25,000 to 40,000, whereas the incidence of the later-onset phenotype may be about 10 times more frequent in various populations.
- Screening of patients in hemodialysis, transplantation, cardiology, and stroke clinics have identified previously unrecognized (and mutation confirmed) patients with Fabry disease. The frequency of these patients varies: in hemodialysis and transplant clinics, approximately 0.2% to 1%, in patients with left ventricular hypertrophy or hypertrophic cardiomyopathy, approximately 0.1% to 2%, in patients with cryptogenic strokes, 0% to 1%.

### Future Directions:
- Various therapeutic approaches are being developed, including pharmacologic chaperones, substrate reduction therapy, stop-codon read-through approaches for nonsense mutations, as well as gene therapy.
- Based on therapeutic studies of other lysosomal diseases (ie, Pompe disease and mucopolysaccharidoses types I, II, and VI), it is becoming increasingly convincing that early intervention may prevent many of the clinical manifestations, including those resulting from fibrosis secondary to vascular occlusions.

- Newborn screening will presumably expand in Asia and the United States, as earlier intervention has been shown to be clinically beneficial in the Fabrazyme phases 3 and 4 studies.
- In addition, experimental approaches are being evaluated for the treatment of Fabry disease. Chaperone therapy uses small molecules that bind to the misfolded enzyme to stabilize it in the endoplasmic reticulum (ER). The binding of the chaperone molecule helps the mutant enzyme fold into its correct shape. This allows the enzyme to be properly trafficked from the ER and targeted to the cellular lysosomes in various organs, thereby increasing enzyme activity and cellular function and reducing substrate and stress on cells. The advantage of chaperone therapy is that it can be given orally and that it can reach a variety of tissues and cell types.
- Gene therapy is still in its early stages, as some studies in mice have been promising. However, there has been no trial in humans.

**BIBLIOGRAPHY:**

1. Opitz JM, Stiles FC, Wise D, et al. The genetics of angiokeratoma corporis diffusum (Fabry's disease) and its linkage relations with the Xg locus. *Am J Hum Genet.* 1965;17:325-342.
2. α-Galactosidase A deficiency: Fabry disease. In: Scriver CR, Beaudet AL, Sly WS, eds. *The Metabolic and Molecular Basis of Inherited Disease.* New York, NY: McGraw-Hill; 2001:3733-3774.
3. Eng CM, Ioannou YA, Desnick RJ. Alpha-galactosidase A deficiency: Fabry disease. In: Valle D, et al., ed. *Scriver's The Online Metabolic and Molecular Basis of Inherited Disease (OMBBID).* McGraw-Hill Companies, Inc.; 2010.
4. Wilcox WR, Oliveira JP, Hopkin RJ, et al. Females with Fabry disease frequently have major organ involvement: lessons from the Fabry Registry. *Mol Genet Metab.* 2008;93:112-128.
5. Desnick RJ, Brady RO. Fabry disease in childhood. *J Pediatr.* 2004;144:S20-S26.
6. Nakao S, Takenaka T, Maeda M, et al. An atypical variant of Fabry's disease in men with left ventricular hypertrophy. *N Engl J Med.* 1995;333:288-293.
7. Nakao S, Kodama C, Takenaka T, et al. Fabry disease: detection of undiagnosed hemodialysis patients and identification of a "renal variant" phenotype. *Kidney Int.* 2003;64:801-807.
8. Elliott P, Baker R, Pasquale F, et al. Prevalence of Anderson-Fabry disease in patients with hypertrophic cardiomyopathy: the European Anderson-Fabry Disease survey. *Heart.* 2011;97:1957-1960.
9. Stenson PD, Mort M, Ball EV, et al. The Human Gene Mutation Database: 2008 update. *Genome Med.* 2009;1:13.
10. Thurberg BL, Rennke H, Colvin RB, et al. Globotriaosylceramide accumulation in the Fabry kidney is cleared from multiple cell types after enzyme replacement therapy. *Kidney Int.* 2002;62:1933-1946.
11. Najafian B, Svarstad E, Bostad L, et al. Progressive podocyte injury and globotriaosylceramide (GL-3) accumulation in young patients with Fabry disease. *Kidney Int.* 2011;79:663-670.
12. Thadhani R, Wolf M, West ML, et al. Patients with Fabry disease on dialysis in the United States. *Kidney Int.* 2002;61:249-255.

13. Linthorst GE, Bouwman MG, Wijburg FA, Aerts JM, Poorthuis BJ, Hollak CE. Screening for Fabry disease in high-risk populations: a systematic review. *J Med Genet*. 2010;47:217-222.

14. Spada M, Pagliardini S, Yasuda M, et al. High incidence of later-onset fabry disease revealed by newborn screening. *Am J Hum Genet*. 2006;79:31-40.

15. Hwu WL, Chien YH, Lee NC, et al. Newborn screening for Fabry disease in Taiwan reveals a high incidence of the later-onset GLA mutation c.936+919G>A (IVS4+919G>A). *Hum Mutat*. 2009;30:1397-1405.

16. Mechtler TP, Stary S, Metz TF, et al. Neonatal screening for lysosomal storage disorders: feasibility and incidence from a nationwide study in Austria. *Lancet*. 2012;379:335-341.

17. Eng CM, Banikazemi M, Gordon RE, et al. A phase 1/2 clinical trial of enzyme replacement in fabry disease: pharmacokinetic, substrate clearance, and safety studies. *Am J Hum Genet*. 2001;68:711-722.

18. Shabbeer J, Yasuda M, Benson SD, Desnick RJ. Fabry disease: identification of 50 novel alpha-galactosidase A mutations causing the classic phenotype and three-dimensional structural analysis of 29 missense mutations. *Hum Genomics*. 2006;2:297-309.

19. Saito S, Ohno K, Sakuraba H. Fabry-database.org: database of the clinical phenotypes, genotypes and mutant alpha-galactosidase A structures in Fabry disease. *J Hum Genet*. 2011;56:467-468.

20. Garman SC, Garboczi DN. Structural basis of Fabry disease. *Mol Genet Metab*. 2002;77:3-11.

21. Benjamin ER, Flanagan JJ, Schilling A, et al. The pharmacological chaperone 1-deoxygalactonojirimycin increases alpha-galactosidase A levels in Fabry patient cell lines. *J Inherit Metab Dis*. 2009;32:424-440.

22. Wu X, Katz E, Della Valle MC, et al. A pharmacogenetic approach to identify mutant forms of alpha-galactosidase A that respond to a pharmacological chaperone for Fabry disease. *Hum Mutat*. 2011;32:965-977.

23. Desnick RJ, Brady R, Barranger J, et al. Fabry disease, an under-recognized multisystemic disorder: expert recommendations for diagnosis, management, and enzyme replacement therapy. *Ann Intern Med*. 2003;138:338-346.

24. Eng CM, Germain DP, Banikazemi M, et al. Fabry disease: guidelines for the evaluation and management of multi-organ system involvement. *Genet Med*. 2006;8:539-548.

25. Lee K, Jin X, Zhang K, et al. A biochemical and pharmacological comparison of enzyme replacement therapies for the glycolipid storage disorder Fabry disease. *Glycobiology*. 2003;13:305-313.

26. Sakuraba H, Murata-Ohsawa M, Kawashima I, et al. Comparison of the effects of agalsidase alfa and agalsidase beta on cultured human Fabry fibroblasts and Fabry mice. *J Hum Genet*. 2006;51:180-188.

27. Eng CM, Guffon N, Wilcox WR, et al. Safety and efficacy of recombinant human alpha-galactosidase A–replacement therapy in Fabry's disease. *N Engl J Med*. 2001;345:9-16.

28. Wilcox WR, Banikazemi M, Guffon N, et al. Long-term safety and efficacy of enzyme replacement therapy for Fabry disease. *Am J Hum Genet*. 2004;75:65-74.

29. Germain DP, Waldek S, Banikazemi M, et al. Sustained, long-term renal stabilization after 54 months of agalsidase beta therapy in patients with Fabry disease. *J Am Soc Nephrol*. 2007;18:1547-1557.

30. Banikazemi M, Bultas J, Waldek S, et al. Agalsidase-beta therapy for advanced Fabry disease: a randomized trial. *Ann Intern Med*. 2007;146:77-86.

31. Schiffmann R, Murray GJ, Treco D, et al. Infusion of alpha-galactosidase A reduces tissue globotriaosylceramide storage in patients with Fabry disease. *Proc Natl Acad Sci USA*. 2000;97:365-370.

32. Schiffmann R, Kopp JB, Austin HA 3rd, et al. Enzyme replacement therapy in Fabry disease: a randomized controlled trial. *JAMA*. 2001;285:2743-2749.

33. Hughes DA, Elliott PM, Shah J, et al. Effects of enzyme replacement therapy on the cardiomyopathy of Anderson-Fabry disease: a randomised, double-blind, placebo-controlled clinical trial of agalsidase alfa. *Heart*. 2008;94:153-158.

34. Benjamin ER, Khanna R, Schilling A, et al. Co-administration with the pharmacological chaperone AT1001 increases recombinant human alpha-galactosidase A tissue uptake and improves substrate reduction in Fabry mice. *Mol Ther*. 2012;20:717-726.

35. Desnick RJ, Schuchman EH. Enzyme replacement and enhancement therapies: lessons from lysosomal disorders. *Nat Rev Genet*. 2002;3:954-966.

36. Desnick RJ, Schuchman EH. Enzyme replacement and enhancement therapies: lessons from lysosomal disorders. *Nat Rev Genet*. 2002;3(12):954-966.

37. Chien YH, Chiang SC, Zhang XK, et al. Early detection of Pompe disease by newborn screening is feasible: results from the Taiwan screening program. *Pediatrics*. 2008;122:e39-e45.

38. Wang RY, Cambray-Forker EJ, Ohanian K, et al. Treatment reduces or stabilizes brain imaging abnormalities in patients with MPS I and II. *Mol Genet Metab*. 2009;98:406-411.

39. McGill JJ, Inwood AC, Coman DJ, et al. Enzyme replacement therapy for mucopolysaccharidosis VI from 8 weeks of age–a sibling control study. *Clin Genet*. 2010;77:492-498.

40. Tylki-Szymanska A, Jurecka A, Zuber Z, Rozdzynska A, Marucha J, Czartoryska B. Enzyme replacement therapy for mucopolysaccharidosis II from 3 months of age: a 3-year follow-up. *Acta Paediatr*. 2012;101:e42-e47.

## Supplementary Information

**OMIM REFERENCES:**

[1] Alpha-Galactosidase A; GLA (#300644)

[2] Fabry Disease (#301500)

**Alternative Names:**

- α-Galactosidase A Deficiency
- Anderson-Fabry Disease
- Angiokeratoma Corporis Diffusum Universale
- Angiokeratoma Diffuse
- Ceramide Trihexosidase Deficiency
- GLA Deficiency
- Hereditary Dystopic Lipidosis

*Key Words:* α-Galactosidase A, angiokeratoma, classic phenotype, enzyme replacement therapy, globotriaosylceramide, glycosphingolipids, genotype or phenotype correlations, later-onset phenotype, microvascular endothelial disease

*Disclosure:* The Mount Sinai School of Medicine, the Department of Genetics and Genomic Sciences and some faculty members in the department (including the Chair Emeritus and Dean for Genetic and Genomic Medicine, Dr. Robert J. Desnick), receive financial benefit from the Genzyme Corporation for the sale of Fabrazyme®, and from Shire HGT for the sale of Replagal, enzyme replacement drugs developed by them for the treatment of Fabry disease. Dr. Desnick is a consultant for the Genzyme Corporation and Synageva Biopharmaceuticals, receives grants from the Genzyme Corporation, and has founder's stock in Amicus Therapeutics.

# 89 The Porphyrias

Peter Tishler

## ACUTE PORPHYRIAS

### KEY POINTS

- *Disease summary:*
  - All porphyrias are diseases resulting from abnormalities of heme biosynthesis.
  - The four acute porphyrias, in descending order of prevalence, and their inborn enzymatic errors are intermittent acute porphyria (IAP; ~50% reduction in porphobilinogen deaminase), variegate porphyria (VP; ~50% reduction in protoporphyrinogen oxidase), hereditary coproporphyria (HCP; ~50% reduction in coproporphyrinogen oxidase), and delta-aminolevulinic acid (ALA) dehydratase deficiency porphyria (ADP; >95% reduction in ALA dehydratase).
  - IAP, VP, and HCP are inherited as autosomal dominant syndromes; ADP is an autosomal recessive syndrome.
  - Carriers of the gene for IAP, VP, and HCP may have no manifestations or chronic but low-level manifestations (the majority), or acute attacks that may be life threatening.
  - Homozygotes for the gene causing ADP may be symptomatic frequently, commencing often in childhood. Heterozygotes may be liable for developing lead toxicity.
  - Precipitants of the acute attack are intercurrent illness, certain medications, environmental agents (eg, impurities in drinking water, organic solvents), dietary restriction, or hormonal fluctuations in the menstrual cycle. Often the cause is unknown.
- *Hereditary basis*
  - IAP, HCP, and VP—autosomal dominant, with low penetrance resulting from variable environmental stimuli. ADP—autosomal recessive; apparently exceedingly rare. Penetrance may approach 100%.
- *Differential diagnosis (Table 89-1)*
  - Manifestations are often nonspecific, and misdiagnosis is common.
  - Abdominal pain consistent with the pain of an acute porphyria is common in constipation, acute gastroenteritis, functional bowel disease, celiac disease, inflammatory bowel disease, pseudomembranous colitis (*Clostridium difficile* toxin), gall bladder disease, pancreatitis, etc.
  - The sympathomimetic manifestations resemble those in pheochromocytoma, thyrotoxicosis, delirium tremens, and neuroleptic malignant syndrome.
  - Ascending polyneuropathy is seen in Guillain-Barré syndrome.
  - The cutaneous manifestations of HCP and VP resemble those of porphyria cutanea tarda (PCT).
  - The possibility that an acute porphyria is responsible for the manifestations of an acute event can be resolved definitively by finding highly abnormal quantities of porphyrin precursors porphobilinogen (PBG) and/or ALA in a spot urine obtained during this attack. Marked elevations of PBG and/or ALA are the rule during an acute attack. Normal urinary PBG and/or ALA excretion rules out an acute porphyric attack.

## Diagnostic Criteria and Clinical Characteristics

### Historical Information:

- A relative with proven acute porphyria
- Intolerances to certain medications, such as oral contraceptives
- Episodic burgundy-colored urine that is not hematuria
- Episodes of abdominal or other pain of uncertain etiology, including premenstrual abdominal pain
- Episodes of ascending peripheral neuropathy
- Seasonal blistering of the skin in sun-exposed areas

### Clinical Characteristics:

- Chronic manifestations
  - Intermittent, recurrent body pain, usually in the abdomen or low back
  - Blistering and fragility of the skin of sun-exposed areas in some patients with VP, HCP

- Acute manifestations (acute attacks)
  - Significant pain, usually but not exclusively abdominal or low back
  - Nausea, vomiting, obstipation, ileus
  - Hypertension, tachycardia (sympathetic hyperactivity); orthostatic hypotension
  - Hyponatremia (usually syndrome of inappropriate antidiuretic hormone secretion [SIADH])
  - Varied psychiatric manifestations, including delirium, psychosis
  - Seizures
  - Loss of deep tendon reflexes, precursor to ascending poly-neuropathy (especially motor) leading to quadriplegia and respiratory paralysis

*Screening:* See Fig. 89-1. During a potential acute attack in a patient with an unknown diagnosis—test a spot urine for PBG (PBG Test Kit, Fisher Thermo Scientific, 800-766-7000; available in some hospital laboratories). If positive, or if the patient is a child,

**Table 89-1  Genetic Differential Diagnosis**

| Syndrome | Gene Symbol | Associated Findings[a] |
|---|---|---|
| Intermittent acute porphyria (IAP) | *PBGD* | Pain, hypertension, tachycardia, ascending polyneuropathy, hyponatremia, delirium. Urine ALA, PBG usually ↑↑ |
| Hereditary coproporphyria (HCP) | *CPO* | As in IAP, also occasional cutaneous blistering. Urine ALA, PBG ↑↑ during attack, often negative otherwise |
| Variegate porphyria (VP) | *PPO* | Same as HCP |
| ALA dehydratase deficiency porphyria (ADP) | *ALAD* | Similar to IAP, but manifestations more severe; tends to occur in young people. Urine ALA ↑↑, PBG normal |
| Lead toxicity | - | Similar to IAP. Urine ALA may be ↑, PBG normal. Elevated blood Pb concentration; decreased ALA dehydratase, reversed with Zn, SH-reducing agents |
| Tyrosinemia | *FAH* | Infantile severe hepatocellular dysfunction, cirrhosis, renal dysfunction, neurologic crises; urine ALA ↑↑, PBG normal. Blood screening (eg, newborn): elevated tyrosine, succinylacetone |

Gene names: *PBGD*, porphobilinogen deaminase (aka hydroxymethylbilane synthase); *CPO*, coproporphyrinogen oxidase; *PPO*, protoporphyrinogen oxidase; *ALAD*, delta-aminolevulinic acid dehydratase; *FAH*, fumarylacetoacetate hydrolase
[a]See Clinical Characteristics for details

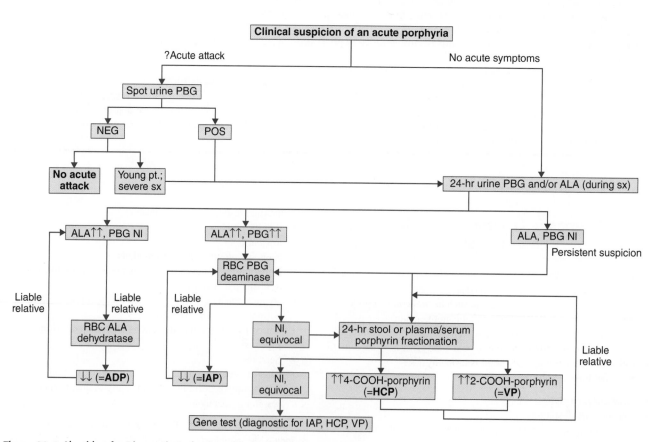

**Figure 89-1** Algorithm for Diagnostic Evaluation of Patients With Suspected Acute Porphyria.

follow with a quantitative analysis of a 24-hour urine for both PBG and ALA. For IAP, HCP, and VP, the acute attack is virtually always associated with daily excretion of greater than 20 mg, (increased ~4×), and usually greater than 50 mg (increased ~10×), of PBG, ALA. For ADP, ALA is similarly increased; PBG is not increased.

During a potential acute attack in a patient with a known acute porphyria: quantitative analysis of a 24-hour urine for PBG and/or ALA, for comparison with similar data when the patient was previously asymptomatic. Their excretion increases greater than or equal to twofold if elevated at baseline (IAP, ADP) or greater than or equal to fourfold if normal at baseline (VP, HCP).

To evaluate a patient with nonacute symptoms and no diagnosis 24-hour urine (best collected when patient has symptoms) PBG and/or ALA (>20 mg/d usually for IAP; similar elevation in ALA only in ADP; potentially ~normal for VP, HCP); 24-hour stool or plasma fractionation for specific porphyrins (marked elevations at all time of 4-carboxyl porphyrin [coproporphyrin] in HCP, and of 2-carboxyl porphyrin [protoporphyrin] in VP).

To screen members of a family in which an individual(s) has already been found to have a porphyria: use the studies that were diagnostic in the index case.

### Biochemical Corroboration of Type of Porphyria:

IAP—Erythrocyte porphobilinogen deaminase (hydroxymethylbilane synthase) assay. A few patients have normal activity of the erythrocyte enzyme, but a reduction in activity of the visceral (eg, hepatic) enzyme

ADP—Erythrocyte ALA dehydratase assay

HCP, VP—Quantitative stool (preferable) or plasma porphyrin fractionation

Reference Laboratories—Porphyria Laboratory, University of Texas Medical Branch, Galveston, TX; Tel 409-772-4661

Commercial laboratory—ARUP, Mayo, Quest

**Counseling** IAP, HCP, and VP are autosomal dominant diseases, with a 50% risk for inheriting the gene from an affected parent. Individuals with the gene rarely experience manifestations until after puberty. Penetrance varies with exposure to environmental stimuli, but is in the 10% to 30% range. There is no genotype-phenotype correlation.

ADP is an autosomal recessive, with a 25% risk to each offspring of heterozygous carrier parents. The likelihood of parental consanguinity may be increased. Affected individuals may be ascertained in childhood or early adulthood. Penetrance is not established, but it may approach 100%. A genotype-phenotype correlation may exist. Heterozygotes may be at increased risk for manifestations of lead toxicity.

Emphasis in counseling must include medications or drugs that may precipitate manifestations (databases of safe and unsafe drugs are available on line—eg, www.apfdrugdatabase.com), and possible exacerbating effects of incurrent illness or fasting. All care providers must be aware of the diagnosis, of the potential implications of certain medications, and of the need to deal expeditiously with individuals in whom an acute attack is identified. The risk for hepatocellular carcinoma may be increased.

## Management and Treatment

**General:** Patients *must*

1. Be educated concerning the causes and effects of the porphyria.
2. Avoid care providers who fail to become familiar with their porphyrias.

3. Have a low threshold for consulting their care providers if an acute porphyric attack may be developing, or if they have an intercurrent illness that may precipitate manifestations. Exacerbations may also vary with phase of the menstrual cycle.
4. Avoid severe dietary restriction, smoking, more than the occasional intake of an alcoholic beverage, or prolonged exposure to organic chemicals such as solvents.
5. Wear a MedicAlert bracelet or pendant.

Care providers *must*

1. Be well informed about causes, effects, and treatments of porphyria.

Patients and their care providers *must*

1. Exercise informed judgment regarding the use of drugs or medications; regularly consult an online porphyria drug database—for example, www.apfdrugdatabase.com.
2. Join the American Porphyria Foundation (www.porphyriafoundation.com) to remain current on new treatments and other developments.

### Specific Therapies for Acute Manifestations:

1. Remove the patient from the source of problems, if possible—for example, hospitalize. Discontinue potentially offending medications.
2. For individuals with early manifestations of an acute attack (eg, new pain): pharmacologic intake of carbohydrate—daily intake of greater than or equal to 300 g/d of carbohydrate in any form (PO, IV) to abort the attack. Oral Polycose (Polycose Glucose Polymers; Ross, Division of Abbott Laboratories) provides carbohydrate efficiently. Gonadotropin-releasing hormone analogs may be used to prevent premenstrual attacks.
3. Second line, for individuals with an advanced attack (changes in mental status, seizures, loss of peripheral deep tendon reflexes, ascending paralysis, sympathetic hyper-reactivity, and hyponatremia): hospitalize immediately. Carbohydrate, as above; intravenous heme arginate or hematin (Panhematin, Recordati Rare Diseases, 100 Corporate Drive, Lebanon, NJ 08833), 3 to 4 mg/kg/d, for 4 to 6 days, following clinical manifestations (including deep tendon reflexes, test of respiratory function) and daily urinary excretion of ALA and PBG; free water restriction (for SIADH); beta-blockers in modest dose (for sympathetic hyperactivity).

## Molecular Genetics and Molecular Mechanism

**Syndrome/Gene/Locus:** See Table 89-2.
ADP/ALA dehydratase/9q34
IAP/PBG deaminase/11q23-q24.2
HCP/coproporphyrinogen oxidase/3q11.2-q12
VP/protoporphyrinogen oxidase/1q21-q25

Clinical manifestations result from increased demand for heme, for example, for metabolism of a drug. Normally, this demand induces synthesis of ALA synthase, the rate-limiting enzyme, leading to increased heme production. With any of the acute porphyrias, symptoms may result from toxicity of excess product (? ALA) and/or deficiency of heme. In IAP, PBG deaminase (reduced ~50%) becomes rate limiting, leading to accumulation of ALA and PBG and potential heme deficiency. In HCP and VP, the enzymes

**TABLE 89-2  *Genes Associated With The Acute Porphyrias***

*Heme Pathway*

| Substrate/Product | Enzyme | Gene | Porphyria Type |
|---|---|---|---|
| Glycine + Succinate | ALA synthetase | ALAS1, ALAS2 | |
| ALA | ALA dehydratase | ALAD | ADP |
| PBG | PBG deaminase | PBGD | IAP |
| [Hydroxymethylbilane] | Uroporphyrinogen III synthase | UROS | |
| 8-COOH porphyrinogen * (uroporphyrinogen) | Uroporphyrinogen decarboxylase | UROD | |
| 4-COOH porphyrinogen * (coproporphyrinogen) | Coproporphyrinogen oxidase[†] | CPO | CP |
| 2-COOH  porphyrinogen * (protoporphyrinogen) | Protoporphyrinogen oxidase[†] | PPO | VP |
| 2-COOH porphyrin * (protoporphyrin IX) Heme | Ferrochelatase[†] | FECH | |

Each substrate is metabolized by the enzyme directly below it to a product, which is in turn metabolized similarly.

* Porphyrinogens, which are of the III isomeric series, autoxidize to porphyrins in urine, plasma, stool.

[†] Mitochondrial enzymes.  All other enzymes are cytosolic.

that are approximately 50% deficient are not rate limiting; the accumulation of ALA and PBG or the production of heme deficiency may result from porphyrin-mediated inhibition of PBGD. Excess porphyrins act as photosensitizers, causing the cutaneous manifestations in some individuals with CP and VP.

**Genetic Testing:** DNA sequence analysis is available for the genes for IAP, HCP, VP at the Porphyria DNA Testing Laboratory, Department of Genetics and Genomic Sciences, Mount Sinai School of Medicine (porphyria@mssm.edu.edu). Gene testing is most valuable in assessing asymptomatic relatives of affected individuals whose diagnosis has been made via biochemical means (*vide supra*), or in symptomatic individuals with suspected IAP and normal erythrocyte PBGD.

**Resources:** Expert help with the diagnosis and management of patients, including the interpretation of laboratory test results, can be accessed by contacting the American Porphyria Foundation, 4900 Woodway Drive, Suite 780, Houston Tx 77056. Tel 866-APF-3635; Fax 713-840-9552; www.porphyriafoundation.com.

### BIBLIOGRAPHY:

1. Desnick RJ, Bishop DF, Anderson KE. et al. Disorders of heme biosynthesis: X-linked sideroblastic anemia and the porphyrias. In: Valle D, et al., eds. *The Online Metabolic & Molecular Bases of Inherited Disease*. New York, NY: McGraw-Hill; 2006. http://www.ommbid.com. Part 13, Chapter 124.

2. Anderson KE, Bloomer JR, Bonkovsky HL, et al. Recommendations for the diagnosis and treatment of the acute porphyrias. *Ann Intern Med.* 2005;142:439-450.

3. Kauppinen R. Porphyrias. *Lancet.* 2005; 365:241-250.

4. Thunell S, Pomp E, Brun A. Guide to drug porphyrogenicity prediction and drug prescription in the acute porphyrias. *Br J Clin Pharmacol.* 2007;64:668-679.

5. Thunell S. Genomic approach to acute porphyria. *Physiol Res.* 2006;55(suppl 2):643-666.

6. Thunnell S. Hydroxymethylbilane synthase (HMBS) deficiency. *GeneReviews.* 2010; www.ncbi.nlm.nih.gov/bookshelf/br.fcgi?book=gene&part=aip

## Supplementary Information

### OMIM REFERENCES:

[1] Porphyria, Acute Intermittent; (#176000)

[2] Porphyria Variegata; (#176200)

[3] Porphyria, Acute Hepatic; (#612740)

[4] Coproporphyria, Hereditary; HCP (#121300)

[5] Hydroxymethylbilane Synthase; HMBS (#609806)

[6] Protoporphyrinogen Oxidase; PPOX (#600923)

[7] Delta-Aminolevulinate Dehydratase; ALAD (#125270)

[8] Coproporphyrinogen Oxidase; CPOX (#612732)

**Key Words:** Porphyria, acute, porphobilinogen, delta-aminolevulinic acid, PBG, ALA, porphyrin

# CUTANEOUS PORPHYRIAS

## KEY POINTS

- *Disease summary:*
  - All porphyrias, including the four porphyrias with cutaneous manifestations in sun or light-exposed skin, are diseases resulting from abnormalities of heme biosynthesis.
  - Porphyria cutanea tarda (PCT), the most common, is characterized by cutaneous bullae, friability, and scarring. In a minority of patients, PCT is inherited via a primary, approximately 50% reduction in activity of the enzyme uroporphyrinogen decarboxylase (UROD), either primarily or (rarely) secondarily. The remainder occurs in association with iron overload from coexistent *HFE* gene mutations, viral liver disease, exposure to chemicals, or other causes. Patients may develop liver cancer. Phlebotomy is the first-line treatment.
  - Erythropoietic protoporphyria (EPP) has both cutaneous and hepatic manifestations, commencing in early childhood: photosensitivity, with pain, burning, erythema, and edema; and hepatocellular disease and hepatic failure. The gene defect leads to either a deficiency in the enzyme ferrochelatase (FECH), or (rarely) a gain of function in erythrocyte ALA synthase 2 (ALAS2). Treatment with beta-carotene is modestly effective.
  - Congenital erythropoietic porphyria (CEP) and hepatoerythropoietic porphyria (HEP) are similar lifelong syndromes, most often with erosive cutaneous manifestations leading to necrosis of skin and skin appendages (eg, nose, auricle, and finger) and anemia. CEP results from an inherited deficiency in the enzyme uroporphyrinogen III synthase (UROS) either primarily or (very rarely) secondarily (mutation in the transcription factor *GATA1*). HEP is a deficiency (usually >90%) of UROD, the enzyme also deficient in hereditary PCT. Bone marrow transplantation can be curative.
- *Hereditary and Nonhereditary basis:*
  - **PCT**—Autosomal dominant in a minority of cases (type II PCT). The majority are sporadic (type I). The common causal factor is excessive visceral iron storage, resulting from heterozygosity or homozygosity for the HFE *C282Y* gene mutation or viral liver disease. A very rare form (type III) is also familial, but its basis is unknown.
  - **EPP**—Autosomal dominant. Small numbers are inherited as X-lined dominant (a gain-of-function mutation in *ALAS2*) or autosomal recessive (unknown source), and rare cases have no known hereditary basis.
  - **CEP, HEP—Autosomal recessive.**
- *Differential diagnosis (Table 89-3):*
  - The cutaneous lesions of these three different types of porphyrias—PCT, EPP, and CEP or HEP—are dissimilar.
  - **PCT**—Lesions, including bullae, are virtually identical in variegate porphyria (VP) and coproporphyria (HCP). VP and HCP are also characterized by acute attacks, and differences in porphyrin excretion and gene pathology.
  - **EPP**—Bullae are rare, but manifestations resemble those seen with hydroa vacciniforme (recurrent vesicles in sun-exposed skin in children), phototoxic drug reactions (pain, burning, erythema, blistering), solar urticaria (pruritic, edematous, erythematous patches at any time of life), contact dermatitis (pruritis, erythema, edema, possibly vesicles and bullae), and angioedema (painful, pruritic welts).
  - **CEP**—Lesions are almost always uniquely severe and destructive, and are accompanied by discolored teeth (erythrodontia) and anemia. CEP causes a nonimmune hydrops fetalis; the pink/red/brown amniotic fluid contains a markedly increased concentration of porphyrin. A minority of patients may have milder manifestations similar to PCT.
  - **HEP**—Similar to CEP, but patients are less likely to have erythrodontia or anemia.

## Diagnostic Criteria and Clinical Characteristics

*Historical Information:* A detailed family history is essential.

☞**PCT:** Adult onset of blistering, friability and scarring of sun-exposed skin during warm seasons; facial hypertrichosis; exposure to polyhalogenated chemicals, hepatitis or HIV viruses, iron in diet (eg, in vitamins), alcohol excess, estrogens; renal failure and/or on hemodialysis; diagnosis of hemochromatosis.

☞**EPP:** Onset in infancy; pain, burning, stinging, redness, swelling, petechiae; relation to sun exposure and avoidance; cholelithiasis and/or hepatic dysfunction.

☞**CEP, HEP:** Onset usually in infancy; cutaneous blistering, fragility, infections, scarring; discolored teeth; colored urine; anemia; acquired deformities of skin appendages; with adult onset, blistering, fragility, and some scarring only; other intercurrent illnesses—for example, hepatitis.

*Clinical Characteristics:*

☞**PCT:** Aged-appearing sun-exposed skin, with vesicles, bullae, scarring, lacerations; facial hypertrichosis; hepatomegaly in older patients

☞**EPP:** Exposure to ultraviolet (UV) light immediately induces the manifestations as described; long-term, leathery, thickened skin, hyperkeratosis; in some patients, manifestations of biliary obstruction (jaundice, abdominal pain), hepatic dysfunction or failure

☞**CEP, HEP:** Hydrops fetalis with pink, red, or brown-colored amniotic fluid; red or brown urine on diaper; early-onset cutaneous vesicles, bullae, scarring, hyper- or hypopigmentation; deformities of skin appendages; corneal clouding; reddish teeth that fluoresce

*Table 89-3* **Genetic Differential Diagnosis**

| Syndrome | Gene Symbol | Associated Findings[a,b] |
|---|---|---|
| Porphyria cutanea tarda (PCT) | *UROD* | Cutaneous bullae, fragility/friability No acute neurovisceral Sx. Urine uroporphyrin ↑↑, ALA/PBG normal |
| Hereditary coproporphyria (HCP) | *CPO* | Same cutaneous manifestations, when present, as PCT; acute attacks. ALA/PBG ↑↑ during attack. Stool coproporphyrin ↑↑ |
| Variegate porphyria (VP) | *PPO* | Like HCP except stool protoporphyrin ↑↑ |
| Erythropoietic protoporphyria (EPP) | *FECH, ALAS2* | Painful cutaneous erythema, edema, petechiae, stinging, burning; usually starts in infancy. Occasionally, hepatic dysfunction/failure. RBC-free protoporphyrin ↑↑ |
| Congenital erythropoietic porphyria (CEP) | *UROS, GATA1* | Variable—(a) hydrops fetalis; (b) early-onset of cutaneous bullae, vesicles, friability, scarring, deformities; erythrodontia; hemolytic anemia; (c) later-onset (rare) milder skin findings similar to PCT. Anemia. Urine uroporphyrin I, urine, fecal coproporphyrin I ↑↑ |
| Hepatoerythropoietic porphyria (HEP) | *UROD* | Early- and later-onset skin, hematologic findings similar to CEP. Urine, fecal isocoproporphyrin ↑↑ |

Gene names: *UROD*, uroporphyrinogen decarboxylase; *CPO*, coproporphyrinogen oxidase; *PPO*, protoporphyrinogen oxidase; *FECH*, ferrochelatase; *ALAS2*, delta-aminolevulinic acid synthase 2; *UROS*, uroporphyrinogen III synthase; *GATA1*, transcription factor GATA1.

[a]See Clinical Characteristics for details.

[b]All cutaneous manifestations occur on sun- or light-exposed skin.

ALA, delta-aminolevulinic acid; PBG, porphobilinogen.

with Wood lamp; splenomegaly; later-onset (youth, adulthood) cutaneous vesicles, bullae, friability, scarring, hypertrichosis

# Screening and Counseling

***Screening (Table 89-4):***
☞**PCT:**
Establishing the diagnosis: 24-hour urinary porphyrin fractionation (uroporphyrin ↑↑, often >1000 µg/d), or plasma porphyrin (↑↑; fluorescence emission peak of ~620 nm, consistent with uroporphyrin)
Determining risk factors for manifestations: ferritin (elevated, reflecting increased hepatic iron stores), viral (hepatitis C and B, HIV) studies (associated particularly with hepatitis C infection), fasting serum Fe/iron-binding capacity, *HFE* genotyping (associated with one or two copies of the *C282Y* and possibly the *H63D* mutation), alpha-fetoprotein (hepatoma screen)
Family member screening: history, examination, urine or plasma total porphyrin, and (if elevated) porphyrin fractionation
Analyses of the UROD enzyme and/or gene are available.
☞**EPP:**
Establishing the diagnosis: plasma total porphyrin (↑↑; fluorescence emission peak of ~634 nm, consistent with protoporphyrin); erythrocyte total porphyrin (↑↑, almost exclusively free protoporphyrin)
Determining secondary phenomena, risk factors: complete blood count (CBC), liver function tests (LFTs), hepatitis virus studies, *HFE* genotyping if indicated, hepatic imaging, serum 25-hydroxy vitamin D
Family member screening: primarily history, examination; plasma total porphyrins

Analyses for mutant enzymes are not available. Genotyping of *FECH* and *ALAS2* is available.
☞**CEP:**
Establishing the diagnosis: examination of skin and appendages is almost always diagnostic of CEP or HEP; amniotic fluid (from hydrops fetalis) or plasma total porphyrin analysis (↑↑, with fluorescence emission peak at ~620 nm); 24-hour stool porphyrins (coproporphyrin I ↑↑)
Anemia evaluation: hemolysis studies
Determining risk for CEP in a fetus: amniotic fluid total porphyrin analysis (↑↑ porphyrins with fluorescence peak of ~620 nm) or *UROS* gene mutation analysis of amniocytes or chorionic villus cells
Family member screening: history, examination, plasma total porphyrins
☞**HEP:** As per CEP except for results of 24-hour stool porphyrin analysis (isocoproporphyrin ↑↑)
***Corroboration of Type of Porphyria:***
☞**PCT:** Aforementioned studies are usually sufficient. If necessary, erythrocyte UROD enzyme assay or *UROD* genotyping (diagnostic in type II PCT only) is done.
☞**EPP:** Aforementioned studies are usually sufficient. Gene testing is done, if necessary.
☞**CEP:** Clinical examination and the aforementioned studies are usually sufficient. For adults who have a mild illness, differentiation from PCT can be made on the basis of the isomeric form of fecal coproporphyrin (~entirely the I series for CEP, predominantly the III series for PCT). Gene testing is available.
☞**HEP:** Clinical examination and the aforementioned studies are usually sufficient. Differentiation of HEP from PCT and CEP in patients with mild illness is made by finding ↑↑ fecal isocoproporphyrin. Activity of the erythrocyte enzyme UROD is reduced 40% to 60% in subjects with hereditary PCT, greater than 75% in HEP. Gene testing is available.

**Table 89-4** *Algorithm for Diagnostic Evaluation of Patient With Suspected Cutaneous Porphyria*

Sources for biochemical or enzyme analysis or gene testing: see Resources.

*Counseling:*

☞**PCT:** Type II PCT (autosomal dominant): The risk is 50% to each and every offspring for inheriting the gene, the penetrance of which is unknown. A fraction of individuals with sporadic PCT do in fact have type II PCT; *UROD* genotyping is diagnostic if this is important to family members. Symptomatic individuals should avoid all exogenous risk factors predisposing to the clinical syndrome. All should comply with treatment, the aim of which is to remove excess iron, normalize porphyrin economy, and minimize the liability for hepatoma.

☞**EPP:** Most cases result from a mutation in one of the *FECH* genes. A change in the second *FECH* gene (a hypomorphic *FECH* IVS3-48C allele, with a prevalence of ~10%) is also required for manifestations, however. Thus, the overall likelihood that each offspring of an affected parent will develop symptomatic EPP is approximately 2.5%. If both parents carry a mutant *FECH* gene but are asymptomatic (lacking the hypomorphic allele) a double dose of the mutation may be required for symptomatic disease. This liability is less than or equal to 25% (autosomal recessive), depending on penetrance, for each offspring. For EPP from the *ALAS2* mutation, the liability is 50% to each and every offspring for inheriting the mutation and, probably, the syndrome.

☞**CEP, HEP:** Each offspring of heterozygous parents has a 25% liability of being a homozygote for the gene, and presumably affected.

Avoiding sun or light exposure is a critical but usually insufficient means of retarding the progression of disease.

## Management and Treatment

- Patients and their care providers should join the American Porphyria Foundation, to keep current on issues and progress.
- Patients should wear a MedicAlert bracelet or pendant.
- Neither care providers nor patients should confuse the cutaneous porphyrias with the acute porphyrias, particularly with regard to the use of medications (few are harmful in the cutaneous porphyrias) and treatment.
- **Patients should avoid light**, avoidance being proportional to the level of cutaneous pathology. This is absolutely critical. Wearing protective clothing should be helpful; the use of topical sunscreens is of dubious value.

☞**PCT:** General: multivitamins. Avoid ingesting iron in nonessential quantities, alcohol intake, smoking, other pathogenic environmental agents (often occupational; eg, polyhalogenated hydrocarbons). Monitor liver chemistries, including alpha-fetoprotein, and hepatic imaging. Treat coexistent hepatitis C (usually after phlebotomy treatment of the PCT, if still indicated) or HIV.

First-line treatment (also for hemochromatosis): phlebotomy, of 1 U biweekly. Monitor skin findings, and serum ferritin + 24-hour

*Table 89-5  Genes Associated With the Cutaneous Porphyrias*

| Heme Pathway | Gene | Porphyria Type |
|---|---|---|
| Glycine + succinate | | |
| ↓ ALA synthase | ALAS1 | |
| | ALAS2 | EPP[a] |
| ALA | | |
| ↓ ALA dehydratase | ALAD | PBG |
| ↓ PBG deaminase | PBGD | |
| Hydroxymethylbilane | | |
| ↓ Uroporphyrinogen III synthase | UROS | CEP |
| | GATA1 | |
| 8-COOH porphyrinogen (uroporphyrinogen III)[b] | | |
| ↓ Uroporphyrinogen decarboxylase | UROD | PCT, HEP[c] |
| 4-COOH porphyrinogen (Coproporphyrinogen III)[b] | | |
| ↓ Coproporphyrinogen oxidase[d] | CPO | |
| 2-COOH porphyrinogen (protoporphyrinogen IX)[b] | | |
| ↓ Protoporphyrinogen oxidase[d] | PPO | |
| 2-COOH porphyrin (protoporphyrin IX) | | |
| ↓ Ferrochelatase[d] | FECH | EPP |
| Heme | | |

[a]Gain-of-function mutation.

[b]Porphyrinogens autoxidize to porphyrins in urine, plasma, stool.

[c]The enzyme deficiency in all tissues in type II PCT is 40% to 60% and in HEP is greater than 75%. In type I PCT, enzyme deficiency is found in liver only.

[d]Mitochondrial enzymes. All other enzymes are cytosolic.

urinary uroporphyrin excretion to gauge iron and porphyrin removal, respectively. Stop phlebotomy when the serum ferritin decreases to low or subnormal level and uroporphyrin excretion decreases to a near-normal level. Repeat these tests, initially at intervals of 3 to 6 months, to ascertain recurring abnormalities and the need for reinstituting phlebotomy. Clinical or chemical abnormalities often do not recur, and the interval between these surveillance testings can be lengthened.

Occasional patients cannot be phlebotomized. The second line active treatment is oral hydroxychloroquine (200 mg twice weekly), administered with the same surveillance. Iron chelators are used rarely. Patients with PCT related to hemodialysis may achieve remission with erythropoietin and/or small volume phlebotomies.

☞**EPP:** General: multivitamins, vitamin D (if serum vitamin D levels are low), oral iron (only for documented iron deficiency). Photosensitivity: oral beta-carotene (Lumitine, 30-300 mg/d, adjusted over several weeks according to response of symptoms). Liver disease: avoid alcohol or illicit drug intake. Immunize for hepatitis. Monitor liver chemistries, alpha-fetoprotein, hepatic imaging. Patients with worsening liver function or photosensitivity require close observation. Provide prompt medical attention for abdominal pain, jaundice, acholic stools, and change in mental status. No treatment of protoporphyric hepatic failure has yet been proven optimal, but liver transplantation can be considered.

☞**CEP:** Avoidance of light applies even to neonates, who may be subjected to UV light therapy. Protect skin from trauma, and treat dermatologic infections (often with bacteremia) appropriately.

Marrow suppression with frequent transfusions (and removal of excess iron by phlebotomy) and bone marrow transplantation have been effective therapies in a limited number of patients.

☞**HEP:** Routine treatments are those for CEP. Phlebotomy is not effective. Affected individuals may be liable for the development of hepatoma, as is the case with PCT.

## Molecular Genetics and Molecular Mechanism

***Syndrome/Gene/Locus:*** See Table 89-5.

PCT, HEP/uroporphyrinogen decarboxylase/1p34

EPP/ferrochelatase/18q21.3; delta-aminolevulinate synthase 2/Xp11.21

CEP/uroporphyrinogen III synthase/10q25.2-q26.3; GATA1/Xp11.23

***Common Denominator:*** The common factor causing the cutaneous pathology is the interaction of light, either natural or artificial (UV), with porphyrins that are deposited in large quantities in pericapillary areas. This interaction leads to the development of reactive oxygen species that are toxic and destructive.

☞**PCT, HEP:** The excess hepatic iron stores may underlie the development of occasional hepatoma in PCT (and possibly HEP), since this contributes to hepatic oncogenesis in hemochromatosis and hepatitis C infection. The long-term hepatic deposition of uroporphyrin may further inflict injury.

☞**EPP:** Protoporphyrin accumulates from either the inhibition of its further metabolism (from the combination of FECH deficiency and the "hypomorphic" *FECH* IVS3-88C allele) or its overproduction (from the *ALSA2* gain-of-function mutation). The large quantities of protoporphyrin produced or deposited (from erythroid cells) in the liver are excreted through the biliary tree into the bowel. Protoporphyrin may precipitate in the bile ducts, leading to ductal occlusion or gallstone formation. Much of this excreted protoporphyrin is redeposited in the liver via the enterohepatic circulation, leading to permanent accumulation of protoporphyrin and liver damage (mechanism unknown).

☞**CEP:** The porphyrin precursor hydroxymethylbilane is shunted to the nonenzymatic and nonmetabolizable I isomeric series, with formation of large quantities of uroporphyrinogen or uroporphyrin I and coproporphyrinogen or coproporphyrin I. The porphyrins that accumulate in marrow damage and destroy erythroid cells, as evidenced by hemolysis.

*Resources:* Expert help with the diagnosis, management, and support of patients is available at

The American Porphyria Foundation
4900 Woodway Drive, Suite 780
Houston Tx 77056
Tel 866-APF-3635
Fax 713-840-9551
www.porphyriafoundation.com
For EPP, additional information is available through the EPP Research and Education Fund
Channing Laboratory, Brigham and Women's Hospital
181 Longwood Avenue
Boston, MA 02115
Tel 617-525-8259 (Dr. Micheline Mathews-Roth)
www.brighamandwomens.org/EPAPRF

**Biochemical Analysis**

Porphyria Laboratory
University of Texas Medical Branch
Galveston TX.
Tel 409-772-4661
Fax 409-772-6287
kanderso@utmb.edu (Dr. Karl E. Anderson)
Dr. Anderson can provide guidance on analyte and/or enzyme testing.

**Gene Testing**

Porphyria DNA Testing Laboratory
Department of Genetics and Genomic Sciences

Mount Sinai School of Medicine
New York NY
Tel. 212-241-7518
Fax 212-659-6780
porphyria@mssm.edu.edu (Robert J Desnick, MD, PhD)

**BIBLIOGRAPHY:**

1. Desnick RJ, Bishop DF, Anderson KE., et al. Disorders of heme biosynthesis: X-linked sideroblastic anemia and the porphyrias. In: Valle D, et al., eds. *The Online Metabolic & Molecular Bases of Inherited Disease.* New York, NY: McGraw-Hill; 2006. www.ommbid.com. Part 13, Chapter 124.

2. Anstey AV, Hift RJ. Liver disease in erythropoietic protoporphyria: insights and implications for management. *Gut.* 2007;56:1009-10018.

3. Lecha M, Puy H, Deybach JC. Erythropoietic protoporphyria. *Orphanet J Rare Dis.* 2009;4:19.

4. Desnick RJ, Astrin KH. Congenital erythropoietic porphyria: advances in pathogenesis and treatment. *Br J Haematol.* 2002;117: 779-795.

5. Phillips JD, Steensma DP, Pulsipher MA, Spangrude GJ, Kushner JP. Congenital erythropoietic porphyria due to a mutation in GATA1: the first *trans*-activating mutation causative for a human porphyria. *Blood.* 2007;109:2618-2621.

6. Granata BX, Parera VE, Melito VA, Teijo MJ, Batlle AM, Rossetti MV. The very first description of a patient with hepatoerythropoietic porphyria in Argentina. Biochemical and molecular studies. *Cell Mol Biol (Noisy-le-grand).* 2009:55:61-65.

## Supplementary Information

**OMIM REFERENCES:**

[1] Porphyria Cutanea Tarda; (#176100)

[2] Protoporphyria, Erythropoietic; (#177000)

[3] Protoporphyria, Erythropoietic, X-Linked Dominant, XLDPP; (#300752)

[4] Porphyria, Congenital Erythropoietic; (#263700)

[5] Porphyria, Hepatoerythropoietic; (#176100)

[6] Delta-Aminolevulinate Synthase 2; ALAS2; (#301300)

[7] Uroporphyrinogen III Synthase; UROS; (#606938)

[8] Ferrochelatase; FECH; (#612386)

*Key Words:* Porphyria, cutaneous, congenital, light-sensitive

# 90 Hyperhomocysteinemia

James Weisfeld-Adams and Brian Kirmse

## KEY POINTS

- *Disease summary:*
  - Homocysteine (Hcy) is a sulfur-containing amino acid whose metabolism stands at an intersection of two biochemical pathways. A remethylation pathway converts Hcy to methionine, and requires the presence of folate and vitamin $B_{12}$, while a trans-sulfuration pathway converts Hcy to cystathionine and cysteine in a reaction requiring vitamin $B_6$.
  - Important monogenic forms of hyperhomocysteinemia (HHcy) include the following:
  - Cystathionine beta-synthase (CBS) deficiency, also known as classic homocystinuria, is associated with a skeletal and ocular phenotype similar to Marfan syndrome, as well as variable developmental delay and a strong predisposition to thromboembolism; around 50% of cases respond to supplementation with vitamin $B_6$.
  - Disorders of $B_{12}$ metabolism: several disorders of intermediary cobalamin metabolism (CblC, CblD, CblE, CblF, and CblG diseases) as well as transcobalamin deficiency can cause moderate-to-severe HHcy; treatment is centered around daily hydroxocobalamin.
  - Mutations and common polymorphisms of methylenetetrahydrofolate reductase (*MTHFR*) cause HHcy of variable severity in both the homo- and heterozygous states.
  - Multifactorial HHcy is also associated with a range of common adult diseases including thrombophilia, coronary artery disease, stroke, neuropsychiatric disease, and osteoporosis.
- *Hereditary basis:*
  - CBS deficiency, most cobalamin disorders and MTHFR deficiency follow autosomal recessive inheritance. Milder forms of HHcy follow complex or multifactorial patterns of inheritance.
- *Twin studies:*
  - In a large Danish twin study, the impact of the *MTHFR* locus was estimated to explain 53% of the total phenotypic variation in Hcy concentrations in persons 18 to 39 years old, and 24% in persons 40 to 65 years old, that is, almost all additive genetic variance. Hcy concentrations have a high heritability that decreases with age.
- *Genome-wide association studies (GWAS):*
  - Significant genome-wide associations have been found between total homocysteine (tHcy) and single-nucleotide polymorphisms (SNPs) located near *GPR51* (9q22) and *MTHFR* (1p36). A GWAS looking at the coronary artery disease phenotype noted an association with MTHFD1L, which is important in methionine-homocysteine metabolism.
- *Pharmacogenomics:*
  - Common *MTHFR* polymorphisms (677C>T and 1298A>C) confer increased sensitivity to fluoropyrimidines (eg, 5-FU) and antifolates (eg, methotrexate).

## Diagnostic Criteria and Clinical Characteristics

**Definitions and Epidemiology:** Severe HHcy is generally restricted to individuals with inherited disorders of Hcy metabolism, is defined as tHcy greater than 100 mmol/L. The most recognized etiology of severe HHcy is CBS deficiency, causing classic homocystinuria. In 1975, the first description of CBS deficiency and its association with thrombophilia leading to early stroke and heart attack in untreated patients led the medical community to suspect milder elevations of Hcy as a contributing factor to atherosclerosis pathogenesis. In the general population, this suspicion has been corroborated through large epidemiologic trials, although Hcy is not currently viewed as an important risk factor.

Mild HHcy is variably defined as tHcy of 12 to 30 mmol/L, and in some literature as 15 to 30 mmol/L while moderate HHcy is defined as tHcy 30 to 100 mmol/L. Mild-to-moderate HHcy of multifactorial etiology appears to be highly prevalent in the general population. The prevalence has been estimated at 5% to 10%, but may be significantly higher (30%-40%) among elderly individuals. HHcy is more common among males and persons with increased muscle mass. HHcy has been observed in the context of disruption of function affecting enzymes of folate metabolism (MTHFR, methionine synthase [MS], methionine synthase reductase [MSR]). Of these, MTHFR is the most significant from a population-wide perspective. Severe HHcy from homozygosity for mutations in *MTHFR* are rare, although the common 677C>T polymorphism is known to cause increased thermolability of the enzyme which may lead to mild HHcy, particularly in the folate-depleted state.

Factors that may influence plasma tHcy include *MTHFR* genotype, acquired folate, $B_6$, or $B_{12}$ deficiencies (dietary inadequacy or malabsorption), medications (insulin, anticonvulsants, lipid-lowering agents, metformin, vitamin $B_6$ antagonists, penicillamine, nitrous oxide), and lifestyle factors including exercise, tobacco consumption, caffeine intake, and alcohol use.

### Clinical Characteristics of Monogenic Disorders Resulting in Hyperhomocysteinemia (Table 90-1):

☞**CBS DEFICIENCY:** This is a rare disease causing severe HHcy with an incidence of 1 in approximately 340,000 live births, though is much common in certain regions (incidence 1:3000 in indigenous Qatari population; 1:65,000 in Ireland and parts of New South Wales, Australia). The enzyme, CBS, is active in several tissues (liver, brain, pancreas, cultured fibroblasts). When CBS is nonfunctional, accumulating Hcy molecules readily form

**Table 90-1 Monogenic Disorders Resulting in Hyperhomocysteinemia**

| Disease | Gene | Locus | OMIM Entries | Common Mutations/ Polymorphisms | Genotype-Phenotype Correlations and Allele Frequency in Certain Populations |
|---|---|---|---|---|---|
| MTHFR deficiency | MTHFR | 1p36.3 | 607093 236250 | 677C>T 1298A>C | Mexico 0.57 Southern Italy 0.51 China 0.45 African American 0.1 South Indian Tamil 0.39 Ireland 0.37 |
| CBS deficiency | CBS | 21q22-23 | 236200 | R336C ($B_6$ nonresponsive) T191M ($B_6$ nonresponsive) G307S ($B_6$ nonresponsive) I278T ($B_6$ responsive) | Homozygosity is estimated 1/3000 in Qatari population Accounts for >50% mutant alleles in Spain, Portugal, Columbia, Venezuela Accounts for >70% of mutant alleles in Ireland Homozygosity is estimated 1/20,500 in Danish population |
| CblC | MMACHC | 1p34.1 | 277400 | 271dupA R111X R132X R161Q | 40% of alleles, esp Mediterranean populations, associated with early-onset disease Early-onset disease Late-onset disease Late-onset disease |
| CblD | MMADHC | 2q23.2 | 277410 611935 | Several described in case reports | Limited information |
| CblE | ?MTR | 5p15.3 | 236270 | S545L | Associated with milder predominantly hematologic phenotype in European patients |
| CblG | MTR | 1p43 | 250940 | Several case reports | Limited information available |

dimeric complexes with methionine, cysteine, and other Hcy molecules, including proteins comprising sulfide-containing amino acids.

Infants with CBS deficiency are typically normal at birth. The spectrum of clinical findings in the *untreated* individual is wide and affects a variety of organ systems, outlined below:

- *Vascular:* Arterial and venous thromboembolism are common in CBS deficiency, and account for the majority of morbidity and mortality. Thrombophlebitis and pulmonary embolism are the most common vascular complications. Thrombosis of medium and large arteries is a frequent cause of death. When CBS deficiency is compounded by the presence of alleles at other loci linked to increased risk of vascular disease (677C>T mutation of *MTHFR* gene; *R506Q* mutation of factor V Leiden gene), tendency toward thromboembolism increases further.
- *Ocular:* Ectopia lentis, myopia, and glaucoma are frequent manifestations, with cataracts, retinal detachment, and optic atrophy occurring as later complications. Ectopia lentis, which is usually inferolateral in orientation (differentiating it from the type observed in Marfan syndrome), is detectable by 5 to 10 years of age and serves as a useful diagnostic clue. After dislocation has occurred, iridodonesis (tremulous movements of the iris with eye or head movement) may be observed.
- *Osseous:* Osteoporosis is invariably detectable after puberty, and often earlier. Affected individuals may develop scoliosis and

vertebral collapse. CBS deficiency is associated with tall stature with thinning and elongation of long bones and enlarged epiphyses and metaphyses, often most evident at the knees. Many patients have pes cavus, genu valgum or pectus carinatum/excavatum. Joint mobility is typically restricted. Body habitus is often described as marfanoid. Radiologic findings include flattened intervertebral discs, growth arrest lines in the distal tibia, enlarged carpal bones, and short fourth metacarpals.

- *Neurodevelopmental:* About 60% of untreated patients have variable degrees of mental retardation and developmental delay. Seizures, subclinical EEG abnormalities and psychiatric symptoms are all common in untreated patients. Neurocognitive morbidity is greatly reduced when treatment is initiated early. Cerebrovascular disease is significantly more prevalent than in the general population.
- *CBS deficiency in pregnancy:* One study of 15 pregnancies in 11 women with CBS deficiency (six pyridoxine responsive, five pyridoxine nonresponsive) reported the birth of 10 healthy infants. One infant had multiple anomalies at birth and another was later diagnosed with Beckwith-Wiedemann syndrome (BWS). Two women suffered pre-eclampsia and another suffered from superficial venous thrombosis. Two pregnancies ended in spontaneous first trimester miscarriage. No relationship was established between biochemical derangements observed during pregnancy and pregnancy outcomes.

☞**DISORDERS OF VITAMIN B$_{12}$ (COBALAMIN) METABOLISM:** Vitamin B$_{12}$ is an essential cofactor for the enzyme methionine synthase, which catalyzes the conversion of Hcy to methionine. Several inherited disorders of vitamin B$_{12}$ metabolism result in hyperhomocysteinemia with or without methylmalonic acidemia (MMA). CblC (homocystinuria with methylmalonic acidemia) is the commonest of this group, and has been ascribed to mutations in the *MMACHC* gene, located at 1p34.1, causing impaired production of methylcobalamin (MeCbl) and adenosylcobalamin (AdoCbl). CblC, D, and F diseases are characterized biochemically by HHcy, hypomethioninemia, and MMA. CblE and CblG diseases cause HHcy without MMA. Although variable, clinical manifestations of CblC are unlike those of either isolated homocystinuria or isolated MMA. The commonest presentation is in early infancy, manifesting as a progressive neurologic syndrome with hematologic, ophthalmologic, and cardiac features. More rarely, symptomatic onset of CblC occurs later in childhood or in adulthood with neuropsychiatric disturbance or dementia. Adult-onset patients may also have megaloblastic anemia, glomerulopathy, and myelopathy. Brain magnetic resonance imaging (MRI) may reveal leukodystrophy. In CblC, tHcy is typically elevated into the 30 to 100 mmol/L range when well and on treatment, but may be greater than 100 mmol/L when ill.

☞**SEVERE MTHFR DEFICIENCY:** When present in the homozygous state, severe mutations of *MTHFR* (such as 1129C>T) cause severe HHcy, infantile-onset neurologic deterioration with seizures, mental retardation, and developmental delay.

☞**POLYMORPHISMS IN MTHFR:** The C677T variant of *MTHFR* has been associated with a decreased activity of *MTHFR*, an increased level of Hcy and altered distribution of folate. The 1298A>C polymorphism has been related to reduced MTHFR activity, but its effects are considered to be less potent than those of the 677C>T variant.

### Clinical Characteristics of Mild Hyperhomocysteinemia:

☞**CARDIOVASCULAR AND CEREBROVASCULAR DISEASE:** HHcy of the magnitude observed in individuals with CBS deficiency was first associated with vascular disease almost 50 years ago, and prompted work leading to later observations that milder HHcy might also have a role in atherosclerosis. Since then, a growing body of evidence has emerged implicating HHcy, either alone or acting in association with other thrombophilic risk factors, as an important risk factor for ischemic heart disease, stroke, and other vascular occlusive disease. It has been suggested that Hcy may affect the evolution of vascular disease by a variety of mechanisms including increased propensity to thrombosis, impaired thrombolysis, increased production of hydrogen peroxide, platelet dysfunction, endothelial dysfunction, and increased oxidation of low-density lipoprotein.

The extent of the causal role of milder HHcy in the pathogenesis of atherosclerosis is a subject of intense debate. In 1995, a meta-analysis demonstrated that elevated plasma tHcy was associated with an increased risk of atherosclerotic vascular disease in the coronary, cerebral, and peripheral circulations. It was estimated that about 10% of coronary heart disease in the general population might be attributable to HHcy. The authors also estimated that a 5 mmol/L increase in tHcy was associated with an increase in vascular risk of about one-third, which is of similar magnitude to an increase in plasma cholesterol of 0.5 mmol/L. Other specific studies conducted since have shown that HHcy is associated with increased risk of vascular disease multiplicative to other risk factors, that relative risk of myocardial infarction (MI) is 3.1 when Hcy

levels exceed the 95th percentile of control values, and that there is a strong, graded relationship between tHcy and mortality. Evidence from patients with cardiovascular disease showed that up to 40% of patients diagnosed with premature coronary artery disease, peripheral vascular disease, or recurrent venous thrombosis have HHcy at presentation. Several large meta-analyses have demonstrated the association of HHcy and risk of cerebral ischemia, with the finding that lowering tHcy by 3 mmol/L decreases risk of cerebral ischemia by 19% to 24%. More recently, HHcy has been associated with atherothrombosis risk in a growing number of specific patient populations (thrombosis in diabetic patients, hypercoagulable state in renal transplant patients and hemodialysis patients).

In contrast to these findings, numerous studies suggest that the link between Hcy and vascular disease may be less significant than previous commentators have suggested. Examples include a retrospective study showing that there is no statistical difference in tHcy between individuals who developed MI and those who did not, and a prospective finding of no association between tHcy and MI. Recently, a meta-analysis of observational studies suggested that elevated tHcy is at most a modest independent predictor of ischemic heart disease and stroke risk in healthy populations. Due to the volume of conflicting data on this subject, and since many studies have shown that successful Hcy-lowering strategies do not significantly lower cardiovascular risk (see later), many commentators suggest that relevance of Hcy is only as a marker for disease and may be an "innocent bystander" in disease pathogenesis.

☞**NEUROPSYCHIATRIC DISEASE:** In animal models and cell culture, Hcy demonstrates neurotoxicity. Postulated mechanisms include choline depletion, N-methyl-D-aspartate (NMDA) receptor activation, and DNA damage. Neuropsychiatric symptoms and signs are frequent findings in individuals with inborn errors of Hcy metabolism. Nutritional causes of HHcy (especially folate and B$_{12}$ deficiencies) can also cause neurologic sequelae in children and adults. Babies breastfed by mothers with B$_{12}$ deficiency, for example due to a vegan diet, can suffer serious and irreversible central nervous system (CNS) damage. In recent years, several neurologic diseases have been associated with abnormal Hcy metabolism and HHcy. Since the majority of these diseases have their highest prevalence among elderly persons, HHcy may be of pronounced importance in the elderly.

Patients with dementia and memory impairment show lower levels of folate and B$_{12}$, and higher tHcy in plasma and cerebrospinal fluid (CSF). tHcy levels are associated with the severity of cognitive, physical, and social impairments in demented persons. A trial that enrolled 1092 dementia-free subjects from the Framingham cohort with extended follow-up confirmed that increased plasma tHcy is a strong, graded, and independent risk factor for the development of dementia of Alzheimer type (AD). An increment of tHcy of 5 mmol/L increased the risk of AD by approximately 40%. The association appeared to be independent of age, sex, APOE genotype, plasma vitamin levels, and other risk factors for AD. The association may be related to a proposed vascular pathogenesis for AD, since several studies have shown that HHcy may also be an important factor in the pathogenesis of cerebral ischemia, and may compound the evolution of other pathologies which cause or contribute to cognitive impairment. Animal studies have implicated Hcy in causing apoptosis in hippocampal neurons. Human studies suggest that beta-amyloid deposition is associated with high levels of *S*-adenosyl-L-homocysteine (SAH) in the brain, and that disease progression correlates with SAH levels.

In Parkinson disease (PD), tHcy has been found to be significantly higher among patients compared to controls. These elevations in tHcy may be related to the methylated catabolism of L-dopa, the main pharmacologic treatment of PD. In one small study there was no direct relationship found between cognitive impairment and/or dementia and tHcy. One recent study found that markers of neurodegeneration in PD are related to markers of methylation (SAM, SAH), and that improved cognitive function is related to higher methylation potential (SAM:SAH ratio) in PD patients.

Several studies have demonstrated an association between HHcy and multiple sclerosis (MS). tHcy values are generally higher in MS patients compared to controls (mean 14.9 and 10.8 mmol/L, respectively in one study), while another study in the Netherlands showed no such association. In individuals with established MS, cognitive impairment appears to be more severe in patients with HHcy. Depression in MS may also correlate with higher tHcy levels.

An Italian study found that CSF and plasma tHcy were significantly higher in patients with amyotrophic lateral sclerosis (ALS) compared to controls, but that tHcy had no relationship with age of onset and rate of progression. The authors concluded that tHcy in plasma and CSF may serve as useful biomarkers for ALS, and may be related to pathophysiology of the disease.

☞BONE DISEASE AND OSTEOPOROSIS: A strikingly increased prevalence of osteoporosis among individuals with CBS deficiency suggests that HHcy may contribute to bone weakening, although the direct mechanisms for this process have not been well elucidated. McKusick suggested that disrupted collagen cross-linking may be responsible for the osseous manifestations observed in CBS deficiency, and later work provided evidence for this. A study of almost 2000 elderly adults (825 males, 1174 females) in the Framingham study reviewed historic plasma tHcy data and followed study participants for proximal femoral fractures for over 12 years. Mean age at baseline was 70 years, and the majority of participants were Caucasian. Lifestyle factors, gender, and age were factored into the statistical analysis. The study found that individuals in the upper quartile for tHcy at enrollment had a significantly increased rate of fractures compared to those in the lowest quartile ($4\times$ higher and $1.9\times$ higher, for men and women, respectively). The authors acknowledged that the relationship between HHcy and hip fractures might not be causal, and suggested that the fractures might in fact be caused by other nutritional and metabolic factors, for which tHcy serves as a marker.

## Screening and Counseling

**Screening for Monogenic Disorders of Homocysteine Metabolism:** Most infants are now diagnosed with CBS deficiency through state administered newborn screening programs. Currently all 50 states screen newborns for CBS deficiency. Hypermethioninemia forms the basis of the existing NBS protocols for CBS deficiency, using variable upper limits of normal methionine. Definitive diagnosis of CBS deficiency requires demonstration of reduced CBS activity in cultured fibroblasts or liver tissue. Molecular diagnosis with characterization of the causative mutations is now becoming routine. Prenatal diagnosis is possible with CBS assays on cultured amniocytes, or if mutations are known, with direct analysis of the *CBS* gene.

Although not as universal as CBS deficiency screening, some state newborn screening programs are capable of detecting infants with certain disorders of cobalamin metabolism, including cobalamin C disease.

**Screening for Mild Hyperhomocysteinemia:** There is currently no agreed upon role for screening older adults for HHcy, although this is an area of debate. According to the American Heart Association (AHA), screening for tHcy may be useful in patients with a personal or family history of cardiovascular disease and no other well-established risk factors (smoking, high blood cholesterol, high blood pressure, physical inactivity, obesity, and diabetes). Although evidence for the benefit of lowering Hcy levels is lacking, the AHA advise ensuring adequate dietary intake of folic acid and vitamins $B_6$ or $B_{12}$ for persons with personal and family history of cardiovascular disease.

**Counseling:** CBS deficiency, CblC, and severe MTHFR deficiency are all autosomal recessive disorders. Each sibling of an affected individual has a 25% chance of being similarly affected, a 50% chance of being an asymptomatic carrier, and a 25% chance of being unaffected and not a carrier. Once siblings are known to be unaffected, their risk of carrier status is two-thirds. Each offspring of a proband whose partner is a carrier has a 50% chance of being affected and a 50% chance of being an asymptomatic carrier.

Prenatal diagnosis of CBS deficiency is available through measurement of enzyme activity in cultured amniocytes but not in chorionic villi; measurements of tHcy are also available in cell-free amniotic fluid. If disease-causing alleles are known in an affected family member, molecular testing can be performed after chorionic villus sampling (CVS) or amniocentesis, or can be used to confirm carrier status of other family members. Preimplantation genetic diagnosis (PGD) may be available for families in which the disease-causing mutations have been identified.

Prenatal diagnosis for pregnancies at increased risk for CblC, CblD, CblE, or CblG is possible by analysis of DNA extracted from fetal cells obtained at CVS or amniocentesis. Both disease-causing alleles of an affected family member must be identified before prenatal testing can be performed.

☞GENOTYPE-PHENOTYPE CORRELATION:

**MTHFR Polymorphisms:** *MTHFR* is located at 1p36. Several common polymorphisms have been described. The most highly prevalent polymorphism is 677C>T, occurring in homozygosity in 10% to 15% of American Caucasians and 25% of American Hispanics. It is associated with mild-moderate HHcy, which is exacerbated by a folate-depleted state. In a Norwegian study, greater than 70% of persons with Hcy greater than 40 $\mu$mol/L were homozygous for 677C>T. This polymorphism has been shown to be an independent risk factor for CAD in some studies, and is especially relevant in folate-depleted patients. Another study found that the 677C>T polymorphism is not, in isolation, a causal risk for CAD. Persons homozygous for the 677C>T polymorphism appear to have altered susceptibility to certain malignancies, with increased risk for some (eg, gastric carcinoma) and diminished risk for others (eg, colorectal carcinoma) compared to individuals with wild-type *MTHFR*. Maternal WT *MTHFR* appears to be associated with lower risk of spontaneous miscarriage than either polymorphism, although one study reported that 677C>T is only a risk factor for fetal loss in a selected Chinese population. Risk of cardiovascular and thromboembolic disease in MTHFR deficiency appears to be compounded by additional risk factors, notably hyperlipidemia and presence of factor V Leiden. It has also been associated with neural tube defects, pre-eclampsia, and recurrent pregnancy loss. In folate-replete patients, the presence of homozygous 677C>T reduces risk of colorectal cancer by around 50%. The 1298A>C polymorphism is less potent at reducing MTHFR activity than 677C>T.

**CBS Deficiency:** The CBS deficiency gene is located at 21q22.3, with over 130 mutations described. Most mutations are private, and only a handful are of epidemiologic relevance. The mutation I278T accounts for approximately 25% of disease alleles, and is associated with pyridoxine responsiveness, even in cases of compound heterozygosity. The presence of a single G307S allele (found in highest frequency in Ireland and other regions with a high population of persons of Celtic ancestry) is usually associated with absent response to pyridoxine therapy.

**Disorders of Cobalamin (Vitamin $B_{12}$) Metabolism:** *MMACHC*, the gene encoding the MMACHC protein which is deficient or nonfunctioning in CblC disease, and is located at 1p34.1, with many mutations described. The mutation 271dupA, accounting for around 40% of disease alleles in one study, is invariably associated with the early-onset phenotype. In another study, in 12 patients with late-onset disease, 9 had primarily neurodegenerative disease onset. Of those nine, four were 394C>T homozygotes, two were 394C>T/271dupA compound heterozygotes, and three were 271dupA/other missense mutation heterozygotes.

Coelho et al. identified the gene responsible for CblD in 2008, and described nine mutations in seven patients with CblD; some mutations interfered with MeCbl production, others disrupted AdoCbl production, and others disrupted both. The authors concluded that the gene activities relating to production of MeCbl and AdoCbl were localized to different domains of the gene product.

☞**Genome-Wide Association Studies:** One recent study confirmed the association of *MTHFR* on chromosome 1p36 with plasma Hcy and identified an additional genome-wide significant locus on chromosome 9q22 associated with plasma Hcy. A search for GWASs on stroke, MI, thrombosis, and AD performed to date did not highlight any genomic regions known to be implicated in Hcy metabolism. A GWAS looking at the coronary artery disease phenotype noted an association with *MTHFD1L*, which is important in methionine-homocysteine metabolism.

## Management and Treatment

***Monogenic Disorders Resulting in Hyperhomocysteinemia:*** In general, inherited monogenic disorders of Hcy metabolism resulting in severe HHcy should be managed in conjunction with a physician or center with experience in these disorders. A multidisciplinary approach (including advice from a specialist metabolic nutritionist) may be required.

☞**CBS Deficiency (Classical Homocystinuria):** The primary treatment goal is to reduce tHcy levels to close to normal. Even suboptimal reductions in tHcy are beneficial, with prevention or minimization of mental retardation, delayed lenticular dislocation, and reduced cardiovascular risk. Early diagnosis and treatment are of clear benefit and support the role of CBS deficiency in the expanded NBS protocol.

In about 50% of affected individuals, tHcy control can be achieved to a variable extent with $B_6$ (pyridoxine) supplements. Dosing requirements are highly variable. In $B_6$-unresponsive patients (and to a lesser extent in $B_6$-responsive patients), a low methionine, high cystine diet is required throughout life. Folate should also be supplemented in all patients, since its depletion can compound HHcy. Oral administration of betaine is another strategy to overcome refractory HHcy in patients with

CBS deficiency, or when compliance with protein-restricted diets is not achievable. Betaine remethylates Hcy and causes markedly elevated methionine concentrations.

Individuals with CBS deficiency require referral to specialty clinics for detection and monitoring of cardiovascular, neurologic, ophthalmologic, and hematologic complications, and require consultation with a metabolic nutritionist with experience of the disorder. Oral contraceptives should be avoided in affected women since they may further elevate the risk of thromboembolism. If surgery is unavoidable, generous fluid volumes (100%-150% maintenance) are required perioperatively. Women with CBS deficiency may benefit from treatment with low molecular weight (LMW) heparin through the third trimester of pregnancy and for 6 weeks postpartum.

☞**Cobalamin C Disease (CBLC):** The mainstay of treatment in CblC and the other Cbl disorders is daily intramuscular hydroxocobalamin (OH-Cbl) injections. Although OH-Cbl ameliorates biochemical abnormalities to a variable extent in most patients, the clinical benefits are less well defined. Some centers also treat these patients, to a varying degree, with protein restriction, folate or folinic acid, carnitine and methionine supplementation.

☞**MTHFR:** There may be some benefit in the neurologic and developmental status of those patients with severe MTHFR deficiency who are treated early with betaine to augment the remethylation of Hcy to methionine. The decision to screen for and/or treat patients with homozygosity for mild *MTHFR* polymorphisms (677C>T and 1298A>C) is controversial, since this finding does not confer increased cardiovascular risk, except perhaps in the setting of a folate-depleted state. With adequate dietary folate intake, MTHFR status has not, to date, had any measurable effect on tHcy or risk of cardiovascular disease. The Vitamins and Thrombosis (VITRO) study showed that lowering tHcy to normal with folate, $B_6$, and $B_{12}$ in individuals in the upper quartile of values when screened, did not significantly reduce the risk for VTE. Pregnant women with homozygosity for these polymorphisms in isolation and no other risk factors for thrombophilia are unlikely to be at significantly increased risk of recurrent pregnancy loss (RPL) or venous thromboembolism (VTE); some practitioners have tried LMW heparin in women with RPL and homozygosity for *MTHFR* polymorphisms with some success, although there is currently insufficient evidence to support its routine use. The Hordaland Homocysteine Study found that the 677C>T polymorphism in homozygosity is a risk factor for placental abruption. Folate supplementation, recommended for all pregnant women due to its proven association with reduced incidence of neural tube defects (NTDs), has also been shown to reduce the risk of NTDs in fetuses of women homozygous for the common 677C>T polymorphism.

***Multifactorial Hyperhomocysteinemia:*** The association of HHcy with a myriad of different pathologies in recent years has led to intense scrutiny of the possible benefits of nutritional supplementation for these diseases, and has produced confusing results. Conventional management of HHcy has included folate, $B_6$ and $B_{12}$ supplementation. Although this approach is successful in lowering tHcy levels in a majority of individuals, elucidation of its effect on clinical vascular pathology and other pathology has only recently begun, and with highly variable results. In many studies, successful Hcy lowering has not successfully translated into measurable clinical benefit, suggesting that Hcy may be an "innocent bystander" in the pathogenesis of many of the disorders it has associations with. Conversely, several studies support a potential role for folate, $B_6$ and $B_{12}$ in reversing endothelial injury in the setting of HHcy. In

1996, the Food and Drug Administration (FDA) mandated fortification of enriched grain products with folate. This intervention has reduced the rate of folate deficiency (<7 nmol/L) in the United States from 22.0% to 1.7% and has reduced the rate of HHcy (defined in this case as tHcy>13 mmol/L) from 18.7% to 9.8%.

☞**Cardiovascular and Cerebrovascular Disease:** Although many intervention trials yielded disappointing results, others have suggested some clinical benefit in Hcy-lowering therapies in the setting of cardiovascular disease. In a recent meta-analysis performed on behalf of the Cochrane Library, the outcomes of eight randomized controlled trials (equivalent to 24,210 participants) were reviewed. There was no evidence that Hcy-lowering interventions, in the form of supplements of vitamins $B_6$, $B_9$, or $B_{12}$ given alone or in combination, at any dosage compared with placebo or standard care, prevent MI, stroke, or reduce total mortality in participants at risk for, or with existing cardiovascular disease. The study suggested that Hcy lowering may, however, be of some benefit in certain select patient groups.

☞**Alzheimer Disease and Cognition:** In the Hordaland Homocysteine Study measuring tHcy and folate, over 2000 patients were subject to memory assessment using a standardized scale at baseline, and 6 years later. The authors concluded that increased plasma tHcy and lower folate are independent risk factors for memory deficit both cross-sectionally and prospectively ($p < .001$), and that favorable changes in folate and tHcy over time are associated with better cognitive performance. Another study looking at nondemented patients between 50 and 70 years with HHcy and normal $B_{12}$ levels showed that the treatment group (folate 0.8 mg daily for 3 years) performed better in tests of processing speed and complex memory tasks than the placebo group.

A trial undertaken in New Zealand with 276 elderly participants with tHcy greater than 13 mmol/L did not support the hypothesis that tHcy lowering with supplements (cocktail of folate 1 mg + $B_{12}$ 500 mg + $B_6$ 10 mg vs placebo) improves cognitive performance. In a separate study, 185 elderly patients with ischemic vascular disease in a randomized, placebo-controlled, double-blind study with three active treatments: folate (2.5 mg), $B_{12}$ (500 mg), $B_6$ (25 mg), and riboflavin (25 mg). Changes in plasma tHcy were measured at 3, 6, and 12 months and changes in cognitive functions at 6 and 12 months. In line with many of the studies of CAD and Hcy, the authors found that, although tHcy levels decreased in the group receiving folate plus $B_{12}$, there were no statistically significant beneficial effects on cognition. It was acknowledged that over shorter follow-up periods, the beneficial effects of supplementation on cognitive performance may be less apparent.

☞**Venous Thromboembolism:** The VITRO study investigated the effect of supplementation of B vitamins on the risk reduction of deep vein thrombosis (DVT) and pulmonary embolism (PE). Patients between 20 to 80 years old with a first confirmed proximal DVT or PE and without known major risk factors and a tHcy concentration above the 75th percentile of a reference group were asked to participate, and followed for 2.5 years. The treatment group was given folate 5 mg, $B_6$ 50 mg, and $B_{12}$ 0.4 mg daily. The results showed that, for individuals in the upper quartile of tHcy values, there was no significant difference in the incidence of second DVT/PE in the treatment group compared to the placebo group (incidence 0.054 vs 0.064, respectively).

☞**Pharmacogenetics:** Polymorphisms in *MTHFR* appear to have potentially important pharmacogenetic roles as genetic determinants of the efficacy and toxicity of antifolate (eg, methotrexate, MTX) and fluoropyrimidine-based therapies. Both the 677C>T and 1298A>C polymorphisms may confer increased chemosensitivity to 5-FU. The 677C>T polymorphism appears to confer increased sensitivity to MTX in breast cancer cells but not in colon cancer cells, suggesting that this polymorphism differentially modulates the sensitivity of cancer cells to MTX, depending on the specific cell type. Other studies overall demonstrated a significant association between the 677C>T polymorphism and worse clinical outcome after MTX-containing therapy. Overall, the precise nature of the influences of *MTHFR* polymorphisms on responses to these agents remains uncertain at this time.

**Bibliography:**

1. Jacques PF, Bostom AG, Williams RR, et al. Relation between folate status, a common mutation in methylenetetrahydrofolatereductase, and plasma homocysteine concentrations. *Circulation.* 1996;93(1):7-9.
2. Levy HL, Vargas JE, Waisbren SE, et al. Reproductive fitness in maternal homocystinuria due to cystathionine beta-synthase deficiency. *J Inherit Metab Dis.* 2002;25(4):299-314.
3. Lerner-Ellis JP, Tirone JC, Pawelek PD, et al. Identification of the gene responsible for methylmalonicaciduria and homocystinuria, cblC type. *Nat Genet.* 2006;38(1):93-100.
4. McCully KS. Vascular pathology of homocysteinemia: implications for the pathogenesis of arteriosclerosis. *Am J Pathol.* 1969;56:111-128.
5. Wald DS, Law M, Morris JK. Homocysteine and cardiovascular disease: evidence of causality from a meta-analysis. *BMJ.* 2002;325:1202-1209.
6. Evans RW, Shaten BJ, Hempel JD, Cutler JA, Kuller LH. Homocyst(e)ine and risk of cardiovascular disease in the Multiple Risk Factor Intervention Trial. *Arterioscler Thomb Vasc Biol.* 1997;17(10):1947-1953.
7. Seshadri S, Beiser A, Selhub J, et al. Plasma homocysteine as a risk factor for dementia and Alzheimer's disease. *N Engl J Med.* 2002;346(7):476-483.
8. Mudd SH, Skovby F, Levy HL, et al. The natural history of homocystinuria due to cystathionine β-synthase deficiency. *Am J Hum Genet.* 1985;37:1-31.
9. McLean RR, Jacques PF, Selhub J, et al. Homocysteine as a predictive factor for hip fracture in older persons. *N Engl J Med.* 2004;350:2042-2049.
10. Kluijtmans LA, Kastelein JJ, Lindemans J, et al. Thermolabile methylenetetrahydrofolate reductase in coronary artery disease. *Circulation.* 1997;96(8):2573-2577.
11. Hazra A, Kraft P, Lazarus R, et al. Genome-wide significant predictors of metabolites in the one-carbon metabolism pathway. *Hum Mol Genet.* 2009;18(23):4677-4687.
12. den Heijer M, Willems HP, Blom HJ, et al. Homocysteine lowering by B vitamins and the secondary prevention of deep vein thrombosis and pulmonary embolism: a randomized, placebo-controlled, double-blind trial. *Blood.* 2007;109(1):139-144.
13. Martí-Carvajal AJ, Solà I, Lathyris D, Salanti G. Homocysteine lowering interventions for preventing cardiovascular events. *Cochrane Database Syst Rev.* 2009;7(4):CD006612.
14. McMahon JA, Green TJ, Skeaff CM, et al. A controlled trial of homocysteine lowering and cognitive performance. *N Engl J Med.* 2006;354:2764-2767.

## Supplementary Information

**Key Words:** Homocysteine, methionine, folate, vitamin $B_{12}$, MTHFR, hyperhomocysteinemia

# 91 Hyperammonemia

Saumya S. Jamuar and Harvey L. Levy

## KEY POINTS

- *Disease summary:*
  - Hyperammonemia in adults has many different causes. Most are nongenetic. Infrequent but important genetic causes are defects in the urea cycle which are life threatening and treatable.
  - Urea cycle disorders (UCDs) are caused by defects in the metabolic cycle which converts ammonia to urea.
  - The adult phenotype may present dramatically or subtly with hyperammonemia of varying degree that can produce cerebral edema. The clinical features include psychosis, altered mental status, vomiting, and focal neurologic signs, or lethargy progressing to obtundation and coma. Acute episodes are often precipitated by surgery, pregnancy, or more likely the postpartum, trauma, and infection.
  - Chronic features include cognitive and learning deficits, intermittent headaches, intermittent visual disturbances, and focal neurologic signs. There may also be a lifelong aversion to dietary protein.
- *Hereditary basis:*
  - All the UCDs are inherited in an autosomal recessive manner with the exception of ornithine transcarbamylase (OTC) deficiency which is X-linked.
- *Differential diagnosis:*
  - Liver failure
  - Sepsis
  - Valproate therapy

## Diagnostic Criteria and Clinical Characteristics

### Diagnostic Criteria:

- High ammonia (>100 µmol/L)
- Abnormal plasma amino acid profile
  - Low or high citrulline
  - Presence of argininosuccinic acid
  - Low or high arginine
- Low or high orotic acid in urine
- In the absence of
  - Liver failure
  - Overwhelming sepsis
  - Metabolic acidosis

*Clinical Characteristics:* UCDs interrupt the conversion of ammonia to urea (Fig. 91-1). Ammonia is generated as a by-product of protein catabolism and elevated ammonia levels (>100 µmol/L) appear to be extremely toxic to the central nervous system. UCD in adults can present with chronic symptoms of intermittent headaches, intermittent visual disturbances, cognitive and learning deficits, and focal neurologic signs. These adults have self-selective dietary protein aversion. Acute episodes can be triggered by increased dietary intake of protein or secondary to increased protein breakdown related to catabolic states, such as infection, trauma, surgery, pregnancy, or the postpartum. These symptoms may resolve spontaneously or may progress to hyperammonemic encephalopathy. Patients may present acutely with vomiting, anorexia, lethargy, altered mental status, seizures, focal neurologic signs, or psychosis. Hepatomegaly may be present on clinical examination. Hyperammonemia can produce cerebral edema and patients, if untreated, continue to deteriorate, become comatose, and may die from cerebral herniation. Upon recovery, patients may be left with significant neurologic deficits.

While the urea cycle disorders usually present in infancy or childhood, often dramatically, all have a late-onset form that presents in adulthood with hyperammonemia and is related to partial (hypomorphic) rather than complete enzyme deficiencies. Due to random X-chromosome inactivation, approximately 15% of female carriers with a defect in OTC develop hyperammonemia. Arginase (ARG) deficiency typically presents as a chronic neurologic problem with cognitive reduction and spastic diplegia. Unlike the dramatic clinical presentation of the other urea cycle disorders, patients with argininosuccinate lyase (ASL) deficiency can develop trichorrhexis nodosa (or brittle hair) and often have chronic liver disease.

*Differential Diagnoses:* The most frequent cause of hyperammonemia in adults is acute and/or chronic hepatic failure. Other causes of hyperammonemia include certain drugs, notably valproic acid, and urinary tract infection with a urease-producing organism such as *Proteus mirabilis* or *Klebsiella pneumoniae*. Certain chemotherapeutic agents such as 5-fluorouracil, cyclophosphamide, and asparaginase have been shown to reduce urea cycle function and cause hyperammonemia. Rare causes of hyperammonemia in adults include Hashimoto thyroiditis and multiple myeloma.

## Screening and Counseling

*Screening:* In evaluating an adult with hyperammonemia, it is important to exclude nongenetic causes such as liver failure or sepsis. First-line investigations include

- Ammonia (blood in sodium heparin tube sent STAT to laboratory on ice)
- Liver function tests
- Electrolytes and blood gases
- Plasma amino acids
- Urine orotic acid

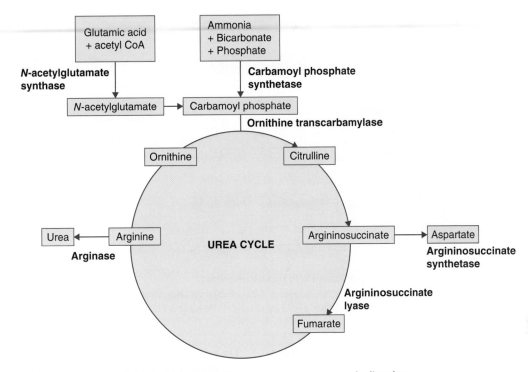

*Figure 91-1* Urea Cycle. Enzymes are labeled in bold. Defect in the enzymes causes urea cycle disorders.

*Note:* Ammonia can be spuriously elevated if there is delay in sample analysis. This is the most frequent cause of hyperammonemia in a relatively well individual.

UCDs presenting as hyperammonemic encephalopathy are clinically indistinguishable from each other (Table 91-1). Plasma amino acids are very important in differentiating the various enzyme deficiencies, as highlighted in the algorithm (Fig. 91-2). As depicted in the pathway (Fig. 91-1), the UCDs may be divided into two categories, proximal and distal, depending on the level of citrulline. Low citrulline levels point to the possibility of a proximal disorder like *N*-acetylglutamate synthase (NAGS), carbamoyl phosphate synthetase (CPS1) or OTC deficiency. Orotic acid, an intermediate in the pyrimidine biosynthetic pathway, is elevated in OTC deficiency but normal or perhaps low in CPS1 and NAGS deficiency. CPS1 and NAGS deficiency are biochemically indistinguishable and require measurement of enzyme activity or molecular genetic testing. Significantly elevated levels of citrulline, argininosuccinic acid, and arginine are suggestive of a distal disorder such as argininosuccinate synthetase (ASS) deficiency, argininosuccinate lyase (ASL) deficiency, or arginase (ARG) deficiency, respectively.

Molecular genetic testing is used for diagnosis, carrier testing, and prenatal diagnosis and is available clinically for all the urea cycle disorders listed in Table 91-1 (see Gene Tests www.genetests.com for directory of laboratory that offer testing). If molecular testing is uninformative, enzyme activity of individual enzymes can be

## Table 91-1 *Genetic Differential Diagnosis*

| Syndrome (alternative names) | Gene Symbol | Inheritance Pattern | Associated Findings |
|---|---|---|---|
| *N*-acetylglutamate synthase deficiency (*NAGS*) | NAGS | AR | |
| Carbamoyl phosphate synthetase deficiency (*CPS1*) | CPS1 | AR | Acute or chronic encephalopathy. Dietary protein aversion |
| Ornithine transcarbamylase deficiency (*OTC*) | OTC | XL | |
| Argininosuccinate synthetase deficiency (*citrullinemia type 1*) | ASS1 | AR | |
| Argininosuccinate lyase deficiency (*argininosuccinic acidemia*) | ASL | AR | Encephalopathy, chronic liver disease, trichorrhexis nodosa |
| Arginase deficiency (*hyperargininemia*) | ARG1 | AR | Spastic diplegia, neurologic features. Rarely hyperammonemia |

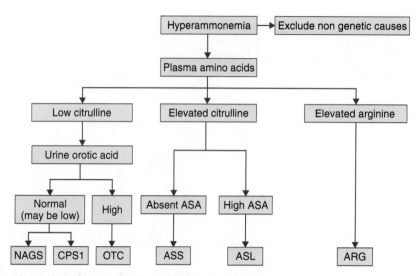

**Figure 91-2** Algorithm for Diagnostic Evaluation of Patient With Hyperammonemia.
ASA, argininosuccinic acid; NAGS, *N*-acetylglutamate synthase deficiency; CPS1, carbamoyl phosphate synthetase deficiency; OTC, ornithine transcarbamylase deficiency; ASS, argininosuccinate synthetase deficiency; ASL, argininosuccinate lyase deficiency; ARG, arginase deficiency

measured in red blood cells (ASL and ARG), fibroblasts (ASS and ASL), and liver (NAGS, CPS1, and OTC).

**Counseling:** NAGS, CPS1, ASS1, ASL, and ARG deficiencies are inherited in an autosomal recessive manner. Affected individuals are at 50% risk of having an affected child if the partner carries a mutant gene for the trait and 100% risk if the partner is also affected. Regardless of the genotype of the partner, all unaffected offspring of an affected individual are carriers. If the sib of a proband is known to be unaffected, the chance of his/her being a carrier is two-thirds (~66%).

OTC deficiency is inherited in an X-linked manner. A male proband will pass the disease-causing mutation to all of his daughters and none of his sons. A female proband has a 50% chance of transmitting the disease-causing mutation to each child. A significant number of carrier females have hyperammonemia secondary to skewed X-inactivation and may present during pregnancy or the postpartum period. Carrier females may have cognitive deficits even in the absence of hyperammonemia. If a male is affected by late-onset disease, the risk of symptoms in his carrier female offspring is much lower since the mutation is expected to produce partial OTC deficiency. Risk of OTC deficiency to the sibs of the proband depends on the carrier status of the parents.

☞**GENOTYPE-PHENOTYPE CORRELATION:** All the UCDs that present in adulthood are highly pleiomorphic disorders and genotype-phenotype correlation has not been ascertained. Genetic and environmental modifiers may play an important role in influencing the clinical phenotype.

## Management and Treatment

Adults with hyperammonemia secondary to UCD include those with a known diagnosis of UCD and those with the first presentation of UCD. Hyperammonemia is a dire emergency. Profound cerebral edema with brainstem herniation and death can occur within a short time after presentation.

**The principles of management for both types of patients include**
1. **Minimize protein intake:** As ammonia is a by-product of protein breakdown, protein should be withdrawn from the diet during the initial period of hyperammonemia. Protein should be reintroduced in small increments after 24 to 48 hours to prevent endogenous protein breakdown. Diet should be planned in conjunction with a metabolic dietician.
2. **Reverse or minimize catabolism:** This can be achieved by infusing high dextrose-containing (10% or greater) fluids. Intravenous intralipids can be added to increase the total caloric intake. Caloric intake should be at least 60 to 70 kcal/kg/d. Total daily fluids should be restricted in the presence of signs of cerebral edema. Glucose levels should be kept between 120 and 170 mg/dL. Intravenous insulin infusion can be used for control of hyperglycemia. Accurate records of intake and output should be kept to monitor hydration. Infection as a potential but severe catabolic stressor should be considered early (when clinical signs are apparent) and managed vigorously. Avoid valproic acid for seizure management, as it decreases urea cycle function and accentuates hyperammonemia.
3. **Promote waste nitrogen excretion:** To help facilitate the excretion of waste nitrogen, the following medications and procedures should be used:
   • Ammonia scavenging medications
     • *Oral medications*
       • **Sodium benzoate**—conjugates with glycine to form hippuric acid which bypasses the urea cycle and is excreted in urine.
       • **Sodium phenylacetate**—conjugates with glutamine to form phenylacetylglutamine which bypasses the urea cycle and is excreted in the urine.
     • *Intravenous medication*
       • **Ammonul**—combination of sodium benzoate and sodium phenylacetate. The dose of 5.5 g/m² is given as a bolus over 60 to 90 minutes followed by the same dose as a continuous infusion over 24 hours given daily till ammonia levels are in the nontoxic range.

*Table 91-2 Molecular Genetic Testing*

| Gene | Testing Modality | Mutation Type | Detection Rate |
|------|------------------|---------------|----------------|
| NAGS | Sequencing | Single base substitutions, insertion | Unknown |
| CPS1 | Sequencing | Single base substitutions (77%), small deletions (13%), insertions (7%), indels (2%), large deletions (1%) | Unknown |
| OTC | Sequencing | Single base substitutions (86%), small deletions and insertions (8%), large deletions (6%) | ~80% |
| ASS1 | Sequencing | Single base substitutions, small deletions, insertions | Unknown |
| ASL | Sequencing | Single base substitutions, small deletions, and insertions | Unknown |
| ARG1 | Sequencing | Single base substitutions, small deletions | Unknown |

If the ammonia continues to rise above 175 μmol/L consider hemodialysis. Arginine can be used to prevent arginine deficiency and any prime residual OTC activity but must not be used in ARG deficiency where there is already an excess of arginine. In OTC and CPS1 deficiencies, enteral citrulline may pull aspartate into the cycle and increase nitrogen clearance. In ASS and ASL deficiencies, it will exacerbate increases in citrulline and ASA, respectively, and therefore should not be used in the latter two disorders. Importantly, lactulose which is used to control hyperammonemia associated with hepatic failure or sepsis is ineffective in controlling the hyperammonemia caused by a UCD.

**Management of Complications:**

☞CEREBRAL EDEMA: Oncotic agents such as albumin will increase the overall nitrogen load but may, in selected cases, be considered. Mannitol has not been found to be helpful for edema secondary to hyperammonemia and steroids should not be used. Hyperventilation is recommended, but only under close appropriate supervision.

☞RECOVERY: As ammonia falls below 60 to 75 μmol/L and clinical status returns to baseline, patient can be switched to oral medications and protein can be gradually reintroduced to the diet in consultation with the metabolic dietician. It is important to note that there may be a rebound hyperammonemia initially with the efflux of intracellular ammonia into the relatively ammonia-depleted blood. Thus it is important to continue closely monitoring ammonia levels until they remain stable in the normal range.

☞SPECIAL SITUATIONS: MANAGEMENT DURING PREGNANCY: Pregnancy in a female with a UCD can produce profound, life-threatening hyperammonemia, especially in the postpartum period. The presentation is usually characterized by psychotic features rapidly progressing to obtundation and coma. Death due to marked cerebral edema and brain herniation have been reported. The plasma ammonia levels are markedly elevated with values exceeding 1000 μmol/L.

Optimally, the woman is known to have a UCD before the pregnancy and should be followed during pregnancy with very frequent measurements of plasma ammonia. At the first indication of elevated ammonia, the measures described earlier in the management and treatment of hyperammonemia should be initiated. These measures should be immediately initiated when a woman not known to have a UCD presents clinically with psychosis or marked lethargy and is found to have an elevated ammonia level.

The postpartum period seems most likely to result in profound hyperammonemia and death. Consequently, a woman with a UCD should be followed postpartum with at least daily measurements of ammonia and treatment according to the level of hyperammonemia. Since there can be a latent rise in ammonia postpartum, the woman should remain in the hospital with close monitoring of her ammonia level for at least 1 week and not discharged until her levels have remained normal.

**Contraindications:**

Steroids and valproic acid are contraindicated in patients with known or suspected UCD as they may exacerbate the hyperammonemia. Steroids cause increased protein breakdown and increase the nitrogen load. Valproic acid inhibits NAGS resulting in decreased clearance of ammonia.

## Molecular Genetics and Molecular Mechanism

**Syndrome/Gene/Locus:**

N-acetylglutamate synthase deficiency/*NAGS*/17q21.31
Carbamoyl phosphate synthetase deficiency/ *PS1*/ q34
Ornithine transcarbamylase deficiency/*OTC*/Xp11.4
Argininosuccinate synthetase deficiency/*ASS*1/9q34.11
Argininosuccinate lyase deficiency/*ASL*/7q11.21
Arginase deficiency/*ARG1*/6q23.2

**Genetic Testing:** Molecular genetic testing involves sequencing of the putative gene and is available clinically for all the UCDs as listed in Table 91-2 (see Gene Tests www.genetests.com for directory of laboratory that offer testing). For definitive diagnostic testing, molecular genetic testing is preferred over enzyme activity assays.

**BIBLIOGRAPHY:**

1. Online Mendelian Inheritance in Man. http://www.omim.org. Accessed December, 2011.

2. Scriver CR, Sly WS, Childs B, et al. *The Metabolic and Molecular Bases of Inherited Disease.* 8th ed. New York, NY: McGraw-Hill Professional; 2000.

3. Urea Cycle Disorders Overview—GeneReviews—NCBI Bookshelf [Internet]. http://www.ncbi.nlm.nih.gov/books/NBK1217/ Accessed December, 2011.

4. Acute Illness Protocols, New England Consortium of Metabolic Programs. http://www.newenglandconsortium.org Accessed December, 2011.

5. Summar ML, Barr F, Dawling S, et al. Unmasked adult-onset urea cycle disorders in the critical care setting. *Crit Care Clin.* 2005;21(4):S1-S8.

## Supplementary Information

**OMIM References:**

[1] *N*-Acetylglutamate Synthase Deficiency: NAGS (#237310)

[2] Carbamoyl Phosphate Synthetase Deficiency: CPS1 (#237300)

[3] Ornithine Transcarbamylase Deficiency: OTC (#311250)

[4] Argininosuccinate Synthetase Deficiency: ASS1 (#215700)

[5] Argininosuccinate Lyase Deficiency: ASL (#207900)

[6] Arginase Deficiency: ARG1 (#207800)

***Key Words:*** Urea cycle disorders, hyperammonemia, *N*-acetylglutamate synthase deficiency, carbamoyl phosphate synthetase deficiency, ornithine transcarbamylase deficiency, argininosuccinate synthetase deficiency, argininosuccinate lyase deficiency, arginase deficiency

# 92 Hereditary Systemic Amyloidosis

Merrill D. Benson

## KEY POINTS

- *Disease summary:*
  - The hereditary systemic amyloidoses are a group of diseases caused by mutations in several structural proteins. The most common is transthyretin (TTR) amyloidosis, which is characterized mainly by peripheral neuropathy but also associated, in many cases, with restrictive cardiomyopathy. Systemic amyloidoses associated with mutations in fibrinogen Aα-chain, lysozyme, apolipoprotein A-I, and apolipoprotein A-II, are mainly associated with renal amyloidosis but may also affect other organ systems. As with all types of amyloidosis, organ dysfunction is caused by deposition of protein fibrils (~10 nm in diameter) which, as they accumulate, displace normal tissue structures. As amyloid deposition progresses organ failure ensues often leading to death within a 10- to 15-year period. Since clinical diagnosis is often delayed until the disease is relatively advanced, death within 5 to 10 years after tissue diagnosis is not uncommon.

- *Differential diagnosis:*
  - Some of the hereditary amyloidoses have overlapping clinical phenotypes while others have unique phenotypes which, when recognized, simplifies diagnosis. For those forms of hereditary amyloidosis with overlapping features it is very important to differentiate these from AL (Ig light-chain) and AA (reactive, secondary) amyloidosis. AL amyloidosis is most commonly associated with either nephrotic syndrome or cardiomyopathy. Both of these phenotypes are common with some forms of hereditary amyloidosis. AA amyloidosis, most commonly presents as nephrotic syndrome with progressive renal failure, a feature that is common to several hereditary amyloidoses.

- *Monogenic forms:*
  - Each of seven types of hereditary amyloidosis arises from single gene mutations. The most common is transthyretin (TTR) amyloidosis, which is caused by mutations in the *TTR* gene (Table 92-1). Mutations in apolipoprotein A-I (*APOA1*), fibrinogen Aα-chain (*FGA*), lysozyme (*LYZ*), apolipoprotein A-II (*APOA2*), gelsolin (*GSN*), and cystatin C (*CST3*) genes also may cause systemic amyloidosis (Table 92-2). All forms of hereditary amyloidosis are inherited as autosomal dominant traits but the degree of penetrance in any one disease is variable.

- *Family history:*
  - Since all of the hereditary amyloidoses are autosomal dominant, family history can be a very important factor in making a correct diagnosis. However, many patients, especially with TTR amyloidosis, present as sporadic cases without an informative family history. Often this is due to the fact that the disease is relatively late onset in any one particular family. A family history of a relative with blindness due to vitreous opacities is very suggestive of TTR amyloidosis.

- *Twin studies:*
  - None

- *Environmental factors:*
  - No definite environmental factors have been shown to be at play in hereditary amyloidosis. There is considerable variation within kindreds and geographic areas but these differences most likely are due to genetic background rather than environmental factors.

- *Genome-wide associations:*
  - None

- *Pharmacogenomics:*
  - None

## Diagnostic Criteria and Clinical Characteristics

***Diagnostic Criteria for Hereditary Amyloidosis:*** The diagnosis of hereditary amyloidosis depends on tissue biopsy demonstrating amyloid deposition. For TTR amyloidosis, nerve and cardiac biopsies can be most definitive; however, abdominal fat pad biopsy, rectal biopsy, salivary gland biopsy, or upper gastrointestinal (GI) biopsies are less invasive and may give the diagnosis of amyloidosis. Identification of type of hereditary amyloidosis is determined by DNA analysis. DNA sequencing for *TTR* mutations is available from a number of commercial laboratories and also is routinely done in amyloid research laboratories. DNA analysis for lysozyme, fibrinogen Aα-chain, apolipoprotein A-I, apolipoprotein A-II, gelsolin, and

cystatin-C may be available at amyloid research centers. Any patient presenting with neuropathy should have a cardiac evaluation with EKG and echocardiogram since this is the most common secondary expression of TTR amyloidosis. Apolipoprotein A-I amyloidosis typically has renal insufficiency without significant proteinuria. A renal biopsy showing amyloid deposition in the interstitial and medullary areas without glomerular involvement is very suggestive of this form of amyloidosis. With gelsolin amyloidosis the lattice corneal dystrophy can be appreciated by careful ophthalmologic examination many years in advance of the facial neuropathy.

**Diagnostic evaluation should include the following (Fig. 92-1):**

- Family history
- Tissue biopsy with Congo red staining

465

*Table 92-1  Transthyretin Amyloidosis*

| Mutation | Codon Change | Clinical Features[a] | Geographic Kindreds |
|---|---|---|---|
| Cys10Arg | TGT - CGT | Heart, eye, PN | USA (PA) |
| Leu12Pro | CTG - CCG | LM | UK |
| Asp18Glu | GAT - GAA | PN | South America, USA |
| Asp18Gly | - GGT | LM | Hungary |
| Asp18Asn | - AAT | Heart | USA |
| Val20Ile | GTC - ATC | Heart, CTS | Germany, USA |
| Ser23Asn | AGT - AAT | Heart, PN | USA |
| Pro24Ser | CCT - TCT | Heart, CTS, PN | USA |
| Ala25Ser | GCC - TCC | Heart, CTS, PN | USA |
| Ala25Thr | - ACC | LM, PN | Japan |
| Val28Met | GTG - ATG | PN, AN | Portugal |
| Val30Met | GTG - ATG | PN, AN, eye, LM | Portugal, Japan, Sweden, USA (FAP I) |
| Val30Ala | - GCG | Heart, AN | USA |
| Val30Leu | - CTG | PN, heart | Japan |
| Val30Gly | - GGG | LM, eye | USA |
| Val32Ala | GTG - GCG | PN | Israel |
| Phe33Ile | TTC - ATC | PN, eye | Israel |
| Phe33Leu | - CTC | PN, heart | USA |
| Phe33Val | - GTC | PN | UK, Japan, China |
| Phe33Cys | - TGC | CTS, heart, eye, kidney | USA |
| Arg34Ser | AGA - AGC/T | PN, heart | USA |
| Arg34Thr | AGA - ACA | PN, heart | Italy |
| Arg34Gly | AGA - GGA | Eye | UK |
| Lys35Asn | AAG - AAC | PN, AN, heart | France |
| Lys35Thr | - ACG | Eye | USA |
| Ala36Pro | GCT - CCT | Eye, CTS | USA |
| Asp38Ala | GAT - GCT | PN, heart | Japan |
| Trp41Leu | TGG - TTG | Eye, PN | USA |
| Glu42Gly | GAG - GGG | PN, AN, heart | Japan, USA, Russia |
| Glu42Asp | - GAT | Heart | France |
| Phe44Ser | TTT - TCT | PN, AN, heart | USA |
| Ala45Thr | GCC - ACC | Heart | USA |
| Ala45Asp | - GAC | Heart, PN | USA |
| Ala45Ser | - TCC | Heart | Sweden |
| Gly47Arg | GGG - CGG/AGG | PN, AN | Japan |
| Gly47Ala | - GCG | Heart, AN | Italy, France |
| Gly47Val | - GTG | CTS, PN, AN, heart | Sri Lanka |
| Gly47Glu | - GAG | Heart, PN, AN | Turkey, USA, Germany |
| Thr49Ala | ACC - GCC | Heart, CTS | France, Italy |
| Thr49Ile | - ATC | PN, heart | Japan, Spain |
| Thr49Pro | - CCC | Heart, PN | USA |
| Ser50Arg | AGT - AGG | AN, PN | Japan, France/Italian, USA |
| Ser50Ile | - ATT | Heart, PN, AN | Japan |
| Glu51Gly | GAG - GGG | Heart | USA |
| Ser52Pro | TCT - CCT | PN, AN, heart, kidney | UK |
| Gly53Glu | GGA - GAA | LM, heart | Basque, Sweden |

*(Continued)*

**Table 92-1** *Transthyretin Amyloidosis (Continued)*

| Mutation | Codon Change | Clinical Features[a] | Geographic Kindreds |
|---|---|---|---|
| Gly53Ala | GGA - ALA | LM | UK |
| Gly53Arg | - AGA | LM | USA |
| Glu54Gly | GAG - GGG | PN, AN, eye | UK |
| Glu54Lys | - AAG | PN, AN, heart, eye | Japan |
| Glu54Leu | GAG - CTG | | UK |
| Leu55Pro | CTG - CCG | Heart, AN, eye | USA, Taiwan |
| Leu55Arg | - CGG | LM | Germany |
| Leu55Gln | - CAG | Eye, PN | USA |
| Leu55Glu | CTG - CAG | Heart, PN, AN | Sweden |
| His56Arg | CAT - CGT | Heart | USA |
| Gly57Arg | GGG - AGG | Heart | Sweden |
| Leu58His | CTC - CAC | CTS, heart | USA (MD) (FAP II) |
| Leu58Arg | - CGC | CTS, AN, Eye | Japan |
| Thr59Lys | ACA - AAA | Heart, PN, AN | Italy, USA (Chinese) |
| Thr60Ala | ACT - GCT | Heart, CTS | USA (Appalachian) |
| Glu61Lys | GAG - AAG | PN | Japan |
| Glu61Gly | - GGG | Heart, PN | USA |
| Glu62Lys | - AAG | PN | Italy |
| Phe64Leu | TTT - CTT/TTG | PN, CTS, heart | USA, Italy |
| Phe64Ile | - ATT | | |
| Phe64Ser | - TCT | LM, PN, eye | Canada, UK |
| Gly67Glu | GGG - GAG | | |
| Ile68Leu | ATA - TTA | Heart | Germany |
| Tyr69His | TAC - CAC | Eye, LM | Canada, USA, Sweden |
| Tyr69Ile | - ATC[b] | Heart, CTS, AN | Japan |
| Lys70Asn | AAA - AAC | Eye, CTS, PN | USA |
| Val71Ala | GTG - GCG | PN, eye, CTS | France, Spain |
| Ile73Val | ATA - GTA | PN, AN | Bangladesh |
| Tyr75Ile | ACC - ATC | Heart | France |
| Ser77Tyr | TCT - TAT | Kidney | USA (IL, TX), France |
| Ser77Phe | - TTT | PN, AN, heart | France |
| Tyr78Phe | TAC - TTC | PN, CTS, skin | France |
| Ala81Thr | GCA - ACA | Heart | USA |
| Ala81Val | GCA - GTA | Heart | UK |
| Ile84Ser | ATC - AGC | Heart, CTS, eye | USA (IN), Hungary (FAP II) |
| Ile84Asn | - AAC | Heart, eye | USA |
| Ile84Thr | - ACC | Heart, PN | Germany, UK |
| His88Arg | CAT - CGT | Heart | Sweden |
| Glu89Gln | GAG - CAG | PN, heart | Italy |
| Glu89Lys | - AAG | PN, heart | USA |
| His90Asp | CAT - GAT | Heart | UK |
| Ala91Ser | GCA - TCA | PN, CTS, heart | France |
| Glu92Lys | GAG - AAG | Heart | Japan |
| Val93Met | GTG - ATG | | Africa (France) Mali |
| Val94Ala | GTA - GCA | Heart, PN, AN, kidney | Germany, USA |
| Ala97Gly | GCC - GGC | Heart, PN | Japan |
| Ala97Ser | - TCC | PN, heart | Taiwan, USA |

*(Continued)*

*Table 92-1  Transthyretin Amyloidosis (Continued )*

| Mutation | Codon Change | Clinical Features[a] | Geographic Kindreds |
|----------|--------------|----------------------|---------------------|
| Ile107Val | ATT - GTT | Heart, CTS, PN | USA |
| Ile107Met | - ATG | PN, heart | Germany |
| Ile107Phe | ATT - TTT | PN, AN | UK |
| Ala109Ser | GCC - TCC | PN, AN | Japan |
| Leu111Met | CTG - ATG | Heart | Denmark |
| Ser112Ile | AGC - ATC | PN, heart | Italy |
| Tyr114Cys | TAC - TGC | PN, AN, eye, LM | Japan, USA |
| Tyr114His | - CAC | CTS, skin | Japan |
| Tyr116Ser | TAT - TCT | PN, CTS, AN | France |
| Ala120Ser | GCT - TCT | Heart | Afro-Caribbean |
| Ala120Thr | GCT - ACT | PN, CTS | Japan |
| Val122Ile | GTC - ATC | Heart | USA |
| ΔVal122 | - ΔΔΔ | Heart, PN | USA (Ecuador), Spain |
| Val122Ala | - GCC | Heart, eye, PN | USA |

[a]Clinical features: AN, autonomic neuropathy; CTS, carpal tunnel syndrome; eye, vitreous deposits; LM, leptomeningeal; PN, peripheral neuropathy.

[b]Double nucleotide substitution.

*Clinical Characteristics:* TTR amyloidosis (Table 92-1) is characterized mainly by neuropathy and cardiomyopathy, two features which are commonly seen with AL amyloidosis. Other forms of hereditary amyloidosis are listed in Table 92-2. Fibrinogen Aα-chain amyloidosis presents with nephrotic syndrome, a common feature with AL and AA amyloidosis. Apolipoprotein A-I and A-II amyloidoses present with renal insufficiency and may be mistaken for AL or AA amyloidosis. Gelsolin amyloidosis, on the other hand, is characterized by lattice corneal dystrophy and cranial nerve palsy. This diagnosis should not be easily missed. Cystatin-C amyloidosis is characterized by repeated intracranial hemorrhages due to cerebral amyloid vascular deposition. It is a systemic form of amyloidosis, however, and amyloid deposits may be found in various organ systems on biopsy, or at autopsy. Lysozyme amyloidosis is commonly characterized by renal insufficiency but also may present with hepatomegaly due to amyloid deposition.

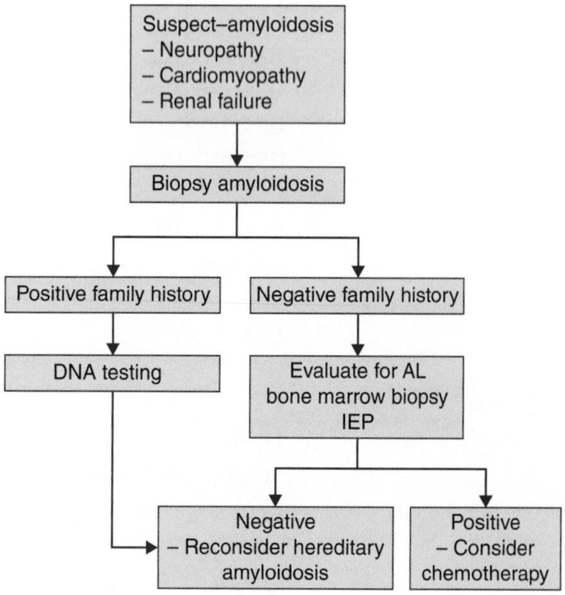

## Screening and Counseling

*Screening:* For members of families with known hereditary amyloidosis DNA testing and medical counseling can be of great value. Each type of hereditary amyloidosis tends to give the same age of onset and clinical phenotype in subsequent generations, but considerable variability can occur and the individual at risk of developing amyloidosis needs to be aware of this possibility. All of the hereditary amyloidoses are adult onset, autosomal dominant diseases, and testing of individuals younger than 18 years is not usually recommended. For the adult who is in the age range of his or her family's clinical onset of amyloidosis, DNA testing is very important. Due to the clinical variations of amyloidosis, definitive diagnosis is often delayed and is only made after long course of medical tests including cardiac catheterizations which could be averted if diagnosis had been considered at an earlier stage. Some individuals who are gene positive for an amyloidosis mutation use the data in family planning. Prenatal testing for TTR amyloidosis has been proven as a possible option but has not generally been widely used.

*Counseling:* For any patient with hereditary amyloidosis, it is standard practice to counsel that individual about the autosomal dominant inheritance pattern and that the disease usually has a fixed pattern within each family, although considerable variation may be encountered. Often family members will seek DNA screening to test for the presence of the identified gene mutation.

*Figure 92-1* Scheme for diagnosis of amyloidosis.

*Table 92-2 Mutant Proteins Associated With Autosomal Dominant Systemic Amyloidosis*

| Protein/Gene/Location | cDNA Change[a] | Amino Acid Change[b] | Codon Change | Clinical Features | OMIM |
|---|---|---|---|---|---|
| Transthyretin/18q12.1 | Greater than 100 mutations[c] (See Table 92-1) | | | | 176300 |
| Apolipoprotein AI/11q23.3 | 148G→C | Gly26Arg | GGC26CGC | PN,[d] nephropathy | 107680 |
| | 172G→A | Glu34Lys | GAA34AAA | Nephropathy | |
| | 251T→G | Leu60Arg | CTG60CGG | Nephropathy | |
| | 220T→C | Trp50Arg | TGG50CGG | Nephropathy | |
| | del250-284insGTCAC | del60-71insVal/Thr | del60-71ins GTCAC | Hepatic | |
| | 263T→C | Leu64Pro | CTC64CCC | Nephropathy | |
| | del280-288 | del70-72 | del70-72 | Nephropathy | |
| | 284T→A | Phe71Tyr | TTC71TAC | Hepatic, nephropathy | |
| | 294insA(fs)[e] | Asn74Lys(fs)[e] | AAC74AAAC(fs)[e] | Nephropathy | |
| | 296T→C | Leu75Pro | CTG75CCG | Hepatic | |
| | 341T→C | Leu90Pro | CTG90CCG | Cardiomyopathy, cutaneous, laryngeal | |
| | 532insGC(fs)[e] | Ala154(fs)[e] | GCC154GGC(fs)[e] | Nephropathy | |
| | 535ΔC | His155Met(fsx46) | CAT155ATG(fs)[e] | Nephropathy | |
| | 581T→C | Leu170Pro | CTG170CCG | Laryngeal | |
| | 590G→C | Arg173Pro | CGC173CCC | Cardiomyopathy, cutaneous, laryngeal | |
| | 593T→C | Leu174Ser | TTG174TCG | Cardiomyopathy | |
| | 595G→C | Ala175Pro | GCX175CCX[f] | Laryngeal | |
| | 604T→A | Leu178His | TTG178CAT | Cardiomyopathy, laryngeal | |
| Gelsolin/9q33.2 | 640G→A | Asp187Asn | GAC187AAC | PN,[d] Lattice corneal dystrophy | 105120 |
| | 640G→T | Asp187Tyr | GAC187TAC | PN[d] | |
| Cystatin-C/20p11.21 | 280T→A | Leu68Gln | CTG68CAG | Cerebral hemorrhage | 105150 |
| Fibrinogen Aα/4q31.3 | 1718G→T | Arg554Leu | CGT554CTT | Nephropathy | 134820 |
| | 1634A→T | Glu526Val | GAG526GTG | Nephropathy | |
| | 1629delG | Glu524Glu(fs)[e] | GAG524GA_ | Nephropathy | |
| | 1622delT | Val522Ala(fs)[e] | GTC522G_C | Nephropathy | |
| | 1676A→T | Glu540Val | GAA540GTA | Nephropathy | |
| | del1636-1650insCA1649-1650 | | | Nephropathy | |
| | 1712C→A | Pro552His | CCT552CAT | Nephropathy | |
| | 1670C→A | Thr538Lys | ACA538AAA | Nephropathy, neuropathy | |
| | 1632delT | Thr525fs | ACT525AC_ | Nephropathy | |
| Lysozyme/2q15 | 221T→C | Ile56Thr | ATA56ACA | Nephropathy, petechiae | 105200 |
| | 253G→C | Asp67His | GAT67CAT | Nephropathy | |
| | 244T→C | Trp64Arg | TGG64CGG | Nephropathy | |

*(Continued)*

*Table 92-2* **Mutant Proteins Associated With Autosomal Dominant Systemic Amyloidosis (Continued )**

| Protein/Gene/ Location | cDNA Change[a] | Amino Acid Change[b] | Codon Change | Clinical Features | OMIM |
|---|---|---|---|---|---|
| Transthyretin/18q12.1 | **Greater than 100 mutations[c] (See Table 92-1)** | | | | *176300* |
| Apolipoprotein AII/1q23.3 | 223T→A | Phe57Ile | TTT57ATT | Nephropathy | |
| | 413T→A | Trp112Arg | TGG112AGG | Nephropathy, GI | |
| | 301T→G | Stop78Gly | TGA78GGA | Nephropathy | 107670 |
| | 302G→C | Stop78Ser | TGA78TCA | Nephropathy | |
| | 301T→C | Stop78Arg | TGA78CGA | Nephropathy | |
| | 301T→A | Stop78Arg | TGA78AGA | Nephropathy | |
| | 302G→T | Stop78Leu | TGA78TTA | Nephropathy | |

[a]cDNA numbering is from initiation codon (ATG).

[b]Amino acids numbered for N-terminus of mature protein.

[c]List of most TTR mutations ( ).

[d]PN, peripheral neuropathy.

[e]fs, frameshift.

[f]Deduced.

☞**GENOTYPE-PHENOTYPE CORRELATION:** See Table 92-2 for an extensive listing of known correlates. The table below summarizes organ involvement for the major genes associated with hereditary amyloidosis:

| Gene Area | Organ Involvement |
|---|---|
| Transthyretin | Peripheral neuropathy, cardiomyopathy, leptomeningeal involvement, vitreous amyloidosis |
| Fibrinogen Aα-chain | Nephrotic syndrome |
| Apolipoprotein A-I | Renal failure, liver deposition |
| Apolipoprotein A-II | Renal failure |
| Gelsolin | Corneal dystrophy, facial paralysis |
| Cystatin-C | Intracranial hemorrhage |
| Lysozyme | Renal failure |

## Management and Treatment

***Management:*** Clinical management of hereditary amyloidosis depends on which type of disease and organ system is involved. The neuropathy of TTR amyloidosis is treated with analgesics. Cardiomyopathy requires treatment of congestive heart failure with diuretics. Use of negative ionotropic agents (β-blockers, calcium channel blockers) should be avoided. Liver transplantation has been done as a specific treatment for TTR amyloidosis and also fibrinogen Aα-chain and apolipoprotein A-I amyloidosis. Plasma TTR is synthesized exclusively by the liver and liver transplantation prevents the circulation of mutated TTR. Unfortunately, in some cases, the disease may progress with deposition of amyloid fibrils from wild type TTR. Some patients benefit with prolonged survival, especially patients with the Val30Met *TTR* mutation. Apolipoprotein A-I is synthesized by both the liver and intestinal tract and liver transplantation decreases the amount of variant apolipoprotein A-I in the circulation by only approximately 50%. Very often renal transplantation is required for apolipoprotein A-I. Fibrinogen Aα-chain amyloidosis can be treated with liver transplantation since only the liver makes fibrinogen and only the mutated fibrinogen forms amyloid fibrils. Unfortunately many patients have advanced renal insufficiency before they receive a liver transplant and therefore, require both liver and kidney transplant. Organ transplantations have been done for TTR amyloidosis (heart), apolipoprotein A-I (liver and kidney), and apolipoprotein A-II (kidney) with good extension of life span. There is no specific therapy for gelsolin or cystatin C amyloidosis. Table 92-2 lists candidate gene chromosome location, number of mutations, and associated disease phenotypes.

Transthyretin: Liver transplantation has been shown as a specific treatment for this type of amyloidosis. Approximately 2000 liver transplantations have been catalogued in Familial Amyloidotic Polyneuropathy World Transplant Registry and Domino Liver Transplant Registry (http://www.fapwtr.org/). The majority have been for Val30Met *TTR* mutation patients and the 5-year survival of approximately 80%. For all of the other *TTR* mutations (non-Val30Met) survival at 5 years has only been approximately 55%. Biochemical studies of tissues from patients dying with these mutations have been consistent with the progression of amyloid cardiomyopathy and neuropathy after liver transplantation due to continued amyloid deposition from wild-type TTR.

Fibrinogen Aα-chain: Liver transplantation has been shown to be a specific therapy for AFib amyloidosis. Amyloid deposits are composed of peptides from only the mutated form of fibrinogen Aα-chain and, therefore, wild-type fibrinogen Aα-chain does not contribute to deposition. In this respect we can consider liver transplantation to be curative for this particular form of amyloidosis. AFib has less than 100% penetrance and, therefore, liver transplantation should not be considered until a definitive tissue diagnosis of amyloidosis has been made.

Apolipoprotein A-I: Liver transplantation has been performed for many patients with this particular form of amyloidosis but studies have shown that only approximately 50% of plasma AApoAI is synthesized by the liver and, therefore, the disease progression may be expected from mutated AApoAI synthesized by the intestinal tract. Even so, many patients have had favorable response although renal transplantation has often become necessary.

***Therapeutics:*** Transthyretin: Small organic molecules that stabilize the structure of the TTR tetramer in plasma by binding to the thyroxin pocket include diflunisal (Dolobid) and tafamidis (Vyndaqel). Vyndaqel has been shown to have slowed progression of stage I polyneuropathy in a blinded placebo-controlled study. It has now been approved for stage I and stage II neuropathy in Europe. It has not, however, been approved by the US Food and Drug Administration. Diflunisal is currently under study in an NIH- and FDA-sponsored 2-year trial to test efficacy in patients with a variety of *TTR* mutations. This study should produce data within the next year.

***Pharmacogenetics:*** At this time there are no pharmacogenetic considerations in the treatment of hereditary amyloidosis.

## Molecular Genetics and Molecular Mechanism

### Genetic Testing:

☞CLINICAL AVAILABILITY OF TESTING: Genetic testing for *TTR* mutations is readily available. For the other genes that are associated with hereditary amyloidosis, genetic testing may be available through amyloid research laboratories. Perhaps the greatest value of genetic testing is alerting the physician that hereditary amyloidosis may be at the root of all of the patient's problems. This will often make lengthy and expensive diagnostic testing unnecessary. In amyloidosis secondary to TTR, early liver transplantation is recommended by many amyloid centers since the slowing of neuropathy or cardiomyopathy progression will lead to better outcomes. Early liver transplantation for amyloidosis secondary to fibrinogen Aα-chain can make renal dialysis and renal transplantation unnecessary if accomplished early in the course of disease.

***Future Directions:*** Presently medical therapies (TTR stabilizers and TTR antisense oligonucleotides) are being pursued for amyloidosis secondary to TTR to replace or augment orthotopic liver transplantation. Orthotopic liver transplantation for amyloidosis secondary to fibrinogen Aα-chain may be developed to preclude need for renal dialysis and kidney transplantation. Tafamidis (Vyndaqel) has been approved in Europe for slowing the progression of ATTR neuropathy when patients are treated in the early stages of disease. Diflunisal (Dolobid) is another TTR "stabilizer" which is currently the subject of a controlled international study and the study results are expected within the next year. On the horizon are clinical studies of TTR antisense oligonucleotide (ASO) to downregulate hepatic synthesis of transthyretin. siRNA is also being tested in early stage I studies for safety and efficacy of reducing plasma levels of TTR.

### BIBLIOGRAPHY:

1. Benson MD. Amyloidosis. In: Scriver CR, Beaudet AL, Sly WS, et al., eds. *The Metabolic and Molecular Bases of Inherited Disease.* 8th ed. New York, NY: McGraw Hill Book Co.; 2001:5345-5378.

2. Benson MD. Amyloidosis. In: Koopman WJ. *Arthritis and Allied Conditions—A Textbook of Rheumatology.* 15th ed. Philadelphia, PA: Lippincott Williams & Wilkins, A Waverly Company; 2004: 1933-1960.

3. Benson MD. Amyloidosis and other protein deposition diseases. In: Rimoin DL, Connor JM, Pyeritz RE, Korf BR. Emery and Rimoin's *Principles and Practice of Medical Genetics.* 5th ed. Philadelphia, PA, Churchill Livingstone publishers; 2005:1821-1834.

4. Benson MD. Other systemic forms of amyloidosis. In: Morie A, Gertz, S. Vincent Rajkumar, ed. *Amyloidosis: Diagnosis and Treatment.* Humana Press—Springer Science + Business Media, LLC; 2010:205-225.

5. Benson MD. Amyloidosis and other protein deposition diseases. In: Rimoin DL, Connor JM, Pyeritz RE, Korf BR, eds. Emery and Rimoin's *Principles and Practice of Medical Genetics—electronic chapter 79, 6th ed. (update).* Philadelphia, PA, Churchill Livingstone publishers; 2013:2144-2161.

## Supplementary Information

### OMIM REFERENCES:

[1] Cystatin C—Cerebral Amyloid Angiopathy (Iceland: type); (#105150)

[2] Apo AII—AFib (Ostertag type); (#105200)

[3] TTR—Oculoleptomeningeal Amyloidosis; (#105210)

[4] Gelsolin—Finnish Type Amyloidosis; (#105120)

### Alternative Names:

• Familial Amyloidosis
• Familial Amyloidotic Polyneuropathy
• Ostertag Amyloidosis

***Key Words:*** Amyloid, amyloidosis, familial amyloidotic polyneuropathy (FAP)

# 93 Glycogen Storage Disorders

Ingrid Cristian and Melissa Wasserstein

## KEY POINTS

- *Disease summary:*
  - Glycogen storage diseases (GSDs) are a group of inherited disorders of glycogen degradation or synthesis. Because glycogen is stored mainly in the liver, skeletal muscle, and heart muscle, the clinical spectrum of the GSDs is defined by involvement of these organs.
  - Currently, there are 10 well-defined types initially enumerated in order by which the enzymatic defect was identified. As the genetics of the glycogen pathway became clearer, different types of GSD have been grouped together, as is the case with type VIII and X which are now considered part of type VI.
  - Types 0, I, III, VI, IX, and XI mainly involve the liver, causing hypoglycemia and hepatomegaly. Type IV disease also involves the liver, but typically causes cirrhosis and liver failure in the absence of significant hypoglycemia. Types II, V, and VII mostly affect the muscle. Patients with type II classically have cardiomyopathy and skeletal muscle weakness, whereas muscle pain, fatigue, and exercise intolerance characterize the latter two types.

- *Hereditary basis:*
  - Most GSDs follow an autosomal recessive inheritance. Some patients with GSD V who were thought to be manifesting heterozygotes (only one mutation found in the *PYGM* gene) recently were found to carry a putative mutant allele when studies were performed on the cDNA in skeletal muscle.
  - GSD type IX is subdivided depending on the affected subunit of the phosphorylase kinase. When the α subunit is affected, this disorder follows an X-linked inheritance, whereas β and γ subunit deficiency follow an autosomal recessive inheritance pattern.

- *Differential diagnosis:*
  - The initial approach to diagnosing a GSD is based on the primary presenting feature. For example, patients with hypoglycemia and hepatomegaly should be evaluated for the hepatic GSDs (I, III, VI, IX) whereas patients with myopathy and muscular weakness in the absence of hypoglycemia should be evaluated for the muscular GSDs (II, V, VII).
  - The differential diagnosis of hypoglycemia is extensive and includes excessive insulin production or poorly controlled diabetes, disorders of cortisol production, and liver disease. The differential diagnosis of hypoglycemia with hepatomegaly is more limited, and includes mitochondrial hepatopathies, congenital disorders of glycosylation, fructose 1,6 bisphosphatase deficiency, Beckwith-Wiedemann syndrome, and fatty acid oxidation defects.
  - The differential diagnosis of myopathy and hypotonia includes spinal muscular atrophy, mitochondrial or respiratory chain disorders, limb-girdle muscular dystrophy, Duchenne-Becker muscular dystrophy, hypothyroidism, and fatty acid oxidation defects, such as very long chain acyl coenzyme A dehydrogenase (VLCAD).

## Diagnostic Criteria and Clinical Characteristics

**Diagnostic Criteria:** There are no universal diagnostic criteria for the various glycogen storage diseases but the following clinical information should direct the diagnosis:

**Clinical Characteristics:** GSD type Ia usually presents within the first few months of life with hypoglycemia, hepatomegaly, lactic acidosis (>2.5 mmol/L), hyperuricemia (>5 mg/dL), hyperlipidemia (TGL >250 mg/dL, cholesterol >200 mg/dL) and typical doll-like faces with fat cheeks, protuberant abdomen, and short stature. GSD type Ib has a similar clinical presentation as GSD type Ia but with additional findings, including neutropenia, recurrent bacterial infections, and inflammatory conditions such as inflammatory bowel disease. Individuals with GSD type Ia and 1b usually become hypoglycemic after about 3 hours of fasting. Glucagon or epinephrine does not cause an increase in blood glucose but lactate levels do increase.

GSD type II can vary and be divided into patients with a classic infantile form and a later-onset form. The classic form is characterized by failure to thrive, severe muscle weakness that includes progressive involvement of the respiratory muscles, hypertrophic cardiomyopathy, and death in infancy if untreated. The later-onset phenotype may present during childhood, adolescence, or adulthood with progressive proximal muscle weakness. The most common presentation of later-onset GSD type II is difficulty rising from a sitting position or climbing stairs, although many patients progress to wheelchair dependence and/or dependence on ventilatory support because of respiratory muscle weakness. Generally, they do not have cardiomyopathy. In all forms, serum creatine kinase may be elevated although a normal value cannot exclude the diagnosis since it can be normal in adults.

GSD type III is similar to GSD type I but usually has a later onset in childhood, and is differentiated by a normal glucagon response if performed within 2 hours after a meal. GSD type IIIa adult patients have skeletal muscle involvement with weakness, occasional pain, and increase in creatine kinase. Cardiomyopathy can occur as well. In adulthood, hepatic transaminases (AST/ALT >1000 U/L) increase but the hypoglycemia usually resolves.

GSD type IV has many different liver and neuromuscular presentations, varying with age of onset. In infants and children there is a classic liver form that presents with progressive liver disease and hepatic fibrosis by the age of 18 months, an infantile neuromuscular form with hypotonia, and a juvenile liver and muscular form which may present with cardiomyopathy. In adults there is a mild nonprogressive liver form; patients may have hepatosplenomegaly but generally do not develop cirrhosis. The adult polyglucosan body disease is an allelic form and may present with progressive central and peripheral nervous system dysfunction such as neurogenic bladder, gait difficulties, sensory loss, and mild cognitive dysfunction (executive function).

GSD type V usually presents in the second to third decade of life with exercise intolerance characterized by cramps and fatigue during the first few minutes of any type of exercise and intense sustained exercise (anaerobic). Symptoms are relieved during rest, as the body uses free fatty acids as a source of energy instead of glycogenolysis to release glucose for fuel. Myoglobinuria with consequent acute renal failure can occur following intense exercise and usually is reversible. GSD type V and VII have similar clinical manifestations. In patients with GSD type VII there may be, in addition, a compensated hemolysis with mild indirect hyperbilirubinemia and reticulocytosis due to partial deficit of erythrocyte glycolysis. Hyperuricemia may be more pronounced in GSD type VII.

Individuals with GSD type VI compared to individuals with GSD type I and III resist an even longer fasting period before they have hypoglycemia, and if present it is usually triggered by an intercurrent illness. They have hepatomegaly and their triglycerides, cholesterol, and liver transaminases may be mildly elevated but the creatine kinase, uric acid, and lactic acid are normal. GSD type VI and IX are difficult to differentiate clinically. If a female has the earlier-mentioned manifestations she is more likely to have type VI since the most common form of type IX has an X-linked inheritance pattern.

GSD type XI is rare and presents in infants. Since a glucose and galactose transporter is defective, there is fasting hypoglycemia and postprandial hyperglycemia and hypergalactosemia. Patients have hepatorenal accumulation of glycogen with secondary proximal renal tubule dysfunction although progression to renal failure is uncommon. Other findings include hyperlipidemia, hyperuricemia, osteopenia, with rickets later in life, and cataracts due to the hypergalactosemia.

GSD type 0 is considered to be a glycogen storage disorder because it involves glycogen metabolism and can present with hypoglycemia. However, GSD 0 is a defect in the synthesis of glycogen, leading to decreased hepatic glycogen content. Children may have fasting hypoglycemia but most adults are asymptomatic or have mild symptoms. See Table 93-1 for system involvement of the different GSDs.

## Screening and Counseling

*Screening:*

☞PRESYMPTOMATIC SCREENING:

- For individuals of Ashkenazi Jewish (AJ) descent (Eastern European) screening for prevalent disorders is available, which includes identification of R83C and Q347X in the *G6PC* gene (GSD type Ia). Screening for these two mutations yields a carrier detection rate of 95% in the Ashkenazi population. See Table 93-2 for genes and common mutations.
- Pilot screening programs are being implemented to test newborns for Pompe disease. Early treatment of infantile Pompe disease is of benefit in prolonging survival and improving cardiac and motor function.

☞SYMPTOMATIC SCREENING:

- Hypoglycemia + hepatomegaly (hepatic): screen for GSD type 0, I, III, IV, VI, IX, and XI

- Myopathy +/− rhabdomyolysis (muscular): screen for GSD type II, III, IV, V, and VII

*Counseling:* All GSDs except type IX (phosphorylase kinase deficiency, α subunit) are inherited in an autosomal recessive pattern. As such, parents are usually both carriers and have a 25% chance of having an affected child, 50% chance of having a carrier (asymptomatic), and 25% chance of having an unaffected child. Risks are not cumulative and each conception carries the same risk regardless of how many affected or unaffected individuals are present in each family.

GSD type IX is subdivided depending on which subunit of the phosphorylase kinase enzyme is affected. When the α subunit is affected this disorder follows an X-linked inheritance. In X-linked inheritance, females who carry an X-chromosome gene mutation have a 50% chance with each pregnancy to pass it on to the child. Females are usually not affected and if so have a milder presentation. Males cannot pass the gene mutation to their sons and always will pass it to their daughters.

☞GENOTYPE-PHENOTYPE CORRELATION: In general, nonsense mutations have a more severe phenotype in comparison to missense and some splice-site mutations. For GSD types 0, Ib, III, IV, VII, and XI there is no clear correlation between the genotype and phenotype.

In GSD type Ia there is genetic heterogeneity but patients homozygous for the splicing mutation, seen frequently in Eastern Asians (c.648G>T, also known as G727T) may have an increased risk to develop hepatocellular carcinoma and a mild phenotype with regard to hypoglycemia. This observation has been described although it has not been a universal finding. Also inconsistently, patients homozygous for a null mutation in the *G6PC* gene (p.G188R) manifest mild neutropenia similar to patients with GSD type Ib.

Two common mutations in the *GAA* gene, c.525delT and deletion of exon 18 when present can predict an infantile Pompe phenotype (type II). The splice-site mutation, IVS1-13T>G, is usually found in adult Pompe disease.

In GSD type VI there is a founder mutation in the Mennonite population (c.1620+1G>A) which deletes completely or partially exon 13 and still conserves the reading frame which may explain the milder phenotype in this population.

Finally, in GSD type IX usually *PHKB* mutations have a mild phenotype, *PHKG2* mutations are associated with a severe phenotype, and *PHKA2* mutations have a broad spectrum of presentation.

## Management and Treatment

*Hepatic GSD:* Perform a fasting blood sugar, lactate, uric acid, triglycerides, and if suggestive, either targeted mutation analysis, sequence analysis or liver biopsy with glycogen quantification and specific enzyme activity. Liver biopsy specimen should not be preserved by methods other than freezing and has to be shipped adequately. Enzyme analysis in whole blood is available for phosphorylase kinase (GSD type IX).

*Muscular GSD:* Perform an electrocardiogram and chest radiograph in infants (GSD type II), creatine kinase (acute and resting state), uric acid, complete blood count to check hemoglobin, indirect bilirubin, urine to determine myoglobinuria, lactate dehydrogenase, electromyography, forearm ischemic lactate test (failure of lactate increase with increased ammonia), and if suggestive,

*Table 93-1* **System Involvement**

| Type of GSD | Enzyme Deficiency | Primary Affected Tissue | Manifestation |
|---|---|---|---|
| 0 | Glycogen synthase | Liver | Hypoglycemia, short stature, osteopenia. |
| Ia (von Gierke disease) | Glucose-6-phospha-tase | Liver | Hypoglycemia, hepatomegaly, short stature, lactic acidemia, hyperuricemia, hyperlipidemia, kidney enlargement. Hypoglycemia usually presents in early infancy and is severe. |
| Ib | Glucose-6-phosphate translocase | Liver | Same features as type Ia as well as neutropenia and neutrophil dysfunction predisposing to severe infections and inflammatory bowel disease. Hypoglycemia usually presents in early infancy and is severe. |
| II (Pompe disease) | Lysosomal acid α-glucosidase (acid maltase deficiency) | Skeletal/cardiac muscle | Infantile: Undetectable or very low enzyme activity; manifests with progressive hypotonia, muscle weakness, hypertrophic and dilated cardiomyopathy and respiratory insufficiency. Fatal in early childhood if untreated.<br>Childhood/Juvenile/Adult: Higher residual enzyme activity presents with progressive proximal muscle weakness with eventual respiratory insufficiency. |
| IIIa (Cori/Forbes disease) | Amylo-1,6 glucosidase (debranching) | Liver Muscle | Hepatomegaly with increased transaminases and fibrosis, hypoglycemia and short stature which improve/resolve with age, muscle weakness with onset in third or fourth decade of life, and ventricular hypertrophy. Absence of renal enlargement. |
| IIIb (Cori/Forbes disease) | Amylo-1,6 glucosidase (debranching) | Liver | Similar to type IIIa with symptoms limited to liver, due to deficiency of only the hepatic enzyme as opposed to liver/muscle enzymatic deficiency seen in type IIIa. |
| IV (Andersen disease) | Amylo-1,4 to 1,6 transglucosidase (branching enzyme) | Liver Muscle CNS | Several variants. *Hepatic*: classic form: hepatomegaly and liver cirrhosis, death in early childhood and a nonprogressive hepatic form; *neuromuscular*: fatal perinatal form, congenital form: hypotonia and death in early infancy; adult form: myopathy resembling muscular dystrophy with central/peripheral nervous system involvement. |
| V (McArdle disease) | Muscle isoform of glycogen phosphorylase | Muscle | Usually young adults with exercise intolerance and recurrent myoglobinuria after exercise. Elevated creatine kinase at rest and rising further during exercise. |
| VI (Hers disease) | Liver isoform of glycogen phosphorylase | Liver | Hepatomegaly, possible hypoglycemia with illness and prolonged fasting, hyperlipidemia and ketosis, and short stature. Symptoms improve with age. |
| VII (Tarui disease) | Muscle phosphofructokinase | Muscle | Similar to type V, but fatigue and pain with exercise start usually in childhood and compensated hemolytic anemia. |
| IX | Liver and muscle phosphorylase kinase | Liver, skeletal/cardiac muscle | Variable presentation (six subtypes) depending on which subunit is affected. Hepatomegaly, mild hypoglycemia, hypotonia, weakness, and exercise intolerance may be possible. |
| XI (Fanconi-Bickel syndrome) | Glucose transporter 2 | Liver Kidney | Hypoglycemia and hepatomegaly with postprandial hyperglycemia and hypergalactosemia, proximal renal tubular dysfunction, short stature, hyperlipidemia, osteopenia. |

*Table 93-2* *Genes and Most Prevalent Mutations*

| Type of GSD | Gene | Chromosome | OMIM Entries | Common Mutations | Prevalence in Certain Populations |
|---|---|---|---|---|---|
| Ia | G6PC | 17q21 | 232200 | R83C<br>Q347X<br>130X | All three mutations: 60%-70% in affected Caucasians<br>R83C: 98% in affected Ashkenazi Jewish (AJ),[a] 33% in affected Caucasians, 26% in affected Chinese |
| Ib | SLC37A4 | 11q23 | 232220 and 602671 | 400X<br>G339C<br>W118R | 400X + G339C: 50% in affected Caucasians<br>W118R: 50% in affected Japanese |
| II | GAA | 17q25.2 | 232300 and 606800 | 525delT<br>del exon 18<br>IVS1-13T>G | All three mutations: 60% in affected Caucasians<br>525delT: 9% of US cases of early onset<br>del exon 18: 5% of US cases of early onset<br>IVS1 -13T>G: 50% of late-onset disease |
| III | AGL | 1p21 | 232400 and 610860 | IVS21+1G >A<br>W1327X | IVS21 +21G>A 28% in affected Italians |
| IV | GBE1 | 3p14 | 232500 and 607839 | No common mutation | |
| V | PYGM | 11q13 | 232600 and 608455 | R50X<br>G205S<br>W798R | > 90% of affected in the general population |
| VI | PYGL | 14q21 | 232700 | No common mutation | IVS13+1G>A in the Mennonite (founder mutation) |
| VII | PFKM | 12q13.3 | 232800 and 606800 | IVS5+1g>a<br>delC2003 | 95% of affected in Ashkenazi Jewish |
| IX | PHKA1<br>PHKA2<br>PHKB<br>PHKG2 | Xq13<br>Xp22.2<br>16q12 | 311870 and 300559<br>300798 and 306000<br>172490 and 261750<br>172471 and 613027 | No common mutation | |
| XI | SLC2A2 | 3q26.1 | 227810 and 138160 | R301X<br>R365X | Most are "private" mutations |
| O | GYS2 | 12p12.2 | 240600 and 138571 | No common mutation | |

[a]Ashkenazi Jewish (AJ) population refers to Jews of Central and Eastern European ancestry.

mutation analysis or muscle biopsy to visualize glycogen and determine muscle enzyme activity. Muscle biopsy is recommended 1 month after an acute exacerbation since myofiber necrosis and inflammatory infiltrates may confuse diagnosis. There are supportive laboratory biomarkers that may be increased in patients with Pompe disease such as elevation of the urinary and plasma concentrations of the tetrasaccharides, $Hex_4$ and $Glc_4$. The concentrations of $Glc_4$ and $Hex_4$ have been shown to correlate with the treatment effects of enzyme replacement therapy and are used to follow metabolic control.

When a diagnosis is confirmed, a multidisciplinary approach is required for most of the glycogen storage disorders including nutritionists, medical geneticists, cardiologists, pulmonologists, neurologists, and other healthcare professionals.

☞MANAGEMENT OF THE HEPATIC GSDs: In GSD type I, the mainstay of treatment is to prevent hypoglycemia and maintain normal acid-base status. It is imperative to maintain good metabolic control in order to avoid severe complications of hypoglycemia. Good glycemic control usually results in good control of lactate, lipids, and uric acid, so prevention of hypoglycemia is imperative. This is obtained by constant infusion of glucose using small frequent meals rich in complex carbohydrates supplemented with uncooked cornstarch. Nocturnal continuous gastric drip feedings are often used in infants younger than 1 year of age, who are often cornstarch intolerant. The amount of uncooked cornstarch varies in each patient and should be carefully designed on an individual basis. Fructose and galactose should be restricted. Recommended biochemical targets and detailed nutrition plans are established in the 2002 Guidelines for management published by the European Study Group. Medications such as xanthine oxidase inhibitors, angiotensin-converting enzyme (ACE) inhibitors, lipid-lowering medications, and supplementation of vitamins and minerals are individualized depending on biochemical markers. Ultrasonography initially should be performed yearly (0-10 years of age) and biannually after 10 years of age to screen for liver adenomas. Liver adenomas can cause mechanical complications and also can undergo malignant transformation, therefore serum α-fetoprotein and carcinoembryonic antigen may be used as markers. In addition, if an adenoma is detected a computed tomography (CT) scan or magnetic resonance imaging (MRI) is recommended. Conservative management with frequent imaging (every 3 months) or surgical interventions are options depending on individual circumstances. Management of GSD type Ib is similar; in addition, granulocyte colony-stimulating factor may be used. Nutritional therapy for GSD type III includes a high protein diet with frequent feeding and complex carbohydrates similar to type 1. Restriction of sucrose, fructose, and lactose is not necessary. Hypoglycemia should also be avoided therefore continuous nocturnal intragastric feeding and raw cornstarch may be required. In addition, cardiology consultation is required because of the risk of cardiomyopathy.

Although patients with GSD type VI may not need any treatment, if hypoglycemia is present, the same management options as for GSD types I and III may be used. GSD type IX usually has a benign course and affected individuals typically do not require specific treatment. Some patients may have hypoglycemia and are encouraged to follow a high, complex carbohydrate diet with frequent feeds. In GSD type 0, symptoms are relieved by frequent feedings, a diet high in protein and cornstarch. In contrast with type I, less carbohydrate is encouraged to prevent postprandial hyperglycemia and subsequent lactic acidosis. Initial management of GSD type XI patients usually requires hydration, electrolyte correction, and replacement of vitamin D. Long-term management includes restriction of galactose and frequent small meals with uncooked cornstarch. If galactose is not restricted, symptoms and signs similar to galactosemia can be present, such as cataracts. Some patients with GSD type IX also have significant liver disease and fibrosis.

Liver transplantation has been performed in patients with GSD types Ia, Ib, III, IV, and VI. The risks of liver transplantation are high and should only be considered when other interventions are not successful and the risk of hepatocellular carcinoma, cirrhosis, or progressive liver dysfunction outweighs these risks. The only effective treatment for GSD type IV patients with progressive liver disease is liver transplantation.

☞**MANAGEMENT OF THE MUSCULAR GSDS:** The American College of Medical Genetics published guidelines for management of GSD type II (Pompe disease) in 2006. Recombinant

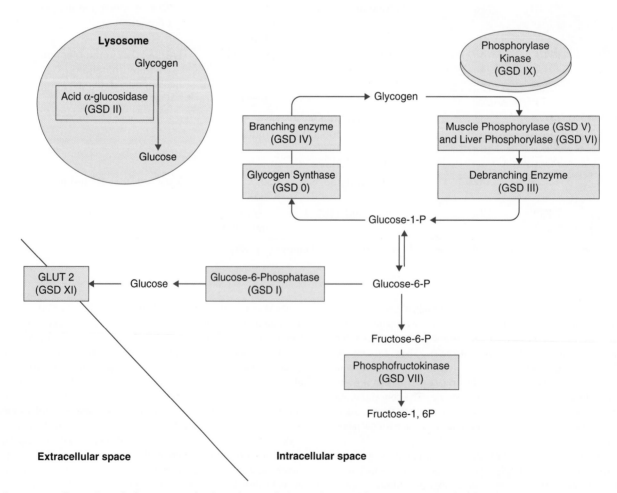

*Figure 93-1* Illustration of Glycogen Synthesis and Degradation Pathway with Respective Metabolic Defects.

human enzyme replacement therapy (acid α-glucosidase) which is marketed under the trade names Myozyme and Lumizyme, are currently FDA approved for the infantile form and the late-onset (noninfantile) form, respectively. Enzyme replacement therapy (ERT) studies for late-onset Pompe disease are ongoing showing variable outcomes but overall treatment seems to stabilize the chronic progressive disorder in some patients. Outcome is improved when ERT is started early before irreversible changes occur. Cross-reacting immunologic material (CRIM) status plays a significant role in determining response to treatment; infants who are CRIM-negative are more likely to have immunologic reactions against ERT and require immunomodulatory therapy. Physical therapy is required to maintain range of motion and decrease contractures for all patients. In advanced respiratory disease, support with biphasic positive airway pressure (BiPAP), continuous positive airway pressure (CPAP), and even mechanical ventilation may be necessary.

In GSD type V, aerobic conditioning programs increase exercise capacity. Systematic reviews have not shown consistent significant evidence from any specific nutritional or pharmacologic intervention. Creatine monohydrates, vitamin $B_6$, carbohydrate-rich diet, protein-rich diet, and ingestion of sucrose before exercising have been studied and may improve symptoms in some patients.

For GSD type VII, no specific management is available but avoiding strenuous exercise is encouraged to prevent muscle cramps and myoglobinuria. Patients with type IX should also follow these recommendations.

## Molecular Genetics and Molecular Mechanism

See Figure 93-1 for illustration of glycogen synthesis and degradation pathway with respective metabolic defects.

Glycogen, as the storage system for glucose, is utilized as a source of energy in the liver and muscle. Multiple enzymes are involved in this process which either participate in the synthesis (glycogenesis) or breakdown of glycogen (glycogenolysis). In the various GSDs there are specific enzymatic deficiencies, which are encoded by different genes that lead to accumulation of products prior to the block and absence of other products distal to the block, most importantly glucose. The glycogenesis pathway involves the glycogen synthase and the branching enzyme (GSD types 0 and IV, respectively). Together they produce glycogen which is reserved for times when systemic glucose is required or high-intensity muscle contraction is occurring. When glucose is required the glycogenolysis pathway is activated which involves glycogen phosphorylase and the debranching enzyme (GSD types V, VI, IX, and III, respectively).

GSD type II is a prototype of the lysosomal storage diseases; there is deficiency of the enzyme essential in releasing glucose from glycogen in lysosomes. GSD type XI is a defect in the transportation of monosaccharides across the membranes, such as glucose.

***Genetic Testing:*** Testing is clinically available in several laboratories. Most GSDs are diagnosed based on clinical parameters combined with targeted mutation analysis or DNA sequencing. Enzyme assays were used more commonly in the past but have been replaced by DNA sequencing, due to its advantages such as the less invasive nature, the ability to detect carriers, and offer prenatal counseling.

For details on specific laboratories offering testing: http://www.ncbi.nlm.nih.gov/gtr/ or http://www.genetests.org/

## BIBLIOGRAPHY:

1. Kishnani PS KD, Chen YT. Glycogen storage diseases. In: Valle D, ed. Online Metabolic and Molecular Bases of Inherited Disease New York, NY: McGraw-Hill; 2009.

2. Garcia-Consuegra I, Rubio JC, Nogales-Gadea G, et al. Novel mutations in patients with McArdle disease by analysis of skeletal muscle mRNA. *J Med Genet.* 2009;46(3):198-202.

3. Bembi B, Cerini E, Danesino C, et al. Diagnosis of glycogenosis type II. *Neurology.* 2008;71(23 suppl 2):S4-S11.

4. Wolfsdorf JI, Weinstein DA. Glycogen storage diseases. *Rev Endocr Metab Disord.* 2003;4(1):95-102.

5. Shin YS. Glycogen storage disease: clinical, biochemical, and molecular heterogeneity. *Semin Pediatr Neurol.* 2006;13(2):115-120.

6. Ozen H. Glycogen storage diseases: new perspectives. *World J Gastroenterol.* 2007;13(18):2541-2553.

7. Burton BK. Newborn screening for Pompe disease: an update, 2011. *Am J Med Genet C Semin Med Genet.* 2012;160(1):8-12.

8. Kishnani PS, Hwu WL, Mandel H, Nicolino M, Yong F, Corzo D. A retrospective, multinational, multicenter study on the natural history of infantile-onset Pompe disease. *J Pediatr.* 2006;148(5):671-676.

9. Matern D, Seydewitz HH, Bali D, Lang C, Chen YT. Glycogen storage disease type I: diagnosis and phenotype/genotype correlation. *Eur J Pediatr.* 2002;161(suppl 1):S10-S19.

10. van Adel BA, Tarnopolsky MA. Metabolic myopathies: update 2009. *J Clin Neuromuscul Dis.* 2009;10(3):97-121.

11. Burr ML, Roos JC, Ostor AJ. Metabolic myopathies: a guide and update for clinicians. *Curr Opin Rheumatol.* 2008;20(6):639-647.

12. Winchester B, Bali D, Bodamer OA, et al. Methods for a prompt and reliable laboratory diagnosis of Pompe disease: report from an international consensus meeting. *Mol Genet Metab.* 2008;93(3):275-281.

13. Heller S, Worona L, Consuelo A. Nutritional therapy for glycogen storage diseases. *J Pediatr Gastroenterol Nutr.* 2008;47(suppl 1): S15-S21.

14. Rake JP, Visser G, Labrune P, Leonard JV, Ullrich K, Smit GP. Guidelines for management of glycogen storage disease type I–European Study on Glycogen Storage Disease Type I (ESGSD I). *Eur J Pediatr.* 2002;161(suppl 1):S112-S119.

15. Davis MK, Weinstein DA. Liver transplantation in children with glycogen storage disease: controversies and evaluation of the risk/benefit of this procedure. *Pediatr Transplant.* 2008;12(2):137-145.

16. van der Ploeg AT, Clemens PR, Corzo D, et al. A randomized study of alglucosidase alfa in late-onset Pompe's disease. *N Engl J Med.* 2010;362(15):1396-1406.

17. Kishnani PS, Goldenberg PC, DeArmey SL, et al. Cross-reactive immunologic material status affects treatment outcomes in Pompe disease infants. *Mol Genet Metab.* 2010;99(1):26-33.

18. Quinlivan R, Martinuzzi A, Schoser B. Pharmacological and nutritional treatment for McArdle disease (Glycogen Storage Disease type V). *Cochrane Database Syst Rev.* 2010;(12):CD003458.

## Supplementary Information

***Key Words:*** Glycogen storage disease, liver, muscle, metabolic myopathies, inborn errors of metabolism

# 94 Cholesteryl Ester Storage Disease

Erin P. Hoffman, Michael F. Murray, and Monica A. Giovanni

## KEY POINTS

- *Disease summary:*
  - Cholesteryl ester storage disease (CESD) is a lysosomal storage disorder (LSD) caused by a deficiency of lysosomal acid lipase (LAL), an enzyme necessary for the breakdown of cholesteryl esters and triglycerides.
  - CESD is part of the LAL deficiency spectrum. In general, mutations that allow for residual LAL enzyme function result in CESD, while Wolman disease (WD), the infantile fatal form of LAL deficiency, stems from null mutations with no residual enzyme function.
  - Features of CESD are predominantly a consequence of the intracellular accumulation of cholesteryl esters and triglycerides in liver, spleen, lymph nodes, and other tissues. Biopsy can show sea-blue histiocytes, large Kupffer cells with increased vacuoles, lipid droplets, or cholesterol crystals.
  - Individuals with CESD commonly present with an abnormal lipid profile, which can include increased total cholesterol, high low-density lipoprotein (LDL), low high-density lipoprotein (HDL), and high-normal to high triglycerides; liver and/or spleen enlargement; or other types of liver disease such as steatosis, fibrosis, or cirrhosis.
  - Individuals with CESD are at risk for premature atherosclerosis, liver disease, bleeding complications, and intestinal malabsorption.

- *Hereditary basis:*
  - CESD is an autosomal recessive disorder caused by mutations in *LIPA*.
  - Variability can be seen in the severity of phenotypes even within families, though both CESD and WD would not be expected within the same sibship.

- *Differential diagnosis:*
  - There is overlap in the clinical features of CESD and other LSDs, such as Gaucher disease (GD) and Niemann-Pick disease (NPD). Individuals with NPD may have a similar lipid profile to individuals with CESD, and hepatosplenomegaly is a common feature of all three diseases. Individuals with CESD would not be expected to have the bone disease common to GD or the lung disease common to NPD. Biochemical analysis can distinguish between LSDs.
  - Hyperlipidemia can be caused by both genetic and environmental factors. It is important to distinguish between CESD and other genetic causes of hyperlipidemia, such as familial hypercholesterolemia (FH). The lipid profile of FH can include high total cholesterol and LDL levels, with low HDL and normal or high triglyceride levels. FH is inherited in an autosomal dominant manner. It is essential to consider the lipid profile, the inheritance pattern, and the nonlipid associated phenotype when distinguishing between potential genetic etiologies of hyperlipidemia.
  - Hepatomegaly and splenomegaly are common features of other storage disorders, such as other LSDs and glycogen storage disorders (GSD). CESD can be distinguished from other storage disorders based on associated features and biochemical analysis.
  - Liver disease in CESD can be misdiagnosed as nonalcoholic fatty liver disease or cryptogenic cirrhosis. In the absence of an identifiable cause of liver disease, CESD should be considered.
  - A high index of suspicion for CESD can potentially lead to a specific diagnosis in cases of "idiopathic" liver disease.

## Diagnostic Criteria and Clinical Characteristics

**Diagnostic Criteria:** Deficient LAL activity is diagnostic and can be demonstrated by enzyme assay performed on peripheral blood or fibroblast sample.

**Clinical Characteristics:** (see Table 94-1) Hepatomegaly or splenomegaly is commonly a presenting feature and may be present since childhood or adolescence. It is not uncommon for diagnosis to be delayed for years after organomegaly is noted. Some individuals initially present with a catastrophic event such as a variceal bleed, stroke, or myocardial infarct.

Cardiovascular disease is common due to premature atherosclerosis caused by increased LDL cholesterol (see Table 94-2), placing affected individuals at increased risk for severe complications such as stroke.

Liver disease due to increased lipid deposition is common. Manifestations can include hepatomegaly, cirrhosis, fibrosis, nonalcoholic fatty liver disease, and altered liver function with or without jaundice. Biopsy shows signs of CESD, which can include sea-blue histiocytes, large Kupffer cells with increased vacuoles, lipid droplets, or cholesterol crystals.

Splenomegaly with resultant hypersplenism and associated cytopenias including anemia and thrombocytopenia can occur.

Intestinal malabsorption due to lipid deposition in the wall of the intestinal tract can lead to diarrhea, weight loss, and associated nutritional deficits.

Varicosities may be present and are at risk for hemorrhage. In particular, varicosities of the esophagus and the limbs have been noted.

Xanthomas are not common but when present are similar to those seen in familial hypercholesterolemia, particularly around the eyes.

*Table 94-1* **System Involvement**

| System | Manifestation | Wolman (W), CESD (C), or Both (B) |
|--------|---------------|-----------------------------------|
| GI | Hepatocellular dysfunction with elevated enzymes | B |
| | Hepatosplenomegaly (HSM) | B |
| | Hepatic steatosis, fibrosis, or cirrhosis | B |
| | Mesenteric lipodystrophy | B |
| | Malabsorption | B |
| | Diarrhea | B |
| | Esophageal varicosities | C |
| Cardiovascular | Atherosclerosis | C |
| Pulmonary | Pulmonary hypertension | C |
| Hematologic | Anemia | B |
| | Thrombocytopenia | B |
| Endocrine | Punctate adrenal calcification, adrenal failure | B |
| Dermatologic | Xanthomas | C |

## Screening and Counseling

*Screening:* CESD should be considered in the presence of unexplained liver disease, hepatomegaly or splenomegaly, premature vascular disease, or unexplained abnormal serum lipid levels (see Table 94-2). Clinical suspicion of NPD, GD, or GSD that cannot be confirmed by biochemical analysis should also arouse suspicion for CESD. LAL enzyme assay will rule in or rule out CESD.

*Counseling:* CESD is inherited in an autosomal recessive manner. Parents of an affected individual are obligate carriers. Siblings of a proband have a 25% chance of being affected, a 50% chance of being unaffected carriers, and a 25% chance of being unaffected and not a carrier. All children of an affected individual will be carriers.

LAL deficiency is thought to be completely penetrant with wide phenotypic variability. LAL deficiency can be fatal in infancy or diagnosed incidentally in late adulthood. The infantile phenotype is known as Wolman disease, with CESD consisting of all later-onset phenotypes (see Table 94-1). Variability stems from different mutations resulting in varying amounts of residual enzyme activity. Severity can be variable even within families, though both WD and CESD would not be expected in the same sibship.

## Management and Treatment

*Management:* There is no consensus regarding screening for CESD. Patients should be monitored for the major causes of morbidity and mortality.

*Treatment:* There is no proven treatment for CESD. Symptoms should be treated as needed. Attempts can be made to reduce cholesterol through standard methods such as the use of statins, cholestyramine, lipophilic vitamins, and a diet low in cholesterol and triglycerides. Liver transplant can be considered for liver failure. Enzyme replacement strategies similar to those in other LSDs are being researched.

## Molecular Genetics and Molecular Mechanism

CESD is caused by mutations in *LIPA* located at 10q23.2-q23.3. Lysosomal acid lipase is responsible for the degradation of LDL cholesteryl esters and triglycerides in lysosomes. Free cholesterol is then transferred to the endoplasmic reticulum, where it performs regulatory functions. HMG-CoA reductase activity is suppressed, thereby reducing the cellular synthesis of cholesterol. Additionally, LDL receptor gene transcription is suppressed, leading to reduced uptake of LDL. The absence of sufficient LAL activity therefore results in heightened synthesis of endogenous cholesterol, increased LDL receptor gene expression, and lysosomal accumulation of cholesteryl esters and triglycerides.

The G894A mutation in *LIPA* accounts for approximately 50% of mutations in individuals of European ancestry with CESD.

*Table 94-2* **Typical Lipid Profile in CESD**

**Typical Lipid Profile in CESD**

| Total Cholesterol (mg/dL) | LDL Cholesterol (mg/dL) | HDL Cholesterol (mg/dL) | Triglycerides (mg/dL) |
|---------------------------|-------------------------|-------------------------|------------------------|
| Normal <200 | Normal <130 | Normal >50 | Normal <150 |
| Range in reported cases: 106-428 | Range in reported cases: 147-292 | Range in reported cases: 8-44 | Range in reported cases: 60-443 |
| Average in reported cases: 293 | Average in reported cases: 226 | Average in reported cases: 26 | Average in reported cases: 214 |
| 88% of reported cases: > normal range | 100% of reported cases: > normal range | 100% of reported cases: < normal range | 76% of reported cases: > normal range |

Table compiled from a review of 26 cases published in the literature 1995-2009.

*Table 94-3 Molecular Genetic Testing*

| Gene | Testing Modality | Mutation Type | Detection Rate |
|------|------------------|---------------|----------------|
| *LIPA* | Sequence analysis | Single-nucleotide changes, small insertions or deletions | >95% |
| *LIPA* | MLPA | Whole exon deletions or duplications | <5% |

Nearly all individuals with CESD in the published literature are compound heterozygous or homozygous for G894A. This mutation leads to alternative splicing and exon skipping, resulting in an in-frame deletion of 24 amino acids from the final protein, rendering it enzymatically ineffective. Correct splicing does occasionally occur in spite of this mutation, however, with approximately 5% of the protein produced of full length and therefore enzymatically active.

*Genetic Testing:* Sequencing and deletion or duplication analysis of *LIPA* is clinically available (see Table 94-3). Targeted mutation analysis and prenatal diagnosis are also clinically available if familial mutations are known.

Enzyme assay is diagnostic. Genetic sequencing of a proband may be undertaken to aid in informing family members of carrier status and for the purposes of family planning to enable prenatal diagnosis or preimplantation genetic diagnosis.

## BIBLIOGRAPHY:

1. Anderson RA, Bryson GM, Parks JS. Lysosomal acid lipase mutations that determine phenotype in Wolman and cholesterol ester storage disease. *Mol Genet Metab*. 1999;68:333-345.

2. Ameis D, Brockmann G, Knoblich R, et al. A 5' splice-region mutation and a dinucleotide deletion in the lysosomal acid lipase gene in two patients with cholesteryl ester storage disease. *J Lipid Res*. 1995;36:241-250.

3. Assmann G, Seedorf U. Acid dipase deficiency: Wolman disease and cholesteryl ester storage disease. In: Scriver CR, Beaudet AL, Sly WS, Valle D, eds. *The Metabolic and Molecular Basis of Inherited Disease*. 8th ed. New York, NY: McGraw-Hill; 2001:3551.

4. Drebber U, Andersen M, Kasper HU, Lohse P, Stolte M, Dienes HP. Severe chronic diarrhea and weight loss in cholesteryl ester storage disease: a case report. *World J Gastroenterol*. 2005;11(15):2364-2366.

5. Elleder M, Ledvinova J, Cieslar P, Kuhn R. Subclinical course of cholesterol ester storage disease (CESD) diagnosed in adulthood: report on two cases with remarks on the nature of the liver storage process. *Virchows Archiv A Pathol Anat Histopathol*. 1990;416:357-365.

6. Gasche C, Aslanidis C, Kain R, et al. A novel variant of lysosomal acid lipase in cholesteryl ester storage disease associated with mild phenotype and improvement on lovastatin. *J Hepatol*. 1997;27:744-750.

7. Hooper AJ, Tran HA, Formby MR, Burnett JR. A novel missense LIPA gene mutation, N98S, in a patient with cholesteryl ester storage disease. *Clin Chim Acta*. 2008;398:152-154.

8. Klima H, Ullrich K, Aslanidis C, Fehringer P, Lackner KJ, Schmitz G. A splice junction mutation causes deletion of a 72-base exon from the mRNA for lysosomal acid lipase in a patient with cholesteryl ester storage disease. *J Clin Invest*. 1993;92:2713-2718.

9. Muntoni S, Wiebusch H, Funke H. Homozygosity for a splice junction mutation in exon 8 of the gene encoding lysosomal acid lipase in a Spanish kindred with cholesterol ester storage disease (CESD). *Hum Genet*. 1995;95:491-494.

10. Pisciotta L, Fresa R, Bellocchio A, et al. Cholesteryl ester storage disease (CESD) due to novel mutation in the *LIPA* gene. *Mol Genet Metab*. 2009;97:143-148.

11. Seedorf U, Wiebusch H, Muntoni S, et al. A novel variant of lysosomal acid lipase (Leu336Pro) associated with acid lipase deficiency and cholesterol ester storage disease. *Arterioscler Thromb Vasc Biol*. 1995;15:773-778.

12. Tadiboyina VT, Liu DM, Miskie BA, Wang J, Hegele RA. Treatment of dyslipidemia with lovastatin and ezetimibe in an adolescent with cholesterol ester storage disease. *Lipids Health Dis*. 2005;4:26.

13. vom Dahl S, Harzer K, Rolfs A, et al. Hepatosplenomegalic lipidosis: what unless Gaucher? Adult cholesteryl ester storage disease (CESD) with anemia, mesenteric lipodystrophy, increased plasma chitotriosidase activity and a homozygous lysosomal acid lipase −1 exon 8 splice junction mutation. *J Hepatol*. 1999;31:741-746.

## Supplementary Information

### OMIM REFERENCES:

[1] Lysosomal Acid Lipase Deficiency (#278000)

[2] Lipase A, Lysosomal Acid; LIPA (*613497)

[3] Wolman Disease With Hypolipoproteinemia and Acanthocytosis (#278100)

### Alternative Names:

- Cholesterol Ester Storage Disease
- Lysosomal Acid Lipase (LAL) Deficiency
- Wolman Disease (Infantile Form)
- Acid Lipase Disease
- Acid Lipase Deficiency
- Acid Cholesteryl Ester Hydrolase Deficiency
- Cholesteryl Ester Hydrolase Deficiency Storage Disease

*Key Words:* Hyperlipidemia, hepatomegaly, splenomegaly, liver disease, steatosis, fibrosis, cirrhosis, premature atherosclerosis, pulmonary hypertension, esophageal varices, xanthomas

# 95 The Organic Acidemias

Deborah Marsden

## KEY POINTS

- *Disease summary:*
  - Organic acidemias are disorders of intermediary metabolism of one or more amino acid constituents of protein, due to a deficiency of an enzyme in the respective catabolic pathway, or an essential enzyme cofactor.
  - The accumulation of the toxic intermediates (organic acids) can result in life-threatening organ damage, primarily of the brain, liver, and kidneys.
  - There is a phenotypic spectrum, ranging from severe neonatal presentation to later onset of milder symptoms in childhood or adulthood. Clinical phenotype depends largely on the amount of residual enzyme activity, determined by the mutations.
- *Hereditary basis:*
  - Autosomal recessive
- *Differential diagnosis:*
  - Sepsis
  - Drug or chemical intoxication
  - Mitochondrial disease

## Diagnostic Criteria and Clinical Characteristics

Urine organic acid analysis demonstrates accumulation of specific metabolites. Plasma acylcarnitine analysis detects characteristic acylcarnitine conjugates of accumulated metabolites, but is not always diagnostic, for example, propionylcarnitine (C3) accumulates in both propionic acidemia (PA) and methylmalonic acidemia (MMA), and hydroxyisovalerylcarnitine (C5OH) accumulates in several disorders (Table 95-1). The diagnosis can usually be confirmed by measurement of the enzyme activity in fibroblasts or white blood cells. Mutation analysis is clinically available for most organic acidemias, though it is not usually a first-line test because of the large number of mutations in each disorder. In some instances, there are mutation hot spots, or an increased frequency of certain mutations due to a founder effect, such as in the Inuits of Greenland and in Japanese with PA and the Old Order Amish with glutaric aciduria type 1 (GA1). In these cases, targeted mutation analysis is feasible.

Severe metabolic acidosis with ketosis is the hallmark of the organic acidemias. Lactic acidosis may occur, either as a primary cause from the inhibition of a relevant enzyme, for example, acetyl coenzyme A (CoA) carboxylase (MCD, Table 95-1) or secondary to decreased perfusion. Hyperammonemia (secondary to inhibition of the urea cycle) is also common and can be distinguished from a primary urea cycle by the urine organic acid pattern and also the presence of acidosis rather than respiratory alkalosis. Hypoglycemia is variable.

The outcomes are often dependent on the severity and timing of the initial episode of decompensation: early neonatal disease is usually associated with a more severe phenotype. Developmental delay is common. Movement disorder (dystonia) can occur in MMA, PA, and GA1, due to infarction of the basal ganglia. In MMA, this can occur at any age, though in GA1 it is a typical outcome of severe acidosis in the first 2 years of life. Pancreatitis is relatively common in PA and other branched-chain organic acidemias.

## Screening and Counseling

Newborn screening by tandem mass spectrometry analysis of acylcarnitines from a dried blood spot sample may detect many organic acidemias presymptomatically, allowing for therapeutic intervention and averting acute crises. Some, however, may present within 2 to 5 days of life before screening results are available.

- Autosomal recessive inheritance. Both parents are carriers of a mutation in the relative gene. Subsequent children have a 25% risk of being affected, 50% risk of being carriers.
- Higher incidence in consanguineous families.
- Prenatal or preimplantation diagnosis is available for most disorders when the specific mutations carried by the parents are known.

## Management and Treatment

The management of acute metabolic acidosis is critical to prevent or limit major neurologic sequelae. Rehydration with high dextrose concentration intravenous fluids is the primary therapy, although in some very severe cases, hemo- or peritoneal dialysis may be used. Dextrose will interrupt the catabolic process; the addition of intravenous lipid will provide additional calories. In severe acidosis, use of bicarbonate may be necessary. Secondary hyperammonemia generally responds to treatment of the underlying organic acidemia.

Cofactor supplementation should be used where appropriate, such as vitamin $B_{12}$ in MMA and biotin in multiple carboxylase deficiency and biotinidase deficiency (Table 95-1); carnitine supplementation is used to conjugate the toxic intermediates (forming acylcarnitines) that can be rapidly cleared and to prevent secondary carnitine deficiency, which can lead to secondary inhibition of fatty acid oxidation, and hypoglycemia. In an acute neonatal presentation, where the underlying disorder has not yet been

*Table 95-1  **Examples of Other Organic Acidemias***

| Organic Acidemia | Amino Acid Precursor(s) | Enzyme Deficiency | Diagnostic Analytes | Newborn Screening Available | Associated Findings |
|---|---|---|---|---|---|
| 3-Methylcrotonyl CoA carboxylase deficiency<br><br>(3-MCC) | Leucine | 3-Methylcro-tonyl CoA carboxylase | 3-Methylcrotonylglycine (U)<br>3-Hydroxyisovaleric acid (U)<br>C5-Hydroxycarnitine (P) | Y<br>False positives occur due to maternal disease | Variable onset<br>May be asymptomatic<br>Seizures<br>Metabolic acidosis |
| 3-Hydroxy-3-methyl-glutaryl CoA lyase deficiency (HMG CoA lyase) | Leucine | 3-HMG CoA lyase | 3-Hydroxy-3-methyglu-taric acid (U)<br>3-Methylglutaconic acid (U)<br>C5-Hydroxycarnitine (P) | Y | Infantile onset<br>Hypoglycemia |
| Mitochondrial acetoacetyl CoA thiolase deficiency (beta-ketothiolase deficiency) | Isoleucine | Acetyl CoA acetyltrans-ferase | Tiglylglycine (U)<br>3-Hydroxyisovaleric acid (U)<br>C5-Hydroxycarnitine (P) | Y | Variable onset<br>Metabolic acidosis<br>Ketosis |
| Multiple carboxylase deficiency (MCD) (acetyl CoA car-boxylase, propionyl CoA carboxylase, 3-methylcrotonyl CoA carboxylase) | | Holocar-boxylase synthetase<br>Biotin-dependent apoenzyme | 3-Hydroxyisovaleric acid (U)<br>3-Methylcrotonylglycine (U)<br>Propionylglycine (U)<br>Lactic acid (P, U)<br>C5-Hydroxycarnitine (P) | Y | Neonatal onset<br>Metabolic acidosis<br>Ketosis<br>Seizures<br>Alopecia<br>Skin rash<br>Psychomotor retardation |
| Biotinidase defi-ciency (late-onset multiple carboxyl-ase deficiency) | | Biotinidase | 3-Hydroxyisovaleic acid (U)<br>3-Methylcrotonylglycine (U)<br>Propionylglycine (U)<br>Decreased biotinidase activity (P) | Y | Later-onset<br>Seizures |
| Glutaric aciduria type 1 (GA1) | Lysine Hydroxylysine Tryptophan | Glutaryl CoA dehydroge-nase | Glutaric acid<br>3-Hydroxyglutaric acid | Y | Infantile-onset more severe<br>Macrocephaly<br>Basal ganglia infarction<br>Movement disorder |

confirmed, a "cocktail" of vitamin cofactor may be used initially, and modified once a diagnosis has been confirmed.

Chronic management requires dietary whole protein restriction, appropriate cofactor supplementation, and a specific amino acid formula (depleted of the toxic precursor amino acids) to provide adequate protein and calorie intake for normal growth and development. A nutritionist experienced in managing metabolic diets is an essential member of the management team.

Organ transplant may be an option in some patients, such as MMA, where chronic renal failure is a common complication. Some patients have undergone combined liver and kidney transplants, although ongoing metabolic damage can still occur.

***Classic Organic Acidemias:***
- PA
  - Due to a deficiency of the biotin-dependent enzyme, pro-pionyl CoA carboxylase (PCC), in the catabolic pathway of the amino acids, isoleucine, valine, methionine, and threonine (also odd chain fatty acids and cholesterol).
  - Diagnostic metabolites are urine 3-hydroxypropionate, meth-ylcitrate, tiglylglycine, and propionylglycine. Plasma acylcar-nitine analysis shows increased propionylcarnitine (C3).
  - Long-term complications include cognitive delay, basal ganglia infarction (and movement disorder), recurrent pan-creatitis, and cardiomyopathy.

- MMA
  - Due to a deficiency of the vitamin B$_{12}$ (adenosylcobalamin)-dependent enzyme, methylmalonyl CoA mutase (MCM), in the same amino acid catabolic pathway as PA.
  - Diagnostic metabolites are urine methylmalonic acid, 3-hydroxypropionic acid, and methylcitric acid. Plasma acyl-carnitine analysis shows increased propionylcarnitine (C3).
  - Complications include progressive renal failure, basal ganglia stroke, and developmental delay.
  - Variant forms of MMA are due to defects of the uptake or intracellular metabolism of vitamin B12 (disorders of cobalamin metabolism).
- Cobalamin A (CblA) and cobalamin B (CblB) are defects of adenosylcobalamin, the cofactor for MCM. Features are similar to, but generally milder than MMA due to MCM deficiency. Treatment is with hydroxocobalamin (vitamin B$_{12}$).
  - Cobalamin C is a defect of both adenosylcobalamin and methylcobalamin (the cofactor for methionine synthase). Patients have accumulation of both methylmalonic acid and homocysteine. Features include developmental delay, maculopathy (that can lead to severe visual impairment), hypotonia, and spasticity. Acute metabolic acidosis does not occur. Treatment is with hydroxocobalamin and betaine (to reduce the homocysteine level).
  - Other defects of cobalamin metabolism have been described, but are extremely rare (CblD, CblF, CblG).
- Isovaleric acidemia (IVA)
  - Due to a deficiency of the enzyme isovaleryl CoA dehydrogenase in the catabolic pathway of the branched-chain amino acid, leucine. The characteristic odor of "sweaty feet" is notable.
  - Three different phenotypes have been described: severe, acute neonatal onset; intermittent later onset; and asymptomatic (identified by newborn screening).
  - Diagnostic metabolites are urine isovalerylglycine and 3-hydroxyisovaleric acid. Plasma acylcarnitine analysis shows increase of isovalerylcarnitine (C5).
  - Long-term outcome is usually good if recurrent episodes of severe metabolic acidosis are prevented by dietary management and early intervention for acute symptoms.

Other examples of organic acidemias are included in Table 95-1.

# Molecular Genetics and Molecular Mechanism

**Syndrome/Gene/Locus:**

1. 3-MCC is caused by mutations in *MCCC1* or *MCCC2* which encodes the alpha and beta subunits of 3-methylcrotonyl CoA carboxylase, respectively.
2. HMG CoA lyase deficiency is caused by mutations in *HMGCL* which encodes 3-hydroxy-3-methylglutaryl CoA lyase.
3. Beta-ketothiolase deficiency is caused by mutations in *ACAT1* which encodes mitochondrial acetyl CoA acetyltransferase.
4. MCD is caused by mutations in *HLCS* or *BTD* which encodes holocarboxylase synthetase and biotinidase, respectively.

5. GA1 is caused by mutations in *GCDH* which encodes glutaryl CoA dehydrogenase.
6. PA is caused by mutations in *PCCA* or *PCCB* which encodes the alpha and beta subunits of propionyl CoA carboxylase, respectively.
7. MMA is caused by mutations in *MUT* which encodes methylmalonyl CoA mutase.
8. IVA is caused by mutations in *IVD* which encodes isovaleryl CoA dehydrogenase.

**Genetic Testing:** Clinical molecular genetic testing is available for all of the organic acidemias discussed earlier and listed in Table 95-1 (see Gene Tests http://www.genetests.com).

All are single gene defects located on different chromosomes.

Propionyl CoA carboxylase is a two-subunit enzyme. The alpha and beta subunits are encoded on different chromosomes: PCCA on 13q22.3; PCCB on 3q22.3.

**Future Directions:** While the genetics of MDS was previously characterized by cytogenetic abnormalities, the recent discovery of somatic mutations has provided new knowledge regarding the pathophysiology of the disease and has the promise to lead to novel therapeutic interventions. Mutations in genes encoding regulators of the epigenome represent an important new paradigm in MDS genetics. Further research is needed to define the prevalence of these mutations in various subtypes of MDS and understand the biologic consequences of these mutations. This, in turn, could help improve the ability to diagnose the disease, evaluate for progression, monitor response to treatment, and assess prognosis.

## BIBLIOGRAPHY:

1. Desviat LR, Pérez B, Pérez-Cerdá C, Rodríguez-Pombo P, Clavero S, Ugarte M. Propionic academia: mutation update and functional and structural effects of the variant alleles. *Mol Genet Metab.* 2004;83(1-2):28-37.
2. Watkins D, Rosenblatt DS. Inborn errors of cobalamin absorption and metabolism. *Am J Med Genet C Semin Med Genet.* 2011;157(1):33-44.
3. Kasahara M, Horikawa R, Tagawa M, et al. Current role of liver transplant for MMA: a review of the literature. *Pediatr Transplant.* 2006;10(8):943-947.
4. Vockely J, Ensenauer R. Isovaleric acidemia: new aspects of genetic and phenotypic heterogeneity. *Am J Med Genet C Semin Med Genet.* 2006;142C(2):95-103.
5. Valle D, Beaudet AL, Vogelstein B, et al, eds. The Online Metabolic and Molecular Bases of Inherited Disease (http://www.ommbid.cm). The Organic Acidemias, ch 93, 94, 95.

# Supplementary Information

**OMIM REFERENCES:**

[1] Propionic Acidemia; PCCA (#232000); PCCB (#232050)

[2] Methylmalonic Acidemia; MUT (#251000); MMAA (#251100); MAAB (251110); MMACHC (#277400)

[3] Isovaleric Acidemia; IVD (#243500)

*Key Words:* Organic acidemia, amino acid, metabolic acidosis, cobalamin, cofactor, basal ganglia, methylmalonic, propionic, isovaleric

# 96 Primary Carnitine Deficiency

Nicola Longo and Marzia Pasquali

## KEY POINTS

- *Disease summary:*
  - Primary carnitine deficiency (OMIM 212140) is a disorder of the carnitine cycle that impairs fatty acid oxidation. It is caused by mutations in the SLC22A5 gene encoding the OCTN2 carnitine transporter. Primary carnitine deficiency has a frequency of about 1:40,000, with 1% of the population being carrier for this condition. It has a very high frequency in the Faroe Islands (prevalence 1:1300 people, incidence 1:720) due to a founder effect.
  - The lack of the plasma membrane carnitine transporter results in urinary carnitine wasting, low serum carnitine levels (0-5 μM, normal 25-50 μM), and decreased intracellular carnitine accumulation. Affected patients can have a predominant metabolic (hypoglycemia, hepatic encephalopathy) or cardiac (cardiomyopathy, arrhythmia) presentation. Some people remain asymptomatic for long time, but are at risk for sudden cardiac death.

- *Hereditary basis:*
  - Primary carnitine deficiency is transmitted as an autosomal recessive disorder caused by mutations in the SLC22A5 gene on 5q31.1. Penetrance in affected individuals is thought to be very high, although quite a few people are identified as adults due to expanded newborn screening.

- *Differential diagnosis:*
  - Primary carnitine deficiency needs to be differentiated from secondary carnitine deficiency. This can occur in disorders of the carnitine cycle (carnitine-acylcarnitine translocase [CACT] or carnitine palmitoyl transferase 2 [CPT-2] deficiency) and fatty acid oxidation (MCAD, VLCAD, LCHAD, TFP deficiency), organic acidemias (propionic, methylmalonic, isovaleric, and glutaric acidemia, 3-methylcrotonylglycinuria, multiple carboxylase deficiency, and other more rare), renal disease (renal Fanconi syndrome, chronic renal failure, dialysis), lysinuric protein intolerance (LPI), chronic ketosis or ketogenic diet, extreme prematurity, prolonged use of intravenous nutrition not supplemented by carnitine, and drug therapy (valproic acid, phenobarbital, phenytoin, carbamazepine, drugs containing pivalic acid).

## Diagnostic Criteria and Clinical Characteristics

**Diagnostic Criteria:**

**At least one of the following**

- Markedly reduced plasma free and total carnitine (usually free carnitine <10 μM and total carnitine <15 μM)
- Low long-chain acylcarnitines (C16, C18, C18:1) in the plasma acylcarnitine profile
- Low-normal plasma free carnitine levels while receiving carnitine supplements

**And the absence of**

- Abnormal acylcarnitine species indicative of other fatty acid oxidation defect or organic acidemia
- Abnormal urine organic acid with prominent ketonuria or metabolites suggestive of an organic acidemia
- Clinical history (prematurity, use of specific drugs, intravenous hyperalimentation, renal disease, etc) suggestive of secondary carnitine deficiency
- Maternal disease causing carnitine deficiency (in breast-fed infants): maternal primary carnitine deficiency, glutaric acidemia type 1, medium-chain acyl CoA dehydrogenase (MCAD) deficiency, cystic fibrosis

**Clinical Characteristics:** Deficiency of carnitine can impair fatty acid oxidation at time of fasting. Typically, symptoms are triggered by fasting, an infection, fever, or an acute gastroenteritis, increasing the requirement of calories from fatty acid oxidation. Carnitine deficiency can remain asymptomatic for long time if patients are not stressed. Patients can present with a predominant metabolic or cardiac presentation or with both (Table 96-1). Patients become lethargic and minimally responsive and can have hepatomegaly (hepatic encephalopathy). Laboratory studies can show hypoglycemia with minimal or no ketones in urine (hypoketotic hypoglycemia) and hyperammonemia with variably elevated liver function tests. Creatine kinase (CK) can also be mildly elevated. Cardiac involvement can occur either as cardiomyopathy or as sudden arrhythmia. Cardiomyopathy (dilated or hypertrophic) is more frequent in patients older than 1 year of age associated sometimes with hypotonia.

Patients require immediate treatment with intravenous glucose and carnitine supplements should be started as soon as possible and continued for life. Some patients remain asymptomatic for long time even without therapy, but are at risk of sudden death due to cardiac arrhythmia.

## Screening and Counseling

**Screening:** Primary carnitine deficiency can be identified by newborn screening by MS/MS. Affected patients have low levels of free carnitine (C0) with low levels of other acylcarnitines (specially long chain). The ratio ([C0+C2+C3+C16+C18+C18:1]/citrulline) can be more effective in identifying affected infants than evaluation of C0 alone, especially in samples collected shortly after birth (<24 hours), when carnitine levels can still be normal due to transplacental carnitine transfer. Affected newborns are usually completely asymptomatic at time of diagnosis; confirmation should be obtained by measuring plasma carnitine levels (free and total), estimating the urinary carnitine reabsorption (with simultaneous measure of carnitine and creatinine in plasma and urine)

*Table 96-1* **System Involvement**

| System | Manifestation |
| --- | --- |
| Metabolic/hepatic | Hypoglycemia, liver failure, sudden death |
| Cardiovascular | Cardiomyopathy, arrhythmia, sudden death |
| Muscular | Hypotonia, muscle pain |
| Cerebral | Loss of consciousness, coma |

and with appropriate functional (transport) studies in fibroblasts or DNA testing.

Low free carnitine in newborns can be caused by maternal carnitine deficiency due to maternal primary carnitine deficiency or secondary to undetected maternal disorders (organic acidemias, fatty acid oxidation defect, and cystic fibrosis). Other causes of low carnitine in newborns are extreme prematurity and the administration of intravenous hyperalimentation not supplemented with carnitine.

*Counseling:* Primary carnitine deficiency is inherited in an autosomal recessive manner. At conception, each sib of an affected individual with primary carnitine deficiency has a 25% chance of being affected, a 50% chance of being an asymptomatic carrier, and a 25% chance of being unaffected and not a carrier. Carriers can have mildly reduced plasma carnitine levels without any symptom. Prenatal testing is possible for at-risk pregnancies by functional studies (measurement of carnitine transport in amniocytes) or molecular genetic testing if both parental mutations are known.

The biochemical phenotype (ie, low plasma carnitine levels) is fully penetrant. A majority of people with primary carnitine deficiency develop symptoms in childhood if untreated. Asymptomatic adult patients are at risk for sudden death if untreated.

☞GENOTYPE-PHENOTYPE CORRELATION: There is no correlation between type of mutation and type and timing of presentation in symptomatic children, with individuals within the same family being affected early or not at all. Environmental factors, such as infections, fasting, or diet, can affect timing of clinical presentation. In asymptomatic adult, there is some genotype-phenotype correlation, with people remaining asymptomatic for long time having at least one missense mutation encoding for a transporter with residual activity.

*Table 96-2* **Algorithm for Screening and Management of Patient With Primary Carnitine Deficiency**

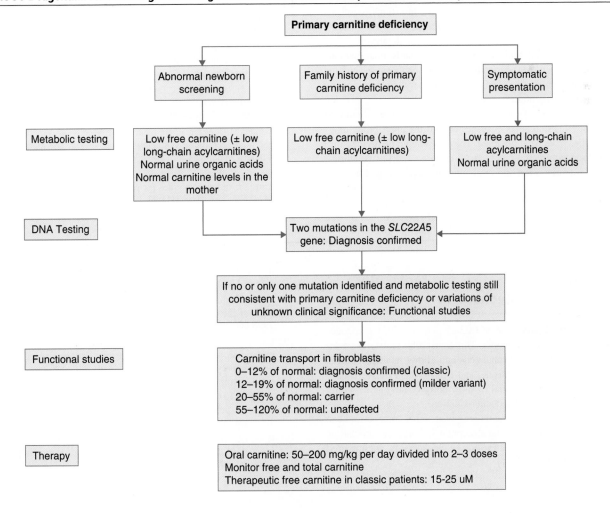

*Table 96-3 Molecular Genetic Testing*

| Gene | Testing Modality | Mutation Type | Detection Rate |
|---|---|---|---|
| *SLC22A5* | Sequencing | Missense, nonsense, small dup/del/ins | 85% |
| *SLC22A5* | MLPA, microchip | Single exon del/dup | ? |

## Management and Treatment

When primary carnitine deficiency is suspected, free and total carnitine levels should be measured (Table 96-2). If free carnitine is less than 10 μM, repeat the measurement, obtain plasma acylcarnitine profile and urine organic acids, and start patient on carnitine (100 mg/kg/d). Patients need to be medically evaluated to exclude other causes of carnitine deficiency (prematurity, insufficient dietary intake, chronic renal disease, etc). If low carnitine is the only consistent abnormality, diagnosis should be confirmed by obtaining a skin biopsy and measuring carnitine transport in fibroblasts. In alternative, DNA testing can be obtained. With the latter, identification of two mutations previously associated with the disease or clearly pathogenic (nonsense, frameshifts, deletions, insertions) confirms the diagnosis. Mutations are not identifiable in a few patients (Table 96-3) and functional studies can clarify the diagnosis.

In newborns, low carnitine levels can be due to maternal carnitine deficiency. In these cases, low carnitine can persist if infants are breast-fed, unless the mother corrects her low carnitine by exogenous supplementation.

*Treatment:* Carnitine supplements (100-300 mg/kg/d) should be started when the diagnosis is suspected and the appropriate diagnostic studies have been obtained. The dose should be divided into three to four administrations in small children and in two administrations in adults. Free and total carnitine levels should be periodically monitored. The blood sample should be obtained at least 8 hours after the last dose of carnitine. Despite therapy, plasma free carnitine usually remains below the normal range. Values of free carnitine of 15 to 25 μM are considered therapeutic.

## Molecular Genetics and Molecular Mechanism

*Syndrome/Gene/Locus:* The SLC22A5 gene on 5q31.1 encodes the OCTN2 carnitine transporter. This transporter reabsorbs carnitine in the brush border of renal cells and allows its accumulation in organs, such as liver, muscle, and heart, which derive energy from fat. Carnitine is essential to allow entry of fatty acids within mitochondria for their subsequent oxidation.

When carnitine supplements are given, other transporters can participate in carnitine intestinal absorption and organ accumulation. The liver has additional carnitine uptake mechanisms, not impaired in carnitine deficiency.

The juvenile visceral steatosis (JVS) mouse is a natural model of primary carnitine deficiency.

*Genetic Testing:*

☞**CLINICAL TESTING:** Plasma free and total carnitine, plasma acylcarnitine profile: finds low levels of both free and total carnitine with normal acylcarnitine profile (long-chain acylcarnitine are also usually low, but most laboratories do not have a lower range of normal): widely available.

Functional studies: carnitine transport in cultured fibroblasts (clinically available): patients' cells typically have less than 10% of normal transport activity. Heterozygotes typically have 25% to 50% of normal activity. This testing is clinically available.

DNA testing: there are no common mutations and gene sequencing should be obtained. This identifies 80% to 90% of causative mutations. Del/dup analysis is available, but the percentage of patients with this type of variations is low. DNA sequencing is clinically available.

Utility of testing: testing is necessary to confirm the diagnosis, exclude other types of carnitine deficiency, and direct therapy with carnitine supplements.

**BIBLIOGRAPHY:**

1. Nezu J, Tamai I, Oku A, et al. Primary systemic carnitine deficiency is caused by mutations in a gene encoding sodium ion-dependent carnitine transporter. Nat Genet. Jan 1999;21(1):91-94.

2. Koizumi A, Nozaki J, Ohura T, et al. Genetic epidemiology of the carnitine transporter OCTN2 gene in a Japanese population and phenotypic characterization in Japanese pedigrees with primary systemic carnitine deficiency. Hum Mol Genet. Nov 1999;8(12):2247-2254.

3. Wilcken B, Wiley V, Sim KG, Carpenter K. Carnitine transporter defect diagnosed by newborn screening with electrospray tandem mass spectrometry. J Pediatr. Apr 2001;138(4):581-584.

4. Amat di San Filippo C, Taylor MR, Mestroni L, Botto LD, Longo N. Cardiomyopathy and carnitine deficiency. Mol Genet Metab. Jun 2008;94(2):162-166.

5. Lund AM, Joensen F, Hougaard DM, et al. Carnitine transporter and holocarboxylase synthetase deficiencies in The Faroe Islands. J Inherit Metab Dis. Jun 2007;30(3):341-349.

6. Scaglia F, Wang Y, Singh RH, et al. Defective urinary carnitine transport in heterozygotes for primary carnitine deficiency. Genet Med. Nov-Dec 1998;1(1):34-39.

7. Tamai I, Ohashi R, Nezu J, et al. Molecular and functional identification of sodium ion-dependent, high affinity human carnitine transporter OCTN2. J Biol Chem. Aug 7 1998;273(32):20378-20382.

8. Schimmenti LA, Crombez EA, Schwahn BC, et al. Expanded newborn screening identifies maternal primary carnitine deficiency. Mol Genet Metab. Apr 2007;90(4):441-445.

9. Christodoulou J, Teo SH, Hammond J, et al. First prenatal diagnosis of the carnitine transporter defect. Am J Med Genet. Dec 2 1996;66(1):21-24.

10. Lamhonwah AM, Olpin SE, Pollitt RJ, et al. Novel OCTN2 mutations: no genotype-phenotype correlations: early carnitine therapy prevents cardiomyopathy. Am J Med Genet. Aug 15 2002;111(3):271-284.

11. Wang Y, Korman SH, Ye J, et al. Phenotype and genotype variation in primary carnitine deficiency. Genet Med. Nov-Dec 2001;3(6):387-392.

12. Rose EC, Amat di San Filippo C, Erlingsson UCN, Ardon O, Pasquali M, Longo N. Genotype-phenotype correlation in primary carnitine deficiency. Hum Mutat. Jan 2012;33(1):118-123.

13. Kuwajima M, Kono N, Horiuchi M, et al. Animal model of systemic carnitine deficiency: analysis in C3H-H-2 degrees strain of mouse associated with juvenile visceral steatosis. Biochem Biophys Res Commun. Feb 14 1991;174(3):1090-1094.

14. Li FY, El-Hattab AW, Bawle EV, et al. Molecular spectrum of SLC22A5 (OCTN2) gene mutations detected in 143 subjects evaluated for systemic carnitine deficiency. Hum Mutat. Aug 2010;31(8):E1632-E1651.

## ACKNOWLEDGMENTS:

Funding: Supported in part by grant R01 DK 53824 from the National Institutes of Health.

Nicola Longo, Marzia Pasquali

Division of Medical Genetics, Department of Pediatrics and Pathology, University of Utah, Biochemical Genetics and Newborn Screening Laboratories, ARUP Laboratories, Salt Lake City, UT, USA

# Supplementary Information

## OMIM REFERENCES:

[1] Carnitine Deficiency, Systemic Primary; CDSP (#212140)

[2] Solute Carrier Family 22 (Organic Cation Transporter), Member 5; SLC22A5 (#603377)

## Alternative Names:

- Systemic Carnitine Deficiency; SCD
- Carnitine Deficiency, Systemic, due to Defect in Renal Reabsorption of Carnitine
- Carnitine Uptake Defect; CUD
- Systemic Primary Carnitine Deficiency

***Key Words:*** Carnitine deficiency, fatty acid oxidation, cardiomyopathy, arrhythmia, sudden death, hypoglycemia, hepatic encephalopathy, hyperammonemia, carnitine transport, OCTN2, SLC22A5

# 97 Phenylketonuria

Amel Karaa, Monica A. Giovanni, and Harvey L. Levy

## KEY POINTS

- *Disease summary:*
  - Phenylketonuria (PKU) is a genetic inborn error of metabolism characterized by the presence of a nonfunctional hepatic (and to a lesser extent renal) enzyme phenylalanine hydroxylase (PAH) that converts the amino acid phenylalanine (PHE) into tyrosine. When there is loss of PAH activity, phenylalanine accumulates leading to brain toxicity and is also secondarily metabolized into phenylketones that are excreted in urine giving the disease its name. PKU is divided into classic PKU with PHE levels greater than 1200 µmol/L and variant PKU with hyperphenylalaninemia lower than 1200 µmol/L. In 1% to 2% of the cases elevated PHE is caused by a deficiency in the PAH cofactor tetrahydrobiopterin (BH4) due to reduced synthesis or deficient recycling.
  - The prevalence of PKU varies worldwide and ranges from 1/2600 (in Turkey) to 1/200,000 (in Thailand) live births. In the United States prevalence is estimated at 1/15000. PKU affects all ethnic groups and both sexes equally.
  - Untreated PKU can result in developmental delay, progressive intellectual disability, seizures, eczema, behavioral and psychiatric issues. In countries with established newborn screening, most affected patients are detected and treated at birth. Adolescents and adults with PKU who have been partially treated, treated for only a short period or noncompliant with their treatment might exhibit a wide array of clinical symptoms ranging from cognitive reduction to intellectual disability; some might present with neuropsychiatric decline.
  - Teratogenicity in maternal PKU occurs when the fetus is exposed to high PHE; only rarely does the fetus have PKU. Teratogenicity results from PHE actively crossing the placenta producing a 1.3 to 2-fold increase in the fetus causing multiple fetal abnormalities.
  - Early diagnosis and prompt dietary treatment with tight control and monitoring of the PHE level will prevent the complications of this disease in the person with PKU and, when begun before or early in pregnancy will prevent teratogenicity from maternal PKU.
- *Hereditary basis:*
  - PKU is a monogenic disorder with an autosomal recessive pattern of inheritance.
- *Differential diagnosis:*
  - Secondary PAH dysfunction from deficient cofactor can occur from defects in the pathways of BH4 metabolism:
    - *Impaired synthesis of BH4* usually due to deficiency of guanosine triphosphate cyclohydrolase (GTPCH) or 6-pyruvoyl tetrahydropterin synthase (PTPS).
    - *Impaired recycling of BH4* due to deficiency of dihydropteridine reductase (DHPR) or deficient pterin-4 acarbinolamine dehydratase (PCD).
  - These are autosomal recessive conditions resulting in hyperphenylalaninemia ranging from slightly abnormal (>120 µmol/L) to as high as 2500 µmol/L. Clinical manifestations overlap with PKU and include microcephaly, intellectual disability, seizures, gait instability, drowsiness, irritability, abnormal movements, recurrent hyperthermia without infections, hypersalivation, and swallowing difficulties.

## Diagnostic Criteria and Clinical Characteristics

***Diagnostic Criteria:*** Patients with hyperphenylalaninemia have a consistently elevated PHE levels above 120 µmol/L (>2 mg/dL). PKU is diagnosed when BH4 cofactor is normal and can be divided as in Table 97-1.

In several countries including the United States of America, most cases are identified at birth by newborn screening (NBS). To confirm the diagnosis in the newborn and to establish diagnosis in suspected older individuals, biochemical testing that includes plasma amino acids as well as measurement of pterins in urine and assay for dihydropteridine reductase activity in blood are indicated. The latter are required to exclude hyperphenylalaninemia as a secondary consequence of an inborn error of biopterin metabolism.

### Clinical Characteristics (Table 97-2):

☞**In Children:** Fetuses exposed to high levels of PHE in utero due to maternal PKU will have an abnormal development regardless of whether or not they carry a PKU mutation. About 90% will develop intellectual disability of varying degrees and 25% will have congenital anomalies, primarily congenital heart disease.

In contrast, children who have PKU are born normal and develop symptoms postnatally as they develop hyperphenylalaninemia from exposure to PHE in their diet (breast milk, formula, soy, and cow milk). These symptoms will differ in spectrum and severity depending on the mutation they carry, the amount of PHE they are exposed to and other factors not fully understood. In general if the child is promptly treated with the appropriate diet, their development will be normal in the majority of the cases.

☞**In Adults:** Clinical features at this age depend on how well PKU was treated from birth. Well-treated infants and children will have normal intelligence or near-normal intelligence as adults but their neuropsychological abilities might be lower than their peers. It is a matter of debate as to whether adults with PKU should be on a restricted diet but most PKU centers advocate "diet for life." It is interesting to point out that some untreated, poorly treated, or late treated adults will still have normal development; this group is estimated at 10% of all PKU patients.

Table 97-1 *Classification of Hyperphenylalaninemia*

| | | Phenylalanine Levels in the Blood | | Dietary PHE Tolerance/Day[a] | % Residual Enzyme Activity |
|---|---|---|---|---|---|
| | | µmol/L | mg/dL | | |
| *Normal Levels* | | 50-110 | <2 | Normal diet | 100 |
| **Variant-PKU** | Mild hyperphenyl-alaninemia | 120-600 | 3-10 | Normal diet | >5 |
| | Mild phenylketonuria | 600-1200 | 10-20 | 400-600 mg | 1-5 |
| **Classic-PKU** | | >1200 | >20 | <250-350 mg | <1 |

[a]Patients tolerate this much dietary phenylalanine per day to keep plasma concentration of PHE at a safe level of no more than 360 µmol/L (6 mg/dL).

Symptoms in adult not observing a strict diet will depend on

- Fluctuating and high levels of PHE in the blood adversely affect cognitive, neuropsychological, and psychiatric function. Abstract reasoning, executive functioning, and attention are deficient in these individuals but can improve with strict dietary control. Adults who relax their diet might suffer from tremors, brisk deep tendon reflexes, poor motor coordination, spastic paresis, late-onset epilepsy, and ataxia. These can be of variable degrees of severity and are associated with white matter abnormalities on magnetic resonance imaging (MRI) thought to be due to reduction in myelin. These findings disappear when the diet is reintroduced. Psychiatric problems have also been reported in untreated or off-diet adults in the third and fourth

Table 97-2 *System Involvement*

| System | Manifestation | Incidence |
|---|---|---|
| Central nervous system | Severe intellectual disability (IQ <50) | |
| | Epilepsy | 25% |
| | EEG abnormalities | 80% |
| | Pyramidal signs | |
| | Tremor | 30% |
| | Spasticity of the limbs | 5% |
| | Paraplegia or hemiplegia | |
| | Decreased myelin formation | |
| | Behavior problems (hyperactivity, purposeless movements, stereotypy, aggressiveness, anxiety, social withdrawal) | >90% |
| Integumentary system | Musty body odor (phenylacetic acid) | |
| | Eczema | 20%-40% |
| | Dry skin | |
| | Decreased skin, hair, and iris pigmentation | |
| | Scleroderma | |
| | Cataract | |
| Skeletal | Osteopenia | |
| Hematologic | Vitamin $B_{12}$ deficiency | |
| Metabolic | Elevated urinary *O*-hydroxyphenylacetic acid, phenylpyruvic acid, phenylacetic acid, phenylacetylglutamine, and phenylpyruvic acidemia | |
| Maternal PKU complications (PHE >1200 µmol/L) | IUGR | 40% |
| | Microcephaly | 73% |
| | Congenital heart defects | 12% |
| | Intellectual disability | 92% |

decade of life. These include depression, anxiety, social withdrawal, agoraphobia, other phobias, low self-esteem, and neurotic behaviors. These tend to be reversible as well on a strict PKU diet.

- Nutritional deficiency can develop from restrictive diet that lacks animal proteins. This is most often vitamin $B_{12}$ deficiency but also deficiencies in vitamin $B_6$, folic acid, and iron. Vitamin $B_{12}$ deficiency can cause peripheral neuropathy, glossitis, anemia, dementia, and psychiatric disturbances that can be sometimes confused with manifestations from PKU.
- Osteoporosis is commonly seen in patients with PKU. The cause is unknown, but it is believed to be related to failure in achieving an optimal peak bone mass in early adult life as a result of deficiencies in protein, calcium, and vitamin D. It is possible that there is a PKU-inherent bone defect.

☞IN PREGNANT WOMEN WITH PKU: PHE plays a major role during embryogenesis and fetogenesis; elevation of PHE is teratogenic and will cause several deleterious effects including facial dysmorphisms, cardiac anomalies, intellectual disability, microcephaly, and intrauterine growth retardation (IUGR). This is especially critical in the first 5 weeks of gestation when the nervous, cardiac system and the cranium are developing. In women with PKU, strict control of PHE level before conception or within the first 4 to 6 gestational weeks is the only measure to improve pregnancy outcome in maternal PKU. There also seems to be genetic and environmental heterogeneity in the outcome in maternal PKU.

## Screening and Counseling

*Screening:* Most cases are now identified at birth by NBS. False-positive results can occur because of technical factors such as a thick blood spot, an improperly processed sample, or from physiologic variants of the newborn including liver immaturity, protein overload (TPN, cow's milk diet), and in premature infants who are heterozygous for PAH deficiency. False-negative test results can be seen if the sample is taken too early (<24 hours after birth) as PHE level starts to rise slowly after birth and might be within normal range during the first day.

Plasma amino acid analysis should be undertaken in all infants with a positive NBS and newly presenting patients if there is any family history of hyperphenylalaninemia or PKU or in the face of acute symptoms evoking the diagnosis of PKU. Some authors advocate screening of women who had previous offspring with idiopathic microcephaly, IUGR, congenital heart disease, or with intellectual disability or low IQ.

Genetic testing for carrier status of PAH deficiency may be conducted in anticipation of prenatal diagnosis or preimplantation genetic diagnosis (PGD) although these procedures are controversial due to the treatability of PKU with minimal residual abnormalities.

*Counseling:*

☞INHERITANCE, PENETRANCE: PKU is an autosomal recessive condition. Parents of a proband are obligate heterozygotes and carry one mutant *PAH* allele but are asymptomatic with PHE level within the normal range. Each sibling of a proband (or fetus when the parents have a child with PKU) has a 25% chance of being affected (homozygous), a 50% chance of being an asymptomatic carrier of a disease-causing allele (heterozygous), and a

25% chance of having two normal alleles. Children born of one parent with PKU and one parent with two normal alleles are obligate heterozygotes.

☞GENOTYPE-PHENOTYPE CORRELATION: There is a well-established correlation between genotype and biochemical phenotype (levels of PHE and dietary PHE tolerance). There is a much weaker correlation however between genotype and clinical phenotype (neurologic impairment and behavioral changes). This is in part secondary to the multifactorial nature of the disease encompassing environmental, dietary, and other molecular mechanisms such as protein and chaperones influence on the metabolic pathway. Genotypes associated with BH4 responsiveness help tailor the treatment with prompt and early initiation of BH4 supplements.

## Management and Treatment

The manifestations of PKU are due to the deleterious effects of elevated PHE; thus the treatment focuses on reducing PHE levels in the blood by decreasing intake in the diet (restrictions in meat, milk, eggs, cheese, nuts, and breads). The indication for treatment depends on the PHE level on a normal protein-containing diet and age (Table 97-3).

It is commonly accepted that dietary restrictions in individuals with a PHE level less than 600 μmol/L are of little value as these individuals usually have normal cognition and development. However, they need to be monitored in childhood and treatment needs to be considered if the PHE levels rise above 600 μmol/L.

For patients diagnosed at birth, the diet should be initiated within the first weeks of life and maintained at least through late childhood and into adolescence. The diet is composed of natural foods that are low on PHE, such as fruits and vegetables and low protein medical foods, and supplemented with PHE-free formula of elemental amino acids and containing vitamins, minerals, and trace elements. PKU diet is highly successful but compliance remains a problem especially in adolescence and adulthood due to its restrictive nature. Continuation of the diet through adulthood, although controversial, is recommended in most centers to prevent neuropsychological deterioration.

BH4 supplementation might reduce PHE levels in milder forms of the disease (up to 75% in mild PKU) and rarely in classic PKU (10% of cases).

Practitioners should be aware that several over-the-counter (OTC) and commonly used medications contain PHE; a list of these medications with the PHE content is available at http://www.pkunews.org/diet/asptable.htm.

A dietician knowledgeable in PKU management should be part of the care team. Adolescents and adults with PKU should be encouraged to maintain a lifelong diet with nutritional supplements (these should include calcium and vitamin D). Blood PHE should be monitored at least every month with yearly clinical examination

**Table 97-3 Recommendations of Target PHE Levels for Age**

| Age in Years | PHE Level in Blood (μmol/L) |
|---|---|
| 0-12 | 120-360 |
| 13-15 | 120-600 |
| >15 | 120-900 |

*Table 97-4 Molecular Genetic Testing*

| Gene | Testing Modality | Mutation Type | Detection Rate |
|------|------------------|---------------|----------------|
| PAH | Targeted mutation analysis | 60.5% missense, 13.5% deletions, 11% splice, 6% silent, 5% nonsense, 2% insertion, 0.7% unknown. | 30%-50% |
| | Mutation scanning | | 99% |
| | Sequence analysis | | 99% |
| | Deletion/duplication analysis | | <1% |

during which a plasma amino acid profile as well as measurements of vitamins $B_{12}$, $B_6$, D, folic acid, iron, ferritin, methylmalonic acid, homocysteine, albumin, and a complete blood count (CBC). Dual-energy x-ray absorptiometry (DEXA) scan should be offered every 2 to 5 years.

Information regarding maternal PKU should be provided at every visit to women of childbearing age and the need for preconception PHE level control should be emphasized. Pregnant PKU patients should be managed by a multidisciplinary team composed of a metabolic disorder specialist, a dietician, and a high-risk obstetrician every 3 to 4 weeks with weekly PHE levels and should have a detailed fetal survey at 17 to 18 weeks of gestation. The recommended blood PHE levels during pregnancy are 120 to 240 µmol/L blood, much stricter than a typical PKU adult on diet due to positive PHE gradient in utero exposing the fetus to higher PHE levels. It is recommended that pregnant PKU patients have strict control of PHE levels before conception or within the first 4 to 6 gestational weeks to prevent or minimize teratogenic effects. Caution must be taken to prevent a diet too restrictive which could cause maternal nutritional deficit leading to fetal growth restriction. Other alternative therapies include

1) Phenylalanine ammonia lyase (PAL), an alternative PHE-metabolizing enzyme that converts PHE into harmless metabolites without the need for cofactor is being developed in a pegylated form ("PEGL-PAL") to lessen immunogenicity. This drug therapy is currently in clinical trials.
2) Large neutral amino acid (LNAA) supplementation (tyrosine, tryptophan, methionine, leucine, isoleucine, and valine) theoretically competes with PHE at the LAT1 LNAA transporter, thus reducing the amount of PHE that crosses the blood-brain barrier.
3) Liver transplant completely reverses PKU. Due to risks of transplant surgery and the need for immune suppressive therapy however, it is seldom used.
4) Gene therapy has been unsuccessful so far but many trials are underway.

# Molecular Genetics and Molecular Mechanism

**Syndrome/Gene/Locus:** *PAH* gene is located on chromosome 12q23.2. The PAH protein product, the enzyme phenylalanine hydroxylase catalyzes the conversion of phenylalanine to tyrosine; it requires the cofactor tetrahydrobiopterin (BH4), oxygen, and iron. The PAH gene contains 13 exons coding for 31 normal allelic variants and 564 pathogenic variants (PAH locus Knowledge database).

**Genetic Testing:** Comprehensive mutation analysis for *PAH* is clinically available in many laboratories throughout the United States and the world. Mutation scanning and sequence analysis has a detection rate of 99% (Table 97-4).

The diagnosis of PKU is usually made by biochemical studies; genetic testing is used for predictions based on genotype-phenotype correlations, and for carrier testing as well as prenatal and preimplantation genetic diagnosis.

**BIBLIOGRAPHY:**

1. Donlon JL, Levy HL, Scriver CR. Hyperphenylalaninemia: phenylalanine hydroxylase deficiency. The Online Metabolic and Miolecular bases of Inherited Disease. Part 8 (Chapter 77).
2. Blau N, van Spronsen FJ, Levy HL. Phenylketonuria. *Lancet.* 2010;376(9750):1417-1427.
3. Mitchell JJ, Scriver CR. Phenylalanine hydroxylase deficiency. 2010, Gene Reviews.
4. Hoeks MP, den Heijer M, Janssen MC. Adult issues in phenylketonuria. *Neth J Med.* 2009;67(1):2-7.
5. Bouchlariotou S, Tsikouras P, Maroulis G. Undiagnosed maternal phenylketonuria: own clinical experience and literature review. *J Matern Fetal Neonatal Med.* 2009;22(10):943-948.
6. Hanley WB. Finding the fertile woman with phenylketonuria. *Eur J Obstet, Gynecol Reprod Biol.* 2008;137(2):131-135.
7. Gentile JK, Ten Hoedt AE, Bosch Am. Psychosocial aspects of PKU: hidden disabilities—a review. *Mol Genet Metab.* 2010;99(suppl 1):S64-S67.
8. Koch R, Hanley W, Levy H, et al. The Maternal Phenylketonuria International Study: 1984-2002. *Pediatrics.* 2003;112(6 pt 2):1523-1529.
9. Maillot F, Cook P, Lilburn M, Lee PJ. A practical approach to maternal phenylketonuria management. *J Inherit Metab Dis.* 2007;30(2):198-201.
10. Fernandez John, Georges Van den JMS, Walter JH. *Inborn Metabolic Diseases: Diagnosis and Treatment.* 4th ed. Springer Medizin Verlag, 2006
11. PAHdb Phenylalanine Hydroxylase Locus Knowledge base. http://www.pahdb.mcgill.ca/.
12. Hanley WB. Adult phenylketonuria. *Am J Med.* 2004;117(8):590-595.
13. van Spronsen FJ, Burgard P. The truth of treating patients with phenylketonuria after childhood: the need for a new guideline. *J Inherit Metab Dis.* 2008;31(6):673-679.
14. Gambol PJ. Maternal phenylketonuria syndrome and case management implications. *J Pediatr Nurs.* 2007;22(2):129-138.

## Supplementary Information

**OMIM References:**

[1] Phenylketonuria; PKU (# 261600)

[2] Phenylalanine Hydroxylase; PAH (# 612349)

**Alternative Names:**

- PKU
- Hyperphenylalaninemia
- Følling Disease

*Key Words:* PKU, hyperphenylalaninemia, phenylalanine, maternal PKU, intellectual disability

# 98 Prenatal Testing, Noninvasive Screening, Invasive Testing, and Carrier Screening

Melissa Savage, Karen Hanson, Ronald Wapner, and W. Andrew Faucett

## KEY POINTS

- *Summary:*
  - Pregnancies found to be at greater than population (high) risk for a genetic disorder are offered invasive diagnostic testing by chorionic villus sampling (CVS) or amniocentesis. These diagnostic tests have a small risk of inducing a pregnancy loss but will diagnose a specific genetic disorder with greater than 99% accuracy.
  - Karyotype, FISH, or microarray are testing options for diagnosis of fetal genetic disorders on chorionic villus or amniotic fluid specimens.
  - Ancestry and family history are tools used to determine which pregnancies are at risk for specific genetic disorders and should help guide carrier screening.
  - The carrier state of some Mendelian disorders is frequent enough in the general population that offering screening to all pregnant couples and those presenting preconception is recommended.
  - Screening tests can be used during pregnancy, at as early as 10 weeks, to identify pregnancies at increased risk for common fetal trisomies such as those causing Down syndrome and Edwards syndrome (trisomy 21 and 18).

- *Uses:*
  - Invasive testing—CVS and amniocentesis
    - Provide a definitive diagnosis for pregnancies identified as having an increased risk of a genetic disorder.
    - Invasive testing is most commonly performed on women who are at an increased risk for a chromosome abnormality based on age-related risk, abnormal noninvasive screening results, and/or abnormal ultrasound findings.
    - Invasive testing is offered for disease-specific testing when the parent(s) are confirmed carrier(s), affected with a dominant genetic disorder, or known to carry a balanced translocation.
    - American College of Obstetrics and Gynecology, Guidelines, 2007
    - All women, regardless of age, should have the option of invasive testing.
    - Maternal age of 35 years alone should no longer be used as a cutoff to determine who is offered screening versus who is offered invasive testing.

## General Descriptions

### Types of Screening:

☞CARRIER SCREENING:

**Purpose: to identify carrier couples of Mendelian disorders**

- Population screening for carriers of common Mendelian disorders
  - Some disorders occur frequently enough throughout the general population that carrier testing is offered to all pregnant couples, for example, cystic fibrosis (Table 98-1).
- Population screening based on ethnicity and race
  - The carrier state of certain genetic disorders occurs at an increased rate in specific ethnic or racial populations (Table 98-1). Since many of these disorders are inherited in an autosomal recessive fashion, identification of couples in which both parents are phenotypically normal but carry a mutated gene for the same disorder allows early decisions about future reproduction.
- Preferably, carrier screening should be performed preconception or as early in pregnancy as possible. Turnaround time averages are 1 to 2 weeks.
- Carrier screening is usually performed in a sequential manor—that is, if the mother tests positive, then the father of the pregnancy is tested. The exception to this is when time constraints, require a rapid analysis of both partners. If the parents are of different ethnicities, the father can be offered screening for those disorders not recommended in the mother based on her ethnicity.
- Screening couples based on family history
  - Specific testing for disorder found in family history (ie, cystic fibrosis, Duchenne muscular dystrophy).
  - Testing can be targeted to look for specific disease mutation found in family member if known.

*Table 98-1  Carrier Screening*

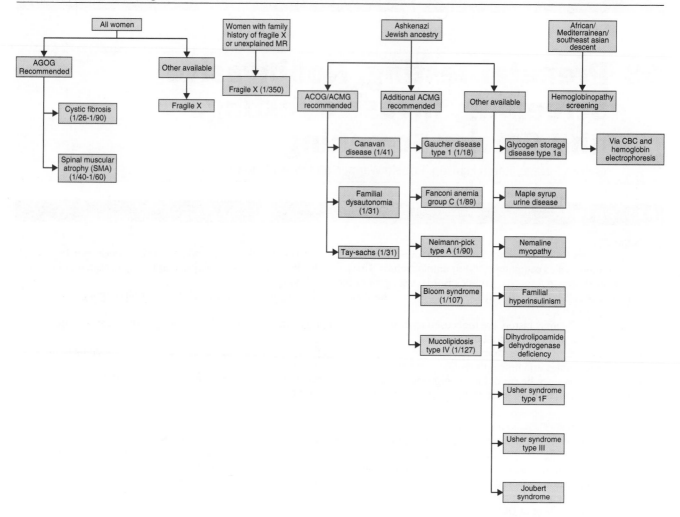

- If it is determined that a fetus is at risk based on carrier screening results, the patient should be offered CVS or amniocentesis to test for that specific disorder.

☞NONINVASIVE MATERNAL SERUM SCREENING AND/OR ULTRASOUND:

**Purpose: 1. To identify pregnancies at increased risk for common aneuploidies or genetic disorders**

- Prenatal maternal serum screening tests and ultrasound are used to target women at high risk (> general population) for fetal aneuploidy (especially Down syndrome and trisomies 13 and 18) and birth defects. Women found to be at high risk can then be offered invasive diagnostic testing.
- Abnormal maternal serum screening results may also indicate an increased risk for an adverse pregnancy (eg, spontaneous abortion, preterm delivery, low birth weight), or other genetic syndromes.
- Most women who have an abnormal first- or second-trimester maternal serum screening will have normal pregnancies.
- Certain ultrasound anomalies are associated with specific genetic disorders and if found, patients should be offered testing

for that disorder (ie, testing for DiGeorge syndrome in a patient with a heart defect).

**Purpose: 2. To avoid the conception of a pregnancy with a genetic disorder**

- Preimplantation genetic diagnosis (PGD)—for some couples at high risk to have a pregnancy affected with a genetic disorder, PGD may be performed so that only genetically unaffected embryos are implanted. In this approach, in vitro fertilization (IVF) is required and one or two cells (blastomeres) are removed at either day 3 or day 5 postfertilization. Single cell analysis is then performed and results may be available with 24 to 48 hours. Because PGD is not perfect, invasive testing should be offered as confirmation.

*Types of Diagnostic Testing:*

☞INVASIVE TESTING:

- **Chorionic villus sampling (CVS)**
  - Performed between 10 and 12 to 14 weeks' gestation (depending on comfort level or experience of the technician)
  - CVS can be performed abdominally or cervically, depending on the location of the placenta.

- During the procedure, a needle (abdominally) or catheter (cervically) is inserted into the placenta and some of the cells that make up the placenta, called the chorionic villi, are removed.
- CVS cannot detect open neural tube defects (ONTDs). Therefore, in the event a CVS is performed, a second-trimester maternal alpha-fetoprotein (AFP) blood test should be performed and along with an anatomy scan, as together they can detect 90% of ONTDs.
- **Amniocentesis**
  - Is performed beginning at 15 to 16 weeks' gestation and can be performed until delivery.
  - Amniocentesis is performed abdominally.
  - During the procedure, a needle is inserted into the abdomen and some of the amniotic fluid is removed.
  - Amniocentesis can detect ONTDs with a 95% detection rate.
- **Laboratory testing of CVS or amniocentesis samples**
  - Karyotype
    - Looks at the chromosomes under a light microscope and uses the banding pattern of the chromosomes to determine if there are aberrations. It is able to detect deletions or duplications greater than 5 to 10 MB in size.
    - Is the gold standard testing performed on all CVS and amniocentesis samples.
    - Turnaround time averages 7 to 10 days.
  - Fluorescence in situ hybridization testing (FISH)
    - Uses fluorescent probes that attach to specific regions of the genome (ie, chromosome 21 or region 22q11.2) to determine copy number of that particular chromosome or region.
    - Is able to detect targeted smaller deletions or duplications than karyotype can, but you have to know exactly what you are looking for (which region to test).
    - Commonly used to provide quick results for the common aneuploidies (13, 18, 21, X, and Y) as turnaround time is 1 to 3 days.
    - Also used when testing for a specific microdeletion or duplication syndrome is warranted, such as testing for 22q11.2 deletion in the presence of a heart defect.
  - Microarray analysis
    - Able to detect very small missing or extra pieces of a chromosome. Unlike FISH, however, microarray can be used to evaluate the entire genome rather than a specific region.
    - Several different microarray technologies are available and generally they are used to detect microdeletion or duplication syndromes.
    - Microarray testing, in concert with genetic counseling, can be offered in cases with abnormal ultrasound and a normal karyotype, as well as in cases of fetal demise with congenital anomalies for which no karyotype is available.
    - Turnaround time for microarray testing averages 1 to 2 weeks.
  - Disease-specific testing
    - Used when the fetus is at risk for an inherited genetic disorder, such as Tay-Sachs disease or fragile X.
    - Turnaround time depends on the disorder being tested but generally averages 1 to 3 weeks.

☞**CARRIER TESTING:**
- For some disorders the gene frequency is only high enough to warrant screening within specific ethnic groups (eg, sickle cell disease, thalassemia, Tay-Sachs disease).
- A few disorders are common enough that offering screening to all pregnant women is recommended (eg, cystic fibrosis and spinal muscular atrophy).
- For some disorders such as sickle cell disease, a single mutation accounts for all the disease-causing mutations. For others, multiple mutations of a gene may be involved requiring screening of a panel of mutations (eg, cystic fibrosis).
- The relative frequency of the disease-causing mutations may vary between ethnic groups so that the percentage of carriers detected by a standard panel may vary by ethnicity. For most disorders all carriers will not be detected.
- Table 98-1 illustrates the common screening approaches to identify couples at risk for Mendelian disorders.

☞**SCREENING TESTS:**
- Used to modify and refine risk for age-related chromosome abnormalities by measuring the level of analytes in the maternal blood stream.
- Presently, first-trimester screening using human chorionic gonadotropin (hCG), pregnancy-associated plasma protein A (PAPP-A), and ultrasound measurement of the nuchal translucency (NT) is the most frequently used approach.
- Table 98-2 describes different approaches to prenatal screening.
- Targeted ultrasound is also recommended and is best performed after 18 weeks' gestation to detect major structural defects.

☞**NEWER TECHNOLOGIES:**
- Fetal cells in maternal circulation: Fetal cells circulating in the maternal blood stream are a source of fetal DNA and RNA which in turn can be used for detecting fetal aneuploidy. Currently, this technology is not in clinical practice and has been most often used to help determine fetal sex.

## Testing Methodologies

*Invasive Testing:* CVS is typically offered between 10 and 12 to 14 weeks of pregnancy, and has an approximate 1/100 to 1/200 risk for miscarriage, depending on experience of the technician. The benefits of CVS testing include receiving results in the first trimester or early second trimester and the option of early pregnancy termination. CVS is generally performed on women at an increased risk for chromosome abnormalities based on age, an abnormal first-trimester screen, ultrasound abnormalities found in the first trimester, or at risk for a specific disorder based on family history or carrier status.

**Amniocentesis** is typically offered after 15 to 16 weeks' gestation and has an approximate risk for miscarriage of 1/200 to 1/400. The benefits of amniocentesis include simultaneous testing for both chromosome abnormalities and open neural tube defects. Amniocentesis is most often performed on women at increased risk for chromosome abnormalities because of age, abnormal maternal serum screening, abnormal ultrasound findings, or at increased risk for a specific disease due to family history or carrier status.

**Genomic testing** on CVS or amniotic fluid samples (ie, microarray testing) is recommended on all fetuses with abnormal

*Table 98-2 Different Approaches to Prenatal Screening*

| Type of Screening test | Detection Rate(s) (DS: Down Syn) | Timing | Comments (NT: Nuchal Translucency) |
|---|---|---|---|
| 1st trimester screen | DS: 64-70% | 11-13.6 weeks | Need 2nd trimester screening for NTDs (serum AFP or US) |
| 1st trimester combined screen | DS: 80-84% Tri 18/13: 98% | 11-13.6 weeks | Need a certified ultra-sonographer to measure NT<br>Allows for option of 1st trimester invasive testing |
| 2nd trimester triple screen | DS: 60-65% Tri 18/13: 50% Open NTD: 80% | 15-20 weeks | Triple screen has been replaced by quad screen in most centers |
| 2nd trimester quad screen | DS: 80% Tri 18/13: 60-80% Open NTD: 80% | 15-21.9 weeks | Only screening option for 'late presenters' |
| Integrated screen | DS: 96% Tri 18/13: 90% Open NTD: 80% | 1st Tri: 11-13.6 weeks 2nd Tri: 15-21.9 weeks | Results of 1st trimester screen combined with results of 2nd trimester screen, results not given to patient until 2nd trimester<br>*serum integrated screen – NT is not included in first trimester screen, detection rate lower |
| Sequential screen | Overall: DS: 90% Tri 18/13: 90% Open NTD: 90% | 1st Tri: 11-13.6 weeks 2nd Tri: 15-21.9 weeks | Preliminary result given in 1st trimester if screen positive, final result given after 2nd trimester screen |
| Contingent screen | DS: 96% Tri 18/13: 90% Open NTD: 80% | 1st Tri: 11-13.6 weeks 2nd Tri: 15-21.9 weeks | 1st trimester screen results given if results are below a specific threshold (1/2000 risk or lower), otherwise results not given until combined with 2nd trimester results |

ultrasounds and normal karyotypes. Microarray has the capacity to detect aneuploidy, hundreds of microdeletion or duplication syndromes, uniparental disomy (UPD), and some Mendelian conditions. Because microarray testing may also detect findings of uncertain clinical significance, genetic counseling is recommended prior to testing.

*Carrier Testing:* **Carrier testing** should be offered to all women of reproductive age to determine their risk to have a child with a potentially serious genetic disorder. The specific tests ordered are determined by ethnicity and/or family history. Most carrier testing does not detect 100% of the mutations associated with a specific disease and therefore, patients who screen negative are often given a modified carrier risk based on their test results and/or ethnicity.

*Noninvasive Screening Tests:*

☞SERUM SCREENING TESTS: Blood tests which look for pregnancy-specific analytes. Levels of analytes are combined in an algorithm to determine a specific risk. Risk cutoffs vary by laboratory and center. Women found to be at high-risk (> general population risk) and are offered additional testing.

The American College of Obstetrics and Gynecology, Guidelines, 2007, state that ideally, patients seen early in pregnancy should be offered aneuploidy screening that combines first- and second-trimester testing (integrated or sequential).

The risk of fetal aneuploidy is determined by many factors including the age of the mother, maternal blood levels of biochemical markers, and fetal ultrasound imaging. Initial risk of aneuploidy

is based on the age of the mother at delivery and increases with advancing maternal age. This "a-priori" risk is then modified by likelihood ratios calculated from the levels of maternal serum analytes.

In Down syndrome pregnancies, first trimester levels of maternal hCG are elevated and PAPP-A is reduced. In the second trimester, AFP levels and estriol levels are reduced and hCG and inhibin A are elevated.

Maternal serum screening risks (or age-related risks in women who have not had screening performed) are frequently combined with any ultrasound abnormalities using likelihood ratios to provide the most accurate approximation risk for chromosome abnormalities. In general, a risk of 1:270 or higher is considered an indication for invasive testing.

☞NUCHAL TRANSLUCENCY MEASUREMENT (FIRST TRIMESTER): It needs to be performed between 11 weeks and 13.6 weeks' gestation by a certified ultrasonographer. Increased nuchal measurement alone is associated with an increased risk for trisomy 21, cystic hygroma, other genetic syndromes, and cardiac defects. Most often, NT measurement is combined with serum screening to improve detection rate of fetal aneuploidy. An NT measurement above 3.5 mm in the first trimester (the 99th percentile) is considered high risk for fetal aneuploidy.

☞NUCHAL FOLD MEASUREMENT (SECOND TRIMESTER): In the second trimester, ultrasound identification of increased nuchal skin fold (>6 mm), a short femur, or cerebral ventriculomegaly increase the risk of trisomy 21.

☞**SERUM ALPHA-FETOPROTEIN MEASUREMENT:** Low AFP is associated with an increased risk for trisomy 21 and high AFP is associated with an increased risk for open neural tube defects and abdominal wall defects. In women who are offered first-trimester prenatal screening and testing, second-trimester AFP, along with targeted ultrasound, is used to screen for ONTDs.

☞**SERUM ESTRIOL:** Isolated low levels of serum estriol are associated with uterine dysfunction and often, fetal death. Low levels of estriol in conjunction with a normal fetal ultrasound are associated with a rare genetic syndrome known as Smith-Lemli-Opitz.

☞**TARGETED ULTRASOUND:** Ultrasound scan performed at 18 to 20 weeks' gestation will detect many birth defects as well as more subtle signs of fetal aneuploidy. Fifty percent of women carrying a fetus with trisomy 21 and 80% of women carrying a fetus with trisomy 13 or 18 will have an anomaly on ultrasound. Women with an abnormal ultrasound can be offered additional testing.

## Counseling Considerations

**Invasive Testing:** All women considering invasive prenatal testing should be offered genetic counseling. Informed consent needs to be signed at the time of the procedure. Women should be informed of risks, benefits, and limitations and made aware of their options given an abnormal result, including terminating the pregnancy, continuing the pregnancy, or placing the baby for adoption.

- Karyotype: Discussion should include a description of major chromosome abnormalities, variability of conditions, and limitations of detection. Discussion of mosaic results should occur for CVS procedures.
- FISH testing: As an addendum to routine karyotype to detect common aneuploidies quicker than karyotype. If done for a single condition, discussion of condition, variability, detection rate, and prognosis should be discussed.
- Microarray: Discussion should include benefits and limitations (most microarray testing cannot detect mosaicism or balanced translocations). The possibility of uncertain results needs to be communicated to patients, as well as the variability of the conditions being tested for and the possibility that a parent could learn that they are affected with a genetic disorder.

**Carrier Testing:** Women of reproductive age considering carrier testing should have access to genetic counseling and educational materials. Ancestry and a targeted family history can help determine which carrier tests should be offered. Carrier testing does not detect all the genetic mutations associated with a specific disorder. Therefore, patients need to understand that their risk to be a carrier for a specific disease may be substantially reduced by carrier screening, but this risk is never zero.

In addition, patients need to be aware that certain carrier tests can identify them as at risk or affected with a genetic condition. For example, women who are carriers of a premutation for fragile X can have premature ovarian failure and Jewish carrier screening can identify people affected with late-onset Tay-Sachs disease.

**Noninvasive Testing:** Screening tests are not diagnostic. Patients should be offered access to genetic counseling and educational materials. All patients with abnormal (screen positive) results on noninvasive testing or ultrasound, positive carrier screening or family history, or with an age of 35 or older, etc, should be offered genetic counseling to discuss options including invasive prenatal diagnosis (CVS in first trimester or amniocentesis in second trimester). Choice of screening test dependent on timing of pregnancy, timing of results and availability of the option of pregnancy termination, center resources (such as trained or certified ultrasonographer), and patient resources (insurance coverage vs self-pay).

**BIBLIOGRAPHY:**

1. ACOG, 2007. Screening for fetal chromosomal abnormalities: all women regardless of age should be offered aneuploidy screening before 20 weeks' gestation.
2. ACMG, 2009. Screening for fetal aneuploidy and neural tube defects: all women regardless of age should be offered invasive prenatal diagnostic testing if they decline they should be offered non-invasive screening before 20 weeks' gestation.
3. Driscoll DA, Gross SJ. Professional Practice and Guidelines Committee. First trimester diagnosis and screening for fetal aneuploidy. *Genet Med.* Jan 2008;10(1):73-75.
4. Gross S, Pletcher B, Monaghan K. ACMG Practice Guidelines: carrier screening in individuals of Ashkenazi Jewish descent. *Genet Med.* 2008;10:54-56.
5. Krantz DA, Hallahan TW, Sherwin JE. Screening for open neural tube defects. *Clin Lab Med.* Sep 2010; 30(3):721-725.
6. Palomaki GE, Lee JE, Canick JA, McDowell GA, Donnenfeld AE. ACMG Laboratory Quality Assurance Committee. Technical standards and guidelines: prenatal screening for Down syndrome that includes first trimester biochemistry and/or ultrasound measurements. *Genet Med.* Dec 2009;11(12):873.
7. Pletcher BA. Preconception and prenatal testing of biologic fathers for carrier status. *Genet Med.* 2006;8(2):134-135.
8. Prior TW. ACMG Practice Guidelines: carrier screening for spinal muscular atrophy. *Genet Med.* 2008;10:840-842.
9. Sherman S, Pletcher BA, Driscoll DA. Fragile X syndrome: diagnostic and carrier testing. *Genet Med.* 2005;7(8):584-587.
10. South ST, Chen Z, Brothman AR. Genomic medicine in prenatal diagnosis. *Clin Obstet Gynecol.* Mar 2008;51(1):62-73.
11. Watson MS, Cutting GR, Desnick RJ, et al. Cystic fibrosis population carrier screening: 2004 revision of American College of medical Genetics mutation panel. *Genet Med.* 2004;6:387-391.
12. ACOG. ACOG Practice Bulletin No. 88. Invasive prenatal testing for aneuploidy. *Obstet Gynecol.* Dec 2007;110(6):1459-1467.
13. ACOG committee opinion No. 298: prenatal and preconceptional carrier screening for genetic diseases in individuals of Eastern European Jewish descent. *Obstet Gynecol.* 2004:104(2):425-428.
14. ACOG committee opinion No. 338: screening for fragile X syndrome. *Obstet Gynecol.* 2006;107:1483-1485.
15. ACOG committee opinion No. 432: spinal muscular atrophy. *Obstet Gynecol.* 2009;113(5):1194-1196.
16. ACOG committee opinion No. 442: preconception and prenatal carrier screening for genetic diseases in individuals of Eastern European Jewish descent. *Obstet Gynecol.* 2009;114(4):950-953.
17. ACOG committee opinion No. 446: array comparative genomic hybridization in prenatal diagnosis. *Obstet Gynecol.* 2009;114(5):1161-1163.
18. ACOG committee opinion No. 486: update on carrier screening for cystic fibrosis. *Obstet Gynecol.* 2011;117:1028-1031.

# 99 Recurrent Pregnancy Loss

Haruki Nishizawa and Hiroki Kurahashi

## KEY POINTS

- *Disease summary:*
  - Recurrent pregnancy loss (RPL) is traditionally defined as three or more consecutive losses of recognized pregnancies in the first or early second trimester (<20 weeks of gestation). Sporadic spontaneous pregnancy loss occurs randomly in one-sixth of clinically recognized pregnancies. However, RPL must be distinguished from sporadic cases as these occasionally respond to treatment. Around 1% of couples attempting pregnancy experience RPL.

- *Hereditary basis:*
  - Structural chromosomal abnormalities such as translocations and inversions are often identified in one partner of a couple experiencing RPL. The fetuses from these couples frequently carry chromosome copy number abnormalities which lead to miscarriage. Hereditary thrombophilia in females is also occasionally associated with RPL.

- *Differential diagnosis:*
  - RPL is a heterogeneous condition. In addition to parental chromosomal abnormalities and hereditary thrombophilia, hormonal and metabolic disorders, uterine anatomic abnormalities, certain infections, and autoimmune disorders have been accepted as etiologic factors in RPL. However, up to 50% of these cases still remain unexplained after standard gynecologic, hormonal, and karyotypic investigations.

## Diagnostic Criteria and Clinical Characteristics

*Diagnostic Criteria:* RPL is traditionally defined as three or more consecutive losses of a recognized pregnancy in the first or early second trimester (<20 weeks of gestation).

*Clinical Characteristics:*

☞**CHROMOSOME ABNORMALITIES:** In 2% to 4% of couples experiencing RPL, a balanced structural abnormality is found in one partner. Chromosomal translocations are the most common structural abnormalities associated with early RPL. Robertsonian translocations involve the centric fusion of two acrocentric chromosomes (numbers 13, 14, 15, 21, and 22). Balanced carriers of Robertsonian translocations have no clinical symptoms, but often produce chromosomally unbalanced gametes. These numerical abnormalities in the autosome usually result in early fetal death, or occasionally in the birth of children with trisomy 13 or 21 (Fig. 99-1).

Other reciprocal translocations also cause RPL. During gametogenesis, paternal and maternal chromosomes undergo homologous pairing and recombine to segregate correctly in meiosis I. In balanced carriers of reciprocal translocations, normal and translocated chromosomes form an abnormal meiotic configuration that often leads to partially unbalanced gametes (Fig. 99-2). Large chromosomal imbalances result in fetal death, while chromosomally unbalanced children might be born if regions involved are small.

Other structural abnormalities such as inversions or insertions can also cause RPL.

☞**HORMONAL AND METABOLIC DISORDERS:** Maternal endocrine and metabolic disorders occasionally contribute to the etiology of RPL. Females with diabetes mellitus, thyroid hormone disorders, and hyperprolactinemia are implicated as being at high risk of RPL. Luteal phase defects might possibly contribute to RPL through impaired placentation, but this is still controversial. Further, polycystic ovary syndrome is occasionally associated with RPL.

☞**UTERINE ANATOMIC ABNORMALITIES:** Uterine anatomic abnormalities are common causes of RPL, and 10% to 15% of females suffering from this disorder have congenital uterine abnormalities such as double uterus (bicornuate, septate, or didelphic). Uterine synechiae or fibroids may also be associated with RPL. Cervical incompetence is a well-known cause of midtrimester RPL. Its diagnosis is based on a history of late miscarriage preceded by spontaneous rupture of membranes or painless cervical dilatation.

☞**INFECTIOUS CAUSES:** Evidence has now accumulated that chorioamnionitis caused by ureaplasma species often contributes to late pregnancy loss. It is possible that females carrying such microorganisms might manifest RPL.

☞**THROMBOPHILIA:** Thrombophilia, whether inherited or acquired, has been thought to contribute to a substantial percentage of RPL cases. It has been well documented that the hypercoagulation status in pregnant women preferentially causes pregnancy loss as a result of a placental thromboembolism. Protein C or S deficiency, antithrombin III deficiency, or activated protein C resistance are the common inherited causes of thrombophilia. Although such genetic susceptibilities to thrombophilia are more prevalent in women with late fetal losses, they are also a major cause of early miscarriage. The Leiden mutation (1691G>A) in the factor V gene or the PTm mutation (20210G>A) in the 3'UTR of the factor II (prothrombin) gene are also well-known risk factors for RPL in Caucasians, but these variants are rare in other populations. Recently, promoter polymorphisms for the annexin A5 gene have been reported to be associated with RPL (Table 99-1). Annexin A5 is a placental anticoagulant, and is decreased in the placentas of risk allele carriers. Antiphospholipid antibodies are a well-known cause of acquired thrombophilia and their presence often leads to a form of RPL known as antiphospholipid syndrome (see later).

☞**IMMUNOLOGIC DISORDERS:** Antiphospholipid syndrome (APS) is an autoimmune disorder characterized by recurrent fetal losses and/or vascular thrombosis in the presence of significant levels of antiphospholipid antibodies. Some instances of APS occur as a part of a systemic autoimmune disease such as systemic

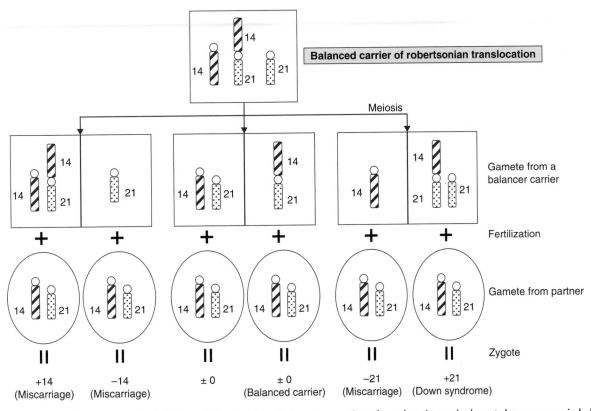

**Figure 99-1** Chromosome Segregation in Balanced Translocation Carriers. Segregation of translocation and relevant chromosomes in balanced carriers for a t(14;21) Robertsonian translocation. Conceptuses are most often aneuploidy, resulting in miscarriage. Occasionally carriers give birth to a child with a normal or balanced karyotype, although some newborns are affected by trisomy 21.

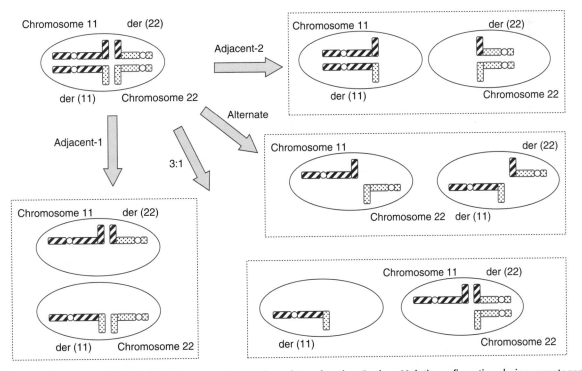

**Figure 99-2** Meiotic Configuration During Gametogenesis in Balanced Translocation Carriers. Meiotic configuration during gametogenesis in balanced carriers of a t(11;22) reciprocal translocation. In adjacent 1 or 2, conceptuses harbor a partial trisomy and partial monosomy resulting in early pregnancy loss. Occasionally carriers give birth with a normal or balanced karyotype, while <1/10 newborns are affected by +der(22) syndrome (Emanuel syndrome) through a 3:1 segregation.

*Table 99-1* **RPL-Associated Susceptibility Variants**

| Candidate Gene (Chromosome Location) | Associated Variant [effect on protein] (DB SNP) | Relative Risk | Frequency of Risk Allele | Putative Functional Significance | Associated Disease Phenotype |
|---|---|---|---|---|---|
| *F5* (1q24.2) | **G1691A** [nonsynonymous amino acid substitution R506Q] (rs6025) | 2.01 in early and 7.83 in late recurrent fetal losses | 3%-5% among Caucasians but 0% among non-Caucasians | Activated protein C resistance | Thrombophilia |
| *F2* (11p11.2) | **G20210A** [3' untranslated region] (rs1799963) | 2.56 in early recurrent and 2.30 in late non-recurrent fetal losses | 1%-2% among Caucasians | Increased efficiency of mRNA 3' end formation | Thrombophilia |
| *ANXA5* (4q27) | **M2 haplotype (−19G>A, 1A>C, 27T>C, 76G>A)** [promoter region] (rs28717001, rs28651243) | 3.88 | 8.2% among Germans | Decreased expression | Thrombophilia? |
| *SYCP3* (12q23.2) | **IVS7-18-21delACTT** | NA | NA | Nondisjunction in meiosis I | Aneuploidy |

lupus erythematosus. "Primary APS" is the diagnosis in those patients without a recognized autoimmune disease. It has been suggested also that antiphospholipid antibodies interfere with the syncytialization of trophoblasts or cause placental infarction leading to the RPL. The contribution of alloimmunity, a maternal immunologic reaction against the fetus (ie, paternal antigen), to RPL has been proposed. It has been reported that partners tend to share human leukocyte antigen (HLA). The number of circulating natural killer (NK) cells is suggested to be associated with RPL. Deficiencies in HLA-G, which inhibit NK cell activation, have also been reported in couples with RPL. However, the possible involvement of each of these immunologic defects in RPL remains controversial.

☞UNEXPLAINED RPL: It is recognized that more than 50% of early spontaneous abortions are cytogenetically abnormal, most being numerical abnormalities. Couples who experienced pregnancy loss due to trisomy for different chromosomes in each miscarriage (heterotrisomy) are at a slightly increased risk of recurrent aneuploidy. The age of the female is an important factor in this regard, but several lines of evidence now suggest that a small proportion of couples with RPL have a predisposition to aneuploid gametes. Mutations in *SYCP3* gene, which encodes a component of synaptonemal complex in meiosis I, have also been reported in females with unexplained RPL (Table 99-1).

## Screening and Counseling

**Screening:** Couples who experience more than two consecutive pregnancy losses should be screened for suspected RPL. Females with RPL should be examined by ultrasonography or hysterosalpingography for the detection of anatomic abnormalities of the genital tract. They should also have blood drawn to test for immunologic risk factors, including NK cell activity, antinuclear

antibodies, and antiphospholipid antibodies, such as lupus anticoagulant. Standard coagulation tests should be performed also as activated partial thromboplastin time (aPTT) might be prolonged in cases with APS. Screening for thrombophilia, via the measurement of plasma levels of antithrombin III and proteins C and S, or activated protein C resistance should be performed. Blood tests for hyperthyroidism, diabetes mellitus, hyperprolactinemia, and for infections, such as Chlamydia, should also be evaluated. Cytogenetic analyses should be undertaken for these individuals, as well as for their partners, and any abortuses.

**Counseling:** As with cytogenetic abnormalities, reproductive risk in couples is based on the karyotype, but the risk assessment depends on various factors which are complex. In Robertsonian translocations, the meiotic configuration indicates only three segregation patterns (Fig. 99-1). The outcome (fetal loss, normal or abnormal live births) depends on the relevant chromosomes. In other structural abnormalities such as reciprocal translocations or inversions, the segregation pattern is affected by the location of the breakpoints. Further, the risk calculation also depends on function of the genes that are located at predicted unbalanced chromosomal regions in the fetuses. Hence, the risk calculation for pregnancy loss cannot be generalized, and should be estimated in each case.

In terms of counseling, it is important to remember that a couple with a structural abnormality is at considerable risk of a liveborn anomalous infant.

In cases of couples without any cytogenetic abnormalities, risk assessments are based on empiric data only.

Couples who experience pregnancy loss struggle with complex emotions and frequently seek information and guidance from their obstetrician or gynecologist. Among the RPL couples with no abnormal findings, women receiving specific antenatal counseling and psychologic support had a higher subsequent pregnancy success rate when compared with women who were given no specific antenatal care.

## Management and Treatment

**Anticoagulants:** Low-dose aspirin (50 mg/d) with or without heparin has become the standard treatment for RPL associated with APS as well as inherited thrombophilia. Regarding heparin, the difference between low molecular weight heparin and unfractionated heparin needs further investigation.

Treatment of women with unexplained RPL using anticoagulants had occasionally been tried, but the effectiveness of this therapy is controversial.

**Immunomodulator Agents:** The use of intravenous immunoglobulins, anti-TNF-α drugs, or glucocorticoids can dampen excessive immune responses and may be occasionally used for APS-associated RPL.

Transfusion of paternal or third-party donor leukocytes prior to conception has been tried, but no beneficial effects have been proven.

**Progestational Agents:** The administration of progesterone has been performed orally, intramuscularly, or virginally to prevent early pregnancy loss as a result of a luteal phase defect. This induces secretory changes in the endometrium and ensures implantation of the embryo.

**Preimplantation Diagnosis:** Couples with a balanced structural abnormality can benefit from in vitro fertilization followed by preimplantation diagnosis. PGD involves a blastomere biopsy, aspiration of one or two blastomeres from eight-cell embryos (3-day old), and FISH, which is usually performed on the interphase nuclei. A blastocyst biopsy at 5 to 6 days is also performed followed by genotyping for the relevant chromosomes using microsatellite polymerase chain reaction (PCR) to determine the segregation pattern (Figs. 99-1 and 99-2). Likewise, PGD is also used to screen for aneuploidy in some unexplained RPL cases as well as in older females to prevent age-related aneuploidy conceptuses.

## Molecular Genetics and Molecular Mechanism

**Syndrome/Gene/Locus:** RPL can be a polygenic disease in which multiple genetic variations are involved, whilst animal studies indicate that RPL can also be a Mendelian disease, which results from a single gene mutation. A number of papers have been published that report a case-control study for RPL, but only a few genetic variations reproducibly show any association with this disease (Table 99-1). All of these variants are related to thrombophilia that leads to RPL through a placental thromboembolism.

**Genetic Testing:** Cytogenetic screening should be performed for couples with RPL. No role yet exists for genetic testing in the diagnosis of RPL.

**Future Directions:** Genomic information can be used to determine the therapeutic intervention in cases of unexplained RPL.

For example, although a recent large cohort study suggests no role for anticoagulation therapies such as low molecular weight heparin or low-dose aspirin for unexplained RPL, selection of appropriate patients using genetic analysis might enhance the therapeutic efficacy of these treatments. The establishment of personalized medical approaches to the treatment of RPL is likely in the near future.

**BIBLIOGRAPHY:**

1. American College of Obstetricians and Gynecologists. ACOG practice bulletin. Management of recurrent pregnancy loss. Number 24, February 2001. *Int J Gynaecol Obstet.* Aug 2002;78(2):179-190.

2. Jauniaux E, Farquharson RG, Christiansen OB, et al. Evidence-based guidelines for the investigation and medical treatment of recurrent miscarriage. *Hum Reprod.* 2006;21:2216-2222.

3. Rey E, Kahn SR, David M, et al. Thrombophilic disorders and fetal loss: a meta-analysis. *Lancet.* 2003;361:901-908.

4. Martinelli I, Taioli E, Cetin I, et al. Mutations in coagulation factors in women with unexplained late fetal loss. *N Engl J Med.* 2000;343:1015-1018.

5. Miyakis S, Lockshin MD, Atsumi T, et al. International consensus statement on an update of the classification criteria for definite antiphospholipid syndrome (APS). *J Thromb Haemost.* 2006;4:295-306.

6. Bogdanova N, Horst J, Chlystun M, et al. A common haplotype of the annexin A5 (ANXA5) gene promoter is associated with recurrent pregnancy loss. *Hum Mol Genet.* 2007;16:573-578.

7. Bolor H, Mori T, Nishiyama S, et al. Mutations of the *SYCP3* gene in women with recurrent pregnancy loss. *Am J Hum Genet.* 2009;84:14-20.

8. Kaandorp SP, Goddijn M, van der Post JA, et al. Aspirin plus heparin or aspirin alone in women with recurrent miscarriage. *N Engl J Med.* 2010;362:1586-1596.

9. Kurahashi H, Inagaki H, Ohye T, et al. The constitutional t(11;22): implications for a novel mechanism responsible for gross chromosomal rearrangements. *Clin Genet.* 2010;78:299-309.

## Supplementary Information

**OMIM REFERENCES:**

[1] Annexin A5; ANXA5 (#131230)

[2] Synaptonemal Complex Protein 3; SYCP3 (#604759)

**Alternative Names:**
- Recurrent Spontaneous Abortion
- Recurrent Spontaneous Miscarriage
- Recurrent Abortion
- Recurrent Miscarriage

**Key Words:** Recurrent pregnancy loss, thrombophilia, chromosome, translocation, aneuploidy

# 100 Folate and Neural Tube Defects

Faith Pangilinan and Lawrence C. Brody

## KEY POINTS

- *Disease summary:*
  - Neural tube defects (NTDs) occur in 0.5 to 2/1000 pregnancies worldwide and are the second most common birth defect after congenital heart defects.
  - The neural tube is an embryonic structure that forms from the folding of ectodermal tissue to into a hollow canal. The floor of this canal (neural plate) combined with migrating neural crest cells will give rise to the major structures of the central nervous system.
  - In humans, the cranial and caudal ends of the tube are the last regions to close. Closure of the neural tube is completed within 5 weeks of fertilization.
  - When the neural tube fails to close, the subsequent development of all underlying structures is disrupted. Lack of closure in the cranial region results in failure of the brain to develop (anencephaly). Lack of closure in the caudal region produces damage to the spinal cord (spina bifida; most commonly myelomeningocele, but also includes meningocele and lipomeningocele).
  - Other forms of NTDs include encephalocele, craniorachischisis, and iniencephaly.
- *Differential diagnosis:*
  - None.
- *Monogenic forms:*
  - NTDs are a feature of several rare inherited syndromes (most notably, Meckel-Gruber syndrome). The vast majority of NTDs occur as isolated defects. Isolated NTDs exhibit hallmarks of a complex disease with multiple environmental and genetic factors.
- *Family history:*
  - The risk to siblings is approximately 2% to 5%.
- *Twin studies:*
  - In one study, NTD twin concordance was more frequent in monozygotic twins than in dizygotic twins.
- *Environmental factors:*
  - Lower levels of folate are observed in mothers with an NTD pregnancy, and periconceptional folic acid supplementation can reduce the risk of an NTD pregnancy by up to 75%. Other risk factors include maternal use of valproic acid (a folate antagonist used to manage migraines, epilepsy, and bipolar disorder), maternal diabetes, and maternal obesity. Antifolate compounds such as methotrexate are known as teratogens. Use of antifolates during pregnancy is contraindicated but exposure to methotrexate during pregnancy has not been associated with NTDs.
- *Genome-wide associations:*
  - The research community is forming a consortium to perform a GWAS of NTDs.

## Diagnostic Criteria and Clinical Characteristics

### Diagnostic Criteria for Neural Tube Defects:

**Diagnostic evaluation should include at least one of the following**

- Spina bifida occulta (closed defect): The posterior elements of the vertebral arch fail to close. There is an absence of a sac of neural tissue protruding from the back. This defect may or may not include an affected spinal cord. If not, it often goes undetected. Asymptomatic spina bifida occulta is an incidental finding arising from lower back imaging studies.
- Spina bifida cystica (open defect): Myelomeningocele is the most common and severe subtype. It involves protrusion of the spinal cord, nerve roots, meninges, and cerebrospinal fluid (CSF). Most lesions are lumbar, and higher lesions are associated with more severe clinical outcomes.
- Anencephaly (open defect): Failure of the neural tube to close at the cranial end results in failure of the brain to

develop normally. These infants usually survive only a few hours after birth.

**And the absence of**

- By definition, isolated neural tube defects are not associated with additional congenital defects. The presence of multiple congenital defects in addition to a neural tube defect may be the product of a single gene defect or chromosomal abnormality. A patient presenting with NTD and polydactyly, cleft palate, or renal cysts may be affected with Meckel-Gruber syndrome. This autosomal recessive disorder is the most common Mendelian cause of NTDs. A number of additional single gene syndromes and trisomies also include NTDs.

### Clinical Characteristics of Spina Bifida:

- Neurologic deficits can include a range of motor and sensory defects dependent on the site of the lesion, and may include paralysis.
- Arnold-Chiari malformation is nearly always present in spina bifida. This involves herniation of the lower brain stem and

**Table 100-1 Disease-Associated Susceptibility Variants**

| Candidate Gene | Associated Variant | Relative Risk | Frequency of Risk Allele[a] | Putative Functional Significance | Associated Disease Phenotype |
|---|---|---|---|---|---|
| *MTHFR* (methylenetetrahydrofolate reductase) | rs1801133 (A222V) | ~1.8 | 0.3 | Thermolabile variant | Case NTD risk |
| *MTHFD1* (methylenetetrahydrofolate dehydrogenase [NADP+ dependent] 1, methenyltetrahydrofolate cyclohydrolase, formyltetrahydrofolate synthetase [cytosolic]) | Maternal rs2236225 (R653Q) | ~1.5 | 0.45 | Codon variant | Maternal NTD risk |
| *MTHFD1L* (methylenetetrahydrofolate dehydrogenase [NADP+ dependent] 1-like [formyltetrahydrofolate synthetase domain containing 1] [mitochondrial]) | rs3832406 (7×ATT repeat) | ~1.2 | 0.65 | Splice variant | Case NTD risk |
| *TCblR* (transcobalamin II receptor; vitamin B$_{12}$ receptor) | rs150384171 (E88del) | ~9 | 0.02 | Codon deletion | Case NTD risk |
| *RFC1* (reduced folate carrier 1) | rs1051266 (H27R) | 1.9 | 0.44 | Codon variant | Case NTD risk |
| *MTRR* (methionine synthase reductase) | rs1801394 (I22M) | 2.1 | 0.54 | Codon variant | Maternal NTD risk |

[a]Allele frequency in the population reported in genetic studies. These are predominantly of European origin. Allele frequencies and degree of risk are expected to vary in other populations.

cerebellum into the spinal canal. It may obstruct the flow of CSF in the fourth ventricle, resulting in hydrocephalus.

- Syringomyelia involves dilation of the central canal of the spinal cord. Progression can lead to scoliosis, upper-extremity weakness, or sensory changes.
- Musculoskeletal problems can include bone and joint deformities, muscle atrophy, and ostopenia. These conditions increase the risk of fractures as growth occurs.
- Lower extremities may exhibit such problems as hip subluxation or dislocation, hip flexion contractures, knee flexion contractures, spasticity, and congenital and acquired foot abnormalities.
- Spinal deformities may include scoliosis, kyphosis, and an abnormal bony spine.
- Bowel and/or bladder incontinence is possible depending on the site of the lesion.

## Screening and Counseling

**Screening:** Three prenatal tests can detect NTDs.
1. Maternal serum alpha-fetoprotein (MSAFP): Alpha fetoprotein (AFP) is secreted by the fetal yolk sac and liver. Elevated levels of AFP can be detected in the maternal circulation after 15 weeks of pregnancy if an open NTD is present.
2. High-resolution ultrasound: Depending on the size of the defect and position of the fetus, an open or closed NTD may be detected at 15 to 24 weeks of pregnancy.
3. Amniocentesis (AFP): Sampling the amniotic fluid allows detection of AFP after 15 weeks of pregnancy.

**Counseling:** Inheritance and penetrance: Neural tube defects are usually isolated defects, with a pattern of multifactorial, multivariate inheritance with low penetrance. The majority of cases occur in the absence of family history. Empirical recurrence risks (1%-2%) are used for families in which a previous pregnancy was affected by an NTD. Use of folic acid supplements during pre- and postconception intervals are recommended. Diabetes mellitus, valproic acid use, and a positive family history in second-degree relatives are associated with increased risk. Families without known risk factors are counseled that their risk of having pregnancy affected with an NTD is one in a thousand.

☞**GENOTYPE-PHENOTYPE CORRELATION:** Because genetic risk factors so far identified for NTDs are common variants (allele frequencies above 0.01) usually observed in the absence of disease, there is currently no genotype-phenotype correlation to report other than the risk (odds ratio [OR] 1.2-9) observed with these variants (Table 100-1).

## Management and Treatment

**Management:** The management and treatment of those with NTDs is largely based on the specific anatomic lesion present in the individuals. Initial treatment is primarily surgical followed by therapy and interventions designed to avoid complications and retain and restore as much neurologic function as possible. Parental training and involvement in care is also an important component of the medical management plan.

- Prenatal surgery poses risk to the mother and greatly increases the risk of premature delivery. However, this procedure, which is done before 26 weeks of gestation, is thought to improve the chances of preventing the rapid decline in nerve function that occurs after birth.

- Surgery 24 to 48 hours after birth can return protruding tissues to their normal position and close the vertebral opening with muscle and skin.
- Although surgery can be helpful to close the lesion, irreparable nerve damage has often already occurred, requiring a team of specialists for ongoing care.
  - Lifelong physical therapy can begin in the neonate to maximize developmental potential. This includes increasing range of motion, promotion of active and passive exercise, and facilitating achievement of developmental milestones.
  - Ongoing evaluation for surgery to address a tethered spinal cord is also necessary. The spinal cord can be bound to the scar at the site of closure, limiting its normal growth and development and affecting muscle function in the legs, bowel, or bladder.
  - Management of bladder and/or bowel incontinence may include urodynamic studies, catheterization, medication, biofeedback, and behavior modification.
- Ongoing assessments determine the need for assistive devices such as crutches, a walker, or a wheelchair.

**Therapeutics:**
- As detailed earlier, a lifelong course of surgery, physical therapy, and orthopedic management are often needed. Therapeutic regimens are tailored to the specific status of the NTD patient and not the underlying malformation.

## Molecular Genetics and Molecular Mechanism

**Genetic Testing:** Because the genetic component of NTDs consists of many risk variants, each of small effect, there is little utility in testing for genetic risk factors at the current time. This is because such testing for the known genetic loci will have limited positive and negative predictive value. Pre- and periconceptional folic acid supplementation is currently the measure to prevent NTDs supported by evidence at the level 1 threshold (randomized, case-control studies). There is a 1% to 2% incidence of NTDs when valproic acid is used during pregnancy. These cases may be occurring in individuals carrying a specific set of single-nucleotide polymorphisms (SNPs) that alter the metabolism of this drug. At this time, no loci of pharmacogenetic importance have been identified in connection with this risk. Alternative therapies should be considered for those currently on anticonvulsants.

**Future Directions:** NTDs are one of the few diseases for which a population-wide, primary prevention strategy has been applied. In North America, the addition of folic acid to milled grains has reduced the incidence of NTDs. Similar food fortification programs are under consideration in many additional countries. Folic acid fortification has been opposed by those with general concerns over "food modification." Additionally, supplemental folic acid also has the potential to accelerate the growth of neoplastic tissues. These concerns are being weighed by public health officials in countries considering folic acid fortification.

The observed recurrence rate within sibships suggests that NTDs have a strong genetic component. Studies performed to date have focused on candidate genes related to folate and vitamin $B_{12}$ metabolic pathways (one-carbon metabolism). NTD risk

alleles have been identified (Table 100-1), but these alleles do not explain the majority of NTD cases. Only 100 of the 22,000 human genes have been screened for NTD risk alleles. Future studies will use the genome-wide association approach to survey the entire human genome for loci that modify NTD risk profile. Such a study should uncover both folate and nonfolate responsive loci.

These additional epidemiologic studies should identify a set of genetic markers associated with NTD risk. Models that incorporate multiple risk loci into an overall risk score can be developed. These models could be used to provide more accurate risk estimates. The search for additional genes associated with NTDs may identify new biologic pathways involved in the biology of neural tube closure. The knowledge of these pathways may suggest new strategies for the prevention of NTDs.

**BIBLIOGRAPHY:**

1. Greene ND, Stanier P, Copp AJ. Genetics of human neural tube defects. *Hum Mol Genet.* 2009;18(R2):R113-R129.
2. Monograph in epidemiology and biostatistics Volume 20. In: Elwood JM, Little J, Elwood JH, eds. *Epidemiology and Control of Neural Tube Defects.* Oxford, UK: Oxford University Press; 1992.
3. Deak KL, Siegel DG, George TM, et al. Further evidence for a maternal genetic effect and a sex-influenced effect contributing to risk for human neural tube defects. *Birth Defects Res A Clin Mol Teratol.* 2008;82(10):662-669.
4. Joo JG, Beke A, Papp C, et al. Neural tube defects in the sample of genetic counselling. *Prenat Diagn.* 2007;27(10):912-921.
5. MRC Vitamin Study Research Group. Prevention of neural tube defects: results of the Medical Research Council Vitamin Study. *Lancet.* 1991;338(8760):131-137.
6. Berry RJ, Li Z, Erickson JD, et al. Prevention of neural-tube defects with folic acid in China. China-U.S. Collaborative Project for Neural Tube Defect Prevention. *N Engl J Med.* 1999;341(20):1485-1490.
7. Czeizel AE, Dudas I. Prevention of the first occurrence of neural-tube defects by periconceptional vitamin supplementation. *N Engl J Med.* 1992;327(26):1832-1835.
8. Lammer EJ, Sever LE, Oakley GP Jr. Teratogen update: valproic acid. *Teratology.* 1987;35(3):465-473.
9. Elwood JM, Little J, Elwood H. Maternal illness and drug use in pregnancy. In: Elwood JM, Little J, Elwood H, eds. *Epidemiology and Control of Neural Tube Defects.* Oxford, UK: Oxford University Press; 1992:414-455.
10. Becerra JE, Khoury MJ, Cordero JF, Erickson JD. Diabetes mellitus during pregnancy and the risks for specific birth defects: a population-based case-control study. *Pediatrics.* 1990;85(1):1-9.
11. Watkins ML, Scanlon KS, Mulinare J, Khoury MJ. Is maternal obesity a risk factor for anencephaly and spina bifida? *Epidemiology.* 1996;7(5):507-512.
12. Werler MM, Louik C, Shapiro S, Mitchell AA. Prepregnant weight in relation to risk of neural tube defects. *JAMA.* 1996;275(14):1089-1092.
13. Lloyd ME, Carr M, McElhatton P, Hall GM, Hughes RA. The effects of methotrexate on pregnancy, fertility and lactation. *QJM.* 1999;92(10):551-563.
14. Ryan KD, Ploski C, Emans JB. Myelodysplasia—the musculoskeletal problem: habilitation from infancy to adulthood. *Phys Ther.* 1991;71(12):935-946.
15. Bjerkedal T, Czeizel A, Goujard J, et al. Valproic acid and spina bifida. *Lancet.* 1982;2(8307):1096.

## Supplementary Information

**OMIM REFERENCES:**

[1] Neural Tube Defects, Folate-Sensitive (Spina Bifida, Folate-Sensitive, Included); (#601634)

[2] Neural Tube Defects (Spina Bifida, Included); (#182940)

[3] Meckel-Gruber Syndrome (Types 1-10); (#s 249000, 603194, 607361, 611134, 611561, 612284, 267010, 213885, 614209, 614175)

**Alternative Names:**
- Spinabifida, Myelomeningocele, Meningocele, Lipomeningocele
- Anencephaly
- Encephalocele
- Craniorachischisis
- Iniencephaly

***Key Words:*** Neural tube, neural crest, folic acid, multifactorial disease

# 101 Liver Disease in Pregnancy

Charlotte Frise and Lucy MacKillop

## KEY POINTS

- *Disease summary:*
  - *Hypertensive disorders of pregnancy*
    - A spectrum of clinical disorders including pre-eclampsia, eclampsia, HELLP syndrome (hemolysis, elevated liver enzymes, low platelets), and pregnancy complicated by hepatic infarction and/or rupture.
    - Pre-eclampsia complicates approximately 5% of all pregnancies. Many women with pre-eclampsia have mildly abnormal liver function tests, but 5% to 20% of pre-eclamptic pregnancies develop HELLP syndrome.
    - Risk factors for the development of pre-eclampsia include primiparity, older maternal age, increased body mass index, long birth interval, medical disorders including diabetes mellitus, chronic renal failure and antiphospholipid syndromes, family history of pre-eclampsia, or fetal factors including multiple pregnancy, or the presence of a hydatidiform mole.
    - Uncomplicated pre-eclampsia is defined as the development of hypertension and proteinuria in pregnancy. Oedema is often seen. Pre-eclampsia can also be associated with abdominal pain, headaches, visual changes, and renal and liver impairment, but the liver impairment is usually mild.
    - HELLP syndrome is a subgroup of women with pre-eclampsia and is a severe variant of the condition. Hypertension and proteinuria may be absent in up to 15% of women presenting with features of HELLP syndrome. Severe disseminated intravascular coagulation and multiorgan failure can be associated with this condition and lead to significant maternal and fetal morbidity and mortality.
    - Hepatic hemorrhage or failure occurs in approximately 1% of pregnancies complicated by HELLP syndrome and are associated with significant mortality as fulminant liver failure may result.
    - All of these conditions are thought to have a common etiology, and result from abnormal placentation early in gestation, when the spiral arteries fail to form low-resistance vessels as they do in normal pregnancy. Diffuse endothelial activation occurs which can result in multiorgan dysfunction later in the course of the pregnancy.
    - Adverse fetal outcomes associated with hypertensive disorders in pregnancy include intrauterine growth restriction, placental abruption, and intrauterine death.
  - *Acute fatty liver of pregnancy*
    - This disorder is a rare and potentially life-threatening condition that occurs in pregnancy and usually presents toward the end of the third trimester.
    - Liver dysfunction results from microvesicular steatosis (in contrast to macrovesicular steatosis which is seen in other liver disorders such as nonalcoholic fatty liver disease).
    - More common in primigravidae, in multiple pregnancies, or pregnancies with male fetuses.
    - Important symptoms that suggest a diagnosis of acute fatty liver of pregnancy (AFLP) include abdominal pain (particularly in the right upper quadrant), nausea, vomiting, and polydipsia on a background of malaise and anorexia.
    - This disorder is considered part of the same spectrum as pre-eclampsia and HELLP syndrome and so the features may overlap. Severe hypertension or proteinuria is rare, however.
  - *Intrahepatic cholestasis of pregnancy*
    - Intrahepatic cholestasis of pregnancy (ICP) is the most frequent cause of cholestasis in pregnancy and is more commonly seen in certain populations (incidence in Chile and Scandinavia is 12% and 1.5%, respectively).
    - The disorder is characterized by the development of pruritus (in the absence of a rash) which can be severe, and deranged liver function tests, in association with elevated serum bile acid concentration.
    - It has also been associated with adverse fetal outcomes including meconium-stained amniotic fluid, spontaneous preterm labor, and intrauterine death.
    - ICP typically presents with pruritus in the third trimester of pregnancy, but has been reported to develop as early as 8 weeks' gestation. Symptoms such as dark urine, steatorrhea, and jaundice can also develop. Pruritus can develop before biochemical parameters become abnormal, so it is important to repeat the liver function tests and serum bile acid concentration if clinical suspicion persists.
    - Women with ICP are more likely to have a family history of gallstones and ICP. Some women may have previously developed similar symptoms when taking the oral contraceptive pill. ICP is more common in women who have hepatitis C and the condition can develop earlier in these pregnancies compared to hepatitis C antibody-negative women (mean 29 weeks compared to 34 weeks).
- *Differential diagnosis:*
  - Other nonpregnancy-specific causes for acute liver dysfunction should also be considered including drug-related liver dysfunction (antibiotics, paracetamol), infective causes (exposure to viral hepatitides particularly hepatitis E), structural causes including Budd-Chiari syndrome and choledocholithiasis, or antibody-associated causes such as autoimmune hepatitis or primary biliary cirrhosis.
- *Monogenic forms:*
  - No monogenic forms of HELLP, AFLP, or ICP have been identified.

- *Family history:*
  - The risk of pre-eclampsia in a primigravida is increased three- to fourfold if there is a family history of the condition.
  - Daughters and siblings of women with ICP have up to a 12-fold increased risk of developing the condition.
- *Environmental factors:*
  - In some populations it has been demonstrated that there is a seasonal variation in the number of cases of ICP. For example, in Portugal more cases were seen in winter months compared to summer.
  - Investigation of the concentrations of selenium, copper, and zinc has also shown these to be lower in women with ICP.

## Diagnostic Criteria and Clinical Characteristics

### Diagnostic Evaluation:

- A thorough history for symptoms such as
  - Abdominal pain (particularly epigastric or right upper quadrant), headaches, visual disturbance (suggestive of pre-eclampsia or HELLP)
  - Nausea, vomiting, anorexia, malaise, abdominal pain, polyuria, polydipsia (suggestive of AFLP)
  - Pruritus, most commonly affecting palms and soles, cholestatic symptoms including dark urine or steatorrhea, and systemic symptoms such as anorexia or malaise (suggestive of ICP)
- Drug history—medications associated with cholestasis, symptoms with previous use of oral contraceptive pill, or in vitro fertilization
- Clinical assessment including
  - Blood pressure and urinalysis
  - Examination particularly for hepatic tenderness, hepatomegaly, ascites, or encephalopathy
  - Skin examination to look for other causes of pruritus (rashes, infections such as scabies)
- Blood tests including
  - Full blood count (hemolysis or thrombocytopenia may be evident in HELLP; leukocytosis is common in AFLP).
  - Renal function (acute renal failure can occur in HELLP or AFLP).
  - Liver function tests are deranged, to differing extents in each disorder (Table 101-1).
  - Increased serum bile acid concentration in ICP.
  - Hypoglycemia and abnormal coagulation parameters are associated with AFLP, but coagulopathy is rarely seen in ICP.

- Viral serology for hepatitis A, B, C, and E, Epstein-Barr virus, cytomegalovirus, herpes simplex virus, and human immunodeficiency virus.
- Liver antibodies including antimitochondrial antibodies (suggestive of primary biliary cirrhosis) and antismooth muscle antibodies.
- Urine analysis for protein-creatinine ratio or 24-hour collection for total protein.
- Abdominal ultrasound is performed to exclude other causes of deranged liver function. Gallstones are more commonly seen in parous women and in women with ICP.

☞**HELLP SYNDROME:** There has been no consensus about diagnostic criteria for HELLP syndrome, and studies have used a variety of measures and thresholds to make the diagnosis. Suggested parameters and thresholds are listed here.

#### Hemolysis
- Microangiopathic hemolytic anemia and schistocytes on film
- Elevated lactate dehydrogenase greater than 600 IU/L ($>2 \times$ ULN)
- Elevated bilirubin
- Low haptoglobin
- Significant drop in hemoglobin

#### Elevated liver enzymes
- Aspartate aminotransferase (AST) greater than 70 IU/L ($>2 \times$ ULN)

#### Thrombocytopenia
- Platelet count less than 100,000/mm³

☞**ACUTE FATTY LIVER OF PREGNANCY:** A set of diagnostic criteria was constructed by Ch'ng and used to diagnose AFLP in a prospective study of all women with liver dysfunction in pregnancy in their local population. This has subsequently been shown to correlate well with both clinical assessment and the presence of

**Table 101-1** *A Comparison of the Typical Changes in Liver Function Tests in the Different Pregnancy-Specific Disorders*

|  | *Obstetric Cholestasis* | *HELLP Syndrome* | *Acute Fatty Liver of Pregnancy* |
|---|---|---|---|
| **Bilirubin (μmol/L)** | 14 (6-34) | 13 (4-155) | 50 (19-61) |
| **Aspartate transaminase (u/L)** | 210 (30-519) | 66 (41-4123) | 278 (86-542) |
| **Gamma GT (u/L)** | 29 (8-278) | 24 (6-209) | 50 (22-209) |
| **Increased serum bile acids** | Majority[a] | Small proportion | Small proportion |

[a]Obstetric cholestasis (OC) unlikely if bile acids are normal on repeat testing.

microvesicular steatosis on liver biopsy where the sensitivity was 100% and the specificity was 57%.

**"Swansea criteria":** Six or more of the following features, in the absence of an alternative explanation

- Vomiting
- Abdominal pain
- Polydipsia/polyuria
- Encephalopathy
- Elevated bilirubin
- Hypoglycemia
- Elevated urate
- Leucocytosis
- Ascites or bright liver on ultrasound scan (USS)
- Elevated transaminases
- Elevated ammonia
- Renal impairment
- Coagulopathy
- Microvesicular steatosis on liver biopsy

## Screening and Counseling

*Screening:* At present no screening tools exist to identify women at risk of developing HELLP, AFLP, or ICP.

## Management and Treatment

*Management:*

☞AFLP AND HELLP:

**Supportive and resuscitative measures** to correct the physiologic, metabolic, and hematologic derangement that may be present.

**Emergent delivery of the fetus** is the only curative measure in the treatment of this condition.

**Antihypertensive treatment** if required.

**N-acetylcysteine** is used in paracetamol-related acute liver failure, but is also increasingly being used in nonparacetamol-related acute liver failure, and is used in many tertiary centers in the management of AFLP and HELLP.

**Support on a critical care unit** is important as significant maternal morbidity and mortality can result from these conditions and intensive monitoring is required before and after delivery. Transfer to a specialist center for liver disease should be considered at an early stage particularly in those women with fulminant liver failure or encephalopathy.

**Liver transplantation** has been used in the treatment of severe AFLP and HELLP syndrome, usually associated with bleeding and hepatic capsular rupture.

☞INTRAHEPATIC CHOLESTASIS OF PREGNANCY:

**Ursodeoxycholic acid (UDCA)** is a hydrophilic bile acid which stimulates bile acid secretion by the hepatocyte and can lead to improvement in both maternal symptoms and liver function tests in ICP, as well as other cholestatic liver diseases. There have been no trials to show whether treatment with UDCA has any effect on fetal outcome.

**Rifampicin** has been shown to reduce the severity of pruritus in a variety of cholestatic liver diseases. A proposed

mechanism is that it enhances bile acid detoxification by increased CYP3A4 expression, and this results in a change in the constituents of the bile acid pool. Elimination of toxic compounds occurs as rifampicin appears to enhance expression of the bile salt export pump. Use alongside UDCA has been reported in cholestatic diseases with good effect on pruritus. In the authors' experience, when used in selected pregnant women with ICP who have worsening symptoms despite UDCA treatment, it appears to provide additional symptomatic benefit. Trials of this are awaited.

**Regular fetal monitoring** (ie, with the use of cardiotocography) has not been shown to predict fetal morbidity and mortality or improve outcome.

**Elective delivery** is advocated in some centers, as the intra-uterine deaths associated with ICP tend to occur late in the third trimester, that is, from 37 weeks' gestation onwards, although there have been case reports of earlier ICP-related deaths. Current national UK guidelines advocate discussion about elective delivery after 37 weeks' gestation, with appropriate counseling on the perinatal and maternal morbidity associated with delivery at this time.

## Molecular Genetics and Molecular Mechanism

Disease associated susceptibility variants are summarised in Table 101-2.

*AFLP and HELLP:* In the early 1990s it was noted that isolated long-chain 3-hydroxyacyl coenzyme A dehydrogenase (LCHAD) deficiency in children may be associated with AFLP, HELLP syndrome, and hyperemesis gravidarum in the mothers during pregnancies with affected fetuses. The commonest mutation in this gene was 1528G>C, which corresponds to an amino acid substitution of E474Q. The cases of AFLP developed in women who were heterozygous for this mutation and carrying a child homozygous for the mutation.

A case-control study published in 2006 analyzed the information about the pregnancies of 50 children with fatty acid oxidation abnormalities and found that maternal liver disease in pregnancy was found in 16% of affected pregnancies, compared to 0.88% of those without affected fetuses (Odds ratio 20.4, CI 7.8-53). Long-chain defects were 50 times more likely than controls to develop maternal liver disease, and short- and medium-chain defects were 12 times more likely to develop maternal liver disease.

*AFLP:*

☞CPT1A: This gene encodes the liver enzyme carnitine palmitoyltransferase 1A. This has a key role in fatty acid oxidation in the mitochondria. Long-chain fatty acids can only enter mitochondria when bound to carnitine, and this enzyme is responsible for the carnitine binding. Mutations in this gene have been associated with CPT1 deficiency, as the activity of the enzyme is either severely reduced or absent.

This mutation has been reported in one family where the mother had AFLP in two consecutive pregnancies. Neither child nor the mother had the common *LCHAD* G1528C mutation, but both children were subsequently shown to have absent activity of CPT1, but mutational analysis was not undertaken. The diagnosis of AFLP was also based on clinical features rather than a liver biopsy, and so it is difficult to say with certainty that the diagnosis here was AFLP rather than HELLP syndrome. This has not been extensively

*Table 101-2 Disease-Associated Susceptibility Variants*

| Candidate Gene (Chromosome Location) | Product Encoded by Gene | Variant | Odds Ratio | Putative Functional Significance | Associated Disease Phenotype |
|---|---|---|---|---|---|
| *HADHA* (2p23.3) | LCHAD | E474Q | | | AFLP, HELLP |
| *CPT1A* (11q13.2) | Carnitine palmitoyltransferase 1A | | | | AFLP |
| *ABCB4* (7q21.1) | MDR3 (multidrug-resistance protein 3) | C711A | 2.27 | Moves phosphatidylcholine into lumen | ICP |
| | | Deletion intron 5 | 14.68 | | |
| *ATP8B1* (18q21-q22) | F1C1 (aminophospholipid translocase) | | | Moves phosphatidylserine into hepatocyte from lumen | ICP |
| *ABCB11* (2q24) | BSEP (bile salt export pump) | E279G | | Exports bile salts into lumen | ICP |
| | | D482G | | | |
| | | V444A | | | |
| *NR1H4* (12q23.1) | FXR (bile acid receptor) | −1g>t | | | ICP |
| | | M1V | | | |
| | | W80R | | | |
| | | M173T | 3.2 | | |
| *ABCC2* (10q24) | MRP2 (multidrug-resistance protein 2) | | | Exports organic anions into bile | ICP |

studied in women with AFLP and so it is too early to draw conclusions about the role of CPT1A and the relevance of dysfunction of this enzyme in women with AFLP.

*ICP:*

☞**ABCB4:** This is the most studied gene in ICP. This gene encodes the multidrug-resistance protein 3, a membrane-associated protein which is a member of the superfamily of ATP-binding cassette transporters. The substrate is phosphatidylcholine which is transported from the inner to outer leaflet of the hepatocyte canalicular membrane by this protein. Once outside the hepatocyte, this phospholipid may bind bile acids and reduce their toxicity.

Homozygous mutations in this gene have been reported in cholestatic disorders including progressive familial intrahepatic cholestasis (PFIC), and in some cases of ICP. One study looked at a subgroup of women with a severe phenotype of ICP, and identified a number of haplotypes that were more common in women with the condition compared to controls. In particular the C711A polymorphism and a deletion of intron 5 were more commonly seen in women with severe ICP (odds ratio 2.27 and 14.68, respectively). Twelve further genetic variants and four splicing mutations of this gene have been identified in cases of ICP.

☞**ATP8B1:** This gene encodes a protein which is thought to be used in aminophospholipid transport across cell membranes. Mutations in this gene have been associated with PFIC and benign recurrent intrahepatic cholestasis (BRIC). Variations in this gene

have been identified in a few cases of ICP. One group studied 16 women with ICP and normal gamma GT, and then studied 182 patients and 120 controls looking for the presence of the variants detected. Two heterozygous transitions that resulted in amino acid substitutions were identified (resulting in D70N and R867C) in the 16 affected women. One variant was present in 3 of 182 cases, and the other was present in 1 of the 182 cases. Neither mutation was present in 120 controls.

☞**ABCB11:** This gene is another member of the ATP-binding cassette transporter family and encodes the bile salt export pump (BSEP) found on the canalicular membrane of hepatocytes. Homozygous mutations have been associated with PFIC and BRIC and have been identified in small numbers of patients with ICP. Two mutations associated with PFIC (*E279G* and *D482G*) have also been identified in a small number of cases of ICP, as have the BSEP variants N591S and V444A polymorphisms.

☞**NR1H4:** This gene encodes a ligand-activated transcription factor, which functions as a receptor for bile acids (known as farnesoid X receptor or FXR). When bound to bile acids this protein regulates the expression of genes involved in bile acid synthesis and transports by binding to DNA response elements in their promoter regions.

A recent study in the United Kingdom and Sweden identified four variants (W80R, −1g>t, M1V, M173T) in FXR in women with ICP. Functional defects in either translational efficiency or activity were demonstrated for the latter three.

☞**ABCC2:** Homozygous mutations in *ABCC2* are responsible for Dubin-Johnson syndrome as the gene encodes MRP2, responsible for exporting organic anions including bilirubin into the bile. A recent South American study reported a single polymorphism of this gene to be associated with ICP.

***Future Directions:*** The identification of associations with a wide range of genetic variants, in differing populations, suggests that these conditions are genetically heterogeneous. Studies of larger populations are therefore required to establish the exact susceptibility that these genetic variants lead to. As more is learnt about the genotypes that predispose to liver disease in pregnancy, and genetic testing becomes more accessible and widespread, more information will be available to appropriately counsel women who are at risk of these potentially life-threatening pregnancy-specific conditions.

## Bibliography:

1. Brites D, Rodrigues CMP, van-Zeller H, Brito A, Silva R. Relevance of serum bile acid profile in the diagnosis of intrahepatic cholestasis of pregnancy in an high incidence area: Portugal. *Eur J Obstet Gynecol Reprod Biol.* 1998;80:31-38.

2. Reyes H, Baez M, Gonzalez MC, et al. Selenium, zinc and copper plasma levels in intrahepatic cholestasis of pregnancy, in normal pregnancies and healthy individuals, in Chile. *J Hepatol.* 2000;32:542-549.

3. Ch'ng CL, Morgan M, Hainsworth I, Kingham JGC. Prospective study of liver dysfunction in pregnancy in Southwest Wales. *Gut.* 2002;51:876-880.

4. Geenes V, Williamson C. Intrahepatic cholestasis of pregnancy. *World J Gastroenterol.* 2009;15:2049-2066.

5. Goulis DG, Walker IA, de Swiet M, Redman CW, Williamson C. Preeclampsia with abnormal liver function tests is associated with cholestasis in a subgroup of cases. *Hypertens Pregnancy.* 2004;23:19-27.

6. Knight M, Nelson-Piercy C, Kurinczuk JJ, Spark P, Brocklehurst P, UK Obstetric Surveillance System (UKOSS). A prospective national study of acute fatty liver of pregnancy in the UK. *Gut.* 2008;57:951-956.

7. Goel A, Ramakrishna B, Zachariah U, et al. How accurate are the Swansea criteria to diagnose acute fatty liver of pregnancy in predicting hepatic microvesicular steatosis? *Gut.* 2011;60:138-139.

8. Marschall H-U, Wagner M, Zollner, et al. Complementary stimulation of hepatobiliary transport and detoxification systems by rifampicin and ursodeoxycholic acid in humans. *Gastroenterology.* 2005;129:476-485.

9. Royal College of Obstetricians and Gynaecologists. Obstetric Cholestasis. Green-top Guideline No. 43. London: RCOG; 2011.

10. Treem WR, Rinaldo P, Hale D, et al. Acute fatty liver of pregnancy and long-chain 3-hydroxyacyl-coenzyme A dehydrogenase deficiency. *Hepatology.* 1994;19:339-345.

11. Browning MF, Levy HL, Wilkins-Haug LE, Larson C, Shih VE. Fetal fatty acid oxidation defects and maternal liver disease in pregnancy. *Obstet Gynecol.* 2006;107:115-120.

12. Innes AM, Seargeant L, Balachandra K, et al. Hepatic carnitine palmitoyltransferase 1 deficiency presenting as maternal illness in pregnancy. *Pediatr Res.* 2000;47:43-45.

13. Wasmuth HE, Glantz A, Keppler H, et al. Intrahepatic cholestasis of pregnancy: the severe form is associated with common variants of the hepatobiliary phospholipid transporter ABCB4 gene. *Gut.* 2007;56:265-270.

14. Mullenbach R, Bennett A, Tetlow N, et al. ATP8B1 mutations in British cases with intrahepatic cholestasis of pregnancy. *Gut.* 2005;54:829-834.

15. Dixon PH, Williamson C. The molecular genetics of intrahepatic cholestasis. *Obstet Med.* 2008;1:65-71.

16. Van Mil SW, Milona A, Dixon PH, et al. Functional variants of the central bile acid sensor FXR identified in intrahepatic cholestasis of pregnancy. *Gastroenterology.* 2007;133:507-516.

17. Sookoian S, Castano G, Burgueno A, Gianotti TF, Pirola CJ. Association of the multidrug-resistance-associated protein gene (*ABCC2*) variants with intrahepatic cholestasis of pregnancy. *J Hepatol.* 2008;48:125-132.

## Supplementary Information

### OMIM References:

[1] Preeclampsia/Eclampsia 1; PEE1 (#189800)

[2] Long-Chain 3-hydroxyacyl-CoA Dehydrogenase Deficiency (#609016)

[3] Cholestasis, Intrahepatic, of Pregnancy; ICP (#147480)

[4] Nuclear Receptor Subfamily 1, Group H, Member 4; NR1H4 (#603826)

***Key Words:*** Obstetric cholestasis, Intrahepatic cholestasis of pregnancy, acute fatty liver of pregnancy, HELLP, hemolysis, elevated liver enzymes, and low platelets

# 102 Pre-eclampsia

Louise Wilkins-Haug

## KEY POINTS

- *Disease summary:*
  - Pre-eclampsia is a multisystem disorder unique to pregnancy and occurs in 4% to 7% of women.
  - This condition is clinically characterized by elevated blood pressure and proteinuria.
  - The manifestations of pre-eclampsia are thought to occur following an interrelated cascade of abnormal placental implantation, hypoxia, release of antiangiogenic factors, placental/fetal/maternal immunologic dysfunction, and dysfunction/destruction of maternal vascular endothelial cells.
  - The constellation of hemolysis, elevated liver enzymes, and low platelets (HELLP syndrome) represents a variant of pre-eclampsia that may present without significant proteinuria.
  - Eclampsia is the progression to grand mal seizures in a woman with pre-eclampsia.

- *Differential diagnosis:*
  - Chronic hypertension, gestational hypertension

- *Monogenic forms:*
  - None identified.

- *Family history:*
  - A mother with pre-eclampsia confers a 20% to 40% risk to her daughter for pre-eclampsia; sisters of pre-eclamptic woman face an 11% to 37% risk of pre-eclampsia. Risks for eclampsia appear to be similar if not slightly higher.

- *Twin studies:*
  - 60% concordance in monozygotic twins.

- *Environmental factors:*
  - Dietary deficiencies of calcium and antioxidant vitamins C and E have been suspected to play a role in pre-eclampsia on an epidemiologic basis. However, numerous trials of repletion have not shown a benefit.

- *Genome-wide associations:*
  - Genome-wide association studies (GWAS) in Iceland, Australia, New Zealand, and Finland have indicated a possible susceptibility locus on chromosome 2 although complete agreement does not exist as to the specific location. Further refinement with transcription-targeted candidate genes initially derived from androgenic (fetus-free) placentas and applied to whole genome screening successfully further refined a pre-eclampsia-linked site to 2q22. Upregulated in decidua from pre-eclamptic women, a candidate gene within this region, activin (*ACVR2*) was given the highest priority as a possible gene for pre-eclampsia. However, other loci have been reported from GWAS of populations including 10q21.3, 2p25.1, 9p21, 2p11.2, and 4q34 reflecting the multifactorial nature of pre-eclampsia and limitations of GWAS applications.

- *Pharmacogenomics:*
  - None applicable.

## Diagnostic Criteria and Clinical Characteristics

### Diagnostic Criteria for Pre-eclampsia:
- Greater than 20 weeks of gestation
- Blood pressure elevation greater than 140 mm Hg systolic or greater than 90 mm Hg diastolic obtained 6 hours apart
- Proteinuria defined as urinary excretion of greater than or equal to 0.3 g protein in a 24-hour collection

### And the absence of
- Previously elevated blood pressure (>140/90) before 20 weeks of gestation

### Diagnostic Criteria for Severe Pre-eclampsia:
- Greater than 20 weeks of gestation
- Blood pressure elevation greater than 160 mm Hg systolic or greater than 100 mm Hg diastolic obtained 6 hours apart
- Oliguria less than 500 cc in 24 hours
- Cerebral or visual disturbances
- Pulmonary edema or cyanosis
- Epigastric or right upper quadrant pain
- Impaired liver function
- Thrombocytopenia
- Fetal growth restriction

### Diagnostic evaluation should include at least one of the following
- Blood pressure obtained 6 hours apart, taken sitting or in left lateral position
- 24-hour collection of urine
- Hematocrit, platelet count
- Liver function analysis for transaminases
- Laboratory assessment of renal function
- Laboratory assessment of coagulopathy
- Assessment of oxygenation

*Clinical Characteristics:* This condition is clinically characterized by elevated blood pressure and proteinuria. While not considered essential for the diagnosis, women often have increased hand, ankle, and facial edema. Progression from mild-to-severe pre-eclampsia represents a continuum of the disease although timing and rate of progression is unpredictable. Some women will present initially with severe pre-eclampsia that is characterized by central nervous system (CNS) changes (headache, blurred vision), liver involvement (right upper quadrant pain, elevated transaminases), renal involvement (marked proteinuria, oliguria), and/or fetal growth restriction. Additional laboratory manifestations can include elevation of the hematocrit reflecting an underlying hemoconcentration, lowered platelet count, and evidence of hemolysis. The constellation of HELLP syndrome represents a variant of pre-eclampsia that may present without significant proteinuria. Progression to seizures is a hallmark of eclampsia with increased deep tendon reflexes and clonus being early signs of CNS irritation. Pre-eclampsia may present initially in the postpartum period in a small number of patients.

Clinically, two broad categories of pre-eclampsia exist—early onset (<34 weeks) and late onset (>34 weeks). Early-onset disease is characterized broadly as a disorder of aberrant placentation with a normal maternal response and late-onset disease is described as a condition of normal placentation in the setting of a maternal system with aberrant endothelial responses. Early-onset pre-eclampsia is notable for a higher rate of familial cases, a higher risk of recurrence in subsequent pregnancies, identification of placental vascular abnormalities, and associated fetal growth restriction. Late-onset pre-eclampsia is more common (80%) and is characterized by maternal risk factors such as diabetes, increased blood pressure (but not hypertension) early in pregnancy, cardiovascular disease, increased body mass index (BMI), and older maternal age.

The maternal vascular changes of pre-eclampsia are characterized by hemoconcentration mediated by intense vasospasm. Women with pre-eclampsia tend to be intravascularly depleted and hemoconcentrated yet with endothelial damage which renders their vascular system throughout their bodies more permeable to capillary leak. This may manifest clinically as peripheral or total body edema, pulmonary edema, and CNS edema. Renal consequences of the vasospasm lead to decreased renal flow, lack of the normal expected increase in glomerular filtration rate with pregnancy, and ultimately a decreased urine output. Uteroplacental blood flow is similarly affected with uteroplacental insufficiency resulting from placental infarct with resultant fetal growth restriction, decreased amniotic fluid, placental abruption, and nonreassuring fetal surveillance.

## Screening and Counseling

*Screening:* Many of the risk factors for developing pre-eclampsia are not modifiable including first pregnancy, multifetal pregnancies, prior pre-eclampsia, maternal age greater than 35 years, and African-American race. However, maternal conditions such as obesity, chronic hypertension, diabetes, vascular and connective tissue disease, and antiphospholipid antibody syndrome may be conditions in which improvement in maternal health prior to entering pregnancy may lower the risk of pre-eclampsia. Smoking is consistently protective for the risk of pre-eclampsia in studies.

No effective and cost-efficient screening for pre-eclampsia has been established. Effective screening for pre-eclampsia among low-risk women has been proposed based on early detection of aberrant production of antiangiogenic factors from the abnormally forming placenta such as plasma-associated protein A (PAPP-A)

and soluble fms-like tyrosine kinase 1 (sFlt-1). While these markers are indeed abnormal prior to the onset of clinical symptoms, their use for widespread screening of low-risk women with an aim to intervention has yet to be established.

*Counseling:* Early-onset pre-eclampsia (before 30 weeks) carries the highest risk of recurrence, with women facing a 40% risk for recurrence in a subsequent pregnancy. Later but still preterm pre-eclampsia (32-36 weeks) is associated with 25% risk of pre-eclampsia in the second pregnancy. HELLP carries as high as a 26% risk of recurrence as well as a risk of other adverse pregnancy outcomes including growth restriction, abruption, and preterm delivery. Interventions to alter the rate of recurrence such as low-dose aspirin, low-dose molecular weight heparin, calcium supplementation, and folate supplementation have been suggested though none has been consistently shown to be effective in large studies likely due to the multifactorial nature of pre-eclampsia.

Women who have experienced a pregnancy with pre-eclampsia face an increased lifelong risk of cardiovascular complications. This risk applies to both morbidity and mortality. Following one pregnancy with pre-eclampsia a woman's risk for subsequent hypertension is fourfold higher and her risks for ischemic heart disease and stroke are twofold higher. These risks may be manifest within 15 years from the pregnancy with pre-eclampsia. If two pregnancies with pre-eclampsia occur, the risks for cardiovascular disease are higher and a threefold risk for type 2 diabetes has been noted. While these risks were modulated to some degree when corrected for BMI, they persisted. Whether the mother's underlying cardiometabolic profile and genetic background when entering the original pregnancy places her at risk for the pre-eclampsia as well as the later cardiovascular events or the pre-eclampsia is an initial and causative event remains a controversial area.

## Management and Treatment

*Management:* A hallmark of pre-eclampsia is that the disease typically resolves with delivery of the infant and placenta. Uncommonly, women will continue to have pre-eclampsia or present with pre-eclampsia for the first time in the postpartum period. In these later situations, other causes of hypertension should be thoroughly investigated.

During pregnancy, the gestational age at onset of pre-eclampsia dictates the management plan. As most pre-eclampsia presents late in pregnancy, then delivery of the pregnancy is considered the treatment for the disorder. Use of magnesium sulfate intravenous (or intramuscular) is usually undertaken for women to decrease the risk of seizures associated with severe pre-eclampsia. While the risk of progressing from severe pre-eclampsia to eclampsia (undergoing a grand mal seizure) remains small (~3%), this can be lowered to less than 1% with magnesium sulfate. The maternal morbidity and mortality following a seizure remains substantial typically associated with maternal cerebrovascular events. Antihypertensive medications are utilized as needed to either lower the maternal blood pressure in the acute setting or on a longer-term basis. Common acute antihypertensive management is accomplished with IV labetalol or hydralazine.

In the situation in which pre-eclampsia presents in the preterm gestation, a decision weighing the maternal and fetal risks ensues. If the pre-eclampsia is mild in nature then prolongation of the pregnancy is possible with close maternal and fetal surveillance. When severe pre-eclampsia exists after 34 weeks, maternal risks typically indicate that delivery should proceed. When severe pre-eclampsia presents, for the pregnancy under 34 weeks' gestation, management should be individualized in concert with providers having experience in high-risk pregnancy management in order to fully evaluate the risks and outcomes for the mother and the infant. Conservative management of women with HELLP has not been evaluated in large-scale studies.

***Pharmacogenetics:*** None applicable.

## Molecular Genetics and Molecular Mechanism

Pre-eclampsia is multifactorial and polygenic and to date neither candidate gene studies based on a functional approach nor GWASs have provided definitive answers. Currently, genetics is thought to account for perhaps 10% to 15% of pre-eclampsia risk although as the various pathways to clinical pre-eclampsia are elucidated, the role of genetics and genetic variation will likely play a larger role.

Approximately 70 candidate genes have been assessed and were reviewed by Ward and Lindheimer (2009). Functional pathways that have been considered of importance in pre-eclampsia have included those of clotting abnormalities (factor V Leiden, prothrombin, MTHFR), hemodynamics (renin, angiotensinogen, AVE, angiotensin receptor), cytokines (IL-6, TNF-alpha), oxidative stress (xanthine and superoxide dismutase), lipid metabolism, (LPL), and angiogenesis (VEGF). Table 102-1 lists the seven most widely studied genes for which more than 100 studies have been completed and fewer than half provided positive significant associations with the candidate gene and pre-eclampsia. Recently enthusiasm has emerged for candidate genes involved in immune regulation, in particular complement activation. Sequencing of the genes for three complement regulatory proteins—membrane cofactor protein, complement factor I, and complement factor H revealed increased rates of heterozygosity among women who had systemic lupus who ultimately developed pre-eclampsia and among women without systemic lupus who also developed pre-eclampsia. If replicated these findings would focus the target of placental damage on excessive complement production with resultant abnormal placental development, release of antiangiogenic factors and downstream endothelial damage that ultimately leads to the maternal symptoms.

Epigenetic alterations also have been implicated in the genetic etiology of pre-eclampsia. Parallels exist between the two most commonly associated loci (10q22 and 2p12) including similar paralogous genes and genes (*LOXL3*, *DOK1*, *HK2*, *TACR1*) known to be imprinted with specific parental patterns of expression. A variant of *STOX1* (storkhead box 1) gene located at 10q22 in particular displays evidence of epigenetic effects with transcription occurring in the early placenta and aberrant levels associated with pre-eclampsia. In particular, the maternally transmitted Y153H variant of *STOX1* has been associated with early-onset pre-eclampsia as characterized by cases with fetal growth restriction, high rates of familiar recurrence, and placental pathology. This would be expected from the known mechanism of this gene which plays a role in conversion of the invasive diploid trophoblast cells to the polyploidy, noninvasive giant cells during the process of fetomaternal vascular connection. Alterations of this process due to variants of this gene could lead to premature halting of placental implantation and the described cascade of hypoxia, antiangiogenesis, and endothelial damage which eventually leads to the maternal symptoms.

***Genetic Testing:*** None clinically available.

***Future Directions:*** Future work refining the subtypes of pre-eclampsia and investigating the unique genetic contributions to the different presentations of pre-eclampsia will be valuable in the efforts to understand the pathophysiology as well as develop predictive tools and interventions.

*Table 102-1* **Candidate Genes for Pre-eclampsia**

| Gene (Polymorphism) | Function | Chromosome | Biologic Association |
| --- | --- | --- | --- |
| *MTHFR* (C677T) | Methylenetetrahydrofolate reductase | 1p36.3 | Vascular diseases |
| *F5* (Leiden) | Factor V Leiden | 1q23 | Thrombophilia—may coexist with other thrombophilic gene |
| *AGT* (M235T) | Angiotensinogen | 1q42-q43 | Blood pressure regulation, linked to essential hypertension |
| HLA (various) | Human leukocyte antigens | 6p21.3 | Immunity |
| *NOS3* (Glu 298 Asp) | Endothelial nitric oxide | 7q36 | Vascular endothelial function |
| *F2* (G20210A) | Prothrombin (factor II) | 11p11-q12 | Coagulation—weekly associated, studied with other thrombophilic genes |
| *ACE* (I/D$^{at}$Intron 16) | Angiotensin-converting enzyme | 17q23 | Blood pressure regulation |

Adapted from Ward and Lindheimer, 2009.

**BIBLIOGRAPHY:**

1. Moses EK, Fitzpatrick E, Freed KA, et al. Objective prioritization of positional candidate genes at a quantitative trait locus for pre-eclampsia on 2q22. *Mol Hum Reprod.* 2006;12(8):505-512.

2. Ward K. Searching for genetic factors underlying pre-eclampsia: recent progress and persistent challenges. *Minerva Ginecol.* 2008; 60(5):399-419.

3. Chappell S, Morgan L. Searching for genetic clues to the causes of pre-eclampsia. *Clin Sci (Lond).* 2006;110(4):443-458.

4. Oudejans CB, van Dijk M, Oosterkamp M, Lachmeijer A, Blankenstein MA. Genetics of preeclampsia: paradigm shifts. *Hum Genet.* 2007;120(5):607-612.

5. Oudejans CB, van Dijk M. Placental gene expression and pre-eclampsia. *Placenta.* 2008;29(suppl A):S78-S82.

6. Nejatizadeh A, Stobdan T, Malhotra N, Pasha MA. The genetic aspects of pre-eclampsia: achievements and limitations. *Biochem Genet.* 2008;46(7-8):451-479.

7. Salmon JE, Heuser C, Triebwasser M, et al. Mutations in complement regulatory proteins predispose to preeclampsia: a genetic analysis of the PROMISSE cohort. *PLoS Med.* 2011;8(3):e1001013.

8. Diagnosis and Management of Preeclampsia, ACOG Practice Bulletin. No 33, Jan 2002.

9. Chelbi ST, Vaiman D. Genetic and epigenetic factors contribute to the onset of preeclampsia. *Mol Cell Endocrinol.* 2008;282(1-2):120-129.

10. Medica I, Kastrin A, Peterlin B. Genetic polymorphisms in vasoactive genes and preeclampsia: a meta-analysis. *Eur J Obstet Gynecol Reprod Biol.* 2007;131(2):115-126.

11. Yinon Y, Kingdom JC, Odutayo A, et al. Vascular dysfunction in women with a history of preeclampsia and intrauterine growth restriction: insights into future vascular risk. *Circulation.* 2010;122(18):1846-1853.

12. Carty DM, Delles C, Dominiczak AF. Preeclampsia and future maternal health. *J Hypertens.* 2010;28(7):1349-1355.

## Supplementary Information

**OMIM REFERENCES:**

| Location | Phenotype | Phenotype MIM Number | Gene/Locus | Gene/Locus MIM Number |
|---|---|---|---|---|
| 2p13 | Pre-eclampsia/eclampsia 1 | 189800 | | |
| 10q21.3-q22.1 | Pre-eclampsia/eclampsia 4 | 609404 | *STOX1* | 609397 |
| 9p13 | Pre-eclampsia/eclampsia 3 | 609403 | | |
| 2p25 | Pre-eclampsia/eclampsia 2 | 609402 | | |

**Alternative Name:**

• Toxemia of Pregnancy

***Key Words:*** Pre-eclampsia, eclampsia, aberrant placentation, HELLP syndrome

# 103  Genetic Basis of Female Infertility

Stephanie Dukhovny and Louise Wilkins-Haug

## KEY POINTS

- *Disease summary:*
  - Infertility is defined as failure to conceive in the setting of regular intercourse within 1 year for women younger than 35 years within 6 months for women older than 35 years. The prevalence of infertility is between 7% and 15%. There are many causes of infertility, with estimates of female factor infertility as an explanation in up to 37% of couples and both male and female factor infertility in 35% of couples. Causes of female infertility include ovulatory disorders, chromosomal abnormalities, endometriosis, pelvic adhesions, tubal blockage and other tubal abnormalities, and hyperprolactinemia. There is growing evidence that genetic abnormalities are present in as many as 10% of infertile females and 15% of infertile males. There is also evidence to suggest that chromosomal abnormalities and single gene mutations contribute to the cause of infertility in a proportion of couples seeking infertility therapy. In 2002 the Italian community of professionals working in reproductive medicine sought to set out guidelines for the appropriate use of genetic testing in infertile couples.

- *Differential diagnosis:*
  - Genetic causes of female infertility include ovulatory disorders such as Kallmann syndrome, fragile X syndrome, as well as karyotype abnormalities, and primary ciliary dyskinesia. Infertility can also be noted as a minor manifestation in many other genetic conditions including galactosemia, mucopolysaccharidosis, Prader-Willi, cystic fibrosis, pseudohypoparathyroidism type 1a, progressive external ophthalmoplegia, autoimmune polyglandular syndrome type I, ovarian leukodystrophy, ataxia telangiectasia, Demirhan syndrome, and blepharophimosis-ptosis-epicanthus inversus syndrome.

- *Monogenic forms:*
  - In addition to the single gene defects noted earlier, additional rare genetic abnormalities have been identified in infertile women. These include mutations in the follicle-stimulating hormone (FSH), luteinizing-hormone (LH), and gonadotropin-releasing hormone (GnRH) receptors, and mutations in the androgen receptor causing androgen insensitivity syndrome.

- *Family history:*
  - A three-generation pedigree for genetic disorders should be obtained from any patient who is undergoing evaluation or treatment for infertility. A family history of males or females with intellectual disability may indicate transmission of fragile X syndrome, and testing for this disorder is indicated.

- *Twin studies:*
  - Twin studies have demonstrated a greater concordance between monozygotic than dizygotic twins in reference to age of menopause. The prevalence of premature ovarian failure is three- to fivefold greater in both monozygotic and dizygotic twins. There are reports in the literature of "ovarian discordancy" in monozygotic twins, and also of sister → sister ovarian tissue transplantation in these cases.

- *Genome-wide associations:*
  - Genome-wide association studies (GWASs) have been used to elucidate the genetic etiology of premature ovarian failure. Candidate genes have been identified; however, the small size of these studies has limited the statistical power of their results. Array comparative genomic hybridization (a-CGH) analysis is also being researched on cohorts of women with premature ovarian failure for analysis of copy number variants (CNVs) over the genome. A number of potential candidate genes including *PTHB1* and *ADAMTS19* have been identified in this fashion, although larger follow-up studies are needed to confirm these findings.

## Diagnostic Criteria and Clinical Characteristics

**Clinical Characteristics:** Infertility is defined as failure to conceive in the setting of regular intercourse within 1 year for women younger than 35 years, within 6 months for women older than 35 years.

*Genetic Causes of Female Infertility:*

☞**OVULATORY DISORDERS:** When infrequent (oligo-ovulation) or absent (anovulation) ovulation is present, the number of available oocytes available for fertilization is decreased. There are genetic causes for oligo-ovulation, anovulation, and premature ovarian failure. Individual syndromes and specific genes have been identified and include

Kallmann syndrome: Kallmann syndrome has a male preponderance and is traditionally characterized by isolated GnRH deficiency and anosmia. Recent research, however, has demonstrated the genetic pathways involved in this disorder and affected females are now being identified. Women with Kallmann syndrome present with amenorrhea and infertility. It is estimated that 1/50,000 women are affected. Kallmann syndrome can occur in both a sporadic and inherited fashion. The disease has been reported to be inherited in X-linked, autosomal dominant, and autosomal recessive manners. There are currently six genes proven to be associated with Kallmann syndrome. Although it is rare, Kallmann syndrome should be considered when evaluated a woman with hypogonadotropic hypogonadism.

Fragile X syndrome: Fragile X syndrome is a result of expansion of a trinucleotide repeat (CGG) in the *FMR1* gene located in Xq27.3. Normal individuals have 6 to 55 repeats. Affected individuals have greater than 200 repeats. Premutation carriers have 55 to 200 repeats. Women who are permutation carriers are at risk for premature ovarian failure, defined as cessation of menses prior to age 40. The risk for premature ovarian failure in women who are permutation carriers is estimated to be approximately 21%. Testing for fragile X syndrome is recommended during the workup for women with oligomenorrhea, premature ovarian failure, in women with a poor response to assisted reproductive technology, as well as in women with a premature decrease in ovarian reserve.

☞**KARYOTYPE ABNORMALITIES:** Chromosomal abnormalities are seen in a higher frequency in women with infertility than in the general population. Chromosomal abnormalities have been estimated most recently to be seen in approximately 1.5% of infertile women. Chromosomal abnormalities can occur in autosomes or in the sex chromosomes. Examples of autosomal abnormalities include translocations and inversions. The most common sex chromosome abnormality associated with female infertility is Turner syndrome in which the karyotype may demonstrate 45,X or mosaicism with the presence of both normal and monosomy X-cell lines, such as 45,X/46,XX, and 45,X/47,XXX. Other sex chromosomal aberrations such as gonadal dysgenesis with a Y-cell line can also be seen in women with complete Turner syndrome and Swyer syndrome (46,XY gonadal dysgenesis) present with primary amenorrhea. Peripheral blood karyotype analysis is recommended during the workup of women with primary ovarian failure, decreased ovarian reserve, and in men and women with recurrent fetal loss. Of note, karyotypically normal women produce oocytes with an abnormal karyotype, and this percentage increases with advanced maternal age as a result of nondisjunction, or an unequal distribution of the chromosomes in the oocyte during oocyte maturation, at the time of ovulation, and/ or fertilization. This in turn increases the risk of aneuploidy in the fetus.

☞**OTHER CONDITIONS:** Primary ciliary dyskinesia, a genetically heterogeneous disorder results in loss of function of the ciliary apparatus, can lead to compromised female fertility in some reports. Infertility can also be noted as a minor manifestation in many other genetic conditions including galactosemia, mucopolysaccharidosis, Prader-Willi, cystic fibrosis, pseudohypoparathyroidism type 1a, progressive external ophthalmoplegia, autoimmune polyglandular syndrome type I, ovarian

leukodystrophy, ataxia telangiectasia, Demirhan syndrome, and blepharophimosis-ptosis-epicanthus inversus syndrome.

## Screening and Counseling

*Screening:* As noted earlier, all women presenting with infertility and significantly decreased ovarian reserve at a young age should have a peripheral blood karyotype, testing for fragile X premutation carrier status. If amenorrhea is present, testing for Kallmann syndrome can be considered.

*Counseling:* Genetic counseling should be offered to all women undergoing assisted reproductive technology. Counseling allows for thorough review of family history, as well as counseling for advanced maternal age and genetic risks associated with ICSI and other embryo manipulation. Patients found to have premature ovarian failure as a result of FMR1 premutation have the risks of having offspring with fragile X syndrome associated with the full *MFR1* mutation, as well as the risk of fragile X-associated tremor or ataxia syndrome (FXTAS) in the permutation carrier herself.

## Management and Treatment

*Management:* The management of an infertile couple diagnosed with a genetic disorder as a cause for female infertility would vary greatly based on the nature of the diagnosis. In the case of premature ovarian failure, diagnosis aids female relatives that may be at a higher risk for infertility and may be interested in family planning prior to ovarian failure occurring. Preimplantation genetic diagnosis (PGD) is available for fragile X syndrome as well as for many other single gene defects. PGD with in vitro fertilization (IVF) should be discussed with couples who are discovered during their infertility workup to both carry recessive genetic mutations, putting them at risk for affected offspring.

*Genetic Testing:* Peripheral blood karyotype analysis and FMR1 gene testing is widely available and highly reliable (>99%). Testing for genes associated with Kallmann syndrome is currently limited to clinically available testing for *KAL1*, *FGFR1*, and *CHD7*. The mutation detection frequency for all three of these genes is greater than 95%. However, these genes are responsible for less than 30% of patients with a clinical diagnosis of Kallmann syndrome. Genetic testing is available for many other syndromic disorders in which infertility is a minor component. It is also important to note that cystic fibrosis carrier screening is recommended by the American College of Obstetrics and Gynecology for all women of reproductive age.

*Future Directions:* As the function of more genes is identified the etiology of what is now considered unexplained infertility may be further elucidated. Additionally, the possibility for single or multiple gene defects is being researched for more common conditions such as polycystic ovarian syndrome and endometriosis. Technology such as a-CGH is currently being used in the setting of preimplantation genetic diagnosis. However, the efficacy of such treatment is unclear; randomized trials of preimplantation genetic screening (PGS) with FISH technology in infertile women undergoing IVF treatment has shown lower delivery rates than IVF without PGS. A randomized controlled trial is needed to evaluate if a-CGH technology for preimplantation genetic screening will improve delivery rates in women undergoing IVF for infertility.

## Bibliography:

1. Foresta C, Ferline A, Gianaroli L, Dallapiccola B. Guidelines for the appropriate use of genetic tests in infertile couples. *Eur J Hum Genet*. 2002;10:303-312.

2. Fechner A, Fong S, McGovern P. A review of Kallmann syndrome; genetics, pathophysiology, and clinical management. *Obstet Gynecol Surv*. 2008;63(3):189-194.

3. Pallais JC. Kallmann Syndrome. http://www.ncbi.nlm.nih.gov/books/NBK1334/. Accessed March 2011.

4. Schwartz CE, Dean J, Howard-Peebles PN, et al. Obstetric and gynecologic complications in fragile X carriers: a multicenter study. *Am J Med Genet*. 1994;51:400-402.

5. Krimov CB, Moragianni VA, Cronister A, et al. Increased frequency of occult fragile X-associated primary ovarian insufficiency in infertile women with evidence of impaired ovarian function. *Hum Reprod*. 2011;26(8):2077-2083.

6. Riccaboni A, Lalatta F, Caliari I, Bonetti S, Sornigliana E, Ragni G. Genetic screening in 2,710 infertile candidate couples for assisted reproductive techniques: results of application of Italian guidelines for the appropriate use of genetic tests. *Fertil Steril*. 2008;89(4):800-808.

7. Angell RR. Aneuploidy in older women: higher rates of aneuploidy in oocytes from older women. *Hum Reprod*. 1994;9(7):1199-1201.

8. Persani L, Rossetti R, Cacciatore C. Genes involved in human premature ovarian failure. *J Mol Endocrinol*. 2010;45:257-279.

9. De Roux N, Young J, Misrahi M, et al. A family with hypogonadotropic hypogonadism and mutations in the gonadotropin-releasing hormone receptor. *N Engl J Med*. 1997;337(22):1597-1602.

10. Layman LC, Cohen DP, Jin M, et al. Mutations in gonadotropin-releasing hormone receptor gene cause hypogonadotropic hypogonadism. *Nat Genet*. 1998;18:14-15.

11. Aittomaki K, Lucena JLD, Pakarinen P, et al. Mutation in the follicle-stimulating hormone receptor gene causes hereditary hypogonadotropic ovarian failure. *Cell*. 1995;82;959-968.

12. Gosden RG, Treloar SA, Martin NG, et al. Prevalence of premature ovarian failure in monozygotic and dizygotic twins. *Hum Reprod*. 2007;22(2):610-615.

13. Silber SJ, DeRosa M, Pineda J, et al. A series of monozygotic twins discordant for ovarian failure: ovary transplantation (cortical versus microvascular) and cryopreservation. *Hum Reprod*. 2008;23(7):1531-1537.

14. Kang H, Lee SK, Kim MH, et al. Parathyroid hormone-responsive B1 gene is associated with premature ovarian failure. *Hum Reprod*. 2008;23:1457-1465.

15. Knauff EA, Frank L, van Es MA, et al. Genome-wide association study in premature ovarian failure patients suggest AMADTS19 as a possible candidate gene. *Hum Reprod*. 2009;24:2372-2378.

16. Lawler AM, Gearhart JD. Genetic counseling for patients who will be undergoing treatment with assisted reproductive technology. *Fertil Steril*. 1998;70(3):412-413.

17. The American College of Obstetrics and Gynecology Committee Opinion Update on Carrier Screening for Cystic Fibrosis. No 486, Apr 2011.

18. Harper JC, Sengupta SB. Preimplantation genetic diagnosis: state of the art 2011. *Hum Genet*. 2012;131(2):175-186.

# 104 Polycystic Ovary Syndrome

Aline Ketefian and Mark Goodarzi

## KEY POINTS

- *Disease summary:*
  - Polycystic ovary syndrome (PCOS) is a highly prevalent and complex genetic disorder affecting reproductive aged women. Its characteristics include clinical and/or biochemical androgen excess, ovulatory dysfunction, and polycystic ovaries (PCOs). Women with PCOS are at increased risk for infertility, obesity, insulin resistance, glucose intolerance, type 2 diabetes mellitus (T2DM), dyslipidemia, and cardiovascular disease.
- *Hereditary basis:*
  - There is an increased prevalence of PCOS among family members. Approximately 20% to 40% of first-degree female relatives of women with PCOS are affected by the condition, compared to a prevalence of 6% to 10% in the general population. A twin-family study showed 71% concordance in monozygotic twins, compared to 38% concordance in dizygotic twins and other sisters. The phenotypic components of PCOS, including hirsutism, hyperandrogenemia, oligomenorrhea, acne, and insulin resistance, are also increased in families of women with PCOS.
- *Differential diagnosis:*
  - It is important to exclude thyroid dysfunction, hyperprolactinemia, nonclassical congenital adrenal hyperplasia, androgen-secreting neoplasms (ovarian and adrenal), Cushing syndrome, use of exogenous androgens, acromegaly, primary hypothalamic amenorrhea, primary ovarian failure, hyperandrogenism/insulin resistance/acanthosis nigricans (HAIRAN) syndrome (often with lipodystrophy), and syndromes characterized by insulin receptor gene mutations.

## Diagnostic Criteria and Clinical Characteristics

**Diagnostic Criteria:** There are currently three different definitions of PCOS.

- In 1990, the National Institutes of Health (NIH)—National Institute of Child Health and Human Development Consensus Conference of PCOS recommended that the major criteria include (in order of importance) hyperandrogenism and/or hyperandrogenemia, oligo-anovulation, and the exclusion of other possible etiologies of these signs and symptoms (see Differential Diagnosis, earlier and Table 104-1).
- In 2003, the Rotterdam consensus expanded the diagnostic criteria, recommending that PCOS be defined by the presence of two out of the following three features (after exclusion of other endocrinopathies): clinical and/or biochemical hyperandrogenism, oligo-anovulation, and PCO on ultrasound. This definition therefore includes all patients meeting the 1990 National Institute of Health (NIH) criteria, but in addition includes (1) ovulatory women with clinical and/or biochemical hyperandrogenism and PCO, and (2) women with PCO and ovulatory dysfunction but without androgen excess.
- In 2006, the Androgen Excess-PCOS Society again emphasized hyperandrogenism, recommending that PCOS be defined principally by clinical and/or biochemical hyperandrogenism, with either oligo-anovulation or PCO, or both, after exclusion of other possible etiologies.

### Clinical Characteristics:

- Menstrual disorders: Women with PCOS often present with menstrual abnormalities, which can include amenorrhea, oligomenorrhea, and menorrhagia. These menstrual abnormalities reflect absent or irregular ovulation.
- Androgen excess: Signs and symptoms of androgen excess are common in women with PCOS. These include hirsutism (present in 60%) (development of coarse facial and body hair in a male-type pattern), acne (present in 15%-25%), androgenic alopecia (present in up to 5%), oily skin, and excessive sweating. Circulating androgen levels (total and free testosterone, and dehydroepiandrosterone sulfate [DHEAS]) are elevated in 50%-75% of these women.
- Obesity: Obesity is common in PCOS, particularly centripetal obesity. However, obesity per se is not intrinsic to PCOS, as up to 40% to 50% of women with PCOS are not obese.
- Metabolic sequelae: Women with PCOS are at increased risk for insulin resistance and its associated conditions, including metabolic syndrome, nonalcoholic fatty liver disease, acanthosis nigricans, and obesity-related disorders such as sleep apnea. Insulin resistance occurs in 50% to 70% of PCOS women, and the degree of insulin resistance is typically beyond that predicted by BMI. Insulin resistance often leads to compensatory hyperinsulinemia and impaired glucose tolerance. These conditions increase the risk of long-term metabolic consequences, including T2DM and cardiovascular disease. Of note, hyperinsulinemia plays a key role in many of the phenotypic features of PCOS.
- Hypertension: Women with PCOS have an increased risk of both hypertension and prehypertension. Hyperandrogenemia and/or the insulin resistance syndrome may contribute to elevated systolic and diastolic blood pressure.
- Dyslipidemia: Abnormalities in the lipid profile occur in approximately 70% of women with PCOS in the United States. The most common abnormalities are hypertriglyceridemia, decreased high-density lipoprotein (HDL), and increased low-density lipoprotein (LDL) cholesterol levels. These changes, combined with the other metabolic abnormalities, promote an inflammatory atherothrombotic state, with impaired endothelial function and vasoreactivity, and increased atherosclerosis. Women with PCOS thus have an increased risk of cardiovascular events and cerebrovascular accidents when compared to women without PCOS.

*Table 104-1* **Genetic Differential Diagnosis**

| Syndrome | Gene Symbol | Associated Findings |
|---|---|---|
| Nonclassical congenital adrenal hyperplasia | CYP21A2 | Androgen excess, ovulatory dysfunction, PCO, elevated 17-hydroxyprogesterone level |
| Type A insulin resistance | INSR | Onset in adolescence, severe hyperinsulinemia and insulin resistance, androgen excess, acanthosis nigricans, PCO, ovulatory dysfunction, normal/near-normal body mass index (BMI) |
| Rabson-Mendenhall syndrome | INSR | Onset congenital, growth retardation, severe hyperinsulinemia and insulin resistance, severe androgen excess, acanthosis nigricans, PCO, ovulatory dysfunction, abnormal dentition |
| Leprechaunism | INSR | Onset congenital, typically fatal in infancy, severe hyperinsulinemia and insulin resistance, severe androgen excess, acanthosis nigricans, PCO |
| True cortisone reductase deficiency | HSD11B1 | Onset in adolescence or early adulthood, androgen excess, ovulatory dysfunction, bilateral adrenal enlargement, very low ratio of urinary tetrahydrocortisol to tetrahydrocortisone (typically <0.1) |
| Apparent cortisone reductase deficiency | H6PD | Onset in adolescence or early adulthood, androgen excess, ovulatory dysfunction, bilateral adrenal enlargement, very low ratio of urinary tetrahydrocortisol to tetrahydrocortisone (typically <0.1) |
| Glucocorticoid resistance | GR | Broad spectrum of clinical disease, from asymptomatic to severe androgen excess; ambiguous genitalia at birth, precocious adrenarche, ovulatory dysfunction, hypertension, hypokalemic alkalosis, chronic fatigue, increased urinary free cortisol |

Gene names: *CYP21A2*, cytochrome P450, family 21, subfamily A, polypeptide 2; *INSR,* insulin receptor; *HSD11B1*, 11-beta-hydroxysteroid dehydrogenase, type 1; *H6PD*, hexose-6-phosphate dehydrogenase; GR, glucocorticoid receptor.

- Polycystic ovaries: Ovarian hyperandrogenism, hyperinsulinemia, and altered intraovarian paracrine signaling are thought to disrupt proper follicular development in polycystic ovaries. This leads to arrested follicular growth and the accumulation of small follicles within the periphery of the ovaries, which appear polycystic in morphology. In women with PCOS, there is an alteration in the normal progression from the recruitment of a group of smaller follicles to the selection of a follicle that becomes dominant and undergoes ovulation.
- Gonadotropin abnormalities: About 70% of women with PCOS have hypersecretion of luteinizing hormone (LH). Elevated LH pulse amplitude and frequency leads to LH levels that are abnormally high in comparison to follicle stimulating hormone (FSH) levels (LH:FSH ratio of two to three). This occurs due to reduced steroid hormone negative feedback from the ovaries because of ovarian androgen excess. Obesity reduces the LH:FSH ratio.
- Infertility: Subfertility in PCOS is primarily caused by oligo-anovulation. In addition, some women with PCOS have impaired oocyte development and increased risk of miscarriage, thought to be secondary to higher degrees of hyperandrogenism and hyperinsulinemia. With the use of ovulation induction agents, women with PCOS have increased risks of ovarian hyperstimulation syndrome and multifetal pregnancy.
- Obstetric morbidity: PCOS in pregnancy increases the risk of pre-eclampsia, pregnancy-induced hypertension, gestational T2DM, and possibly preterm delivery. These complications lead to a greater risk of perinatal mortality and a higher rate of admission to the neonatal intensive care unit.
- Malignancy: Women with PCOS are at increased risk for endometrial cancer, given the high prevalence of risk factors including chronic oligo-anovulation (resulting in unopposed estrogen), obesity, and T2DM. These women may also be at increased risk for ovarian and breast cancer, however, these risks are not well documented.

## Screening and Counseling

*Screening:*

- At this time, there are no established recommendations regarding screening family members of women with PCOS. Evaluation should be initiated in the setting of symptoms that suggest PCOS. Early detection is critical so that treatment can be initiated before the syndrome becomes advanced.
- Evaluation for PCOS begins with a careful history and physical examination. Laboratory evaluation is detailed in Table 104-2.
- Important aspects of the history include the menstrual history, onset and duration of symptoms of androgen excess, medications, and family history of PCOS, T2DM, and cardiovascular disease.
- On physical examination, it is important to note signs of androgen excess (acne, hirsutism and distribution of hair growth, alopecia). A modified Ferriman-Gallwey score can be used to note the location and degree of hirsutism. Virilization (clitoromegaly, voice deepening, increased muscle mass) is not typically associated with PCOS, and suggests very high androgen levels, such as with an androgen-secreting tumor. It is important to note any signs of insulin resistance, such as acanthosis nigricans, hypertension, obesity (BMI >30 kg/m$^2$), and centripetal fat distribution (waist circumference >35 in).

*Table 104-2 Algorithm for Diagnostic Evaluation of Patients With Suspected PCOS*

| Laboratory Test | Role | Notes |
|---|---|---|
| TSH | To evaluate for thyroid disease | If present, reassess for PCOS once treated. |
| Prolactin | To evaluate for hyperprolactinemia | Mild elevations are common in PCOS. If high levels are present, reassess for PCOS once evaluated and treated. |
| 17-hydroxyprogesterone (17OHP) | To evaluate for nonclassical congenital adrenal hyperplasia | A morning level in the follicular phase >2 ng/mL is abnormal and should be followed by an acute adrenal stimulation test using 250 $\mu$g of corticotropin, with measurement of 17OHP before and 60 minutes after administration. |
| Total and free testosterone | To document biochemical hyperandrogenemia, primarily ovarian in origin | Testosterone measurements are not absolutely necessary if the patient already has hirsutism. If total testosterone is >200 ng/dL, consider ovarian androgen-secreting tumor, though this cutoff has poor sensitivity and specificity. |
| DHEAS | To document biochemical hyperandrogenemia of adrenal origin | Most helpful in cases of rapid virilization (suggesting a possible androgen-secreting tumor) as a marker of adrenal androgen production. If DHEAS is >7000 ng/mL, consider a tumor, though this cutoff has poor sensitivity and specificity. |
| Fasting lipid profile | To evaluate for abnormalities in triglycerides, HDL, and LDL levels | Triglycerides >150 mg/dL and HDL <50 mg/dL are abnormal. |
| 2-hour oral glucose tolerance test (OGTT) | To evaluate for glucose intolerance and T2DM and evaluate for HAIRAN syndrome | Fasting glucose 110-125 mg/dL or 2-hour glucose 140-199 mg/dL indicates impaired fasting glucose and impaired glucose tolerance, respectively. Fasting glucose ≥126 mg/dL or 2-hour glucose ≥200 mg/dL indicates DM. |
| Luteal phase (day 22-24) progesterone level | To evaluate for ovulation in patients reporting regular cycles | A level above 3 ng/mL indicates ovulation. |
| Low-dose dexamethasone suppression test or 24-hour urinary free cortisol level | To screen for Cushing syndrome in patients with suggestive clinical signs or symptoms | |
| Gonadotropin levels (LH, FSH) | To determine the cause in patients with amenorrhea | Low levels indicate hypogonadotropic hypogonadism, while elevated levels in the menopausal range indicate primary ovarian failure. |

- Ultrasound examination determines the presence of PCO (either ≥12 follicles measuring 2-9 mm in diameter, or ovarian volume >10 cm³). The presence of one polycystic ovary is sufficient to meet the criteria for PCO.

***Counseling:*** PCOS is a complex disorder comprised of both genetic and environmental components. Women with PCOS should be counseled that approximately 20% to 40% of first-degree relatives are typically affected by the condition, and their daughters would have the same increased risk. The signs and symptoms of PCOS usually arise during or close to the onset of puberty. Premature adrenarche and hyperinsulinemia in adolescence often herald the onset of PCOS. Low birth weight may also be a risk factor for PCOS.

A Dutch twin-family study observed a 71% concordance in monozygotic twins, compared to 38% concordance in dizygotic twins and other nontwin sisters. Body weight differs between the phenotypes in affected sisters. Sisters with irregular cycles and hyperandrogenemia are typically heavier than sisters with regular cycles and hyperandrogenemia, while unaffected sisters have lower body weights.

The phenotypic components of PCOS, including hirsutism, hyperandrogenemia, oligomenorrhea, acne, and insulin resistance, are also increased in families of women with PCOS. First-degree male relatives have elevated DHEAS levels, and increased prevalence of insulin resistance, endothelial dysfunction, and metabolic syndrome.

## Management and Treatment

Treatment of PCOS addresses the signs and symptoms that are prominent in the individual, as well as the reduction of long-term risks. Those who are seeking pregnancy are treated with ovulation induction.

*Menstrual Disorders:* Given the lack of consistent ovulation and production of progesterone from the corpus luteum, estrogen causes proliferation of the endometrial lining, unopposed by the secretory effect of progesterone. Thus, unopposed endometrial growth can, over time, result in endometrial abnormalities including hyperplasia and carcinoma. Weight loss of as little as 5% to 10% of total body weight can restore ovulation and menstrual cycle regularity, and is an important aspect of management. Without ovulatory cycles, it is imperative to protect the endometrium with a hormonal regimen containing a progestin. Several options exist, including combination estrogen-progestin oral contraceptives (OCs), progestins alone (given either continuously or cyclically), and the progestin-containing intrauterine device. The benefits of combination OCs go beyond endometrial protection alone and include reduction of free testosterone levels via increased circulating levels of sex hormone-binding globulin (SHBG) and suppression of ovarian androgen secretion.

*Hirsutism:* Combination OCs suppress circulating androgen levels and are therefore helpful in the treatment of hirsutism. Studies have found an additive benefit when combination OCs are used in conjunction with other treatments, typically an agent that blocks androgens peripherally, including spironolactone, finasteride, flutamide, or cyproterone acetate. These agents (particularly finasteride) are teratogenic and contraception (typically in the form of an OC) must be used if they are to be utilized. Of note, if an OC that contains drospirenone (a weak antimineralocorticoid) is combined with spironolactone, potassium levels can rise. For facial hirsutism, topical eflornithine (an inhibitor of the enzyme ornithine decarboxylase) has been shown to improve symptoms in 30% of women after 2 months of use. Medical treatment is often combined with mechanical hair removal, such as shaving, plucking, waxing, chemical depilation, and more longer-lasting treatments including electrolysis and laser therapy.

*Other Symptoms of Androgen Excess:* Acne is typically treated with OCs and topical or oral antibiotics. Androgenic alopecia can be treated with combination OCs in conjunction with antiandrogens or topical medications that stimulate hair growth, such as minoxidil.

*Prevention of T2DM and Cardiovascular Disease:* Lifestyle modifications including diet and exercise regimens are a cornerstone for decreasing the long-term risk of T2DM and cardiovascular complications. In the setting of impaired glucose tolerance, diet and exercise have been shown to reduce diabetes risk as much as or better than the use of medications. Weight loss may also improve the metabolic complications already present in PCOS. Caloric restriction, rather than a particular type of dietary regimen, is the most important factor in weight loss in women with PCOS. Although currently there are insufficient data to recommend insulin-sensitizing agents such as metformin to prevent T2DM in all women with PCOS, those with glucose intolerance or metabolic syndrome may benefit from metformin to improve insulin sensitivity and glucose tolerance. For those women who have lipid abnormalities that persist after lifestyle modifications have been implemented, a statin medication should be initiated in women whose overall risk factor profile indicates a high long-term risk of cardiovascular events. Insulin sensitizers may also have benefit in this regard.

*Infertility:* Before medical treatment for infertility is attempted, preconception counseling should stress the importance of lifestyle modifications, including weight loss in overweight or obese women. Modest weight loss (5%-10% of body weight) may lead to the resumption of ovulatory cycles. In addition, weight reduction decreases the risks of the obstetrical complications of obesity. When ovulation induction is necessary, clomiphene citrate is typically the first-line agent. Metformin has not been shown to be superior to clomiphene for achieving ovulation, pregnancy, or live birth rates. Metformin takes longer than clomiphene to induce ovulatory cycles but has lower rates of multiple pregnancy. In clomiphene-resistant women, addition of metformin might increase efficacy. Aromatase inhibitors such as letrozole appear to have similar efficacy as clomiphene in small trials, but have not been extensively studied for ovulation induction. Gonadotropins are second-line agents if clomiphene either alone or in combination with metformin has failed to induce ovulation. Gonadotropins have higher rates of multiple pregnancy and ovarian hyperstimulation syndrome, but the risks of these complications can be reduced by using lower doses. Laparoscopic ovarian drilling is another second-line intervention; ovulation and pregnancy rates are similar to gonadotropins, but long-term effects on ovarian function are unknown. In vitro fertilization is the last line of intervention if other methods have failed.

## Molecular Genetics and Molecular Mechanism

Although more than 100 candidate genes have been examined, only the following genes have been found to be associated with PCOS or its component traits in multiple cohorts:

- Substantial evidence of an association of a single gene with PCOS is for allele 8 of the dinucleotide repeat microsatellite marker D19S884, which lies within intron 55 of the fibrillin-3 gene (*FBN3*), locus 19p13.2. The function of this marker is unknown. *FBN3* is a member of the fibrillin family of extracellular matrix proteins. Allele 8 of D19S884 is also associated with higher levels of fasting insulin and homeostasis model assessment of insulin resistance (HOMA-IR) in women with PCOS, and higher levels of fasting proinsulin and proinsulin to insulin ratio in brothers of women with PCOS.

- A single-nucleotide polymorphism (SNP), rs12473543, in the pro-opiomelanocortin gene (*POMC*) at locus 2p23.3 is associated with PCOS. This is an intronic SNP, and the functional significance in PCOS is unknown. POMC encodes a polypeptide hormone that is alternatively cleaved to form up to 10 different peptide hormones in a tissue-specific manner, including hormones that are involved in different processes including steroidogenesis, energy metabolism, obesity, and lipolysis.

- SNPs rs1015240 and rs6494730 in the fem-1 homolog b gene (*FEM1B*) are protective against PCOS. This gene is located at locus 15q22, and is the human homolog of one of the nematode Caenorhabditis elegans feminizing (fem) genes. Its function in humans is unknown, but it is predicted to encode for ankyrin repeat proteins.

- SNP rs1640262 in the small glutamine-rich tetratricopeptide repeat-containing protein alpha (SGTA) gene at locus 19p13 is also protective against PCOS. SGTA encodes a member of the androgen receptor chaperone–cochaperone complex that may play a role in androgen signaling as a cochaperone.

- SNPs rs14224941 and rs3768688 in the activin A receptor type IIA gene (*ACVR2A*) are nominally associated with PCOS. *ACVR2A* is located at locus 2q22.3 and encodes a receptor that is required for binding activin and for expression of the type I activin receptors.

- SNP rs898611 in the 17-beta-hydroxysteroid dehydrogenase type 6 gene (*HSD17B6*), located at locus 12q13.3, is associated with increased BMI, increased HOMA-IR, increased fasting insulin, and decreased fasting glucose to insulin ratio. In addition, haplotypes in *HSD17B6* are associated with BMI and insulin. HSD17B6 is an enzyme that has both epimerase and oxidative activities and converts 3-alpha-androstanediol to dihydrotestosterone and androsterone to epiandrosterone.

- Five SNPs in the fat mass- and obesity-associated gene (*FTO*) and two SNPs in the melanocortin 4 receptor gene (*MC4R*) are associated with BMI in PCOS families (FTO SNPs rs1421085, rs17817449, rs8050136, rs9939609, and rs9930506; MC4R SNPs rs17782313 and rs12970134). *FTO* is located at locus 16q12.2 and may play a role in nucleic acid methylation. *MC4R* is located at locus 18q22 and encodes a member of the melanocortin receptor family that interacts with adrenocorticotropic- and melanocyte-stimulating hormones.

- A genome-wide association study (GWAS) of PCOS in Han Chinese women identified associations between PCOS and three loci: 2p16.3, 2p21, and 9q33.3. At 2p16.3, SNP rs13405728 is in linkage disequilibrium with the general transcription factor IIA, 1-like gene (*GTF2A1L*), and the LH/choriogonadotropin receptor gene (*LHCGR*). *GTF2A1L* encodes a germ cell-specific protein involved in the binding of TATA-binding protein to DNA. *LHCGR* encodes the receptor for LH and human chorionic gonadotropin. At 2p21, the SNPs associated with PCOS are rs13429458 and rs12478601, both located in the thyroid adenoma-associated gene (*THADA*). *THADA* was initially identified in thyroid adenomas, and a variant is associated with T2DM. At 9q33.3, SNPs rs10818854 and rs2479106 are associated with PCOS. Both are located in the DENN/MADD domain-containing protein 1A gene (*DENND1A*), which encodes a protein that regulates endoplasmic reticulum aminopeptidase 1 and plays a role in clathrin-mediated endocytosis.

*Genetic Testing:* At this time, genetic testing for PCOS is not widely available or recommended.

### BIBLIOGRAPHY:

1. Goodarzi MO, Dumesic DA, Chazenbalk G, Azziz R. Polycystic ovary syndrome: etiology, pathogenesis and diagnosis. *Nat Rev Endocrinol*. 2010;7:219-231.

2. Vink JM, Sadrzadeh S, Lambalk CB, Boomsma DI. Heritability of polycystic ovary syndrome in a Dutch twin-family study. *J Clin Endocrinol Metab*. 2006;91:2100-2104.

3. Azziz R, Woods KS, Reyna R, Key TJ, Knochenhauer ES, Yildiz BO. The prevalence and features of the polycystic ovary syndrome in an unselected population. *J Clin Endocrinol Metab*. 2004;89:2745-2749.

4. Revised 2003 consensus on diagnostic criteria and long-term health risks related to polycystic ovary syndrome. Rotterdam ESHRE/ASRM-Sponsored PCOS Consensus Workshop Group. *Fertil Steril*. 2004;81:19-25.

5. Azziz R, Carmina E, Dewailly D, et al. Positions statement: criteria for defining polycystic ovary syndrome as a predominantly hyperandrogenic syndrome: an Androgen Excess Society guideline. *J Clin Endocrinol Metab*. 2006;91:4237-4245.

6. Moran LJ, Noakes M, Clifton PM, Tomlinson L, Galletly C, Norman RJ. Dietary composition in restoring reproductive and metabolic physiology in overweight women with polycystic ovary syndrome. *J Clin Endocrinol Metab*. 2003;88:812-819.

7. Legro RS, Barnhart HX, Schlaff WD, et al. Clomiphene, metformin, or both for infertility in the polycystic ovary syndrome. Cooperative Multicenter Reproductive Medicine Network. *N Engl J Med*. 2007;356:551-566.

8. Urbanek M, Woodroffe A, Ewens KG, et al. Candidate gene region for polycystic ovary syndrome on chromosome 19p13.2. *J Clin Endocrinol Metab*. 2005;90:6623-6629.

9. Jones MR, Mathur R, Cui J, Guo X, Azziz R, Goodarzi MO. Independent confirmation of association between metabolic phenotypes of polycystic ovary syndrome and variation in the type 6 17β-hydroxysteroid dehydrogenase gene. *J Clin Endocrinol Metab*. 2009;94:5034-5038.

10. Ewens KG, Jones MR, Ankener W, et al. FTO and MC4R gene variants are associated with obesity in polycystic ovary syndrome. *PLoS One*. 2011;6:e16390.

11. Chen ZJ, Zhao H, He L, et al. Genome-wide association study identifies susceptibility loci for polycystic ovary syndrome on chromosome 2p16.3, 2p21, and 9q33.3. *Nat Genet*. 2011;43:55-59.

## Supplementary Information

### OMIM REFERENCES:

[1] Polycystic Ovary Syndrome 1; PCOS1 (%184700)

[2] Fibrillin 3; FBN3 (*608529)

[3] Pro-opiomelanocortin; POMC (*176830)

[4] Caenorhabditis Elegans, Homolog of, B; FEM1B, FEM1 (*613539)

[5] Small Glutamine-Rich Tetratricopeptide Repeat-Containing Protein, Alpha; SGTA (*603419)

[6] Activin A Receptor, Type IIA; ACVR2A (*102581)

[7] 17-Beta-Hydroxysteroid Dehydrogenase VI; HSD17B6 (*606623)

[8] Fat Mass- and Obesity-Associated Gene; FTO (*610966)

[9] Melanocortin 4 Receptor; MC4R (*155541)

[10] General Transcription Factor IIA, 1-like; GTF2A1L (*605358)

[11] Luteinizing Hormone/Choriogonadotropin Receptor; LHCGR (+152790)

[12] Thyroid Adenoma-Associated Gene; THADA (*611800)

[13] DENN/MADD Domain-Containing Protein 1A; DENND1A (*613633)

### Alternative Names:

- Stein-Leventhal Syndrome
- Polycystic Ovarian Syndrome
- Polycystic Ovarian Disease

*Key Words:* Androgen excess, hirsutism, polycystic ovaries, ovulatory dysfunction, oligo-anovulation, insulin resistance

# 105 Uterine Leiomyomata

Stacey L. Eggert and Cynthia C. Morton

## KEY POINTS

- *Disease summary:*
  - Uterine leiomyomata (UL) are benign tumors of the uterine myometrium.
  - UL are classified by tumor location within the uterus: subserosal, intramural, and submucosal.
  - The prevalence of UL is estimated around 75% for women of reproductive age.
  - Approximately 25% of women of reproductive age have symptoms related to UL. These symptoms include menorrhagia, pelvic pressure, infertility, and a range of complications during pregnancy.
  - UL are hormonally dependent tumors and are not observed prior to puberty. Estrogen, progesterone, and other small growth factors promote tumor growth. UL may regress at menopause.
  - Rarely, estimated at 0.1%, UL may progress to their malignant counterpart, uterine leiomyosarcoma (LMS).
- *Differential diagnosis:*
  - Adenomyosis, solid adnexal mass, focal myometrial contraction, and LMS
- *Monogenic forms:*
  - Hereditary leiomyomatosis and renal cell cancer (HLRCC) is a disorder that predisposes the carrier to renal cell cancer and UL. HLRCC is caused by mutations in the *FH* gene encoding fumarate hydratase, an enzyme involved in the citric acid cycle.
- *Family history:*
  - There is evidence of genetic liability for UL. First-degree relatives of an affected individual are 2.2 times more likely to also have UL.
- *Twin studies:*
  - Monozygotic (MZ) twins have about twice the rate of hospitalization due to UL when compared to dizygotic (DZ) twins, and the correlation for hysterectomy in MZ twins is about twice that observed in DZ twins.
- *Environmental factors:*
  - Early-life exposure to diethylstilbestrol (DES), a synthetic estrogen, has been associated with the development of UL. Other conditions that affect estrogen levels in the body, including parity and obesity, are also linked to UL growth.
- *Genome-wide associations:*
  - A genome-wide linkage analysis for nonsyndromic UL has identified multiple linkage peaks with significant LOD scores. Fine mapping in two replication populations detected several markers in 17q25.3 associated with UL diagnosis. The associated markers are in linkage disequilibrium with each other including the genes *FASN*, *CCDC57* and *SLC16A3*. Functional studies are required to elucidate the possible role of these genomic regions in UL predisposition.
- *Pharmacogenomics:*
  - Pharmacogenomics do not yet play a role in UL management.

## Diagnostic Criteria and Clinical Characteristics

### Diagnostic Criteria for UL:

**Diagnostic evaluation should include**

- UL may be detected during a routine pelvic examination as a pelvic mass or enlarged uterus.
- Imaging studies, such as ultrasonography, magnetic resonance imaging (MRI), and computed tomography (CT) may be indicated to confirm the diagnosis.
- Family medical history is warranted to distinguish between nonsyndromic UL and HLRCC.

**Clinical Characteristics:** The most common symptoms of UL are abnormal uterine bleeding and pelvic pressure. Many women with UL present with varying degrees of menorrhagia, or heavy menstrual bleeding. If the tumors are exerting pressure on nearby organs, such as the bowel or bladder, women may also have problems with bowel movements and urinary frequency.

Reproductive issues include recurrent miscarriage and infertility. Complications during pregnancy include premature labor, pain, bleeding, fetal malpresentation, and an increased risk of a cesarean section.

## Screening and Counseling

**Screening:** As of now, there is no screening method for nonsyndromic UL beyond routine pelvic examinations.

Molecular genetic testing is available for families with HLRCC. Family members may be screened for mutations in *FH* that are known to cause HLRCC.

**Counseling:** Relatives of women with UL are more likely to also have UL. However, because UL is so prevalent in the general population, counseling with risk assessment is limited.

There are more than 150 families with HLRCC and mutations in *FH*. These mutations are inherited in an autosomal dominant manner and children who have one parent with HLRCC have a 50% chance of inheriting the mutation.

## Management and Treatment

***Gonadotropin-Releasing Hormone Agonists:*** Gonadotropin-releasing hormone agonists (GnRHa), such as Lupron, Synarel, and Zoladex, induce a low-estrogen environment in the body which decreases UL size. The reduction in size is contingent on continuous exposure to the agonists, and tumors regrow rapidly when therapy has ceased. Long-term use of GnRHa has adverse side effects, specifically for bone density. GnRHa therapy is only used to decrease tumor size temporarily. It is typically administered several months prior to surgery to improve anemia thought to be secondary to menorrhagia, and to allow for a more minimally invasive procedure.

***MRI-Guided Focused Ultrasound Therapy:*** Focused ultrasound therapy (FUS) uses high-frequency, high-energy sound waves to denature proteins in UL cells, thereby causing cell death and tumor destruction. An MRI scanner is used to locate and target UL in the uterus. FUS is a low-risk and noninvasive procedure, however, it is not widely available and its effect on future fertility is unknown.

***Uterine Artery Embolization:*** Uterine artery embolization (UAE) involves guiding a catheter from a small incision in the groin, through a leg artery, to the arteries in the uterus. Embolic agents are delivered through the catheter to block blood supply to the tumors, which results in UL volume reduction. UAE does not eliminate tumors but instead relieves symptoms by reducing their size. It is minimally invasive with a short recovery time but is not recommended presently for women who plan to become pregnant.

***Myomectomy:*** A myomectomy is a surgical procedure in which individual UL are excised and removed from the uterus. While some submucous UL can be removed through the vagina with a hysteroscope, most UL are removed through the abdomen with either an abdominal myomectomy or a laparoscopic myomectomy. The laparoscopic approach is quickly replacing the traditional abdominal incision because it is less invasive and associated with a quicker recovery time. Myomectomies are the only treatment for UL that is recommended for women who want to become pregnant, however, approximately half of all myomectomy patients will experience tumor recurrence and 10% require additional surgery.

***Hysterectomy:*** Hysterectomy is the only essentially curative treatment for UL. It involves the surgical removal of the entire uterus. Hysterectomies are the most common treatment for UL and UL are the most common indication for hysterectomies in the United States. Hysterectomies can be performed with a minimally invasive approach, such as vaginally or laparoscopically. As the definitive treatment for UL, hysterectomy leaves the patient unable to bear children.

## Molecular Genetics and Molecular Mechanism

Cytogenetic studies support a genetic component to UL development. Approximately 40% of UL tumors have nonrandom cytogenetic abnormalities and several subgroups are recognized, including t(12;14)(q14-15;q23-24), del(7)(q22q32), trisomy 12, rearrangements involving 6p21 and 10q22, and deletions of 1p and 3q. Positional cloning and fluorescence in situ hybridization (FISH) experiments of two of the subgroups revealed the involvement of high mobility group protein genes (HMG) in UL:

*HMGA2* at 12q15 in the t(12;14) subgroup and *HMGA1* at 6p21 in tumors with rearrangements in 6p. These genes encode proteins that are DNA architectural factors which can influence transcription by changing chromatin conformation. Increased expression of *HMGA1* and *HMGA2* is found in tumors with 6p21 rearrangements and t(12;14), respectively. Trisomy 12 is also a major cytogenetic subgroup in UL and these results taken together suggest that increased expression of HMGA proteins is a key molecular event in UL pathobiology. Further, variants in the 5' UTR of *HMGA2* have been associated with UL diagnosis in a cohort of white sister pairs. Cytogenetic abnormalities have been correlated with tumor size, location, and pathology, which indicate that these events play a fundamental role in tumor development. It is expected that many more genes associated with UL will be discovered by studying the cytogenetic abnormalities found in these tumors.

Several factors have been found to predispose women to develop UL. Age, obesity, parity, and race have all been associated with UL biology. Black women are disproportionately affected by UL, with prevalence rates three to four times higher than white women even after controlling other known risk factors. Affected black women have more numerous and larger UL in comparison to affected white women. The average age of diagnosis of black women is younger than that in white women and black women are more likely to report severe UL symptoms. Further, analyses of twin studies and familial aggregation indicate a genetic component to UL predisposition. These findings support a genetic component to the disease that is heritable and conveys a predisposition to develop UL. Finding pathogenetic sequences that predispose women to UL will provide insight into the development of the tumors and could lead to a screening strategy or improved therapy.

***Genetic Testing:*** There is no role, yet, for genetic testing for nonsyndromic UL. Genetic testing of the *FH* gene is performed for families with HLRCC.

***Future Directions:*** Additional linkage and genome-wide association studies (GWAS) will undoubtedly provide valuable information regarding genes involved in UL predisposition. Functional studies will uncover the potential role of *HMGA2* and the genomic region in 17q25.3 in UL development. When disease-associated alleles have been discovered, genotype-phenotype correlations can be made and UL cases may be stratified by genotype. UL predisposition alleles may also lead to new screening strategies and tumor therapy.

**BIBLIOGRAPHY:**

1. Advincula AP, Xu X, Goudeau S IV, Ransom SB. Robot-assisted laparoscopic myomectomy versus abdominal myomectomy: a comparison of short term surgical outcomes and immediate costs. *J Minim Invasive Gynecol.* 2007;14:698-705.

2. Goodwin SC, Spies JB, Worthington-Kirsch R, et al. Uterine artery embolization for treatment of leiomyomata: long term outcomes from the FIBROID registry. *Obstet Gynecol.* 2008;111(1):22-33.

3. Hodge JC, Morton CC. Genetic heterogeneity among uterine leiomyomata: insights into malignant progression. *Hum Mol Genet.* 2007;16:R7-R13.

4. Huyck KL, Panhuysen CI, Cuenco KT, et al. The impact of race as a risk factor for symptom severity and age at diagnosis of uterine leiomyomata among affected sisters. *Am J Obstet Gynecol.* 2008;198:168 e161-e169.

5. Jin C, Hu Y, Chen XC, et al. Laparoscopic versus open myomectomy—a meta-analysis of randomized controlled trials. *Eur J Obstet Gynecol Reprod Biol.* 2009;145:14-21.

6. Kjerulff KH, Langenberg P, Seidman JD, et al. Uterine leiomyomas. Racial differences in severity, symptoms and age at diagnosis. *J Reprod Med*. 1996;41:483-490.

7. Lobel MK, Somasundaram P, Morton CC. The genetic heterogeneity of uterine leiomyomata. *Obstet Gynecol Clin N Am*. 2006;33:13-39.

8. Pritts EA, Parker WH, Olive DL. Fibroids and infertility: an updated systematic review of the evidence. *Fertil Steril*. 2009;91(4):1215-1223.

9. Stewart EA, Gostout B, Rabinovici J, et al. Sustained relief of leiomyoma symptoms by using focused ultrasound surgery. *Obstet Gynecol*. 2007;110:279-287.

10. Eggert SL, Huyck KL, Somasundaram P, et al. Genome-wide linkage and association analyses implicate *FASN* in predisposition to uterine leiomyomata. *Am J Hum Genet*. 2012;91:621-628.

## Supplementary Information

**OMIM REFERENCES:**

[1] Uterine Leiomyoma (#150699)

[2] Hereditary Leiomyomatosis and Renal Cell Cancer (#605839)

**Alternative Names:**

- Fibroids
- Fibromyomas
- Fibromas
- Myofibromas
- Myomas

*Key Words:* HLRCC, uterine fibroids, leiomyomata, FH, HMGA

# 106 **Psoriasis and Psoriatic Arthritis**

Darren D. O'Rielly and Proton Rahman

## KEY POINTS

- *Disease summary: Psoriasis and psoriatic arthritis (PsA) are complex genetic disorders involving multiple genes and epigenetic factors that contribute to disease manifestation and progression.*
  - Typical psoriasis lesions are well demarcated, scaly erythematous plaques that occur in various sizes and shapes. Psoriasis most often manifests on the extensor surfaces of the elbows and knees, as well as the scalp and sacral lesions.
  - PsA is an inflammatory arthritis associated with psoriasis. Approximately 30% of patients with psoriasis will at some point develop psoriatic arthritis. The psoriasis precedes the onset of arthritis in approximately 70% of patients, occurs concurrently in 15% of patients, and follows the onset of psoriasis in the remaining 15% of patients.
  - The diagnosis of PsA is dependent on clinical, laboratory, and radiologic assessments. The recently published classification criteria, ClASsification criteria for Psoriatic ARthritis (CASPAR) is now widely accepted for classifying this entity.
- *Differential diagnosis:*
  - The differential diagnosis of psoriasis includes atopic dermatitis, contact dermatitis, pityriasis rosea, pityriasis alba, seborrheic dermatitis, nummular eczema, and lichen planus. The differential diagnosis for PsA includes rheumatoid arthritis, ankylosing spondylitis, Reiter syndrome, inflammatory bowel disease (IBD) arthropathy, and systemic lupus erythematous.
- *Monogenic forms:*
  - There are no monogenic forms for psoriasis and PsA. The genes associated with psoriasis and PsA appear to be multiple with each displaying modest effect size.
- *Family history:*
  - An affected first-degree relative confers a relative risk between 4 and 10 for psoriasis. PsA displays stronger heritability than psoriasis, as an affected first-degree relative confers a relative risk between 30 and 47.
- *Twin studies:*
  - Twin studies in psoriasis demonstrate that there is a threefold increase in concordance in monozygotic versus dizygotic twins. The one twin study in PsA did not reveal significant heritability.
- *Environmental factors:*
  - Trauma, streptococcal infection or HIV infection may precipitate or worsen psoriasis and PsA.
- *Genome-wide associations:* Numerous genes are associated with the pathogenesis of both psoriasis and PsA (Tables 106-1 and 106-2; Figs. 106-1 and 106-2).
- *Pharmacogenomics:*
  - Polymorphisms exist that affect the pharmacokinetic and pharmacodynamic profiles of many drugs used in the treatment of psoriasis and PsA (Table 106-3). Pharmacogenetic data specific to psoriasis and PsA are lacking.

## Diagnostic Criteria and Clinical Characteristics

**Clinical Characteristics:** Psoriasis is an inflammatory hyperproliferative skin disorder that affects approximately 2% of the North American population. The peak age of onset of psoriasis is between the second and third decade, although it can occur at any age. The most common variant of this skin condition is psoriasis vulgaris, which encompasses approximately 85% to 90% of patients with psoriasis. The typical psoriasis lesions are well demarcated, scaly erythematous plaques that occur in various sizes and shapes. Psoriasis most often manifests on the extensor surfaces of the elbows and knees, as well as the scalp and sacral lesions.

PsA is an inflammatory arthritis associated with psoriasis. In fact, approximately 30% of patients with psoriasis will at some point develop psoriatic arthritis. The presenting features for PsA include pain and stiffness in the peripheral joints, spine or entheseal insertions, which is accentuated with rest and alleviated with moderate activity. Moll and Wright have described five patterns of PsA based on their own clinical observations. The five clinical patterns include "classic PsA" confined to distal interphalangeal (DIP) joints of the hands and feet, symmetric polyarthritis indistinguishable from rheumatoid arthritis (RA), asymmetric oligoarthritis, arthritis mutilans, and spondyloarthropathy. Subsequent reports validated these subgroups; however, there is considerable overlap and evolution between them. The psoriasis precedes the onset of arthritis in approximately 70% of patients, occurs concurrently in

*Table 106-1  Genome-Wide Susceptibility Loci Associated With Psoriasis*

| Gene/Locus | Chromosome Location | Variant | Function |
|---|---|---|---|
| HLA-C | 6p21.3 | rs12191877<br>rs10484554<br>rs2395029 | Antigen presentation |
| IL-12B | 5q33.3 | rs3212227<br>rs6887695<br>rs2082412<br>rs3213094 | Stimulates growth and differentiation of Th1 or Th2 cells; stimulates the production of IFN-$\gamma$ and TNF-$\alpha$ from T and NK cells |
| IL-23R | 1p31.3 | rs7530511<br>rs11209026<br>rs11465804<br>rs12131065<br>rs2201841 | Receptor for the proinflammatory cytokine, IL-23, which stimulates IFN-$\gamma$ production, proliferation of memory Th1 cells, and has a role in the novel Th17 pathway |
| IL-23A/STAT2 | 12q13.2 | rs2066808 | Stimulates IFN-$\gamma$ production, proliferation of memory Th1 cells, and has a role in the novel Th17 pathway |
| TNFAIP3 | 6q23.3 | rs610604 | Regulates TNF-$\alpha$-induced NF$\kappa$B activation reducing inflammation |
| TNIP1 | 5q32-33.1 | rs17728338 | Regulates TNF-$\alpha$-induced NF$\kappa$B activation reducing inflammation |
| IL-13/IL-4 | 5q31 | rs20541<br>rs848 | Involved in B-cell differentiation and Th2 differentiation and function |
| LCE gene cluster | 1q21 | rs6701216<br>rs4085613 | Involved in epidermal differentiation |

PsV, psoriasis vulgaris; HLA, human leukocyte antigen; IL, interleukin; STAT, signal transducers and activator of transcription; TNFAIP3, TNF-$\alpha$-induced protein 3; TNIP1, TNFAIP3 interacting protein 1; LCE, late cornified envelope.

*Table 106-2  Susceptibility Loci Associated With Psoriatic Arthritis*

| Gene/Locus | Chromosome Location | Variant | Function |
|---|---|---|---|
| HLA-C | 6p21.3 | rs10484554<br>rs2395029 | Antigen presentation |
| TNF-$\alpha$ | 6p21.3 | −238G>A in promoter region | A cytokine involved in inflammation, immune response regulation, and apoptosis |
| MICA | 6p21.3 | MICA*002 | Functions as a stress-induced antigen recognized by NK cells, NKT cells, and most of the subtypes of T cells |
| IL-12B | 5q33.3 | rs6887695<br>rs3212227 | Stimulates growth and differentiation of Th1 or Th2 cells; stimulates the production of IFN-$\gamma$ and TNF-$\alpha$ from T and NK cells |
| IL-23R | 1p31.3 | rs11209026 | Receptor for the proinflammatory cytokine, IL-23, which stimulates IFN-$\gamma$ production, proliferation of memory Th1 cells, and has a role in the novel Th17 pathway |
| IL-1 gene cluster | 2q13 | rs3811047 | A potent proinflammatory cytokine, involved in immune responses and inflammatory processes |
| KIR2DS1/KIR2DS2 (+ HLA-Cw*0602) | 19q13.4 | CNV | Located on NK cells and recognizes antigen-presenting molecules; produce large quantities of cytokines (IL-1, TNF-$\alpha$) |

PsA, psoriatic arthritis; HLA, human leukocyte antigen; TNF-$\alpha$, tumor necrosis factor $\alpha$; MICA, major histocompatibility complex class I-related gene A; IL, interleukin; CNV, copy number variant; KIR, killer inhibitory receptor.

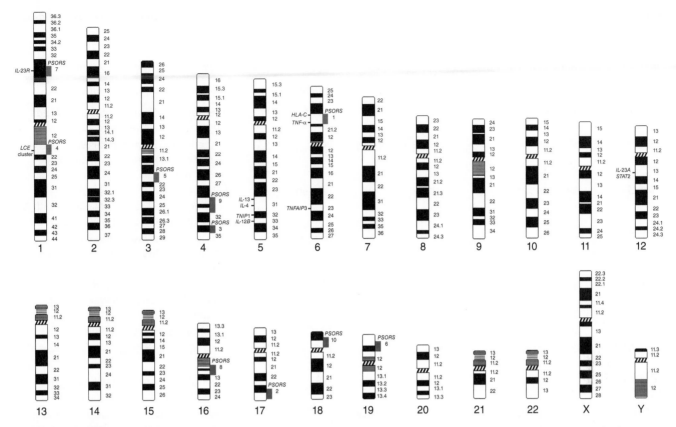

**Figure 106-1** Location of genes and loci associated with risk for psoriasis. Abbreviations: HLA, human leukocyte antigen; IL, interleukin; TNF-α, tumor necrosis factor-α; TNFAIP3, TNF-α-induced protein 3; TNIP1, TNFAIP3 interacting protein 1; LCE, late cornified envelope; STAT2, signal transducer and activator of transcription 2; PSORS; psoriasis susceptibility.

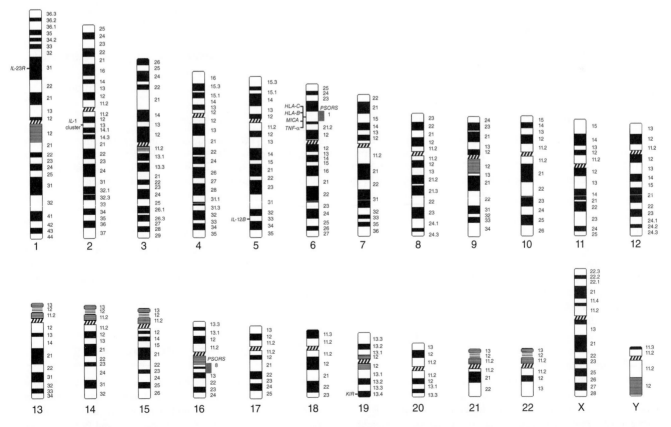

**Figure 106-2** Location of genes and loci associated with risk for psoriatic arthritis. Abbreviations: HLA, human leukocyte antigen; IL, interleukin; TNF-α, tumor necrosis factor-α; MICA, major histocompatibility complex class I-related gene A; KIR, killer inhibitory receptor; PSORS; psoriasis susceptibility.

*Table 106-3 Candidate Genes Associated With Pharmacogenetics of Inflammatory Arthritis (Primarily Rheumatoid Arthritis)*

| Gene | Associated Medications | Goal of Testing | Variants | Genotype/Phenotype Correlation |
|------|------------------------|-----------------|----------|-------------------------------|
| CYP2C9 | NSAIDs | Safety and efficacy | *2, *3 | Increased risk of gastrointestinal bleeding; lower dose required |
| SLC19A1 | Methotrexate | Safety and efficacy | 80G>A | Uptake lowest in individuals with GG genotype than those with GA or AA genotypes |
| TYMS | Methotrexate | Efficacy | Tandem repeat | Alleles with only 2 repeats associated with improved response; alleles with 3 repeats associated with MTX resistance |
| MTHFR | Methotrexate | Safety | 677C>T | CT/TT genotype associated with increased ADRs and higher rate of MTX toxicity |
| MTHFR | Methotrexate | Safety | 1298A>C | AC/AA genotype associated with higher rate of MTX toxicity; lower dose required |
| ATIC | Methotrexate | Safety | 347C>G | GG genotype associated with ADRs |
| DHODH | Leflunomide | Efficacy | 19C>A | Frequency of remission increased with C allele |
| CYP1A2 | Leflunomide | Safety | *1F | CC genotype associated with a higher rate of toxicity; lower dose required |
| TPMT | Azathioprine | Safety and efficacy | *2, *3A, *3C | Variants associated with decreased efficacy and increased toxicity; lower dose is required |
| NAT2 | Sulfasalazine | Safety | *4 | Decreased risk of severe ADRs |
| TNF-α | Etanercept Infliximab | Efficacy | −308G>A | GG is associated with positive response |
| TNFRII | Etanercept Infliximab Adalimumab | Efficacy | 676T>G | TG genotype is associated with negative response; TT genotype is associated with positive response |
| FCGR3A | Infliximab | Efficacy | 158F>V | FF genotype is associated with positive response |
| HLA-DRB1 | Etanercept | Efficacy | *0404 & *0101 combination | Genotype is associated with positive response |
| IL-1RN | Infliximab | Efficacy | *2 | Increased efficacy |

CYP2C9, cytochrome P450 2C9 complex; SLC19A1, solute carrier family 19 member 1; TYMS, thymidylate synthase; ADRs, adverse drug reactions; ATIC, 5-aminoimidazole-4-carboxamide ribonucleotide formyltransferase/IMP cyclohydrolase; DHODH, dihydro-orotate dehydrogenase; CYP1A2, cytochrome P450 1A2 complex; TPMT, thiopurine methyltransferase; NAT2, N-acetyltransferase 2; TNF-α, tumor necrosis factor α; TNFRII, tumor necrosis factor receptor 2; FCGR3A, Fc fragment of IgG, low affinity IIIa, receptor; IL-1RN, interleukin-1 receptor.

15% of patients, and follows the onset of psoriasis in the remaining 15% of patients. Moreover, there does not appear to be a clear association between the severity of psoriasis and severity of inflammatory arthritis.

**Differential Diagnosis:** The differential diagnosis of psoriasis includes atopic dermatitis, contact dermatitis, pityriasis rosea, pityriasis alba, seborrheic dermatitis, nummular eczema, and lichen planus. The differential diagnosis for PsA includes rheumatoid arthritis, ankylosing spondylitis, Reiter syndrome, IBD arthropathy, and systemic lupus erythematosus.

**Classification Criteria for Psoriatic Arthritis:** The diagnosis of PsA is dependent on clinical, laboratory, and radiologic assessments. The recently published classification criteria, CASPAR, is now widely accepted for classifying this entity. The CASPAR criteria consists of established inflammatory articular, spinal or entheseal disease, and at least three points from the following features:

current psoriasis (assigned a score of 2 points), a history of psoriasis, a family history of psoriasis, nail dystrophy, dactylitis, rheumatoid factor negativity, dactylitis and juxta-articular new bone formation. At present, there are no validated serologic or biomarkers that will help predict the development of inflammatory arthritis in psoriasis patients.

## Screening and Counseling

**Mode of Inheritance:** There are no monogenic forms for psoriasis and PsA. Both psoriasis and PsA are complex multifactorial diseases that are caused by underlying genetic and environmental factors. The genes associated with psoriasis and PsA appear to be multiple with each displaying modest effect size.

**Family History:** An affected first-degree relative confers a relative risk between 4 and 10 for psoriasis. Twin studies in psoriasis demonstrate that there is a threefold increase in concordance in monozygotic versus dizygotic twins (concordance 35%-72% vs 12%-23%, respectively). PsA displays stronger heritability than psoriasis, as an affected first-degree relative confers a relative risk between 30 and 47 for PsA. There is only one twin study in PsA, which did not reveal significant heritability for PsA. However, this study requires validation with larger number of twin pairs.

**Heterogeneity of Psoriasis and PsA Based on Age of Onset of Psoriasis:** In 1985, Henseler and Christophers described two types of psoriasis. Type 1 psoriasis was defined by the onset of psoriasis prior to age 40, and type 2 psoriasis was defined by age of onset of psoriasis after the age of 40. Type 1 psoriasis was more familial, had more severe psoriasis, and stronger *HLA* associations (*HLA-Cw6, HLA-DR7, HLA-B13,* and *HLA-Bw57*) as compared to type 2 psoriasis. PsA can also be stratified according to the age of onset of psoriasis. In PsA patients in whom psoriasis started prior to the age of 40, the PsA patients were more likely to have a family history of psoriasis, skin lesions preceding joint lesions, more actively inflamed joints at presentation, and stronger *HLA* associations (*HLA-B17, HLA-Cw6*) as compared to PsA patients with psoriasis after the age of 40.

**Epigenetic Effect:** Parent-of-origin effect has been demonstrated clinically in psoriasis and PsA. In both of these entities there is an excess of paternal transmission. The proportion of proband's affected fathers was 0.6 as compared to the expected of 0.5. Similar trends were noted in offspring and second-degree relatives of the proband.

**Genotype-Phenotype Correlations:** *HLA-Cw*0602* may have potential clinical utility as it is associated with early onset of psoriasis, higher incidence of guttate or streptococcal-induced flares of psoriasis and more severe skin involvement. Women carrying *HLA-Cw*0602* are more likely to experience remission with pregnancy. Meanwhile in PsA, *HLA-B39* alone, *HLA-B27* (only in the presence of *HLA-DR7*), and *HLA-DQ3* (only in the absence of *HLA-DR7*), conferred an increased risk for disease progression. The *HLA-DRB1*04* allele and the *IL-4R* gene have been associated with radiographic progression in PsA. Patients with PsA carrying both *HLA-Cw6* and *HLA-DRB1*07* alleles have a less severe course of arthritis.

## Management and Treatments

Numerous modalities now exist to manage psoriasis including ultraviolet light, topical and systemic therapies. The choice of modalities for the management of psoriasis depends on the extent of psoriasis, relative effectiveness of the modality, and coexisting comorbidities. Another important factor is patient preference as patient compliance is one of the greatest barriers to effective treatment in psoriasis.

**Treatment of Psoriasis:**

☞**ULTRAVIOLET LIGHT:** Ultraviolet light is a well-established and widely utilized treatment for psoriasis. The ultraviolet light can be administered as ultraviolet B radiation (UVB; 290-320 nm), narrow-band UVB (311 nm), or phototherapy (PUVA; 320-400 nm). Standard UVB is used to treat extensive psoriasis alone or in combination with topical tar. The narrow UVB is more effective than the standard UVB in treating psoriasis, but also more expensive. PUVA treatment involves use of psoralen (administered orally or via bath) followed by UVA radiation. UVA penetrates deeper into the dermis than UVB; however, there is an increased risk of non-melanoma skin cancer and melanoma with UVA.

☞**TOPICAL AGENTS:** The topical therapies for psoriasis include emollients, corticosteroids, topical vitamin D analogs, retinoids, and tar. Corticosteroids are widely used and are considered the mainstay of therapy. Various potencies of topical steroids are available depending on the location of the lesion and severity of psoriasis. Typically, low-potency corticosteroid creams are used on the face and intertriginous areas whereas more potent topical corticosteroids are used for thick plaques on extensor surfaces. Topical vitamin D analogs such as calcipotriene and tacalcitol are also used to treat psoriasis. Although they are effective as monotherapy, combination with topical steroids is more effective.

☞**SYSTEMIC AGENTS:** Systemic therapies are usually reserved for psoriasis patients with moderate-to-severe psoriasis. The two most common systemic medications are methotrexate (a folic acid antagonist) and cyclosporine (a T-cell suppressor). Methotrexate is increasingly being used first as first-line systemic therapy in psoriasis. Methotrexate is administered once a week (either orally or subcutaneously) and serious side effects include cytopenias and hepatotoxicity. Meanwhile cyclosporine is given orally on a daily basis at a dose of 3 to 5 mg/kg per day, and requires close monitoring as it can result in renal toxicity and hypertension.

☞**BIOLOGIC AGENTS:** Biologic agents are now increasingly being used to treat moderate to severe psoriasis, particularly in patients that have failed systemic therapy. The biologic agents presently available for the treatment of psoriasis include alefacept, etanercept, adalumumab, infliximab, and ustekinumab. Alefacept is a recombinant protein that binds to the CD2 on memory effector T-lymphocytes, inhibiting their activation in psoriatic plaques. It is administered weekly for 12 weeks as an IM injection. Additional 12-week courses can be administered if a minimum of 12 weeks has passed since the last treatment and the CD4 count has returned to normal. Etanercept, adalumumab, and infliximab are all TNF-α inhibitors. Etanercept is a human TNF-α receptor antagonist whereas adalumumab is a human anti-TNF-α antibody and infliximab is a chimeric anti-TNF-α antibody. Etanercept is administered subcutaneously weekly, adalumumab is administered subcutaneously once every 2 weeks, and infliximab is given intravenously every 6 to 8 weeks. Ustekinumab is a human anti-IL-12 and anti-IL-23 monoclonal antibody that is given subcutaneously every 3 months after two loading doses.

**Treatment of Psoriatic Arthritis:** When considering treatment for psoriasis, it is important to be aware of the presence of arthritis. Ideally, systemic treatment should be selected so that it is beneficial for both psoriasis and inflammatory arthritis. Treatment decisions in PsA are driven partly by the extent and severity of the involvement of the following components of PsA: peripheral arthritis, skin and nail disease, axial involvement, dactylitis, and enthesitis. Peripheral arthritis may be managed by nonsteroidal anti-inflammatory drugs (NSAIDs) alone; however, a large proportion of patients are treated with disease-modifying antirheumatic drugs (DMARDs). Most of the evidence for the use of DMARDs in PsA has been borrowed from the experience from RA. If the PsA is resistant to DMARD(s) therapy, biologic agents (anti-TNF-α agents) are initiated. For patients with predominant axial disease, dactylitis, or enthesitis, they are initially treated with NSAIDs. If the symptoms are refractory to NSAID therapy, anti-TNF-α agents are initiated, as there is no convincing role for DMARD therapy for axial disease, enthesitis, or dactylitis.

☞**DISEASE-MODIFYING AGENTS:** As in psoriasis, methotrexate is the initial DMARD of choice for most rheumatologists. Other DMARDs that are commonly used in PsA include sulfasalazine, leflunomide, and azathioprine. Sulfasalazine is a sulfa-based drug that is taken orally twice a day. Leflunomide is a pyrimidine antagonist that is given orally daily. Azathioprine is a purine antagonist that is given orally daily.

☞**BIOLOGIC AGENTS:** Presently, there are four anti-TNF-α agents approved for the treatment of PsA (ie, adalimumab, etanercept, infliximab, and golimumab). In a recent meta-analysis of the use of anti-TNF-α agents in PsA, Saad et al. determined that the anti-TNF-α agents studied (ie, adalimumab, etanercept, and infliximab) were equally effective in the treatment of inflammatory arthritis, as measured by the American College of Rheumatology criteria for 20% improvement (ACR20). In contrast, a difference was documented for the treatment of psoriasis as measured by psoriasis area severity index (PASI) 75 (>75% PASI improvement). In clinical trials in PsA, monoclonal antibodies (ie, adalimumab, infliximab, and golimumab) appear to be more effective in treating psoriasis than a receptor antagonist (ie, etanercept).

*Pharmacogenetics:* There is great interindividual variability in drug efficacy as well as adverse drug reactions (ADRs) with almost any treatment for psoriasis or PsA. Currently, pharmacogenetic studies in psoriasis and PsA cohorts are lacking; however, these inter-related diseases share similar pathology and therapeutic regimen with RA, and as a result, candidate genes for psoriasis and PsA have been suggested from RA studies (Table 106-3).

## Genetic studies in Psoriasis and Psoriatic Arthritis

*Genome-Wide Linkage Studies:* A number of genome-wide linkage studies that have been completed in psoriasis and one in PsA. Generally these studies have been underpowered due to modest effect size of the causative genes, lack of dense microsatellite coverage, and relatively small sample sizes. This has resulted in lack of replication of many loci that were identified and the inability to consistently identify specific risk variants using this approach. The most consistently associated locus in psoriasis is within the major histocompatibility complex (MHC) region at chromosome 6p21.3 referred to as psoriasis susceptibility region 1 (*PSORS1*). It is estimated that this region accounts for one-third to one-half of the genetic susceptibility to psoriasis. Numerous other susceptibility loci also have been identified using the linkage approach, designated as *PSORS2* to *PSORS10*. Four of these loci are of particular interest as they contain potentially relevant genes in psoriasis: *PSORS3* (4q34) (which contains a gene that regulates the production of type 1 interferon), *PSORS4* (1q21) (which encodes S-100 proteins that are involved in chemotaxis), *PSORS6* (19p13) (which harbors the *JUNB* gene which is an essential component of the AP-1 transcription factor), and *PSORS9* (4q31) (which contains an important cytokine in psoriasis, IL-15). Only one genome-wide linkage study has been completed in PsA. In that Icelandic study, suggestive linkage was noted on chromosome 16q, and a significant LOD score was achieved, when the linkage analysis was conditioned on paternal transmission.

*Association Studies:*

☞**PSORIASIS AND PsA AND GENES WITHIN THE MHC REGION:** Polymorphisms in the genes encoded in the MHC region have consistently been associated with psoriasis and PsA. In psoriasis, the association has primarily been with class I antigens: *HLA-B13*, *HLA-B17* (along with its splits *B39* and *B57*), *HLA-Cw\*06*, and *HLA-Cw\*07*. Among these alleles, the *HLA-Cw\*06* represents the strongest association with a relative risk of 20. PsA is also associated with multiple HLA antigens, many of which are similar to psoriasis as the two diseases are inter-related. However, specific associations do exist for PsA. These include *HLA-B27* which is associated with greater spinal involvement, and *HLA-B38* and *HLA-B39* which are associated with peripheral polyarthritis.

☞**NON-*HLA* GENES WITHIN THE MHC:** The MHC is a very gene-dense region and as a result multiple non-*HLA* genes within the MHC region with possible biologic significance have been associated with psoriasis (eg, *OTF3*, *SPR1*, *SEEK1*, corneodesmosin [*CDSN*], and *TNF-α*). However, replication studies have been inconsistent and it has been difficult to determine whether these are independent causative alleles as they are likely to be in linkage disequilibrium (LD) with *PSORS1*. Similar issues exist for PsA studies within this region. The two most studied non-*HLA* genes within this region are *TNF-α* and *MICA*. A recent meta-analysis confirmed an association between *TNF-α-238* polymorphism and PsA. The association with *PSORS1C1* is probably due to LD with *HLA-Cw\*0602*. MICA protein product is expressed on cell surface and functions as a stress-induced antigen. The trinucleotide repeat polymorphism *MICA-A9* that corresponds to *MICA\*002* was shown to be associated with PsA independent of *HLA Cw\*06*, *MICB*, or *TNF-α*.

☞**ASSOCIATION STUDIES OUTSIDE THE MHC REGION:** The most robust non-*MHC* genes in psoriasis have been identified as a result of three genome-wide association scans and a large pooling study. The high-powered GAIN genome-wide association study provided strong support for the association of at least seven loci for psoriasis including *HLA-C*, three genes involved in IL-23 signaling (*IL-23A*, *IL-23R*, *IL-12B*), two genes that regulate nuclear factor-κB (NFκB) signaling (*TNFAIP3*, *TNIP1*), and two genes involved in the modulation of Th2 immune responses (*IL-4*, *IL-13*) (Fig. 106-1, Table 106-1). Associations between higher genomic copy number for β-defensin genes on chromosome 8, and *LCE3B* and *LCE3C* members of the late cornified envelope (*LCE*) gene cluster on 1q21, and psoriasis have been demonstrated.

To date an adequately powered genome-wide association study on PsA has not yet completed, but they are presently underway. Association studies in PsA have primarily involved candidate gene association studies. These studies have identified a number of genes outside the MHC region, including the *IL-1* gene cluster, killer-cell immunoglobulin-like receptor (*KIR*) genes, *IL12B*, and *IL-23R* (Fig. 106-2, Table 106-2). The *IL12B* gene encodes the common IL-12p40 subunit of two heterodimeric cytokines, IL-12 and IL-23, and *IL23R* encodes a subunit of the receptor for IL23A/IL23. These cytokines belong to the TH17 pathway of effector CD4+ T-helper cells produced directly from naive CD4 T cells and reflect the important role of this pathway in the pathogenesis of psoriasis and PsA. That the effect sizes of the associations observed in patients with PsA are similar to or smaller than those reported in patients with psoriasis, suggests that the primary association is with psoriasis susceptibility.

The *IL-1* gene cluster is of interest in the pathogenesis of PsA as IL-1 is a potent proinflammatory cytokine and treatment with an IL-1 receptor antagonist (IL-1ra) has been shown to reduce swollen joints in RA patients. The contribution of the *IL-12B* and *IL-23R* genes to the pathogenesis of PsA is similar to that previously described for psoriasis. *KIR* alleles are certainly an attractive candidate for exerting a direct effect on pathogenesis of both psoriasis and PsA (Table 106-2). Recent studies show a strong association of *KIR2DS1* and *KIR2DS2* with PsA. This association was exacerbated in the absence of ligands for the corresponding inhibitory NK cell receptors, *KIR2DL1* and *KIR2DL2/3*, respectively compared to subjects lacking both *KIR2DS1* and *KIR2DS2*. Thus, it appears that an activating KIR, such as *KIR2DS1*, might be detrimental in terms of developing PsA if the ligand for either *KIR2DL1* or *KIR2DL2/3* is absent.

*Future Directions:* There have been major progress in understanding the genetics implicated in the pathogenesis of psoriasis and PsA as numerous susceptibility loci have been discovered and the pace of discovery has accelerated. Within the past 2 years, the number of independent genetic loci confidently associated with psoriasis has increased from 1 to at least 10; although the effect size appears to be quite modest for most of the identified associations. As the identified loci explain only a fraction of the heritability estimates, additional genetic loci (including rare variants and CNVs) remain to be identified. Follow-up studies with larger numbers of single-nucleotide polymorphisms (SNPs), execution of genome-wide scans in larger sample sets, meta-analyses of genome-wide scan results, and large-scale analyses of rarer variants should result in identification of additional susceptibility loci for psoriasis and PsA.

In contrast to susceptibility studies, few pharmacogenetic studies have been conducted in psoriasis or PsA cohorts and thus less progress has been made in understanding the genetics related to drug efficacy and/or toxicity. While convincing pharmacogenetic targets in psoriasis and PsA are still lacking, candidate genes for psoriasis and PsA have been suggested primarily from RA studies. Similar to genetic susceptibility studies, pharmacogenetic studies are often too small and the results of which can be inconsistent and misleading. The effect sizes are modest, so there is limited clinical predictive value. Studies similar to those mentioned previously for psoriasis and PsA susceptibility will be a prerequisite to accurately assess the impact of genetic variants on drug efficacy and/or toxicity. A priori knowledge of pharmacogenetic mechanisms associated with psoriasis and PsA pharmacotherapy has the potential to identify and therefore stratify patients into clinically important treatment categories (ie, responders vs nonresponders; tolerant vs intolerant). There is now an increasing trend to use more targeted therapies for the management of PsA. In particular, there has been an emergence of anticytokine therapy, including TNF-α and IL-23. Genetic variants from these cytokines may be of value in predicting therapeutic response.

## Bibliography:

1. Langley RG, Krueger GG, Griffiths CE. Psoriasis: epidemiology, clinical features, and quality of life. *Ann Rheum Dis*. 2005;64 (suppl 2):ii18-ii23.

2. Wright V, Moll JMH. Psoriatic arthritis. *Seronegative Polyarthritis*. Amsterdam: New York: Elsevier Scientific Publishing Co.; 1976:169-223.

3. Taylor W, Gladman D, Helliwell P, et al. CASPAR Study Group. Classification criteria for psoriatic arthritis: development of new criteria from a large international study. *Arthritis Rheum*. 2006;54:2665-2673.

4. Rahman P, Elder JT. Genetic epidemiology of psoriasis and psoriatic arthritis. *Ann Rheum Dis*. 2005;64:ii37-ii39.

5. Henseler T, Christophers E. Psoriasis of early and late onset: characterization of two types of psoriasis vulgaris. *J Am Acad Dermatol*. Sep 1985;13(3):450-456.

6. Duffin KC, Chandran V, Gladman DD, et al. Genetics of psoriasis and psoriatic arthritis: update and future direction. *J Rheumatol*. 2008;35(7):1449-1453.

7. Saad AA, Symmons DP, Noyce PR, et al. Risks and benefits of tumor necrosis factor-alpha inhibitors in the management of psoriatic arthritis: systematic review and metaanalysis of randomized controlled trials. *J Rheumatol*. 2008;35(5):883-890.

8. Nair RP, Stuart PE, Nistor I, et al. Sequence and haplotype analysis supports HLA-C as the psoriasis susceptibility 1 gene. *Am J Hum Genet*. 2006;78(5):827-851.

9. Gladman DD, Anhorn KAB, Schachter RK, et al. HLA antigens in PsA. *J Rheumatol*. 1986;13:586-592.

10. Nair RP, Duffin KC, Helms C, et al. Genome-wide scan reveals association of psoriasis with IL-23 and NF-kappaB pathways. *Nat Genet*. 2009;41:199-204.

11. Zhang XJ, Huang W, Yang S, et al. Psoriasis genome-wide association study identifies susceptibility variants within LCE gene cluster at 1q21. *Nat Genet*. 2009;41(2):205-210.

12. Kooloos WM, Huizinga TW, Guchelaar HJ, Wessels JA. Pharmacogenetics in treatment of rheumatoid arthritis. *Curr Pharm Des*. 2010;16(2):164-175.

## Supplementary Information

**OMIM References:**

[1] Psoriasis Susceptibility 1; PSORS1 (#177900)

[2] Major Histocompatibility Complex, Class I, B; HLA-B (*142830)

[3] Major Histocompatibility Complex, Class I, C; HLA-C (*142840)

[4] Major Histocompatibility Complex Class I Chain-Related Gene A; MICA (*600169)

[5] Tumor Necrosis Factor; TNF (*191160)

[6] Interleukin-1 α; IL1A (*147760)

[7] Interleukin-1 β; IL1B (*147720)

[8] Interleukin-12B; IL12B (*161561)

[9] Interleukin-23R; IL23R (*607562)]10] Interleukin-23A; IL23A (*605580)

[10] Tumor Necrosis Factor-α-Induced Protein 3; TNFAIP3 (*191163)

[11] TNFAIP3-Interacting Protein 1; TNIP1 (*607714)

[12] Thiopurine-S-Methyltransferase; TPMT (*187680)

[13] 5,10-Methylenetetrahydrofolate reductase; MTHFR (*607093)

***Key Words:*** Psoriasis, psoriatic arthritis, genome-wide association studies, genome-wide linkage studies, pharmacogenetics

# 107 Hereditary Melanoma and Other High-Risk Skin Cancer Susceptibility Syndromes

Michele Gabree and Hensin Tsao

## KEY POINTS

- *Disease summary:*
  - The genetics of hereditary skin cancer susceptibility syndromes is complex and expression is influenced by confounding environmental factors, including solar ultraviolet radiation, as well as other genetic factors.
  - Hereditary melanoma is characterized by the presence of multiple diagnoses of cutaneous melanoma within a family. In addition, an increased risk for other types of cancer, including pancreatic cancer, has been observed in some families with hereditary melanoma.

- *Hereditary basis:*
  - Germline mutations in the *CDKN2A* gene are estimated to account for approximately 20% to 40% of hereditary melanoma. Mutations in the *CDK4* gene are uncommon and have been detected in a small number of hereditary melanoma families.
  - Although the penetrance is complicated by environmental and confounding genetic factors, *CDKN2A* and *CDK4* gene mutations are generally considered to be associated with an autosomal dominant pattern of inheritance with variable penetrance.
  - Geographic location has been associated with variable *CDKN2A* expression. A study of *CDKN2A* carriers with positive family histories of melanoma estimated the risk of developing melanoma by age 80 in *CDKN2A* carriers to be 58% in Europe, 76% in the United States, and 91% in Australia. This difference has been attributed to environmental influences as well as other inherited factors.

- *Other cancer susceptibility syndromes associated with high skin cancer risk:*
  - In addition to *CDKN2A* and *CDK4*, other hereditary syndromes have been associated with a highly increased susceptibility for skin cancer (Table 107-1).

## Diagnostic Criteria and Clinical Characteristics

***Criteria for Genetics Referral:*** Due to the variable expressivity, standard diagnostic criteria do not exist for hereditary melanoma. Genetic counseling for hereditary melanoma predisposition syndromes should be considered for the individuals who meet the criteria below.

Criteria for individuals in areas with a high incidence of melanoma (including the United States):

- Three or more relatives on the same side of the family with melanoma
- Greater than or equal to three primary melanomas in one individual
- Pancreatic cancer and melanoma on the same side of the family

Criteria for individuals in areas with a low incidence of melanoma:

- Two or more relatives on the same side of the family with melanoma
- Greater than or equal to two primary melanomas in one individual
- Pancreatic cancer and melanoma on the same side of the family

Although sometimes observed in hereditary melanoma families, the following features are unlikely to be associated with a hereditary melanoma susceptibility syndrome in the absence of a family history of melanoma:

- Early age of onset of melanoma
- Multiple dysplastic nevi
- Melanoma in situ

***Clinical Characteristics:***

☞**MELANOMA:** The incidence of melanoma varies based on geographic location. Both genetic and environmental factors influence an individual's risk to develop melanoma.

☞**PANCREATIC CANCER:** Although the presence of pancreatic cancer in addition to melanoma increases the likelihood of detecting a *CDKN2A* gene mutation, pancreatic cancer has been reported as a feature in a minority of hereditary melanoma families.

☞**OTHER TYPES OF CANCER:** A slightly increased risk for other types of cancer, including central nervous system tumors, ocular tumors, nonmelanoma skin cancer, respiratory tumors, soft tissue tumors, and cancer of the lip, mouth, and pharynx, has been observed in some *CDKN2A* mutation-positive families.

☞**DYSPLASTIC NEVI:** Clinically dysplastic nevi are a feature of some families who harbor a *CDKN2A* gene mutation. Regardless of *CDKN2A* mutation status, the presence of dysplastic nevi is a risk factor for melanoma.

Table 107-1 Other High-Risk Hereditary Skin Cancer Susceptibility Syndromes[4,5]

| Syndrome | Associated Gene Symbols | Inheritance | Associated Findings | Clinical Phenotype | Genetic Testing |
|---|---|---|---|---|---|
| Xeroderma pigmentosum (XP) | XPA, ERCC3 (XPB), XPC, ERCC2 (XPD), DDB2 (XPE), ERCC4 (XPF), ERCC5 (XPG), ERCC1, and POLH (XP-V) | Autosomal recessive | Sun sensitivity, melanoma and nonmelanoma skin and ocular cancers, neurologic abnormalities | Cutaneous: melanoma and nonmelanoma skin cancer at UV-exposed areas of the body, severe sunburn, persistent erythema, facial freckling < age 2, xerosis, poikiloderma<br>Noncutaneous:<br>Ocular: photophobia, keratitis, increased eye lid pigmentation, atrophy of the eye lid skin<br>Nervous system: progressive sensorineural hearing loss, cognitive impairment, abnormal deep tendon stretch reflexes, acquired microcephaly | Clinical testing available for XPA and XPC<br>Limited availability for other XP-related genetic testing outside of research testing. |
| Nevoid basal cell carcinoma syndrome (BCNS; see Chap. 113) | PTCH1<br>PTCH2[a]<br>SUFU[a] | Autosomal dominant, approximately 40% of cases are de novo[4] | Basal cell carcinoma, jaw keratocysts, skeletal abnormalities, characteristic facial features, ectopic calcification, cardiac and ovarian fibromas, medulloblastoma | One major criteria and molecular confirmation, two major criteria, or one major and two minor criteria (adapted from):<br>Major criteria: Basal cell carcinoma (BCC) < age 20 or excessive number of BCCs; odontogenic keratocysts of the jaw (histologically proven) < age 20; palmar or plantar pits; lamellar calcification of the falx cerebri; medulloblastoma; first-degree relative with BCNS.<br>Minor criteria: rib abnormalities; macrocephaly; ocular abnormalities; cleft lip/palate; other skeletal abnormalities (including vertebral abnormalities, kyphoscoliosis, polydactyly); ovarian or cardiac fibromas; lymphomesenteric cysts | |

[a]Rarely associated with BCNS.

Gene names: XPA, xeroderma pigmentosum, complementation group A; ERCC3 (XPB), excision repair cross-complementing rodent repair deficiency, complementation group 3 (xeroderma pigmentosum group B complementing); XPC, xeroderma pigmentosum, complementation group C; ERCC2 (XPD), excision repair cross-complementing rodent repair deficiency, complementation group 2; DDB2 (XPE), damage-specific DNA binding protein 1, 127kDa; ERCC4 (XPF), excision repair cross-complementing rodent repair deficiency, complementation group 4; ERCC5 (XPG), excision repair cross-complementing rodent repair deficiency, complementation group 5; ERCC1, excision repair cross-complementing rodent repair deficiency, complementation group 1; POLH (XP-V), polymerase (DNA directed), eta; PTCH, protein patched homolog 1; SUFU, suppressor of fused homolog (Drosophila).

## Screening and Counseling

**Screening:** Screening recommendations are based on personal and family history. When a *CDKN2A* mutation has been identified in an individual, increased melanoma surveillance is recommended, as summarized in Table 107-2. Consideration of pancreatic cancer surveillance is also warranted for *CDKN2A* mutation-positive individuals.

Because the majority of families with hereditary melanoma will test negative for a *CDKN2A* mutation, increased surveillance is recommended for all individuals with a personal and/or family history of melanoma. In addition, individuals who test negative for a familial *CDKN2A* mutation also remain at increased risk for melanoma due to other genetic and environmental factors, and should be monitored accordingly; however, it is important to note that the risk for melanoma in mutation-negative family members is lower than the risk for developing melanoma in an individual with a *CDKN2A* mutation.

Pancreatic cancer surveillance currently may include a combination of endoscopic ultrasound, magnetic resonance imaging (MRI), serum tumor markers, and magnetic resonance cholangio-pancreatography (MRCP), if indicated. It is important to note that pancreatic cancer surveillance has not been proven to be effective at improving the outcome of pancreatic cancer. The risks, benefits, and limitations of pancreatic cancer surveillance should be discussed with a gastroenterology specialist.

**Counseling:** The clinical utility of *CDKN2A* genetic testing remains a source of debate due to relatively low likelihood of detecting a *CDKN2A* mutation as well as the complexity of assessing the influence of confounding environmental and other inherited factors on melanoma risk. In addition, the current lack of effective pancreatic cancer surveillance also complicates the utility and implications of testing.

Prior to genetic testing, patients should undergo genetic counseling with a healthcare provider who has expertise in hereditary melanoma genetics. Genetic counseling for hereditary melanoma susceptibility syndromes should include (1) minimum three-generation pedigree, including melanoma and nonmelanoma cancer diagnoses, (2) assessment of family history, including discussion on likelihood of a hereditary melanoma syndrome, (3) discussion of technical accuracy of test and possible test results, (4) discussion of the risks, benefits, and limitations of genetic testing, including effect on clinical management, impact and implications for family members, and risk of genetic discrimination.

*CDKN2A* genetic testing is most informative for an individual affected with melanoma and/or pancreatic cancer. The possible test results for an affected individual and example screening recommendations are included in Table 107-2. The test result of an unaffected individual who is found to be negative for a *CNKN2A* mutation is considered to be uninformative, unless a *CDNK2A* mutation has been identified in another family member. Individuals who test negative for a familial *CDKN2A* gene mutation are still at an increased risk for melanoma based on other factors and should be monitored accordingly. In addition, it is important to consider that within a family, some melanoma cases may be due to *CDKN2A* mutations while other melanoma may be sporadic; therefore a negative *CDKN2A* test in one individual with melanoma does not preclude a positive test for other family members.

Recently, a statistical risk model utilizing Bayesian analysis was developed to assess the risk for carrying a *CDKN2A* gene mutation based on ethnicity and personal/family history of melanoma. This model, called melaPRO is a user-friendly program which can currently be obtained free of charge through the CancerGene software package (which also includes risk estimates for other hereditary cancers such as breast and ovarian cancer) at the following website: http://www4.utsouthwestern.edu/breasthealth/cagene/.

Many companies offer direct-to-consumer (DTC) marketing for genetic tests, which bypasses the health professional by providing information from a company directly to the patients. DTC tests vary, and may include well-known high-risk loci, such as *CDKN2A*, as well as genomic profiling (through short-nucleotide repeat [SNP] analysis) for regions of possible disease susceptibility. Genomic

---

*Table 107-2 **Genetic Testing Results and Medical Management for Individuals With Hereditary Melanoma***

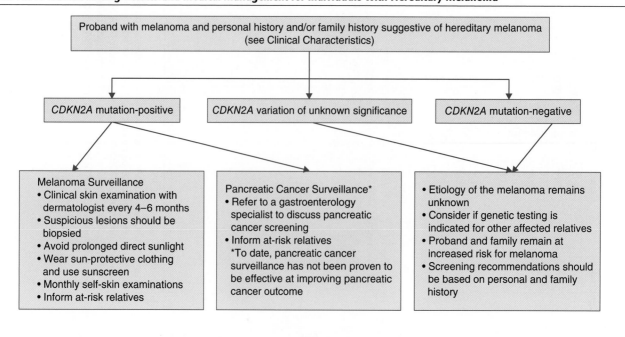

profiling results often lack validation and may differ based on the company used; therefore, caution should be used when interpreting the results of a DTC test.

Multi-gene panel tests are now clinically available and include known high risk melanoma genes such as *CDKN2A* and *CDK4* as well as other rare genes associated with melanoma. In addition, whole genome and whole exome tests are also now being utilized to test for hereditary syndromes. Individuals undergoing these tests may not have a phenotype associated with hereditary skin cancer. Therefore, this may lead to the detection of a skin cancer susceptibility gene mutation in individuals who do not have a personal or family history of skin cancer. In addition, individuals with hereditary skin cancer may be found to have mutations in genes not known to be associated with skin cancer susceptibility. Research is needed to further understand the implications of these tests on cancer risk and clinical management.

## Molecular Genetics and Molecular Mechanism

*Syndrome/Gene/Locus:*

☞**CDKN2A/Cyclin-Dependent Kinase Inhibitor 2A/9p21:** The cyclin-dependent kinase inhibitor (*CDKN2A*) locus includes four exons: exon1β, exon 1α, exon2, and exon 3. Through alternate splicing, the *CDKN2A* locus encodes for two distinct proteins, p16 and p14ARF. Both proteins function as tumor suppressors with roles in the regulation of the cell cycle and apoptosis. The p16 protein binds to cyclin-dependent kinase 4 (CDK4), inhibiting the CDK4 protein from phosphorylating the retinoblastoma protein. The p14ARF protein is involved in p53 regulation and *CDKN2A* mutations that disrupt *p14ARF* function consequently impair the function of the p53 protein. Mutations in *CDKN2A* and *CDK4* allow the cell cycle to proceed without regulation, which may ultimately result in tumor development.

*Genetic Testing:* Genetic testing for *CDKN2A* and *CDK4* is clinically available As discussed earlier, the utility of this testing remains controversial.

### Bibliography:

1. Tsao HT, Neindorf KB. Genetic testing in hereditary melanoma. *J Am Acad Dermatol.* 2004;51:803-808.

2. Leachman SA, Carucci J, Kohlmann W, et al. Selection criteria for genetic assessment of patients with familial melanoma. *J Am Acad Dermatol.* 2009;61:677.e1-e14.

3. Bishop DT, Demenais F, Goldstein AM, et al. Geographical variation in the penetrance of CDKN2A mutations for melanoma. *J Natl Cancer Inst.* 2002;94(12):894-903.

4. Bree AF, Shah MR. Consensus statement from the first international colloquium on basal cell nevus syndrome (BCNS). *Am J Med Genet Part A.* 2011;155:2091-2097.

5. Cleaver JE, Lam ET, Revet I. Disorders of nucleotide excision repair: the genetic and molecular basis of heterogeneity. *Nat Rev Genet.* 2009;10(11):756-768.

6. de Snoo FA, Bishop DT, Bergman W, et al. Increased risk of cancer other than melanoma in CDKN2A founder mutation (p16-Leiden)-positive melanoma families. *Clin Cancer Res.* 2008;14(21):7151-7157.

7. Goldstein AM, Chan M, Harland M, et al. High-risk melanoma susceptibility genes and pancreatic cancer, neural system tumors, and uveal melanoma across GenoMEL. *Cancer Res.* 2006;66(20):9818-9828.

8. de Snoo FA, Riedijk SR, van Mil AM, et al. Genetic testing in familial melanoma: update and implications. *Psycho-Oncology.* 2008;17:790-796.

9. Wang W, Niendorf KB, Patel D, et al. Estimating CDKN2A carrier probability and personalizing cancer risk assessments in hereditary melanoma using MelaPRO. *Cancer Res.* 2010;70(2):552-559.

10. Robson ME, Storm CD, Weitzel J, et al. American Society of Clinical Oncology policy statement update: genetic and genomic testing for cancer susceptibility. *J Clin Oncol.* 2010;28(5):893-901.

11. Udayakumar D, Tsao H. Melanoma genetics: an update on risk-associated genes. *Hematol Oncol Clin N Am.* 2009;23:415-419.

## Supplementary Information

### OMIM References:

[1] Cyclin-Dependent Kinase Inhibitor 2A; CDKN2A (#600160)

[2] Cyclin-Dependent Kinase 4; CDK4 (#123829)

[3] Basal Cell Nevus Syndrome; BCNS (#109400)

[4] Xeroderma Pigmentosum, Complementation Group A; XPA (#278700)

[5] Xeroderma Pigmentosum, Complementation Group B; XPB (#610651)

[6] Xeroderma Pigmentosum, Complementation Group C; XPC (#278720)

[7] Xeroderma Pigmentosum, Complementation Group D; XPD (#278730)

[8] Xeroderma Pigmentosum, Complementation Group E; XPE (#278740)

[9] Xeroderma Pigmentosum, Complementation Group F; XPF (#278760)

[10] Xeroderma Pigmentosum, Complementation Group G; XPG (#278780)

[11] Xeroderma Pigmentosum, Variant Type; XPV (#278750)

[12] Xeroderma Pigmentosum IX; XPI (#278810)

### Alternative Names:
- Familial Melanoma
- Familial Atypical Mole Malignant Melanoma Syndrome
- Dysplastic Nevus Syndrome
- Gorlin Syndrome (BCBN)

*Key Words:* Melanoma, dysplastic nevi, pancreatic cancer, nonmelanoma skin cancer, basal cell carcinoma, medulloblastoma

# 108 Neurofibromatosis Type 1

Douglas R. Stewart

## KEY POINTS

- *Disease summary:*
  - Neurofibromatosis type 1 (NF1) is a common (~1/3000), progressive neurocutaneous disorder primarily of increased tumor predisposition, but also pigmentary abnormalities, osseous dysplasia, and impaired cognitive function that arises secondary to mutations in the tumor suppressor gene *NF1*.
  - NF1 is a pleiotropic disorder, affecting different organ systems (central and peripheral nervous systems, bone, vasculature) with wide variation in severity of clinical features, even among members of the same family. There is limited genotype-phenotype correlation (see Counseling).
  - NF1 affects all ethnic groups and both sexes equally.
  - As a population, individuals with NF1 have a reduced lifespan.
- *Hereditary basis:*
  - NF1 is a monogenic disorder with an autosomal dominant pattern of inheritance. It is 100% penetrant, typically by late adolescence. Approximately half of the individuals affected with NF1 have a family history of the disorder.
- *Differential diagnosis:*
  - The diagnosis is rarely mistaken in a patient with numerous café-au-lait macules, neurofibromas, and axillary freckling. Certain features, especially when present in isolation or in a younger patient, may present a diagnostic challenge (Table 108-1). Consideration of a missense *NF1* mutation, or a de novo *NF1* mutation present in a segmental or mosaic state (see Counseling) should be made when confronted with either café-au-lait macules only or neurofibromas only, especially in a limited distribution. A diagnosis of Legius syndrome should be considered in older individuals with pigmentary findings only and absence of neurofibromas.

## Diagnostic Criteria and Clinical Characteristics

**Diagnostic Criteria for NF1:** The NIH Consensus Criteria for the diagnosis of NF1 were developed in 1987.

**Neurofibromatosis type 1 is present in a patient who has two or more of the following:**

1. Six or more café-au-lait macules over 5 mm in greatest diameter in prepubertal individuals and over 15 mm in greatest diameter in postpubertal individuals
2. Two or more neurofibromas of any type *or* one plexiform neurofibroma
3. Freckling in the axillary or inguinal regions
4. Optic glioma
5. Two or more Lisch nodules (iris hamartomas)
6. A distinctive osseous lesion such as sphenoid wing dysplasia or thinning of the long bone cortex with or without pseudarthrosis
7. A first-degree relative (parent, sibling, offspring) with NF1 by the above criteria

The criteria were reviewed in 1997 and were left unchanged. More recently, Huson has suggested that the diagnostic criteria be changed to (1) include *NF1* pathogenic mutations, (2) recognize segmental NF1, and (3) distinguish numerous café-au-lait macules arising from DNA mismatch repair and ring chromosome syndromes (Table 108-1).

In adults, the diagnosis of NF1 can usually be made based on history and physical examination findings. A Wood (ultraviolet) lamp is necessary for a thorough skin examination. Biopsy and pathologic examination of skin "lumps and bumps" is occasionally required. Referral to ophthalmology for a slit-lamp examination of the irides for Lisch nodules is prudent.

In younger children without a family history of NF1, multiple examinations over several years may be needed to establish the diagnosis (see Counseling). Although café-au-lait macules are present in greater than 95% of children by age 1 year, there is typically delay before the appearance of other features. In this situation, genetic testing of *NF1* may be useful to expedite diagnosis. By age 5 years, approximately 50% of children with NF1 will have three or more of the seven diagnostic features.

**Clinical Characteristics:**

☞**NEUROFIBROMA:** This is the hallmark lesion of NF1, and is a soft, fleshy benign tumor of the Schwann cell. They may develop from essentially any nerve in the body, although they have a predilection for the back, abdomen, arms, and face. They may number in the thousands and vary in size from pinhead to large pedunculated masses. It is difficult to predict neurofibroma burden. They typically appear in adolescence and the number of lesions often increases with puberty and pregnancy, suggesting hormonal influence. They are usually asymptomatic but may itch (Table 108-2).

☞**PLEXIFORM NEUROFIBROMA:** These are complex, likely congenital tumors that may grow unpredictably and impose considerable morbidity, especially in childhood. They involve multiple nerve fascicles or extend along the length of a single nerve. They may occur anywhere. Their natural history is variable; they may grow rapidly in childhood and adolescence, resulting in organ compromise and significant cosmetic problems, or they may be essentially asymptomatic and quiescent. When palpable, plexiform neurofibromas are typically described as a "bag of worms"; the overlying skin is often hyperpigmented and excessively hirsute.

☞**MALIGNANCY:** Traditionally, individuals with NF1 as a population were thought to have a 10 to 15 year reduction in expected lifespan, due to an increased number of peripheral and central nervous system (CNS) malignancies. More recent work

*Table 108-1  Differential Diagnosis of Isolated Disease Features in NF1*

| Syndrome | Gene Symbol | Associated Findings |
|---|---|---|
| **Pigmentary abnormalities, especially numerous café-au-lait macules** | | |
| Mosaic or segmental NF1 | *NF1* | Mild (mosaic) or isolated (segmental) manifestations of classical NF1 |
| Missense mutation in *NF1* | *NF1* | Varied; *NF1* gene testing often helpful |
| Legius/NF1-like syndrome | *SPRED1* | Lipomas, macrocephaly, learning disabilities |
| Neurofibromatosis type 2 | *NF2* | Bilateral vestibular schwannomas, schwannomas elsewhere, lens opacities. Typically few café-au-lait macules |
| Constitutional mismatch repair-deficiency syndrome (homozygosity or compound heterozygosity for mutations in listed genes) | *MLH1, MSH2, MSH6, PMS2* | Hematologic malignancy and brain tumors in childhood; also early-onset GI malignancies<br>Family history of HNPCC/Lynch syndrome<br>Skin findings only in autosomal recessive form |
| Bannayan-Riley-Ruvalcaba | *PTEN* | Pigmentation of glans and shaft of penis in boys; café-au-lait macules typically not widely distributed |
| McCune-Albright syndrome with polyostotic fibrous dysplasia | *GNAS* | "Coast of Maine" or jagged appearance to café-au-lait macules; bony abnormalities |
| LEOPARD syndrome | *PTPN11, RAF1, BRAF* | Multiple lentigines, pulmonic stenosis, growth retardation, sensorineural deafness; no tumors |
| Ring chromosome phenotype | Various chromosomes | Short stature, microcephaly, moderate-to-severe mental retardation are also seen |
| **Neurofibromas** | | |
| Mosaic or segmental NF1 | *NF1* | Mild (mosaic) or isolated (segmental) manifestations of classical NF1 |
| Spinal neurofibromatosis | *NF1* | Neurofibromas of spine but few dermal neurofibromas or pigmentary abnormalities, often do not meet consensus criteria for diagnosis of NF1 (see Diagnostic Criteria and Clinical Manifestations) |
| Neurofibromatosis type 2 | *NF2* | Bilateral vestibular schwannomas, schwannomas elsewhere, lens opacities. Typically few café-au-lait macules |

Gene names: *NF1*, neurofibromin 1; *SPRED1*, sprouty-related EVH1 domain-containing 1; *NF2*, neurofibromin 2 (merlin); *MLH1*, mutL homolog 1, colon cancer, nonpolyposis type 2 (*Escherichia coli*); *MSH2*, mutS homolog 2, colon cancer, nonpolyposis type 1 (*E coli*); *MSH6*, mutS homolog 6 (*E coli*); *PMS2*, PMS2 postmeiotic segregation increased 2 (*Saccharomyces cerevisiae*); *PTEN*, phosphatase and tensin homolog; *GNAS,* GNAS complex locus; *PTPN11*, protein tyrosine phosphatase, nonreceptor type 11; *RAF1*, v-raf-1 murine leukemia viral oncogene homolog 1.

suggests the decrease in life span to be approximately 8 years less than their counterparts in the general population. The most common malignancies in NF1 are malignant peripheral nerve sheath tumors (MPNSTs) and high-grade astrocytomas. Patients with NF1 face an 8% to 13% lifetime risk for the development of a MPNST. These primarily arise from the malignant transformation of plexiform neurofibromas, although they may occur anywhere. They metastasize early and are difficult to treat. Low-grade astrocytomas (WHO grade I: optic pathway gliomas and pilocytic astrocytomas) in NF1 are common, especially in children and generally have a favorable prognosis. However, higher-grade lesions (WHO II-IV: glioblastomas) are malignant. Most glioblastomas are diagnosed without an antecedent lower-grade tumor being detected. There is one report of an increased risk for breast cancer in women with NF1. Children but not adults are at an increased risk for the development of juvenile myelomonocytic leukemia (JMML). A link between JMML and juvenile xanthogranuloma has been suggested but not substantiated.

☞CAFÉ-AU-LAIT MACULES AND INTERTRIGINOUS FRECKLING: Nearly all individuals with NF1 harbor distinct pigmentary abnormalities. There are usually multiple (>6), smooth-bordered ("coast of California"), oval café-au-lait macules, typically on the buttocks, lower abdomen, arms, and thighs. The café-au-lait macules are present by 1 year of age in greater than 99% of individuals with NF1. Most individuals will have freckling in the bilateral axillae and groin by the age of 10 years. Absence of these features should prompt reconsideration of the diagnosis of NF1. Importantly, patients with Legius syndrome may have numerous café-au-lait macules and intertriginous freckling only.

☞LEARNING DISABILITIES: Learning problems and attention deficit hyperactivity disorder are common in children with NF1 and may persist into adulthood. There is no specific pattern of learning disabilities unique to NF1. Severe cognitive impairment is unusual, and should prompt reconsideration of the diagnosis, although individuals with an *NF1* microdeletion may be more cognitively impaired than individuals with NF1 who do not have an

*Table 108-2* **System Involvement**

| System | Manifestation | Frequency[a] |
|---|---|---|
| Central and peripheral nervous systems | Neurofibromas | >95% of adults; individuals with *NF1* exon 17 3-bp in-frame deletion do not have dermal neurofibromas |
| | Plexiform neurofibromas | Up to 50% with use of medical imaging |
| | Migraine-like headaches and other chronic pain | Unknown, but common |
| | Malignant peripheral nerve sheath tumor (MPNST) | 8%-13% lifetime risk |
| Central nervous system | Learning disabilities and attention deficit hyperactivity disorder (severe cognitive impairment rare) | 30%-60% |
| | Optic pathway glioma | 15% in childhood with use of imaging; ~5% of these are symptomatic (visual impairment and precocious puberty) |
| | Epilepsy | ~5% |
| | Pilocytic (low-grade) astrocytoma | 5% |
| | High-grade astrocytoma | 1%-5% |
| | Aqueductal stenosis | 1.5% (typically <30 years) |
| Endocrine | Pheochromocytoma | <5% |
| | Precocious puberty | ~1% in children; typically secondary to optic pathway glioma encroachment on hypothalamus |
| Gastrointestinal | Gastrointestinal stromal tumor | Unknown, but <5% |
| Hematologic | Juvenile myelomonocytic leukemia | <1% in children |
| Ophthalmologic | Lisch nodules | 90%-95% |
| Skeletal | Macrocephaly | ~45% |
| | Short stature (10-25th percentile) | ~30% |
| | Scoliosis | 10% |
| | Generalized osteopenia | Unknown, but common |
| | Scoliosis requiring surgery | 5% (primarily in childhood) |
| | Tibial and forearm dysplasia | <5% |
| | Sphenoid wing dysplasia | ~1% |
| Skin | Café-au-lait macules | >99% |
| | Intertriginous (skin-fold) freckling (axilla, groin, submammary) | 67%-85% |
| Vasculature | Cherry ("senile") angioma | Common, increases with age |
| | Cerebral, renal, peripheral, and pulmonary vasculopathy | Renal artery stenosis ~1%; others rare |
| | Glomus tumor of the fingertips | Unknown, but <5% |

Data from Huson 2008, Ferner 2007, Williams et al. 2009, and Friedman 1999.

[a]Frequency reflects adult population, except where noted.

*NF1* microdeletion. It is controversial whether focal areas of high signal intensity on T2-weighted brain magnetic resonance imaging (MRI) (unidentified bright objects [UBOs]) are correlated with learning disabilities. Studies in the NF1 mouse model of the benefits of lovastatin or simvastatin on learning problems yielded mixed results.

☞LISCH NODULES: These tumor-like melanocyte proliferations on the surface of the iris appear in mid-childhood and are useful in the diagnosis of NF1. They are easily detected with a slit lamp. Individuals with blue or green eyes tend to have more Lisch nodules than those with brown eyes. Multiple Lisch nodules are rarely observed outside of NF1. They rarely, if ever, have clinical consequences.

☞OPTIC PATHWAY GLIOMAS: These are low-grade astrocytomas found in 15% of children with NF1. Although overall they have a favorable prognosis, in a minority of children they may progress and cause visual loss, field defects, or precocious puberty. For this reason it is important that children with NF1 be regularly evaluated by an experienced pediatric ophthalmologist (see Screening). Use of routine brain MRI to screen children for optic pathway gliomas (OPGs) is not recommended since it does not affect outcome.

☞Quality-of-Life: Several studies have demonstrated that quality-of-life is reduced in NF1. Although the burden of neurofibromas, plexiform neurofibromas, pigmentary differences, and learning problems is easily understood, other factors such as anxiety, depression, chronic pain, and migraine headaches are also likely to be important. Individuals with NF1 may have chronic pain related to a plexiform neurofibroma; however, symptoms frequently do not have an obvious anatomic correlate and need to be taken seriously.

## Screening and Counseling

**Screening:** After childhood, other than blood pressure checks, no special screening is recommended on a routine basis. Importantly, routine screening imaging of the spine and brain in adults is not warranted. Age- and gender-appropriate studies (eg, cholesterol, Pap smears) following general population recommendations should be pursued (Table 108-3).

**Counseling:** NF1 has an autosomal dominant pattern of inheritance. Each child of an affected parent has a 50% risk of inheriting the disorder. Approximately 50% of individuals have a de novo *NF1* gene mutation and are therefore the first person in their family to be affected, while the other 50% have a parent with the disorder. There is 100% penetrance of NF1 by early adulthood but significant variability of manifestations is seen both within and between families. Careful clinical evaluation of both parents of a newly diagnosed proband is prudent, as diagnosis of a mildly affected parent will inform medical management and recurrence risk. Germline mosaicism, where an apparently unaffected parent had multiple children with NF1, has been reported.

Prenatal diagnosis is available if an affected parent's *NF1* mutation is known (see Genetic Testing). Successful preimplantation genetic diagnosis (PGD) of NF1 has been reported. Importantly, there are multiple documented families segregating more than one *NF1* mutation. Caution should therefore be used when assuming all affected family members share the same mutation.

Mosaic and segmental NF1 are diagnostic challenges and may complicate recurrence risk prediction and genetic counseling. It is prudent to counsel up to a 50% recurrence risk. Individuals with spinal NF and/or a missense mutation in *NF1* may harbor some features of the disorder but may not meet strict diagnostic consensus criteria.

There are two known examples of genotype-phenotype correlation in NF1. Individuals with a microdeletion of *NF1* tend to have more neurofibromas, an increased risk of MPNST, facial dysmorphism, cardiac abnormalities, and more severe learning problems. Individuals with a 3-bp in-frame deletion in exon 17 have no dermal neurofibromas.

Despite its prevalence, many individuals with NF1 may not know anyone else with the disorder. Referral to national support groups should be considered.

## Management and Treatment

**Benign Tumors:** Although they rarely, if ever, undergo malignant transformation, neurofibromas can impose a substantial cosmetic burden. To date, no effective chemotherapy exists to control neurofibroma growth. Surgery and/or electrodessication may be helpful; however, there is a risk for scarring and recurrence. Oral or topical antihistamines may help with itching. Plexiform neurofibromas are a significant surgical challenge since scarring, recurrence, or functional neurologic deficit may result. Pheochromocytomas can be fatal and should be considered in a patient with hypertension, palpitations, anxiety, and diaphoresis. Patients can be screened with adrenal imaging plus plasma-free metanephrines and/or 24-hour urine collection for analysis of metanephrines, catecholamines, and vanillylmandelic acid. Patients should be asked about fingertip pain and cold sensitivity to screen for glomus tumors of the fingers. Surgery is generally curative for these exquisitely painful tumors.

**Malignancy:** Patients with the development of new, severe, persistent pain, and/or a rapidly growing tumor should be promptly imaged by MRI to assess for MPNST. Consider mammography for women starting at age 40 years. Sudden cognitive or personality changes may reflect the development of an astrocytoma and should be promptly imaged. Migraine headaches are common and do not necessarily signal CNS malignancy.

**Quality-of-Life:** Depression, anxiety, chronic pain, learning disabilities, un- and underemployment, barriers to care due to lack of medical insurance plus cosmetic concerns, and general lack of awareness by the medical community add to the burden of this uniquely stigmatizing disorder. Quality-of-life may be improved by treating underlying depression, anxiety, and pain. Referral to a pain or headache center, psychotherapy, and vocational counseling may help. Early intervention programs for children are essential. It is important to consider new symptoms, however pedestrian, with an open mind and within the framework of a tumor-predisposition syndrome.

*Table 108-3 Screening*

| Childhood | Adulthood |
| --- | --- |
| Yearly pediatric ophthalmologist examination to assess for optic pathway glioma (until at least age 7 years); routine screening imaging not recommended | Yearly blood pressure check |
| Screening for learning disabilities | Consider starting mammography for women in 40s |
| Screen for evidence of precocious puberty (height and weight and development) | Ask about development of fingertip pain and cold sensitivity (screen for glomus tumors) |
| Yearly blood pressure check | Monitor for depression, anxiety, chronic pain |
| Monitor for scoliosis | Monitor for new, persistent severe pain, or neurologic deficit worrisome for MPNST |
| Head circumference (rapid increase may indicate tumor or hydrocephalus) | Refer adults of reproductive age for genetic counseling to discuss recurrence risks |

*Table 108-4 Molecular Genetic Testing*

| Gene | Testing Modality | Mutation Type | Detection Rate |
|------|------------------|---------------|----------------|
| NF1 | Multiple: genomic and cDNA sequencing, MLPA (multiplex ligation-dependent probe amplification) for exon deletion, fluorescent in situ hybridization (FISH) | Microdeletion, single/multiple exon deletion, missense, nonsense (stop), frame-shift | >95% |

# Molecular Genetics and Molecular Mechanism

*Syndrome/Gene/Locus:* *NF1* is a RAS-regulatory tumor suppressor gene located on chromosome 17q11.2. The protein product of NF1, neurofibromin, catalyzes the conversion of active RAS-GTP to inactive RAS-GDP. Many NF1-associated tumors feature biallelic inactivation of *NF1*, increased cellular levels of RAS-GTP, and dysregulated RAS-dependent cellular signaling.

*Genetic Testing:* Comprehensive mutation detection in *NF1* is clinically available but is costly given the large size of the gene and multiple mutation types. A mutation detection rate of greater than 95% has been reported (Table 108-4).

It is important to remember that a diagnosis of NF1 can generally be made based on history and physical examination. Genetic testing is useful in younger children with one diagnostic feature, in familial cases to facilitate preimplantation and/or prenatal diagnosis, and in atypical presentations.

## BIBLIOGRAPHY:

1. Maertens O, De Schepper S, Vandesompele J, et al. Molecular dissection of isolated disease features in mosaic neurofibromatosis type 1. *Am J Hum Genet.* Aug 2007;81(2):243-251.

2. Ferner RE. Neurofibromatosis 1 and neurofibromatosis 2: a twenty first century perspective. *Lancet Neurol.* Apr 2007;6(4):340-351.

3. Brems H, Chmara M, Sahbatou M, et al. Germline loss-of-function mutations in SPRED1 cause a neurofibromatosis 1-like phenotype. *Nat Genet.* Sep 2007;39(9):1120-1126.

4. Wimmer K, Etzler J. Constitutional mismatch repair-deficiency syndrome: have we so far seen only the tip of an iceberg? *Hum Genet.* Sep 2008;124(2):105-122.

5. Friedman JM. Evaluation and management. In: Friedman JM, Gutmann DH, MacCollin M, Riccardi V, eds. *Neurofibromatosis: Phenotype, Natural History, and Pathogenesis.* Baltimore: Johns Hopkins Press; 1999.

6. Ars E, Kruyer H, Gaona A, et al. A clinical variant of neurofibromatosis type 1: familial spinal neurofibromatosis with a frameshift mutation in the NF1 gene. *Am J Hum Genet.* Apr 1998;62(4):834-841.

7. Upadhyaya M, Huson SM, Davies M, et al. An absence of cutaneous neurofibromas associated with a 3-bp inframe deletion in exon 17 of the NF1 gene (c.2970-2972 delAAT): evidence of a clinically significant NF1 genotype-phenotype correlation. *Am J Hum Genet.* Jan 2007;80(1):140-151.

8. Neurofibromatosis. Conference statement. National Institutes of Health Consensus Development Conference. *Arch Neurol.* May 1988;45(5):575-578.

9. Gutmann DH, Aylsworth A, Carey JC, et al. The diagnostic evaluation and multidisciplinary management of neurofibromatosis 1 and neurofibromatosis 2. *JAMA.* Jul 2 1997;278(1):51-57.

10. Huson SM. The neurofibromatoses: classification, clinical features and genetic counseling. In: Kaufmann D, ed. *Neurofibromatoses.* Basel: Karger; 2008:1-21.

11. Sorensen SA, Mulvihill JJ, Nielsen A. Long-term follow-up of von Recklinghausen neurofibromatosis. Survival and malignant neoplasms. *N Engl J Med.* Apr 17 1986;314(16):1010-1015.

12. Brems H, Beert E, de Ravel T, Legius E. Mechanisms in the pathogenesis of malignant tumours in neurofibromatosis type 1. *Lancet Oncol.* May 2009;10(5):508-515.

13. Evans DG, O'Hara C, Wilding A, et al. Mortality in neurofibromatosis 1: in North West England: an assessment of actuarial survival in a region of the UK since 1989. *Eur J Hum Genet.* Nov 2011;19(11):1187-1191.

14. Sharif S, Moran A, Huson SM, et al. Women with neurofibromatosis 1 are at a moderately increased risk of developing breast cancer and should be considered for early screening. *J Med Genet.* Aug 2007;44(8):481-484.

15. Williams VC, Lucas J, Babcock MA, Gutmann DH, Korf B, Maria BL. Neurofibromatosis type 1 revisited. *Pediatrics.* Jan 2009;123(1):124-133.

16. Krab LC, de Goede-Bolder A, Aarsen FK, et al. Effect of simvastatin on cognitive functioning in children with neurofibromatosis type 1: a randomized controlled trial. *JAMA.* Jul 16 2008;300(3):287-294.

17. Page PZ, Page GP, Ecosse E, Korf BR, Leplege A, Wolkenstein P. Impact of neurofibromatosis 1 on quality of life: a cross-sectional study of 176 American cases. *Am J Med Genet A.* Sep 15 2006;140(18):1893-1898.

18. Radtke HB, Sebold CD, Allison C, Haidle JL, Schneider G. Neurofibromatosis type 1 in genetic counseling practice: recommendations of the National Society of Genetic Counselors. *J Genet Couns.* Aug 2007;16(4):387-407.

19. Tonsgard JH, Yelavarthi KK, Cushner S, Short MP, Lindgren V. Do NF1 gene deletions result in a characteristic phenotype? *Am J Med Genet.* Nov 28 1997;73(1):80-86.

20. Lenders JW, Eisenhofer G, Mannelli M, Pacak K. Phaeochromocytoma. *Lancet.* Aug 20-26 2005;366(9486):665-675.

21. Messiaen LM, Callens T, Mortier G, et al. Exhaustive mutation analysis of the NF1 gene allows identification of 95% of mutations and reveals a high frequency of unusual splicing defects. *Hum Mutat.* 2000;15(6):541-555.

# Supplementary Information

**OMIM REFERENCE:**

[1] Neurofibromatosis Type 1; NF1 (#162200)

**Alternative Names:**

- Neurofibromatosis
- von Recklinghausen Disease
- NF1 Microdeletion Syndrome

*Key Words:* Neurofibromin, neurofibroma, plexiform neurofibroma, café-au-lait macule, freckling, Lisch nodule, malignant peripheral nerve sheath tumor

# 109 Tuberous Sclerosis Complex

Darcy A. Krueger, Katie Wusik, David N. Franz, and Elizabeth K. Schorry

## KEY POINTS

- *Disease summary:*
  - Tuberous sclerosis complex (TSC) is a multiorgan disorder characterized by benign growths called hamartomas that can occur anywhere throughout the body. Hypopigmented macules, facial angiofibromas, shagreen patches, ungual fibromas, and dental pitting are characteristic of the disease. Central nervous system involvement is associated with highest morbidity and clinically manifests as epilepsy, learning disabilities or cognitive impairment, autism and other behavioral disorders, psychiatric disorders, and sleep abnormalities. The hallmarks of cerebral involvement are cortical tubers, subependymal nodules (SENs), and subependymal giant cell astrocytomas (SEGAs). Angiomyolipomas (AMLs) of the kidney, lymphangioleiomyomatosis (LAM) of the lung, and rhabdomyomas of the heart also cause significant morbidity.

- *Hereditary basis:*
  - TSC is an autosomal dominant genetic disorder with near 100% penetrance, but clinical severity is highly variable. It is genetically heterogeneous, with mutations in one of two genes (TSC1 or TSC2) causing the disorder. About one-third of cases are familial, the remainder is sporadic. Genetic mosaicism, including germline mosaicism, also exists. Genetic testing is available for affected individuals. Mutation in either gene (*TSC1*, *TSC2*) is detected in 85% of cases.

- *Differential diagnosis:*
  - The combination of multiple features of TSC is rarely mistaken for other disorders. However, individual features may overlap with those of other syndromes. Hypopigmented macules (ash leaf macules) can occur from many different etiologies; vitiligo, piebaldism, hypomelanosis of Ito, and incontinentia pigmenti are among the differential diagnosis. Renal AMLs and pulmonary LAM can occur sporadically but certainly occur in high association with TSC. Cortical migration defects can occur as an isolated, idiopathic finding unrelated to TSC. Other neurocutaneous disorders, such as neurofibromatosis 1 or 2, have distinct skin manifestations and tumor types which should not be mistaken for TSC.

- *Management:*
  - Treatment with the mammalian target of rapamycin (mTOR) inhibitors such as sirolimus and everolimus results in significant shrinking of SEGAs and renal AMLs, and can be an alternative to surgery in some cases. Benefit in lung disease (LAM) has also been demonstrated. Additional studies are ongoing to determine their efficacy for epilepsy and neurocognition in TSC.

## Diagnostic Criteria and Clinical Characteristics

**Diagnostic Criteria\*:**

Clinically definite tuberous sclerosis: two major or one major + two minor features

Clinically probable tuberous sclerosis: one major + one minor feature

Clinically possible tuberous sclerosis: one major or two minor features

\*Genetic confirmation of known disease-causing mutation in either *TSC1* or *TSC2* gene is also considered sufficient for confirmed diagnosis of TSC. However, failure to identify a disease-causing mutation in *TSC1* or *TSC2* does not exclude the diagnosis if clinical criteria are met.

**Clinical Characteristics:** Any organ system can be affected in patients with tuberous sclerosis, with central nervous system, skin, kidney, lung, and heart being most common. Many of the features are age dependent.

☞**CENTRAL NERVOUS SYSTEM:** Cortical and subcortical tubers are essentially migration defects occurring in utero and are the hallmark of tuberous sclerosis. SENs are also characteristic and in 15% to 20% of affected individuals can exhibit spontaneous growth in childhood or early adulthood. While benign, these

| Major features | Minor features |
|---|---|
| 1. Cortical tubers | 1. Dental enamel pits |
| 2. Subependymal nodules | 2. Hamartomatous rectal polyps |
| 3. Subependymal giant cell astrocytomas | 3. Bone cysts |
| 4. Hypomelanotic macules (3 or more) | 4. Cerebral white matter radial migration |
| 5. Shagreen patch lines | |
| 6. Facial angiofibromas or forehead plaque | 5. Gingival fibromas |
| 7. Multiple retinal nodular hamartomas | 6. Nonrenal hamartoma |
| 8. Nontraumatic ungual or periungual fibromas | 7. Retinal achromatic patches |
| 9. Cardiac rhabdomyoma | 8. "Confetti" skin lesions |
| 10. Pulmonary LAM and/or renal angiomyolipomas | 9. Multiple renal cysts |

SEGAs can impede central spinal fluid flow through the foramen of Monro, leading to hydrocephalus. Seizures occur in more than 90% of patients, often presenting during infancy as infantile spasms. In adulthood, partial motor and complex partial seizures that often generalize are typical and can be difficult to manage with conventional anticonvulsant therapies. Learning difficulties and cognitive impairment are present in the majority of patients, although many can have normal IQ. Obsessive-compulsive behaviors, anxiety, mood disorders, aggressive behaviors, autism, and sleep disorders also frequently are associated with tuberous sclerosis.

☞**SKIN:** Hypopigmented macules are present at birth but may be more noticeable as patients get older. Likewise connective tissue nevus (shagreen patch) may not be visible initially. Facial angiofibromas (adenoma sebaceum) usually appear by mid- or late-childhood and can continue to grow or accumulate during adulthood. Ungual fibromas can affect hands or feet and are most likely to appear during adolescence or as early adults. Dental pitting is nearly universally present in all adults with TSC.

☞**KIDNEY:** AMLs are discrete lesions containing fat, smooth muscle, and abnormal blood vessels and may appear as small lesions scattered throughout the kidneys or as larger, isolated lesions. Significant risk of hemorrhage (Wunderlich syndrome) is associated with AMLs greater than 4 to 6 cm in diameter. Lesions are also associated with renal hypertension and renal insufficiency or failure. Renal cysts, including polycystic kidney disease, can be associated with TSC, especially if a large deletion of 16p is present such that both *TSC2* and *PKD1* gene loci are affected. Renal cell carcinoma can occur, but is very rare.

☞**LUNG:** A rare but potentially fatal progressively destructive pulmonary disease known as LAM can affect up to 40% of female patients of childbearing age with TSC. It is rare for pediatric female or adult male patients to develop LAM, but cases do occur. Clinically, patients can present with progressive dyspnea on exertion, chylothorax, and pneumothorax.

☞**HEART:** Rhabdomyomas, benign growths arising from the cardiac chambers, may be diagnosed prenatally by fetal magnetic resonance imaging (MRI) or ultrasound. The majority will regress spontaneously within the first or second year of life, but it is not unusual for some to persist throughout adulthood. Disruption of conduction pathways may also result, leading to arrhythmias or other abnormalities noted on electrocardiography.

☞**OTHER ORGANS:** Extrarenal and pulmonary hamartomas can occur in any organ, including the eye, liver, uterus, and thyroid. Bone cysts, gingival and dermal fibromas also occur.

## Screening and Counseling

*Counseling:* TSC is inherited in an autosomal dominant fashion. Each child of an affected parent has a 50% risk of inheriting the condition. Variable expressivity is observed, even among family members with the same mutation. Therefore, it is not possible to predict the severity of symptoms in offspring.

Two-thirds of individuals with TSC have the condition as a result of a de novo mutation. Siblings of individuals with a confirmed de novo mutation have a mildly increased risk (~2%) of having TSC due to germline mosaicism.

☞**PENETRANCE:** With thorough clinical examination including physical, ophthalmologic, and dermatologic examinations, and appropriate imaging studies including computed tomography (CT) or MRI of the brain and ultrasound of the kidneys, penetrance of TSC is thought to be close to 100% in adulthood.

☞**GENOTYPE-PHENOTYPE CORRELATION:** *TSC1* and *TSC2* mutations occur with equal frequency in familial cases; however,

in sporadic cases and in the overall TSC clinic population, *TSC2* is much more common by a 4:1 ratio. As a group, individuals with mutations in *TSC2* can have more severe disease than those with mutations in *TSC1*; however, the full spectrum of expression can be seen with either *TSC1* or *TSC2* mutations. Greater degree of cognitive impairment and increased numbers of hypomelanotic macules, renal AML, facial angiofibromas, and cortical tubers are seen in individuals with *TSC2* mutations. A small subset of patients (2%-3%) will have a large deletion of *TSC2* which also includes *PKD1*. These deletions result in a combined phenotype of polycystic kidney disease and TSC.

## Management and Treatment

*Epilepsy:* Recognition of seizures and aggressive management with anticonvulsants by a neurology specialist is tantamount, as uncontrolled epilepsy in patients with TSC is associated with increased risk of permanent neurocognitive and neurobehavioral decline. Ketogenic diet, vagus nerve stimulation, and/or epilepsy surgery should be considered for patients when medical management fails.

*Subependymal Giant Cell Astrocytomas:* MRI of the brain should be performed every 1 to 2 years in asymptomatic patients. Evidence of interval growth of subependymal lesions on serial imaging is sufficient for diagnosis of giant cell astrocytoma. Symptomatic patients should be imaged more frequently. Referral to neurosurgeon for evaluation and surgical planning is appropriate, especially for large or rapidly growing lesions and for patients with symptoms due to accompanying hydrocephalus (ventricle enlargement, headache, nausea/vomiting, tremor, vision disturbances, ataxia, or unexplained behavior or changes in activity). The deep location is problematic for surgical removal, as lesions incompletely resected will invariably recur. Treatment with mTOR inhibitors (ie, sirolimus, everolimus) has emerged as an alternative to surgery for many patients.

*Psychiatric Disorders:* Bipolar disorder, anxiety, attention-deficit hyperactive disorder, and obsessive-compulsive behaviors are often overlooked and a high degree of suspicion is needed. Treatment with selective serotonin receptor inhibitors (fluoxetine, escitalopram) is often helpful for these disorders. Aggressive behaviors, especially when associated with autism or cognitive impairment, can benefit from treatment with atypical antipsychotics (ie, risperidone, quetiapine), mood stabilizers (lithium, valproic acid, lamotrigine), and central-acting antiadrenergic medications (ie, clonidine, guanfacine). Sleep difficulties are often amenable to melatonin or anticholinergics (ie, amitriptyline, trazodone).

*Angiomyolipomas:* Patients should be routinely screened and treated for hypertension, which can aggravate underlying renal dysfunction. Annual renal ultrasound or abdominal MRI should be performed to ensure no sudden change or abnormal growth in AMLs. Excision or biopsy should be avoided in order to preserve best residual renal function. AMLs larger than 4 to 6 cm in diameter have increased risk of hemorrhage and should be treated with minimally invasive procedures such as selective arterial embolization or focal cryotherapy. Treatment with mTOR inhibitors can significantly reduce AML size and presumably decrease risk of spontaneous hemorrhage.

*Lymphangioleiomyomatosis:* High-resolution chest CT without contrast should be performed at baseline in all postpubertal females with TSC, and every 3 years thereafter if asymptomatic. Symptomatic patients should undergo imaging more frequently,

*Table 109-1* **Screening in TSC**

| Screening Test | Frequency |
|---|---|
| MRI of the brain | Every 1-2 years in asymptomatic patients. More frequent screening in symptomatic patients. |
| EEG | At least once in any patient with clinical seizures, cognitive impairment, or altered mental status. Does not have to be repeated on a scheduled basis, only as often as clinically indicated. |
| Renal ultrasound or abdominal MRI | Annually. |
| High-resolution lung CT scan without contrast | Baseline in all postpubertal females. Every 3 years in asymptomatic patients. More frequent screening in symptomatic patients. |
| Pulmonary function test (PFT) | At least annually in postpubertal females. |
| Molecular testing | If needed for diagnosis or for evaluation of family members. |

depending on the severity of disease, as well as pulmonary function testing at least annually. Lung biopsy is no longer necessary in patients with known TSC or AML. Remainder of treatment is generally supportive, including supplement oxygen and bronchodilator therapy. High-dose estrogen (oral contraceptives or hormone replacement therapy) is thought to contribute to disease pathogenesis and should be avoided. Pleural fusion using mechanical abrasion is recommended for patients with pneumothorax. Early clinical trials suggest LAM disease progression is slowed by treatment with mTOR inhibitors.

***Facial Angiofibromas and Ungual Fibromas:*** Lesions are benign but can be associated with bleeding, discomfort, or significant cosmetic concerns. Referral to dermatologic specialist for dermal abrasion or laser therapy treatment of fibromas is appropriate, although benefit tends to wear off over time and requires periodic repeating. Similarly, treatment of bleeding or pain/discomfort from larger lesions can be excised surgically. A summary of recommended screening for individuals with TSC can be found in Table 109-1.

# Molecular Genetics and Molecular Mechanism

***Syndrome/Gene/Locus:***
TSC/hamartin (*TSC1*)/9q34
TSC/tuberin (TSC2)/16p13.3

Hamartin and tuberin form a heterodimer which inhibits the mTOR complex via a GTPase-activating protein, Rheb. mTOR is a master switch for cell growth and protein synthesis. Individuals with TSC have a constitutional *TSC1* or *TSC2* mutation. A second hit at the allele with the constitutional mutation, causing loss of heterozygosity, drives Rheb into a GTP-bound state, resulting in activation of mTOR. The gene acts as a tumor suppressor, and loss of heterozygosity (LOH) is necessary for formation of some TSC lesions. LOH, primarily of *TSC2*, has been demonstrated in the majority of renal AMLs, and cardiac rhabdomyomas studied, but only rarely in pulmonary LAM lesions, cortical tubers, or SNEs. This implies differing pathogenesis for some types of TSC lesions.

***Genetic Testing:*** DNA sequence analysis and MLPA analysis are clinically available for *TSC1* and *TSC2* (see Gene Tests http://www.ncbi.nlm.nih.gov/sites/GeneTests/lab?db=GeneTests). See Table 109-2. Current clinical testing has a sensitivity of 80% to 85% for detecting a mutation in those with a known diagnosis of TSC. Identification of a pathogenic mutation in an individual with a probable or possible diagnosis of TSC (those who meet some but not all of the diagnostic criteria) would confirm his or her diagnosis. Negative test results would not exclude a diagnosis of TSC. Identification of a mutation in a known affected individual confirms the diagnosis of TSC but does not currently affect management. Knowledge of an affected individual's mutation would permit (1) prenatal and/or preconception testing to be performed, (2) family members (parents, siblings, children, etc) to have testing to learn their disease status and information about their recurrence risk. Prenatal diagnosis is available either by amniocentesis or chorionic villous sampling when there is a known parental mutation. Preimplantation genetic diagnosis (PGD) is possible, but has been rarely utilized.

Fifteen to twenty percent of individuals with TSC do not have an identifiable mutation in *TSC1* or *TSC2*. Many of those with no identifiable mutation may have somatic mosaicism undetectable with current methodology. Of those with mutations, approximately 65% to 80% have *TSC2* mutations and 20% to 35% have *TSC1* mutations. *TSC2* mutations can be of many different types, including truncating mutations, missense mutations, and large deletions. Almost all pathogenic deletions of *TSC1* are truncating mutations.

*Table 109-2* **Molecular Genetic Testing**

| Gene | Testing Modality | Mutation Type | Mutation Frequency |
|---|---|---|---|
| *TSC1* | Sequencing | Small deletions, insertions, nonsense | <25% |
| *TSC1* | MLPA | Large deletion/duplication | Rare |
| *TSC2* | Sequencing | Small deletions, insertions, nonsense, missense | 47%-55% |
| *TSC2* | MLPA | Large deletion/duplication (including contiguous gene deletion of *TSC2* and *PKD1*) | 10%-18% (2%-3%) |
| No mutation | | | 15%-20% |

**BIBLIOGRAPHY:**

1. Goh S, Butler W, Thiele E. Subependymal giant cell tumors in tuberous sclerosis complex. *Neurology.* 2004;63(8):1457-1461.

2. Krueger D, Franz D. Current management of tuberous sclerosis complex. *Paediatr Drugs.* 2008;10(5):299-313.

3. Prather P, de Vries P. Behavioral and cognitive aspects of tuberous sclerosis complex. *J Child Neurol.* 2004;19(9):666-674.

4. Yamakado K, Tanaka N, Nakagawa T, Kobayashi S, Yanagawa M, Takeda K. Renal angiomyolipoma: relationships between tumor size, aneurysm formation, and rupture. *Radiology.* 2002;225(1):78-82.

5. Moss J, Avila NA, Barnes PM, et al. Prevalence and clinical characteristics of lymphangioleiomyomatosis (LAM) in patients with tuberous sclerosis complex. *Am J Respir Crit Care Med.* 2001;164(4):669-671.

6. McCormack F. Lymphangioleiomyomatosis. *Med Gen Med.* 2007;8(1):15.

7. Cheadle J. Reeve MP, Sampson JR, Kwiatkowski DJ. Molecular genetic advances in tuberous sclerosis. *Hum Genet.* 2000;107(2):97-114.

8. Roach E, Sparagana S. Diagnosis of tuberous sclerosis complex. *J Child Neurol.* 2004;19(9):643-649.

9. Osborne J, Jones AC, Burley MW, et al. Non-penetrance in tuberous sclerosis. *Lancet.* 2000;355(9216):1698.

10. Au K, Williams AT, Roach ES, et al. Genotype/phenotype correlation in 325 individuals referred for a diagnosis of tuberous sclerosis complex in the United States. *Genet Med.* 2007;9(2):88-100.

11. Dabora S, Jozwiak S, Franz DN, et al. Mutational analysis in a cohort of 224 tuberous sclerosis patients indicates increased severity of TSC2, compared with TSC1, disease in multiple organs. *Am J Hum Genet.* 2001;68(1):64-80.

12. Crino P, Nathanson K, Henske E. The tuberous sclerosis complex. *N Engl J Med.* 2006;355(13):1345-1356.

13. Jozwiak S, Goodman M, Lamm S. Poor mental development in patients with tuberous sclerosis complex: clinical risk factors. *Arch Neurol.* 1998;55(3):379-384.

14. Franz DN, Leonard J, Tudor C, et al. Rapamycin causes regression of astrocytomas in tuberous sclerosis complex. *Ann Neurol.* 2006;59:490-498.

15. Krueger D, Care MM, Holland K, et al. Everolimus for supependymal giant-cell astrocytomas in tuberous sclerosis complex. *N Engl J Med.* 2010;363:1801-1811.

16. Williams J, Racadio JM, Johnson ND, Donnelly LF, Bissler JJ. Embolization of renal angiomyolipomata in patients with tuberous sclerosis complex. *Am J Kidney Dis.* 2006;47(1):95-102.

17. Bissler J, McCormack FX, Young LR, et al. Sirolimus for angiomyolipomata in tuberous sclerosis or lymphangioleiomyomatosis. *N Engl J Med.* 2008;358(2):140-151.

18. McCormack F, Inoue Y, Moss J, et al. Efficacy and safety of sirolimus in lymphangioleiomyomatosis. *N Engl J Med.* 2011;364(17):1595-1606.

19. Bittencourt RC, Huilgol SC, Seed PT, Calonje E, Markey AC, Barlow RJ. Treatment of angiofibromas with a scanning carbon dioxide laser: a clinicopathologic study with long-term follow-up. *J Am Acad Determatol.* 2001;45(5):731-735.

20. Henske E, Scheithauer BW, Short MP, et al. Allelic loss is frequent in tuberous sclerosis kidney lesions but rare in brain lesions. *Am J Hum Genet.* 1996;59(2):400-406.

21. Niida Y, Stemmer-Rachamimov AO, Logrip M, et al. Survey of somatic mutations in tuberous sclerosis complex (TSC) hamartomas suggests different genetic mechanisms for pathogenesis of TSC lesions. *Am J Hum Genet.* 2001;69(3):493-503.

22. Rendtorff N, Bjerregaard B, Frödin M, et al. Analysis of 65 tuberous sclerosis complex (TSC) patients by TSC2 DGGE, TSC1/TSC2 MLPA, and TSC1 long-range PCR sequencing, and report of 28 novel mutations. *Hum Mutat.* 2005;26(4):374-383.

## Supplementary Information

**OMIM REFERENCES:**

[1] Tuberous Sclerosis; TS (#191100)

[2] Polycystic Kidney Disease, Infantile Severe, With Tuberous Sclerosis; PKDTS (#600273)

[3] Multiple Endocrine Neoplasia Type I; MEN1 (#131100)

[4] Lymphangioleiomyomatosis; LAM (#606690)

[5] Focal Cortical Dysplasia of Taylor; FCDT (#607341)

[6] Polycystic Kidney Disease 1; PKD1 (#601313)

[7] Polycystic Kidneys; PKD (#173900)

**Alternative Names:**

- Tuberous Sclerosis
- Tuberous Sclerosis Complex

***Key Words:*** Angiofibromas (adenoma sebaceum), angiomyolipomas, ash leaf macule, cortical tuber, subependymal nodule, SEGA, cardiac rhabdomyoma, lymphangioleiomyomatosis, periungual fibromas, seizures, autism

# 110 Epidermolysis Bullosa

Benjamin S. Daniel and Dedee F. Murrell

## KEY POINTS

- *Disease summary:*
  - Inherited epidermolysis bullosa (EB) is a heterogenous group of genodermatoses characterized by blisters and erosions after minimal trauma. There are four main types of EB, namely epidermolysis bullosa simplex (EBS), junctional epidermolysis bullosa (JEB), dystrophic epidermolysis bullosa (DEB), and mixed Kindler syndrome. Diagnosis is made by a combination of electron microscopy (EM) and immunofluorescence findings. Management consists of avoiding trauma and preventing complications. In lethal cases, supportive measures are instituted as well as providing emotional and financial support for families or carers.
- *Hereditary basis:*
  - Autosomal recessive and autosomal dominant
- *Differential diagnosis:*
  - Bullous pemphigoid, pemphigus vulgaris, linear IgA disease, arthropod bites, bullous lupus erythematosus, epidermolysis bullosa acquisita

## Diagnostic Criteria and Clinical Characteristics

*Epidermolysis Bullosa Simplex:* EBS is inherited in an autosomal dominant fashion with prevalence between 6 and 30 per 1 million live births. The actual prevalence may be higher than this as there are many patients who are undiagnosed. It is the most common type of EB but the least severe. It accounts for about 50% to 85% of all EB cases. The age of onset ranges between birth and the third decade of life.

In the majority of cases, fragility of the keratinocytes results in blister formation in the basal cell layer of the epidermis. It is distinguished from suprabasal EBS in which blisters form in the suprabasal levels. Most cases are due to missense mutations of keratin 14 and 5 which is important for the structural integrity of epidermal keratinocytes. Other genes implicated in EBS include plectin, plakophilin1, desmoplakin, and alpha-6 beta-4 (α6β4) integrin, see Table 110-1.

### ☞CLINICAL MANIFESTATIONS:

- Erosions and blistering with minimal trauma or friction which usually heal without scarring, though hyperpigmentation can occur. EBS usually improves with age.
- Complications include pain, infections, malnutrition, anemia, fluid and electrolyte imbalance, and an increased risk of skin cancer if severe EBS.
- There are many clinical variants of EBS including localised EBS, EBS generalized (Dowling Meara), EBS generalized (non-Dowling Meara), EBS with muscular dystrophy, EBS with mottled pigmentation, and EBS with pyloric atresia, see Table 110-2.

### ☞DIAGNOSIS:

- Light and electron microscopy: demonstrates blister formation in the basal cell layer of the epidermis.
- Antigen epitope mapping: demonstrates the level of separation and hence the type of EB.
- Immunohistochemistry: shows an absence of keratin intermediate filaments.
- Molecular diagnosis: screen for mutations in keratins 5 and 14. Mutations in other genes such as *PLEC1*, *DSP*, *Col17A1*, and *ITGB4* can be investigated.

### ☞TREATMENT:

- Prevention of blisters
- Adequate footwear
- Dressings and wound care
- Adequate nutrition
- Emotional, psychologic, and financial support

*Junctional Epidermolysis Bullosa:* JEB is an autosomal recessive condition characterized by separation between the lamina lucida and lamina densa in the dermal-epidermal junction. There are three main subtypes of JEB. JEB-Herlitz type (HJEB) is a lethal blistering disease with a poor life expectancy. Patients often develop blisters within 1 week of birth and die by the age of 2 years. Sepsis, severe blistering, and respiratory failure are the main causes of death. Laminin 332 is an anchoring filament protein that has been implicated in HJEB. It consists of three subunits (alpha-3, beta-3, and gamma-2) which are coded by *LAMA3*, *LAMB3*, and *LAMC2* genes, respectively. One or more mutations in any of these genes result in an absence of laminin 332 and hence HJEB. There are at least 35 mutations in the *LAMB3* gene. The most commonly reported are *R635X* and *R42X* mutations. Though diagnosis is often made after birth, technologic advances have facilitated prenatal diagnosis of HJEB. Management of HJEB is predominantly supportive, with palliative and preventative measures typically instituted soon after diagnosis.

Non-Herlitz JEB (nH-JEB) is due to laminin 332 and/or collagen XVII abnormalities. Mutations are usually nonsense, missense, insertions, or deletions. Patients present with blisters at or soon after birth and have mucosal involvement, nail changes, and alopecia. Healing with scarring and pigment change is common. Though risk of death is high in infancy, nH-JEB is less severe than HJEB and complications are less.

Genes affected in nH-JEB are *COL17A1*, *LAMA3*, *LAMB3*, and *LAMC2*.

EM and immunofluorescence epitope mapping (IFM) findings

- Skin cleavage within the lamina lucida of the dermal-epidermal junction
- Reduced number and size of hemidesmosomes
- Absence of type XVII collagen or laminin332

*Table 110-1  Genes Affected in Epidermolysis Bullosa*

| EB Type | Protein | Target Gene |
|---|---|---|
| EBS | Plakophilin-1 | *PKP1* |
| | Desmoplakin | *DSP* |
| | Keratin 5 | *KRT5* |
| | Keratin 14 | *KRT14* |
| | Plectin | *PLEC1* |
| JEB | Laminin-332 | *LAMA3, LAMB3, LAMC2* |
| | Type XVII collagen | *COL17A1* |
| | α6β4 integrin | *ITGA6, ITGB4* |
| DEB | Type VII collagen | *COL7A1* |
| Kindler syndrome | Fermitin family homologue 1 (Kindlin-1) | *FERMT1 (KIND1)* |

Management is aimed at preventing blisters, promoting wound healing with appropriate dressings, and adequately dealing with complications as they arise.

***Dystrophic Epidermolysis Bullosa:*** DEB accounts for about 40% of EB. It is due to mutations in the gene *COL7A1* which encodes type VII collagen. There are five subtypes of DEB classified according to the inheritance pattern. Both males and females are equally affected. Skin cleavage occurs in the sublamina densa and is associated with reduced or absent numbers of anchoring fibrils.

Severe generalized recessive DEB was previously referred to as Hallopeau-Siemens type. Blistering typically begins at birth and can affect all surfaces especially the bony prominences. Severe scarring occurs on all cutaneous surfaces. Scarring involving the hands and feet results in mitten deformities and contractures which often requires surgical intervention. Patients with recessive dystrophic epidermolysis bullosa (RDEB) often have a reduced life expectancy, with metastatic squamous cell carcinoma (not sun-related) and renal

*Table 110-2  Epidermolysis Bullosa Types and Subtypes*

| | |
|---|---|
| Epidermolysis bullosa simplex (EBS) | Localised EBS |
| | EBS Dowling Meara |
| | EBS generalized (Non-Dowling Meara) |
| | EBS with pyloric atresia |
| | EBS with muscular dystrophy |
| | EBS autosomal recessive |
| | EBS lethal acatholytic |
| Junctional epidermolysis bullosa (JEB) | JEB-Herlitz type |
| | JEB–non-Herlitz type |
| | JEB with pyloric atresia |
| Dystrophic epidermolysis bullosa (DEB) | DDEB generalized |
| | DDEB bullous dermolysis of the newborn |
| | RDEB severe generalized |
| | RDEB generalized other |
| | RDEB bullous dermolysis of the newborn |

failure the main causes of death. Extracutaneous complications involve the nails (dystrophic or absent nails which usually starts in childhood and may progress to permanent anonychia), hair (scarring alopecia), gastrointestinal (oesophageal strictures, anal fissures), renal (chronic renal impairment), and teeth (caries, dystrophic teeth).

*Recessive DEB-other* is similar to *severe generalized recessive DEB* except for less severe blistering and scarring. In dominant DEB (DDEB), blistering is mild and patients have less complications compared to patients with the recessive disease. Nail and hair abnormalities are common in DDEB. Unlike EBS, patients develop severe scarring which can cause significant pain requiring analgesia and dressings.

☞**DIAGNOSIS:** EM: reveals structurally abnormal anchoring fibrils. The number of anchoring fibrils may be reduced or absent.

☞**MOLECULAR DIAGNOSIS:**
- Collagen VII abnormality
- Mutation of *COL7A1*—the gene responsible for collagen VII

Management of DEB consists of preventing mechanical trauma and blister formation, providing dressings, and preventing complications. Monitoring of blood tests and multidisciplinary team involvement has shown to be useful in patients with RDEB.

***Kindler Syndrome:*** Kindler syndrome is an autosomal recessive mechanobullous disorder characterized by congenital blistering predominantly in acral areas followed by progressive skin atrophy and poikiloderma. Photosensitivity and mucosal inflammation are also common.

Kindler syndrome is due to mutations in the gene *FERMT1* which encodes the adhesion protein fermitin family homolog 1 (*FFH1*). *FFH1* is found near the dermal-epidermal junction and is responsible for signalling and interactions between the actin cytoskeletal system and the extracellular matrix.

Management consists of preventing complications such as anemia, strictures, and dental abnormalities (eg, gingivitis). Patients should be advised to avoid excess sunlight exposure to prevent photosensitive reactions and have regular skin checks. Kindler syndrome is associated with an increased risk of nonmelanoma skin cancers.

## Screening and Counseling

Diagnosis of EB is made by transmission EM and IFM on a freshly induced blister. EM and IFM determine the level of skin affected, while identifying structural abnormalities and changes in protein numbers.

Molecular testing in EB should be performed after EM and IFM have been performed to narrow down the candidate gene. DNA is predominantly obtained from the patient's blood, though buccal swabs and skin biopsies are sometimes used. The sensitivity of molecular testing varies depending on the subtype of EB, the gene involved, and the screening technique. Before molecular testing is performed, detailed discussion with the patient's relatives is recommended. The results can significantly impact relationships and influence reproductive decision making. Because some subtypes of EB are lethal and have severe complications (eg, JEB-Herlitz type and RDEB), prenatal diagnosis and genetic counseling have been employed. More accurate prenatal diagnostic tests have become available with improved technology and are usually used in high-risk cases. Currently chorionic villus and amniotic fluid sampling are used to collect foetal DNA between weeks 10 and 12 gestation or at 15 to 16 weeks, respectively. Because termination of pregnancy can be a distressing and/or moral issue for some couples, preimplantation genetic diagnosis is an alternative in which unaffected embryos are implanted into the uterus. This procedure, however, is not widely available, may not result in a viable pregnancy, and is associated with complications.

## Management and Treatment

Management of EB is aimed at prevention rather than cure. It is about providing support (emotional, financial, and social) and medical care for the patients and their families. Preventing trauma-induced blisters, wound infections, and complications such as anemia, esophageal strictures, dental abnormalities, and malnutrition is the key. Pain control, appropriate dressings, and skin checks are also important. Some types of EB are associated with an increased risk of skin cancers (especially aggressive squamous cell carcinomas), so regular skin checks are recommended.

Patient support groups and financial support for dressings reduce the burden on carers.

### BIBLIOGRAPHY:

1. Fine JD, Eady RA, Bauer EA, et al. The classification of inherited epidermolysis bullosa (EB): report of the Third International Consensus Meeting on Diagnosis and Classification of EB. *J Am Acad Dermatol*. 2008;58(6):931-950.
2. Sprecher E. Epidermolysis bullosa simplex. *Dermatol Clin*. 2010;28(1):23-32.
3. Bruckner-Tuderman L. Dystrophic epidermolysis bullosa: pathogenesis and clinical features. *Dermatol Clin*. 2010;28(1):107-114.
4. Lai-Cheong JE, McGrath JA. Kindler syndrome. *Dermatol Clin*. 2010;28(1):119-124.
5. Tosti A, de Farias DC, Murrell DF. Nail involvement in epidermolysis bullosa. *Dermatol Clin*. 2010;28(1):153-157.
6. Tosti A, Duque-Estrada B, Murrell DF. Alopecia in epidermolysis bullosa. *Dermatol Clin*. 2010;28(1):165-169.
7. Castiglia D, Zambruno G. Molecular testing in epidermolysis bullosa. *Dermatol Clin*. 2010;28(2):223-229, vii-viii.
8. Fassihi H, McGrath JA. Prenatal diagnosis of epidermolysis bullosa. *Dermatol Clin*. 2010;28(2):231-237, viii.
9. Sybert VP. Genetic counseling in epidermolysis bullosa. *Dermatol Clin*. 2010;28(2):239-243, viii.

## Supplementary Information

### OMIM REFERENCES:

[1] Epidermolysis Bullosa Simplex, Localized (#131800)
[2] Epidermolysis Bullosa Simplex, Dowling-Meara Type (#131760)
[3] Epidermolysis Bullosa Simplex, Generalized (#131900)
[4] Epidermolysis Bullosa Simplex With Pyloric Atresia (#612138)
[5] Epidermolysis Bullosa Simplex With Muscular Dystrophy (#226670)
[6] Epidermolysis Bullosa Simplex, Autosomal Recessive (#601001)
[7] Junctional Epidermolysis Bullosa, Non-Herlitz Type (#226650)
[8] Junctional Epidermolysis Bullosa, Herlitz Type (#226700)
[9] Junctional Epidermolysis Bullosa With Pyloric Atresia (#226730)
[10] Epidermolysis Bullosa Dystrophica, Autosomal Recessive; RDEB (#226600)
[11] Epidermolysis Bullosa Dystrophica, Autosomal Dominant; DDEB (#131750)
[12] Kindler Syndrome (#173650)

*Key Words:* Epidermolysis bullosa, epidermolysis bullosa simplex, junctional epidermolysis bullosa, dystrophic epidermolysis bullosa, dominant dystrophic epidermolysis bullosa, recessive dystrophic epidermolysis bullosa

# 111 Atopic Dermatitis

Sara J. Brown and W. H. Irwin McLean

## KEY POINTS

- *Disease summary:*
  - Atopic dermatitis (AD) is a complex trait, resulting from the interaction of multiple genetic and environmental factors.
  - The specific clinicopathologic definition of "atopic" dermatitis is debated; however, atopic dermatitis, synonymous with atopic eczema, is characterized by elevated levels of circulating IgE and coassociation with the other atopic disorders, asthma, allergic rhinitis, and food allergies.
  - AD is an itchy inflammatory skin disease that follows a chronic relapsing and remitting course. It usually begins in childhood and approximately 90% of cases resolve before adulthood. Diagnosis is based on clinical features (Table 111-1).
  - Moderate-to-severe AD is associated with significant morbidity as a result of pruritus and sleep deprivation. There is an associated reduction in quality of life of the affected child and their close family which is similar in severity to type I diabetes.

- *Differential diagnosis:*
  - Irritant dermatitis, allergic contact dermatitis, seborrheic dermatitis, impetigo (*Staphylococcus aureus* infection) and scabies; severe congenital immunodeficiency and Netherton syndrome may also present as a widespread eczematous rash with failure to thrive

- *Monogenic forms:*
  - No monogenic form of AD is known to exist, however, common loss-of-function mutations in the gene encoding the skin barrier protein filaggrin (*FLG*) cause the dry scaly skin condition ichthyosis vulgaris and approximately 70% of ichthyosis vulgaris cases have AD.

- *Family history:*
  - Atopic diseases show strong familial clustering, but a child whose parents have AD is more likely to develop AD than a child whose parents have asthma or allergic rhinitis, suggesting that skin-specific genes may influence phenotype.

- *Twin studies:*
  - Monozygotic twins have a 70% to 80% concordance rate for AD, compared to approximately 20% in dizygotic twins.

- *Environmental factors:*
  - The prevalence of AD has risen dramatically over the past 20 to 30 years, illustrating the importance of environmental effects, but the key environmental factors remain to be defined. The "hygiene hypothesis" proposes that lack of early life exposure to infectious agents has increased the prevalence of atopic disease.

- *Candidate gene studies:*
  - Many different candidate genes have been investigated for association with AD because of their biologic roles in systemic atopic inflammation, cutaneous inflammation, or skin barrier function (Table 111-2). A Few have been replicated in independent studies, most notably *FLG*, the gene encoding the skin barrier protein filaggrin, in which loss-of-function mutations increase AD risk (odds ratio ~4).

- *Genome-wide associations:*
  - Two independent genome-wide association studies have been published to date. Some disease-associated genetic variants (single-nucleotide polymorphisms [SNPs]) provide insight into disease pathogenesis but testing for SNPs is not yet clinically validated to diagnose or guide management of AD.

- *Pharmacogenomics:*
  - Carriage of one or more loss-of-function mutations in *FLG* increases the risk of severe and persistent AD. Testing for common thiopurine methyltransferase (*TPMT*) variants to guide the choice of azathioprine dose has proven validity in AD.

## Diagnostic Criteria and Clinical Characteristics

***Diagnostic Criteria for AD:*** There are various sets of diagnostic criteria which may be used in research studies; however, the most widely validated clinical diagnostic criteria are the UK Working Party's diagnostic criteria, a refinement of the more complex Hanifin and Rajka diagnostic criteria.

***Clinical Characteristics of AD:*** AD is an itchy inflammatory skin condition which follows a chronic, relapsing, and remitting course. There is a characteristic epidermal barrier dysfunction which is widespread and has been demonstrated in nonlesional as well as lesional skin.

Clinical examination reveals

- Ill-defined areas of redness (erythema) and scaling
- Excoriations
- Acute phase vesiculation, crusting, and weeping
- In the chronic phase lichenification (skin thickening) may predominate

AD is predominantly a pediatric disorder; the majority of cases begin in infancy or early childhood and 90% resolve before adolescence. A minority of cases show adult-onset but

*Table 111-1* **The UK Working Party's Diagnostic Criteria for Atopic Dermatitis**

For the clinical diagnosis of AD, an individual must have

- An itchy skin condition in the last 12 months
- Plus three or more of the following:
  1. Onset before the age of 2 years (not applicable in a child under 4 years)
  2. History of flexural involvement
  3. History of generally dry skin
  4. Personal history of other atopic disease (asthma or allergic rhinitis), or history in first-degree relative if the child is under 4 years
  5. Visible flexural dermatitis

recurrence of AD in adulthood after childhood AD has resolved is not uncommon.

AD lesions may occur anywhere on the skin surface, but the distribution tends to vary with age. Infantile AD characteristically affects the facial skin whereas later in childhood the flexural skin of the limbs and neck are predominantly affected. Hand eczema may be particularly problematic in adulthood if there are occupational or environmental irritants to the hand skin.

Generalized xerosis (dry skin) or ichthyosis (scaling skin) is a hallmark of AD; ichthyosis vulgaris, palmar hyperlinearity, and keratosis pilaris are clinical signs indicating the presence of *FLG* loss-of-function mutations which strongly predispose to atopic disease.

☞**EXTRACUTANEOUS FEATURES:**

- 30% to 50% of AD cases have asthma and/or allergic rhinitis.
- Up to 20% of AD cases have coexistent food allergy.
- Ocular abnormalities associated with AD include conjunctival inflammation, keratoconus, and cataract.
- Epidemiologic evidence shows an association between AD and childhood attention-deficit hyperactivity disorder, but the mechanistic basis for this observation is currently unknown.

☞**COMPLICATIONS OF AD:**

- Bacterial infection with *S aureus* or streptococci contributes to exacerbations of disease.
- Viral infection with herpes simplex results in eczema herpeticum, characterized by a rapid evolution of monomorphic "punched-out" lesions, with severe pain and a high fever.

- Growth delay may be associated with AD as a result of the disease itself and/or as a complication of corticosteroid treatment.
- Psychosocial problems may result from chronic pruritus and sleep disturbance, affecting the patient and their close family.

☞**INVESTIGATIONS:** The diagnosis of AD is usually based on clinical features, however, some investigations may be useful to confirm the atopic diathesis and exclude other forms of eczema.

**Serum IgE (total and specific)**—to test for "atopy" and to investigate possible food allergies, however, these investigations have low sensitivity and specificity

**Skin prick tests**—may be used to confirm reactivity suggested by elevated IgEs, but care must be taken in interpreting the results because of false-positive and false-negative results

**Patch testing**—may be used to demonstrate a delayed-type hypersensitivity in cases of localized AD where contact allergy may be relevant

**Swab for bacterial and virologic assessment**—to guide treatment when infection is suspected

**Skin biopsy**—this is rarely required because of the characteristic appearance of AD, although an erythrodermic case may lack some diagnostic features. Histologic examination reveals signs of inflammation in the epidermis and dermis, with spongiosis (intraepidermal vesicles), a dermal inflammatory infiltrate and in chronic cases, epidermal acanthosis (thickening).

## Management and Treatment

Mild-moderate AD may be managed in the community; the treatment of moderate-severe disease benefits from a multidisciplinary approach including specialist nurse input and patient education.

*First-Line Treatments:* The main principles of treatment for AD are listed below:

- *Avoid* detergents, soap, shampoo, bubble bath
- Use an *emollient*
- Apply an appropriate strength of *topical corticosteroid* cream or ointment
- *Treat infection* when necessary, using topical antiseptics and/or oral antibiotics

Oral antihistamine medication may be used primarily for its sedative effect at night. Nonsedating antihistamines provide little benefit for the pruritus of AD.

*Table 111-2* **Some Candidate Genes Associated with AD in Two or More Independent Studies**

| Gene Showing Association with AD | Locus | Rationale for Candidate Gene Study |
|---|---|---|
| Interleukin-4 (*IL4*) | 5q31-33 | Interleukin 4 promotes the switch to Th2 immune response and IgE production |
| Interleukin-4 receptor (*IL4R*) | 16p12.1-11.2 | |
| Interleukin-13 (*IL13*) | 5q31-33 | Interleukin 13 promotes B-cell switch to IgE production |
| Mast cell chymase (*CMA1*) | 14q11.2 | Mast cell chymase promotes increased microvascular permeability and accumulation of inflammatory cells |
| Serine protease inhibitor kazal-type 5 (*SPINK5*) | 5q31 | Mutations in *SPINK5* gene cause Netherton syndrome |
| Filaggrin (*FLG*) | 1q21 | *FLG* null mutations cause ichthyosis vulgaris |

*Second-Line Treatments:* **Bandaging** with dry or wet bandages (wet wraps) or medicated bandages, for example, those containing zinc oxide paste, may be used to control pruritus, excoriation, and lichenification.

Topical **calcineurin inhibitors** (pimecrolimus or tacrolimus ointment or cream) may be substituted for topical corticosteroids when side effects limit their use. There is a theoretical increased risk of lymphoma and skin malignancy which should be discussed with patients; to date there has been no evidence of an increase in these malignancies in 10 years' clinical use of topical calcineurin inhibitors.

*Third-Line Treatments:*

☞SYSTEMIC IMMUNOSUPPRESSION: Recalcitrant cases of severe AD may require treatment with oral immunosuppressive medication, including **ciclosporin**, **azathioprine**, **methotrexate**, or **mycophenolate mofetil**, but the risk of toxicity limits their long-term use. Individual patient response varies considerably, but at present there are no genetic tests or biomarkers to predict responsiveness to these systemic immunosuppressive treatments.

Screening for thiopurine methyltransferase (TPMT) activity is indicated prior to commencing treatment with azathioprine, to guide dosage, and there is evidence that this approach reduces toxicity.

☞PHOTOTHERAPY: A subset of AD patients improve with environmental UV exposure and several phototherapeutic modalities, including **UVB**, **narrow-band UVB**, **UVA1,** and **psoralen-UVA** have shown experimental efficacy. However, care must be taken, particularly in pediatric patients, because of the long-term risk of photoaging and cutaneous malignancy.

☞BIOLOGIC THERAPY: It is hoped and anticipated that an improved understanding of the immunopathogenesis of AD will lead to targeted, specific biologic therapies for this disease.

Various biologic agents have been used in case series and small open-label trials for severe, treatment-resistant AD. These include TNF-alpha inhibitors (infliximab, etanercept), a monoclonal antibody against the Fc portion of IgE (omalizumab), a recombinant humanized monoclonal antibody that binds CD-11a and inhibits T-cell function (efalizumab), an anti-IL-5 recombinant humanized monoclonal antibody (mepolizumab), recombinant interferon-gamma, a monoclonal antibody against the CD20 antigen on B cells (rituximab), and a human lymphocyte function-associated antigen-3/IgG1 fusion protein that binds CD2 on T cells and induces apoptosis (alefacept). However, at present there are no approved biologic therapies for AD, in contrast to their success in another inflammatory skin disease, psoriasis.

☞PRIMARY PREVENTION: Children at high risk of developing AD, particularly those with a genetic predisposition, may be targeted for primary prevention by environmental manipulations including soap and detergent avoidance and intensive emollient application. However, evidence is currently lacking as to whether this will reduce the incidence of AD or prevent the development of other atopic diseases.

## Molecular Genetics and Molecular Mechanisms

*Genetic Factors in AD:* There is a strong genetic component in AD demonstrated by twin studies, which show a concordance rate of approximately 80% in monozygotic twins compared with approximately 20% in dizygotic twin pairs.

AD as well as asthma and allergic rhinitis show clustering within families and common features of the systemic immune response link AD with other atopic diseases. Children whose parents have eczema show a higher risk of developing eczema than children whose parents have asthma or hay fever and eczema can occur with increased severity along Blaschko lines, consistent with genetic mosaicism.

These observations support the concept that risk may be mediated through skin-specific genes, as well as via systemic immune or "atopy" risk genes. Recent thinking has focused on the importance of epithelial barrier dysfunction in atopic eczema, directed by evidence from genetics as well as biochemical and physiologic studies.

*Genome-Wide Studies:* **Genome-wide linkage** screens have been reported in families with atopic eczema from five different populations and regions on chromosomes 3q, 3p, 17q, and 18q have shown evidence of linkage in two or more studies. Interestingly, only two of these four regions have shown linkage to asthma or other atopic disorders in more than one study indicating that separate genes may be responsible for eczema.

The regions on 1q21, 3q21, 17q25, and 20p linked to AD overlap with known psoriasis susceptibility loci and the colocalization of eczema and psoriasis genes supports the concept that tissue-specific genes influence the eczema phenotype via control of epidermal function, immunity, and inflammation.

The 1q21 locus includes the epidermal differentiation complex, a dense cluster of genes including filaggrin, involucrin, loricrin, and S100 proteins, which are involved in the terminal differentiation of keratinocytes.

**DNA microarray analyses** have demonstrated that four genes encoded on 1q21 (the epidermal differentiation complex) show different levels of expression in eczema lesional skin compared with controls. These findings suggest that S100A7 and S100A8 (showing increased expression) plus filaggrin and loricrin (showing reduced expression) may be responsible at least in part for the epidermal barrier dysfunction that is characteristic of atopic eczema.

An independent microarray analysis has shown increased expression of genes encoding CC chemokines in eczematous skin, which may contribute to the attraction of Th2 cells and eosinophils. However, the functional significance of these plus other genes and partial DNA sequences identified by DNA microarray analysis remains to be elucidated.

Two **genome-wide association studies (GWASs)** on AD have been published to date. The first showed association of a common variant on chromosome 11q13.5 (rs7927894) with AD and this SNP has been replicated in an independent case-control study. rs7927894 is located in an intergenic region between two annotated genes: chromosome 11 open reading frame 30 (*C11orf30*) and leucine-rich repeat containing 32 (*LRRC32*). *C11orf30* encodes the EMSY protein, which has been shown to bind the BRCA2 breast cancer susceptibility protein and may therefore play a role in epithelial differentiation. The second nearby gene, *LRRC32* is a cell surface molecule expressed on regulatory T cells and therefore may play a role in the T-cell–mediated inflammation of AD. However, the strongest effect in this first GWAS was shown to be the *FLG* locus on chromosome 1q21.

The second GWAS, from a Han Chinese population identified previously undescribed susceptibility loci at 5q22.1 (*TMEM232* and *SLC25A46*, rs7701890) and at 20q13.33 (*TNFRSF6B* and *ZGPAT*, rs6010620) and replicated the previously reported locus at 1q21.3 (*FLG*, rs3126085). This study indicated new genetic susceptibility factors and previously unidentified biologic pathways in AD.

**Candidate Genes:** Many different candidate genes have been investigated as risk factors for AD because of their known biologic roles in systemic atopic inflammation (Th2-dominated), local cutaneous inflammation, or epidermal barrier function; a selection of the replicated candidates is shown in Table 111-2.

Of these candidates, loss-of-function mutations in *FLG* are the strongest and the most widely replicated risk factors for AD. Meta-analysis has shown that *FLG* loss-of-function mutations are associated with an odds ratio of approximately 4 for AD, emphasizing the important role of skin barrier dysfunction in AD pathogenesis.

**Copy Number Variation:** Copy number variation (CNV) is defined as "a DNA segment that is 1 kb or larger and presents at variable copy number in comparison with a reference genome." CNV occurs extensively throughout the genome and is an important component of genetic variation that has only recently been widely studied.

Two genetic loci involved with epidermal barrier formation have been reported to affect AD risk: An extra 24 base pair repeat within the small proline-rich protein 3 gene (*SPRR3*) is significantly associated with AD; and intragenic copy number variation in *FLG* has a significant dose-dependent effect on AD risk.

**Clinical Relevance of Genetic Studies:** At present there are no widely available genetic tests that can predict a patient's long-term prognosis with respect to AD. Nevertheless application of current understanding of genetic risk factors may have clinical relevance.

- AD patients with ichthyosis vulgaris (indicated by the clinical features of scaling on extensor surfaces, plus palmar hyperlinearity, plus keratosis pilaris) are likely to be heterozygous or homozygous for *FLG* loss-of-function mutations and therefore have a poorer prognosis, since *FLG* mutations are associated with early onset, persistent and severe AD. These patients are also at increased risk of asthma, hay fever, and peanut allergy and enquiry should be made for symptoms of these diseases.
- The effect of CNV within *FLG* on AD risk implies that therapeutic efforts to increase the amount of filaggrin within the epidermis by a modest degree (5%-10%) may be clinically effective. At present there are no specific treatments to increase filaggrin expression, but these are anticipated; in the meantime, studies are ongoing to assess the efficacy of intensive emollient therapy early in life to improve skin barrier function and prevent the onset of AD.
- Atypical eczematous skin signs raise the possibility of other genetic disorders, including immunodeficiency syndromes and Netherton syndrome, indicating need for specialist dermatologic assessment and further investigation.

**Pharmacogenetics in AD:** At present the only clinically useful pharmacogenetic application for AD patients is the screening of TPMT activity prior to commencing azathioprine treatment. There is marked interindividual variability in the metabolism of azathioprine, resulting from a common genetic polymorphism in TPMT, which is part of one pathway for 6-MP metabolism. About 11% of the population has low TPMT activity and is vulnerable to myelosuppression with azathioprine treatment, but 1 in 300 individuals has undetectable TPMT activity and is susceptible to rapid-onset, prolonged, life-threatening pancytopenia if treated with conventional doses of azathioprine.

Azathioprine is contraindicated in individuals with very low TPMT activity; in other patients the starting dose for treatment of AD (0.5-3 mg/kg) may be adjusted according to the TPMT result, with a lower dose for those with lower TPMT activity. There is evidence that this approach reduces the risk of toxicity, but careful monitoring for side effects including myelosuppression and hepatotoxicity is still required.

**Future Directions:** The study of genetic factors in the pathogenesis of AD has significantly improved the understanding of key mechanisms in this disease. However, further work is needed to fully elucidate genetic mechanisms as well as important gene-environment interactions in this complex trait.

Following on from this improved understanding will be opportunities to translate genetic mechanisms into novel treatments, targeted at key biologic pathways, and tailored to the predominant pathomechanism in each individual patient.

### BIBLIOGRAPHY:

1. Williams HC, Burney PG, Pembroke AC, et al. Validation of the U.K. diagnostic criteria for atopic dermatitis in a population setting. U.K. Diagnostic Criteria for Atopic Dermatitis Working Party. *Br J Dermatol*. 1996;135:12-17.
2. Schultz Larsen F. Atopic dermatitis: a genetic-epidemiologic study in a population-based twin sample. *J Am Acad Dermatol*. 1993;28:719-723.
3. Larsen FS, Holm NV, Henningsen K. Atopic dermatitis. A genetic-epidemiologic study in a population-based twin sample. *J Am Acad Dermatol*. 1986;15:487-494.
4. Thomsen SF, Ulrik CS, Kyvik KO, et al. Importance of genetic factors in the etiology of atopic dermatitis: a twin study. *Allergy Asthma Proc*. 2007;25:535-539.
5. Wadonda-Kabondo N, Sterne JA, Golding J, et al. Association of parental eczema, hayfever, and asthma with atopic dermatitis in infancy: birth cohort study. *Arch Dis Child*. 2004;89:917-921.
6. Hladik F, Jurecka W, Hayek B, et al. Atopic dermatitis with increased severity along a line of Blaschko. *J Am Acad Dermatol*. 2005;53:S221-S224.
7. Jakasa I, Verberk MM, Esposito M, et al. Altered penetration of polyethylene glycols into uninvolved skin of atopic dermatitis patients. *J Invest Dermatol*. 2007;127:129-134.
8. Cookson W. The immunogenetics of asthma and eczema: a new focus on the epithelium. *Nat Rev Immunol*. 2004;4:978-988.
9. Taieb A, Hanifin J, Cooper K, et al. Proceedings of the 4th Georg Rajka International Symposium on Atopic Dermatitis, Arcachon, France, September 15-17, 2005. *J Allergy Clin Immunol*. 2006;117:378-390.
10. Irvine AD, McLean WH. Breaking the (un)sound barrier: filaggrin is a major gene for atopic dermatitis. *J Invest Dermatol*. 2006;126:1200-1202.
11. Hudson TJ. Skin barrier function and allergic risk. *Nat Genet*. 2006;38:399-400.
12. Lee YA, Wahn U, Kehrt R, et al. A major susceptibility locus for atopic dermatitis maps to chromosome 3q21. *Nat Genet*. 2000;26:470-473.
13. Cookson WO, Ubhi B, Lawrence R, et al. Genetic linkage of childhood atopic dermatitis to psoriasis susceptibility loci. *Nat Genet*. 2001;27:372-373.
14. Bradley M, Soderhall C, Luthman H, et al. Susceptibility loci for atopic dermatitis on chromosomes 3, 13, 15, 17 and 18 in a Swedish population. *Hum Mol Genet*. 2002;11:1539-1548.
15. Haagerup A, Bjerke T, Schiotz PO, et al. Atopic dermatitis—a total genome-scan for susceptibility genes. *Acta Derm Venereol*. 2004;84:346-352.
16. Enomoto H, Noguchi E, Iijima S, et al. Single nucleotide polymorphism-based genome-wide linkage analysis in Japanese atopic dermatitis families. *BMC Dermatol*. 2007;7:5.
17. Hoffjan S, Epplen JT. The genetics of atopic dermatitis: recent findings and future options. *J Mol Med*. 2005;83:682-692.

18. Mischke D, Korge BP, Marenholz I. et al. Genes encoding structural proteins of epidermal cornification and S100 calcium-binding proteins form a gene complex ("epidermal differentiation complex") on human chromosome 1q21. *J Invest Dermatol.* 1996;106:989-992.

19. Sugiura H, Ebise H, Tazawa T, et al. Large-scale DNA microarray analysis of atopic skin lesions shows overexpression of an epidermal differentiation gene cluster in the alternative pathway and lack of protective gene expression in the cornified envelope. *Br J Dermatol.* 2005;152:146-149.

20. Nomura T, Sandilands A, Akiyama M, et al. Unique mutations in the filaggrin gene in Japanese patients with ichthyosis vulgaris and atopic dermatitis. *J Allergy Clin Immunol.* 2007;119:434-440.

21. Saito H. Much atopy about the skin: genome-wide molecular analysis of atopic eczema. *Int Arch Allergy Immunol.* 2005;137:319-325.

22. Esparza-Gordillo J, Weidinger S, Fölster-Holst R, et al. A common variant on chromosome 11q13 is associated with atopic dermatitis. *Nat Genet.* 2009;41:596-601.

23. O'Regan GM, Campbell LE, Cordell HJ, et al. Chromosome 11q13.5 variant associated with childhood eczema: an effect supplementary to filaggrin mutations. *J Allergy Clin Immunol.* 2010;125:170-4 e1-e2.

24. Sun LD, Xiao FL, Li Y, et al. Genome-wide association study identifies two new susceptibility loci for atopic dermatitis in the Chinese Han population. *Nat Genet.* 2011;43:690-694.

25. Brown SJ, McLean WH. Eczema genetics: current state of knowledge and future goals. *J Invest Dermatol.* 2009;129:543-552.

26. Brown SJ, McLean WH. One remarkable molecule: filaggrin. *J Invest Dermatol.* Mar 2012;132(3 pt 2):751-762.

27. Rodríguez E, Baurecht H, Herberich E, et al. Meta-analysis of filaggrin polymorphisms in eczema and asthma: robust risk factors in atopic disease. *J Allergy Clin Immunol.* 2009;123:1361-1370.e7.

28. Redon R, Ishikawa S, Fitch KR, et al. Global variation in copy number in the human genome. *Nature.* 2006;444:444-454.

29. Brown SJ, Kroboth K, Sandilands A, et al. Intragenic copy number variation within filaggrin contributes to the risk of atopic dermatitis with a dose-dependent effect. *J Invest Dermatol.* 2012;132:98-104.

30. Brown SJ, Relton CL, Liao H, et al. Filaggrin haploinsufficiency is highly penetrant and is associated with increased severity of eczema: further delineation of the skin phenotype in a prospective epidemiological study of 792 school children. *Br J Dermatol.* 2009;161:884-889.

31. Brown SJ, Sandilands A, Zhao Y, et al. Prevalent and low-frequency null mutations in the filaggrin gene are associated with early-onset and persistent atopic eczema. *J Invest Dermatol.* 2008;128:1591-1594.

32. Barker JN, Palmer CN, Zhao Y, et al. Null mutations in the filaggrin gene (FLG) determine major susceptibility to early-onset atopic dermatitis that persists into adulthood. *J Invest Dermatol.* 2007;127:564-567.

33. McGrath JA. Profilaggrin, dry skin, and atopic dermatitis risk: size matters. *J Invest Dermatol.* 2012;132:10-11.

34. Anstey AV, Wakelin S, Reynolds NJ. Guidelines for prescribing azathioprine in dermatology. *Br J Dermatol.* 2004;151:1123-1132.

## Resources:

**NICE Guidelines for Atopic Eczema** (UK) http://www.nice.org.uk/CG57

**DermNet NZ** (New Zealand) http://dermnetnz.org/dermatitis/dermatitis.html

**Atopic Dermatitis: The Epidemiology, Causes, and Prevention of Atopic Eczema**

HC Williams (ed), Cambridge University Press, ISBN-13: 978-0521570756

**Key Advances in the Clinical Management of Atopic Eczema**

RJ Hay & MHA Rustin (eds), Royal Society of Medicine Press, ISBN-13: 978-1853155529

**Paediatric Dermatology (Oxford Specialist Handbooks in Paediatrics)**

S Lewis-Jones (ed), OUP Oxford, ISBN-13: 978-0199208388

**Gene Cards®** The Human Gene Compendium http://www.genecards.org/

**Online Mendelian Inheritance in Man** (OMIM) http://www.ncbi.nlm.nih.gov/omim

# 112 Graft-Versus-Host Disease

Jennifer Huang and Arturo Saavedra

## KEY POINTS

- *Disease summary:*
  - Graft-versus-host disease (GVHD) occurs most commonly in the setting of allogeneic hematopoietic stem cell transplantation (HSCT), and is the most common cause of nonrelapse mortality in HSCT recipients.
  - GVHD is subdivided into acute and chronic forms, but an overlap syndrome also exists.
  - Since the widespread use of reduced-intensity conditioning and donor lymphocyte infusions, clinical presentation, rather than time of onset, is most helpful in differentiating acute from chronic GVHD.
  - While acute GVHD causes inflammation of the skin, gastrointestinal tract, and liver, chronic GVHD results in fibrosis of multiple organ systems.
  - In both acute and chronic GVHD, donor T cells attack genetically defined proteins on host cells, most commonly major human leukocyte antigens (HLAs) and minor histocompatibility antigens (mHAs).
  - The pathogenesis of acute GVHD is described as a three-phase process involving (1) activation of host antigen-presenting cells due to underlying tissue damage, (2) activation of donor T cells, and (3) cytokine and cell-mediated tissue injury.
  - The pathogenesis of chronic GVHD is less clearly defined, but thought to be due to alloreactive Th2 type CD4+ T cells, similar to other autoimmune diseases.
  - Genetic polymorphisms of various cytokines in both donors and recipients have been implicated in predicting risk and severity of acute and chronic GVHD.

- *Differential diagnosis:*
  - Acute GVHD: eruption of lymphocyte recovery, various bacterial and viral infections, drug toxicity or allergy, graft rejection
  - Chronic GVHD: scleroderma, drug toxicity or allergy, various bacterial and viral infections, lichen planus, lichenoid drug eruption, eczema, ichthyosis

- *Pathogenesis:*
  - Acute GVHD
    - Phase 1: activation of antigen-presenting cells, most importantly dendritic cells, as a result of tissue damage caused by underlying disease and HSCT conditioning regimen. Cytokines involved TNF-$\alpha$, IL-1, IL-6, bacterial lipopolysaccharide, IL-10 (protective).
    - Phase 2: donor T-cell activation, including costimulatory signaling, in response to host histoincompatible antigens presented by activated antigen-presenting cells, Th1 differentiation. Cytokines involved: IL-2, IFN-$\gamma$.
    - Phase 3: complex cascade of cellular mediators (cytotoxic T cells, natural killer cells) and soluble inflammatory cytokines (TNF-$\alpha$, IFN-$\gamma$, IL-1), further promote tissue inflammation and injury.
  - Chronic GVHD
    - The pathogenesis of chronic GVHD is not well understood, but is thought to be the result of an autoimmune process with Th2 differentiation of CD4+ T cells.
    - Animal studies have shown that T cells react to specific MHC class II molecules shared by donor and recipient.
    - As in acute GVHD, donor alloreactive CD4 and CD8 T cells, and dendritic cells target and attack host mHA on autosomal and Y chromosomes.
    - Both dysregulation of central and peripheral T-cell tolerance has been proposed.
    - Injury of the thymus from the conditioning regimen and acute GVHD prevents negative selection of autoreactive T cells.
    - Deficiency of T-regulatory cells has been shown to contribute to the pathogenesis of other autoimmune diseases.

- *Impact of GVHD on immune reconstitution:*
  - Due to MHC expression, the thymus and bone marrow are primary targets in acute GVHD, resulting in depletion of T and B cells.
  - In acute GVHD, expansion of alloreactive T cells results in skewing of T-cell repertoire (clonal exhaustion and immune senescence) and subsequent apoptosis of both alloreactive and nonalloreactive T cells.
  - Although the cause is yet undetermined, there is diminished homeostatic peripheral expansion of CD4+ T cells in GVHD.

- *Risk factors:*
  - Acute GVHD: HLA and/or mHA mismatch, older donor or recipient age, gender mismatch, reduced intensity conditioning, donor lymphocyte infusions
  - Chronic GVHD: history of acute GVHD, HLA mismatch, donor-recipient mismatches for mHAs such as HA-1, HA-2, and HA-5, peripheral blood source of stem cells

- *Genetic polymorphisms-associated acute GVHD, chronic GVHD, and transplant related mortality (TRM):*
  - Genetic polymorphisms of multiple cytokines have studied in relation to GVHD. However, most studies are single centered based on small patient populations. Although there are other cytokine polymorphisms implicated in the pathogenesis of GVHD, listed below are the ones most well studied.
  - TNF-$\alpha$: located on chromosome 6, near the HLA region. Therefore, in HLA-matched sibling transplants, TNF-$\alpha$ genotype is the same in donor and recipient. Single-nucleotide polymorphisms (SNPs) which upregulate TNF-$\alpha$ have been shown to increase risk of acute GVHD and TRM. SNPs in the TNF receptor II (*TNFRII*) gene which downregulate TNFRII, resulting in increased soluble TNF-$\alpha$, has been shown to increase incidence of chronic GVHD.

- IL-1: of the 10 genes within the IL-1 family, SNPs in 3 (IL-1α, IL-1β, IL1Ra) have been correlated with acute GVHD, chronic GVHD, and TRM.
- IL-6: SNPs in the promoter region of IL-6, which upregulate production, have been shown to increase the risk of acute GVHD, chronic GVHD, and TRM.
- IL-10: normally inhibits T-cell proliferative responses and proinflammatory cytokine production. Most studies show that SNPs which downregulate IL-10 production increase the risk for acute and chronic GVHD, but there are conflicting data in other studies.
- *Plasma biomarkers:*
  - The combination of values for IL-2Rα, TNFR1, HGF, and IL-8 has been shown to predict occurrence of acute GVHD.
  - High levels of elafin may predict severity of cutaneous GVHD.

## Diagnostic Criteria and Clinical Characteristics

### Diagnostic Criteria for Acute GVHD:

**Diagnostic evaluation should include at least one of the following:**

- History and physical examination
  - Previous allogeneic HSCT or organ transplant
  - Characteristic clinical features (see later)
- Biopsy of affected organs
  - Skin: apoptosis of basal keratinocytes at dermoepidermal junction, interface vacuolar change, follicular prominence
  - Gastrointestinal tract: patchy ulcerations, apoptotic bodies in base of crypts, crypt abscesses, loss and flattening of surface epithelium
  - Liver: endothelialitis, lymphocytic infiltration of portal areas, pericholangitis, bile duct destruction
- Radiologic studies
  - Gastrointestinal tract: luminal dilatation with thickening of small bowel wall, air or fluid levels suggestive of ileus

### Clinical Characteristics of Acute GVHD:

☞**GENERAL INFORMATION:** Although acute GVHD usually occurs 20 to 40 days after HSCT, reduced-intensity conditioning may delay onset of acute GVHD.

**Clinical features should include at least one of the following:**

- Skin: pruritic morbilliform rash that initially involves palms and soles but can become diffuse, often sparing the scalp. Can progress to generalized erythroderma, bullae, and desquamation.
- Gastrointestinal tract: voluminous secretory diarrhea, bloody diarrhea, vomiting, anorexia, abdominal pain.
- Liver: cholestatic hyperbilirubinemia.

### Diagnostic Criteria for Chronic GVHD:

**Diagnostic evaluation should include at least one of the following:**

- Presence of at least one diagnostic clinical sign (Table 112-1) *or*
- Presence of at least one distinctive clinical manifestation (Table 112-2) confirmed by biopsy or other relevant tests of the same or another organ
- Other causes of similar manifestations, especially infections, must be excluded

### Clinical Characteristics of Chronic GVHD:

☞**GENERAL INFORMATION:** Although chronic GVHD usually occurs more than 100 days after HSCT, it can occur at any time post-HSCT. Multiple organs can be involved and is most often characterized by fibrosis of the affected organ.

## Prevention and Screening

### Prevention:

- Since two-thirds of patients with chronic GVHD have a history of acute GVHD, efforts to prevent acute GVHD are important in minimizing morbidity and mortality after HSCT.
- Modification of donor, recipient, and transplant-related factors may reduce the risk of GVHD: younger, related male donor, use of bone marrow (vs peripheral blood), limiting CD34+, and T-cell infusions.
- Studies using cyclosporine and thalidomide have not shown to reduce the risk of GVHD.
- Although not well studied, high-dose steroid therapy for presumptive acute cutaneous GVHD may potentially be a risk factor for the development of chronic cutaneous GVHD. Therefore, without a definitive diagnosis of acute GVHD, high-dose steroids should be used with caution.

**Table 112-1  *Diagnostic Clinical Signs of Chronic GVHD***

| Skin | Poikiloderma |
| --- | --- |
| | Lichen planus-like features |
| | Morphea-like features |
| | Lichen sclerosus-like features |
| Mouth | Lichen-type features |
| | Hyperkeratotic plaques |
| | Restriction of mouth opening from sclerosis |
| Genitalia | Lichen planus-like features |
| | Vaginal scarring or stenosis |
| Gastrointestinal tract | Esophageal web |
| | Strictures or stenosis on the upper to mid third of the esophagus |
| Lungs | Bronchiolitis obliterans diagnosed by biopsy |
| Muscles, fascia, joints | Fasciitis |

**Table 112-2 *Distinctive Clinical Signs of Chronic GVHD***

| | |
|---|---|
| Skin | Depigmentation |
| Nails | Dystrophy |
| | Longitudinal ridging, splitting, or brittle features |
| | Onycholysis |
| | Pterygium unguis |
| | Nail loss (usually symmetric; affects most nails) |
| Scalp and body hair | New-onset scarring or nonscarring scalp alopecia (after recovery from chemoradiotherapy) |
| | Scaling, papulosquamous lesions |
| Mouth | Xerostomia |
| | Mucocele |
| | Mucosal atrophy |
| | Pseudomembranes |
| | Ulcers |
| Eyes | New-onset dry, gritty, or painful eyes |
| | Cicatricial conjunctivitis |
| | Keratoconjunctivitis sicca |
| | Confluent areas of punctate keratopathy |
| Genitalia | Erosions |
| | Fissures |
| | Ulcers |
| Lung | Bronchiolitis obliterans diagnosed with PFTs and radiology |
| Muscles, fascia, joints | Myositis or polymyositis |

- Other preventive strategies have been anecdotal
  - Extracorporeal photopheresis of recipient prior to infusion of donor stem cells: depletion of host antigen-presenting cells
  - Treatment of donor stem cells with monoclonal or polyclonal antibodies against various T-cell epitopes: anti-CD52, anti-CD6, antithymocyte globulin

### Screening:

- Patients should be assessed carefully throughout the hospital stay and at each clinic visit for signs and symptoms of acute or chronic GVHD.
- Often, the diagnosis can be made clinically but appropriate biopsies may be necessary to confirm the diagnosis.
- Peripheral eosinophilia may predict the onset of acute and/or chronic GVHD. Recent studies also suggest that peripheral eosinophilia is associated with increased survival. Further study is needed in this area.
- Currently testing for genetic polymorphisms for risk assessment or plasma biomarkers for diagnostic evaluation is not available.

## Management and Treatment

***Management:*** Early detection, early treatment, and adequate supportive care are critical to minimizing morbidity and mortality of disease.

- Long-term survival of patients with grade 0-1 disease approaches 50% while those with grade IV disease is as low as 11%
- Supportive care
  - Skin: topical emollients and meticulous wound care
  - Gastrointestinal: bowel rest and hyperalimentation, antimotility agents such as loperamide, octreotide for control of secretory component, transfusions as needed for bloody diarrhea, treating secondary causes of gastrointestinal symptoms such as infectious colitis, cytomegalovirus (CMV), adenovirus, intestinal thrombotic microangiopathy
  - Hepatic: ursodeoxycholic acid may help prevent hepatic GVHD
  - Infectious complications: standard prophylaxis with trimethoprim-sulfamethoxazole and acyclovir, routine serum viral load monitoring for CMV, adenovirus, Epstein-Barr virus (EBV), serial monitoring of serum galactomannan and β-glucan levels to detect incipient invasive fungal disease. Steroid refractory disease: empiric prophylaxis with broad-spectrum antibiotics and extended-spectrum antifungal agents (voriconazole, posaconazole, echinocandins)

### Therapeutics:

- Acute GVHD
  - Standard initial therapy: prednisone 2 mg/kg/d
  - Adjunctive therapy with systemic corticosteroids with several biologic agents has not been shown to improve outcome, although oral beclomethasone as topical therapy may augment treatment for gastrointestinal disease
  - There is no established consensus for treatment of steroid refractory disease. Options include
    - Antithymocyte globulin
    - OKT3: anti-CD3 antibody
    - Anti-IL-2 receptor a chain (CD25) antibodies: inolimomab, basiliximab
    - Alemtuzumab: anti-CD52 antibody
    - Denileukin diftitox: IL-2 receptor antagonist
    - TNF-α inhibitors: etanercept, infliximab
    - Chemotherapeutics: pentostatin, mycophenolate mofetil, sirolimus
    - Extracorporeal photopheresis
    - Haploidentical mesenchymal stem cell infusion
    - Intra-arterial administration of steroid or methotrexate for gastrointestinal or hepatic disease
- Chronic GVHD
  - Standard initial therapy: prednisone and cyclosporine or tacrolimus
  - Options for second-line therapy
    - Mycophenolate mofetil: associated with higher rates of opportunistic infection
    - Rituximab: higher efficacy with musculoskeletal and skin involvement
    - Sirolimus: increased toxicity when used in conjunction with calcineurin inhibitor
    - Extracorporeal photopheresis
    - High-dose methylprednisolone
    - Pentostatin
    - Hydroxychloroquine
    - Oral beclomethasone: topical activity in gastrointestinal involvement
    - Thalidomide low dose IL-2

**Genetic Testing:** Currently testing for genetic polymorphisms for risk assessment of GVHD is not available, since the relevance of these polymorphisms is still unclear.

**Future Directions:**

- Although various genetic polymorphisms have been found to modify the risk for development of GVHD, larger collaborative studies are needed to establish a unifying approach to assessing one's risk for GVHD.

- Further research in the pathogenesis of chronic GVHD is essential in further establishing practice guidelines for prevention and treatment of disease.

- Multi-institutional studies are needed to investigate therapeutic options for steroid-resistant acute and chronic GVHD.

## BIBLIOGRAPHY:

1. Ferrara JLM, Levine JE, Reddy P, et al. Graft-versus-host disease. *Lancet.* 2009;373:1550-1561.

2. Reddy P, Arora M, Guimond M, et al. GVHD: a continuing barrier to the safety of allogeneic transplantation. *Biol Blood Marrow Transplant.* 2008;15(1S):162-168.

3. Filipovich AH. Diagnosis and manifestations of chronic graft-versus-host disease. *Best Pract Res Clin Haematol.* 2008;21(2):251-257.

4. Dickinson AM, Holler E. Polymorphisms of cytokine and innate immunity genes and GVHD. *Best Pract Res Clin Haematol.* 2008;21(2):149-164.

5. Toubai T, Sun Y, Reddy P. GVHD pathophysiology: is acute different from chronic? *Best Pract Res Clin Haematol.* 2008;21(2):101-117.

6. Markey KA, MacDonald KPA, Hill GR. Impact of cytokine gene polymorphisms on graft-versus-host disease. *Tissue Antigens.* 2008;72(6):507-516.

7. Ball LM, Egeler RM. Acute GVHD: pathogenesis and classification. *Bone Marrow Transplant.* 2008;41(S2):S58-S64.

8. Ho VT, Cutler C. Current and novel therapies in acute GVHD. *Best Pract Res Clin Haematol.* 2008;21(2):223-237.

9. Paczesny S, Levine JE, Braun TM, et al. Plasma biomarkers in GVHD: a new era? *Biol Bone Marrow Transplant.* 2008;15(S1):33-38.

10. Tyndall A, Dazzi F. Chronic GVHD as an autoimmune disease. *Best Pract Res Clin Haematol.* 2008;21(2):281-289.

11. Hansen JA. Genomic and proteomic analysis of allogeneic hematopoietic cell transplant outcome. Seeking greater understanding the pathogenesis of GVHD and mortality. *Biol Blood Marrow Transplant.* 2008;15(S1):e1-e7.

12. Lee JW, Deeg HJ. Prevention of chronic GVHD. *Best Pract Res Clin Haematol.* 2008;21(2):259-270.

13. Kim DH, Popradi G, Xu W, et al. Peripheral blood eosinophilia has a favorable prognostic impact on transplant outcomes after allogeneic peripheral blood stem cell transplantation. *Biol Blood Marrow Transplant.* 2009;15(4):471-482.

14. Jacobsohn DA, Schechter T, Seshadri R, et al. Eosinophilia correlates with the presence or development of chronic graft-versus-host disease in children. *Transplantation.* 2004;77(7):1096-1100.

## Supplementary Information

### OMIM REFERENCE:

[1] There are no causative genes identified in acute or chronic GVHD.

### Alternative Names:

- GVHD
- Graft-versus-host reaction
- GVHR

**Key Words:** Acute graft-versus-host disease, chronic graft-versus-host disease, GVHD, graft-versus-host reaction, GVHR, hematopoietic stem cell transplant, bone marrow transplant, cytokine polymorphisms

# 113 Nevoid Basal Cell Carcinoma Syndrome

Kimberly R. McDonald and Christopher A. Friedrich

## KEY POINTS

- *Disease summary:*
  - Nevoid basal cell carcinoma syndrome (NBCCS) is characterized by multiple basal cell carcinomas and odontogenic keratocysts.
  - A characteristic appearance including facial milia, frontal bossing, wide nasal bridge, coarse facial features, high-arched eyebrows and palate, mandibular prognathism, and macrocephaly may be present. Palmar and plantar pits, skeletal abnormalities of the ribs, and vertebrae and ectopic calcification of the falx cerebri are often found and useful in diagnosis.
  - Individuals are also at increased risk for developing other cysts and neoplasms including medulloblastoma and cardiac and ovarian fibromas.

- *Hereditary basis:*
  - NBCCS is inherited in an autosomal dominant fashion, with approximately 70% to 80% of patients receiving an affected gene from a parent and the remaining 20% to 30% representing de novo mutations. Penetrance is near complete.

- *Differential diagnosis:*
  - While other inherited disorders such as susceptibility to basal cell carcinoma (BCC), Bazex syndrome and Rombo syndrome should be considered in the setting of multiple BCCs, NBCCS should be highly suspected in cases of odontogenic keratocysts or early-onset medulloblastoma, see Table 113-1.

## Diagnostic Criteria and Clinical Characteristics

***Diagnostic Criteria for Nevoid Basal Cell Carcinoma Syndrome:*** Diagnosis may be made in the presence of two major and one minor criterion or one major and three minor criteria.

Major criteria:
- Multiple BCCs
  - Greater than five in a lifetime or one under age 30
- Odontogenic keratocyst
- Palmar or plantar pits
  - Two or more
- Ectopic calcification
  - Lamellar calcification of the falx or calcification of the falx at less than 20 years
- First-degree relative with NBCCS

Minor criteria:
- Congenital skeletal anomaly
- Macrocephaly
  - Occipitofrontal head circumference greater than 97th percentile
- Ovarian or cardiac fibromas
- Childhood medulloblastoma
- Lymphomesenteric or pleural cysts
- Cleft lip or palate
- Preaxial or postaxial polydactyly
- Ocular anomalies

***Clinical Characteristics:***

☞**APPEARANCE:** Many patients have a characteristic appearance with coarse facial features, frontal bossing, high-arched eyebrows and palate, wide nasal bridge, mandibular prognathism, macrocephaly, and facial milia. Shoulders are downward sloping and some patients may be very tall.

☞**BASAL CELL CARCINOMAS:** Early skin lesions may have the appearance of nevi. Carcinomas are histologically indistinguishable from a typical BCC. These occur most frequently in the third and fourth decades of life, and are more common in individuals of lighter skin color and those with more exposure to ultraviolet light. However, approximately 10% of individuals with NBCCS never manifest BCCs.

☞**OTHER SKIN FINDINGS:** Facial milia are present in 50% to 60% of patients. Skin tags may appear in childhood, especially around the neck, and are histologically similar to BCC. Meibomian cysts, sebaceous cysts, and dermoid cysts are frequent.

☞**ODONTOGENIC KERATOCYSTS:** Keratocysts are cystic lesions of the bone lined with a thin, uniform layer of keratinized epithelium. Lesions are locally destructive and aggressive, leading to tooth disruption or jaw fracture if left untreated. Approximately 90% of those with NBCCS develop multiple odontogenic keratocysts and peak occurrence is within the second and third decades. Three-fourths occur in the mandible.

☞**PALMAR AND PLANTAR PITS:** Pits are highly characteristic of NBCCS and useful in diagnosis, present in about 80% of those affected. They are more easily visualized after soaking the hands and feet in warm water for 10 to 15 minutes. Pits are shallow, 1 to 3 mm, white or pink depressions at areas of partial or complete absence of the stratum corneum.

☞**ECTOPIC CALCIFICATION:** Calcification of the falx cerebri, sella turcica, tentorium cerebelli, or petroclinoid ligament may take place; calcification of the falx is nearly always present after age 20. This is visible on skull x-rays.

☞**CONGENITAL SKELETAL ANOMALIES:** Many patients demonstrate rib abnormalities such as bifid, splayed, extra or absent ribs. Bifid, wedged or fused vertebrae may also be present. Sprengel and pectus deformities are less common.

☞**CARDIAC FIBROMA:** Cardiac fibromas occur in a small percentage of individuals with NBCCS and are generally present at the time of birth. These may lead to obstruction or conduction abnormalities.

☞**OVARIAN FIBROMA:** Approximately 20% of females with the syndrome develop ovarian fibromas, which usually calcify and are asymptomatic but may cause torsion of the ovary.

*Table 113-1* **Genetic Differential Diagnosis**

| Syndrome | Gene Symbol | Associated Findings |
|---|---|---|
| Susceptibility to basal cell carcinoma | *BCC1, BCC2, BCC3, BCC4, BCC5, BCC6* | Basal cell carcinoma |
| Bazex syndrome | *BZX* | Basal cell carcinoma, congenital hypotrichosis, follicular atrophoderma |
| Rombo syndrome | Unknown | Basal cell carcinoma, atrophoderma, milia, hypotrichosis, trichoepitheliomas, peripheral vasodilation with cyanosis |
| Multiple familial trichoepithelioma | *CYLD* | Trichoepitheliomas that may degenerate into basal cell carcinoma |
| Brooke-Spiegler syndrome | *SBS* | Trichoepitheliomas that may degenerate into basal cell carcinoma, cylindromas, and spiradenomas |

Gene names: *BCC*, basal cell carcinoma; *BZX*, Bazex syndrome; *CYLD*, CYLD gene; *SBS*, Spiegler-Brooke syndrome.

☞**MEDULLOBLASTOMA:** Incidence of medulloblastoma in individuals with NBCCS is approximately 5%. Tumors usually have desmoplastic histology, a histologic variant generally believed to carry a more favorable prognosis than other subtypes of medulloblastoma. In contrast to sporadic medulloblastoma with peak age of onset 6 to 10 years, most of those cases in NBCCS occur by age 2.

☞**OCULAR ANOMALIES:** May include cataract, glaucoma, strabismus, microphthalmia, orbital cyst, pigmentary changes of the retinal epithelium, coloboma, hypertelorism, or telecanthus.

☞**LYMPHOMESENTERIC AND PLEURAL CYSTS:** Cysts may be present but usually calcify and are asymptomatic.

## Screening and Counseling

**Screening:** Diagnosis of a proband is based on the clinical criteria listed earlier. Radiographs including anteroposterior (AP) and lateral x-rays of the skull, an orthopantogram, chest x-ray, and spine x-ray should be obtained in any patient suspected of having NBCCS. Hand and foot x-rays may also aid in verification of diagnosis. Skin biopsy of a BCC, if present, may be tested for mutations in the case of suspected mosaicism; an identical mutation in two separate carcinomas confirms the diagnosis of NBCCS, see Table 113-2. Molecular genetic testing of lymphocyte DNA can be used to confirm diagnosis in questionable or atypical cases, see Table 113-3.

**Counseling:** NBCCS is inherited as an autosomal dominant trait, with a 50% risk of inheriting the condition for each child of an affected individual. Approximately 70% to 80% of probands receive an affected gene from a parent, with the remaining 20% to 30% representing de novo mutations.

Family members may demonstrate variable expression, and mosaicism with milder clinical features may be present in the proband or first individual possessing the mutation, but penetrance is believed to be near 100%.

*Table 113-2* **Recommended Diagnostic Evaluation of Patient With Nevoid Basal Cell Carcinoma Syndrome**

| Test | Possible Finding |
|---|---|
| Skull x-rays, AP and lateral | Calcification of falx cerebri, tentorium cerebelli, or petroclinoid ligament, complete or partial bridging of the sella turcica |
| Orthopantogram | Jaw keratocyst |
| Chest x-ray | Bifid, fused, splayed, extra or absent rib |
| Spine x-ray | Bifid, wedged or fused vertebrae |
| Hand and foot x-rays | Flame-shaped lytic bone lesions |
| Head circumference, baseline | Macrocephaly |
| Ophthalmologic examination | Cataract, coloboma, microphthalmia, pigmentary changes of retinal epithelium, nystagmus, strabismus, hypertelorism, telecanthus |
| Ultrasound of ovaries | Ovarian fibroma |
| Echocardiography | Cardiac fibroma |
| Dermatologic examination | Basal cell carcinoma |
| **To confirm diagnosis or if atypical presentation or suspected mosaicism:** | |
| Biopsy of basal cell carcinoma (BCC) | Histologically indistinguishable from sporadic BCC; confirms diagnosis if identical mutation in two separate lesions |
| Molecular genetic testing | Mutation of *PTCH1, PTCH2,* or *SUFU* |

**Table 113-3 Molecular Genetic Testing**

| Gene | Testing Modality | Mutation Type | Detection Rate |
|------|------------------|---------------|----------------|
| PTCH1 | Sequence analysis | Sequence variants | 50%-85% |
| | Deletion/duplication analysis | Exonic, multiexonic, and whole gene deletions | 6% |
| | Linkage analysis | Not applicable | Not applicable |

Predictive testing for asymptomatic family members as well as prenatal testing may be offered if a specific mutation has been identified within the family.

No definite genotype-phenotype correlation has been described thus far.

## Management and Treatment

**Basal Cell Carcinomas:** Prevention should be emphasized with avoidance of excessive sun exposure and irradiation as possible. Once BCCs develop, early treatment with surgical excision, Mohs micrographic surgery, cryotherapy, laser treatments, or topical treatments (tretinoin, 5-FU, and imiquimod if lesions are superficial) should take place. Prevention with systemic retinoids is sometimes attempted, but these are not useful for treatment of existing lesions and may be poorly tolerated. Skin examination should be performed by a dermatologist at least annually and preferably every 2 to 3 months to evaluate for new lesions. Vismodegib was approved by the FDA in 2012 for treatment of BCC that has metastasized or that cannot be treated surgically.

**Odontogenic Keratocysts:** Surgical excision is required if present, but recurrence is frequent following surgery. After reaching 8 years of age, patients should have an orthopantogram every 12 to 18 months to identify any new lesions.

**Cardiac Fibromas:** Echocardiogram should be obtained within the first year of life. If fibromas are present, monitoring should be performed by a pediatric cardiologist, with intervention as necessary if arrhythmias or obstruction develop.

**Ovarian Fibromas:** Ultrasound of the ovaries should be done prior to pregnancy. If surgical intervention is necessary due to size or torsion it is preferable to attempt preservation of ovarian tissue.

**Medulloblastoma:** Due to increased risk, developmental assessment and physical examination may be warranted every 6 months during the first several years of life. Peak incidence is at 2 years of age. Serial neuroimaging has not been evaluated for use in surveillance, but some recommend a cranial magnetic resonance imaging (MRI) annually until the age of eight. Computed tomography (CT) should be avoided due to delivery of large amounts of radiation. If medulloblastoma occurs, radiation therapy should be avoided if possible.

**Macrocephaly:** Head circumference should be monitored throughout childhood. Any rapid increase should be followed with evaluation for hydrocephalus and treatment as needed if present.

## Molecular Genetics and Molecular Mechanism

**Syndrome/Gene/Locus:**
PTCH1/protein patched homolog 1/9q22.3

PTCH2/protein patched homolog 2/1p32
SUFU/suppressor of fused homolog/10q24-q25

Mutations of *PTCH1* have been well studied and documented as causes of NBCCS. However, the related *PTCH2* and *SUFU* genes have been implicated in a small number of cases of the syndrome as well.

Protein patched homolog 1 is an integral membrane protein that serves in the sonic hedgehog signaling pathway as a receptor for the hedgehog protein, SHH. Protein patched homolog 1 represses the activity of the coreceptor smoothened (SMO), also a transmembrane protein, when SHH is not present. When SHH binds to the PTCH1/SMO complex, signaling via the SHH pathway takes place. If a mutation occurs in *PTCH1*, repression of SMO no longer takes place and the SHH pathway is constitutively overexpressed.

Protein patched homolog 2 is very similar to *PTCH1* and is also a transmembrane protein that functions as a tumor suppressor in the hedgehog signaling pathway.

Suppressor of fused homolog encodes a negative regulator of the hedgehog signaling pathway. The product of this gene interacts with the three different GLI transcription factors involved in the pathway, downregulating transcription of their target genes. Transcription of *SUFU* is regulated by the same transcription factors with which its product interacts.

**Genetic Testing:** Sequence analysis and deletion or duplication analysis of PTCH is available at several laboratories both in the United States and in other countries. Presence of a pathologic allele confirms NBCCS, but absence of such an allele does not rule out the diagnosis. Diagnosis, again, is based on clinical criteria and analysis of *PTCH2* and *SUFU* are not included in routine laboratory testing. Linkage analysis may be performed within a family affected by NBCCS as well. If a pathogenic mutation is identified within a family, predictive testing may be offered to asymptomatic family members and prenatal testing may be performed.

**BIBLIOGRAPHY:**

1. Anderson DE, Taylor WB, Falls HF, Davidson RT. The nevoid basal cell carcinoma syndrome. *Am J Hum Genet*. 1967;19:12-22.
2. Cowan R, Hoban P, Kelsey A, Birch JM, Gattamaneni R, Evans DG. The gene for the naevoid basal cell carcinoma syndrome acts as a tumour-suppressor gene in medulloblastoma. *Br J Cancer*. 1997;76:141-145.
3. Evans DG, Ladusans EJ, Rimmer S, Burnell LD, Thakker N, Farndon PA. Complications of the naevoid basal cell carcinoma syndrome: results of a population based study. *J Med Genet*. 1993;30:460-464.
4. Evans GE, Farndon PA, Pagon RA, et al (Ed). Nevoid Basal Cell Carcinoma Syndrome. Genereviews (Internet). Seattle: University of Washington. 1993-2002, rev 2011.
5. Fan Z, Li J, Du J, et al. A missense mutation in PTCH2 underlies dominantly inherited NBCCS in a Chinese family. *J Med Genet*. 2008;45:303-308.

6. Gorlin, RJ. Multiple nevoid basal cell epithelioma, jaw cysts and bifid rib: a syndrome. *New Engl J Med.* 1960;262:908-912.

7. Gorlin RJ. Nevoid basal cell carcinoma (Gorlin) syndrome. *Genet Med.* 2004;6:530-539.

8. Kimonis VE, Goldstein AM, Pastakia B, et al. Clinical manifestations in 105 persons with nevoid basal cell carcinoma syndrome. *Am J Med Genet.* 1997;69:299-308.

9. Pastorino L, Ghiorzo P, Nasti S, et al. Identification of a SUFU germline mutation in a family with Gorlin syndrome. *Am J Med Genet.* 2009;149A:1539-1543.

10. Ratcliffe JF, Shanley S, Ferguson J, Chenevix-Trench G. The diagnostic implication of falcine calcification on plain skull radiographs of patients with basal cell naevus syndrome and the incidence of falcine calcification in their relatives and two control groups. *Br J Radiol.* 1995;68:361-368.

11. Southwick GJ, Schwartz RA. The basal cell nevus syndrome: disasters occurring among a series of 36 patients. *Cancer.* 1979;44:2294-2305.

12. U.S. National Institutes of Health. http://clinicaltrials.gov/ct2/show/NCT00957229. Accessed January 14, 2012.

13. Wicking C, Shanley S, Smyth I, et al. Most germ-line mutations in the nevoid basal cell carcinoma syndrome lead to a premature termination of the PATCHED protein, and no genotype-phenotype correlations are evident. *Am J Hum Genet.* 1997;60:21-26.

## Supplementary Information

**OMIM REFERENCES:**

[1] Basal Cell Nevus Syndrome; BCNS (#109400)

[2] Patched, Drosophila, Homolog of, 1; PTCH1 (#601309)

[3] Patched, Drosophila, Homolog of, 2; PTCH2 (#603673)

[4] Suppressor of Fused, Drosophila, Homolog of; SUFU (#607035)

**Alternative Names:**
- Gorlin Syndrome
- Basal Cell Nevus Syndrome
- Gorlin-Goltz Syndrome
- Multiple Basal Cell Nevi
- Basal Cell Cancer Syndrome

*Key Words:* Basal cell carcinoma, odontogenic keratocyst, medulloblastoma, cardiac fibroma, ovarian fibroma, macrocephaly, palmar pits, plantar pits, lymphomesenteric cyst, pleural cyst, falx cerebri calcification, polydactyly

# SECTION XIV PULMONOLOGY

## 114 Cystic Fibrosis

Ahmet Z. Uluer and Henry L. Dorkin

### KEY POINTS

- *Disease summary:*
  - Cystic fibrosis (CF) is the most common genetically inherited autosomal recessive disease in Caucasians that leads to multisystem organ dysfunction with the majority of morbidity and mortality related to respiratory and gastrointestinal (GI) systems.
  - CF arises secondary to mutations in the cystic fibrosis transmembrane conductance regulator (*CFTR*) gene on the long arm of chromosome 7; CFTR is translated into a multidomain chloride ion channel belonging to ATP-binding cassette (ABC) transporter superfamily.
  - Greater than 1800 *CFTR* mutations are known and may be classified by their functional defect; each mutation leads to varying impact on salt and water balance.
  - The pathogenesis of CF involving the lungs includes a vicious cycle of infection, inflammation, and bronchiectasis.
  - The clinical course of CF is typically chronic or progressive punctuated by acute exacerbations and eventual respiratory failure. As patient survival improves, other organ system complications are increasingly identified and require therapy.

- *Hereditary basis:*
  - Autosomal recessive pattern with variable clinical phenotype affected by the specific *CFTR* mutation, modifier genes, and environment

- *Differential diagnosis:*
  - Bronchiectasis from other causes: primary ciliary dyskinesia, tuberculosis, chronic aspiration
  - Primary immune deficiency, for example common variable immune deficiency
  - Other causes of elevated sweat chloride levels: malnutrition, hypothyroidism, adrenal insufficiency

## Diagnostic Criteria and Clinical Characteristics

### Diagnostic Criteria:

- Clinical presentation (one or more typical clinical findings)
- Sweat chloride concentration greater than or equal to 60 mol/L (40-59 mmol/L considered indeterminate, <40 mmol/L considered negative)
- *CFTR* mutation analysis indicating two known CF disease-causing mutations in *trans* configuration (Table 114-1). Mutation analysis may include the attempted identification of polymorphisms, deletions, and duplications
- Newborn screening: Evidence of elevated immune-reactive trypsinogen (IRT) and/or identification of one or more disease-causing *CFTR* mutation triggers sweat chloride testing and more extensive *CFTR* mutation analysis

Other considerations:
- CF-related metabolic syndrome (CRMS) is a new term proposed for patients who are asymptomatic but have either nondiagnostic sweat chloride or *CFTR* mutation analysis concerning for, but not diagnostic of cystic fibrosis.
- *CFTR*-related disorder (CRD) is a term proposed for CRMS patients who are symptomatic in some way.

**Clinical Characteristics:** Progressive pulmonary disease due to chronic infection, airway inflammation, and bronchiectasis is associated with the greatest morbidity and mortality in patients with CF. However, CF is a multisystem disorder (Table 114-2), a result of *CFTR* expression in most organs of the body, with varying clinical presentation that requires a multidisciplinary approach to treatment.

Chronic infection with pathogens such as methicillin-sensitive and methicillin-resistant *Staphylococcus aureus* (MSSA/MRSA), *Haemophilus influenzae, Pseudomonas aeruginosa* (mucoid and non-mucoid), *Burkholderia cepacia* complex species, *Achromobacter, Stenotrophomonas,* and others, complicate sinus and airway infections. Chronic cough and sputum production reflect the persistent infection with such organisms, as well as inflammation that leads to airway obstruction, progression of lung disease, and respiratory failure. The vicious cycle of infection and inflammation leads to radiographic abnormalities such as bronchiectasis, infectious opacities, and hyperinflation. CF patients are also at increased risk for pneumothoraces and hemoptysis. Hemoptysis can range from scant in amount to massive and life threatening. These manifestations eventually lead to chronic respiratory failure and premature death for those not undergoing lung transplantation.

A presentation with meconium ileus is highly suggestive of a diagnosis of CF. There is an increased lifetime risk of bowel obstruction due to ileus recurrence (termed distal intestinal obstruction

**Table 114-1  CFTR Mutation Classification**

| CFTR Mutation Class | Functional Defect |
| --- | --- |
| Class I | No protein |
| Class II | Defective trafficking |
| Class III | Gating defect |
| Class IV | Defective conductance |
| Class V | Reduced CFTR protein |

**Table 114-3  Most Common CFTR Mutations**

| Mutation Type | % of CF Patients With at Least One Copy of CFTR Mutation |
| --- | --- |
| Delta *F508* | 88.5 |
| *G542X* | 4.6 |
| *G551D* | 4.4 |
| *R117H* | 2.7 |
| *N1303K* | 2.5 |
| *W1282X* | 2.4 |
| *R553X* | 1.9 |

Used with permission from Cystic Fibrosis Foundation Patient Registry, 2010 Annual Data Report, Bethesda, Maryland ©2011 Cystic Fibrosis Foundation.

syndrome [DIOS]) in noninfants. Pancreatic insufficiency is present in nearly 85% of patients with increased risk for protein-calorie malnutrition and fat-soluble vitamin deficiency, particularly in the absence of pancreatic enzyme replacement. Recurrent and chronic pancreatitis may be a manifestation in those with pancreatic sufficiency. Liver disease in the form of cirrhosis manifested by obstruction of intrahepatic bile ducts can lead to focal or diffuse involvement. A small number of patients will develop portal hypertension and gastroesophageal varices. Cholelithiasis can lead to biliary duct obstruction, cholecystitis, and jaundice.

Abnormalities in salt-water balance, particularly with sweat gland involvement, increase the risk for hyponatremic dehydration and metabolic alkalosis. There is also an increased risk for developing CF-related diabetes. Although patients require exogenous insulin similar to type 1 diabetes, diabetic ketoacidosis (DKA) is rare due to low levels of circulating endogenous insulin, though insulin resistance also exists. Bone disease may be due to a combination of increased bone turnover and vitamin D malabsorption. An increased risk of acute and chronic kidney disease, as well as hearing loss, are complications of antibiotic treatment in patients with CF, specifically aminoglycosides. Infertility is common due to obstructive azoospermia in men and cervical mucus obstruction or plugging for women.

## Screening and Counseling

*Screening:* Newborn screening is offered in every state in the United States. It typically involves the measurement if immunoreactive trypsinogen, genetic analysis, or some combination of these diagnostic assessments. At present, complete genetic sequencing, intron 8 poly (T) analysis and the number of adjacent TG repeats within that region (increased TG repeat number is

associated with increased risk of disease) are available commercially but are not routinely provided by any state newborn screening program. A combined review panel from the CDC, NIH and other partners is reviewing diagnostic criteria for CF and related metabolic syndromes, with a diagnostic algorithm update due soon (2014). It should be noted that prenatal screening mandates by the American College of Obstetrics and Gynecology (ACOG) consider less than 30 of the over 1800 allele defects which can lead to phenotypic CF (Table 114-3). Thus, while these alleles chosen by the ACOG represent the most common abnormal alleles in the most susceptible population, they are only a limited screen, with diminished sensitivity in ethnic populations other than European Caucasians.

*Counseling:* The disease is transmitted by autosomal recessive inheritance. The diagnosis of CF in one offspring renders the probability of 25% for any subsequent (or previous) pregnancy. There are *CFTR* mutations with variable penetrance (eg, *D1152H* and *R117H*) and polymorphisms that lead to splicing inefficiencies (polyT-TG repeats). In addition, there are hypothesized "modifier" genes, which can either mitigate or accentuate the disease impact of the principal CF mutations.

Genotype-phenotype correlation may help predict those who have a better chance of clinical pancreatic sufficiency, but it is not possible to associate phenotype with a specific genotype with regard to the pulmonary manifestations of the disease at this time. Should such "modifier" genes be identified in the future, they may add to our prognostic ability.

**Table 114-2  CF Organ System Involvement**

| System | Manifestation |
| --- | --- |
| Sinopulmonary | Chronic sinusitis, acute and chronic airway infection |
| Hepatobiliary | Cholelithiasis, liver cirrhosis, portal hypertension |
| Pancreatic insufficiency | Pancreatic steatorrhea, malabsorption, distal intestinal obstruction syndrome (DIOS) |
| Genitourinary | Obstructive azoospermia, infertility |
| Endocrine | CF-related diabetes (CFRD) |
| Rheumatology | CF-related arthropathy |
| Sweat gland | Sweat chloride >60 mmol/L (40-59 mmol/L considered indeterminate) |

## Management and Treatment

Early diagnosis through newborn screening programs allows early detection and intervention in CF and permits better management of GI and pulmonary disease.

Gastrointestinal disease:

1. Pancreatic enzyme supplementation
2. Fat-soluble vitamin supplementation and serum vitamin level monitoring
3. Early detection of CF liver disease and pancreatitis with monitoring of serum enzyme levels
4. Prevention and/or treatment of other GI complications like hyponatremic dehydration, constipation, DIOS, diabetes, and cholelithiasis

Pulmonary disease:

1. Airway clearance using one or several of various methods: percussion and postural drainage, autogenic drainage, positive expiratory pressure (PEP) devices (eg, Acapella valve, flutter valve), oscillating vests, intrapulmonary percussive ventilator (IPV), and exercise
2. Mucolytics (dornase alfa)
3. Oral, aerosolized, and intravenous antibiotics
4. Anti-inflammatories (macrolides, ibuprofen, steroids)
5. Hydration of airway surface liquid (hypertonic saline, inhaled mannitol)
6. *CFTR* modulators (eg, potentiators of chloride transport)
7. Lung transplantation

Early detection of disease, initiation of Cystic Fibrosis Foundation (CFF) care guidelines, and early involvement of a multidisciplinary CF team are goals in pediatric care. The goal is to begin treatment as well as screening and monitoring for the usual impediments to growth and nutrition as well as early detection of pulmonary and other complications of the disease. In adults, attention to depression, osteoporosis, diabetes, reproductive issues, cancer screening, and complications from chronic care (antibiotic-related hearing loss and acute and chronic renal insufficiency) is critical. Patients with CF age and are of course subject to the usual illnesses of adulthood as well as initiation or progression of complications specific to CF (Fig. 114-1).

## Molecular Genetics and Molecular Mechanism

*Syndrome/Gene/Locus:* Mutations in the gene *CFTR* (located on chromosome 7q) were first identified in 1989 and lead to an absent or dysfunctional chloride ion channel. This in turn leads to depletion of the pericellular liquid layer, on which rides the mucociliary blanket. With loss of the pericellular liquid layer thickness, movement of the mucus layer (which traps bacteria and other debris) is impaired, leading to obstruction of the bronchioles. Similar defects affect the bile ducts secondary to impairment of the intrahepatic biliary epithelia and the pancreatic ducts. In the lungs, a cycle of obstruction, infection, and inflammation leads to bronchiectasis, reduced airway clearance, and fibrosis. The major form of death in CF patients is respiratory insufficiency and failure.

*Genetic Testing:*

1. Targeted *CFTR* mutation analysis widely available. Detection rates are based on ethnicity.
2. Full *CFTR* gene sequencing widely available commercially (eg, Ambry, Genzyme).

Since the discovery of the *CFTR* gene in 1989 gene therapy research has received enormous attention but sustained results have remained elusive. However, our understanding of the mechanisms by which *CFTR* mutations lead to a dysfunctional or absent CFTR protein have led to new pharmacogenetic therapies that target the underlying basic defect. Identification of a specific *CFTR* mutation found in 4.4% of patients with CF, referred to as G551D, now

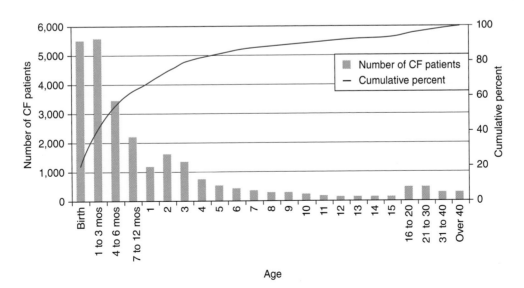

*Figure 114-1* Age at Diagnosis for all CF Patients–2009.
Cystic Fibrosis Foundation Annual Data Report 2009.

determines eligibility for a new FDA-approved therapy called iva-caftor. Ivacaftor (Kalydeco) is a small molecule taken orally that helps to partially correct the dysfunctioning CFTR protein at the cell surface and returns functionality to a mutation that (when left uncorrected) results in an ineffective chloride channel. Its discovery has opened the door for future "personalized" therapies designed to modulate specific *CFTR* mutations. A new website sponsored by the Cystic Fibrosis Foundation in partnership with Johns Hopkins University called CFTR2 (http://www.cftr2.org/) provides guidelines for a better understanding of identified *CFTR* mutations. It is intended for patients or families as well as healthcare providers and is available to the general public.

***Other:*** The CFF was established in 1955, initially as a result of parental frustration with the limited CF disease knowledge of the medical community. Focusing on the handful of clinics that had arisen from the interest of a few physicians (eg, Leroy Matthews in Cleveland, Dorothy Anderson in New York, and Harry Shwachman in Boston), these families set out to help fund a disease-oriented organization that ultimately became the CFF. The organization initially focused on disease awareness, eventually (through fund-raising) supporting research, clinical care, and physician training. Quality improvement, a currently widespread activity, was embarked on in the 1960s by the CFF with a Care Committee composed of senior CF physicians who helped create care guidelines and also site-visited the centers on a regular basis to ensure quality. In the 1980s Consensus Conferences were begun to scrutinize areas of care controversy or limited knowledge, in order to advance understanding in those areas. The Foundation developed a Therapeutic Development Network to support clinical trials with industry and accelerate the speed of drug discovery. Venture-philanthropy, a new discipline, was created using funds raised through fund-raising to increase interest in orphan disease drug research. For further information, see the CFF website (www.cff.org).

**BIBLIOGRAPHY:**

1. Borowitz D, Parad RB, Sharp JK, et al. Cystic Fibrosis Foundation practice guidelines for the management of infants with cystic fibrosis transmembrane conductance regulator-related metabolic syndrome during the first two years of life and beyond. *J Pediatr.* 2009;Suppl-15:S106-S116.

2. Castellani C, Cuppens H, Macek M Jr, et al. Consensus on the use and interpretation of cystic fibrosis mutation analysis in clinical practice. *J Cyst Fibros.* 2008;7(3):179-196.

3. Couper RT, Durie PR. What is cystic fibrosis? *N Engl J Med.* 2002;347(6):439-442.

4. Davis P. Clinical pathophysiology and manifestations of lung disease. In: Yankaskas J, Knowles M, eds. Cystic fibrosis in adults. Philadelphia, PA: Lippincott-Raven Publishers; 1999:45-67.

5. Flume PA, Mogayzel PJ, Robinson KA, et al. Cystic fibrosis pulmonary guidelines. Pulmonary complications: hemoptysis and pneumothorax. *Am J Respir Crit Care Med.* 2010;182:298-306.

6. Kerem E. Mutation specific therapy in CF. *Ped Respir Rev.* 2006;7(suppl 1):S166-S169.

7. Moran A, Brunzell C, Cohen RC, et al. Clinical care guideline for cystic fibrosis-related diabetes. *Diabetes Care.* 2010;33(12):2697-2708.

8. Park JE, Yung R, Stefanowicz D, et al. Cystic fibrosis modifier genes related to Pseudomonas aeruginosa infection. *Genes Immun.* Jul 2011;12(5):370-377.

9. Moskowitz SM, Chmiel JF, Sternen DL, et al. Clinical practice and genetic counseling for cystic fibrosis and *CFTR*-related disorders. *Genet Med.* 2008;10(12):851-868.

10. Parkins MD, Parkins VM, Rendall JC, Elborn S. Changing epidemiology and clinical issues arising in an ageing cystic fibrosis population. *Ther Adv Respir Dis.* Apr 2011;5(2):105-119.

11. Ramsey BW, Davies J, McElvaney NG, et al. A CFTR potentiator in patients with cystic fibrosis and the G551D mutation. *N Engl J Med.* 2011;365(18);1663-1670.

12. Riordan JR, Rommens JM, Kerem B, et al. Identification of the cystic fibrosis gene: cloning and characterization of complementary DNA. *Science.* Sep 8 1989;245(4922):1066-1073.

13. Stern RC. The diagnosis of cystic fibrosis. *N Engl J Med.* Feb 1997;336.7:487-491.

## Supplementary Information

**OMIM REFERENCES:**

[1] Cystic Fibrosis (#219700)

[2] Cystic Fibrosis Conductance Regulator Gene; CFTR (#602421)

***Key Words:*** Cystic fibrosis, bronchiectasis, sweat chloride, cystic fibrosis transmembrane conductance regulator gene

# 115 Alpha-1 Antitrypsin Deficiency

James K. Stoller

## KEY POINTS

- *Disease summary:*
  - Alpha-1 antitrypsin (AAT) deficiency is an autosomal codominant condition characterized by a decrease in the circulating level of AAT, a member of the serine protease inhibitor (serpin) family of proteins. AAT neutralizes several proteolytic enzymes, most notably neutrophil elastase, which can break down matrix proteins of the lung like elastin. Emphysema results from the unopposed proteolytic burden to the lung that is abetted by decreased levels of AAT.
  - The most common severe deficient variant of the AAT allele (ie, the Z allele) is also characterized by intrahepatocyte polymerization and accumulation of the Z-type AAT protein, with resultant cirrhosis and/or hepatoma. In the genetic variants of AAT deficiency that are characterized by intrahepatocyte accumulation of unsecreted AAT (eg, Z, $M_{malton}$), different pathogenetic mechanisms cause the liver versus the lung disease. Liver disease results from a toxic gain of function, which can trigger cirrhosis and/or hepatoma (by incompletely understood mechanisms). Lung disease results from the unopposed proteolytic burden to the lung that exists when levels of AAT are decreased and worsened by increased lung inflammation, as from cigarette smoking.
  - In addition to associations with emphysema and liver disease as clinical manifestations of AAT deficiency, panniculitis and C-ANCA-positive vasculitis have been established to be associated with AAT deficiency.
  - Guidelines recommend testing for AAT deficiency in all symptomatic adults with fixed airflow obstruction on postbronchodilator spirometry, as well as individuals with panniculitis, patients with otherwise unexplained cirrhosis, unexplained bronchiectasis, and siblings of AAT-deficient individuals.
- *Hereditary basis:*
  - AAT deficiency is inherited as an autosomal codominant condition.
  - The gene for AAT, *SERPINA1*, is located on chromosome 14 (14q32.1).
  - Genetic modifiers of pulmonary risk have been proposed and remain the subject of active investigation.
- *Differential diagnosis:*
  - AAT deficiency should be considered in the differential diagnosis of various pulmonary, hepatic, and dermatologic conditions, including emphysema, chronic bronchitis, bronchiectasis, or even asthma in which a component of fixed airflow obstruction exists, panniculitis, cirrhosis, chronic hepatitis, hepatoma, and C-ANCA-positive vasculitis.
  - While AAT deficiency should be considered in all symptomatic adults with fixed airflow obstruction, features of emphysema that might further heighten suspicion include basilar-predominant hyperlucency on chest imaging, early-onset emphysema (eg, before age 55), occurrence of emphysema in a non- or trivial-smoker, or a family history of liver or lung disease.

## Diagnostic Criteria and Clinical Characteristics

***Diagnostic Criteria for Alpha-1 Antitrypsin Deficiency:*** Subjects may be asymptomatic and unaffected. However, affected individuals may have one or more of the following clinical manifestations that have been found to be associated with AAT deficiency:

- Chronic obstructive pulmonary disease (eg, emphysema, chronic bronchitis)
- Bronchiectasis
- Cirrhosis
- Chronic hepatitis
- Hepatoma
- Neonatal jaundice
- Panniculitis
- C-ANCA-positive vasculitis

***Clinical Characteristics:***

☞**CHRONIC OBSTRUCTIVE PULMONARY DISEASE:** Guidelines suggest that all patients with chronic obstructive pulmonary disease (COPD) should be tested for AAT deficiency, which accounts for up to 3% of all cases of COPD. Features that should especially prompt suspicion of and testing for AAT deficiency include early-onset emphysema (eg, age <55 years), COPD in the absence of smoking or trivial smoking, radiographic pattern in which the changes of emphysema (eg, hyperlucency, bullous changes) are more prominent at the lung bases than at the apices, and a family history of liver and/or lung disease (even if other risk factors for these conditions [eg, smoking, alcohol use, etc] are present).

COPD may become manifest in AAT-deficient individuals in their mid-40s. Most individuals with severe AAT deficiency will develop COPD and the rate of decline of forced expiratory volume in 1 second ($FEV_1$) in AAT-deficient individuals is five- to sixfold faster among AAT-deficient active smokers (109 mL/y) and two- to threefold faster than normal (~54-67 mL/y) among AAT-deficient ex- or never-smokers. Studies of the radiographic pattern of emphysema on chest computed tomography (CT) indicate that approximately two-thirds of PI*ZZ individuals have a basilar-predominant pattern of emphysema and that the remainder has a more usual pattern of upper lobe-predominant emphysema.

☞**LIVER DISEASE:** Hepatic manifestations of AAT variants that are associated with intrahepatocyte polymerization (eg, Z, $M_{malton}$) include neonatal jaundice, neonatal cirrhosis, chronic hepatitis, cryptogenic cirrhosis, and hepatoma. The rare null variants that are characterized by complete absence of AAT synthesis do not cause liver disease.

☞**PANNICULITIS:** Panniculitis is manifested by painful areas of skin induration with breakdown and liquefaction, often in areas

*Table 115-1 Genetic Differential Diagnosis*

| Syndrome | Gene Symbol | Associated Findings |
|---|---|---|
| Cystic fibrosis | *CFTR* | Bronchiectasis, sinusitis, failure to thrive, infertility, pancreatic insufficiency |

Gene names: *CFTR*, cystic fibrosis transmembrane conductance regulator.

of physical trauma (eg, buttocks, arms, legs, extravasation sites after intravenous catheter placement).

☞C-ANCA-POSITIVE VASCULITIS: There is a higher than expected prevalence of abnormal AAT alleles (eg, Z, S) in individuals with C-ANCA vasculitis. It is speculated that this association with C-ANCA-positive vasculitis relates to the fact that proteinase-3, the presumed antigen in Wegener granulomatosis, is a substrate for AAT and that the deficiency of AAT allows the antigenicity of proteinase-3 to increase.

## Screening and Counseling

**Screening:** In patients with COPD, the prevalence of severe deficiency of AAT may be up to 3%. Guidelines from the American Thoracic Society/European Respiratory Society (with endorsements by the American College of Chest Physicians and the American Association for Respiratory Care) recommend testing (with a level A recommendation) the following groups: all symptomatic adults with fixed airflow obstruction on pulmonary function tests (whether characterized clinically as emphysema, chronic bronchitis, or even asthma with incomplete reversal of airflow obstruction on postbronchodilator spirometry testing), individuals with unexplained liver disease (including in neonates, children, and adults); asymptomatic individuals with persistent obstruction on pulmonary function tests with identifiable risk factors (eg, cigarette smoking, occupational exposure); adults with necrotizing panniculitis; and siblings of an individual with AAT deficiency. Population-based screening (eg, of all newborns) has not been recommended currently.

Because the pathogenetic mechanisms of lung disease and liver disease differ (ie, inadequate antiprotease protection against proteolytic burden in the lung versus toxic gain of function due to sequelae of unsecreted AAT polymers in the hepatocyte), individuals may present with lung disease alone, liver disease alone, or both lung and liver disease.

Results of population-based screening studies suggest that AAT-deficient individuals detected at birth have a lower likelihood of starting or continuing to smoke than age and gender-matched AAT-replete peers, emphasizing the importance of counseling against smoking in affected individuals.

**Counseling:** AAT deficiency is inherited as an autosomal codominant condition. Genotypes are described according to a protease inhibitor (PI*) nomenclature, with the individual's two allele names following "PI*." For example, normal individuals with both normal M alleles are PI*MM; heterozygotes for the Z allele (PI*MZ) comprise approximately 3% of Americans. Homozygotes for the severe deficiency allele Z are PI*ZZ and account for approximately 1 per 5000 live births in the United States and for approximately 1/1500 births in Sweden. Children of parents who are PI*MM (normal) and PI*ZZ will all be heterozygotes for the severe deficiency Z allele (PI*MZ). Heterozygotes are not deemed to be at significant

risk of developing emphysema. Children of two PI*MZ parents carry a 50% chance of being PI*MZ, and a 25% chance of being PI*MM or PI*ZZ, respectively. Siblings of PI*ZZ individuals should undergo genotyping (ie, determination of allelic combination, usually by polymerase chain reaction testing for the Z and S alleles) or phenotyping (identification of the protein products of component alleles by isoelectric focusing). Normal serum levels of AAT are 20 to 53 μmol (or ~80-220 mg/dL using nephelometry), with severe deficiency characterized by serum levels below a so-called "protective threshold" value. The protective threshold value is considered to be the serum level below which risk for emphysema rises, which is 11 μmol or 57 mg/dL. Most clinicians favor initial AAT testing with both a serum level and either a genotype or phenotype test.

Most but not all severely deficient individuals develop emphysema, risk for which is markedly increased by smoking. For liver disease, the lifetime risk is estimated to be approximately 40% and may be increased in longer-lived nonsmokers, who are more likely to escape the adverse health effects of COPD due to AAT deficiency.

## Management and Treatment

**Workup:** Initial evaluation of patients with AAT deficiency usually includes pulmonary function tests (with spirometry pre- and post-bronchodilator and diffusing capacity measurement), assessment of oxygenation, liver function tests, and plain chest radiograph. Some clinicians recommend further chest imaging with chest computerized tomographic scans (to assess for emphysema) and hepatic ultrasound to assess for cirrhotic changes and hepatoma.

**COPD:** Treatment of COPD in individuals with severe deficiency of AAT includes conventional therapy of COPD with bronchodilators, pulmonary rehabilitation, preventative vaccinations (ie, influenza and pneumococcal), inhaled corticosteroids, and supplemental oxygen when indicated. Lung volume reduction surgery, though effective in patients with AAT-replete COPD with a heterogeneous distribution of emphysema and low postrehabilitation exercise capacity, confers shorter-lived and generally lower lung function benefits in individuals with AAT deficiency. Lung transplantation is indicated when the usual criteria of severe airflow obstruction and functional impairment are present.

Specific therapy of AAT deficiency is so-called augmentation therapy, the intravenous infusion of purified pooled human AAT. Though definitive, confirmatory randomized controlled trials are not available, the weight of evidence suggests that intravenous augmentation therapy can slow the progression of emphysema, with the greatest benefit evident in individual with $FEV_1$ values between 30% and 65% predicted. Official guidelines recommend augmentation therapy for patients with established emphysema and $FEV_1$ values of 30% to 65% predicted while recommending against its prophylactic use (ie, for individuals with normal lung function). The evidence regarding benefit is weaker in those with $FEV_1$ greater than 65% predicted and for those with $FEV_1$ less than 30% predicted. Augmentation therapy offers no benefit for liver disease, which results from a gain-of-toxic function mechanism rather than from unopposed proteolytic damage.

**Liver Disease:** No specific therapy for the liver disease associated with AAT deficiency is available currently and usual therapy (eg, diuretics, beta-blockers, etc) is indicated for patients with cirrhosis. Liver transplantation is indicated for individuals with end-stage liver disease. Investigation is ongoing regarding the potential benefits of drugs (eg, rapamycin, carbamazepine) that enhance autophagy as a way of lessening liver disease associated with intrahepatic AAT accumulation (eg, Z homozygotes).

***Panniculitis:*** Panniculitis is an unusual complication of AAT deficiency. First-line therapy is anti-inflammatory (eg, dapsone). Anecdotal reports suggest that augmentation therapy can help resolve refractory lesions, though use for panniculitis is off-label.

## Molecular Genetics and Molecular Mechanism

***Syndrome/Gene/Locus:*** AAT is coded by *SERPINA1*, which is located on the long arm of chromosome 14 (14q32.1). The gene spans 12.2 kb and is organized into four coding (2, 3, 4, and 5) and three noncoding (1a, 1b, and 1c) exons.

The protein product, AAT, is a 394 amino acid glycoprotein with three carbohydrate side chains (Fig. 115-1). The normal gene codes for the M-type protein with four normal variants are M1, M2, M3, and M4 (Table 115-2). Normal serum levels (in PI*MM

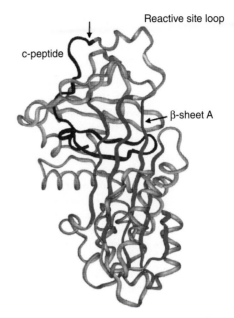

**Figure 115-1**

**Table 115-2  Selected PI Variants With Characteristics Including Type of Mutation, Cellular Defect, and Disease Association**

| PI Allele | Type of Mutation | Cellular Defect | Disease Association |
| --- | --- | --- | --- |
| **Normal alleles** | | | |
| M1V | Val213 | None | Normal |
| M1A | Ala213 | None | Normal |
| M2 | Arg101His on M3 | None | Normal |
| M3 | Glu376Asp on M1V | None | Normal |
| M4 | Arg101His on M1V | None | Normal |
| Christchurch | Glu363Lys | None | Normal |
| V$_{munich}$ | Asp2Ala on M1V | None | Normal |
| **Deficiency alleles** | | | |
| S | Glu264Val on M1V | IC degradation | Lung |
| Z* | Glu342Lys on M1A | IC accumulation | Lung, liver |
| M$_{malton}$ | Phe52del on M2 | IC accumulation | Lung, liver |
| S$_{iiyama}$ | Ser53Phe on M1V | IC accumulation | Lung |
| M$_{heerlen}$ | Pro369Leu on M1A | IC degradation | Lung |
| M$_{procida}$ | Leu41Pro on M1V | IC degradation | Lung |
| M$_{mineral\ springs}$[a] | Gly67Glu on M1V | IC degradation | Lung |
| **Null alleles** | | | |
| Q0$_{granite\ falls}$ | Tyr160Ter on M1A | No mRNA | Lung |
| Q0$_{bellingham}$ | Lys217Ter on M1V | No mRNA | Lung |
| Q0$_{ludwigshafen}$ | Ile92Asn on M2 | Disrupted tertiary structure IC accumulation | Lung[b] |
| Q0$_{hongkong-1}$ | 2-bp del Leu318 fs334ter on M2 | Truncated protein IC accumulation | Lung[b] |
| Q0$_{isola\ di\ procida}$ | 17 kb del on M2 | No mRNA | Lung |
| **Dysfunctional alleles** | | | |
| F | Arg223Cys on M1V | Defective NE inhibition | Lung |
| Pittsburgh | Met358Arg | Antithrombin 3 activity | Bleeding diathesis |
| M$_{mineral\ springs}$[a] | Gly67Glu on M1V | Defective NE inhibition | Lung |
| Z[a] | Glu342Lys on M1A | Defective NE inhibition | Lung, liver |

[a]Note that M$_{mineral\ springs}$ and Z have dysfunctional characteristics described based on altered rates of association and inhibition of neutrophil elastase, as well as deficiency characteristics.

[b]Although liver disease is theoretically possible in these null variants associated with IC accumulation, there are no reports of liver disease.

IC, intracellular; bp, base pair(s); NE, neutrophil elastase; del, deletion; fs, frameshift; ter, terminal codon.

Adapted with permission from BMJ Publishing Group Limited from DeMeo DL, Silverman EK. *Thorax.* 2004;59:259-264; and from Online Mendelian Inheritance in Man, (OMIM®), Johns Hopkins University, Baltimore, MD. 7/04/2011: http://omim.org/entry/107400.

individuals) are 20 to 53 µmol or approximately 80 to 220 mg/dL as measured by nephelometry.

More than 100 allelic variants have been described to date and have been characterized into four groups:

1. Normal variants (characterized by serum AAT levels in the normal range [20-53 µmol, or ~80-220 mg/dL by nephelometry])
2. Deficient variants, characterized by serum levels of AAT below 20 µmol and, for some alleles (eg, Z), decreased functional activity of the AAT molecule
   a. Among the deficient variants, the Z allele, characterized by a single amino acid substitution of lysine for glutamic acid at position 342 (Table 115-2), is the most common, accounting for approximately 95% of cases of clinically recognized AAT deficiency. Serum levels in individuals who are homozygous for the Z allele (PI*ZZ) fall in the range 3 to 8 µmol and are uniformly below the serum protective threshold of 57 mg/dL.
3. Null variants, characterized by absent circulating AAT due to transcriptional or translational errors that interrupt full protein synthesis.
4. Dysfunctional variants, characterized by abnormal function of AAT, for example, with decreased binding to neutrophil elastase (as in the F variant) or AAT Pittsburgh, where the structural abnormality causes the protein to serve as a thrombin inhibitor rather than as an antielastolytic protein, causing a bleeding diathesis. Table 115-2 summarizes the features of various alleles.

The most deficient variant, Z, is associated with intrahepatocyte accumulation of unsecreted Z-type protein because an instability of the Z-type AAT molecule (resulting from the single amino acid substitution at position 342 of a lysine for a glutamic acid) allows polymerization of Z-type molecules within the endoplasmic reticulum of the hepatocyte. The intracellular accumulation of the unsecreted protein causes lowering of serum levels below the serum protective level. Also, the Z-type molecule binds neutrophil elastase less avidly than normal M-type AAT. Another factor contributing to the pathogenesis of emphysema in Z-type AAT deficiency is that Z-type AAT polymers, which can be synthesized within the lung by alveolar macrophages, are chemotactic for polymorphonuclear leukocytes, thereby increasing the inflammatory burden in the lung.

**Genetic Testing:** Testing for AAT deficiency is available with three general types of tests: (1) measuring the serum level of AAT, usually by nephelometry, (2) phenotyping by isoelectric focusing to determine the band patterns that are described by various allelic combinations, and (3) genotyping, generally determined by polymerase chain reaction for the S and Z alleles. DNA sequencing is available in research laboratories.

In addition to commercial assays, free test kits using dried blood spots from which an AAT serum level and genotype are determined are available from several of the manufacturers of augmentation therapy drugs. Finally, free confidential home testing is available through the Alpha-1 Foundation (www.alphaone.org); patients can consent on line to participate in the Alpha-1 Coded Testing Study and then receive a dried blood spot test kit at home. On submitting the specimen, the serum level and genotype are determined at no cost to the patient and then returned confidentially to the patient with explanatory materials and access to genetic counseling.

## BIBLIOGRAPHY:

1. American Thoracic Society/European Respiratory Society Statement: standards for the diagnosis and management of individuals with alpha-1 antitrypsin deficiency. *Am J Respir Crit Care Med.* 2003;168:818-900.
2. Stoller JK, Aboussouan LS. Alpha-1 antitrypsin deficiency. *Lancet.* 2005;365:2225-2236.
3. Aboussouan LS, Stoller JK. Myths and misconceptions about alpha-1 antitrypsin deficiency. *Arch Intern Med.* 2009;169:546-550.
4. Aboussouan LS, Stoller JK. Detection of alpha-1 antitrypsin deficiency: a review. *Respir Med.* 2009;103:335-341.
5. The Alpha-1 antitrypsin Deficiency Registry Study Group, Crystal RG, Buist AS, et al. Survival and rate of FEV1 decline in subjects enrolled in the NHLBI Registry of Patients with Severe Deficiency of Alpha-1 Antitrypsin. *Am J Respir Crit Care Med.* 1998;158:49-59.
6. Parr DG, Stoel BC, Stolk J, Stockley RA. Pattern of emphysema distribution in alpha-1 antitrypsin deficiency influences lung function impairment. *Am J Respir Crit Care Med.* 2004;170:1172-1178.
7. Sveger T. Liver disease in alpha-1 antitrypsin deficiency detected by screening of 200,000 infants. *N Engl J Med.* 1976;294:1316-1321.
8. O'Brien ML, Buist NR, Murphey WH. Neonatal screening for alpha-1 antitrypsin deficiency. *J Pediatr.* 1978;92:1006-1010.
9. Tanash HA, Nilsson PM, Nilsson JA, Piitulainen E. Clinical course and prognosis of never-smokers with severe alpha-1 antitrypsin deficiency (PiZZ). *Thorax.* 2008;63:1091-1095.
10. Eriksson S. Alpha-1 antitrypsin deficiency and liver cirrhosis in adults. An analysis of 35 Swedish autopsied cases. *Acta Med Scand.* 1987;221:461-467.
11. American Thoracic Society COPD Guideline 2004. http://www.thoracic.org/index.php. Accessed September 25, 2011.
12. Stoller JK, Gildea T, Meli Y, Karafa M, Ries A. Lung volume reduction surgery in patients with emphysema and alpha-1 antitrypsin deficiency: experience in the National Emphysema Treatment Trial. *Ann Thorac Surg.* 2007;83:241-251.
13. Heresi G, Stoller JK. Augmentation therapy in alpha-1 antitrypsin deficiency. *Expert Opin Biol Ther.* 2008;8:515-526.
14. Teckman JH. Rapamycin reduces intrahepatic alpha-1 antitrypsin mutant Z protein polymers and liver injury in a mouse model. *Exp Biol Med (Maywood).* 2010;235:700-709.
15. Hidvegi T, Ewing M, Hale P, et al. An autophagy-enhancing drug promotes degradation of mutant alpha-1 antitrypsin Z and reduces hepatic fibrosis. *Science.* 2010;329:229-232.
16. Stoller JK, Piliang M. Panniculitis in alpha-1 antitrypsin deficiency. *Clin Pulm Med.* 2008;15:113-117.
17. Lomas DA, Mahadeva R. Alpha-1 antitrypsin polymerization and the serpinopathies: pathobiology and prospects for therapy. *J Clin Invest.* 2002;110:1585-1590.

## Supplementary Information

### OMIM REFERENCES:

[1] Serpin Peptidase Inhibitor, Clade A, Member 1; SerpinA1 (#107400)

[2] Phenotype Emphysema due to Alpha-1 Antitrypsin Deficiency; (#613490)

### Alternative Names:

- Alpha-1 Antiprotease Inhibitor
- Genetic Emphysema

**Key Words:** Emphysema, COPD, cirrhosis, alpha-1 antitrypsin, panniculitis, bronchiectasis, hepatitis, C-ANCA vasculitis, augmentation therapy

# 116 Asthma

Scott Weiss

## KEY POINTS

- *Disease summary:*
  - Asthma is a disease that is defined by reversible airflow obstruction, airway inflammation, and respiratory symptoms of wheezing and cough. The disorder is closely associated with allergy, or immediate type hypersensitivity to aeroallergens. Roughly 70% of all childhood asthmatics are allergic. Epidemiologically the disease is very common, affecting roughly 6% of the US population. Asthma commonly starts in early childhood. It has a variable early natural history; roughly 30% of children have wheezing with colds or occasionally apart from colds in the first year of life. This decreases to about 15% at age 3, with a similar percentage at age 6. Unfortunately, the phenotype does not breed true, and clinicians cannot predict which of those children wheezing at age 1 will be wheezing at age 3 or age 6. Adult asthma is often a recrudescence of childhood disease and has a less clear-cut relationship to allergy. There is a growing body of evidence that persistent asthma leads to reduced growth in lung function and an increased risk for the development of chronic obstructive lung disease (COLD) in adult life. Major morbidity is incurred from uncontrolled disease by reduced quality of life, days lost from work, hospitalizations, and emergency room visits. More details of the clinical features of asthma are given in references 1 and 2.

- *Differential diagnosis:*
  - In children asthma can be confused with chronic bronchitis, cystic fibrosis, bronchopulmonary dysplasia, and bronchiectasis. Asthma in adults is often confused with COLD. It can be differentiated from chronic obstructive pulmonary disease (COPD) via chest x-ray, and spirometry (lung function tests) before and after a short-acting bronchodilator. Occasionally a computed tomography (CT) scan is helpful in distinguishing these two conditions. In children, asthma must be differentiated from bronchiolitis or bronchitis. This is usually done by the same sort of clinical testing, for example, x-ray and spirometry, and clinical response to anti-inflammatory medication.

- *Monogenic forms:*
  - None described

- *Family history:*
  - Roughly two-thirds of all asthma patients will have a family history of allergies or asthma in a first-degree relative. This does not prove a genetic origin to the disease as this also occurs with any prevalent complex condition of reasonably high prevalence.

- *Twin studies:*
  - Concordance for dizygotic twins ranges from 15% to 40% and for monozygotic twins ranges from 50% to 80%.

- *Environmental factors:*
  - The most important environmental risk factors are aeroallergens (house dust mite, alternaria, cockroach) and smoking. In utero and postnatal passive smoking are important risk factors in children increasing the disease occurrence from 40%-200%. Active smoking is important in adolescents and adults. Additional environmental exposures of importance are viral infections and pets, particularly cats and dogs. In adults, postmenopausal estrogen is a risk factor.

- *Genome-wide associations:*
  - This analytic approach that uses single-nucleotide polymorphisms (SNPs) across the whole genome has identified a three-gene locus on chromosome 17q21 containing *ORMDL3*, *GSDMB*, and *ZPBP2* as the strongest locus for asthma. Other genes identified by this approach include *IL1RL1/IL18*, *TSLP*, *HLADQ*, *IL2RB*, *SLC22A5*, *RORA*, *IL33*, and *SMAD3*.

- *Pharmacogenomics:*
  - Genome-wide association studies (GWASs) have implicated the *GLCCI1* and the *T* gene as determinants of change in lung function with inhaled corticosteroid. Short-acting bronchodilator GWAS has implicated *SPATS2L* as a gene for response to short-acting beta-2 agonists.

## Diagnostic Criteria and Clinical Characteristics

### Diagnostic Criteria for Asthma:

**Diagnostic evaluation should include at least two of the following**

1. History of intermittent or continuous wheezing or shortness of breath (SOB)
2. Exertional symptoms of wheeze and/or SOB
3. Normal chest-x-ray
4. Normal CT scan of the chest
5. Obstructive pattern on spirometry (reduced $FEV_1$, normal forced vital capacity [FVC]) reversal with short-acting bronchodilator. Asthmatics have variable levels of lung function as defined by the $FEV_1$. This is the amount of air that is breathed out in 1 second after a maximal inhalation. This variability occurs spontaneously, but is best elicited in response to drugs. Asthmatics have an exaggerated bronchodilator response to short-acting beta-2 agonist drugs that act through the beta-2 adrenergic receptors on airway smooth muscle to bronchodilate the airway. They also have an exaggerated response to bronchoconstrictor drugs such

*Table 116-1 Pharmacogenetic Considerations in Asthma*

| Gene | Associated Medications | Goal of Testing | Variants | Effect |
|------|------------------------|-----------------|----------|--------|
| GLCCI1 | Glucocorticoids | Not recommended | rs37973 | 6% change in FEV$_1$ on ICS if you have the variant |
| T | Glucocorticoids | Not recommended | rs327412 | Twofold difference in FEV between wild type and mutant allele |
| SPATS2L | Short-acting beta-2 agonists | Not recommended | rs295137 | Median 6% difference in bronchodilator response between CC and CT and TT subjects |

as histamine and methacholine and bronchoconstrict dramatically to low doses of these drugs.

**And the absence of**
1. Any evidence of emphysema or bronchiectasis on chest-x-ray or CT scan
2. Lack of reversibility of lung function with bronchodilator

*Clinical Criteria:* Asthma is a syndrome without a sensitive or specific diagnostic test. In general, the symptoms of wheezing and reversible airflow obstruction are sufficient to make the diagnosis.

## Screening and Counseling

*Screening:* There are no indications for genetic screening at the present time.

*Counseling:* There are no indications for genetic counseling at the present time unless there is inadvertent pick up of a cystic fibrosis carrier (see Chapter 114).

## Management and Treatment

*Management:* Asthma is managed according to the NAEP guidelines for treatment that take into account symptoms, lung function, activity limitation, and severity.

*Therapeutics:* Mild intermittent asthma characterized by intermittent symptoms, little or no activity limitation and normal lung function can be managed with intermittent short-acting beta-2 agonist. Mild persistent asthma requires the use of inhaled corticosteroids and moderate, persistent, or severe asthma requires a progressive escalation in medication to the use of combination therapy with a reliever medication (short-acting beta-2 agonist) and a combination of a long-acting beta-2 agonist and an inhaled corticosteroid. There are special indications for the use of leukotriene antagonists and anti-IgE therapy in severe cases.

*Pharmacogenomics:* Table 116-1 lists glucocorticosteroid genes involved in treatment response. There are no clinical pharmacogenomics indications at this time.

## Molecular Genetics and Molecular Mechanisms

*Genetic Testing:* This is currently not available clinically and testing has no known clinical utility at the present time. Table 116-2 lists the most important asthma disease-associated susceptibility variants based on GWAS.

*Future Directions:* Asthma genomics is still in its infancy and as such it seems likely that it will take more integrative genomics to work out the epistasis and importance of various asthma pathways

*Table 116-2 Disease-Associated Susceptibility Variants (Based on GWAS)[a]*

| Candidate Gene | Associated Variant | Relative Risk | Frequency of Risk Allele | Putative Functional Significance | Associated Disease Phenotype |
|----------------|--------------------|---------------|--------------------------|----------------------------------|------------------------------|
| 17q21 | rs7216389 | 1.45 | 62% in cases | Not known | Asthma |
| Il1/RL1 | rs13408661-G | 1.23 | 84% in cases | Not known | Asthma |
| IL18 | Same as above | 1.23 | Same as above | Not known | Asthma |
| TSLP | rs1837253-C | 1.17 | 35% in cases | Not known | Asthma |
| HLADP | rs987870-C | 1.40 | 86% | Not known | Asthma |
| IL2RB | rs2284033-G | 1.12 | 44% in cases | Not known | Asthma |
| SLC22A5 | rs2073643-T | 1.11 | 55% in cases | Not known | Asthma |
| RORA | rs11071559-C | 1.18 | 14% in cases | Not known | Asthma |
| IL33 | rs1342326-C | 1.20 | 16% in cases | Not known | Asthma |
| SMAD3 | rs744910-G | 1.12 | 51% in cases | Not known | Asthma |

[a]To date 20 other genes have been implicated in 10 or more genetic association studies and fine mapping studies: *IL5, IL13, Il4, CC15, FCER1B, CD14, ACAR2, THF, IL4R, FLG, IL10, VDR, LTA, GSTP1, Il12, STAT3, IL19, CCL5, TGFB1, CFGHCL9*. These genes are involved in Th2 inflammation, human leukocyte antigen (HLA), IgE, cytokines, and immune function.

that might be informative with regard to risk and prediction of clinical events.

## BIBLIOGRAPHY:

1. Litonjua A, Weiss ST. Asthma epidemiology: natural history of asthma. In: Drazen JM, ed. *Up To Date in Pulm and Crit Care Med*. Mar 20 1996.

2. Litonjua A, Weiss ST. Asthma epidemiology: definition, diagnostic criteria, and prevalence of asthma. In: Drazen JM, ed. *Up To Date in Pulm and Crit Care Med*. Mar 4 1996.

3. Strachan DP, Wong HJ, Spector TD. Concordance and interrelationship of atopic diseases and markers of allergic sensitization among adult female twins. *J Allergy Clin Immunol*. Dec 2001;108(6):901-907.

4. Torgerson DG, Ampleford EJ, Chiu GY. Meta-analysis of genome-wide association studies of asthma in ethnically diverse North American populations. *Nat Genet*. Jul 31 2011;43(9):887-892.

5. Moffatt MF, Gut IG, Demenais F, et al. A large-scale, consortium-based genomewide association study of asthma. *N Engl J Med*. Sep 23 2010;363(13):1211-1221.

6. Tantisira KG, Lasky-Su J, Harada M, et al. Genomewide association between GLCCI1 and response to glucocorticoid therapy in asthma. *N Engl J Med*. Sep 29 2011;365(13):1173-1183.

7. Himes BE, Jiang X, Hu R, et al. Genome-wide association analysis in asthma subjects identifies SPATS2L as a novel bronchodilator response gene. *PLoS Genet*. Jul 2012;8(7):e1002824.

8. Postma DS, Kerkhof M, Boezen HM, Koppelman GH. Asthma and chronic obstructive pulmonary disease: common genes, common environments? *Am J Respir Crit Care Med*. Jun 15 2011;183(12):1588-1594.

# 117 Sarcoidosis

Birendra P. Sah and Michael Iannuzzi

## KEY POINTS

- *Disease summary:*
  - Sarcoidosis is a multisystemic disease of unknown etiology that is characterized by granulomatous inflammation. It is presumed to be triggered by a complex interaction between environmental and genetic factors.
  - The incidence of sarcoidosis varies widely throughout the world depending on ethnicity and geographic region. The annual incidence ranges from 1 to 64 cases per 100,000 persons.
  - Although sarcoidosis affects people of all racial and ethnic groups and occurs at all ages, it usually develops before the age of 50 years and it is three times more common among blacks than whites. Blacks also develop more severe and chronic disease.
  - Sarcoidosis can involve any organ system, with the respiratory system most commonly involved. About 50% of cases are detected in asymptomatic individuals due to incidental radiographic abnormalities of bilateral hilar lymphadenopathy with or without pulmonary infiltrates. When symptomatic the most common complaints are cough, dyspnea, chest pain, eye lesions, and/or skin lesions.
- *Differential diagnosis:*
  - Mycobaterial and fungal infections (histoplasmosis, coccidiodomycosis), chronic berylliosis, talcosis, hypersensitivity pneumonitis, autoimmune disorders (Wegener granulomatosis, primary biliary cirrhosis, Crohn disease), lymphoma, and tumor-related granulomatous disease.
- *Monogenic forms:*
  - Blau syndrome (early-onset sarcoidosis), an autosomal dominant disorder, results from mutations in the NACHT domain of *CARD15* (also known as *NOD2*) located on chromosome 16q12.1-13. Blau syndrome usually presents before the age of 4 years and mainly involves skin, joints, and eyes. Lung involvement is notably absent.
- *Family history:*
  - From 3.6% to 9.6% of patients report that their first- or second-degree relatives also have sarcoidosis. Siblings of the affected patient have a fivefold increase in the relative risk of developing sarcoidosis.
- *Twin studies:*
  - A registry-based twin study showed about a 10-fold increased risk for concordant disease in monozygotic twins compared to dizygotic twins.
- *Environmental factors:*
  - Exposures associated with increased risk for sarcoidosis include agricultural employment, mold or mildew, musty odors at work, and pesticide-using industries. Tobacco use is negatively associated with sarcoidosis. In the United States, occupational clustering of sarcoidosis has been reported in ship workers, firefighters, and rescue workers who responded to the attacks on the World Trade Center.
- *Genome-wide associations:*
  - Genome-wide association studies (GWASs) have identified several human leukocyte antigen (HLA) and non-HLA candidate disease genes for sarcoidosis (Tables 117-1 and 117-2).
- *Pharmacogenomics:*
  - Pharmacogenetic studies are indicated for some of the medications used in sarcoidosis treatment (Table 117-3).

## Diagnostic Criteria and Clinical Characteristics

### Diagnostic Criteria for Sarcoidosis:

**Diagnostic evaluation should include (Fig. 117-1 algorithm)**

- Compatible clinical features established through history and physical examination with attention to environmental or occupational exposure and family history.
- A chest radiograph shows bilateral hilar lymphadenopathy with or without pulmonary infiltrate.
- For patients without apparent lung involvement, fluorodeoxyglucose positron emission tomography (FDG-PET) may be useful in identifying sites for diagnostic biopsy.
- Biopsy of the affected organ showing noncaseating granulomas with exclusion of other causes of granulomas such as mycobacterial and fungal infections.
- Pulmonary function tests may show restrictive, obstructive, or mixed ventilatory defect with reduced diffusion capacity of carbon monoxide (DLCO).
- Bronchoalveolar lavage (BAL) may show lymphocytosis with CD4:CD8 greater than 3·5.
- Measurement of the serum angiotensin-converting enzyme (ACE) level may be helpful. ACE is produced by sarcoidal granulomas and its level can be elevated in sarcoidosis. The diagnostic and prognostic usefulness of the serum ACE is limited because of its low sensitivity and specificity. Furthermore, the serum ACE level is influenced by *ACE* gene polymorphisms.

**Table 117-1  *Summary of HLA Association Studies of Sarcoidosis***

| HLA | Risk Alleles | Putative Functional Significance |
|---|---|---|
| *HLA-A* | A*1 | Susceptibility |
| *HLA-B* | B*8 | Susceptibility in several populations |
| *HLA-DQB1* | *0201 *0602 | Protection, Löfgren syndrome, mild disease in several populations Susceptibility/disease progression in several groups |
| *HLA-DRB1* | *0301 | Acute onset/good prognosis in several groups |
| | *01, *04 | Protection in several populations |
| | *1101 | Susceptibility in whites and African Americans. Stage II/III chest x-ray |
| *HLA-DRB3* | *1501 | Associated with Löfgren syndrome |
| | *0101 | Susceptibility/disease progression in whites |

ACE levels may have their greatest usefulness in detecting medical noncompliance in patients with previously elevated ACE levels since serum ACE levels plummet in response to low-dose prednisone.

- Screening for extrapulmonary manifestations: electrocardiography (EKG), liver function test, slit-lamp examination of eyes, serum and 24-hour urine for calcium.

***Clinical Characteristics:*** Sarcoidosis often first comes to attention when abnormalities are detected incidentally on a chest radiograph during a routine screening examination. Constitutional symptoms such as fatigue, night sweats, and weight loss occur in one-third of the patients. Sarcoidosis can affect any organ system but the thorax is the most common site involved in over 90% of patients. Thoracic involvement includes enlarged mediastinal as well as bilateral hilar lymph nodes and lung infiltrates. Common presenting symptoms include dyspnea, dry cough, chest pain, eye lesions, and/or skin lesions.

☞**EXTRAPULMONARY MANIFESTATIONS OF SARCOIDOSIS:**

- *Dermatologic:* Skin lesions are varied and include macules, papules, plaques, hypopigmentation, and hyperpigmentation. Lupus pernio presents as indurated, lumpy, violaceous lesions on the nose, cheeks, lips, and ears. Erythema nodosum (EN) occurs in about 10% of the patients and is most common in white women. EN often occurs with Löfgren syndrome, an acute presentation consisting of arthritis, EN, and bilateral hilar lymphadenopathy. A diagnosis of sarcoidosis is reasonably certain without biopsy in patients who present with Löfgren syndrome.
- *Ocular:* Ocular involvement occurs in about 25% of the patients and includes anterior and posterior uveitis and lacrimal gland enlargement. Chronic anterior uveitis has few symptoms and is more common than acute anterior uveitis which typically presents with photophobia, blurry vision, and pain.
- *Neurologic:* Neurologic manifestations occur in about 5% of patients. Cranial nerve involvement is most common, particularly

seventh cranial nerve but any part of the nervous system may be involved.

- *Cardiac:* Cardiac sarcoidosis most commonly presents as an electrical conduction disturbances such as complete heart block (sudden death), arrhythmias, and cardiomyopathy with loss of muscle function.
- *Lymphatic:* In addition to intrathoracic lymphadenopathy, peripheral lymph node enlargement is common. Intra-abdominal lymphadenopathy may also occur.
- *Liver/Spleen:* Noncaseating granulomas are found on liver biopsy in about 80% of patients. Organomegaly occurs in about 15%. Liver involvement may progress to cholestatic jaundice, hepatic failure, and portal hypertension.
- *Upper respiratory tract:* About 5% of patients will have symptoms of sinusitis, hoarseness, or shortness of breath. Sarcoidosis of the upper respiratory tract (SURT) can result in airway stenosis.
- Other extrapulmonary manifestations include arthralgia, myalgia, hypercalcemia, and renal calculi. Rarely, the gastrointestinal tract, reproductive organs, salivary glands, and the kidneys are affected.

Two-thirds of patients with sarcoidosis generally have a remission within a decade after diagnosis, with few or no consequences. Remission occurs in more than half of patients within 3 years. Unfortunately, up to a third of patients have unrelenting disease, leading to clinically significant organ impairment. A recurrence after 1 or more years of remission is uncommon (affecting <5% of patients), but recurrent disease may develop at any age and in any organ. Less than 5% of patients die from sarcoidosis; death is usually the result of pulmonary fibrosis with respiratory failure or of cardiac or neurologic involvement.

## Screening and Counseling

***Screening:*** Screening of family members of sarcoidosis patients is not recommended as only about 1% of first-degree relatives are also affected with sarcoidosis.

***Counseling:*** Familial clustering of sarcoidosis cases is common. A first-degree relative of a sarcoidosis patient has a 3.6% to 9.6% lifetime risk of also developing sarcoidosis. Siblings of the affected patient have a fivefold relative risk of developing sarcoidosis. There is an 80-fold increased risk of developing sarcoidosis in monozygotic cotwins and sevenfold increased risk in dizygotic twins.

## Management and Treatment

***Management and Therapeutics:*** Spontaneous remission without treatment occurs in 50% of patients. For patients who require treatment, corticosteroids remain the mainstay of treatment. The indications for systemic treatment include severe troubling symptoms, decline in any organ function, neurologic or cardiovascular involvement, posterior uveitis, laryngeal involvements, hypercalcemia, and disfiguring skin lesions such as lupus pernio. Prednisone is started at the dose of 20 to 40 mg daily. The response should be assessed in 2 to 3 months and if there has been a response, the prednisone dose should be tapered to 10 to 15 mg per day, with treatment planned for an additional 6 to 9 months. The common

*Table 117-2 Non-HLA Candidate Gene Associations With Sarcoidosis*

| Candidate Gene | Gene Symbol | Chromosome Location | Association[a,b] | Putative Functional Significance |
|---|---|---|---|---|
| Angiotensin-converting enzyme | ACE | 17q23 | C | Increased risk for ID and DD genotypes Moderate association between II genotype and radiographic progression |
| Annexin A11 | ANXA11 | 10q22.3 | A+ | Depletion or dysfunction of annexin A11 may affect the apoptosis pathway in sarcoidosis |
| Butyrophilin-like 2 | BTNL2 | 6p21 | A | Sarcoidosis is associated with a truncating splice-site mutation in BTNL2 |
| Caspase recruitment domain family 15 | CARD15 (NOD2) | 16q12.1-13 | A | Gene responsible for Blau syndrome |
| CC-chemokine receptor 2 | CCR2 | 3p21.3 | C+/− | Protection/Löfgren syndrome association |
| Clara cell 10 kD protein | CCR10 | 11q 12-13 | C | An allele associated with sarcoidosis and with progressive disease at 3-year follow-up |
| Complement receptor 1 | CR1 | 1q32 | A | The GG genotype for the Pro1827Arg(C[5,507]G) polymorphism was significantly associated with sarcoidosis |
| Cystic fibrosis transmembrane regulator | CFTR | 7q31.2 | A+/− | R75Q increases risk |
| Heat shock protein 70-hom | HSP70-hom | 6p21.3 | C | HSP(-2437)CC associated with susceptibility and LS |
| Inhibitor κ (kappa) β-α | IκB-alpha | 14q13 | C | Association with -297T allele. Association of haplotype GTT at -881, -826, and -297, respectively. Allele -827T in Stage II |
| Interlukin-1α | IL-1α | 2q14 | A | The IL-1α-889 1.1 genotype increased risk |
| Interlukin-4 receptor | IL-4R | 16p11.2 | | No association detected in 241 members of 62 families |
| Interlukin-18 | IL-18 | 11q22 | A+/− | Genotype -607CA increased risk over AA No association with organ involvement |
| Interferon-γ | IFN-γ | 9p22 | A | IFNA17 polymorphism (551T→G) and IFNA10 (60A) IFN-α 17 (551G) haplotype increased risk |
| Natural resistance-associated macrophage protein | SLC11A1 (NRAMP1) | 2q35 | A | Protective effect of (CA)(n) repeat in the immediate 5′ region of the SLC11A1 gene |
| Toll-like receptor 4 | TLR4 | 9q32 | B | Asp299Gly and Thre399Ile mutations associated with chronic disease |
| TLR10-TLR1-TLR6 cluster | - | 4p14 | B | Genetic variation in this cluster is associated with increased risk of chronic disease |
| Transforming growth factor-β | TGF-β | 19q13.2 | B | TGF-2 59941 allele, TGF-β3 4875 A, and 17369 C alleles were associated with chest x-ray detection of fibrosis |
| Tumor necrosis factor-α | TNF-α | 6p21.3 | C+/− | Genotype -307A allele associated with Löfgren syndrome and erythema nodosum and -857T allele with sarcoidosis. -307A not associated in African Americans |
| Vascular endothelial growth factor | VEGF | 6p12 | C | Protective effect of +813 CT and TT genotypes |
| Vitamin D receptor | VDR | 12q12-14 | A− | BsmI allele elevated in sarcoidosis patients |

[a]Type of association: A, susceptibility; B, disease course; C,. both.
[b]−, association refuted; +, association replicated.

IL, interleukin; LS, Löfgren syndrome; TNF, tumor necrosis factor; VEGF, vascular endothelial growth factor.

**Table 117-3 *Pharmacogenetics in Sarcoidosis and Other Autoimmune Disorders***

| Gene | Associated Medications | Goal of Testing | Variants | Effect |
|---|---|---|---|---|
| *TPMT* (thiopurine *S*-methyltransferase) | Azathioprine, 6-mercaptopurine | Safety and efficacy | *2,*3A, *3C | Variants—lower dose WT—higher dose Less frequent WBC monitoring |
| *MTHFR* (5,10-methylenetetrahydrofolate reductase) | Methotrexate | Safety | *1298C | All side effects: nausea/vomiting, rash, abnormal LFTs |
| *FCGR3A* (Fc fragment of IgG, low affinity IIIa, receptor) | Infliximab | Efficacy | *G4985T | Lower efficacy |
| *FASLG* (FAS ligand) | Infliximab | Efficacy | *843TT | Lower efficacy, apoptotic pathway |
| *ABCB1* ATP-binding cassette, subfamily B (MDR/TAP), member 1 | Glucocorticoids | Efficacy | *G2677TT *C3435T *843TT | Lower efficacy Steroid resistance Ethnic variation |

side effects of prednisone include short term—weight gain, glucose intolerance, mood swing, and insomnia; long term—osteoporosis, cataract, glaucoma, and hypertension.

In patients with no response or contraindication to corticosteroids or in those patients who need a long-term prednisone dose higher than 10 mg daily, other immunosuppressive drugs are indicated. Weekly low-dose methotrexate, daily azathioprine, or mycophenolate mofetil are the most commonly used immunosuppressive drugs. Hydroxychloroquine may be useful for extensive skin lesions, peripheral lymphadenopathy, hypercalcemia, and fatigue. Cyclophosphamide has been used to treat severe neurologic symptoms. In certain refractory cases, case reports support the use of infliximab, an antitumor

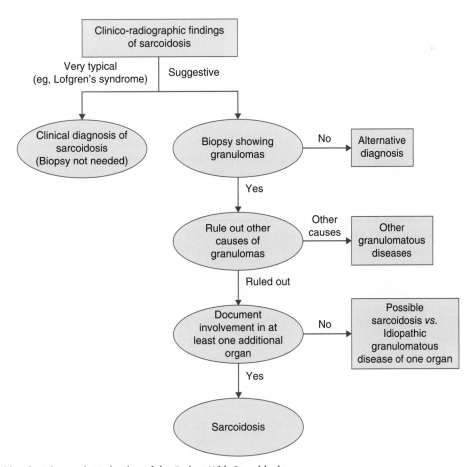

**Figure 117-1** Algorithm for Diagnostic Evaluation of the Patient With Sarcoidosis.

necrosis factor (anti-TNF) antibody. Topical corticosteroids can be used for limited skin involvement and anterior uveitis. Inhaled corticosteroids have not been shown to improve lung function but do lessen cough. Nonsteroidal anti-inflammatory drug (NSAID) is indicated for the treatment of EN, arthralgia, and myalgia.

***Pharmacogenetics:*** Pharmacogenetic testing is indicated for some agents used to treat sarcoidosis (Table 117-3). Thiopurine *S*-methyltransferase (TPMT) is a key metabolic enzyme for azathioprine and 6-mercaptopurine (6-MP). Azathioprine is metabolized to 6-MP and eventually to active 6-thioguanine (6-TG). 6-Mercaptopurine can be inactivated by either TPMT or xanthine oxidase to nontoxic products. Polymorphisms in the *TPMT* gene reduce TPMT activity, shunting metabolism to 6-TG, and increasing toxicity and risk for neutropenia. Testing for TPMT enzyme activity in red blood cells or *TPMT* single-nucleotide polymorphism (SNP) genotyping is both available and widely used before initiating therapy. Approved by the FDA, *TPMT* testing appears to be cost-effective. Methylenetetrahydrofolate reductase (*MTHFR*) polymorphisms are also associated with increased toxicity of methotrexate; testing is not yet widely available.

# Molecular Genetics and Molecular Mechanism

Sarcoidosis is an immune-mediated disease that is thought to be caused by complex interaction between genetic and environmental factors. Familial clustering, increased concordance in monozygotic twins, and variation in the incidence and disease presentation among different ethnic groups all support a genetic contribution to sarcoidosis etiology. Clustering of sarcoidosis cases in families has been observed worldwide. In the ACCESS study, subjects were five times more likely than control subjects to report a sibling or parent affected with sarcoidosis. Twin studies indicate that monozygotic twins are more often concordant for disease than dizygotic twins. In the United States, sarcoidosis affects African Americans more frequently than other ethnic groups. African Americans also have chronic and more severe disease.

The immunopathogenesis of sarcoidosis involves the presentation of an antigen to T lymphocytes that leads to the activation of T-helper 1 (Th1) cells, a final pathway of granulomas formation. During this process cytokines IL-8, IL-15, and IL-16 are released to recruit additional Th1 cells from blood. These cells then release a cascade of Th1 cytokines interferon (IFN)-gamma, IL-2, and IL-12 while simultaneously suppressing the Th2 cytokines (IL-4 and IL-5). Because of this characteristic inflammatory profile, genetic studies on sarcoidosis have focused on identifying candidate genes (both HLA and non-HLA) that may result in dysregulation of the T-cell response. These genes may include genes involved in antigen processing, antigen presentation, macrophage and T-cell activation, and cell recruitment and injury repair.

HLA genes have been the best-studied candidates in sarcoidosis because major histocompatibility complex (MHC) class II proteins are responsible for antigen presentation to T cells (Table 117-1). There is evidence to also support a role for HLA class I genes in sarcoidosis pathophysiology. The first reported HLA association was of HLA class I antigen *HLA-B8* with acute sarcoidosis. Subsequently, HLA class II antigens, encoded by the *HLA-DRB1* and *DQB1* alleles, were also found to be associated with sarcoidosis. *HLA-DRB1*01* and *HLA-DRB1*04* correlate

negatively (protect against disease) with sarcoidosis, whereas *HLA-DRB1*03*, *HLA-DRB1*11*, *HLA-DRB1*12*, *HLADRB1*14*, and *HLA-DRB1*15* are associated with an increased risk of developing sarcoidosis. Specific HLA genotypes may correlate with the course of disease; *HLADRB1*0301* and *HLA-DQB1*0201* are associated with Löfgren syndrome, an acute form of sarcoidosis with a favorable course and high rate (~80%) of spontaneous remission. *HLA-DRB1*1501* and *HLA-DQB1*0602* haplotypes have been associated with a chronic course and severe pulmonary sarcoidosis. *HLA-DRB1*1101* is associated with stage II or stage III radiographic pattern of sarcoidosis. In Japanese, *HLA-DQB1*0601* is present in higher frequency in the patients with splenomegaly and cardiac sarcoidosis.

The antigen-binding properties of the HLA class II peptide-binding groove are determined by polymorphic amino acid residues. These residues form pockets in the groove, interacting with the antigenic peptide side chains. A recent study in Dutch sarcoidosis patients suggested that pocket 9 of *HLA-DQ* and pocket 4 of *HLA-DR* are the most important regions associated with sarcoidosis. Also, Arg74 situated in *DRB1* pocket 4 was found to independently correlate with radiographic stage 1. One study indicated that the *HLADQB1*0201* associated risk for sarcoidosis was modified through exposure to high humidity in the workplace or exposure to water damage.

In addition to *HLA* genes, polymorphisms within non-HLA candidate genes also play a role in the immunopathogenesis of sarcoidosis (Table 117-2). The results of the studies of non-HLA candidate genes have been inconsistent. The most attractive non-HLA candidate genes are caspase recruitment domain family, member 15 (CARD15); natural resistance–associated macrophage protein-1 (*NRAMP1*); *ACE*; and chemokine (C–C motif) receptor-2 (*CCR2*). CARD15, alias nucleotide oligomerization domain protein-2 (*NOD2*), located on chromosome 16, is the gene responsible for Blau syndrome. The *ACE* gene insertion (I) or deletion (D) polymorphism causes variation in the serum ACE level. Studies to support a role for *ACE* gene polymorphisms in susceptibility or severity have been inconsistent. *NRAMP1*, now named *SLC11A1*, is expressed primarily in macrophages and polymorphonuclear leukocytes. It is associated with increased risk of sarcoidosis in Poles. The V64I polymorphism in *CCR2*, a receptor for monocyte chemotactic protein-1, has been reported to be associated with increased risk of sarcoidosis in Japanese and Czech populations. This association has not been replicated in other studies.

***Genome-Wide Association Studies:*** Two GWASs have been conducted in families with sarcoidosis. A German study identified the butyrophilin-like 2 (*BTNL2*) gene, a B7 family member of costimulatory molecules in the MHC II region on chromosome 6p. The *BTNL2* SNP associated with sarcoidosis (rs2076530 G→A) may influence T-lymphocyte activation and regulation. SNPs within *BTNL2* have been associated with increased sarcoidosis risk in both white and black Americans. Subsequent GWAS studies in African-Americans families showed sarcoidosis susceptibility loci at chromosome 3p and 5q11.2 and protective genes in the region of 5p15.2. Phenotypic analysis of these genome-wide scans shows the strongest linkage signals on chromosome 1p36 for radiographic resolution of sarcoidal lesions and on chromosome 18q22 for the presence of cardiac or renal involvement.

The GWAS conducted by Hofmann and colleagues in German patients found annexin A11 (*ANXA11*) gene on chromosome 10q22.3 associated with sarcoidosis. Validation in an independent sample confirmed the association. Depletion or dysfunction of

*ANXA11* may affect the apoptosis pathway in sarcoidosis. Recently the same group reported another associated locus 6p12.1 that comprises several genes, a likely candidate being *RAB23*. *RAB23* is proposed to be involved in antibacterial defense processes and regulation of the sonic hedgehog-signaling pathway.

Recently Hofmann, Fischer, and colleagues conducted a genome-wide linkage analysis in 181 German sarcoidosis families using clustered biallelic markers. This study revealed one region of suggestive linkage on chromosome 12p13.31 at 20 cM (LOD = 2.53; local *p* value = .0003) and another linkage on 9q33.1 at 134 cM (LOD = 2.12; local *p* value = .0009). It is proposed that these regions might harbor as yet unidentified, possibly subphenotype-specific risk factors for the disease (eg, immune-related functions like the tumor necrosis factor receptor 1).

*Genetic Testing:* Genetic testing at present does not play any role in the diagnosis and treatment of sarcoidosis.

*Future Directions:* The cause of sarcoidosis remains unknown. Methods such as multiplexed liquid chromatography and nano–high-performance liquid chromatography coupled to electrospray or matrix-assisted laser desorption or ionization mass spectrometry may aid in the identification of inciting sarcoidal antigens. Gene expression profiling in bronchoalveolar lavage fluid and blood at the time of presentation may help predict disease progression.

### BIBLIOGRAPHY:

1. Iannuzzi MC, Rybicki BA. Genetics of sarcoidosis. *Proc Am Thorac Soc.* 2007;4:108-116.

2. Grunewald J, et al. Genetics of sarcoidosis. *Curr Opin Pulm Med.* 2008;14:434-439.

3. Iannuzzi M, Morgenthau A. Recent advances in sarcoidosis. *Chest.* 2011;139:174-182.

4. Iannuzzi M, Rybicki B, Teirstein A. Sarcoidosis. *N Engl J Med.* 2007;357:2153-2165.

5. Rybicki BA, Iannuzzi MC, Frederick MM, et al. Familial aggregation of sarcoidosis. A case control etiologic study of sarcoidosis (ACCESS). *Am J Respir Crit Care Med.* 2001;164(11):2085-2091.

6. Harrington D, Major M, Rybicki B, Popovich J Jr, Maliarik M, Iannuzzi MC. Familial analysis of 91 families. *Sarcoidosis.* 1994;11:240-243.

7. Brewerton DA, Cockburn C, James DC, James DG, Neville E. HLA antigens in sarcoidosis. *Clin Exp Immunol.* 1977;27: 227-229.

8. Grunewald J, Eklund A, Olerup O. Human leukocyte antigen class I alleles and the disease course in sarcoidosis patients. *Am J Respir Crit Care Med.* 2004;169:696-702.

9. Hofmann S, FrankeA, Fischer A, et al. Genome-wide association study identifies ANXA11 as a new susceptibility locus for sarcoidosis. *Nat Genet.* 2008;40 (9):1103-1106.

10. Hofmann S, Fischer A, Till A, et al. A genome-wide association study reveals evidence of association with sarcoidosis at 6p12.1 *Eur Respir J.* 2011;38:1127-1135.

11. Fischer A, Hofmann S, Schürmann M, Müller-Quernheim J, Schreiber S, Hofmann S. A genome-wide linkage analysis in 181 German sarcoidosis families using clustered biallelic markers. *Chest.* 2010;138:151-157.

12. Veltkamp M, van Moorsel CH, Rijkers GT, Ruven HJ, Grutters JC. Genetic variation in the Toll-like receptor gene cluster (TLR10-TLR1-TLR6) influences disease course in sarcoidosis. *Tissue Antigens.* Jan 2012;79(1):25-32.

13. Sverrild A, Backer V, Kyvik KO, et al. Hereditary in sarcoidosis: a registry-based twin study. *Thorax.* 2008;63:894-896.

## Supplementary Information

### OMIM REFERENCES:

[1] Blau Syndrome—Synovitis, Granulomatosis, With Uveitis and Cranial Neuropathies (#186580)

[2] Early-Onset Sarcoidosis (#609464)

[3] Angiotensin-Converting Enzyme; ACE—Plasma Level (#106180)

[4] Butyrophilin-Like Protein 2; BTNL2 (#606000)

### Alternative Name:

• Besnier-Boeck-Schaumann disease

*Key Words:* Sarcoidosis, genetics, genomics

# 118 Idiopathic Pulmonary Fibrosis

Kenneth D. Macneal, Marvin I. Schwarz, and David A. Schwartz

## KEY POINTS

- *Disease summary:*
  - Idiopathic pulmonary fibrosis (IPF) is the most common form of the idiopathic interstitial pneumonias (IIPs), which are further grouped under the diffuse parenchymal lung diseases (DPLD), and commonly referred to as interstitial lung disease (ILD). IPF is a progressive lung disease that likely involves multiple interacting gene loci and has a median survival rate of 2 to 3 years.
  - Patients with IPF generally report the insidious onset of mild dyspnea, a nonproductive cough, and have evidence of restrictive lung function upon physiologic testing. The disease progresses at various rates and may have episodes of acute exacerbations.
  - Patients with IPF are over 50 years of age and are often current or former cigarette smokers, but the initiating stimulus is unknown.
  - Familial interstitial pneumonia (FIP), a subcategory of IIP, refers to the presence of two first-degree relatives with IIP. It is not known what percentage of an IIP population is familial, but it is estimated that up to 10% of cases have other family members with some form of IIP.
- *Differential diagnosis:*
  - IIPs are diagnosed only after excluding known causes of ILD, such as medications, occupational and environmental factors, systemic autoimmune diseases, granulomatous ILDs such as sarcoidosis and other forms of interstitial lung diseases, for example, Langerhans cell histiocytosis or histiocytosis X, and eosinophilic pneumonia. IPF is further distinguished from other IIPs by the presence of bibasilar reticulonodular opacities and honeycombing consistent with usual interstitial pneumonia (UIP) on a high-resolution computed tomography (HRCT), although some cases of nonspecific interstitial pneumonia (NSIP) have also been associated with IPF.
- *Monogenic forms:*
  - No monogenic forms have been found.
- *Family history:*
  - Putative transmittance for FIP is autosomal dominant with reduced penetrance. No monogenic form is known, but a number of contributing genes have been identified with different associated risks for the offspring.
- *Twin studies:*
  - None.
- *Environmental factors:*
  - No environmental factors have been shown to trigger IPF (although some have been shown to cause pulmonary fibrosis). However, smoking cigarettes, chronic aspiration, some environmental pollutants, and medications have been correlated with the future development of IPF. In particular, smoking relatives of individuals with FIP have more than a twofold increase in the chance of developing ILD.
- *Gene variant associations:*
  - Various associations exist, however the known disease-associated genetic variations in surfactant protein C (SPC) and telomerase genes account for less than 10% of cases of FIP (Table 118-1). Although a promoter variant in *MUC5B* occurs in approximately 20% of individuals in the normal population, this variant is observed in 60% to 70% of individuals with FIP or IPF and is associated with an increase in the production of *MUC5B* in the lung. Testing exists for the genetic variants in SPC, the telomerase genes, and *MUC5B*.
- *Pharmacogenomics:*
  - No treatment specific for any genomic variants of IPF exists.

## Diagnostic Criteria and Clinical Characteristics

### Diagnostic Criteria for Idiopathic Pulmonary Fibrosis:

**Major Criteria—All three required**

1. Abnormal pulmonary function that includes evidence of restriction (reduced vital capacity [VC], often with an increased $FEV_1$/FVC ratio) and impaired gas exchange (increased $P(A-a)O_2$, decreased $PaO_2$ with rest or exercise and decreased DLCO)

2. Bibasilar reticular abnormalities with or without ground-glass opacities on HRCT scan

3. Exclusion of other known causes of ILD such as drug toxicities, environmental and occupational exposures, and connective tissue diseases

**Minor Criteria—at least three out of the four**

1. Age greater than 50 years

2. Insidious onset of otherwise unexplained dyspnea on exertion

3. Duration of illness greater than 3 months

4. Bibasilar, inspiratory crackles (dry or "Velcro"-type in quality)

**Table 118-1 Disease-Associated Susceptibility Variants**

| Candidate Gene (Chromosome Location) | Associated Variant [effect on protein] | Relative Risk of Developing IPF | % of FIP Cases With Variant(s) in Gene | Frequency of Risk Allele in Controls | Putative Functional Significance | Associated Disease Phenotype | Genetic Testing |
|---|---|---|---|---|---|---|---|
| MUC5B (11p15) | SNP [upregulation of MUC5B] rs35705950 | 8.0 heterozygous 27.0 homozygous | 59% | 19% | Promoter for MUC5B gene | IPF and FIP | Yes |
| SFTPC (8p21) | Multiple variations, I73T mutation most common | Rare autosomal dominant | ~1% | Unclear | Inhibits synthesis of surfactant protein C | IPF and FIP | Yes |
| TERT (5p15.3) | Various nonsense, missense codons, and splice-site variations | Rare autosomal dominant | ~5%-10% | Unclear | Loss of functionality of telomere reverse transcriptase | IPF and FIP | Yes |
| TERC (3q21-q28) | Mutation in the pseudoknot region | Rare autosomal dominant | ~2% | Unclear | TERC is unable to provide template for telomere extension | IPF and FIP | Yes |

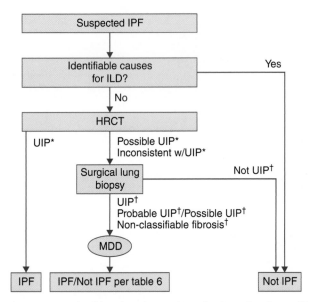

***Figure 118-1*** Algorithm for Diagnostic Evaluation of Patient With Idiopathic Pulmonary Fibrosis
Modified from Fig. 3 in Raghu et al, 2011. MDD, multidisciplinary discussion (among ILD experts)

**Diagnostic evaluation should include at least one of the following (Fig. 118-1 algorithm)**

- HRCT with bibasilar reticular abnormalities with or without ground-glass opacities
- If the HRCT is atypical, a surgical lung biopsy that demonstrates the histologic features of UIP

**And the absence of**

- Any environmental or occupational exposure factors that could be responsible for the clinical radiographic picture

***Clinical Characteristics:*** IPF can present with mild dyspnea with exertion, a nonproductive cough and fatigue. Patients demonstrate restrictive pulmonary function (reduced forced vital capacity and impaired gas exchange). One study indicated that almost 90% of patients with IPF will have acid reflux indicating the potential for aspiration. The onset of IPF is generally insidious and characterized by periods of stability or slow progression and sometimes punctuated by periods of exacerbation and acute respiratory failure.

Once diagnosed, a reduced survival time seen in patients who are older at presentation, have a history of cigarette smoking, have a lower body mass index (BMI), are more physiologically impaired, have a greater radiologic extent of disease, and have comorbid illnesses (ie, emphysema, heart disease).

## Screening and Counseling

***Screening:*** Genetic testing is routinely offered for family members of individuals with FIP (Table 118-1), however given incomplete penetrance, the predictive value of these tests is limited. Symptomatic first-degree relatives of individuals with FIP should undergo pulmonary function testing and obtain an HRCT scan. Some asymptomatic relatives of patients with FIP have evidence of ILD on their HRCT.

***Counseling:*** While the chance of developing disease remains unpredictable, most studies of FIP are consistent with autosomal inheritance with reduced penetrance. Thus the chance of inheriting mutant gene is 50%, but the chance of developing the disease is less than 50%, due to the reduced penetrance. No Mendelian forms are known to exist.

## Management and Treatment

The prognosis of IPF is poor, with only 20% to 30% of patients surviving more than 5 years following diagnosis. A number of therapies have been tested, but none has been shown to reverse the progression of the disease. Oxygen therapy may improve exercise tolerance and lung transplant, once a diagnosis is established, should be considered in eligible patients.

☞**GLUCOCORTICOIDS OR IMMUNOTHERAPY:** While inflammation is modest in IPF, it has been assumed that inflammatory immune pathways are involved and contribute to fibrosis. However, there is no data to support the use of this treatment. Treatments should be directed toward reflux, obstructive sleep apnea, hypoxemia, and possibly physical therapy. Most importantly, patients with suspected IPF should be referred for treatment trials of novel therapeutic agents.

☞**N-ACETYLCYSTEINE:** When given in conjunction with azathioprine and a glucocorticoid, *N*-acetylcysteine was shown to slow the deterioration of FVC ($-60$ mL/y instead of $-190$ mL/y) and DLCO ($-0.11$ instead of $-0.70$ mmol/min per pKa). However, these data have been questioned; more recent work suggests that this treatment regimen may not be effective, and we do not recommend this treatment.

☞**PIRFENIDONE:** Antifibrotic agents such as pirfenidone are being tested as possible treatments for IPF and FIP. Initial studies have shown a slight beneficial effect in patients treated with pirfenidone; however, this does not yet appear to be clinically meaningful in terms of outcome. Another trial is currently in progress.

☞**PHARMACOGENETICS:** Pharmacogenetic interventions have not been shown to influence the development of IPF or FIP.

## Molecular Genetics and Molecular Mechanism

☞**MUC5B:** This gene codes for a specific mucous that lines the epithelium of the lungs. This common polymorphism in the promoter of the gene increases the expression of *MUC5B* (over 30-fold in unaffected individuals), and this overexpression may contribute to the observed fibrosis and honeycombing in the lungs.

☞**SFTPC:** This gene codes for an enzyme that catalyzes an integral step in the synthesis of SPC from its precursors. Private mutations in this gene have been correlated with decreased production of SPC or lack of production altogether.

☞**TERT/TERC:** The *TERT* gene codes for telomere reverse transcriptase which combines with an RNA component (*TERC*) to form telomerase, an enzyme extends the telomeres of chromosomes during replication. Without this enzyme, the telomeres of cells become progressively smaller, which eventually leads to the arrest of cell division and apoptosis. Telomerase is therefore expressed highly in proliferative stem cells, specific germline cells, and immortal cancer cells. It is hypothesized that shortened telomeres may be associated with the development of IPF.

***Genetic Testing:*** Genetic testing (including prenatal testing) is available for variants known to be associated with IPF (Table 118-1), but their predictive value is unknown due to incomplete penetrance. In symptomatic family members of individuals with IPF or FIP, presence of the *MUC5B* promoter polymorphism substantially affects the risk of developing interstitial lung disease. However, early intervention has not been shown to alter the course of this disease.

***Future Directions:*** There is currently a significant amount of research on IPF and FIP with the goals of understanding the genetics, genomics, and pathology of the disease. The specific triggers for the disease in susceptible individuals are still unknown, as are the contributing factors in the development of the disease. It is hoped that research into these areas will lead to the development of more accurate testing, diagnoses of the genomic variants, and novel therapeutic interventions. There are currently a number of drug trials working toward discovering a treatment to cure or slow the progress of IPF and FIP.

## BIBLIOGRAPHY:

1. Raghu G, Collard HR, Egan JJ, et al. An official ATS/ERS/JRS/ALAT statement: idiopathic pulmonary fibrosis: evidence-based guidelines for diagnosis and management. *Am J Respir Crit Care Med.* Mar 15 2011;183(6):788-824.

2. Steele MP, Speer MC, Loyd JE, et al. The clinical and pathologic features of familial interstitial pneumonia (FIP). *Am J Respir Crit Care Med.* Nov 1 2005;172(9):1146-1152.

3. Nogee LM, Dunbar AE 3rd, Wert SE, Askin F, Hamvas A, Whitsett JA. A mutation in the surfactant protein C gene associated with familial interstitial lung disease. *N Engl J Med.* 2001;344(8):573-579.

4. Lawson WE, Grant SW, Ambrosini V, et al. Genetic mutations in surfactant protein C are a rare cause of sporadic cases of IPF. *Thorax.* Nov 2004;59(11):977-980.

5. Armanios MY, Chen JJ, Cogan JD, et al. Telomerase mutations in families with idiopathic pulmonary fibrosis. *N Engl J Med.* Mar 29 2007;356(13):1317-1326.

6. Seibold MA, Wise AL, Speer MC, et al. A common MUC5B promoter polymorphism and pulmonary fibrosis. *N Engl J Med.* Apr 21 2011;364(16):1503-1512.

7. Talbert J, Wise A, Schwartz DA. Pulmonary Fibrosis, Familial. In: GeneReviews at Gene Tests. University of Washington, Seattle (updated 2010 Oct 19). http://www.ncbi.nlm.nih.gov/books/NBK1230/

## Supplementary Information

### OMIM REFERENCES:

[1] Pulmonary Fibrosis, Idiopathic; TERT, TERC, MUC5B (#178500)

[2] Surfactant, Pulmonary-Associated Protein C; SFTPC (#178620)

[3] Condition; Gene Name (OMIM#)

### Alternative Name:

- Familial Pulmonary Fibrosis

***Key Words:*** Idiopathic, pulmonary, fibrosis, familial, interstitial, pneumonia, lung, disease

# 119 Obstructive Sleep Apnea Syndrome

Brian D. Kent, Silke Ryan, and Walter T. McNicholas

## KEY POINTS

- *Disease summary:*
  - Obstructive sleep apnea syndrome (OSAS) is a highly prevalent, but underdiagnosed disorder. Recurrent collapse of the upper airway during sleep causes repetitive episodes of intermittent hypoxia, and recurrent arousals from sleep, leading to daytime sleepiness, poor quality of life, and increased risk of road traffic accidents, cardiovascular morbidity and mortality, and metabolic dysfunction.
- *Hereditary basis:*
  - OSAS is approximately twice as common in males. Up to 40% of the variability in sleep breathing can be accounted for by heritable factors. However, a discrete genetic basis is unlikely in the majority of cases.
- *Environmental factors:*
  - Obesity is the major reversible risk factor for the development of OSAS. Factors such as alcohol use and sedative medications may contribute to disease severity.
- *Differential diagnosis:*
  - Simple snoring, obesity hypoventilation syndrome, periodic limb movements of sleep, narcolepsy, shift work sleep disorder, congenital central hypoventilation syndrome (Ondine's curse).

## Diagnostic Criteria and Clinical Characteristics

**Diagnostic Criteria:** A diagnosis of OSAS is based on the finding of significant respiratory disturbance due to collapse of the upper airway during sleep in the setting of compatible daytime symptomatology. The gold standard for diagnosis of OSAS is the performance of inpatient nocturnal polysomnography (PSG), which provides detailed information on respiration, sleep staging and quality, and a range of other variables including heart rate and rhythm. Sleep-disordered breathing is defined as an apnea-hypopnea index (AHI) of greater than five events per hour as measured by PSG, and can be further classified as mild (AHI 5-15 events per hour), moderate (AHI 15-30 events per hour), or severe (AHI >30 events per hour). Unfortunately, PSG is both resource intensive and time consuming for the patient, and a growing research interest lies in the development and validation of technologies facilitating the ambulatory investigation of subjects with suspected OSAS, but the utility of these methods requires confirmation in large-scale clinical outcome studies. A proposed diagnostic algorithm is presented in Fig. 119-1.

**Clinical Characteristics:** OSAS is a highly prevalent, but under-diagnosed disorder, affecting at least 4% of adult men and 2% of adult women in developed countries. OSAS is intimately and intrinsically linked with obesity, and its prevalence is likely to be increasing as the worldwide obesity epidemic develops. Patients may experience a wide variety of symptoms, ranging from snoring, nocturia, and witnessed apnea during sleep to impaired concentration, depression, and decreased libido. Excessive daytime sleepiness and fatigue are present in approximately 70% of cases. Untreated OSAS leads to reduced quality of life, impaired functional status, and reduced cognitive function. It is significantly associated with the risk of depressive illness, and markedly increases the risk of road traffic accidents.

However, the principal long-term adverse consequence of OSAS is cardiovascular disease, and a growing body of literature suggests untreated severe OSAS leads to significantly increased cardio- and cerebrovascular morbidity and mortality. Particularly strong evidence supports an independent role for OSAS in the genesis of hypertension, above and beyond the effect of traditional risk factors, while a number of studies indicate an independent association with ischemic heart disease, cardiac dysrhythmia, and stroke. Similarly, it appears increasingly likely that OSAS may contribute to the development of metabolic dysfunction, dyslipidemia, and overt diabetes mellitus. A number of contributory factors are thought to underlie cardiometabolic morbidity in OSAS, including the generation of systemic inflammation and oxidative stress by the intermittent hypoxia that characterizes the disorder, and sympathetic excitation accompanying airway obstruction.

## Screening and Counseling

There is no evidence at present to suggest that relations of subjects with OSAS need to be assessed in a different fashion to the general population. Similarly, although familial clustering of OSAS occurs, there is no indication for dedicated genetic counseling.

## Management and Treatment

The administration of nocturnal continuous positive airway pressure (nCPAP) therapy acts to splint the upper airway open during sleep, and improves awake performance, quality of life, neurocognitive function, and driving performance. Furthermore, long-term cardiovascular outcome studies demonstrate significantly reduced morbidity and mortality in nCPAP-treated patients with severe OSAS in comparison to nontreated subjects. Unfortunately, while CPAP is highly effective at controlling OSAS, the device is rather cumbersome, and compliance with therapy is variable. Milder cases of OSAS can be effectively treated by use of individually fitted mandibular advancement dental devices, which prevent retroglossal collapse. While obesity is the key reversible risk factor for OSAS,

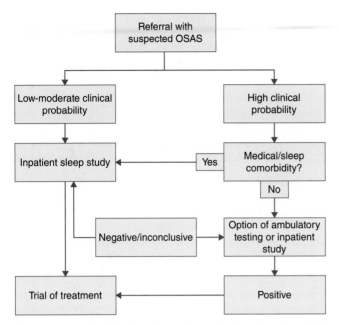

**Figure 119-1** Algorithm for Diagnostic Evaluation of Patient With Suspected OSAS

and weight loss can significantly ameliorate disease severity, most OSAS patients find substantial weight reduction difficult to achieve.

# Molecular Genetics and Molecular Mechanism

The investigation of a potential genetic cause of OSAS has been complicated by the lack of a single specific OSAS phenotype. Rather, the disorder generally arises as the result of a combination of factors—the so-called intermediate phenotypes. Furthermore, much of the genetic investigation has concentrated on the development of the cardiovascular sequelae of the disease. Nonetheless, it has been estimated that up to 40% of variability in sleep disordered breathing can be attributed to inheritable factors.

### Intermediate Phenotypes and Genetic Influences in OSAS:

☞**OBESITY:** Obesity represents the single most important reversible risk factor for the development of OSAS. Obesity is a polyfactorial disorder, requiring the interaction of genetic susceptibility with a sympathetic environment. A number of international collaborative studies using a genome-wide association study (GWAS) approach have succeeded in identifying replicable discrete loci that confer an increased risk of central obesity. A number of investigators have attempted to identify genetic interactions between obesity and OSAS. Loci at 6q23-25 and 10q24-25 independently predicted body mass index (BMI) and AHI in European Americans enrolled in the Cleveland family study. A large-scale candidate gene study in this same population identified significant associations between OSAS and single-nucleotide polymorphisms (SNPs) for C-reactive protein, glial-derived growth factor, and serotonin 2A receptor genes.

☞**CRANIOFACIAL MORPHOLOGY:** Individuals with OSAS have shortened maxillary and mandibular length, narrowed nasopharyngeal airways, and greater pharyngeal soft tissue structure volume than age- and sex-matched controls. A hereditary contribution to this phenotype is suggested by a number of studies suggesting that relatives of OSAS patients have narrower upper airways and soft palates than controls, while recent data using magnetic resonance imaging (MRI) have found significant heritability of upper airway soft tissue characteristics among both OSAS and non-OSAS subjects.

While there is little data on discrete genetic polymorphisms contributing to craniofacial morphology in the general OSAS population, an association between sleep-disordered breathing and craniofacial anatomy is seen in a number of disorders, such as Treacher Collins, Pierre-Robin, and Down syndromes. Similarly, a higher prevalence of OSAS is seen in patients with Marfan syndrome than in matched controls.

☞**UPPER AIRWAY CONTROL:** Reduction of upper airway tone during sleep leaves subjects with OSAS at increased risk of airway collapse and obstruction. Serotonin appears to be the key neurotransmitter in the maintenance of upper airway tone, with the serotonin 2A receptor predominating at hypoglossal motor neurons. Evidence from the Cleveland family study suggests SNPs in the serotonin 2A receptor gene may influence OSAS severity particularly among African-American subjects, although larger confirmatory studies are required.

☞**VENTILATORY CONTROL:** As seen in subjects with congenital central hypoventilation syndrome (Ondine's curse), discrete genetic mutations may lead to abnormalities of nocturnal ventilation. To date, no relevant polymorphisms have been identified in general OSAS populations that could contribute to the ventilatory instability seen in the disorder. Indeed, recent data would suggest that dysregulated respiratory control in subjects with OSAS is likely to be an acquired rather than inherited factor. Nonetheless, some investigators have found relatives of OSAS patients to have blunted hypoxic ventilatory responses compared to controls.

☞**CARDIOVASCULAR DISEASE:** The development of atherosclerosis and overt cardiovascular disease is the key adverse consequence of OSAS. A number of factors are thought to contribute to this increased burden of disease, including systemic inflammation, oxidative stress, endothelial dysfunction, and metabolic dysfunction. A substantial research effort has been focused on identifying genetic factors contributing to this increased risk; unfortunately a significant number of these studies are limited by relatively small size, and several have generated conflicting data.

Intermittent hypoxia resulting from OSAS leads to the generation of systemic inflammation. Polymorphisms in the tumor necrosis factor (TNF)-α gene have been found to be significantly associated with a diagnosis of OSAS in both European and Indian populations, while mutations in the C-reactive protein and interleukin-6 genes have also been suggested to increase the risk of OSAS in European-American and Chinese populations respectively. Oxidative stress may also be generated by intermittent hypoxia, contributing to the development of endothelial dysfunction and subsequent atherosclerosis. SNPs in the antioxidant haptoglobin gene have been shown to be related to cardiovascular disease in subjects with OSAS, while polymorphisms in NADPH oxidase predict AHI and systolic blood pressure in Chinese individuals.

Evidence of an association between SNPs in mediators of endothelial function (specifically, in endothelial nitric oxide synthase, endothelin-1, and endothelin receptor subtype-A genes) and sleep-disordered breathing have been reported in multiple studies. There is no significant evidence of association with OSAS and candidate variants in the β-adrenergic receptors, which mediate sympathetic excitation, lipid metabolism, insulin sensitivity, and blood pressure.

Studies examining the role of angiotensin-converting enzyme (ACE) polymorphisms in the genesis of cardiovascular sequelae have yielded some apparently conflicting results. Data from the Wisconsin Sleep Cohort suggested the ACE insertion or deletion (I/D) polymorphism were associated with the development of hypertension in subjects with mild-moderate OSAS, while the ACE deletion allele appeared to be protective against hypertension in the Cleveland family study. Similarly, investigations of the apolipoprotein E (*APOE*) gene, which plays a key role in lipid metabolism, have failed to produce evidence of a clear association with a diagnosis of OSAS.

***Future Directions:*** In general, research efforts to date in the field of OSAS genetics serve to emphasize the need for large, multicenter collaborative studies to successfully identify polymorphisms contributing to the development of the disorder and its sequelae. The establishment of investigative networks such as the European Sleep Apnoea Database study (ESADA) provides an excellent opportunity for such collaborations.

## BIBLIOGRAPHY:

1. McNicholas WT, Bonsignore MR. Management Committee of EU COST ACTION B26. Sleep apnoea as an independent risk factor for cardiovascular disease: current evidence, basic mechanisms and research priorities. *Eur Respir J.* 2007;29(1):156-178.

2. Redline S, Tosteson T, Tishler PV, Carskadon MA, Milliman RP. Studies in the genetics of obstructive sleep apnea: familial aggregation of symptoms associated with sleep-related breathing disturbances. *Am Rev Respir Dis.* 1992;145:440-444.

3. Young T, Palta M, Dempsey J, et al. The occurrence of sleep-disordered breathing among middle-aged adults. *N Engl J Med.* 1993;328:1230-1235.

4. Riha RL, Gislasson T, Diefenbach K. The phenotype and genotype of adult obstructive sleep apnoea/hypopnoea syndrome. *Eur Respir J.* 2009;33:646-655.

5. Kent BD, Ryan S, McNicholas WT. The genetics of obstructive sleep apnoea. *Curr Opin Pulm Med.* 2010;16(6):536-542.

6. Larkin EK, Patel SR, Elston RC, et al. Using linkage analysis to identify quantitative trait loci for sleep apnea in relationship to body mass index. *Ann Hum Genet.* 2008;72(pt 6):762-773.

7. Larkin EK, Patel SR, Goodloe RJ, et al. A candidate gene study of obstructive sleep apnea in European Americans and African Americans. *Am J Respir Crit Care Med.* 2010;182(7):947-953.

8. Salloum A, Rowley JA, Mateika JH, et al. Increased propensity for central apnea in patients with obstructive sleep apnea: effect of nasal continuous positive airway pressure. *Am J Respir Crit Care Med.* 2010;181:189-193.

9. Riha RL, Brander P, Vennelle M, et al. Tumour necrosis factor-alpha (-308) gene polymorphism in obstructive sleep apnoea-hypopnoea syndrome. *Eur Respir J.* 2005;26:673-678.

10. Buck D, Diefenbach K, Penzel T, et al. Genetic polymorphisms in endothelin-receptor-subtype-a-gene as susceptibility factor for obstructive sleep apnea syndrome. *Sleep Med.* 2010;11:213-217.

11. Lin L, Finn L, Zhang J, et al. Angiotensin-converting enzyme, sleep-disordered breathing, and hypertension. *Am J Respir Crit Care Med.* 2004;170:1349-1353.

12. Patel SR, Larkin EK, Mignot E, et al. The association of angiotensin converting enzyme (ACE) polymorphisms with sleep apnea and hypertension. *Sleep.* 2007;30:531-533.

13. Thakre TP, Mamtani MR, Kulkarni H. Lack of association of the APOE epsilon 4 allele with the risk of obstructive sleep apnea: meta-analysis and meta-regression. *Sleep.* 2009;32:1507-1511.

## Supplementary Information

### OMIM REFERENCE:

[1] Apnea, Obstructive Sleep; (#107650)

### Alternative Names:
- OSA
- OSAS
- Sleep Apnea/Hypopnea Syndrome (SAHS)
- Obstructive Sleep Apnea/Hypopnea Syndrome (OSAHS)

***Key Words:*** Sleep apnea, intermittent hypoxia, cardiovascular disease, obesity

# 120 Pulmonary Arterial Hypertension

James E. Loyd

## KEY POINTS

- *Disease summary:*
  - Pulmonary arterial hypertension (PAH) is a rare condition characterized by proliferative growth of the media and intima of the smallest pulmonary arteries.
  - Widespread obstruction of the smallest pulmonary arteries causes increased resistance to blood flow through the lungs and is usually lethal due to right ventricular failure. Mean survival untreated is less than 3 years.
  - PAH diagnosis is established by measuring increased pulmonary artery pressure (mean >25 mm Hg) at cardiac catheterization, along with exclusion of disorders which cause pulmonary hypertension (Table 120-1).
  - PAH may occur sporadically (idiopathic PAH [IPAH]) or in families (6%). Heritable PAH (HPAH) is the current terminology for familial or sporadic patients in whom a responsible genetic (eg, *BMPR2*) mutation is identified.
  - PAH occurs at all ages and disproportionately affects women, more than twice as commonly as men.
  - Nine therapies are now available for PAH, all in FDA approved in the past 15 years. But, most are expensive, labor intensive (require continuous IV infusion), and limited in overall effect.
  - Lung transplantation is possible for some patients with PAH, but has significant limitations.

- *Differential diagnosis:*
  - Several conditions in addition to PAH are associated with pulmonary hypertension, as listed in Table 120-1. The commonest symptoms are nonspecific, and include dyspnea, chest pain, dizziness, or syncope.

- *Monogenic forms:*
  - Mutations in bone morphogenetic protein receptor type 2 (*BMPR2*) are responsible for approximately 80% of familial PAH cases. More than 300 different *BMPR2* mutations are described. Mutations in other transforming growth factor beta (TGF-β) pathway members known to cause hereditary hemorrhagic telangiectasia (HHT) (ALK-1 or endoglin) are rarely associated with PAH, with or without clinical evidence of HHT. Other members of the TGF-β family are also associated with familial PAH, such as via *SMAD8* mutation.
  - Decreased penetrance (~20%) and variable age of onset (all ages) of PAH due to a *BMPR2* mutation may conceal a true familial basis of disease because it can skip multiple generations. This confounds disease prediction in mutation carriers and limits the value of genetic counseling in this subset. A significant minority of patients (reports vary from 10% to 40%) otherwise believed to have IPAH actually carry a responsible *BMPR2* mutation. Because the prevalence of sporadic PAH far exceeds familial PAH (~94% vs ~6%), the majority of *BMPR2* mutations present in the overall population of PAH patients are actually possessed by patients thought to have sporadic disease and thus assigned the diagnosis of IPAH.

- *Family history:*
  - Family history is positive in 6% of PAH patients. Skip generations due to reduced penetrance (20%) may conceal a familial basis, creating a false impression that familial disease is sporadic. Earlier age of onset in subsequent generations is apparent for many families but it remains unknown whether it has a biologic basis.

- *Twin studies:*
  - Twin studies have not been reported for PAH.

- *Environmental factors implicated in the development of PAH:*
  - a) Drugs and toxins as causes of PAH:
    - Definite: aminorex, fenfluramine, dexfenfluramine, toxic rapeseed oil
    - Likely: amphetamines, L-tryptophan, methamphetamines
    - Possible: cocaine, phenylpropanolamine, St. John's wort, chemotherapeutic agents, selective serotonin reuptake inhibitor (SSRI) antidepressants, exogenous estrogen
  - b) Infections: HIV infection, schistosomiasis
  - c) Other: low oxygen environment or high altitude

- *Genome-wide associations:*
  - Genome-wide association studies (GWASs) are planned for IPAH, but have not been reported to date.
  - Recently, genome-wide studies designed to identify genes which impact the clinical expression of *BMPR2* mutation used novel linkage approaches to identify four loci at 3q22, 3p12, 2p22, and 13q21 (see Table 120-2).

- *Pharmacogenomics:*
  - Acute pulmonary vasodilator response, which predicts response to chronic treatment with calcium channel antagonists, is rarely seen in *BMPR2* mutation PAH patients. The pathophysiologic consequences of this have not been fully elucidated, although such subjects may respond poorly to calcium channel blocker therapy alone. Treatment is otherwise similar.

*Table 120-1  Updated Classification of Pulmonary Hypertension (Dana Point, WHO meeting 2008)*

1. Pulmonary arterial hypertension (PAH)
   1.1 Idiopathic PAH (IPAH)
   1.2 Heritable (IPAH)
       1.2.1. BMPR2
       1.2.2. ALK1, endoglin (with or without hereditary hemorrhagic telangiectasia [HHT])
       1.2.3 Unknown
   1.3 Drugs and toxins induced
   1.4 Associated with
       1.4.1 Connective tissue diseases
       1.4.2 HIV infection
       1.4.3 Portal hypertension
       1.4.4 Congenital heart diseases
       1.4.5 Schistosomiasis
       1.4.6 Chronic hemolytic anemia
   1.5 Persistent pulmonary hypertension of the newborn
1'. Pulmonary veno-occlusive disease (PVOD) and/or pulmonary capillary hemangiomatosis (PCH)
2. Pulmonary hypertension due to left heart disease
   2.1 Systolic dysfunction
   2.2 Diastolic dysfunction
   2.3 Valvular disease
3. Pulmonary hypertension due to lung diseases and/or hypoxia
   3.1 Chronic obstructive pulmonary disease
   3.2 Interstitial lung disease
   3.3 Other pulmonary diseases with mixed restrictive and obstructive pattern
   3.4 Sleep-disordered breathing
   3.5 Alveolar hypoventilation disorders
   3.6 Chronic exposure to high altitude
   3.7 Developmental abnormalities
4. Chronic thromboembolic pulmonary hypertension (CTEPH)
5. PH with unclear and/or multifactorial mechanisms
   5.1 Hematologic disorders: myeloproliferative disorders, splenectomy
   5.2 Systemic disorders, sarcoidosis, pulmonary Langerhans cell histiocytosis, lymphangioleiomyomatosis, neurofibromatosis, vasculitis
   5.3 Metabolic disorders: glycogen storage disease, Gaucher disease, thyroid disorders
   5.4 Others: tumor obstruction, fibrosing mediastinitis, chronic renal failure on dialysis

## Diagnostic Criteria and Clinical Characteristics

*Diagnostic Criteria:* PAH is diagnosed by excluding other causes such as heart disease, lung disease, pulmonary emboli or others (Table 120-1) and confirming pulmonary hypertension by cardiac catheterization (see Fig. 120-1).

*Clinical Characteristics:* Symptoms of PAH are usually nonspecific, including dyspnea, chest pain, or syncope during exertion, as well as Raynaud phenomenon and edema. Findings of pulmonary hypertension on physical examination such as increased pulmonic component of the second heart sound, prominent jugular venous pulsation, or murmur of tricuspid regurgitation increase the likelihood of PAH. Women are affected disproportionately, and recent evidence supports the possibility that the gender disparity may be attributable to the effects of estrogen or its metabolites.

## Screening and Counseling

In families with HPAH, screening by echocardiography is recommended at serial intervals of a few years for bloodline family members, who have a crude risk of 1 in 10 (10%) to develop PAH. If the specific *BMPR2* mutation responsible for disease in that family is known, then individuals who do not carry the mutation have a risk similar to the general population (~1 per 500,000). Individuals who

*Table 120-2* **Disease-Associated Susceptibility Variants**

| Candidate Gene (Chromosome Location) | Relative Risk | Putative Functional Significance | Associated Disease Phenotype |
|---|---|---|---|
| BMPR2 (2q33-q34) | >100,000 | Altered BMP pathway signaling | HPAH, PVOD |
| ACVRL1/ALK1 (12q11-q14) | 100 | Altered BMP pathway signaling | HHT, PAH |
| Endoglin (9q33-9q34.1) | 5 | Altered BMP pathway signaling | HHT, PAH |
| SMAD8 (13q12-q14) | Unknown | Altered BMP pathway signaling | HPAH |

do carry a *BMPR2* mutation have a 1 in 5 (20% penetrance) chance of developing PAH during their lifetime, and serial screening with echocardiography is the current recommendation. Counseling topics often include issues related to genetic testing as discussed in a subsequent section, and about family planning.

## Management and Treatment

*Therapeutics:* Several pharmacologic therapies, including prostacyclins, endothelin receptor antagonists, and phosphodiesterase inhibitors (Fig. 120-2), have been approved to treat PAH since the mid 1990s. The routes for these treatments are by inhalation, oral, or continuous infusion delivered subcutaneously or intravenously. Because CTEPH may present with identical symptoms and signs,

and its optimal therapy is surgical thromboendarterectomy, it is especially important to exclude CTEPH.

☞**PHARMACOGENETICS:** PAH patients with *BMPR2* mutations are unlikely to demonstrate vasoreactivity which is believed to predict clinical effectiveness of chronic calcium channel blocker therapy.

## Molecular Genetics and Molecular Mechanism

Missense *BMPR2* mutations escape nonsense-mediated decay so they result in transcripts that may produce proteins that cause dominant negative effects that are relatively more detrimental than

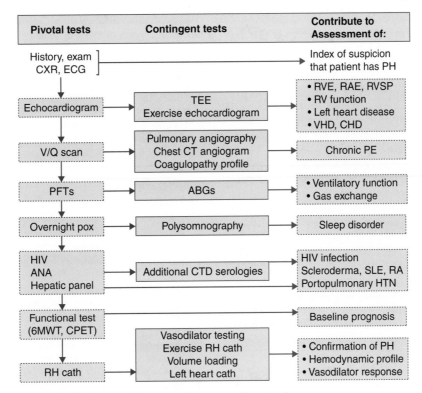

*Figure 120-1* Algorithm for Diagnostic Evaluation of Suspected Pulmonary Hypertension. Adapted from McLaughlin VV. *J Am Coll Cardiol.* 2009.

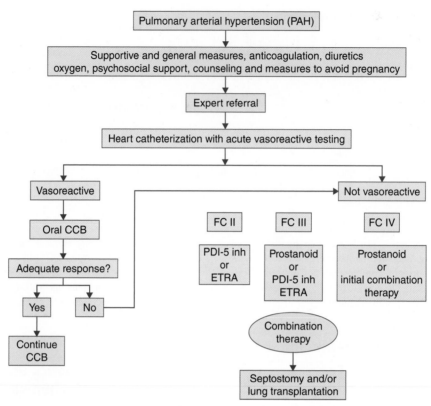

***Figure 120-2*** PAH Treatment Algorithm.
Adapted from Adamali H, SRCCM 2009.

the haploinsufficient effects of truncating mutations in which total BMPR2 protein levels are quantitatively reduced to the level of the single wild-type allele. Functional polymorphisms of TGF-β1 impact clinical expression of multiple lung diseases, including cystic fibrosis and PAH.

***Genetic Testing:*** *BMPR2*-related PAH is inherited in an autosomal dominant manner. The average penetrance of *BMPR2* mutations is approximately 20%. If a parent of a proband has *BMPR2*-related PAH (HPAH), the risk to each sib of inheriting the gene mutation is 50%; however, because of reduced penetrance the risk to a sibling of developing PAH is approximately 10% (50% × ~20%). Similarly, each child of an affected individual is at a 50% risk of inheriting the mutant allele; however, because of reduced penetrance the risk to offspring of developing PAH is approximately 10% (50% × ~20%). Prenatal testing for pregnancies at increased risk is available if the disease-causing mutation has been identified in the family.

A significant minority of IPAH (negative family history) carry responsible *BMPR2* mutations. The identification of a responsible genetic mutation in an IPAH patient provides the first knowledge that the disease may be familial. Revealing that a mutation is responsible for IPAH is often associated with distress for the patient and relatives because it uncovers the risk to family members which had previously gone unrecognized, unlike when disease in a family is apparent.

Discussion of most issues related to genetic counseling and testing for *BMPR2* are discussed on two websites. The Gene Tests website www.genetests.org lists two US sites and one in Spain that tests *BMPR2*. The Pulmonary Hypertension Association at www.phassociation.org lists four sites in the United States and also includes information for patients and healthcare professionals about all aspects of PAH, including diagnosis, treatment, genetic testing, and counseling.

***Future Directions:*** Current efforts are directed toward identifying the genetic or epigenetic modifiers which regulate the clinical expression of *BMPR2* mutation, in order to refine the prediction of disease in mutation carriers. IPAH is phenotypically identical to HPAH, but its molecular basis is not known and is a topic of great interest. The ultimate goal is to translate new understanding into highly effective therapies with major effect.

### BIBLIOGRAPHY:

1. Austin ED, Loyd JE, Phillips JA 3rd. Genetics of pulmonary arterial hypertension. *Semin Respir Crit Care Med.* Aug 2009;30(4):386-398.

2. Simonneau G, Robbins IM, Beghetti M, et al. Updated clinical classification of pulmonary hypertension. *J Am Coll Cardiol.* Jun 30 2009;54(1 suppl):S43-S54.

3. Machado RD, Eickelberg O, Elliott CG, et al. Genetics and genomics of pulmonary arterial hypertension. *J Am Coll Cardiol.* Jun 30 2009;54(1 suppl):S32-S42.

4. Rodriquez-Murillo L, Subaran R, Stewart WCL, et al. Novel loci interacting epistatically with bone morphogenetic protein receptor 2 cause familial pulmonary arterial hypertension. *J Heart Lung Transplant.* Feb 2010;29(2):174-180.

5. Elliott CG, Glissmeyer EW, Havlena GT, et al. Relationship of BMPR2 mutations to vasoreactivity in pulmonary arterial hypertension. *Circulation.* May 30 2006;113(21):2509-2515.

6.  McLaughlin VV, Archer SL, Badesch DB, et al. ACCF/AHA 2009 expert consensus document on pulmonary hypertension. *J Am Coll Cardiol.* Apr 28 2009;53(17):1573-1619.

7.  Austin ED, Cogan JD, West JD, et al. Alterations in estrogen metabolism: implications for higher penetrance of FPAH in females. *Eur Respir J.* Nov 2009;34(5):1093-1099.

8.  Adamali H, Gaine SP, Rubin LJ. Medical treatment of pulmonary arterial hypertension. *Semin Respir Crit Care Med.* Aug 2009;30(4):484-492.

9.  Hoeper MM, Barberà JA, Channick RN, et al. Diagnosis, assessment, and treatment of non-pulmonary arterial hypertension pulmonary hypertension. *J Am Coll Cardiol.* Jun 30 2009;54 (1 suppl):S85-S96.

10. Austin ED, Phillips JA, Cogan JD, et al. Truncating and missense BMPR2 mutations differentially affect the severity of heritable pulmonary arterial hypertension. *Respir Res.* 2009;10:87.

11. Phillips JA 3rd, Poling JS, Phillips CA, et al. Synergistic heterozygosity for TGFbeta1 SNPs and BMPR2 mutations modulates the age at diagnosis and penetrance of familial pulmonary arterial hypertension. *Genet Med.* 2008;10:359-365.

## Supplementary Information

### OMIM References:

[1] Pulmonary Hypertension, Primary, 1; PPH 1 (#178600)

[2] vBone Morphogenetic Protein Receptor, Type 2; BMPR2 (#600799)

[3] Hereditary Hemorrhageic Telangiectasia; Activin A Receptor, Type II-like 1; ACVRL1 (#601284)

[4] Activin Receptor-Like Kinase; ALK1 (#601284)

### Alternative Names:

• Primary Pulmonary Hypertension (~1950-2003)
• Idiopathic Pulmonary Hypertension

**Key Words:** Pulmonary hypertension, pulmonary arterial hypertension, genetics, BMPR2, ALK1, ENG

### Abbreviations and Acronyms:

| | |
|---|---|
| ABG | arterial blood gas |
| ALK1 | activin-like kinase type1 |
| ANA | antinuclear antibody serology |
| BMPR2 | bone morphogenetic protein receptor type 2 |
| CHD | congenital heart disease |
| CPET | cardiopulmonary exercise test |
| CT | computerized tomography |
| CTEPH | chronic thromboembolic pulmonary hypertension |
| CTD | connective tissue disease |
| CXR | chest x-ray |
| ECG | electrocardiogram |
| ENG | endoglin |
| ETRA | endothelin receptor antagonist |
| FC | functional class |
| HHT | hereditary hemorrhagic telangiectasia |
| HIV | human immunodeficiency virus screening |
| HTN | hypertension |
| HPAH | heritable pulmonary arterial hypertension |
| IPAH | idiopathic pulmonary arterial hypertension |
| LFT | liver function test |
| PAH | pulmonary arterial hypertension |
| PCH | pulmonary capillary hemangiomatosis |
| PDE-5i | phosphodiesterase 5 inhibitor |
| PE | pulmonary embolism |
| PFT | pulmonary function test |
| PGI2 | prostacyclin |
| PPH | primary pulmonary hypertension |
| PVOD | pulmonary veno-occlusive disease |
| RA | rheumatoid arthritis |
| RAE | right atrial enlargement |
| RHC | right heart catheterization |
| RVE | right ventricular enlargement |
| TGF | transforming growth factor |
| TEE | transesophageal echocardiography |
| VHD | valvular heart disease |
| VQ scan | ventilation perfusion scintigram |
| WHO | World Health Organization |

### Supplemental References:

1.  Sztrymf B, Coulet F, Girerd B, et al. Clinical outcomes of pulmonary arterial hypertension in carriers of BMPR2 mutation. *Am J Respir Crit Care Med.* Jun 15 2008;177(12):1377-1383.

2.  West J, Cogan J, Geraci M, et al. Gene expression in BMPR2 mutation carriers with and without evidence of pulmonary arterial hypertension suggests pathways relevant to disease penetrance. *BMC Med Genomics.* 2008;1:45.

3.  Newman JH, Phillips JA 3rd, Loyd JE. Narrative review: the enigma of pulmonary arterial hypertension: new insights from genetic studies. *Ann Intern Med.* 2008;148:278-283.

4.  Hamid R, Cogan JD, Hedges LK, et al. Penetrance of pulmonary arterial hypertension is modulated by the expression of normal BMPR2 allele. *Hum Mutat.* 2009;30:649-654.

# 121 Epilepsy

Annapurna Poduri and Chellamani Harini

## KEY POINTS

- *Disease summary:*
  - Epilepsy is a common condition affecting 0.5% to 1% of the world's population in which genetics play an important role. Genetic factors play a predominant role in about 40% of all epilepsies. Common epilepsies are believed to have complex genetic inheritance, influenced by variation in several susceptibility genes with or without an acquired or environmental component. Idiopathic generalized epilepsy (more recently called genetic generalized epilepsy [GGE]) represents 20% to 30% of all epilepsies, and the designation of genetics is based on evidence from family history patterns, twin studies, and known monogenic epilepsies, though the latter represent only a small minority of the epilepsies.

- *Differential diagnosis:*
  - Syncope, nonepileptic seizures, migraine, movement disorders, metabolic disturbances, and sleep disorders

- *Monogenic forms:*
  - Mutated genes may encode components of neuronal voltage-gated ion channels (sodium and potassium channels) or ligand-gated ion channels (acetylcholine and g-aminobutyric acid type A [GABA-A] receptors) or nonion channel genes LGI1 (leucine-rich glioma-inactivated 1).

- *Family history:*
  - There is 8% to 12% risk for developing epilepsy among first-degree relatives of individuals when compared to the risk of approximately 0.5% in the general population. Both generalized and focal epilepsy can be caused by genetic mutations.

- *Twin studies:*
  - There is a high concordance of epilepsy for monozygous twins compared to dizygotic twins for generalized epilepsies (~0.8), evidence for the influence of genetic factors in epilepsy especially GGE.

- *Environmental factors:*
  - The role of environmental factors and other epigenetic factors in epilepsy is suspected but not well characterized, although fever can be a precipitating factor in some epilepsy syndromes.

- *Genome-wide associations:*
  - GWAS failed to identify common genetic variants that contribute to the risk of focal epilepsy.

- *Pharmacogenomics:*
  - None known.

## Diagnostic Criteria and Clinical Characteristics

The diagnosis of epilepsy is made clinically and relies largely on a detailed clinical history. The history should include triggers, prodromal symptoms, complete description of the event, and postevent symptoms but history may need to be confirmed by appropriate tests, including an electroencephalogram (EEG) when the clinical suspicion for epilepsy is high (note, however, that a normal EEG does not rule out a clinical diagnosis of epilepsy).

The differential diagnosis of epilepsy includes syncope, nonepileptic seizures, migraine (epileptic auras arising from the occipital lobe may be mistaken for typical visual migraine auras), movement disorders (paroxysmal dystonia or hyperplexia), metabolic disturbances, sleep disorders (confusional arousals and other parasomnias, rapid eye movement [REM] sleep behavior disorder, cataplexy).

## Screening and Counseling

*Screening:* When assessing a patient for a potential genetic cause of epilepsy, one should undertake a detailed history starting with the gestational and birth history and focusing on the timing of onset of epilepsy and specific seizure types that occurred at each stage. When seeing an adult with epilepsy, particularly if the individual is intellectually disabled, it is important to attempt to obtain detailed records or to speak with a parent or caregiver for information about the early presentation of the seizures. One should ask about the presence of febrile seizures in childhood, accurate seizure phenotype, significant past medical history (PMH) including trauma, meningitis, prematurity, and other potential factors that would predispose to epilepsy. It is also important to ask about comorbidities such as learning disability, intellectual disability, autism, attention deficit hyperactivity disorder (ADHD), and psychiatric comorbidities. A detailed

*Table 121-1 Molecular Genetics of Some Epilepsy Syndromes That Can Be Seen in Adults*

| Disease or Epilepsy Syndrome | Candidate Gene (Chromosome Location) | Clinical Characteristics | Proportion of Patients/ Families With Mutations | Clinical Availability of Testing/Utility of Testing |
|---|---|---|---|---|
| 1. Classic glucose transporter type1 (GLUT1) deficiency<br>2. Early-onset absence epilepsy (EOA)<br>3. GGE | SLC2A1 | 1. Infantile refractory seizures, movement disorders developmental delay<br>2. Absence seizures <4 years<br>3. CAE, JAE, JME, GTCS alone, myoclonic astatic epilepsy (MAE), absences in adults, focal epilepsy, exercise-induced dyskinesia | 1. Unknown<br>2. ~10% of patients<br>3. Unknown | Available Useful in EOA |
| JME | 1. EFHC1<br>2. GABRA1, GABRD, GABRG2<br>3. CLCN2 | 1. Early morning myoclonus, >90% GTCS, 30% absence seizures, rapid generalized spike-wave<br>2. Other GGE phenotypes<br>3. Other GGE phenotypes | Unknown, occurs in rare families | Available/not useful |
| Genetic epilepsy with febrile seizures plus (GEFS+) | 1. SCN1A<br>2. SCN1B<br>3. GABRG2 | Febrile seizures, febrile seizure plus (FS+), meaning febrile seizures that persist beyond the age of 6 years and/or afebrile seizures generalized seizures (GTCS, absence, atonic, myoclonic), focal seizures, SMEI, MAE | 1. 5%-10% of families<br>2. <5% of families<br>3. <1% of families | Available/not useful |
| Epilepsy and mental retardation limited to females | PCDH19<br>X-linked dominant with male sparing; consider even in absence of family history and/or mental retardation | Females with (67%) or without developmental delay, infantile seizure (mean onset 14 months) with regression after seizure onset, sensitivity to fever in most patients, multiple seizure types tonic-clonic, tonic, atonic, absences, myoclonic jerks, focal seizures | 10% of girls with seizure onset <5 years | Available/useful |

*(Continued)*

Table 121-1 *Molecular Genetics of Some Epilepsy Syndromes That Can Be Seen in Adults (Continued)*

| Disease or Epilepsy Syndrome | Candidate Gene (Chromosome Location) | Clinical Characteristics | Proportion of Patients/ Families With Mutations | Clinical Availability of Testing/Utility of Testing |
|---|---|---|---|---|
| Autosomal dominant nocturnal frontal lobe epilepsy (ADNFLE) | CHRNA4, CHRNB2, CHRNA2 | Clusters of brief (5 seconds-5 minutes) stereotyped events with gasps, grunts or vocalizations, motor hyperkinetic seizures with tonic or dystonic features, occur most commonly, in stage 2 sleep | 10%-20% of families | Available/useful |
| Autosomal dominant partial epilepsy with auditory features (ADPEAF) or autosomal dominant lateral temporal lobe epilepsy (ADLTE) | LGI1 | Seizures with auditory symptoms or ictal aphasia | ~50% of the ADLTE patients | Available/not useful |
| Dravet syndrome (severe myoclonic epilepsy of infancy [SMEI]) | 1. SCN1A 2. GABRG2 3. SCN1B | Infantile onset (first year) with febrile, afebrile and/or vaccination-provoked hemiclonic/ GTCS, between 1 and 4 years myoclonic, absences, and partial seizures, with developmental delay or regression, +/− ataxia, pyramidal signs<br>Adults: history of severe epilepsy (multiple seizure types) at a young age with or without fever, as adults with nocturnal convulsive and complex partial seizures less frequent than childhood, intellectual disability (varying severity), +/− ataxia, pyramidal signs | 1. 70%-80% (mutation), 3% CNV involving SCN1A 2. Rare 3. Rare | Available/very useful |
| Focal or generalized epilepsies | Microdeletions of 15q13.3, 16p13.11, 15q11.2 | Epilepsy with or without mental retardation and neuropsychiatric disability (autism, schizophrenia) | Recurrent CNV in 2.9% of patients | Available/probably useful |

family history including epilepsy, febrile seizures, as well as the cognitive and psychiatric comorbidities of epilepsy is also important.

**Counseling:**

☞**INHERITANCE:** Most idiopathic epilepsies are complex genetic disorders. An autosomal dominant mode of inheritance is seen in families with autosomal dominant nocturnal frontal lobe epilepsy (ADNFLE), autosomal dominant lateral temporal lobe epilepsy (ADLTE), and genetic epilepsy with febrile seizures plus (GEFS+). An unusual pattern of inheritance occurs in pedigree with mutations in *PCDH19* in that the mutation is passed down through unaffected males and only females are affected. Certain forms of temporal and frontal lobe epilepsies have autosomal dominant inheritance. Recurrent copy number variants (CNVs) (microdeletions at 15q13.3, 16p13.11, and 15q 11.2) have been identified in patients with generalized as well as focal epilepsies. In addition to accounting for epilepsy, they may in addition predispose to neuropsychiatric conditions. However, due to incomplete penetrance and variable expressivity the phenotypes of these CNV cannot be predicted; thus offspring, who have a 50% chance of inheriting them, have a range of potential outcomes from being asymptomatic to having epilepsy and/or neuropsychiatric disorders. Recall also that epilepsy is present in 0.5% to 1% of the population, and thus the absence of an inherited CNV or mutation does not make an individual completely without risk of epilepsy.

☞**MONOGENIC FORMS:** Monogenic focal epilepsies include ADNFLE, autosomal dominant partial epilepsy with auditory features (ADPEAF), or ADLTE, in which specific molecular basis have been identified in some families and are discussed in the Table 121-1.

Classical GGE phenotypes include juvenile myoclonic epilepsy (JME), juvenile absence epilepsy (JAE), childhood absence epilepsy (CAE), and epilepsy with generalized tonic-clonic seizures (GTCS) alone. There are rare monogenic causes of GGE.

Mutations in *GABRA1*, *GABRG2*, *GABRB3*, *GABRD* encoding respectively the α1, γ2, β3, and δ subunits of the GABA-A receptors, and mutations in *CLCN2*, which encodes the voltage-gated chloride channel CLC-2 have been described in a few families with different GGE phenotypes. Mutations in the *EFHC1* (EF-hand motif containing 1) gene are associated with JME in a minority of familial and sporadic JME patients.

Ten percent of patients with early-onset absence (EOA) epilepsy (with onset occurs under 4 years of age) have glucose transporter type 1 (GLUT1) deficiency. The majority of GGE patients display an oligogenic or polygenic predisposition.

The epilepsy gene *SCN1A* encodes the α1 subunit of the sodium channel and is associated with a variety of phenotypes, even within families with a single mutation, ranging from GEFS+ to severe myoclonic epilepsy of infancy (SMEI).

Mutations in the gene *PCDH19* cause epilepsy in females beginning in infancy; seizures can be fever associated and occur in females only, typically with intellectual disability.

☞**GENOTYPE-PHENOTYPE CORRELATION:** Variable, as discussed earlier in the context of GEFS+ and CNVs.

## Management and Treatment

**Management:** Antiepileptic medications. Ketogenic diet is a treatment for GLUT1 deficiency.

☞**PHARMACOGENETICS:** None

**Future Directions:** Whole exome and whole genome sequencing will likely replace single gene testing for epilepsy as with many other disorders. Clinically, the diagnosis of epilepsy will remain based on careful history, and epilepsy syndrome diagnosis will continue to be based on features such as EEG and family history. With the increasing availability of genetic determinants of epilepsy, we will need to adapt our classifications of epilepsy to incorporate new genetic information. In addition to adding to the richness of the characterization of epilepsy, genetics may in time help us to individualize treatment for individuals with epilepsy.

**BIBLIOGRAPHY:**

1. Berkovic SF, Mulley JC, Scheffer IE, et al. Human epilepsies: interaction of genetic and acquired factors. *Trends Neurosci.* 2006;29:391-397.

2. Depienne C, Trouillard O, Bouteiller D, et al. Mutations and deletions in PCDH19 account for various familial or isolated epilepsies in females. *Hum Mutat.* 2011;32:E1959-E1975.

3. Harkin LA, McMahon JM, Iona X, et al. The spectrum of SCN1A-related infantile epileptic encephalopathies. *Brain.* 2007;130:843-852.

4. Hirose S. Autosomal Dominant Nocturnal Frontal Lobe Epilepsy. *GeneReviews.* Initial posting: May 16, 2002; last update: April 5, 2010.

5. Jansen FE, Sadleir LG, Harkin LA, et al. Recognition and diagnosis in adults: severe myoclonic epilepsy of infancy (Dravet syndrome). *Neurology.* 2006;67:2224.

6. Kasperavičiūtė D, Catarino CB, Heinzen EL, et al. Common genetic variation and susceptibility to partial epilepsies: a genome-wide association study. *Brain.* 2010;133:2136-2147.

7. Mulley JC, Mefford HC. Epilepsy and the new cytogenetics. *Epilepsia.* 2011;52(3):423-432.

8. Mullen SA, Suls A, De Jonghe P, Berkovic SF, Scheffer IE. Absence epilepsies with widely variable onset are a key feature of familial GLUT1 deficiency. *Neurology.* 2010;75:432.

9. Ottman R, Hirose S, Jain S, et al. Genetic testing in the epilepsies—report of the ILAE Genetics Commission. *Epilepsia.* April 1 2010;51(4):655-670.

10. Ottman R. Analysis of genetically complex epilepsies. *Epilepsia.* 2005;46(suppl 10):7-14.

11. Ottman R. Autosomal Dominant Partial Epilepsy with Auditory Features. GeneReviews [Online]. Initial posting: April 20, 2007; last update: July 13, 2010.

12. Scheffer IE. Genetic testing in epilepsy: what should you be doing? *Epilepsy Curr.* Jul 2011;11(4):107-111.

13. Scheffer IE, Turner SJ, Dibbens LM, et al. Epilepsy and mental retardation limited to females: an under-recognized disorder. *Brain.* 2008;131:918-927.

14. Scheffer IE, Berkovic SF. Generalized epilepsy with febrile seizures plus. A genetic disorder with heterogeneous clinical phenotypes. *Brain.* 1997;120:479-490.

15. Suzuki T, Delgado-Escueta AV, Aguan K, et al. Mutations in EFHC1 cause juvenile myoclonic epilepsy. *Nat Genet.* 2004;36(8):842-849.

# 122 Autism Spectrum Disorders

Rachel J. Hundley, Ramzi H. Nasir, and Wen-Hann Tan

## KEY POINTS

- *Disease Summary:*
  - Autism spectrum disorders (ASD) are a heterogeneous group of disorders characterized by impairments in social communication and the presence of restricted interests or repetitive behaviors.
  - With increasing recognition of autism, it may also be diagnosed in adults who have received other diagnoses in the past (e.g. Intellectual Disability).
  - Autism is usually a lifelong condition. However, the range of disability is variable. Some individuals may be able to function in the community with variable levels of supports, whereas others may require more intensive residential based supports.
  - Management of Autism is multidisciplinary and involves addressing the core deficits (communication and restricted/repetitive behaviors) as well as comorbid psychiatric and medical conditions.

- *Differential Diagnosis:*
  - Autism is often confused with intellectual disability. Although the two conditions often co-occur, intellectual disability is not a core diagnostic feature of autism. Other disorders with features that may be confused with autism include social anxiety/selective mutism, obsessive-compulsive disorder, expressive/receptive language delay, Attention Deficit Hyperactivity Disorder, schizophrenia, acute psychological trauma, and rare epilepsy syndromes leading to speech regression and hearing loss.

- *Monogenic Forms:*
  - Monogenic forms of autism include both "syndromic" and "non-syndromic" autism. "Syndromic" autism includes disorders associated with congenital malformations, facial dysmorphic features, abnormal head sizes or linear growth, seizures, and hypotonia and/or muscle weakness. Monogenic "non-syndromic" autism is often due to genes that encode neuronal and synaptic proteins; they are typically not associated with other clinical features, except for intellectual disability.

- *Family history:*
  - Monogenic autism can be inherited in an autosomal dominant, autosomal recessive, and X-linked pattern, but there can be variable expressivity and variable penetrance.
  - Some individuals with autosomal dominant forms of autism have *de novo* mutations and hence would not have any family history of the condition.
  - Female carriers of X-linked syndromic autism may have mild manifestations of some autistic features such as rigid personality and a strong desire for routines. The empiric recurrence risk of having a second child with autism (ie, having a sibling with autism) in cases where the underlying etiology is unknown is about 3%–5%.

- *Environmental factors:*
  - Prenatal exposure to specific teratogens can be associated with syndromic autism. Postnatal exposure to lead in young children may also result in autism. Gene-environment interactions may also play a role in the pathogenesis of autism in some individuals.

- *Genome Wide Association Studies:*
  - These studies have identified numerous chromosomal loci associated with autism. The causative genes at a few of these loci are now known, but the causative genes at many of these loci are still unknown.

- *Pharmacogenomics:*
  - Considering the genetic heterogeneity in autism, pharmacogenomics are of great interest. However, at the time of writing no specific pharmacogenomically driven intervention strategies are approved.

# Diagnostic Criteria and Clinical Characteristics

*Clinical Characteristics:* Autism spectrum disorders (ASDs) are a heterogeneous group of disorders characterized by impairments in social communication and the presence of restricted interests or repetitive behaviors. Although autistic disorder, Asperger syndrome, and pervasive developmental disorder were identified as separate diagnoses within the category of pervasive developmental disorders in the fourth edition of the *Diagnostic and Statistical Manual of Mental Disorders* (DSM) (DSM-IV), the proposed DSM-V uses the term ASD as a single category that encompasses all of these diagnoses. Across individuals with ASD, there is tremendous variability in intellectual skills, adaptive and communicative competency, and behavioral regulation. Other features often associated with ASD include intellectual disability, reduced verbal cognition, anxiety, attention problems, obsessive-compulsive disorder, sleep difficulties, and seizures. Macrocephaly may be present by 2 to 3 years old in about 20% of children with ASD, including those with nonsyndromic ASD. ASDs are usually lifelong.

Approximately 10% of individuals with ASD have an underlying genetic syndrome along with syndrome-specific congenital malformations or dysmorphic features. The remaining 90% of individuals with ASD have "nonsyndromic" ASD and do not have any specific malformations nor dysmorphic features.

Autism is increasingly recognized in children. At times, parents may recognize autistic symptoms in themselves at the time of their child's diagnosis. With increasing recognition of autism, it may also be diagnosed in adults in residential facilities who were previously diagnosed with intellectual disability alone. Such individuals may have remarkable aspects of nonverbal intelligence even though they present with severe deficits in their use of language. Cognitive testing by experienced psychologists and use of augmentative communication strategies may help improve function and demonstrate areas of competency.

*Diagnostic Criteria:* The diagnosis of ASD that is proposed for the DSM-V is based on a dimensional approach and specific behavioral criteria. Currently proposed criteria state that an individual must manifest all four of the following:

A. Persistent deficits in social communication and social interaction across contexts, not accounted for by general developmental delays and manifest by all three of the following:
  1. *Deficits in social-emotional reciprocity,* ranging from abnormal social approach and failure of normal back and forth conversation through reduced sharing of interests, emotions, and affect and respond to total lack of initiation of social interaction
  2. *Deficits in nonverbal communicative behaviors used for social interaction,* ranging from poorly integrated verbal and nonverbal communication through abnormalities in eye contact and body language, or deficits in understanding and use of nonverbal communication, to total lack of facial expression or gestures
  3. *Deficits in developing and maintaining relationships,* appropriate to developmental level (beyond those with caregivers), ranging from difficulties adjusting behavior to suit different social contexts through difficulties in sharing imaginative play and in making friends to an apparent absence of interest in people

B. Restricted, repetitive patterns of behavior, interests, or activities as manifested by at least two of the following:
  1. *Stereotyped* or repetitive speech, motor movements, or use of objects (such as simple motor stereotypies, echolalia, repetitive use of objects, or idiosyncratic phrases)
  2. Excessive adherence to routines, ritualized patterns of verbal or nonverbal behavior, or excessive resistance to change (such as motoric rituals, insistence on same route or food, repetitive questioning or extreme distress at small changes)
  3. Highly restricted, fixated interests that are abnormal in intensity or focus (such as strong *attachment* to or preoccupation with unusual objects, excessively circumscribed or perseverative interests)
  4. Hyper-or hyporeactivity to sensory input or unusual interest in sensory aspects of *environment* (such as apparent indifference to pain or heat or cold, adverse response to specific sounds or textures, excessive smelling or touching of objects, fascination with lights or spinning objects)

C. *Symptoms must be present in early childhood* (but may not become fully manifest until social demands exceed limited capacities).
D. *Symptoms together limit and impair everyday functioning.*

An individual suspected of ASD should be evaluated by a psychologist or a physician who is trained to diagnose ASD using a standardized and validated set of diagnostic developmentally appropriate instruments, such as the *Autism Diagnostic Observation Schedule,* second edition (ADOS-2) and/or the *Autism Diagnostic Interview-Revised* (ADI-R). Diagnostic assessment should also include interviewing the parent, spouse, or caretaker regarding the individual's developmental history, social communication across settings, and behavior.

The ADOS-2 is a semistructured standardized assessment consisting of various activities allowing the experienced clinician to observe social, communication, and play behaviors as they relate to the diagnosis of an ASD. It can be used with toddlers, children, and adults. The ADOS-2 has a module system allowing it to be used with individuals having very little speech to those who are fully verbally fluent. The ADOS-2 results in an algorithm score for classification of ASD or for the narrower definition of autism.

The ADI-R is a comprehensive, standardized interview that is administered to a parent or caretaker who is familiar with the developmental history and current behavior of the individual being evaluated. It is primarily used in research as it generally takes 2 to 3 hours to administer.

Screening tools commonly used for adults include the *Social Responsiveness Scale* (second edition) and the Social Communication Questionnaire (previously known as the Autism Screening Questionnaire). These are completed by a parent, spouse, or caretaker of an individual suspected of having ASD.

*Syndromic ASD:* Mitochondrial disorders—various genetic etiologies resulting in mitochondrial dysfunction. Common biochemical finding—high plasma lactate and alanine concentrations. Variable presentations.

# Etiology of ASD

Only consistently replicated findings are listed. Many loci have been implicated through various genome-wide association studies (GWASs), but in some cases, the findings have been contradictory among different studies.

*Syndromes due to Known Genes*

| Syndrome | Inheritance/Gene (Chromosome) | Key Clinical Features |
| --- | --- | --- |
| Fragile X | X-linked (but females may be affected)/>200 CGG repeats in 5'UTR of *FMR1* (chromosome Xq27.3) | Head circumference >50th percentile; large, soft ears; macro-orchidism; joint hyperextensibility; mitral valve prolapse; strabismus; anxiety/hyperarousal and sensory defensiveness; gaze aversion<br>If 55-200 CGG repeats: premutation<br>Also associated with ASD<br>Males: fragile X-associated tremor/ataxia syndrome (FXTAS)<br>Females: FXTAS and premature ovarian failure (before 40 years old) |
| Rett syndrome | X-linked/*MECP2* (chromosome Xq28) (point mutations or deletions only—"duplication MECP2" is a different syndrome that affects mainly males)<br>X-linked/*CDKL5* (*STK9*) (chromosome Xp22.13) (typically with early-onset seizures)<br>Autosomal dominant/*FOXG1* (chromosome 14q12) | Wide phenotypic variability<br>Classic Rett syndrome in females:<br>  Postnatal deceleration in head growth<br>  Normal development followed by developmental regression after 6 months<br>  Stereotypic hand movements/wringing<br>  Irregular breathing; bruxism; seizures; constipation; scoliosis<br>Variant Rett syndrome in females:<br>  May have normal head circumference<br>  May have "preserved speech"<br>May be normal in females with highly skewed X-inactivation<br>*MECP2* mutation/deletion in males (less often associated with ASD)<br>  Neonatal encephalopathy → early death or PPM-X (manic-depressive psychosis, *p*yramidal signs, *p*arkinsonian features, and *m*acro-orchidism)—no seizures or microcephaly |
| Duplication MECP2 | X-linked/*MECP2* (chromosome Xq28) (classic manifestations only in males. Females: may have "broad autism phenotype"—prefers structure/routines and small groups; risk of depression, anxiety, compulsion) | Normal head circumference<br>Initial hypotonia → later spasticity<br>Delayed or lack of speech; speech regression<br>Seizures (in ~50%)<br>Recurrent infections |
| Tuberous sclerosis | Autosomal dominant/(i) *TSC1* (chromosome 9q34.13); (ii) *TSC2* (chromosome 16p13.3) | Hypomelanotic macules; facial angiofibromas; subependymal glial nodules or cortical/subcortical tubers (brain MRI); retinal hamartomas or achromic patches; renal angiomyolipomas or cysts; seizures |
| PTEN hamartoma syndrome | Autosomal dominant/*PTEN* (chromosome. 10q23.31) (includes Cowden and Bannayan-Riley-Ruvalcaba syndromes) | Macrocephaly; many with normal IQ, some with mild MR; penile or scrotal freckling in males; lipomas; vascular malformations; intestinal polyps; risk of breast, thyroid, endometrial, renal cell carcinoma |
| Cornelia de Lange syndrome | (i) Autosomal dominant/*NIPBL* (chromosome 5p13.2)<br>(ii) X-linked/*SMC1A* (*SMC1L1*) (chromosome Xp11.22)<br>(iii) Autosomal dominant/*SMC3* (chromosome 10q25.2)<br>(iv) Autosomal dominant/*RAD21* (chromosome 8q24.11)<br>(v) X-linked/*HDAC8* (chromosome Xq13.1) | Microcephaly; hypertrichosis; arched eyebrows with synophrys; ptosis; long philtrum; thin upper lip; high palate; micrognathia, prenatal and postnatal growth failure; upper limb defects (including small hands); toes 2-3 syndactyly |

*(Continued)*

*Syndromes due to Known Genes (Continued)*

| Syndrome | Inheritance/Gene (Chromosome) | Key Clinical Features |
|---|---|---|
| Smith-Magenis syndrome | Autosomal dominant/*RAI1* (chromosome 17p11.2) (either mutation in *RAI1* or deletion of chromosomal region) | Short stature; brachydactyly; infantile hypotonia; hyporeflexia; sleep disturbance with inverted melatonin circadian rhythm; self-injurious behavior; temper tantrums; self-hugging; "lick and flip" (licking hands and flipping pages); polyembolokoilamania (insertion of foreign objects into body orifices); onychotillomania (nail yanking); may be "calmer" in adulthood |
| Timothy syndrome | Autosomal dominant/*CACNA1C* (chromosome 12p13.3) | Prolonged corrected QT interval (QTc)<br>Atrioventricular (2:1) heart block<br>Congenital heart defects<br>Syndactyly of fingers and toes<br>Developmental delays (esp. language)<br>Intermittent hypoglycemia |
| Calcium channelopathy | Autosomal dominant/*CACNA1H* (chromosome 16p13.3) | Also associated with childhood absence epilepsy and idiopathic generalized epilepsy |
| Angelman syndrome | Imprinting—loss of maternally inherited *UBE3A* (chromosome 15q11.2) | Mouthing objects; sleep difficulties; fascination with water; abnormal EEG; ataxic/broad-based gait |
| Prader-Willi syndrome | Imprinting—loss of paternally inherited chromosome 15q11.2q13 region.<br>Maternal uniparental disomy of chromosome 15 more likely associated with ASD | Neonatal hypotonia and feeding difficulties → failure to thrive<br>Hyperphagia in childhood → obesity<br>Hypogonadism<br>Small hands and feet |
| ARX spectrum disorders | X-linked (but females may be affected)/*ARX* (chromosome Xp21.3) | Multiple phenotypes—intellectual disability common to all phenotypes<br>May include:<br>Seizures, lissencephaly, agenesis of corpus callosum, abnormal genitalia |
| Duchenne muscular dystrophy | X-linked/*DMD* (chromosome Xp21.1p21.2) | Progressive muscle weakness, more proximal than distal; calf hypertrophy; dilated cardiomyopathy; high CK |
| Smith-Lemli-Opitz syndrome | Autosomal recessive/*DHCR7* (chromosome 11q13.4)<br>- High serum 7-dehydrocholesterol | Microcephaly; ptosis; cleft palate<br>Abnormal genitalia; photosensitivity<br>2-3 toe syndactyly ("Y-shaped") |
| Phenylketonuria (**only if untreated**) | Autosomal recessive/*PAH* (chromosome 12q23.2)<br>- High plasma phenylalanine | Microcephaly; seizures<br>Eczema; decreased pigmentation |

*Syndromes due to Chromosomal Duplications or Deletions*

| Syndrome | Chromosomal Aberration | Key Clinical Features |
|---|---|---|
| Chromosome 2q37 *deletion* | Critical gene—*HDAC4* | Brachymetaphalangy of digits 3-5; short stature; obesity; joint laxity; scoliosis |
| Chromosome 7q11.23 *duplication* | Duplication of the Williams syndrome critical region (*GTF2I* may be the critical gene) | Mild facial dysmorphism (prominent forehead, straight eyebrows, short philtrum, thin vermilion of upper lip); variable degrees of intellectual disability with speech delay |
| Chromosome 15q11q13 *duplication* (ie, 3 copies) | Interstitial duplication of maternally inherited chromosome 15q11q13 region. Duplication of paternally inherited region is often (not always) asymptomatic | Variable penetrance—not all with ASD<br>Hypotonia; seizures; abnormal gait; hypogonadism; emotional lability, tantrums. May be at risk of sudden death (etiology unknown) |
| Chromosome 15q11q13 *triplication* (ie, 4 copies) | Interstitial triplication of chromosome 15q11q13 region<br>- May be equally affected regardless of parent-of-origin | Severe intellectual disabilities; seizures; hypotonia |

**Syndromes due to Chromosomal Duplications or Deletions**

| Syndrome | Chromosomal Aberration | Key Clinical Features |
|---|---|---|
| Isodicentric chromosome 15 (Idic(15)) (also known as: inv dup(15)) syndrome | Marker chromosome (ie, extra structurally abnormal chromosome (ESAC)) in the form of a maternally derived inverted chromosome resulting in *tetrasomy* (*4 copies*) of the PWS/AS critical region on chromosome 15q11q13 (ie, dic(15)(q13)) <br> N.B. If the PWS/AS critical region is not involved (eg, dic[15][q11] in a smaller ESAC) – Usually phenotypically normal | Poor or absent expressive language; poor receptive language <br> Fascinated by sound, water, or spinning/glistening objects <br> Seizures, including infantile spasms <br> Hypotonia <br> Joint hyperextensibility <br> Drooling <br> Regression in socialization skills |
| Chromosome 15q13.3 *deletion* | ~ 2.0 Mb deletion on chromosome 15q13.3 at coordinates 28.5-30.5 Mb (NCBI build 36; hg18) | Variable penetrance—also in controls <br> Seizures <br> ? Cardiac malformations, schizophrenia |
| Chromosome 16p11.2 *deletion* | ~550 kb deletion on chromosome. 16p11.2 at coordinates 29.5-30.1 Mb (NCBI build 36.1; hg18) | Variable penetrance—also in controls <br> Developmental and language delay. No other specific features. |
| Potocki-Lupski syndrome | *Duplication* of chromosome 17p11.2 | Failure to thrive in infancy; sleep apnea; oropharyngeal dysphagia; hyperopia; EEG abnormalities |
| Down syndrome | Duplication of chromosome 21— either full or mosaic trisomy 21 (~96%), or chromosomal translocation (~4%) | Midface hypoplasia, upslanting palpebral fissures, small low-set ears, Brushfield spots (iris), hypotonia (improves with age) |
| Velocardiofacial syndrome | *Deletion* of chromosome 22q11.2 | Congenital heart disease (conotruncal malformations); palate abnormalities (including velopharyngeal insufficiency); hypocalcemia; T-lymphocyte deficiency |
| Phelan-McDermid syndrome | *Deletion* of chromosome 22q13.3 – Association of critical gene *SHANK3* with ASD controversial | Hypotonia; normal/increased growth; prominent ears; large, fleshy hands; dysplastic toenails; mouthing objects |
| Turner syndrome | Loss of 1 copy of X chromosome (45,X) | Short stature; short, webbed neck; cubitus valgus; broad chest; ovarian dysgenesis; congenital lymphedema |
| Klinefelter syndrome | Extra copy of X chromosome in male (47,XXY) | Long limbs; hypogonadism/hypogenitalism; gynecomastia |

**Teratogens**

| Teratogen | Key Clinical Features |
|---|---|
| Valproic acid | Facial dysmorphism; hyperconvex fingernails; contractures of small joints; congenital heart defects; spina bifida |
| Congenital rubella | Cataracts (congenital or early onset); sensorineural hearing loss; congenital heart disease (patent ductus arteriosus, pulmonary stenosis); neonatal hepatosplenomegaly and jaundice |

**Single Genes Associated With Nonsyndromic ASD**

| Gene | Chromosomal Locus (GRCh37) | Function/Key Clinical Features |
|---|---|---|
| *NRXN1* | Chr. 2p16.3 | Links presynaptic with postsynaptic membrane via neuroligins |
| *OXTR* | Chr. 3p25.3 | Oxytocin receptor—involved in social cognition and behavior |
| *CNTN4* | Chr. 3p26.2p26.3 | Neuronal cell adhesion |

(Continued)

*Single Genes Associated With Nonsyndromic ASD (Continued)*

| Gene | Chromosomal Locus (GRCh37) | Function/Key Clinical Features |
|---|---|---|
| *GRIK2* (previously *GLUR6*) | Chr. 6q16.3 | Glutamate receptor—involved in synaptic transmission |
| *RELN* | Chr. 7q22.1 | Neuronal migration in cerebral cortex and cerebellum; ? Associated w/ schizophrenia |
| *MET* | Chr. 7q31.2; associated with specific allele in *MET* promoter. | Hepatocyte growth factor receptor—proto-oncogene; ? No increased cancer risk in ASD individuals |
| *CNTNAP2* | Chr. 7q35q36.1 | Synaptic protein—may be involved in release of neurotransmitters |
| *EN2* | Chr. 7q36.3 | Development of cerebellum |
| *GABRB3* | Chr. 15q12 (within Angelman syndrome critical region) | GABA-A receptor; development of cerebellum |
| *SLC6A4* | Chr. 17q11.2 | Presynaptic serotonin (5-HT) reuptake transporter—clears 5-HT from synapse |
| *ITGB3* | Chr. 17q21.32 | Platelet glycoprotein IIIa—mediates platelet aggregation; ?? No increased risk of bleeding in ASD individuals |

## Screening and Genetic Counseling

All individuals with ASD should be evaluated for clinical features that may suggest a syndromic cause (See Table in Etiology section). Unless a single gene disorder is suspected, chromosomal analysis and microarray comparative genomic hybridization (also known as chromosomal microarray) should be performed on all individuals.

Fluorescent in situ hybridization (FISH) analyses should be performed on parents of the probands who are found to have a chromosomal gain or loss on chromosomal microarray to determine whether the parents are carriers of chromosomal rearrangements, which could increase their risk of having future children with similar chromosomal abnormalities.

The risk of having another child with ASD depends on the underlying etiology. In the absence of an identifiable etiology, it is difficult to provide accurate recurrence risk, which could be as high as 25%. Moreover, in some families, siblings of individuals with ASD present with language delays instead of ASD.

## Management and Treatment

**Management:** Management of ASD will vary based on the strengths and weaknesses of the individual. More able adults with ASD may attend college and successfully maintain employment in a typical environment. However, residual communication or social issues may arise, potentially leading to the need for further support. Others with ASD may require vocational rehabilitation services or closer supervision provided through a supported work experience or sheltered work environment. For those with weaker language skills, treatment may continue to include educational and behavioral therapies designed to promote communication and adaptive skills and to reduce the occurrences of unwanted behaviors. Augmentative communication devices or strategies will continue to be an important component of treatment for individuals who struggle to communicate.

Although individuals with ASD tend to retain their diagnosis from adolescence to adulthood, longitudinal studies of transition from adolescence to adulthood provide some evidence for continued improvement over time, particularly in reduction of symptomatic behaviors, such as restricted, repetitive behaviors and interests. However, studies of adults with ASD have demonstrated that many are dependent on others and face challenges in housing, finding and keeping jobs, and being integrated into their community. One study of adults has documented high rates of internalizing disorders. Very little is known about life expectancy, neurocognitive changes with aging, or quality of life for older adults with ASD. Prognosis is certainly affected by an individual's level of cognitive ability as well as the presence of comorbid concerns such as attention deficit hyperactivity disorder (ADHD), anxiety, depression, irritability, and aggression.

It is important to start early in planning for the transition from adolescence to adulthood. Steps in the transition process may include: (1) maximizing the autonomy of the individual, (2) planning for guardianship or conservatorship if needed, (3) continuation of educational services when possible, and (4) considering different options for adult living and what levels of support may be needed.

**Therapeutics:** Appropriate behavioral interventions are the first-line treatments that may help improve the core deficits in autism (eg, deficits in language, communication, social skills, and atypical behaviors). The strongest evidence-based approaches are those based on the principles of Applied Behavioral Analysis. However, considering the variability in presentation and skills, each patient must have an individualized treatment plan targeting the core areas of deficits and other associated symptoms.

Pharmacologic interventions are second-line treatments for autism. Currently, there are no pharmacologic interventions that target the core deficits in autism. At the time of writing, the only medications approved by the FDA for use in subjects with autism are the atypical antipsychotics risperidone (for the treatment of irritability in children with autism aged 5-16 years) and aripiprazole (treatment of irritability in children with autism aged 6-17 years). No medications are approved by the FDA for treatment of autism in adults. Commonly used "off-label" medications include selective serotonin reuptake inhibitors (SSRI), anxiolytics, antipsychotic medications (atypical and typical), antiepileptic medications, stimulants, and sleep agents for the treatment of various behavioral symptoms and comorbid conditions (eg, irritability, aggression, inattention or distractibility, hyperactivity, impulsivity, depression, anxiety, and sleep disturbances).

Prior to initiating pharmacologic interventions, the medical provider should consult with the behavioral support team to make sure that all appropriate behavioral interventions have been implemented to reduce the targeted behaviors. Additionally, it is important to exclude medical conditions that can present with behavioral changes, such as seizures, pain from gastroesophageal reflux, constipation, otitis media, and toothache. Some behaviors in individuals with autism have health consequences. For example, a restricted diet predisposes one to constipation or nutritional deficiencies; pica predisposes to lead poisoning. Individuals with autism are often unable to express discomfort or maltreatment, so providers should be vigilant to these possibilities.

Pharmacologic agents used in individuals with autism carry inherent risks such as tardive dyskinesia, diabetes mellitus, and hyperlipidemia in antipsychotic agents. FDA-approved manufacturer guidelines explicitly recommend the monitoring of vital signs and specific laboratory parameters that require routine blood draws. In clinical practice, it is often difficult to perform blood draws or reliably check vital signs in individuals with autism. At times, behavioral strategies such as social stories and gradual desensitization may help the individual cooperate with these monitoring assessments. In cases where monitoring cannot be effectively performed, it is important to weigh the costs versus benefits and document informed consent of the inherent risks by the patient or their legal guardian. In institutionalized individuals, appropriate institutional and regulatory policies should be followed in the dispensation and monitoring of psychotropic medication.

In syndromic autism, specific medical complications associated with the syndrome should be taken into account when considering pharmacologic interventions. For example, as noted by the Dup15q Alliance parent support group, there appears to be an increased risk for sudden deaths among some individuals with the chromosome 15q11q13 duplication syndrome (http://www.idic15.org/Doctors.html). It has been speculated that this may be due to the use of GABA-A receptor agonists and alcohol-derived medications. In the absence of further information about this risk, it is important to exercise caution when prescribing these classes of medications, or those that have the potential to cause arrhythmias or respiratory depression.

Complementary and alternative therapies are commonly used in individuals with autism. These include dietary modification (eg,

casein and gluten-free diets), use of hyperbaric oxygen therapies, chelation therapy, treatment with antifungals, and high-dose vitamin supplementation. At the time of writing, there is little scientific evidence to justify the use of such modalities. However, in the absence of a highly effective medical intervention for the core symptoms of autism, it is likely that caregivers and patients will continue to seek alternative interventions. Medical professionals can assist families by reviewing the evidence, potential benefits, and side effects of such interventions.

Another controversial practice is to defer vaccinations in individuals with autism. The weight of scientific evidence demonstrates no correlation between receipt of vaccines and development of autism. Vaccinations are therefore not contraindicated in children or adults with autism.

***Future Directions:*** Current behavioral and pharmacologic interventions do not take into consideration the genetic background of the affected individuals. It is anticipated that as the molecular pathways in various forms of syndromic and nonsyndromic autism become known, targeted therapeutic interventions will be developed and tested. For example, ongoing clinical trials are evaluating the treatment of the core symptoms of autism with arbaclofen, which was developed based on preclinical research in fragile X syndrome, one of the most common forms of syndromic autism.

## BIBLIOGRAPHY:

1. Trialing targeted therapies for autism. *Nat Med.* 2012;18(12): 1746-1747.

2. Bellstedt E., Gillberg IC, Gillberb C. Aspects of quality of life in adults diagnosed with autism in childhood: a population based study. *Autism.* 2011;15:7-20.

3. Betancur C. Etiological heterogeneity in autism spectrum disorders: more than 100 genetic and genomic disorders and still counting. *Brain Res.* 2011;1380:42-77.

4. Dove D, Warren Z, McPheeters ML, Taylor JL, Sathe NA, Veenstra-VanderWeele J. Medications for adolescents and young adults with autism spectrum disorders: a systematic review. *Pediatrics.* Oct 2012;130(4):717-726.

5. Happe F, Charlton RA. Aging in autism spectrum disorders: a mini-review. *Gerontology.* 2012;58:70-78.

6. Holt R, Monaco AP. Links between genetics and pathophysiology in the autism spectrum disorders. *EMBO Mol Med.* Aug 2011;3(8):438-450.

7. Howlin P, Good S, Hutton J, Rutter M. Adult outcome for children with autism. *J Child Psychol Psychiatry.* 2004;45:212-229.

8. Li X, Zou H, Brown WT. Genes associated with autism spectrum disorder. *Brain Res Bull.* Sep 1 2012;88(6):543-552.

9. Lord C, Jones RM. Annual research review: re-thinking the classification of autism spectrum disorders. *J Child Psychol Psychiatry.* May 2012;53(5):490-509.

10. McPartland JM, Volkmar FR. Autism and related disorders. In: Schlaepfer TE, Nemeroff CB, eds. *Handbook of Clinical Neurology, Vol 106. Neurobiology of Psychiatric Disorders.* Amsterdam, The Netherlands: Elsevier B.V.; 2012:407-418.

11. Miles JH. Autism spectrum disorders—a genetics review. *Genet Med.* Apr 2011;13(4):278-294.

12. Myers SM, Johnson CP; American Academy of Pediatrics Council on Children With Disabilities. Management of children with autism spectrum disorders. *Pediatrics.* Nov 2007;120(5):1162-1182.

13. Seltzer MM, Krauss MW, Shattuck PT, Orsmond G, Swe A, Lord C. The symptoms of autism spectrum disorders in adolescence and adulthood. *J Autism Dev Disord.* 2003;33(6):565-581.

14. Scherer SW, Dawson G. Risk factors for autism: translating genomic discoveries into diagnostics. *Hum Genet.* Jul 2011;130(1):123-148.

15. Shattuck PT, Seltzer MM, Greenberg JS, et al. Change in autism symptoms and maladaptive behaviors in adolescents and adults with an autism spectrum disorder. *J Autism Dev Disord.* 2007;37:1735-1747.

16. Veenstra-VanderWeele J, Blakely RD. Networking in autism: leveraging genetic, biomarker and model system findings in the search for new treatments. *Neuropsychopharmacology.* 2012;37(1):196-212.

17. Venkat A, Jauch E, Russell WS, Crist CR, Farrell R. Care of the patient with an autism spectrum disorder by the general physician. *Postgrad Med J.* 2012;88(1042):472-481.

18. SFARI GENE website: http://gene.sfari.org/ (Simons Foundation Autism Research Institute)

# 123 Frontotemporal Lobar Degeneration

David J. Irwin and Vivianna Van M. Deerlin

## KEY POINTS

- *Disease summary:*
  - Frontotemporal lobar degeneration (FTLD) is a nonamnestic primary neurodegenerative disorder that is clinically, neuropathologically, and genetically heterogeneous. Characteristic symptoms include progressive behavioral disturbance and/or language impairment, with variable underlying neuropathologic substrates.
  - Clinically FTLD is comprised of *two major subtypes*:
    - The behavioral variant (bvFTD), a progressive cognitive or behavioral syndrome
    - Primary progressive aphasia (PPA), a degenerative language disorder
    - PPA variants are further subdivided into three variants based on the specific language abnormality present: the nonfluent-agrammatic variant (naPPA), semantic variant (svPPA), and logopenic variant (lvPPA). lvPPA is considered an atypical presentation of Alzheimer disease (AD) and will not be further discussed as an FTLD clinical syndrome.
  - FTLD patients may present with or acquire concomitant motor disorders including parkinsonism or the motor neuron disease, amyotrophic lateral sclerosis (ALS-FTLD). There is also overlap with the extrapyramidal movement disorders progressive supranuclear palsy (PSP) and corticobasal syndrome (CBS).
  - FTLD clinical spectrum disorders occur most commonly in patients before the age of 65 years, and have a similar prevalence to AD in this age group.
  - The only known nongenetic risk factor for FTLD is a history of head trauma.
  - Neuropathologically FTLD can be broadly divided into *two major categories*: tauopathies (FTLD-tau), a class of neurodegenerative diseases which contain aggregations of the abnormally modified microtubule-binding protein tau, and FTLD-TDP, characterized by inclusion bodies formed from the DNA-binding protein, TDP-43.
  - FTLD-tau consists of clinical FTLD-spectrum disorders with neuropathologic diagnoses of Pick disease, corticobasal degeneration (CBD), PSP, argyrophilic grain disease, multisystem tauopathy, or FTLD with parkinsonism linked to chromosome 17 (FTDP-17).
  - FTLD-TDP has four major subtypes (A-D) based on the morphology of TDP-43 positive inclusions and cortical layers involved. All FTLD-spectrum clinical disorders can be associated with each of these subtypes, while most genetic etiologies of FTLD-TDP are generally associated with a specific neuropathologic subtype.
  - A minority of FTLD cases have inclusions composed of the fused in sarcoma (FUS) protein (FTLD-FUS), a RNA-binding protein similar to TDP-43, and in a small number of others the pathologic protein has not yet been identified.
- *Hereditary basis:*
  - Approximately 40% of FTLD patients have a family history of dementia and/or movement disorder and in 10% to 30% of cases an autosomal dominant inheritance pattern is detected. The remaining cases are apparent sporadic cases.
  - Autosomal dominant mutations in five genes have been associated with FTLD: *MAPT*, *GRN*, *C9orf72*, *VCP*, and *CHMP2B*. Of these, mutations in *MAPT*, *GRN*, and a hexanucleotide expansion mutation in *C9orf72* are the most common, while mutations in *VCP* and *CHMP2B* are rare. Together these genes explain only about 30% of familial FTLD cases suggesting that there are still additional genes to be discovered.
  - Mutations in a few additional genes, *TARDBP* and *FUS*, which are primarily associated with ALS phenotypes have been identified in a few FTLD cases.
- *Differential diagnosis:*
  - Includes other primary neurodegenerative conditions (AD, dementia with Lewy bodies [DLB], Parkinson disease dementia), nondegenerative primary central nervous system (CNS) conditions (cerebrovascular disease or vascular dementia, CNS malignancy, CNS trauma, CNS infections, and CNS inflammatory diseases—eg, vasculitis, systemic lupus erythematosus, neurosarcoidosis, multiple sclerosis), primary psychiatric (nonprogressive FTLD "phenocopy") disorders (schizophrenia, late-onset psychosis, autism/Asperger spectrum disorders, decompensated personality disorders, depression, and bipolar disease), and systemic medical conditions (hypothyroidism, drug intoxication, medically induced delirium, vitamin $B_{12}$ deficiency, and other toxic or metabolic CNS insults). AD is a common misdiagnosis, and is encountered in approximately 20% of all FTLD clinical cases at autopsy.

## Diagnostic Criteria and Clinical Characteristics

### Diagnostic Criteria for FTLD:

**Diagnostic evaluation should include (Fig. 123-1 algorithm)**

- Cognitive examination consistent with prominent early behavioral or executive impairment (bvFTD) or language impairment (PPA) with relative sparing of memory and visuospatial function.
- Evaluation of symptoms for progression over time ($\geq 1$ year), as evidenced by serial examination or caregiver history.
- Evaluation of symptoms for associated functional impairment.
- Serum and cerebrospinal fluid (CSF) laboratory studies to exclude toxic, infectious, inflammatory, and metabolic etiologies if suspected.

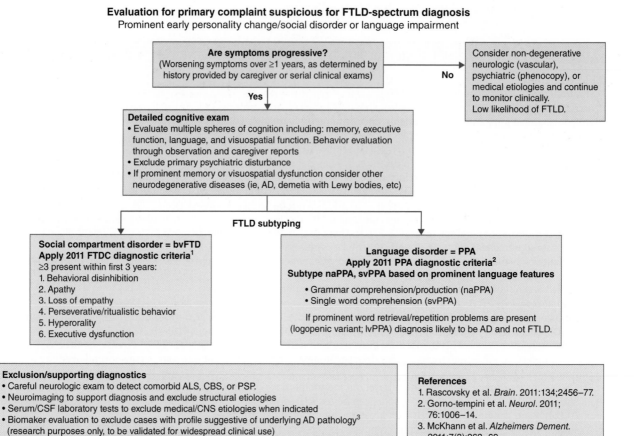

*Figure 123-1* **Diagnostic Algorithm for FTLD.** FTLD clinical syndromes, like all neurodegenerative diseases, require autopsy confirmation as the gold standard for diagnosis; thus, it is necessary to exclude other non-degenerative etiologies that could mimic FTLD during the diagnostic work up. A step-wise approach can be performed to demonstrate progressive changes in language or social cognition suggestive of FTLD. Abbreviations: FTLD (frontotemporal lobar degeneration), AD (Alzheimer's disease), bvFTD (behavioral-variant frontotemporal dementia), PPA (primary progressive aphasia), naPPA (non-fluent agrammatic variant primary progressive aphasia), svPPA (semantic variant primary progressive aphasia), lvPPA (logopenic variant primary progressive aphasia), ALS (amyotrophic lateral sclerosis), CBS (corticobasal syndrome)

- Neuroimaging for regional atrophy or hypometabolism supportive of FTLD-spectrum diagnosis (see later) and exclusion of structural etiologies (eg, malignancy).
- Detailed neurologic examination to detect comorbid motor neuron disease (ALS) or extrapyramidal movement disorder (parkinsonism including PSP and CBS).
- Biomarker (CSF tau and beta-amyloid [Aβ] levels or Aβ ligand neuroimaging) evaluation to exclude patients with biomarkers suggestive of underlying AD neuropathology (recent FTLD and AD criteria indicate these measures have utility for research purposes but need to be validated for widespread clinical use).

**And the absence of**

- Any other neurodegenerative, non-neurodegenerative primary CNS, medical, or psychiatric disorder that better accounts for the observed pattern of clinical deficits.

### Clinical Characteristics:

☞**bvFTD:** It is a cognitive or behavioral disorder associated with atrophy and neurodegeneration in the anterior cingulate gyrus, insular cortex, basal ganglia, and dorsolateral and ventromedial frontal lobes. Clinical features include behavioral disinhibition

and obsessive, ritualistic behaviors. There is a loss of empathy or concern for others and patients can display difficulty multitasking and set-shifting (executive dysfunction). Dietary changes, including carbohydrate craving and hyperorality are common. As the disease progresses to involve more medial frontal areas, apathy and inertia often predominate. Problematic behaviors can be severely detrimental to patient's functioning and extremely difficult for caregivers to manage. Often patients come to medical attention after resultant serious detrimental interpersonal problems such as loss of employment. At autopsy roughly equal numbers of patients have FTLD-tau and FTLD-TDP diagnoses.

☞**naPPA:** It is a primary language disorder characterized by grammatical comprehension and expressive deficits with associated effortful speech. A motor planning deficit and resulting articulation difficulties (apraxia of speech) and executive dysfunction are also common. Single word comprehension and object knowledge are not typically affected. Atrophy is most prominent in the dominant posterior or inferior frontal and anterior insular cortex. Extrapyramidal symptoms of comorbid CBS and PSP are frequent and can precede or emerge after symptoms of naPPA. The majority of naPPA cases have FTLD-tau pathology.

☞**svPPA:** This has the key feature of loss of word meaning and object knowledge. As patients lose the ability to identify objects, they progressively use more imprecise terms to describe them (eg, "animal" or "bird" to describe a "pelican"). Speech is fluent and grammatically correct; however, it is usually empty of meaningful content. These patients also have difficulty reading phonetically irregular words (eg, choir, yacht) due to loss of semantic knowledge required for correct pronunciation (surface dyslexia). Corresponding atrophy is in the dominant anterior temporal lobe. Behavioral features of ritualistic and compulsive behavior with loss of empathy may emerge, corresponding to nondominant anterior temporal lobe involvement. FTLD-TDP is the most common neuropathology associated with svPPA.

☞**PARKINSONIAN DISORDERS:** PSP and CBS are akinetic-rigid syndromes characterized by axial rigidity, early falls and vertical gaze palsy, and asymmetric rigidity, limb apraxia, and cortical sensory loss, respectively. Both, in contrast to idiopathic Parkinson disease, typically have a poor response to dopaminergic treatment. These syndromes can develop cognitive dysfunction consistent with naPPA and other FTLD-spectrum disorders, as earlier, and are considered a part of the FTLD-spectrum of clinical syndromes. Similar extrapyramidal symptoms (bradykinesia and rigidity) are also typical in FTDP-17.

☞**FTLD-ALS:** FTLD clinical syndromes can also accompany or precede clinical signs of ALS, which include upper motor neuron findings of spasticity and hyper-reflexia, and lower motor neuron signs of muscle wasting and fasciculations. In addition, some FTLD patients have subclinical signs of motor neuron disease on electromyographic testing and at autopsy. FTLD-ALS can include bvFTD and all other clinical FTLD syndromes, and is highly predictive of a TDP-43 proteinopathy (FTLD-TDP).

## Screening and Counseling

*Screening:* An algorithm for diagnostic evaluation of patient with a primary complaint of behavioral or language difficulties is shown in Fig. 123-1.

*Counseling:* FTLD is inherited in an autosomal dominant manner. Autosomal dominant pedigrees typically show one or more first-degree relatives with an FTLD-spectrum disorder (including ALS), or first- and second-degree relatives. Because of the variable clinical phenotype seen among FLTD patients, even within the same family, family members may have a variety of neurodegenerative disease phenotypes. Furthermore, older generations may have been diagnosed before FTLD was recognized as a unique disorder or by a physician with limited experience with the spectrum of FTLD phenotypes. *MAPT* and *GRN* mutations may be identified in sporadic-appearing pedigrees as a result of extremely rare de novo mutations or more likely due to decreased penetrance in the parent or an uninformative pedigree (eg, early death of one parent). All children of a known FTLD mutation carrier are at a 50% risk of carrying the mutation. *C9orf72* expansions are seen in apparent sporadic cases, however the mechanism (decreased penetrance versus de novo expansion) is not yet known. *GRN* and *MAPT* mutations are highly penetrant in an age-dependent manner, although a few cases of incomplete penetrance have been published for both genes.

There are no obvious genotype-clinical phenotype correlations for FTLD gene mutations (Table 123-1). Genetic forms may present clinically with bvFTD or na- and svPPA phenotypes. Although some mutations have an earlier age of onset or a specific phenotypic presentation, the variability of individuals with the same mutation, even within the same family, suggests that other genetic and environmental factors impact the onset and presentation of disease. The heterogeneity in clinical presentation likely reflects the different anatomic distribution of the lesions in each individual, which is affected by these and other modifying factors. At the level of the specific *FTLD* gene, there are some characteristic neuropathologic phenotypic correlations. Genetic etiologies and corresponding neuropathology include *MAPT* mutation (tau pathology), *GRN* mutation (FTLD-TDP type A pathology), *CHMP2B* mutation (FTLD with ubiquitinated inclusions), *VCP* mutation (FTLD-TDP type D), and *C9orf72* hexanucleotide expansion (mostly FTLD-TDP type B pathology).

### Table 123-1 *Genetic Differential Diagnosis*

| Syndrome | Gene Symbol | Associated Findings |
|---|---|---|
| FTLD (including bvFTD, naPPA, and svPPA) | *MAPT, GRN, C9orf72, CHMP2B* | May co-occur with ALS or parkinsonism. In familial cases, the underlying genetic defect cannot be predicted by the clinical syndrome. However, if brain autopsy has been done, the type of abnormal protein inclusion identified and the pattern of pathology can help identify the most likely genetic cause. *MAPT* cases usually present at an earlier age of onset than *GRN*. |
| FTLD-ALS | *C9orf72* | Either ALS or FTLD may be the presenting symptom. |
| Progressive supranuclear palsy (PSP) | *MAPT* | In addition to being occasionally caused by *MAPT* mutations, a specific haplotype of *MAPT* is associated with an increased risk for PSP. |
| Inclusion body myopathy and Paget disease of bone | *VCP* | Variable presence of inclusion body myopathy, Paget disease of bone, and FTLD. Patients with *VCP* mutations may also present with pure ALS. |

Gene names (Gene/locus MIM number, chromosomal location): *MAPT*, microtubule-associated protein tau (157140, 17q21.1); *GRN*, granulin precursor (138945, 17q21.32); *C9orf72*, chromosome 9 open reading frame 72 (614260, 9p21.2); *CHMP2B*, chromatin-modifying protein or charged multivesicular body protein (CHMP) family member 2B (609512, 3p11.2); *VCP*, valosin-containing protein (601023, 9p13.3).

## Management and Treatment

*Management:* Management is largely supportive with behavioral modification techniques and increased supervision, the mainstay of treatment. Due to behavioral disinhibition and poor judgment, bvFTD patients require careful monitoring of their contact with strangers and management of finances due to susceptibility to exploitation. Simplifying the environment to limit triggers of problematic behaviors can be effective, as are structured schedules to help with executive difficulties and attention deficits. PPA patients can benefit from slowed conversation speed using small, simple sentences. Occupational and physical therapy can assist with associated motor dysfunction and provide strategies to help prevent falls. Limiting polypharmacy and removing medications that could potentially worsen cognition, such as sedatives and anticholinergic medications commonly used for management of urinary incontinence is also very important.

There are currently no FDA-approved treatments for FTLD and minimal data available to guide physicians in selecting appropriate treatment in this patient population. This is due to difficulties in performing large multicenter randomized double-blinded placebo-controlled trials in this clinically heterogeneous patient population.

Pharmacologic interventions are mainly off-label adaptations of psychiatric medications to manage problematic behaviors and include

☞ANTIDEPRESSANTS: Selective serotonin reuptake inhibitors (SSRIs) have a biologic rationale for use in FTLD, as patients have been found to have a deficit in the serotonergic neurotransmitter system. Symptoms such as impulsivity, compulsions, dietary changes, disinhibition, and associated depression may respond to serotonergic treatment. Trazodone can be an effective option but is often limited by side effects of somnolence.

☞ANTIPSYCHOTICS: This class of medications can be used to treat agitation and aggressiveness, but is limited in use for FTLD patients due to its potential to potentiate extrapyramidal symptoms through D2 receptor blockade. Newer, second-generation medications have lower D2 receptor affinity, but still should be used with caution. Additionally, data on increased risk of death in the elderly has resulted in a FDA-issued black box warning for these agents.

☞ANTIEPILEPTICS (AEDs): This class of medications is often used for mood-stabilizing properties for management of disruptive behaviors.

☞DOPAMINE AGONISTS (DAs): Associated extrapyramidal symptoms may be treated with a trial of L-dopa or dopamine agonists, although a sustained improvement in abnormal movements, as seen in idiopathic Parkinson disease, is not typical and there is a risk of inducing psychosis.

☞STIMULANTS: Methylphenidate, modafinil, or armodafinil may be useful for treating symptoms of apathy and inattention, as it is used in other frontal lobe-mediated apathetic conditions.

☞ACETYLCHOLINESTERASE INHIBITORS (AChEIs): These agents are FDA approved for use in AD, and FTLD patients commonly receive these medications due to difficulty in clinically differentiating these disorders. In contrast to AD, there is minimal cholinergic deficit in FTLD, limiting the biologic rationale for use of this class of medications. Conflicting data exist from small trials, with some reporting these agents may worsen problematic behaviors and the associated social disorder. Most authorities conclude AChEIs should not be used in FTLD.

☞MEMANTINE: This *N*-methyl D-aspartate (NMDA) receptor antagonist and potential neuroprotective agent is approved for use in moderate-to-severe AD, showing particular improvement in agitated behaviors. Its efficacy in FTLD is unclear, although it is generally well tolerated; A multi-center trial has been published since the initial submission of the manuscript. However, a recent multicenter trial of memantine in bvFTD and svPPA patients did not find evidence of benefit for cognitive and behavioral outcomes.

For all medical treatments in FTLD careful consideration of side effect profiles and underlying medical conditions of individual patients must be considered. In addition, slow titrations using the lowest effective dose of medication is crucial. Nonpharmacologic management is first-line treatment, and should be maximized prior to initiation of pharmacologic therapy. Etiology-targeted treatments that effect mechanism of disease (eg, tau/TDP-43 aggregation and neuron loss) are in need for FTLD and development and evaluation efforts are currently in progress.

## Molecular Genetics and Molecular Mechanism

A family history of FTLD or ALS is present in about 40% to 50% of FTLD cases. Autosomal dominant mutations in *MAPT* and *GRN*, both on chromosome 17, together account for about 10% to 20% of FTLD patients. Rare genetic causes of FTLD include mutations in *CHMP2B* and *VCP*, which are associated with a form of Paget disease of bone with FTLD. A pathologic hexanucleotide repeat expansion in *C9orf72* on chromosome 9 is associated with both ALS and FTLD. The frequency of *C9orf72* expansions is highest in familial ALS and FTLD-ALS and in the subset of FTLD cases with FTLD-TDP pathology where these mutations may represent between 20% and 60%. The frequency of *C9orf72* expansions in unselected clinical FTLD cases is less than 10%, similar to the frequency of *MAPT* and *GRN* mutations.

*MAPT* mutations are missense, splice-site, and small deletion mutations in exons 1 and 9 to 13 or flanking intronic regions. About 44 different mutations have been reported, although most are rare. Microtubule-associated protein tau is involved in the assembly of tubulin. Pathogenic *MAPT* mutations cause disease by either altering the ratios of spice variant isoforms expressed or by altering the tubulin-binding properties of the tau protein.

*GRN* (also known as *PGRN*) encodes progranulin a ubiquitously expressed growth factor precursor with 7.5 granulin peptides. Granulin functions are not fully understood, but the precursor and peptides are involved in wide range of biologic functions including inflammation and wound repair. Most *GRN* mutations are nonsense or frameshift mutations that produce null alleles as a result of nonsense-mediated decay of the transcript. Thus, disease is caused by haploinsufficiency of progranulin. At least 69 different *GRN* mutations have been described that encompass the entire coding region of the gene.

*C9orf72* encodes a ubiquitously expressed protein of unknown function. The genetic defect is an expansion of a hexanucleotide repeat (GGGGCC) in the promoter region of *C9orf72* which results in loss of expression of the major transcript. Control individuals have between 2 and 25 repeats. The sizes of the pathogenic expansions are from the low 30 repeats to hundreds of repeats. There are many unanswered questions about this new disease-causative gene including its penetrance, presence of anticipation, the implication

*Table 123-2* **Molecular Genetic Testing**

| Gene | Testing Modality | Mutation Type | Detection Rate |
|---|---|---|---|
| *MAPT* | DNA sequencing of selected exons and flanking intronic regions | Sequence mutations and small deletions | 1%-10% |
| *GRN* | DNA sequencing of whole coding region and 5'UTR | Sequence mutations, splice-site mutations, and insertions or deletions | 5%-10% |
| *C9orf72* | Repeat PCR size analysis/Southern blot | Hexanucleotide repeat expansion | 5%-10% |
| *VCP* | DNA sequencing | Missense mutations | <1% |

of intermediate size repeats, occurrence of de novo expansions, and genotype-phenotype correlations. Nevertheless, what is known is that it is now the most common genetic abnormality in ALS and FTLD-ALS. The expansions are found in familial cases as well as sporadic cases of ALS, FTLD-ALS, and FTLD.

**CHMP2B** encodes the charged multivesicular body protein 2B which is involved in endosomal sorting. A point mutation in *CHMP2B* was identified as the causative gene in a Danish family with linkage to chromosome 3. A few additional families have been identified, but overall *CHMP2B* is considered a rare familial cause of FTLD.

**VCP**: Missense mutations in VCP, encoding valosin-containing protein, are associated with inclusion body myopathy with Paget disease of the bone and/or FTD (IBMPFD). VCP is an adenosine triphosphatase involved in protein degradation in the endoplasmic reticulum. Carriers of *VCP* mutations show variable penetrance and phenotype with myopathy present in a majority of patients and FTLD and Paget disease in some. *VCP* mutations have also been identified in ALS.

**Genetic Testing:** Clinical genetic testing for FTLD is available for *MAPT*, *GRN*, *C9orf72*, and *VCP* in the United States. Testing for all *FTLD* genes is available in Europe.

Although the FTLD diagnosis is made based on the clinical features as shown in Fig. 123-1, genetic testing can be used to support a clinical diagnosis or to exclude an alternate differential diagnosis (Table 123-2). In addition, the identification of a pathogenic mutation in an affected individual enables testing for that specific mutation in family members for confirmation in affected family members and predictive testing in unaffected individuals who are at risk of having the mutation. Counseling for predictive testing of FTLD follows the same guidelines as for Huntington disease. As new drugs are developed and studied that target a specific pathologic protein or pathway, knowledge of the disease-causing mutation will enable personalized targeted therapy since the FTLD mutations are well correlated with pathology.

## BIBLIOGRAPHY:

1. McKhann GM, Knopman DS, Chertkow H, et al. The diagnosis of dementia due to Alzheimer's disease: recommendations from the National Institute on Aging-Alzheimer's Association workgroups on diagnostic guidelines for Alzheimer's disease. *Alzheimers Dement.* May 2011;7(3):263-269.

2. Rascovsky K, Hodges JR, Knopman D, et al. Sensitivity of revised diagnostic criteria for the behavioural variant of frontotemporal dementia. *Brain.* 2011;134(pt 9):2456-2477.

3. Gorno-Tempini ML, Hillis AE, Weintraub S, et al. Classification of primary progressive aphasia and its variants. *Neurology.* Mar 15 2011;76(11):1006-1014.

4. Mackenzie IR, Neumann M, Bigio EH, et al. Nomenclature and nosology for neuropathologic subtypes of frontotemporal lobar degeneration: an update. *Acta Neuropathol.* Jan 2010;119(1):1-4.

5. Mackenzie IR, Neumann M, Bahorie A, et al. A harmonized classification system for FTLD-TDP pathology. *Acta Neuropathol.* 2011;122(1):111-113.

6. Grossman M. Primary progressive aphasia: clinicopathological correlations. *Nat Rev Neurol.* Feb 2010;6(2):88-97.

7. Rabinovici GD, Miller BL. Frontotemporal lobar degeneration: epidemiology, pathophysiology, diagnosis and management. *CNS Drugs.* 2010;24(5): 375-398.

8. Forman MS, Farmer J, Johnson JK, et al. Frontotemporal dementia: clinicopathological correlations. *Ann Neurol.* Jun 2006;59(6):952-962.

9. Huey ED, Putnam KT, Grafman J. A systematic review of neurotransmitter deficits and treatments in frontotemporal dementia. *Neurol.* 2006;66:17-22.

10. Grossman M. Biomarkers in frontotemporal lobar degeneration. *Curr Opin Neurol.* 2010; 23:643-648.

11. Sleegers K, Cruts M, Van Broeckhoven. Molecular pathways in frontotemporal lobar degeneration. *Ann Rev Neurosci.* 2010;33:71-88.

12. Goldman JS, Rademakers R, Huey ED, et al. An algorithm for genetic testing of frontotemporal lobar degeneration. *Neurology.* 2011;76(5):475-483.

13. Gijselinck I, Van Langenhove T, van der Zee J, et al. A C9orf72 promoter repeat expansion in a Flanders-Belgian cohort with disorders of the frontotemporal lobar degeneration-amyotrophic lateral sclerosis spectrum: a gene identification study. *Lancet Neurol.* 2012;11(1):54-65.

14. Chen-Plotkin AS, Martinez-Lage M, Sleiman PM, et al. Genetic and clinical features of progranulin-associated frontotemporal lobar degeneration. *Arch Neurol.* 2011;68(4):488-497.

15. Boxer AL, Knopman DS, Kaufer DI, et al. Memantine in patients with frontotemporal lobar degeneration: a multicentre, randomised, double-blind, placebo-controlled trial. *Lancet Neurol.* 2013;12:149-156.

16. Wood EM, Falcone D, Suh E, et al. Development and validation of pedigree classification criteria for frontotemporal lobar degeneration. *JAMA Neurol.* 2013(in press).

## Supplementary Information

**OMIM REFERENCES:**

[1] Dementia, Frontotemporal, With or Without Parkinsonism; MAPT (#600274)

[2] Pick Disease; MAPT (#172700)

[3] Supranuclear Palsy, Progressive; MAPT (#601104)

[4] Supranuclear Palsy, Progressive Atypical; MAPT (#260540)

[5] Frontotemporal Lobar Degeneration With Ubiquitin-Positive Inclusions; GRN (#607485)

[6] Amyotrophic Lateral Sclerosis With Frontotemporal Dementia; C9orf72 (#105550)

[7] Amyotrophic Lateral Sclerosis 14 With or Without Frontotemporal Dementia; VCP (#613954)

[8] Inclusion Body Myopathy With Early-Onset Paget Disease and Frontotemporal Dementia; VCP (#167320)

[9] Dementia, Familial, Nonspecific, FTD3; CHMP2B (#600795)

**Alternative Names:**
- Pick Disease
- Frontotemporal Dementia (FTD)

- Frontotemporal Dementia Linked to Chromosome 17 With Parkinsonism (FTDP17)
- Frontotemporal Lobar Degeneration With Ubiquitin-Positive Inclusions (FTLD-U)
- Tauopathy
- TDP-43-Opathy
- Primary Progressive Aphasia (PPA)
- Corticobasal Syndrome
- Progressive Supranuclear Palsy
- Frontotemporal Dementia With Amyotrophic Lateral Sclerosis (FTLD-ALS)

***Key Words:*** Dementia, aphasia, neurodegeneration, tau, TDP-43, frontal lobe syndrome, motor neuron disease, parkinsonism

# 124 Alzheimer Disease

Matthew Schu and Robert C. Green

## KEY POINTS

- *Disease summary:*
  - Alzheimer disease (AD) is the most common form of dementia. It is characterized by debilitating and progressive episodic memory loss, difficulty with language and decision making, and (in advanced stages) loss of motor control, incontinence, and mutism.
  - The neuropathologic hallmarks of the AD brain include an abundance of senile plaques largely composed of beta-amyloid (Aβ) deposits and neurofibrillary tangles made up of tau protein. While these features are consistently observed in autopsies of AD patients, the exact role that these proteins play in AD pathogenesis is still unclear.
  - Most patients with AD begin developing symptoms after 60 years of age, although in the rare cases of autosomal dominantly inherited AD symptoms typically manifest at an earlier age.
  - Although risk for AD increases with age, AD is not a symptom of normal aging.

- *Differential diagnosis:*
  - *Treatable diagnoses:* depression, chronic drug intoxication, chronic central nervous system (CNS) infection, thyroid disease, vitamin deficiencies (particularly B$_{12}$ and thiamine), CNS angiitis, and normal-pressure hydrocephalus (NPH)
  - *Other neurodegenerative disorders:* vascular dementia, diffuse Lewy body syndrome, Parkinson disease, Pick disease, Creutzfeldt-Jakob disease, and cerebral autosomal dominant arteriopathy with subcortical infarcts and leukoencephalopathy (CADASIL)

- *Monogenic forms:*
  - Rare cases of very early-onset familial AD (FAD) follow a Mendelian autosomal dominant inheritance pattern.
  - Approximately 70% of FAD cases can be explained by mutations in one of three genes: *PSEN1*, *PSEN2*, and *APP*.

- *Family history:*
  - The average person has a 10% to 12% chance of developing AD in his or her lifetime. First-degree relatives of patients with AD have a 20% to 44% lifetime risk for the disease.

- *Twin studies:*
  - Monozygotic twins show a 60% concordance rate for AD.

- *Environmental factors:*
  - Risk factors include female gender, lower level of education, and history of head trauma.

- *Genome-wide Associations:*
  - Recent large-scale genome-wide association studies (GWASs) have identified multiple genetic loci associated with AD risk (Table 124-1). Of these results however, even the most robust marker for AD susceptibility, the ε4 allele of APOE, is neither necessary nor sufficient for AD diagnosis.

- *Pharmacogenomics:*
  - While several studies have begun stratifying AD patients based on genetic markers to test for differential response to treatment, at present no consistently replicated pharmacogenomic associations have been observed for AD therapies.

## Diagnostic Criteria and Clinical Characteristics

***Diagnostic Criteria for AD:*** Making a diagnosis of AD can be particularly challenging (see Fig. 124-1), since a definitive diagnosis of AD requires autopsy results demonstrating a large number of Aβ neuritic plaques and neurofibrillary (tau protein) tangles in the brain. However, clinical criteria for making the diagnosis were established in 1984 and have proven highly accurate (81% sensitivity, 70% specificity). To meet the clinical criteria, the patient must have gradual progressive cognitive decline (as opposed to acute onset of symptoms) and cognitive impairment must be observed in at least two of the following domains:

- Impaired ability to learn or recall information
- Impaired language skills
- Impaired visuospatial abilities
- Executive dysfunction
- Changes in behavior or personality

More recent criteria for the clinical diagnosis of AD have described AD as part of a continuum of biologic phenomena starting from a preclinical phase then progressing to a phase of mild cognitive impairment and later dementia. Supportive evidence of this model has been demonstrated from a longitudinal study of families with a history of autosomal dominant AD, which showed that physiologic changes in affected brains are observable up to 20 years prior to the onset of dementia and 10 years before the earliest cognitive symptoms manifest. These data suggest that previous diagnoses of AD were made late in the course of disease progression and provide a strong case for earlier diagnosis by applying several methods of biomarker detection discussed later in addition to standard clinical assessments for monitoring cognitive decline.

***Clinical Characteristics:*** AD typically presents in patients between 40 and 90 years of age, but most frequently occurs after the age

*Table 124-1 Molecular Genetic Testing For Alzheimer Disease*

| Gene (Location) | Name | Form of AD | Inheritance Pattern | Penetrance | Available Testing |
|---|---|---|---|---|---|
| APP[a]<br>(21q21.3) | Amyloid precursor protein | FAD | Autosomal dominant | 100% | Clinically available for adults but rare |
| PSEN1<br>(14q24.2) | Presenilin 1 | FAD | Autosomal dominant | 100% | Clinically available for adults and prenatal testing |
| PSEN2<br>(1q42.13) | Presenilin 2 | FAD | Autosomal dominant | 95% | Clinically available for adults but rare |
| APOE<br>(19q13.32) | Apolipoprotein E | Sporadic AD | Complex | N/A | Clinically available for adults through direct-to-consumer testing |

[a]At least one variant within the *APP* gene has been demonstrated to be protective for AD. However, to date clinical genetic tests only exist for the deleterious mutations in *APP* that are associated with the autosomal dominant form of FAD.

of 65. In the early stages, patients and/or their families notice subtle progressive decline in memory, initiative, word-finding, and concentration. As the disease progresses, deficits in memory, language, and reasoning skills become apparent. Some patients also exhibit personality changes and agitation. Depression commonly coexists in patients with dementia. End-stage dementia is characterized by a loss of motor control, incontinence, and mutism. Death typically arises from general lack of mobility, malnutrition, and/or pneumonia.

Promising biomarkers that would allow clinicians to detect evidence of Aβ deposition within the brains of at-risk patients

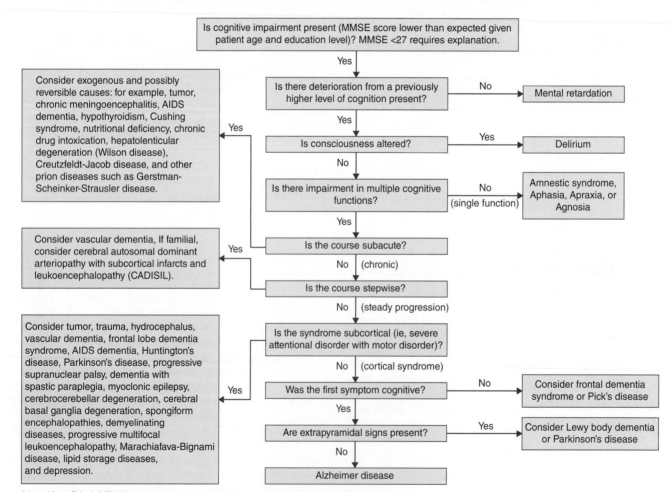

• Adopted from: Folstein MF, Differential diagnosis of dementia. The clinical process. Psychiatric Clinics of North America. 1997 March; 20(1):45-57. Review.

*Figure 124-1 Algorithm for Diagnostic Evaluation of Patient With AD.*

include decreased levels of $A\beta_{42}$ in the cerebrospinal fluid (CSF) and/or positive amyloid imaging results using positron emission tomography (PET). In 2012 the FDA approved the use of florbetapir for PET amyloid imaging as an adjunct to the evaluation of patients with cognitive impairment. Additionally, biomarkers for neuronal degeneration, including elevated tau in the CSF, PET scans showing decreased glucose metabolism in the temporoparietal cortex, and magnetic resonance imagining (MRI) scans showing advanced cerebral atrophy relative to that of age-matched brains, may be supportive of a probable AD diagnosis.

## Screening and Counseling

### Screening:

☞**FAMILIAL AD:** Less than 5% of AD cases are attributed to autosomal dominant FAD. A handful of rare mutations fully explain the transmission of FAD in select lineages, therefore genetic testing for mutations in *APP*, *PSEN1*, and *PSEN2* may help to confirm diagnosis. Mutations in the *APP* and *PSEN1* genes explain the majority of familial FAD cases, while mutations in the *PSEN2* are significantly rarer with most recorded mutations in this gene arising within a single pedigree known as the Volga Germans.

☞**AD AND DOWN SYNDROME:** When carefully monitored, over 50% of aging patients with Down syndrome (DS) show signs of cognitive decline consistent with AD and nearly all brains of DS patients contain substantial numbers of $A\beta$ plaques. The association between AD and DS occurs because the *APP* gene, which encodes the parent protein of $A\beta$, is located on chromosome 21. Trisomy 21 therefore causes an overproduction of $A\beta$ presumably leading to AD progression. Family members of AD patients with DS do not have an increased risk for AD.

☞**SPORADIC AD SUSCEPTIBILITY GENES:** The APOE genotype is the most robust predictive marker for sporadic AD, however variants of APOE are only associated with risk of developing AD. Those homozygous for the ε4 allele have an 8- to 15-fold increase in risk for AD, while ε4 heterozygotes (individuals with only one copy of ε4 allele) have a 2- to 3-fold increase in risk compared to individuals with the more common ε3/ε3 genotype. Meanwhile, the ε2 allele (the rarest of the APOE risk variants) is thought to be protective for AD. Some studies have also shown that affected ε4 carriers also tend to have an earlier age of onset for AD. While these associations have been most widely studied in Caucasians, the ε4 variant is also associated with AD risk in other ethnicities, but the magnitude of this risk effect varies in different populations. Outside of APOE, discoveries from GWAS have greatly expanded the list of known AD susceptibility genes (Table 124-2). These genes further implicate the compliment system and immune response pathways (perhaps via their involvement in $A\beta$ clearance), mechanisms of endocytosis, and protein trafficking pathways in the pathogenesis of AD. Additionally, a recent sequencing experiment involving over 1700 Icelandic participants has revealed a rare coding mutation in *APP* that is not only protective for AD, but also appears to be associated with generally reduced symptoms of cognitive decline in aging carriers. While the individual effect size of any one of these non-APOE variants is much smaller than that of APOE, researchers still hope the combined genotypic knowledge of these susceptibility genes may lead to better risk assessments for individuals who seek genetic testing for AD.

### Counseling:

☞**AUTOSOMAL DOMINANT FAD:** First-degree relatives of patients carrying any one of the rare autosomal dominant mutations for FAD have a 50% chance of harboring the same mutant form of the gene and may wish to seek genetic testing or counseling even before they manifest symptoms. Genetic testing for deleterious mutations in the *APP*, *PSEN1*, and *PSEN2* genes are available for adults who are at risk for FAD, however it should be noted that disclosing test results to asymptomatic individuals has the potential to affect a person's relationships with others, career goals, and emotional well-being. Nonetheless, several studies suggest that revealing deterministic test results to adults at risk for FAD is not typically associated with harmful psychologic distress when screening protocols including education and counseling are adopted. It should be noted though that disclosure of negative test results (absent of FAD mutations) is not predictive of post-testing psychologic burden. In fact, many individuals receiving negative test results still report relatively high levels of distress, perhaps indicative of "survivor guilt" which has been observed in studies of disclosing other deterministic genetic results (such as test results for Huntington disease). Genetic counseling for symptomatic individuals should be performed while the patient's legal guardian or another family member is present.

☞**SPORADIC AD:** While the more common form of the disease does not follow a dominant Mendelian inheritance pattern, late-onset sporadic AD is nonetheless highly heritable. Using genotype and ethnicity-specific risk curves from clinical and epidemiologic data, a comprehensive study of both Caucasian and African-American AD probands and their families found that Caucasian first-degree relatives of AD patients have a roughly 27% chance of developing dementia by age 85, while African-American first-degree relatives have a 44% risk of developing dementia by the same age. In both Caucasian and African-American populations, the data suggest that female children or siblings of AD patients have a higher cumulative risk for dementia, though this difference is more prevalent in Caucasians where female cumulative risk estimates among first-degree relatives are roughly 1.5 times greater than those of their male counterparts (31% in females vs 20% in males). Further stratifying patient samples by APOE genotype reveals that individuals who inherit a least one copy of the ε4 variant of APOE are at increased risk for AD. In the extreme case of homozygous ε4/ε4 first-degree relatives, Caucasians have a greater than 55% risk for developing dementia by the age of 85, while African Americans have 85-year cumulative risk estimates as high as 75%.

Despite these established associations, genetic tests for sporadic AD are more controversial in part because the known genetic markers are not deterministic for developing AD. For example, while the APOE genotype ε4/ε4 is highly over-represented in AD patient populations (occurring at a frequency of 1% in controls but 19% among AD cases) it is well established that not every individual with an ε4-positive genotype will later develop AD. Moreover, testing negative for APOE ε4 does not eliminate the possibility one may develop AD, as roughly 42% of patients with AD do not carry a single copy of the ε4 variant. Interestingly, despite a clear inability of the APOE genotype to predict future onset of AD in asymptomatic individuals, studies show that persons receiving negative APOE ε4 test results (indicative of reduced but nonzero risk for AD) are significantly less likely to experience short-term postdisclosure distress than individuals receiving positive results. In the light of these data and given the growing public interest in

**Table 124-2 Alzheimer Disease-Associated Susceptibility Variants**

| Candidate Gene (Location) | SNP/Variants | OR[a] [population][a] | Frequency of Risk Allele[b] | Putative Functional Significance | Risk Effect of AD |
|---|---|---|---|---|---|
| APOE (19q13.32) | ε2 ε3 ε4 | 3.69 [General, ε4 only] | 0.08[c] 0.77[c] 0.15[c] | Aβ modulation/ pleiotropic | Protective (ε2) Baseline (ε3) Deleterious (ε4) |
| APP (21q21.3) | rs63750847 (A673T) | 0.24[d] [Icelandic] | 0.0045[d] | Aβ modulation | Protective |
| BIN1 (chr2:12789465) | rs744373 | 1.17 [general] | 0.38 | Endocytosis | Deleterious |
| CLU (chr8:27464769) | rs11136000 | 0.88 [Caucasian] | 0.30 | Protein trafficking | Protective |
| ABCA7 (chr19:1046770) | rs3764650 | 1.23 [general] | 0.09 | Protein trafficking | Deleterious |
| CR1 (chr1:207785218) | rs3818361 | 1.17 [Caucasian] | 0.25 | Complement system | Deleterious |
| PICALM (chr11:85868890) | rs3851179 | 0.88 [Caucasian] | 0.29 | Endocytosis | Protective |
| MS4A6A (chr11:59939557) | rs610932 | 0.90 [general] | 0.50 | Immune response | Protective |
| CD33 (chr19:51728212) | rs3865444 | 0.89 [general] | 0.24 | Immune response | Protective |
| MS4A4E (chr11:59972045) | rs670139 | 1.08 [general] | 0.40 | Immune response | Deleterious |
| CD2AP (chr6:47453628) | rs9349407 | 1.12 [general] | 0.19 | Endocytosis | Deleterious |
| SORL1 (chr11:121368171) (chr11:121448504) | rs668387 rs3781835 | 1.08[e] 0.72[f] [Caucasian] | 0.43 0.06 | Aβ modulation | Deleterious Protective |

[a]Unless otherwise indicated, OR estimates and populations reported from Alzgene database (http://www.alzgene.org).

[b]Unless otherwise indicated, frequency estimates from Hapmap 3 CEPH reference population (Utah residents with ancestry from northern and western Europe).

[c]Allele frequencies reported from Leoni et al.

[d]OR, allele frequency, and populations reported in Jonsson et al.

[e]OR, allele frequency, and populations reported in Reitz et al.

[f]OR, allele frequency, and populations reported in Naj et al.

SNP, single nucleotide polymorphism; OR, odds ratio; location, chromosome : base pair (GRCh36/hg19 build).

predictive screens for AD (see Genetic Testing subsection), it is clear that continued efforts in developing effective education and counseling protocols for helping patients interpret and cope with the results of genetic susceptibility tests are needed.

## Management and Treatment

☞**SUPPORTIVE CARE:** Treatment for AD is largely supportive and should be tailored to a patient's unique presentation. Both medication and behavioral therapy may be considered for treating the noncognitive symptoms including depression, agitation, and mood disorder. In most cases, symptoms eventually progress to a level where patients require assisted living or nursing home care.

☞**ACETYLCHOLINESTERASE INHIBITORS:** Four cholinesterase inhibitors (ChEIs) have been approved by the FDA and provide modest cognitive benefits in mild-to-moderate forms of AD,

although none of these agents slows the neuropathologic progression of the disease. Common gastrointestinal (GI)-related side effects of ChEIs include nausea, vomiting, cramps, and diarrhea. In general, the second-generation drugs (donepezil [Aricept], rivastigmine [Exelon], and galantamine [Razadyne]) are more specific and produce less side effects than tacrine (Cognex), which was the first ChEI-approved by the FDA for treatment of AD despite concerns of hepatotoxicity. New drugs in this class are not hepatotoxic, however with all ChEIs' higher dosing increases efficacy and also the incidence of side effects.

☞**MEMANTINE:** The N-methyl-D-aspartate (NMDA) receptor antagonist, memantine (Namenda), is indicated for patients with moderate-to-severe AD. Clinical trials report a low rate of adverse side effects associated with treatment. Recent studies report that memantine is well tolerated in patients already receiving donepezil, however, not all studies report significantly greater efficacy of this drug combination over single-agent therapies.

☞**IMMUNOTHERAPY:** While not yet approved for use, the development of Aβ immunotherapy agents is among the most exciting areas of AD drug research. Early efforts in drug development were limited by severe side effects including meningoencephalitis, vasogenic edema, and cerebral microhemorrhages in both mouse and human models. However, more recently developed therapies, such the off-label use of intravenous immunoglobulin (IVIg) for the treatment of moderate AD, appear to be safer and more effective. Composed of pooled human immunoglobulins collected from thousands of healthy donors, IVIg is already FDA approved for the treatment of various immunocompromised disorders. As early as 2002, it was observed that IVIg contains natural anti-Aβ antibodies and promotes Aβ clearance outside the CNS, prompting further research into the feasibility of developing IVIg as an AD drug. One early trial evaluating the safety of repeated IVIg treatments in patients with mild-to-moderate AD not only showed that the IVIg regimen was well tolerated, but also that treatment correlated with net gains in cognitive function. A subsequent small double-blinded study of 24 placebo-control samples also confirmed the moderate cognitive improvement of patients receiving IVIg therapy. Currently there are a number of ongoing phase III trials involving Aβ immunotherapeutic agents for the treatment of AD, including a pivotal study involving 360 patients investigating the effectiveness of IVIg treatment.

☞**SECRETASE INHIBITORS:** Other compounds under investigation in clinical trials include β-secretase and γ-secretase inhibitors, which are being designed to treat the effects of AD by modulating the production of specific Aβ isoforms. Given that these enzymes cleave the parent proteins of Aβ, inhibiting their activity should in theory result in reduced Aβ production. In practice however, development of either class of inhibitor has faced unique obstacles. On the one hand, studies in mouse models show that knocking down β-secretase can nearly eliminate Aβ production while simultaneously avoiding severe damage to the rest of animal, however, development of small molecules that can bind to the enzyme's active site still pass through the blood-brain barrier has proven elusive. On the other hand, while γ-secretase at first appears to be a more drugable target, one challenge to development of this class of drugs has been that the target cleaves at least one other crucial cellular substrate, thus rendering earlier molecules inhibiting γ-secretase toxic. Despite these setbacks, drug developers seem to have cleverly overcome these obstacles, producing safer γ-secretase inhibitors and more potent and specific γ-secretase inhibitors that are currently being tested in clinical trials.

# Molecular Genetics and Molecular Mechanism

*Description of Basic Gene Functions:* Aβ is a protein byproduct that is found in both normal and AD brains. APP encodes for a transmembrane protein highly expressed in neuronal synapses that is selectively degraded by the β-site cleavage enzyme 1 (BACE-1) and then by the γ-secretase complex to form Aβ. The molecule has two main isoforms ($A\beta_{40}$ and $A\beta_{42}$) consisting of 40 and 42 amino acids, respectively. Both types of Aβ monomers are found in healthy brains and are not particularly neurotoxic by themselves. However, small aggregates of the molecule appear to be highly damaging to synapses in the brain and can lead to disruptive events such as endocytosis of NMDA surface receptors. Furthermore, while the $A\beta_{40}$ isoform is the more prevalent species in healthy brains, the longer $A\beta_{42}$ molecules are more prone to aggregation and more commonly found in the amyloid plaques of AD patient brains.

The roles of many of the currently identified causal and susceptibility genes for AD are supportive of what is known as the *amyloid hypothesis*, a theory that argues atypical production and/or clearance of Aβ is responsible for much of AD pathogenesis. Several protein-coding mutations in the *APP* gene have been linked with increased net production of Aβ and/or a relative increase in the production of $A\beta_{42}$. Interestingly, the aforementioned protective *APP* mutation is also supportive of the amyloid hypothesis, as the mutation occurs near the BACE-1 cleavage site thereby impeding Aβ production in carriers. Meanwhile, aberrant forms of *PSEN1* and *PSEN2* (either of which may alternatively make up the γ-secretase complex) have also been linked to changes in the ratio of $A\beta_{40}$ to $A\beta_{42}$ produced in the brain. As stated earlier, these mutations are associated with the autosomal dominant form of familial AD but are very rare in the general population.

Here it is worth noting that APP is not always degraded into Aβ. Another mechanism of APP proteolysis is initiated when an α-secretase cleaves the protein at a site that would otherwise fall within the interior of the Aβ molecule and thereby eliminating downstream production of Aβ. Additionally, neuronal sortilin-related receptor (SORL1) encodes for a receptor that facilitates trafficking of APP from the plasma membrane to the trans-Golgi apparatus via the retromer recycling endosome. This mechanism of APP processing ultimately reduces net production of Aβ. Multiple studies of SORL1 have found variants in two distinct loci associated with AD risk, which illustrates the complexity of locus heterogeneity that must be considered when identifying genetic associations with AD.

APOE encodes for a chaperone protein involved in lipoprotein transfer and is primarily expressed in the liver and brain. Expression of the gene has pleiotropic effects many of which are consistent with several theories on AD etiology, including (but not limited to) neurodegeneration, synaptic dysfunction, and hyperphosphorylation of tau. However, some of the most highly replicated findings comparing the effect of ApoE4 expression to that of the ApoE3 isoform demonstrate that the ε3 variant has a higher binding capacity for Aβ than ε4, suggesting that the ε3 variant provides superior clearance of Aβ from the extracellular space. Additionally, Table 124-2 lists other genes known to be associated with AD risk but whose exact roles in AD etiology are less well understood.

*Genetic Testing:*

☞**AUTOSOMAL DOMINANT FAD:** Genetic testing for deleterious mutations resulting in the rare autosomal dominant form of AD are available for adults at risk for FAD (Table 124-2), however as noted previously, the disclosure of test results to asymptomatic individuals carries some risk of negatively affecting an individual's interpersonal relationships, career aspirations, and general emotional state. According to current clinical guidelines, genetic testing for dominantly inherited FAD is only advised when it is delivered in the context of genetic counseling from an appropriate expert. Additionally, given the current lack of effective preventative therapies for AD, genetic testing for AD is not recommended for young children and prenatal testing for PSEN1 is not recommended if pregnancy is likely to be continued upon result of a positive test for a dominant FAD mutation.

☞**SPORADIC AD:** With public demand for direct-to-consumer (DTC) genetic testing for a variety of diseases including AD on the rise, understanding the ramifications of disclosing AD risk results is of paramount importance to healthcare providers. Presently, clinical guidelines do not recommend DTC testing for AD susceptibility. Furthermore, APOE testing is frequently not offered in a clinical setting given reservations of clinicians regarding the sensitivity and specificity of testing, the current lack to therapeutic options, and the general difficulty of accurately imparting risk estimates to patients. To evaluate the benefits and risks of APOE testing, a recent series of four separate multicenter randomized clinical trials, known as the Risk Evaluation and Education for Alzheimer's Disease Study (REVEAL), were conducted to explore the psychologic and behavioral outcomes of APOE disclosure. The REVEAL study has investigated several aspects of genetic testing for sporadic AD including the emotional impact of disclosing data regarding AD risk, the most common motivations for obtaining genetic test results for AD, how a patient's personal perception of AD risk is impacted by disclosure of genetic test results, how well patients recall and value test results and share these results with others, and how the disclosure of test results affects subsequent patient health behaviors including the purchasing of long-term health insurance. One key observation from these studies was that when delivered under established protocols that provided sufficient educational and emotional support, disclosure of APOE genotype data did not result in significant psychologic distress to adult children of AD patients. Another theme surfacing from this body of work is that despite the limited predictive power of APOE genotype, the disclosure of APOE status can result in lifestyle and behavioral changes in individuals seeking genetic testing for AD susceptibility. In total, these results highlight the importance of genetic counseling for adults with family members suffering from AD.

***Future Directions:*** Despite recent successes, much of the genetic heritability of AD remains unexplained. The effect sizes of many of the newly discovered AD susceptibility genes are low and will not be useful for predicting the risk of disease. Still, this growing list of AD risk genes offers important clues to researchers seeking to find novel drug targets to treat AD. There have also been early successes in applying gene-gene interaction models to uncover epistatic effects between known risk loci and AD progression and future exploration of gene-environment interactions as well as pharmacogenetic studies may reveal similar encouraging results. Presently, given the lack effective treatment options for AD, genetic testing for sporadic AD risk is mostly done in research settings and is typically not recommended for adults at risk for sporadic AD. However, breakthroughs in drug development for the treatment and/or prevention of AD, like those anticipated in the field of immunotherapy, may drastically change the implications of genetic testing. Given that several studies have shown the accumulation of Aβ plaques typically precedes cognitive symptoms of AD, identifying asymptomatic individuals likely to develop AD will be of paramount importance if new prophylactic treatments against Aβ deposition are developed. When this happens, those seeking to combat this disease will rely heavily upon the exciting advancements currently being made in the fields of neuroimaging and AD genetics.

**BIBLIOGRAPHY:**

1. Bekris LM, Yu CE, Bird TD, Tsuang DW. Genetics of Alzheimer disease. *J Geriatr Psychiatry Neurol*. Dec 2010;23(4):213-227.

2. Bertram L, McQueen M, Mullin K, Blacker D, Tanzi R. The AlzGene Database. Alzheimer Research Forum. http://www.alzgene.org. Accessed February 21, 2012.

3. Bird TD. Alzheimer Disease Overview. 1998 Oct 23 [Updated 2010 Mar 30]. In: Pagon RA, Bird TD, Dolan CR, et al., eds. GeneReviews [Internet]. Seattle, WA: University of Washington, Seattle; 1993.

4. Christensen KD, Roberts JS, Royal CDM, et al. Incorporating ethnicity into genetic risk assessment for Alzheimer's disease: the REVEAL Study experience. *Genet Med*. 2008;10:207-214.

5. Citron M. Alzheimer's disease: strategies for disease modification. *Nat Rev Drug Discov*. May 2010;9(5):387-398.

6. Dodel R, Hampel H, Depboylu C, et al. Human antibodies against amyloid beta peptide: a potential treatment for Alzheimer's disease. *Ann Neurol*. Aug 2002;52(2):253-256.

7. Folstein MF. Differential diagnosis of dementia. The clinical process. *Psychiatr Clin North Am*. Mar 1997;20(1):45-57. Review

8. Goldman JS, Hahn SE, Catania JW, et al. Genetic counseling and testing for Alzheimer disease: joint practice guidelines of the American College of Medical Genetics and the National Society of Genetic Counselors. *Genet Med*. Jun 2011;13(6):597-605.

9. Green RC, Roberts JS, Cupples LA, et al. Disclosure of APOE genotype for risk of Alzheimer's disease. *N Engl J Med*. 2009;361:245-254.

10. Green RC. *Diagnosis and Management of Alzheimer's Disease and Other Dementias*. 2nd ed. New York, NY: Professional Communications, Inc: 2005.

11. Jonsson T, Atwal JK, Steinberg S, et al. A mutation in APP protects against Alzheimer's disease and age-related cognitive decline. *Nature*. Aug 2 2012;488(7409):96-99.

12. Leoni V. The effect of apolipoprotein E (ApoE) genotype on biomarkers of amyloidogenesis, tau pathology and neurodegeneration in Alzheimer's disease. *Clin Chem Lab Med*. Mar 2011;49(3):375-383.

13. McKhann GM, Knopman DS, Chertkowd H, et al. The diagnosis of dementia due to Alzheimer's disease: recommendations from the National Institute on Aging and the Alzheimer's Association workgroup. *Alzheimers Dement*. May 2011;7(3):263-269.

14. Naj AC, Jun G, Beecham GW, Wang LS. Common variants at MS4A4/MS4A6E, CD2AP, CD33 and EPHA1 are associated with late-onset Alzheimer's disease. *Nat Genet*. May 2011;43(5):436-441.

15. Querfurth HW, LaFerla FM. Mechanisms of disease: Alzheimer's disease. *N Engl J Med*. Jan 28 2010;362(4):329-344.

16. Reitz C, Cheng R, Rogaeva E, et al. Meta-analysis of the association between variants in SORL1 and Alzheimer Disease. *Arch Neurol*. Jan 2011; 68(1):99-106.

17. Relkin NR. Current state of immunotherapy for Alzheimer's disease. *CNS Spectr*. Oct 2008;13(10 suppl 16):39-41.

18. Roberts J, Cupples L, Relkin N, Whitehouse P, Green RC. Genetic risk assessment for adult children of people with Alzheimer's disease: the Risk Evaluation and Education for Alzheimer's Disease (REVEAL) Study. *J Geriatr Psychiatr Neurol*. 2005;18: 250-255.

19. Schellenberg GD, Montine TJ. The genetics and neuropathology of Alzheimer's disease. *Acta Neuropathol*. Sep 2012;124(3): 305-323.

20. Sperling RA, Aisen PS, Beckett LA, et al. Toward defining the preclinical stages of Alzheimer's disease: recommendations from the National Institute on Aging-Alzheimer's Association workgroups

on diagnostic guidelines for Alzheimer's disease. *Alzheimers Dement*. May 2011;7(3):280-292.

21. Lautenbach DM, Christensen KD, Sparks JA, Green RC. Communicating genetic risk information for common disorders in the era of genomic medicine. *Ann Rev of Geno and Hum Genet*. 2013;14:491-513.

## Supplementary Information

**OMIM REFERENCES:**

[1] Alzheimer Disease 1, Familial; AD1 (#104300)

[2] Alzheimer Disease 2, Late-Onset; AD2 (#104310)

[3] Amyloid Precursor Protein; APP (#104760)

[4] Presenilin 1; PSEN1 (#104311)

[5] Presenilin 2; PSEN2 (#600759)

[6] Apolipoprotein E; APOE (#107741)

**Alternative Names:**

☞**FAD:**

• Early-Onset Alzheimer Disease (EOAD)

☞**SPORADIC AD:**

• Late-Onset Alzheimer Disease (LOAD)

*Key Words:* Alzheimer disease, APP, PSEN1, PSEN1, APOE, susceptibility gene, amyloid hypothesis

# 125 Huntington Disease

Aaron Sturrock and Blair R. Leavitt

## KEY POINTS

- *Disease summary:*
  - Huntington disease (HD) is a neurodegenerative condition that usually manifests as a triad of movement disorder, cognitive dysfunction, and behavioral or psychiatric abnormalities; however, these features can vary widely between individuals.
  - HD is the most prevalent inherited neurodegenerative disease affecting up to 1 in 10,000 individuals in most populations of European descent.
  - HD is caused by expansion of the trinucleotide CAG (polyglutamine-encoding) repeat sequence in exon 1 of the huntingtin gene (*HTT*) to greater than 35 repeats. The age of disease onset in HD is inversely correlated with the size of the CAG repeat expansion.
  - Following identification of the causative gene defect in 1993, at-risk individuals (with an affected parent) can be offered direct predictive genetic testing prior to the onset of symptoms.
- *Hereditary basis:*
  - HD is a familial condition with autosomal dominant inheritance and is fully penetrant (in most cases with expansions of greater than 40 CAG trinucleotide repeats).
- *Differential diagnosis:*
  - The high prevalence of HD compared to genetic disorders with similar presentation means that, even without a family history, HD is the major diagnostic consideration in the choreic individual.
  - In the event of a negative HD test or atypical presentation, the differential diagnoses become a focus of investigation.
  - Any individual with an otherwise unexplained clinical presentation consistent with HD should be offered the direct genetic test for HD, since it is easily the most common inherited cause of such a presentation. The main inherited disorders with similar clinical presentation (HD phenocopies) are outlined in Table 125-1. Of these, HDL-2 and SCA17 are probably the most common HD phenocopies. For a useful algorithm for the screening of potential HD phenocopies, see Wild and Tabrizi (2007).
  - In the event of a negative HD test or an atypical presentation, it is most important to exclude any treatable (and/or potentially reversible) acquired causes. Wilson disease is a genetic case which is also treatable. Acquired causes of an HD presentation include (1) medication-related tardive dyskinesia or chorea following use of typical neuroleptics or the oral contraceptive pill, and L-dopa-induced dyskinesias, (2) postinfectious, for example, Sydenham chorea (poststreptococcal) or tertiary syphilis, (3) metabolic thyrotoxicosis and chorea gravidarum of pregnancy, (4) inflammatory lupus and antiphospholipid syndrome.

## Diagnostic Criteria and Clinical Characteristics

***Diagnostic Criteria:*** The clinical diagnosis of HD should be made by a clinician with expertise in the evaluation of HD. It requires

- The presence of a defined *motor phenotype* consisting of an otherwise unexplained extrapyramidal movement disorder in an individual with either a positive HD test result or a family history of HD

**And the absence of**

- A clear alternative cause of the clinical presentation

***Clinical Characteristics:*** Classically HD presents with a combined cognitive, psychiatric, and extrapyramidal movement phenotype. Clinical onset for most adults is between ages 35 and 44. The movement disorder usually comprises both involuntary and voluntary components. The involuntary movement disorder may follow a biphasic pattern with initial, increasing hyperkinesia, and chorea reaching a peak usually in the mid-stages of disease. This hyperkinesia gradually diminishes, giving rise to bradykinesia and rigidity which eventually develops into a rigid-akinetic state. The voluntary component of the movement disorder is also progressive. Gait abnormalities present as a broad-based ataxia. Mobility deteriorates until the individual becomes bed-bound. Progressive dysarthria, dysphagia, ocular pursuit abnormalities, and loss of fine motor coordination also characterize the motor phenotype. Eventually the patient becomes mute and unable to tolerate oral nutrition.

Psychiatric manifestations in HD are protean. Depression, irritability, and impulsivity are the most common, but obsessive compulsive and aggressive behaviors, psychosis, mania, anxiety, and substance abuse also occur. The lifetime prevalence of clinically diagnosable depression in HD may be around 40%. The rate of suicide is much higher than in the general population with those approaching clinical diagnosis (ie, those with worsening "soft" clinical signs) and those experiencing increasing functional limitation in early HD, possibly most at risk. Clinicians should be aware of this, and the fact that suicide in such individuals may be a spontaneous, unmediated, act.

The progressive cognitive disorder in HD is "frontal-subcortical" and emerges early in the disease, although individuals may lack insight into deficits. As part of the subcortical dementia, bradyphrenia becomes manifest while procedural memory (ability to learn or recall new motor skills) and visuospatial memory becomes affected. Executive dysfunction may present with impaired planning, organization, attention, and concentration. Cognitive deficits

Table 125-1 *Major Genetic Differential Diagnoses*

| Modality | Gene Symbol | Discriminative Clinical Characteristics |
|---|---|---|
| Spinocerebellar ataxia 17 (SCA17 or HDL-4) | TBP | SCA associated with prominent cerebellar ataxia, epilepsy |
| Huntington disease like-2 (HDL-2) | JPH3 | Often rapidly progressive dementia, usually black African ancestry (may not always be apparent) |
| Dentatorubropallidoluysian atrophy (DRPLA) | ATN1 | Epilepsy; often progressive myoclonic epilepsy (particularly among those with juvenile onset), higher prevalence in those of Japanese ancestry |
| SCA1-3 | ATXN1-3 | SCAs associated with prominent cerebellar ataxia. Optic atrophy (SCA1), childhood onset (SCA2), mixed pyramidal/extrapyramidal features (SCA3), peripheral neuropathy may be present (SCA1-3) |
| Neuroferritinopathy | FTL | Prominent facial dyskinesias and parkinsonism. Imaging may be characteristic |
| Huntington disease like-1 (HDL-1) | PRNP | Very rare, epilepsy, earlier onset, prominent psychiatric/behavioral phenotype |
| Chorea-acanthocytosis | VPS13A | May closely mimic HD but features orofacial self-mutilation secondary to oral dystonia, myopathy, neuropathy, and epilepsy |
| Wilson disease | ATP7B | Dystonia more than chorea, psychiatric and cognitive features may be prominent. Kayser-Fleischer rings of the iris |
| Pantothenate kinase-associated neurodegeneration (PKAN) | PANK2 | Usual onset in infancy, pigmentary retinopathy, generalized dystonia and marked oromandibular involvement. Imaging may be characteristic |
| X-linked (recessive) McLeod syndrome | XK | Cardiomyopathy, myopathy, neuropathy, epilepsy |
| Huntington disease like-3 (HDL-3) | Location 4p15.3 | Very rare. Presentation comparable with juvenile HD |

Disorders in gray are autosomal dominant, the remainder are autosomal recessive unless specified.

are progressive in HD. By the advanced stages of the disorder, initially selective cognitive deficits have progressed to a global decline. Sleep disruption and weight loss are also features of HD, the latter possibly influencing disease progression. The median survival from onset of disease is from 15 to 20 years. A major cause of death in HD is infection (eg, pneumonia).

☞PRODROMAL OR PRESYMPTOMATIC HD: All aspects of the clinical phenotype (cognition, movement disorder, and psychiatric manifestations) may be subtly present among premanifest HD individuals, some years before the individual develops a movement disorder sufficient for a clinical diagnosis of HD. Often these soft signs do not reach threshold criteria required for a clinical diagnosis of, for example, depression or dementia.

☞VARIANT PRESENTATIONS: Disease can occur at any age, with reports of onset in infancy and among individuals in their nineties. Unlike adult-onset HD, juvenile HD (disease onset within the first 20 years of life) is usually characterized by an early rigid or bradykinetic and even dystonic (rather than primarily choreic) phenotype. Additional features of juvenile HD presentation include declining cognitive or scholastic function and seizures. Deterioration is usually rapidly progressive, particularly among the youngest affected individuals. Seizures are often generalized tonic-clonic or myoclonic and may be intractable. Senile chorea is a name sometimes applied to another variant presentation of HD.

In this late-onset form of HD, disease onset is at the age of 50 years or older, and as the term suggests features prominent chorea. The phenotype is usually less severe than most adult cases with slower disease progression.

## Screening and Counseling

*Predictive Testing (Screening):* Predictive testing can be offered to asymptomatic adults at risk of HD due to a parent (symptomatic or asymptomatic) testing positive for the causative gene defect. Following the International Huntington Association guidelines, predictive testing should only be provided with appropriate pre- and post-test counseling, with support provided by a genetic counselor, neurologist, psychiatrist, and social worker all within a specialist HD setting. One central role of counseling will be to dynamically evaluate the individual's psychiatric and emotional response to the test result, regardless of its outcome. Receiving even a negative test result can, in a proportion of individuals, lead to an adverse adjustment reaction (in some cases because of "survivor guilt" issues). Genetic testing for HD is now widely available.

Alternatively, diagnostic gene testing should be performed as a confirmatory or exclusionary investigation in an individual with a clinical presentation compatible with HD, regardless of the family history.

***Counseling:***

☞**INHERITANCE, PENETRANCE:** HD exhibits autosomal dominant inheritance, with each child of an affected parent at 50% risk of inheriting the causative gene defect. In the majority of cases (repeat expansions >40) the disease is fully penetrant. Individuals with repeat expansions ranging from 36 to 39 are considered to exhibit reduced penetrance, in that they may develop the disease later in life, but not necessarily so. Intermediate alleles (IA, 27-35 CAG repeats), are thought to occur in 1% to 4% of individuals in some populations. These individuals are not themselves at risk of developing HD, but the allele is at risk of expansion into the disease-causing range during transmission to offspring. Thus IA individuals may transmit the reduced or fully penetrant allele to their offspring, and is a particular risk for paternal transmission. The normal CAG repeat tract length comprises 26 CAG repeats or fewer. See Fig. 125-1.

Anticipation can occur in HD; expanded alleles transmitted from parent to child often exhibit further expansion in successive generations. However larger expansions, especially those associated with juvenile HD, are almost exclusively associated with paternal transmission. This can also occur for IA, and alleles within the reduced or fully penetrant range.

Sporadic cases of HD, occurring in individuals without a family history may arise for a number of reasons. These include nonpaternity, undisclosed adoption, the failure to identify the disorder in a parent, the presence of an intermediate allele in the father or alternatively death of an affected parent before the onset of disease (particularly so for reduced penetrance alleles).

☞**GENOTYPE-PHENOTYPE CORRELATION:** CAG repeat size is inversely correlated with age-of-disease onset when the full spectrum of expansion is considered, including individuals at both extremes of CAG repeat expansion. CAG repeat length appears to explain about 70% of variability in age-of-disease onset, with other genetic factors likely influencing a significant proportion (10%-20%) of the remaining variability. Importantly, rate of cognitive and motor deterioration appears to be increased with larger CAG repeat sizes.

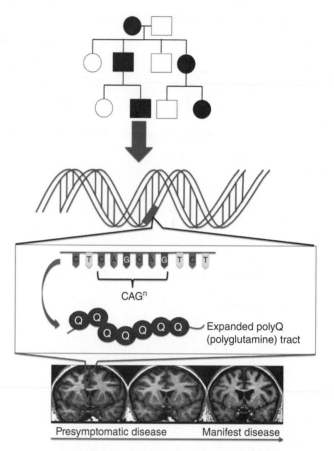

**Figure 125-1** From Inheritance to Neurodegeneration.

## Management and Treatment

While no disease-modifying treatment has been identified in HD, symptom control for many aspects of the condition is possible. Figure 125-2 outlines the general therapies commonly used for specific symptoms.

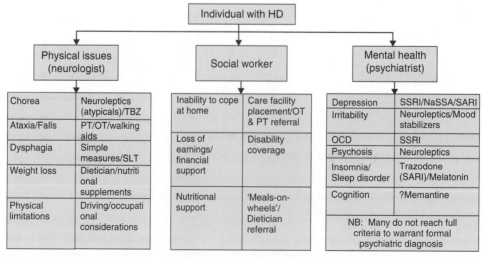

***Figure 125-2*** Algorithm for Management of Patient With HD.

Among the commonly used neuroleptics for control of chorea and psychotic phenomena, atypicals (eg, olanzapine and risperidone) are favored due to their preferable adverse effect profile. It is important to remember that agents used for the treatment of chorea, by virtue of their parkinsonizing abilities, usually lead to increased rigidity with an impact on mobility, falls, and even dysphagia. It should be borne in mind that these symptoms may become more problematic than the chorea itself. The appropriate management of cognitive dysfunction in HD is unclear, although some centers may make "off of label" use of the N-methyl-D-aspartate (NMDA) receptor antagonist memantine for this purpose. A multidisciplinary approach to management of symptomatic HD individuals is essential; in addition to the neurologist, psychiatrist, and social worker, an occupational therapist (OT), physiotherapist (PT), and speech and language therapist (SLT) may be involved.

# Molecular Genetics and Molecular Mechanism

*Syndrome/Gene/Locus:* Huntington disease/*HTT*/4p16.3

HTT encodes the huntingtin protein that, while ubiquitously expressed, reaches highest levels of expression in the brain. Pathology in HD is widely attributed to a toxic gain of function, although a loss of normal huntingtin function has also been implicated. Knockout embryonic stem cells demonstrated that normal huntingtin protein expression was critical for normal nuclear and perinuclear membrane organelles (including mitochondria and endoplasmic reticulum) and for regulation of the iron pathway. Huntingtin protein is required for normal embryonic neural development. Furthermore, wild-type huntingtin is neuroprotective against the mutant form of the protein and may affect additional neuroprotection through upregulation of the prosurvival factor brain-derived neurotrophic factor (BDNF).

*Genetic Testing:* After the exclusion of any potentially acquired causes of chorea (see Differential Diagnoses) through careful history-taking and examination, HD should be the first considered inherited cause in the adult presenting with a choreiform movement disorder, even in the absence of a supportive family history. The disease-causing CAG trinucleotide repeat expansion within the *HTT* gene can be readily detected, with 100% sensitivity, using targeted mutation analysis. Polymerase chain reaction (PCR)-based methods are sufficient in most cases, while Southern blotting can be used to detect larger expansions associated with juvenile onset of disease (which sometimes amplify poorly using PCR).

## Bibliography:

1. Wild EJ, Mudanohwo EE, Sweeney MG, et al. Huntington's disease phenocopies are clinically and genetically heterogeneous. *Mov Disord.* 2008;23(5):716-720.

2. Wild EJ, Tabrizi SJ. Huntington's disease phenocopy syndromes. *Curr Opin Neurol.* 2007;20(6):681-687.

3. Paulsen JS, Hoth KF, Nehl C, Stierman L. Critical periods of suicide risk in Huntington's disease. *Am J Psychiatry.* 2005;162(4):725-731.

4. Warby SC, Graham RK, Hayden MR, et al. GeneReviews: Huntington Disease. http://www.ncbi.nlm.nih.gov/books/NBK1305/. Accessed December 17th, 2011.

5. Sturrock A, Leavitt BR. The clinical and genetic features of Huntington disease. *J Geriatr Psychiatry Neurol.* 2010; 23(4):243-259.

6. International Huntington Association guidelines for the Molecular Genetics Predictive Test. http://www.huntington-assoc.com/guidel.htm. Accessed December 2011.

7. Maat-Kievit A, Losekoot M, Van Den Boer-Van Den Berg H, et al. New problems in testing for Huntington's disease: the issue of intermediate and reduced penetrance alleles. *J Med Genet.* 2001;38:E12.

8. Semaka A, Collins JA, Hayden MR. Unstable familial transmissions of Huntington disease alleles with 27-35 CAG repeats (intermediate alleles). *Am J Med Genet B Neuropsychiatr Genet.* 2010;153B:314-320.

9. Hilditch-Maguire P, Trettel F, Passani LA, Auerbach A, Persichetti F, MacDonald ME. Huntingtin: an iron-regulated protein essential for normal nuclear and perinuclear organelles. *Hum. Mol Genet.* 2000;9:2789-2797.

10. Nasir J, Floresco SB, O'Kusky JR, et al. Targeted disruption of the Huntington's disease gene results in embryonic lethality and behavioral and morphological changes in heterozygotes. *Cell.* 1995;81(5):811-823.

11. Leavitt BR, Guttman JA, Hodgson JG, et al. Wild-type huntingtin reduces the cellular toxicity of mutant huntingtin in vivo. *Am J Hum Genet.* 2001;68:313-324.

12. Zuccato C, Ciammola A, Rigamonti D, et al. Loss of huntingtin-mediated BDNF gene transcription in Huntington's disease. *Science.* 2001;293(5529):493-498.

# Supplementary Information

## OMIM References:

[1] Huntington Disease (HD); HTT (#143100)

[2] Huntington Disease Like-1 (HDL-1); PRNP (#603218)

[3] Huntington Disease Like-2 (HDL-2); JPH3 (#606438)

[4] Huntington Disease Like-3 (HDL-3); Location 4p15.3, Gene Uncertain (#600482)

[5] Chorea-Acanthocytosis (CHAC); VPS13A (#200150)

[6] Dentatorubropallidoluysian Atrophy (DRPLA); ATN1 (#125370)

[7] Neuroferritinopathy (Neurodegeneration With Brain Iron Accumulation 3; NBIA3); FTL (#606159)

[8] Pantothenate Kinase-Associated Neurodegeneration (PKAN or Neurodegeneration With Brain Iron Accumulation 1; NBIA1); PANK2 (#234200)

[9] Spinocerebellar Ataxia 1 (SCA1); ATXN1 (#164400)

[10] Spinocerebellar Ataxia 2 (SCA2); ATXN2 (#183090)

[11] Spinocerebellar Ataxia 3 (SCA3); ATXN3 (#109150)

[12] Spinocerebellar Ataxia 17 (SCA17); TBP (#607136)

[13] Wilson Disease; ATP7B (#277900)

[14] X-Linked McLeod Syndrome; XK (#300842)

*Key Words:* Ataxia, chorea, dystonia, HD multidisciplinary team, HD phenocopy, juvenile HD, predictive testing, rigidity, senile chorea

# 126 Parkinson Disease

John Hardy

## KEY POINTS

- *Disease summary:*
  - Parkinson disease (PD) is marked by tremor, muscle rigidity, and slowed movement and known to have multiple etiologies both genetic and idiopathic. Many genetic risk factors are known but environmental factors are not established.
  - A cardinal pathologic feature is the presence of Lewy bodies in the substantia nigra, although a minority of cases may not exhibit this finding.
  - The disease presents with bradykinesia and often with a resting tremor. At first the disease responds well to L-dopa and related therapies, but as the disease progresses, therapy becomes more problematic with shorter periods of drug efficacy and dyskinesias as an effect of treatment. Cognitive and other complications increase during the disease progression.
  - Anatomic involvement: While the major motor symptoms of the disease result from the damage to the substantia nigra, recent studies from Braak have suggested that the disease may start in the lower brain stem and spread progressively.

- *Differential diagnosis:*
  - It includes progressive supranuclear palsy, multiple system atrophy, and essential tremor.

- *Monogenic forms:*
  - Many monogenic forms exist, both recessive and dominant; see Table 126-1.

- *Family history:*
  - An affected first-degree relative confers an increase in risk of disease, but this varies both with age, and naturally is dependent on the precise etiology in any family.

- *Twin studies:*
  - Monozygotic twins have a 20% to 50% concordance rate in PD, lower in dizygotic twins. Since this is a late-onset disease and a disease in which the onset in twin can vary enormously, precise figures are not available and are, in any event, difficult to interpret.

- *Environmental factors:*
  - None are known, although smoking and caffeine intake are negatively associated with disease occurrence. Whether this relates to the role of dopamine in the reward system and therefore is related to premorbid addictive behavior is not clear. MPTP (1-methyl-4-phenyl-1,2,3,6-tetrahydropyridine) is a neurotoxin which causes permanent symptoms of PD and has been used to study disease models in various animal studies; MPTP has caused human cases when injected but has no association with typical disease presentations.

- *Genome-wide associations:*
  - Many associations exist. Disease-associated genetic variants (single-nucleotide polymorphisms [SNPs]) provide insight into disease pathogenesis; testing for SNPs is not yet clinically validated to diagnose or guide management of PD (Table 126-2).

## Diagnostic Criteria and Clinical Characteristics

***Diagnostic Criteria for Parkinson Disease:*** A clinical diagnosis of PD is based on the clinical findings of tremor, rigidity, and bradykinesia. Postmortem pathologic studies often demonstrate the loss of dopaminergic neurons in the substantia nigra replaced by Lewy bodies, although a minority of cases may not exhibit this finding. Clinical evaluation should document the presence of resting tremor, response to dopamine agents such as L-dopa, asymmetrical onset of symptoms, and the absence of features of other neurologic conditions.

***Clinical Characteristics:*** PD patients often present with the triad of tremor, muscle rigidity, and bradykinesia; additionally psychiatric manifestations are common and less commonly dementia in approximately 20% of cases. The clinical diagnosis is subdivided based on age of onset with juvenile onset including individuals with onset before age 20 years, early onset defined as before age 50 years, and those with onset after age 50 years termed as late onset.

## Screening and Counseling

***Genetic Screening:*** Some genetic testing is available. Recessive screening for *PKRN* and *PINK1* in patients with age of onset below 40 years is often available. In some centers, *LRRK2* and *SNCA* screening is also offered.

***Counseling:*** As PD can be Mendelian, inherited in an autosomal dominant or autosomal recessive manner, or multifactorial, caused by multiple genes and environmental risk factors, counseling for families is difficult. In families with a non-Mendelian form of PD, first-degree relatives of an affected individual are at an increased risk of developing PD as compared with the general population with an odds ratio of 2.7 to 3.5; the cumulative lifetime risk is approximately 3% to 7%.

## Molecular Genetics and Molecular Mechanism

***Mendelian Loci for Parkinson Disease:*** The Mendelian loci for PD are shown in Table 126-1. Most of these were identified by

*Table 126-1* **Mendelian Genes for Parkinson Disease**

| LOCUS1 | Inheritance | Onset | Protein | Path |
|---|---|---|---|---|
| PARK-1/4 | AD | ~45 | SNCA | LB |
| PARK-2 | AR | 7-60 | PKRN | None (usually) |
| PARK-6 | AR | 36-60 | PINK-1 | ? one case with LB |
| PARK-7 | AR | 27-40 | DJ-1 | ? |
| PARK-8 | AD | 45-57 | LRRK2 | Usually LB |
| PARK-9 | AR | Teens | ATP13A2 | ? |
| PARK-14 | AR | Teens | PLA2G6 | LB |
| PARK-15 | AR | Teens | FBX07 | ? |
| PARK-17 | AD | 50-70 | VPS35 | ? |

positional cloning strategies, although *VPS35* was found by exome sequencing. Broadly speaking these loci fall into three groups: the dominant late-onset loci (*SNCA, LRRK2, VPS35*), the aggressive and rapidly fatal early-onset loci (*PLA2G6, ATP13A2*), and the benign early-onset loci (*PKRN, DJ1, PINK1,* and *FBXO7*). The last grouping makes biologic sense as all four genes encode proteins which are part of the quality control response to mitochondrial damage. *ATP13A2* is, like glucocerebrosidase (GBA) (next section) a lysosomal protein and this suggests a form of the disease process which has parallels with lysosomal storage disorders. *VPS35* is involved in vesicle recycling and *SNCA* also has a role in this pathway. Thus the three different forms of disease may relate to mitochondrial homeostasis (certainly), lysosomal metabolism (probably), and vesicle recycling (possibly). Given the rather mixed and uncertain relationships between these grouping and pathology (Table 126-1), it is clear that we do not yet have a clear view of whether these three groups impinge on one, two, or more disease processes.

☞GBA MUTATIONS: A RARE HIGH-RISK LOCUS: Gaucher disease, a lysosomal storage disorder, has homozygous loss-of-function mutations in GBA. It had long been reported that patients with Gaucher disease who had neurologic symptoms had Lewy body pathology, but the significance of this had not been appreciated. Sidransky and colleagues noted an increase in the occurrence of PD in the relatives of patients with Gaucher and this led to a systematic analysis which has shown that these loss-of-function mutations, in a heterozygous state, lead to an increased risk of about fivefold for PD. In most European populations, these mutations have an aggregate frequency of about 1% (increasing to 5% in PD), but in the Ashkenazim this can be up to 8% increasing to 40%. The association is with typical, late-onset PD with Lewy body pathology.

This finding is important on several levels: first, simply in terms of the number of cases it explains; second, because, together with the ATP13A2 (previous section) it implicates lysosomal dysfunction in the etiology of the disease; and third, because it is an example of what we might expect to find as other high-risk, rare loci. As we start to carry out exome and whole genome sequencing to find other genetic risk for PD, we might expect to find other heterozygous loss-of-function mutations, which when homozygous, are lethal or give rise to pediatric disease, particularly perhaps lysosomal disorders.

☞COMMON LOW-RISK LOCI: Genome-wide association studies (GWASs) have revolutionized the process of the identification of common low-risk variants, since they can systematically, and in a hypothesis-free way, identify loci which influence risk. They do, however, require very large numbers of samples and therefore collaborative groups. In PD, *SNCA* and *MAPT* had been identified as loci through candidate gene analysis and their importance became clear when these were the top hits in genome-wide studies. In both cases, the effect seems to be mediated through higher expression levels. With regard to SNCA, this expression effect, of course, is consistent with the fact that duplications and triplications cause Mendelian disease. With increasing sample numbers, more loci have been identified (Table 126-2), two deserve further comment. First, the involvement of the human leukocyte antigen (*HLA*) locus is consistent with neuropathologic studies showing the damaged nigra stained with HLA. This observation presumably suggests that genetic variability in damage response is important in determining whether someone will develop the disease. Second, the *LRRK2* locus appears; in this case, it is not a mutation, but presumably relates to genetic variability in expression of the protein. This observation strongly suggests that the normal function of LRRK2 is important in PD pathogenesis and that the mutation amplify that function.

An important point to remember is that the GWASs identify a common variant associated with disease: It is likely that at these loci there are multiple forms of risk (as we already know there are at SNCA and LRRK2), and that further genetic analysis will identify other risk variants at the loci already identified. As more studies are added to the current ones, more loci will be identified as the power of the analyses increase.

*Table 126-2* **Risk Loci for Parkinson Disease With Approximate Odds Ratios and Likely Type of Variability Which Is Important at the Locus**

| | |
|---|---|
| • SNCA (~1.6) | Expression |
| • MAPT? (~1.4) | Expression |
| • AMCSZ (~1.1) | Not known |
| • HLA-DRB5 (~1.1) | Probably coding |
| • BST1 (~1.2) | Not coding |
| • LAMP3 (~1.1) | Not known |
| • CCDC62 (~1.1) | Not known |
| • STK39 | Not known |
| • LRRK2 (1.1) | Could be coding |

***Genetic Testing:*** *LRRK2, PKRN*, and *GBA* mutation testing are widely available. Other loci are less common and testing is often not available. This situation is likely to change in the next few years.

***Future Directions:*** The recent and current explosion in molecular genetics is likely to continue. There are known to be unresolved further recessive loci and the more risk loci will be found with increasing sample numbers. Perhaps the greatest current need is for an increased understanding of how the genes for the disease all tie together in terms of pathways for disease.

## Bibliography:

1. McInerney-Leo A, Hadley DW, Gwinn-Hardy K, Hardy J. Genetic testing in Parkinson's disease. *Mov Disord*. Jan 2005;20(1):1-10.

2. Hardy J, Lewis P, Revesz T, Lees A, Paisan-Ruiz C. The genetics of Parkinson's syndromes: a critical review. *Curr Opin Genet Dev*. Jun 2009;19(3):254-265.

3. Vilariño-Güell C, Wider C, Ross OA, et al. VPS35 mutations in Parkinson disease. *Am J Hum Genet*. Jul 15 2011;89(1):162-167.

4. Zimprich A, Benet-Pagès A, Struhal W, et al. A mutation in VPS35, encoding a subunit of the retromer complex, causes late-onset Parkinson disease. *Am J Hum Genet*. Jul 15 2011;89(1):168-175.

5. Sidransky E. Gaucher disease: complexity in a "simple" disorder. *Mol Genet Metab*. Sep-Oct 2004;83(1-2):6-15.

6. Goker-Alpan O, Schiffmann R, LaMarca ME, Nussbaum RL, McInerney-Leo A, Sidransky E. Parkinsonism among Gaucher disease carriers. *J Med Genet*. Dec 2004;41(12):937-940.

7. Sidransky E, Nalls MA, Aasly JO, et al. Multicenter analysis of glucocerebrosidase mutations in Parkinson's disease. *N Engl J Med*. Oct 22 2009;361(17):1651-1661.

8. Neumann J, Bras J, Deas E, et al. Glucocerebrosidase mutations in clinical and pathologically proven Parkinson's disease. *Brain*. Jul 2009;132(pt 7):1783-1794.

9. Krüger R, Vieira-Saecker AM, Kuhn W, et al. Increased susceptibility to sporadic Parkinson's disease by a certain combined alpha-synuclein/apolipoprotein E genotype. *Ann Neurol*. May 1999;45(5):611-617.

10. Golbe LI, Lazzarini AM, Spychala JR, et al. The tau A0 allele in Parkinson's disease. *Mov Disord*. May 2001;16(3):442-447.

11. Simón-Sánchez J, Schulte C, Bras JM, et al. Genome-wide association study reveals genetic risk underlying Parkinson's disease. *Nat Genet*. Dec 2009;41(12):1308-1312.

12. Singleton A, Farrer M, Johnson J, et al. Alpha-Synuclein locus triplication causes Parkinson's disease. *Science*. Oct 31 2003;302(5646):841.

13. International Parkinson's Disease Genomics Consortium (IPDGC); Wellcome Trust Case Control Consortium 2 (WTCCC2). A two-stage meta-analysis identifies several new loci for Parkinson's disease. *PLoS Genet*. Jun 2011;7(6):e1002142.

14. McGeer PL, Itagaki S, Boyes BE, McGeer E. Reactive microglia are positive for HLA-DR in the substantia nigra of Parkinson's and Alzheimer's disease brains. *Neurology*. Aug 1988;38(8):1285-1289.

15. Hardy J, Singleton A. Genomewide association studies and human disease. *N Engl J Med*. 2009;360:1759-1768.

16. Hughes AJ, Daniel SE, Ben-Shlomo Y, Lees AJ. The accuracy of diagnosis of parkinsonian syndromes in a specialist movement disorder service. *Brain*. Apr 2002;125(pt 4):861-870.

17. Elbaz A, Bower JH, Maraganore DM, et al. Risk tables for parkinsonism and Parkinson's disease. *J Clin Epidemiol*. 2002;55:25-31.

## Supplementary Information

### OMIM References:

[1] Parkinson Disease 6, Autosomal Recessive Early-Onset; PARK6 Parkinson Disease 6, Late-Onset, Susceptibility To, Included; (#605909)

Gene map locus 1p36

[2] Parkinson Disease 1, Autosomal Dominant; PARK1, Parkinson Disease 1, Autosomal Dominant Lewy Body; (#168601)

Gene map locus 4q21

[3] Synuclein, Alpha; SNCA (*163890)

Gene map locus 4q21

[4] Parkinson Disease 2, Autosomal Recessive Juvenile; PARK2 (#600116)

Gene map locus 6q25.2-q27

[5] Parkinson Disease 3, Autosomal Dominant; PARK3 (%602404)

Gene map locus 2p13

[6] Parkinson Disease 4, Autosomal Dominant; PARK4 (#605543)

Gene map locus 4q21

[7] Parkinson Disease 10; PARK10 (%606852)

Gene map locus 1p32

[8] Parkinson Disease 12; PARK12 (%300557)

Gene map locus Xq21-q25

[9] Parkinson Disease 8, Autosomal Dominant; PARK8 (#607060)

Gene map locus 12q12

***Key Words:*** Parkinson disease, LRRK2, SNCA, PKRN, PINK1, DJ-1, FBXO7, VPS35, Lewy bodies, mitochondria, lysosomes

# 127 Multiple Sclerosis

Riley Bove and Philip L. De Jager

## KEY POINTS

- *Disease summary:*
  - Multiple sclerosis (MS) is a genetically complex disorder, involving many susceptibility loci that probably interact with environmental factors to trigger the disease.
  - MS is a chronic, inflammatory demyelinating disorder of the central nervous system (CNS) typically characterized by demyelinating lesions disseminated "in time and space," meaning that different parts of the CNS are involved and that a patient has had at least two inflammatory events 3 months apart.
  - Demyelinating lesions can occur in the brain, spinal cord, and optic nerves.
  - Clinical presentation includes focal sensory or motor impairment, optic neuritis, transverse myelitis, loss of bowel or bladder function, gait instability, fatigue, depression, cognitive impairment. Vertigo, Uhthoff phenomenon, and Lhermitte sign are common.
  - Disease course is divided into three categories: relapsing remitting MS (RRMS, 85% of first presentations), secondary progressive MS (SPMS, many RRMS patients go on to exhibit a gradual functional and decline reminiscent of neurodegenerative diseases), and primary progressive MS (PPMS, patients who never had a clinical relapse).
  - More rare forms include neuromyelitis optica (NMO), Marburg variant, Schilder disease, Baló concentric sclerosis, and tumefactive MS.

- *Differential diagnosis:*
  - Can be organized by site of CNS involvement and includes:
  - Cerebrum and brain stem: acute demyelinating encephalomyelitis (ADEM), lymphoma, infection (Lyme disease, HIV, progressive multifocal leukoencephalopathy [PML], syphilis), small vessel disease (leukoaraiosis), CADASIL, vasculitis, rheumatologic diseases (systemic lupus erythematosus [SLE]), rheumatoid arthritis (RA), Sjögren syndrome), antiphospholipid antibody syndrome (APLAS), spinocerebellar ataxia, and leukodystrophy
  - Optic neuritis: NMO, sarcoidosis, retinal artery occlusion, retinal detachment, acute glaucoma
  - Spinal cord: sarcoidosis, spinal stenosis, syrinx, epidural abscess, spinal arteriovenous malformation (AVM), infectious myelitis (HIV, HTLV-1, *Mycoplasma*), nutritional ($B_{12}$, copper or zinc) deficiencies, toxicity, hereditary spastic paraparesis, adrenomyeloneuropathy

- *Monogenic forms:*
  - No single gene cause of MS is known to exist.

- *Family history:*
  - The lifetime risk of developing MS for a sibling or a child of an MS patient is 2% to 3%, which is about 30 times greater than the risk to the general population.

- *Twin studies:*
  - Monozygotic twins have a 30% concordance rate for clinical disease; in one study, concordance was 50% if magnetic resonance imaging (MRI) is performed and clinically silent MS-like lesions are considered as evidence of the disease.

- *Environmental factors:*
  - In terms of MS susceptibility, good epidemiologic data support the role of (1) the Epstein-Barr virus (EBV) (particularly in its clinical manifestation as infectious mononucleosis), (2) low vitamin D levels, and (3) smoking. More preliminary evidence supports the role of elevated adolescent body mass index (BMI) and living in Northern latitude during childhood, which may be related to vitamin D. There is some evidence for a gene-environment interaction. For example, individuals who have both the *HLA DRB1\*1501* allele and high levels of antibodies directed against the EBV protein EBNA-1 (two known risk factors), have a ninefold increase in risk over individuals that have neither risk factor.

- *Genome-wide associations:*
  - About 49 well-validated susceptibility loci harboring 54 risk alleles exist. Testing for susceptibility alleles is not yet clinically validated to diagnose or guide management of MS. Genome-wide association studies (GWASs) of disease course and other traits such as resilience and repair are beginning, but there is no variant with a validated role for these traits.

- *Pharmacogenomics:*
  - There are no validated associations with response to a given treatment.

## Diagnostic Criteria and Clinical Characteristics

**Diagnostic Criteria for MS:**
**Diagnostic evaluation should include**

- Neuroimaging of the brain and spinal cord with MRI, with and without gadolinium, to confirm demyelinating lesions in the white and gray matter. Classic findings include acute lesions that enhance with gadolinium; chronic lesions that appear dark on T1 sequence ("black holes"), ovoid-shaped white matter "Dawson fingers" on T2/FLAIR that are perpendicular to the ventricles. In the spinal cord, lesions typically are peripheral and less than one spinal cord segment in length. Imaging also helps to eliminate other elements of the differential diagnosis such as neoplasm and certain infections.

- Lumbar puncture to identify oligoclonal bands and calculate an IgG index (CSF IgG/CSF albumin)/(serum IgG/serum albumin), suggestive of demyelination, and to exclude infectious or neoplastic etiologies.
- Ophthalmologic examination to assess for optic neuritis or eye movement abnormalities.
- Exclusion of rheumatic or granulomatous etiologies with serologic markers (ANA, ESR, ACE) and chest x-ray.
- Visual-evoked potentials (VEP) to identify prior demyelination of the optic pathway.
- Somatosensory-evoked potentials (SSEP) to identify sensory disturbances.

### Diagnostic Criteria for MS (2010 McDonald Criteria):
**# clinical attacks (time), # objective lesions (space)→ additional data needed for dx**

- ≥2, ≥2 → None (clinical evidence alone suffices)
- ≥2, 1 → Dissemination in space (DIS) by MRI *or* second clinical attack at new site
- 1, ≥2 → Dissemination in time by MRI *or* second clinical attack
- 1, 1→ DIS by MRI *and* DIT by MRI; *or* second clinical attack
- 0, ≥1→ >1 year progression and two-thirds of (1) DIS on brain MRI (2) DIS on spinal cord MRI (≥2 T2 lesions), (3) +CSF (oligoclonal bands and/or elevated IgG index). Likely PPMS

### Criteria for Dissemination in Time or in Space on MRI:
**Time (DIT):**
1. A new T2 and/or gadolinium-enhancing lesion on follow-up MRI, with reference to a baseline scan, irrespective of the timing of the baseline MRI, *or*

**Space (DIS):**
- Greater than or equal to one T2 lesion in greater than or equal to two-fourths CNS areas: periventricular, juxtacortical, infratentorial, spinal cord.
- If a subject has a brainstem or spinal cord syndrome, the symptomatic lesions are excluded from the criteria and do not contribute to lesion count.

**Clinical Characteristics:** The clinical hallmark of MS is demyelinating lesions of the CNS disseminated in time and space.

Specific signs and symptoms can include focal sensory or motor impairment, optic neuritis, transverse myelitis, loss of bowel or bladder function, gait instability. Systemic (fatigue), psychiatric (depression, anxiety), and cognitive symptoms are common. Uhthoff phenomenon (sensitivity to increased body temperature, which causes a transient recrudescence of symptoms) and Lhermitte sign (a sensation described as an electric shock radiating caudally upon neck flexion) are common.

## Screening and Counseling

**Screening:** There is currently no validated role for screening of family members of MS patients or other high-risk individuals. Similarly, there is no role today for screening of the general population. There is also, currently, no validated primary prophylaxis therapy for MS. Thus, there is no screening tool today.

**Counseling:** Familial clustering is uncommon. While there is some evidence for the role of rare *CYP27B1* variants of strong effects on MS susceptibility, no clearly Mendelian forms of MS have been discovered to date. The use of common variants of modest effect has not entered the clinical setting. Thus, currently, there is no formal counseling. Informally, neurologists discuss the rate of MS in first-degree relatives, which is approximately 2% to 3%.

## Management and Treatment

**Acute Attacks** are managed with 3 to 5 days of intravenous methylprednisolone (1 g daily), with the goal of halting expansion of the acute inflammatory lesion. Plasmapheresis is considered when symptoms continue to evolve despite the methylprednisolone pulse.

**Disease-modifying treatments** (DMTs) are approved for reducing the likelihood of relapses. They are also indicated to reduce the risk of or delay the time to a second attack in clinically isolated syndrome. There are nine FDA-approved DMTs.

☞**FIRST-LINE TREATMENTS:**

**Beta interferons:** Interferon beta-1a (Avonex and Rebif) and interferon beta-1b (Betaseron and Extavia): These injectable treatments have incompletely understood mechanisms of action that may include enhancing suppressor T-cell function, a decrease in the release of metalloproteinases and proinflammatory cytokines, shutting down the blood-brain barrier, and downregulating antigen presentation. Common adverse events include injection-site reactions, headache, fatigue, and flu-like symptoms which tend to remit after the first few weeks of use. Depression, hepatitis, lymphopenia, and thyroid abnormalities are rarer. Beta interferons are also associated with neutralizing antibody formation which negates the effect of the medication.

**Glatiramer acetate (Copaxone):** This injectable acetate salt of synthetic polypeptides has an incompletely understood mechanism of action that may include enhancement of the regulatory T-cell function that control with myelin-damaging, proinflammatory T cells. Adverse events include injection-site reactions, and localized lipodystrophy at the injection sites. Patients may also experience a transient episode of shortness of breath following injection.

**Dimethyl fumarate (Tecfidera):** This oral methyl ester of fumaric acid has an incompletely understood mechanism of action that may involve upregulation of nuclear factor (erythroid-derived 2)-like 2 (Nrf2), thereby inducing a neuroprotective antioxidant response. Common adverse events include flushing, gastrointestinal symptoms (nausea, vomiting, abdominal pain, diarrhea), which may abate after the first few weeks to months. Leukopenia can also develop and white blood cell counts must be monitored.

☞**SECOND-LINE TREATMENTS:**

**Fingolimod (Gilenya):** This oral therapy is a sphingosine-1-phosphate receptor modulator which alters lymphocyte egress from lymph nodes. Adverse events include bradycardia and arrhythmia on the first day of treatment and includes one case of sudden death. There is also an increased risk of macular edema and basal cell cancer. In the pivotal trials, two subjects died of herpes encephalitis.

**Mitoxantrone (Novantrone):** This DNA intercalating agent originally developed as an antineoplastic agent is approved but no longer used because of its cardiotoxicity and significant risk of treatment-induced leukemia. Other adverse events include myelosuppression, alopecia, amenorrhea, nausea, susceptibility to infection, and bluish discoloration of the sclera and urine.

**Natalizumab (Tysabri):** This humanized antibody against alpha-4 integrin is infused on a monthly basis and prevents T cells and other immune cells from crossing the blood-brain barrier. Adverse events include hypersensitivity reactions, headaches, susceptibility to infection, and most notably progressive multifocal leukoencephalopathy (PML) caused by the JC virus. An anti-JC virus antibody test is available and is used to stratify patients for the likelihood of PML.

**Teriflunomide (Aubagio):** This oral pyrimidine synthesis inhibitor blocks the proliferation and function of activated T and B lymphocytes. Common adverse events include diarrhea, nausea, flu-like symptoms, and alopecia. It has also been associated with hepatotoxicity, ranging from transaminitis to fulminant hepatic failure.

☞**PHARMACOGENETICS:** There are no pharmacogenetic tests for clinical use in MS.

## Molecular Genetics and Molecular Mechanism

With certain genetic factors now well established (such as the *HLA DRB1\*1501* haplotype), specific hypotheses can be tested to see whether subjects with different levels of genetic susceptibility to MS respond differently to environmental exposures or whether certain environmental factors are dependent on a particular genetic architecture. Given that HLA DRB1 is a coreceptor for EBV entry and that the *HLA DRB1\*1501* allele may be able to present EBV antigen that mimic self-antigen, assessing the interaction of these two strong risk factors is of great interest. A recent study suggests that these two risk factors are largely independent and may be multiplicative. Specifically, individuals who have both risk factors (the *HLA DRB1\*1501* allele and high levels of antibodies directed against the EBV protein EBNA-1) have a ninefold increase in risk over individuals that have neither risk factor. This observation has been validated in another cohort that also supports the idea that there may be an interaction between these two risk factors. Interestingly, smoking appears to enhance the risk of MS associated with high anti-EBNA-1 titers, and this effect appears to account for the increased risk of MS due to smoking in some cohorts. The same cohorts were also analyzed using *HLA DRB1\*1501*, but this genetic risk factor did not influence the association between smoking, anti-EBNA-1 titers and MS risk. These and other observations have led to approaches that integrate genetic and environmental risk factors to predict a diagnosis of MS. The one study published to date on this topic suggests that environmental and genetic risk factors offer nonredundant information for a diagnostic algorithm. While our predictive model produces consistent results over several different subject cohorts, this algorithm that uses only 16 genetic variants is not yet performing well enough to be deployed clinically. Nonetheless, it demonstrates the way forward as we begin to integrate different risk factors; future versions of the algorithm will include the 50 to 100 common genetic variants and probably many rare variants that are thought to have a role in MS susceptibility. Furthermore, it will integrate interactions between risk factors as it is likely that environmental factors may have differential effects in different subsets of subjects with MS and that taking the genetic architecture of subjects into account will clarify the role of environmental susceptibility factors.

Can we consider exposure to sunlight and vitamin D levels? Is their role similarly independent from genetic causes or can genetic predisposition account for their effect on MS risk? Researchers recently investigated the role of sun exposure using disease-discordant monozygotic twins. The avoidance of sunlight early in life seems to put people at risk for the future development of MS, independent of genetic susceptibility to MS. Yet more evidence points in the direction of a complex interplay of genetic factors and vitamin D regulation: A recent study identified a novel MS susceptibility locus that includes the 1-alpha-hydroxylase (*CYP27B1*) gene involved in vitamin D metabolism. Diet, sun exposure, and genetics are all involved in vitamin D regulation. Since we know that serum levels of 25 (OH)D affect one's risk of MS, the exact degree to which diet and sunlight influence MS risk, apart from genetics, becomes more difficult to tease out without large sample sizes. Future epidemiologic studies will benefit from knowledge of the genetic architecture of MS and will be better able to explore the independence, or interdependence, of genes and the environment.

*Genetic Susceptibility for MS:* MS susceptibility is a genetically complex trait. Many different genetic loci with incomplete penetrance contribute to an individual's risk of developing MS. The evidence indicates that each of these genes probably only exerts a modest influence. This is consistent with the fact that heritability of MS is modest. The lifetime risk of developing MS for a sibling of an MS patient is approximately 3%, which is similar to the rate for children whose parents have MS and is about 30 times greater than the risk to the general population. The identical twin of an MS patient has, on average, a 30% risk of developing MS, highlighting the important but not overwhelming role that genes play in the onset of MS. While susceptibility and age at which a patient develops symptoms show modest evidence of heritability, there is little evidence that a disease course is strongly heritable, so a patient's course is not very informative when considering what may happen to a family member who is newly diagnosed with MS.

The search for susceptibility loci outside of the major histocompatibility complex (MHC) initially relied on linkage studies of families with multiple cases of MS, without success. Around the turn of the century, it became clear that this lack of success was consistent with theoretical models that highlighted the lack of statistical power of the linkage approach in discovering genetic variants of modest effect for a common disease such as MS. Instead, an association-based approach, such as a simple case-control design, was put forward as the preferred method for gene discovery. This realization led to the formation of the International MS Genetics Consortium (IMSGC), since, to be successful, an association study design requires very large sample sizes and very dense genotyping. In 2007, the collaboration came to fruition, and the first MS genome-wide association scan (GWAS) was performed by the IMSGC, resulting in the identification of two non-MHC susceptibility loci. This groundbreaking discovery was possible because of a combination of newly developed resources such as the HapMap (a catalog of several million common human genetic variation), technologic advances (including novel high-throughput genotyping platforms), and more powerful statistical methodologies. However, the critical strategic breakthrough with this study was the validation of the gene discovery strategy. A simple association study comparing allele frequencies in cases and controls proved successful when sufficient numbers of genetic markers and subjects were analyzed. The way forward was now clear: Larger studies with more markers would enhance statistical power and lead to more discoveries.

*The Major Histocompatibility Complex:* Increasing sample sizes and high-density genotyping panels have also led to new insights into the well-known MHC association with MS susceptibility. Human leukocyte antigen (*HLA*) genes, located within the MHC on chromosome 6p21, were first found to be associated with MS in 1972. Numerous linkage and association studies have since made this the most replicated finding in MS genetics. In particular, the *HLA DRB1*1501* haplotype (also known by the *HLA DR2* and *HLA DR15* tissue types) has consistently demonstrated linkage and association with MS in different human populations. However, other alleles within the MHC may separately affect MS risk. For example, Sardinians have a high concentration of *HLA DR3* and *HLA DR4* alleles, which may account for their high rates of MS, and *HLA DR3* was found to be associated with susceptibility for MS in UK subjects.

Because of strong linkage disequilibrium (LD, the co-occurrence of alleles at two or more loci within individuals more frequently than would be expected by chance) within the MHC, as well as the strong effect size (odds ratio [OR] = 2.7 for one copy of the allele), it remains unclear where the true susceptibility factor resides within the *HLA DRB1*1501* haplotype or whether multiple, linked alleles are required. In a study of African Americans with MS, Oksenberg and colleagues show not only that *HLA DRB1*0301* (*HLA DR3*) and *HLA DRB1*1503* are associated with MS, but also that the *HLA DRB1*1501* allele confers MS risk independent of the tightly linked *HLA DQB1*0602* allele. This pre-eminent role for *HLA DRB1*1501* is also seen in rare individuals of European descent where *HLA DRB1*1501* has been separated from *HLA DQB1*0602*. While the linkage disequilibrium in the MHC and allelic heterogeneity at *HLA DRB1* make it difficult to tease out the causal variant, it is clear that the *HLA DRB1*1501* allele is the strongest known MS susceptibility factor in the human genome and that the magnitude of its effect on MS susceptibility is unique for such a common allele.

More recently, larger sample sizes have enabled the resolution of susceptibility haplotypes that have effects independent of *HLA DRB1*1501* within the four megabases of the MHC. Specifically, it is now clear that the MHC class I region contributes to disease susceptibility. Multiple studies have validated the protective effect of the haplotype tagged by the *HLA A*02* allele. Furthermore, other studies suggest that additional susceptibility alleles exist within the MHC, so further investigation with larger sample sizes will provide more insights into the role of this critical region of the genome. Nonetheless, we have already gained the critical insights that MHC class I molecules, and not just class II molecules, are involved in the onset of MS implicating, for example, CD8+ T cells and natural killer cells in the earliest events in MS.

*Non-MHC MS Susceptibility Alleles:* Several different GWAS have been conducted for MS susceptibility since the original study in 2007, and many of their results have been subsequently validated. Overall, outside of the MHC, the GWASs discovered the type of risk-associated variants that are targeted by this study design: Genetic variants that are relatively common (frequency >0.05) in the general population of European ancestry and have modest effects on disease susceptibility (OR 1.1-1.25). About 49 susceptibility loci identified to date fit this pattern. It is now clear that there are no common variants of strong effect on susceptibility outside of the MHC. The *caveat* to this statement is that current genotyping arrays do not interrogate the entire human genome. Estimates vary, but roughly 80% of the common variation in the human genome has been explored to date for association with MS.

Thus, we may still be surprised by what is lurking in the 20% of the genome that is more difficult to interrogate using current technologies. Nonetheless, the current GWAS strategy is an extremely powerful tool that has yet to deliver its full complement of susceptibility loci; 50 to 100 susceptibility loci may exist and will gradually be identified as study sample sizes increase. Ongoing efforts include a new meta-analysis of all existing MS GWAS that will incorporate data on over 16,000 subjects with MS and 30,000 controls, and replicate results in an additional 18,000 subjects with MS and 18,000 controls. While this effort will have 99% power to discover common alleles with an OR of 1.2, two or three times that number will be needed to identify the alleles with more modest effects (OR >1.1). Thus, much remains to be done in investigating common variants associated with MS.

A complementary area of investigation that will begin to bear fruit in the next few years involves the study of less common and rare variants (population frequency <0.05) in MS. Next generation-sequencing technologies are rapidly maturing and are making the identification and study of such variants practical for the first time. Interest in these approaches is bolstered by the recent validation of variants in this class that share the expected profile of being present in relatively few individuals in the general population but of having strong effects. Both sets of variants were discovered as part of targeted investigations of a given gene: the 92Q allele of *TNFRSF1A* is present in approximately 2% (OR 1.6) and rare variants in *CYP27B1*. Thus, rare variants with large effect sizes on MS susceptibility exist and are discoverable using genome-sequencing approaches. One final class of variant may exist but will not be discovered using current strategies: Rare variants of modest effect will be extremely difficult to discover and validate as these variants would require extremely large sample sizes to be discovered.

The future of gene discovery in MS looks bright, but we already have important insights from the current complement of 19 susceptibility loci: *CBLB, CYP27B1, CD6, CD40, CD58, CD226, CLEC16A, CD80/TMEM39A, IL2RA, IL7R, IL12A, IRF8, KIF21B, MPHOSPH9/CDK2AP1, RGS1, STAT3, TNFRSF1A, SIAE,* and *TYK2*. Almost all of these loci contain genes with well-known immunologic functions, which suggests that the onset of MS is most likely to involve an immune dysregulation that secondarily triggers a degenerative process within the CNS. However, a definitive resolution of this question awaits the discovery of the full complement of susceptibility genes and a better grasp of the functional consequences of each locus on the human body. Given the known functions of the genes found in the MS susceptibility loci identified to date, we can make a few broad statements regarding which aspects of the immune system appear to be preferentially affected by MS risk alleles. For example, it appears that T-cell activation is an important nexus for the effect of many of the variants, including those found in or near costimulatory genes (*CD6, CD40, CD58, CD80, CD226*) and those affecting signaling pathways involved in transmitting activation and proliferation signals (*CBLB, IL2RA, RGS1*). These and other molecules involved in several aspects of the innate immune system (*IRF8, STAT3, TNFRSF1A,* and *TYK2*) suggest that the onset of MS is probably not due to the dysfunction of a single cell type but is instead due to systemic immune dysfunction. This observation is underscored by the fact that many of the susceptibility genes enumerated earlier have different functions at different levels of the immune system, and so tying the function of a risk allele to a single cell type is a useful but limited approximation as we begin to consider the sequence of events leading to the onset of MS.

***Use of Genetic Risk Factors in Predictive Models for Multiple Sclerosis:*** Since the genetic architecture of MS susceptibility is constituted primarily of loci of modest effect, analyzing the behavior of groups of susceptibility alleles could be informative. Recently, an aggregate measure of MS risk that combines weighted ORs from 16 genetic susceptibility loci (the weighted genetic risk score (wGRS) was created and used to predict a diagnosis of MS in three independent cohorts. The results revealed that the wGRS can modestly but robustly predict MS risk, consistent with another recent effort which used a similar strategy and also evaluated family members of MS subjects. A noteworthy but unsurprising observation is that a group of subjects with a clinically isolated demyelinating syndrome appear to have an architecture of genetic risk that is indistinguishable from that of subjects with MS.

With only 16 loci assayed in this version of the wGRS (out of the likely 50-100 loci that should emerge from current studies), it is too early to say whether a purely genetic algorithm will have clinical utility, particularly since we do not yet understand the role that less common variants of large effect (such as *TNFRSF1A* R92Q) may play. It is more likely that a predictive algorithm incorporating these risk alleles as well as other dimensions of information will eventually emerge. In fact, prediction of a case of MS is enhanced by the inclusion of nongenetic risk factors, such as sex, smoking, and anti–Epstein-Barr virus titers. This suggests that an algorithm using MS susceptibility loci might provide useful information if used in the context of a diagnostic algorithm that incorporates other data, such as environmental risk factors or, ultimately, blood biomarker or imaging data. However, genetic data in the context of the diagnostic evaluation of a sporadic MS case may be of marginal utility unless imaging is not available to support the clinical evaluation. A more useful application of this predictive score may ultimately be for individuals who are at higher risk to develop the disease, such as the first-degree relatives of patients with MS. The identification of individuals during the clinically silent phase of the disease could be extremely helpful in guiding the selection of those subjects who would benefit most from early imaging screening and eventually early treatment.

***Genetic Testing:*** No role yet exists for genetic testing in the diagnosis of MS.

***Future Directions:*** During the past 10 years, a dramatic change has occurred in our understanding of MS genetic and environmental risks. A robust method to discover common variants of modest effect, the association study, is now available, and many collaborations are maximizing the yield of this method by increasing the number of genotyped individuals. Many more loci will doubtlessly emerge as system analyses and integrated analyses of genetic and other data are deployed to uncover pathways that have a predilection for being targeted by MS susceptibility alleles.

Overall, the study of the human genome has yielded strong dividends in the field of MS, and a new generation of studies to assess other classes of genetic variation is already starting. The next decade promises to deliver a robust assessment of rare variants, using whole genome sequencing, and to finally validate loci affecting treatment and disease course as investigators begin to perform joint analyses across datasets. Given the technologies and methods available today, it looks likely that this new generation of studies will quickly inform existing efforts to develop algorithms that support clinical decisions. While it is too early to say whether personalized medicine will appear in MS, it is likely that genetic and environmental information will be incorporated into some aspects of the management of the disease in the coming decade.

## BIBLIOGRAPHY:

1. Sadovnick AD, Dircks A, Ebers GC. Genetic counselling in multiple sclerosis: risks to sibs and children of affected individuals. *Clin Genet*. 1999;56:118-122.
2. Patsopoulos NA, Bayer Pharma MS Genetics Working Group, Steering Committees of Studies Evaluating IFNβ-1b and a CCR1-Antagonist, et al. Genome-wide meta-analysis identifies novel multiple sclerosis susceptibility loci. *Ann Neurol*. Dec 2011;70(6):897-912.
3. International Multiple Sclerosis Genetics Consortium. Genome-wide association study of severity in multiple sclerosis. *Genes Immun*. Dec 2011;12(8):615-625.
4. De Jager PL. Identifying patient subtypes in multiple sclerosis and tailoring immunotherapy: challenges for the future. *Ther Adv Neurol Disord*. Nov 2009;2(6):8-19.
5. Sadovnick AD. Genetic background of multiple sclerosis. *Autoimmun Rev*. Jan 2012;11(3):163-166.
6. Ramagopalan SV, Guimond C, Dyment DA, et al. Early life child exposure and the risk of multiple sclerosis: a population based study. *J Neurol Sci*. Aug 15 2011;307(1-2):162-163.
7. Chao MJ, Ramagopalan SV, Herrera BM, et al. MHC transmission: insights into gender bias in MS susceptibility. *Neurology*. Jan 18 2011;76(3):242-246.
8. Ottoboni L, Keenan BT, Tamayo P, et al. An RNA profile identifies two subsets of multiple sclerosis patients differing in disease activity. *Sci Transl Med*. Sep 26 2012;4(153):153ra131.
9. International Multiple Sclerosis Genetics Consortium, Hafler DA, Compston A, et al. Risk alleles for multiple sclerosis identified by a genomewide study. *N Engl J Med*. 2007;357(9):851-62. Epub 2007 Jul 29.
10. Gourraud PA, McElroy JP, Caillier SJ, et al. Aggregation of multiple sclerosis genetic risk variants in multiple and single case families. *Ann Neurol*. 2011;69(1):65-74.

## Supplementary Information

### OMIM REFERENCES:

[1] Condition; Gene Name (OMIM#)

[2] Multiple Sclerosis, Susceptibility to (#126200)

[3] MHC Class II, Multiple Sclerosis, Susceptibility to, 1 (MS1); HLA-DRB1 (#142857, 604304)

[4] MHC Class II, Multiple Sclerosis, Susceptibility to, 1 (MS1); HLA-DQB1 (#604305)

[5] Multiple Sclerosis; MS2 (#612594)

[6] Multiple Sclerosis; MS3 (#612595)

[7] Multiple Sclerosis; MS4 (#612596)

[8] Multiple Sclerosis; MS5/TNFRSF1A (#614810, 191190)

[9] Programmed Cell Death, Multiple Sclerosis, Disease Progression, Modifier of; PDCD1 (#600244)

### Alternative Names:

- Disseminated Sclerosis
- Demyelinating Disorder
- Optic Neuritis
- Transverse Myelitis

# 128 Ataxia-Telangiectasia

Susanne A. Schneider and Kailash P. Bhatia

## KEY POINTS

- *Disease summary:*
  - Ataxia-telangiectasia (AT) is a recessive hereditary genomic instability disorder occurring in between 1 out of 40,000 and 1 out of 100,000 persons worldwide.
  - AT is clinically characterized by early-onset progressive cerebellar ataxia, telangiectasias of the skin and bulbar conjunctiva, progressive apraxia of eye movements, increased susceptibility to sinopulmonary infections, endocrine deficiencies and lymphoreticular malignancies, and other malignant tumors. Atypical forms including adult-onset AT and AT with early-onset dystonia including levodopa-responsive dystonia may occur.
  - Laboratory confirmation of the diagnosis is based on a combination of increased serum α-fetoprotein level, increased in vitro radiosensitivity, decreased or absent intracellular ATM protein levels on western blotting, and mutations in the *ATM* gene.
- *Hereditary basis:*
  - AT is due to *ATM* gene mutations, which follow an autosomal recessive inheritance pattern. More than 600 mutations of the *ATM* gene have already been identified, most of which are unique to single families (private mutations). Genetic screening can be extensive and remains unsuccessful in 5% to 15% of cases.
- *Differential diagnosis:*
  - AT variants have been recognized which include the Nijmegen breakage syndrome due to mutations in the *NBS1* gene on chromosome 8q21, and AT-like disorder (ATLD) due to mutations in the *MRE11*.
  - Ataxia with ocular motor apraxia types 1 and 2 can clinically mimic AT. Other ataxia disorders including Friedreich ataxia and vitamin E-associated ataxia should also be considered.

## Diagnostic Criteria and Clinical Characteristics

### Diagnostic Criteria:

**At least one of the following**

- An increased serum α-fetoprotein level (not specific)
- Increased in vitro radiosensitivity
- Decreased or absent intracellular ATM protein levels on western blotting
- Mutations in the *ATM* gene

### Supportive Criteria:

- Reduced IgG or IgA levels (reduced in 80% and 60% of AT patients)
- 7;14 chromosome translocation

**Clinical Characteristics:** AT should be considered in the context of progressive cerebellar dysfunction with onset in infancy. This can present as

- Gait instability or truncal ataxia
- Dysarthria (slurred speech)
- Oculomotor apraxia
- Presence of telangiectasia (which usually appears several years after the onset of neurologic symptoms), present in 97% of a series of 171 AT cases. The dilated blood vessels are most frequently found in the bulbar conjunctiva, particularly the lateral part. Ear helices, the bridge of the nose and the butterfly area of the face, the back of the hands, axillae, popliteal and antecubital fossae should also be closely examined for dilated vessels.
- Extrapyramidal features appear late through the disease course, but may rarely be present early.
- Dopa-responsive dystonia with confirmed *ATM* gene mutations has recently been described.

- Susceptibility to sinopulmonary infections.
- Increased risk of malignancies (in classic AT about 40%), in particular leukemia and lymphoma accounting for about 85% of malignancies. Young AT patients are typically prone to acute lymphocytic leukemia (ALL) of T-cell origin (rather than of pre-B cell origin otherwise common childhood ALL). Lymphomas are usually B-cell types. Other cancers and tumors, including ovarian cancer, breast cancer, gastric cancer, melanoma, leiomyomas, and sarcomas, may also occur. Cancer may occasionally precede the onset of ataxia.
- Cerebellar atrophy may be detected by neuroimaging, for example, magnetic resonance imaging (MRI).

## Screening and Counseling

### Screening:

- Serum concentration of **α-fetoprotein** is elevated (levels above 10 ng/mL) in 95% of cases with increasing levels over time.
- **Radiosensitivity assays**, such as the colony survival assay (CSA), assess the survival of patient-derived lymphoblastoid cells following irradiation with 1 Gy. The CSA was abnormal in 99% of individuals with at least one identifiable *ATM* mutation.
- **Immunoblotting for ATM protein** is the most sensitive and specific clinical test for establishing a diagnosis of AT. It reveals absent (in about 90% of patients) or markedly reduced levels (about 10%) in AT patients. About 1% of AT patients have a normal amount of ATM protein with absent ATM serine or threonine kinase activity (so-called "kinase-dead").
- **ATM serine or threonine kinase activity** assays evaluate ATM function. ATM serine or threonine kinase activity is absent

when the ATM protein levels are undetectable. Common substrates include p53-serine15, ATM-serine1981, KAP1, and SMC1-serine966.

- **Chromosome analysis:** A 7;14 chromosome translocation is present in 5% to 15% of cells in routine chromosomal studies of peripheral blood after stimulation with phytohemagglutinin. The break points are often located at 14q11 and at 14q32 (the T-cell receptor $\alpha$ and the B-cell receptor loci).

*Counseling:* AT is due to *ATM* gene mutations, which follow an autosomal recessive inheritance pattern. Accordingly, AT patients are expected to carry mutations on each allele, in a homozygous or compound heterozygous state. Both parents are suspected obligate carriers. Each sib of an affected individual carries a 25% risk of being affected, a 50% risk of being an asymptomatic carrier, and a 25% risk of not carrying any mutation. Offsprings of patients are obligate carriers.

AT patients and heterozygotes have an increased risk of cancer, in particular breast cancer (two-fold increased risk compared to the general population), and should be counseled and screened accordingly.

## Management and Treatment

Treatment of AT remains symptomatic and should include supportive therapies like speech therapy and physiotherapy to minimize contractures. By the age of 10 years a wheelchair may be required. Pulmonary infections and chronic bronchiectasis require pulmonary hygiene. Intravenous immunoglobulin (IVIG) replacement therapy may be necessary in those with frequent and severe infections. Malignancies should be screened for and treated according to current standards.

## Molecular Genetics and Molecular Mechanism

*Gene/Locus/Basic Gene Function:* The *ATM* gene is located on chromosome 11q22.3 and contains 66 exons spanning approximately 150 kb of genomic DNA. The ATM protein is a member of the phosphatidylinositol 3-kinase family of proteins that play a key role in DNA damage control by phosphorylating substrates involved in DNA repair and/or cell cycle control. However, the large size of the ATM protein and its multiple subcellular localization suggest that ATM may have more than one function.

*Genetic Testing:* DNA sequence analysis is clinically available (see Gene Tests http://www.genetests.org; http://www.ncbi.nlm.nih.gov/sites/GeneTests/lab/clinical_disease_id/2802?db=genetests) including prenatal and carrier testing.

However, because of the large size of the gene which comprises 66 exons, genetic screening can be extensive and limits the utility of direct mutation screening as a diagnostic tool which

remains unsuccessful in 5% to 15% of cases. More than 600 mutations of the *ATM* gene have already been identified, most of which are unique to single families. Most mutations result in premature protein truncations. In addition to sequence variants larger genomic deletions have been reported.

### BIBLIOGRAPHY:

1. Carrillo F, Schneider SA, Taylor AM, Srinivasan V, Kapoor R, Bhatia KP. Prominent oromandibular dystonia and pharyngeal telangiectasia in atypical ataxia telangiectasia. *Cerebellum.* 2009;8:22-27.

2. Concannon P. ATM heterozygosity and cancer risk. *Nat Genet.* 2002;32:89-90.

3. Chun HH, Gatti RA. Ataxia-telangiectasia, an evolving phenotype. *DNA Repair (Amst).* 2004;3:1187-1196.

4. Farr AK, Shalev B, Crawford TO, Lederman HM, Winkelstein JA, Repka MX. Ocular manifestations of ataxia-telangiectasia. *Am J Ophthalmol.* 2002;134:891-896.

5. Gatti RA, Berkel I, Boder E, et al. Localization of an ataxia-telangiectasia gene to chromosome 11q22-23. *Nature.* 1988;336:577-580.

6. Honda M, Takagi M, Chessa L, Morio T, Mizuatni S. Rapid diagnosis of ataxia-telangiectasia by flow cytometric monitoring of DNA damage-dependent ATM phosphorylation. *Leukemia.* 2009;23:409-414.

7. Matsuoka S, Ballif BA, Smogorzewska A, et al. ATM and ATR substrate analysis reveals extensive protein networks responsive to DNA damage. *Science.* 2007;316:1160-1166.

8. Perlman S, Becker-Catania S, Gatti RA. Ataxia-telangiectasia: diagnosis and treatment. *Semin Pediatr Neurol.* 2003;10:173-182.

9. Sun X, Becker-Catania SG, Chun HH, et al. Early diagnosis of ataxia-telangiectasia using radiosensitivity testing. *J Pediatr.* 2002;140:724-731.

10. Taylor AM, Byrd PJ. Molecular pathology of ataxia telangiectasia. *J Clin Pathol.* 2005;58:1009-1015.

11. Uziel T, Savitsky K, Platzer M, et al. Genomic organization of the ATM gene. *Genomics.* 1996;33:317-320.

12. Woods CG, Taylor AM. Ataxia telangiectasia in the British Isles: the clinical and laboratory features of 70 affected individuals. *Q J Med.* 1992;82:169-179.

## Supplementary Information

### OMIM REFERENCE:

[1] Condition; Ataxia Telangiectasia (OMIM# *607585)

### Alternative Name:
- Louis Bar Disease

*Key Words:* Ataxia, apraxia of eye movements, extrapyramidal features, susceptibility to sinopulmonary infections, lymphoreticular malignancies, breast cancer, dilated blood vessels, $\alpha$-fetoprotein, in vitro radiosensitivity, chromosome translocation, ATM serine or threonine kinase, autosomal recessive

# 129 von Hippel-Lindau Syndrome

Brian Shuch and W. Marston Linehan

## KEY POINTS

- *Disease summary:*
  - Manifestations of von Hippel-Lindau (VHL) disease were first observed in the early 20th century by Drs. von Hippel (retinal angiomas) and Lindau (cerebellar hemangioblastomas).
  - The disease is characterized by the development of multiple tumors including retinal angiomas, central nervous system (CNS) hemangioblastomas, pancreatic cysts and neuroendocrine tumors, renal cell carcinomas (RCC), pheochromocytomas, and epididymal cystadenomas.
  - Prior to comprehensive screening and early intervention, median survival of those with VHL was less than 50 years due to complications of RCC and hemangioblastomas.
  - VHL has an incidence of 1:35,000 and the majority of affected individuals have a family history of the disease.
  - Patients can have a germline missense, nonsense, or partial/complete deletion of the *VHL* gene. Most tumors generally have a second hit in the wild-type allele, which results from loss of heterozygosity, hypermethylation, and occasionally a second mutation.
- *Hereditary basis:*
  - VHL is a highly penetrant autosomal dominant disease due to a germline mutation in the *VHL* gene. Children of affected individuals have a 50% chance of inheriting the affected allele. In kindreds with VHL, up to a quarter have no family history and have been considered as founder mutations. However in cases of apparently de novo mutations, these actually may represent a nontraditional transmission of the *VHL* mutation. Detailed testing of parents of affected individuals can demonstrate genetic mosaicism in VHL.
- *Differential diagnosis:*
  - It is important to distinguish VHL from other multiorgan syndromes that have overlapping tumor types. Syndromes that feature pheochromocytomas include multiple endocrine neoplasia (MEN2a/b), neurofibromatosis type 1, and succinate dehydrogenase deficiency (SDH). Other kidney cancer syndromes associated with multiple tumor types include Birt-Hogg-Dubé (BHD), hereditary leiomyomatosis and renal cell carcinoma (HLRCC), SDH B and C deficiency, and Cowden syndrome.

## Diagnostic Criteria and Clinical Characteristics

***Diagnostic Criteria:*** The presence of two or more characteristic tumors associated with VHL should raise clinical suspicion for this syndrome. Over 75% of VHL individuals are diagnosed in kindreds with a prior family history of the disorder. These patients generally are asymptomatic when genetic testing is performed and routine screening can find manageable disease in one or more affected organ systems. Up to 25% of individuals with VHL have a *de novo* mutation. Many of these patients present with symptomatic, advanced disease due to a delay in diagnosis. The presence of two or more characteristic tumors associated with VHL should raise clinical suspicion for this syndrome.

***Clinical Characteristics:*** VHL-associated tumors generally present after the second decade of life with mean age presentation between 20 and 40 years of age. One exception is retinal angiomas; these tumors can occur as early as 1 year of age. See Table 129-1.

☞**Retinal Angiomas:** These tumors occur in the periphery of the retina and optic nerve and frequently are bilateral and multifocal. Initially they are asymptomatic but as these tumors grow they can cause permanent loss of vision from bleeding, development of macular exudate, and retinal detachment.

☞**Cerebellar, Brainstem, and Spinal Hemangioblastomas:** These highly vascular tumors can occur in the brain stem, cerebellum, and anywhere in the spinal cord. Symptoms are dependent on the location, size, and compressive effects of the lesion. If lesions become compressive to the surrounding tissue, common side effects include headaches, numbness, weakness, dizziness, worsening coordination, weakness, and back pain.

☞**Endolymphatic Sac Tumors:** The endolymphatic sac runs from the inner ear to the dura and controls balance and equilibrium. In patients with VHL, endolymphatic sac tumor (ELST) arises from this structure. When tumors are small they generally do not cause symptoms, however as tumors grow larger, patients can experience either gradual or sudden hearing loss, vertigo, tinnitus, and problems with balance. Large tumors can cause facial paralysis by damaging the seventh cranial nerve and can also erode into the temporal bone.

☞**Renal Cell Carcinoma and Renal Cysts:** Renal cysts generally are asymptomatic. However, while rare, cyst rupture can cause flank pain. Clear cell renal tumors when small cause no symptoms, but when larger they can cause hematuria, flank pain, and abdominal mass. Prior to the current screening methods in VHL patients, approximately 20% to 50% of patients would develop metastasis and die from kidney cancer.

☞**Pheochromocytoma:** Pheochromocytomas are adrenaline-producing chromaffin tumors located in the adrenal gland and may cause hypertension, anxiety, palpitations, diaphoresis, and rage. Prompt diagnosis, proper management, and treatment of pheochromocytoma is important to prevent complications related to catecholamine-induced cardiovascular morbidity such as malignant hypertension, stroke, heart failure, and fatal arrhythmias. While rare in patients with VHL, malignant pheochromocytoma can occur and patients frequently succumb to their disease.

☞**Pancreatic Cysts and Neuroendocrine Tumors:** Pancreatic cysts are the most common VHL manifestation of pancreatic disease. Cysts are generally asymptomatic but extensive

*Table 129-1 Organ System Involvement*

| System | Manifestation | Incidence |
|---|---|---|
| Brain | Cerebellar/Brainstem hemangioblastoma | 44%-72% |
| Spine | Spinal hemangioblastoma | 13%-50% |
| Ophthalmologic | Retinal angiomas | 25%-60% |
| Ear | Endolymphatic sarc tumor | 10%-15% |
| Pancreas | Pancreatic cysts and neuroendocrine tumors | 35%-70% |
| Kidney | Clear cell kidney cancer and renal cysts | 25%-60% |
| Adrenal | Pheochromocytoma | 10%-20% |
| Epididymis | Papillary cystadenomas | 25%-60% |

Adapted from Lonser et al. von Hippel-Lindau disease. *Lancet.* 2003;361:2059-2067.

replacement of the pancreas can cause exocrine dysfunction (steatorrhea) and endocrine dysfunction (diabetes mellitus). Pancreatic neuroendocrine tumors (PNETs) are the most common pancreatic tumor in VHL. When small, PNETs are generally asymptomatic. However, when larger they can obstruct the biliary tract and patients can present with jaundice and pruritus from elevations in bilirubin. Additionally these tumors tend to metastasize to the liver.

☞PAPILLARY CYSTADENOMAS OF THE EPIDIDYMIS (MEN) AND BROAD LIGAMENT (WOMEN): Epididymal cystadenomas are palpable tumors of the head of the epididymis and are common in young men with VHL. They do not generally cause symptoms, but may be tender to palpation on examination. Cystadenomas of the broad ligament are generally incidentally detected on abdominal imaging and rarely cause symptoms.

## Screening and Counseling

*Screening:* Routine ophthalmologic, CNS, and visceral screening are strongly encouraged in those affected with VHL and non-germline-tested individuals who may be asymptomatic carriers (Table 129-2). Close screening and early intervention greatly reduces the risk of permanent morbidity and mortality from VHL-related tumors. Aside from retinal angiomas, most VHL manifestations do not present until the second and third decade of life. Age-stratified screening has been developed to minimize unnecessary anxiety and radiation exposure in children who are less likely to have these manifestations. Clinicians should be aware that outliers can occur and additional testing should be obtained when indicated.

☞GENOTYPE-PHENOTYPE CORRELATION: VHL is commonly divided into type I (no pheochromocytoma) and type II (pheochromocytoma present). Type I disease accounts for the majority of patients with VHL and is characterized by germline *VHL* deletions, insertions, and nonsense mutations. Individuals with type VHL II typically harbor specific missense mutations in *VHL* strongly associated with susceptibility to pheochromocytoma. VHL type II can be further subdivided based on the probability of developing RCC and hemangioblastoma. Type IIa has a very high risk of hemangioblastoma whereas type IIb has a very high risk of hemangioblastoma and RCC. Type IIc is rare and is a predominant pheochromocytoma phenotype. Patients with partial deletion (PD) of *VHL* had greater than a twofold increase in the incidence of kidney cancer (but similar rates of other tumor types) compared to those with complete deletion (CD) of VHL.

*Table 129-2 Algorithm for Screening of Patients With VHL*

**Annual Testing Recommendations**

| Age 1 | Age 2-7 | Age 8-11 | Age 12-18 | Age 19+ |
|---|---|---|---|---|
| Eye exam | Eye exam | Eye exam | Eye exam | Eye exam |
| Physical exam/vitals | Physical exam/Vitals | Physical exam/vitals | Physical exam/vitals | Physical exam/vitals |
| | catecholamine testing | catecholamine testing | catecholamine testing | catecholamine testing |
| | | Abdominal ultasound | Abdominal ultasound | Abdominal CT or MRI |
| | | | MRI brain/spine | MRI brain/spine |

· All magnetic resonance imaging (MRI) and computed tomography (CT) should be obtained with contrast when possible.

· Catecholamine testing can be performed on urine or plasma samples.

· The frequency of MRI brain or spine can be every 1 to 2 years depending on extent of CNS disease. If no kidney or pancreas tumors are present or growth rates are extremely low, the abdominal imaging schedule can be less frequent (every 1-3 years)

· Any sign of hearing loss, vertigo, and tinnitus should prompt MRI or CT of the auditory canal and an audiologic evaluation.

*Table 129-3* *Management Algorithm for VHL-Associated Tumors*

| | |
|---|---|
| Retinal tumors | Small peripheral tumors—laser photocoagulation<br>Larger tumors—consider transconjunctival cryotherapy<br>Asymptomatic optic disc tumor—close observation<br>Symptomatic optic disc tumor—photodynamic therapy or anti-VEGF clinical trial<br>Painful tumors in eye with severe blindness—enucleation |
| Cerebellar, brain-stem, and spinal hemangioblastomas | Symptomatic brainstem/cerebellar tumor—craniotomy and resection<br>Symptomatic spinal tumor—laminectomy and resection<br>Select tumors stereotactic radiosurgery can be performed but worse local control |
| Endolymphatic sac tumors | If asymptomatic, either closely observe or consider surgical excision<br>If signs and symptoms, complete excision |
| Renal cell carcinoma and renal cysts | If tumor <3 cm closely observe with surveillance imaging<br>If solid tumor ≥3 cm partial nephrectomy with enucleation (Robotic/Lap vs Open)<br>Radical nephrectomy If poor kidney function or partial nephrectomy not feasible<br>Renal cysts observed, but removed if feasible during solid tumor management |
| Pheochromocytoma | Document catecholamine excess<br>Localization—MRI/CT<br>Consider functional imaging—$^{131}$—1 MIBG<br>Adrenal blockade ($\alpha/\beta$ and catecholamine synthesis)<br>Partial adrenalectomy when feasible (otherwise total adrenalectomy) |
| Pancreatic neuroendocrine tumors and cysts | Pancreatic cysts are observed<br>Tumor <2 cm, closely observe with surveillance imaging<br>Pancreatic head—If ≥2 cm, enucleation surgery if possible otherwise Whipple<br>Tail/body—If ≥3 cm, distant pancreatectomy vs enucleative surgery |

## Management and Treatment

See Table 129-3.

☞**RETINAL TUMORS:** Early diagnosis is the key as smaller lesions are easier to treat and less likely to cause long-term complications. Patients are evaluated with fundoscopy and pharmacologic dilation of the iris to assess lesion size and location. Treatment of small peripheral tumors is generally performed with laser photocoagulation surgery. Larger tumors may need to be treated with a transconjunctival intervention. Tumors of the optic nerve are difficult to treat and are usually observed since they generally are slow growing. For symptomatic tumors options include photodynamic therapy or enrollment into (antivascular endothelial growth factor [anti-VEGF]) therapeutic trials.

☞**CEREBELLAR, BRAIN STEM, AND SPINAL HEMANGIO-BLASTOMAS:** Due to an irregular and unpredictable pattern of growth, treatment of hemangioblastomas is deferred until symptoms develop. Surgical resection has been the standard of care to remove these lesions. Some centers have performed angioembolization preoperatively due to the high tumor vascularity but our center does not use it routinely. Stereotactic radiosurgery has emerged as an option for hemangioblastomas, however, an NCI prospective trial found poor long-term local control.

☞**ENDOLYMPHATIC SAC TUMORS:** Any subtle hearing loss, vertigo, or tinnitus must be evaluated immediately to preserve function as once lost it is hard to regain. If incidentally detected, the patient can be offered either observation or surgery. Factors influencing this decision depend on the patient's baseline hearing, presence of bilateral tumors, and the risk of facial nerve palsy with surgery. If an ELST is visible on MRI and the patient is symptomatic, surgical excision is indicated, preferably by a neurosurgeon and a head-and-neck surgeon trained in neurotology.

☞**RENAL CELL CARCINOMA AND RENAL CYSTS:** Prior to the current era, patients who presented with large renal tumors were managed with radical nephrectomy, many of whom would progress to bilateral nephrectomy and permanent dialysis. In the past three decades, patients followed with abdominal imaging have had earlier detection and intervention. In patients with bilateral, multifocal renal tumors, preserving renal function and removing all visible tumors at first sign of emergence is not feasible. Observational studies have shown that both renal tumors and cysts generally enlarge on follow-up imaging with variable growth rates, but progression to metastatic disease is rare for tumors smaller than 3 cm. Closely observing lesions to this 3-cm threshold limits the number of surgical procedures, allows for partial nephrectomy, and limits metastasis. Partial nephrectomy has emerged as the treatment of choice in patients with VHL in order to spare normal parenchyma and maximize renal function. to avoid ischemia, enucleation of tumors allows for maximal parenchymal preservation and limits bleeding. Many patients need repeat partial nephrectomy and salvage surgery in order to preserve renal function; therefore these patients should be managed in experienced centers capable of handling complex renal surgery.

Renal cysts rarely are symptomatic and intervention is rarely indicated. However, the walls of these cysts can contain elements of clear cell RCC and during a partial nephrectomy for solid lesions, if safe, these lesions should be removed. Mixed cystic-solid lesions account for approximately 10% of tumors. Our practice is to follow mixed cystic-solid lesions until the solid component approaches the 3-cm threshold.

☞**PANCREATIC NEUROENDOCRINE TUMORS AND CYSTS:** Pancreatic cysts rarely require intervention. However, if extensive and exocrine and endocrine dysfunction occurs, patients may require enzymatic support to manage malabsorption and insulin for blood glucose control. If cysts become very large and symptomatic,

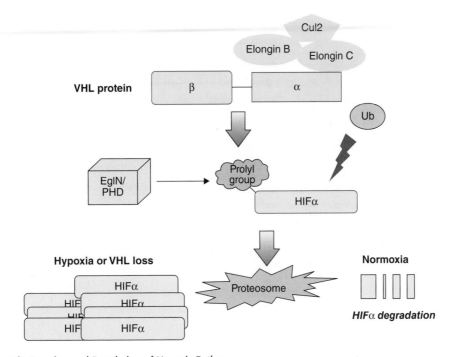

**Figure 129-1** VHL Protein Function and Regulation of Hypoxic Pathway.
In normoxic conditions with functional VHL, a hydroxylation by EglN/PHD allows VHL to ubiquitinate (Ub) HIF leading to proteosomal degradation. No hypoxia or with VHL loss, HIFa does not become ubiquitinated and accumulates, thus leading to transcriptional activation of downstream targets.

percutaneous or endoscopic drainage may be performed. Similar to renal tumors, small PNET can be observed as many have slow growth rates; one review of patients with resected tumors less than 3 cm found that none developed metastatic disease. Smaller lesions with rapid growth rates should also be considered for surgical intervention. Tumors of 1 cm or less should be observed with abdominal CT scans at 12-month intervals. Tumors in the body and tail of the pancreas can be watched until they reach 3 cm in size. In these locations PNETs are amenable to enucleation or distal pancreatectomy. PNETs in the head of the pancreas present complex anatomic challenges. The Whipple procedure (pancreaticoduodenectomy) is frequently required for tumors greater than 3 cm. Thus to permit effective enucleation, pancreatic head tumors are treated when they reach 2 cm in size.

☞**PHEOCHROMOCYTOMAS:** The initial pheochromocytoma workup includes biochemical testing to document excessive catecholamine section. Clinicians can screen patients with the more sensitive test, plasma-free metanephrines, or utilize a more specific test, 24-hour urinary catecholamines. Patient factors (stress and illness), dietary factors (caffeine), and multiple medications can greatly alter testing. Once excess catecholamine production is confirmed, the next step is to localize the tumor. Both abdominal MRI and CT scans are excellent anatomic imaging studies with excellent sensitivity and specificity. If inconclusive, functional imaging such as the I-MIBG scan can aid localization. If patients are symptomatic, endocrine management can alleviate symptoms. Our recommendations are to use combined alpha or beta-blockage with phenoxybenzamine and catecholamine synthesis inhibition with metyrosine.

The surgical management in patients with pheochromocytoma has traditionally been total adrenalectomy. However, for patients with VHL who may have bilateral, multifocal disease, surgically induced adrenal insufficiency leads to long-term consequences such as hypertension, diabetes, osteoporosis, and weight or body habitus changes. Partial adrenalectomy is an option in these patients. Observation of asymptomatic pheochromocytoma associated with VHL may also be an option in select patients. Minimally invasive (laparoscopic and robotic) adrenal surgery may decrease the morbidity of the procedure.

☞**PAPILLARY CYSTADENOMAS OF THE EPIDIDYMIS (MEN) AND BROAD LIGAMENT (WOMEN):** Papillary cystadenomas of the epididymis do not need special monitoring other than routine testicular self-examination. A scrotal ultrasound can be performed to rule out a testicular mass if physical examination is inconclusive. If lesions are painful they can be excised; however, ipsilateral obstruction of the vas deferens can occur after surgery. In women, papillary cystadenomas of the broad ligament are rarely diagnosed and treatment is generally not required.

## Molecular Genetics and Molecular Mechanism

***Syndrome/Gene/Locus:*** Positional cloning from affected VHL kindreds localized the VHL locus to 3p. Later this gene, *VHL*, (located on 3p25.3) was identified and determined to be responsible for both VHL disease and most cases of sporadic clear cell kidney cancer. The *VHL* gene contains three exons with an open reading frame of 852 nucleotides, encoding for the 284 amino acid protein, VHL.

***Description of Basic Gene Functions:*** The VHL protein binds to elongin B and C, Cul2 and Rbx1 to make up the E3-ubiquitin ligase complex. This complex is a critical regulator of the hypoxic

*Table 129-4 Molecular Genetic Testing*

| Gene | Testing Modality | Mutation Type | Detection Rate |
|------|------------------|---------------|----------------|
| *VHL* | Direct sequence analysis | Missense/nonsense mutations, small deletions | >~90% |
| *VHL* | Real-time quantitative PCR | Complete deletions | |

pathway. The hypoxia-inducible factors α (HIFa) are targeted for degradation by the proteasome due to ubiquitination by this complex. For VHL binding, HIF requires modification for binding at specific prolyl residues, a process controlled by a class of proteins call prolyl hydroxylases. Dysregulation of this pathway by loss of VHL function causes a pseudohypoxic state and may lead to tumorigenesis (Fig. 129-1). VHL also may have nonhypoxic roles including the control of apoptosis, the NFKB pathway, epithelial-mesenchymal transformation, and regulation of protein kinase C isoforms.

***Genetic Testing:*** Obtaining *VHL* genetic testing is important as possible asymptomatic carriers are recommended to follow routine screening. A negative test can avoid unnecessary anxiety, radiation exposure, and expense. Many patients have concerns about how a positive result may affect employment and insurability. Direct sequencing of the *VHL* can detect mutations while real-time quantitative polymerase chain reaction (PCR) can detect copy number alterations. Knowledge of a family mutation can limit whole gene sequencing and could reduce costs of testing. With current testing practices the sensitivity of detecting genetic alterations in VHL is over 90% (Table 129-4).

## BIBLIOGRAPHY:

1. Latif F, Tory K, Gnarra J, et al. Identification of the von Hippel-Lindau disease tumor suppressor gene. *Science.* 1993;5112:1317-1320.

2. Choyke PL, Filling-Katz MR, Shawker TH, et al. von Hippel-Lindau disease: radiologic screening for visceral manifestations. *Radiology.* 1990;3(pt 1):815-820.

3. Chen F, Kishida T, Yao M, et al. Germline mutations in the von Hippel-Lindau disease tumor suppressor gene: correlations with phenotype. *Hum Mutat.* 1995;1:66-75.

4. Lonser RR, Glenn GM, Walther M, et al. von Hippel-Lindau disease. *Lancet.* 2003;9374:2059-2067.

5. Maranchie JK, Afonso A, Albert PS, et al. Solid renal tumor severity in von Hippel Lindau disease is related to germline deletion length and location. *Hum Mutat.* 2004;1:40-46.

6. Asthagiri AR, Mehta GU, Zach L, et al. Prospective evaluation of radiosurgery for hemangioblastomas in von Hippel-Lindau disease. *Neuro Oncol.* 2010;1:80-86.

7. Choyke PL, Glenn GM, Walther MM, et al. The natural history of renal lesions in von Hippel-Lindau disease: a serial CT study in 28 patients. *AJR Am J Roentgenol.* 1992;6:1229-1234.

8. Duffey BG, Choyke PL, Glenn G, et al. The relationship between renal tumor size and metastases in patients with von Hippel-Lindau disease. *J Urol.* 2004;1:63-65.

9. Walther MM, Choyke PL, Weiss G, et al. Parenchymal sparing surgery in patients with hereditary renal cell carcinoma. *J Urol.* 1995;3(pt 2):913-916.

10. Steinbach F, Novick AC, Zincke H, et al. Treatment of renal cell carcinoma in von Hippel-Lindau disease: a multicenter study. *J Urol.* 1995;6:1812-1816.

11. Poston CD, Jaffe GS, Lubensky IA, et al. Characterization of the renal pathology of a familial form of renal cell carcinoma associated with von Hippel-Lindau disease: clinical and molecular genetic implications. *J Urol.* 1995;1:22-26.

12. Blansfield JA, Choyke L, Morita SY, et al. Clinical, genetic and radiographic analysis of 108 patients with von Hippel-Lindau disease (VHL) manifested by pancreatic neuroendocrine neoplasms (PNETs). *Surgery.* 2007;6:814-818; discussion 818 e1-e2.

13. Walther MM, Keiser HR, Choyke PL, Rayford W, Lyne JC, Linehan WM. Management of hereditary pheochromocytoma in von Hippel-Lindau kindreds with partial adrenalectomy. *J Urol.* 1999;2:395-398.

14. Hosoe S, Brauch H, Latif F, et al. Localization of the von Hippel-Lindau disease gene to a small region of chromosome 3. *Genomics.* 1990;4:634-640.

15. Gnarra JR, Tory K, Weng Y, et al. Mutations of the VHL tumour suppressor gene in renal carcinoma. *Nat Genet.* 1994;1:85-90.

16. Maxwell PH, Wiesener MS, Chang GW, et al. The tumour suppressor protein VHL targets hypoxia-inducible factors for oxygen-dependent proteolysis. *Nature.* 1999;6733: 271-275.

17. Min JH, Yang H, Ivan M, Gertler F, Kaelin WG Jr, Pavletich NP. Structure of an HIF-1alpha-pVHL complex: hydroxyproline recognition in signaling. Science. 2002;5574:1886-1889.

18. Ivan M, Haberberger T, Gervasi DC, et al. Biochemical purification and pharmacological inhibition of a mammalian prolyl hydroxylase acting on hypoxia-inducible factor. *Proc Natl Acad Sci USA.* 2002;21:13459-13464.

19. Nickerson ML, Jaeger E, Shi Y, et al. Improved identification of von Hippel-Lindau gene alterations in clear cell renal tumors. *Clin Cancer Res.* 2008;15:4726-4734.

## Supplementary Information

### OMIM REFERENCE:

[1] von Hippel-Lindau; VHL (# 608537)

***Key Words:*** Clear cell kidney cancer, partial nephrectomy, hemangioblastoma, pheochromocytoma, cystadenoma, retinal angioma, endolymphatic sac tumor, pancreatic neuroendocrine tumors

# 130 Amyotrophic Lateral Sclerosis

Shawn S. Wallery, Faisal Fecto, and Teepu Siddique

## KEY POINTS

- *Disease summary:*
  - Amyotrophic lateral sclerosis (ALS) is a progressive paralytic and fatal neurodegenerative disease affecting motor neurons in the brain and spinal cord.
  - **Epidemiology:** The prevalence of ALS has been estimated up to 2.7 to 7.4 per 100,000 with an annual incidence of 1.5 to 2.7 per 100,000. There is a male predominance of 1.5:1 and the average age of onset for sporadic ALS is between 55 and 75 years. Familial onset is noted to occur at a younger age, approximately 45 to 50, although this varies between genes. After the age of 70, the gender incidence is equal.
  - **Prognosis:** The average life expectancy after diagnosis is between 2 and 5 years. However, this is highly variable and up to 10% survive for at least 10 years and 5% survive over 20 years. Older-onset patients and those with initial respiratory involvement or bulbar forms of the disease tend to have a worse prognosis.
  - **Clinical presentation:** ALS is well known as a condition with a relentless progression of asymmetric muscular weakness and atrophy. The presentation varies widely depending on the region affected and the predominance of either upper or lower motor neuron (LMN) findings.
  - **Anatomic involvement:** Anatomic involvement of ALS includes primarily the motor neurons of the corticospinal tract in the brain and spinal cord as well as the anterior horn cells. A strong glial reaction typically surrounds the affected upper and lower motor neurons and degenerating descending tracts of ALS patients.
- *Differential diagnosis:*
  - It is highly important to recognize potentially treatable conditions that may mimic ALS.
  - **Upper motor neuron presentation:** Differential diagnoses include any condition affecting central nervous system (CNS) motor systems such as hereditary spastic paraplegia, spinocerebellar ataxias, tumors, cervical disc disease, demyelinating conditions, strokes, myelopathic conditions, and other forms of degenerative diseases.
  - **Lower motor neuron presentation:** Differential diagnoses include any condition affecting the lower motor neuron including focal nerve injuries, mononeuropathies, radiculopathies, plexopathies, and other conditions affecting the anterior horn cells (viral infections, spinal muscular atrophy, and Kennedy disease). Myopathies, primarily adult onset, may often be initially considered as well. Peripheral nerve disorders such as multifocal motor neuropathy, chronic inflammatory demyelinating polyneuropathy and Charcot-Marie-Tooth disease could be mistaken for ALS at the outset.
  - **Bulbar presentation:** Myasthenia gravis should always be considered in patients with a strict bulbar presentation. Any other causes of cranial nerve palsies, dysarthria, or dysphagia may be of consideration.
- *Monogenic forms:*
  - ALS is a genetically heterogeneous disease (Table 130-1).
- *Family history:*
  - Approximately 90% of ALS cases are sporadic and 10% familial. Mode of inheritance can be autosomal dominant (most common), recessive (usually juvenile onset) or X-linked dominant (adult or juvenile onset).
- *Twin studies:*
  - There is evidence for concordance among twins, but conclusions may be limited by the small numbers of patients included in these studies.
- *Environmental factors:*
  - Cigarette smoking and battlefield exposure have been reported as risk factors.
- *Genome-wide associations:*
  - Many genetic associations have been reported although very few have been validated. The validated ones include *PON* gene cluster polymorphisms and ATXN2 intermediate length polyglutamine expansions. In a recent meta-analysis, a locus at 1p34.1 was associated with age at onset. Testing for single-nucleotide polymorphisms (SNPs) is not yet clinically validated to diagnose ALS.
- *Pharmacogenomics:*
  - Although data are limited, slow and fast metabolizers of riluzole have been reported.

## Diagnostic Criteria and Clinical Characteristics

***Diagnostic Criteria for ALS:*** Despite advancements in the diagnosis of many neurologic conditions, ALS remains a diagnosis of exclusion without specific biomarkers or definitive tests. A progressive spread of upper and LMN signs and symptoms are required. The diagnosis of ALS requires

A. the presence of
  - (A:1) Evidence of LMN degeneration by clinical, electrophysiologic, or neuropathologic examination
  - (A:2) Evidence of upper motor neuron (UMN) degeneration by clinical examination

*Table 130-1 Summary of Major Genes and Pathologic Proteins in ALS and FTD[a]*

| Disease Phenotype | Causative Genes | Proteinopathy |
|---|---|---|
| **ALS** | | |
| Adult-onset SOD1-positive | *SOD1* | Ubiquitin, p62, SOD1, UBQLN2 |
| Adult-onset SOD1-negative | *FUS, TARDBP, OPTN, UBQLN2, C9ORF72, PFN1* | Ubiquitin, p62, FUS, TDP43, OPTN, UBQLN2 |
| Juvenile-onset ubiquitin-positive | *FUS, SOD1, UBQLN2, ALS5*[b] | Ubiquitin, p62, FUS, OPTN,[c] UBQLN2 |
| Juvenile-onset (other) | *ALS2, SETX, SPG11* | Unknown |
| **ALS-FTD** | | |
| Adult onset | *C9ORF72, UBQLN2, FUS, TARDBP* | Ubiquitin, p62, TDP43, FUS, OPTN, UBQLN2 |
| Juvenile onset | *ALS5, FUS, UBQLN2* | Unknown |
| **FTLD-U** | | |
| FTLD-TDP | *PGRN, VCP* | Ubiquitin, p62, TDP43, OPTN, UBQLN2 |
| FTLD-FUS | Unknown | Ubiquitin, p62, FUS, UBQLN2 |
| FTLD (other) | *CHMP2B* | Unknown |

[a]In rare cases, and sometimes, ethnically restricted cohorts, mutations in several other genes, including *DCTN1, VAPB, CHMP2B, ANG, PGRN, FIG4, MAPT, DAO, DJ1*, the *PONs, VCP*, and *SQSTM1/p62* have been described in ALS or ALS-like pleiotropic syndromes.

[b]ALS5 pathology is ubiquitin-positive, but other pathologic proteins remain to be identified.

[c]Not present in *SOD1*-positive juvenile-onset ALS.

ALS, amyotrophic lateral sclerosis; ALS-FTD, ALS with frontotemporal lobe dementia; FTLD-U, frontotemporal lobar degeneration with tau-negative ubiquitin-positive inclusions; FTLD-TDP, frontotemporal lobar degeneration with ubiquitin and TDP-43-positive neuronal inclusions; FTLD-FUS, frontotemporal lobar degeneration with fused in sarcoma (FUS)–immunopositive inclusions.

(A:3) Progressive spread of symptoms or signs within a region or to other regions, as determined by history or examination, together with

B. the absence of

(B:1) Electrophysiologic and pathologic evidence of other disease processes that might explain the signs of LMN and/or UMN degeneration

(B:2) Neuroimaging evidence of other disease processes that might explain the observed clinical and electrophysiologic signs

**Diagnostic Categories:**

*Clinically Definite ALS* is defined on clinical evidence alone by the presence of UMN, as well as LMN signs, in three regions.

*Clinically Probable ALS* is defined on clinical evidence alone by UMN and LMN signs in at least two regions with some UMN signs necessarily rostral to (above) the LMN signs.

The terms *Clinically Probable ALS-Laboratory-supported* and *Clinically Possible ALS* are used to describe these categories of clinical certainty on clinical and criteria or only clinical criteria:

*Clinically Probable ALS-Laboratory-supported* is defined when clinical signs of UMN and LMN dysfunction are in only one region, or when UMN signs alone are present in one region, and LMN signs defined by electromyography (EMG) criteria are present in at least two limbs, with proper application of neuroimaging and clinical laboratory protocols to exclude other causes.

*Clinically Possible ALS* is defined when clinical signs of UMN and LMN dysfunction are found together in only one region or UMN signs are found alone in two or more regions; or

LMN signs are found rostral to UMN signs and the diagnosis of *Clinically Probable ALS-Laboratory-supported* cannot be proven by evidence on clinical grounds in conjunction with electrodiagnostic, neurophysiologic, neuroimaging, or clinical laboratory studies. Other diagnoses must have been excluded to accept a diagnosis of clinically possible ALS.

*Clinically Suspected ALS* is a pure LMN syndrome, wherein the diagnosis of ALS could not be regarded as sufficiently certain to include the patient in a research study. Hence, this category is deleted from the revised El Escorial Criteria for the Diagnosis of ALS.

**Clinical Characteristics:** The presentation of ALS varies widely depending on the region affected and the predominance of either upper or lower motor neuron findings. Limb onset represents approximately 68% of initial presentations, bulbar 25%, and respiratory symptoms in approximately 7%. It has been known for some time that at least 2% to 3% of ALS patients develop features of overt and disabling dementia of the frontotemporal variety (FTD). Although not cognitively dysfunctional, up to 50% of unselected ALS patients may have evidence of disturbances in executive functions on detailed neuropsychiatric testing.

☞**PATTERN OF DISEASE IN LMN-PREDOMINANT ALS:** LMN symptoms generally start focally in a single limb with focal weakness and atrophy without sensory symptoms. As the disease progresses, weakness generally progresses within the same limb and to other limbs. Neck weakness may also be present either anteriorly or posteriorly. Fasciculations and cramping may be devastating symptoms. If the LMN symptoms exist without an UMN component, reflexes may be depressed and a pure flaccid syndrome may exist. Speech generally may be less affected, however, swallowing may have great difficulty. This is especially true as tongue weakness, atrophy, and slow mobility become evident. Respiratory symptoms may be prominent as diaphragmatic involvement becomes evident.

☞**PATTERN OF DISEASE IN UMN-PREDOMINANT ALS:** UMN symptoms generally may be first noticed as spasticity, instability with falls, or incoordination. Reflexes are brisk with clonus, a positive Hoffmann sign, and a present Babinski sign. A spastic dysarthria may be the presenting sign or occur during the course of the disease. Dysphagia may also be present. In UMN-predominant ALS, bladder symptoms, primarily urgency, may occur.

☞**PATTERN OF DISEASE IN BULBAR-ONSET ALS:** Bulbar-onset ALS occurs more frequently in older women. Symptoms often appear as dysarthria more than dysphagia and, in the absence of other initial signs or symptoms, may be mistaken for a multitude of other more common conditions such as gastroesophageal reflux disease (GERD), strokes, cranial nerve palsies, and myasthenia gravis. Tongue fasciculations with atrophy may be visualized. Physicians should carefully watch for palatal movements as well as lower facial weakness. Upper facial weakness may also be noticed in watching the speed of eye blinks.

## Screening and Counseling

Genetic testing for specific ALS-causing mutations is most useful for establishing the diagnosis, particularly in juvenile-onset or early-stage disease. It is also useful in assessing risk among family members of an affected relative with an established genetic cause. In contrast, genetic testing for prognostic purposes in ALS is of limited value.

## Management and Treatment

### Disease Modification:

☞**MEDICATION MANAGEMENT:** Riluzole, manufactured by Sanofi-Aventis under the brand name Rilutek, is the only medication FDA-approved for ALS disease modification. The effect is modest at best and it carries common side effects of fatigue, asthenia, nausea, abdominal pain, as well as hepatic side effects of enzyme elevation and even jaundice.

☞**PULMONARY MANAGEMENT:** Attention to pulmonary care is one of the most important factors in reducing overall disease burden, improving quality of life, and reducing the number of hospital visits. Respiratory failure, manifested as hypercapnic respiratory failure, and pulmonary infections are the most common causes of death in patients with ALS.

The institution of noninvasive positive pressure ventilation (NIV) has become a standard of care for every qualifying ALS patient. Consideration for diaphragmatic pacing is now an option for patients with ALS. The NeuRx Diaphragmatic Pacing System (DPS) first received FDA approval as a humanitarian device exemption in the fall of 2011 and is currently the only system approved as a pacing device in ALS. There are not, as of yet, set clinical standards for when pacing may be considered as an option. Thus patients with significant LMN dysfunction may not benefit from pacing if muscle tissue has significant atrophy. Airway clearance is imperative for several reasons. As the disease progresses, patients may experience a progressive inability to cough. The long-term

consideration for placement of a tracheostomy is a highly personal and an often emotionally charged discussion between patients and families.

☞**NUTRITION:** Nutrition is a strong predictor of morbidity and mortality in ALS. Recommendations are for the early placement of gastric feeding tubes prior to forced vital capacity decline below 50% of predicted secondary to patient concerns of safety during placement. Recent unpublished data have demonstrated tubes placed via interventional radiology are safer with fewer complications than traditional percutaneous endoscopic gastrostomy (PEG). As the disease progresses, patients should be encouraged to eat by mouth for pleasure and not as a way to sustain caloric intake.

☞**SYMPTOM MANAGEMENT:** The treatment of ALS revolves primarily around symptomatic management. An improved understanding of disease progression has led to the ability to optimize management. ALS is no longer a "diagnose and ditch" disorder. Improved outcomes have been demonstrated in centers with a multidisciplinary team approach to assess all aspects of disease progression. Important members of the team may include neurology, a pulmonologist experienced in neuromuscular conditions, physical therapy or occupational therapy (PT or OT), speech therapy, respiratory therapy, social work, and palliative care. Contact with an ALS support organization or foundation to assist with educational, emotional, and functional needs for patients and families is essential for optimizing quality of life.

☞**PHARMACOGENETICS:** Although pharmacogenetics data are limited, there is evidence showing patient populations that are slow or fast metabolizers of riluzole, suggesting that therapy should be optimized for individual cases, with slow metabolizers getting lower doses and fast metabolizers getting higher doses.

## Molecular Genetics and Molecular Mechanisms

The penetrance of genetic mutation-linked familial ALS may vary substantially, ranging from classic Mendelian pattern to apparently sporadic disease. The genetic heterogeneity and etiologic diversity in the pathogenesis of ALS has been highlighted in recent years by discovery of genetic alterations in several genes, including *SOD1, TARDBP (TDP43), FUS, OPTN, VCP, SQSTM1/p62, UBQLN2, C9ORF72,* and *PFN1* (Table 130-1). Recent studies have highlighted the causal involvement proteins involved in RNA processing pathways, like TDP43 and fused in sarcoma (FUS). Another major functional convergence is emerging at the level of abnormal protein cycling and disposal (via the ubiquitin-proteasome system and autophagy) with mutations identified in *UBQLN2, SQSTM1/p62, VCP,* and *OPTN.* All cases of ALS have the common pathologic hallmark of cytoplasmic ubiquitinated inclusions in anterior horn motor neurons. Histopathologic studies indicate that *TDP43, FUS,* and *OPTN* may be involved in a common pathogenic pathway shared by sporadic ALS, familial ALS, and ALS-FTD, but the *SOD1*-linked familial ALS is likely to have a pathway that is distinct from the other forms of ALS. It is highly plausible that these alternate pathways eventually converge downstream to turnover of ubiquitinated proteins mediated by UBQLN2 and p62.

### Genetic Testing:
Testing is commercially available for most of the ALS-linked genes, but is usually pursued only if there is a clear family history of autosomal dominant, recessive or X-linked dominant disease. Flaccid paralysis of one lower extremity with absent

Achilles reflex is highly suggestive of a genetic form of ALS, such as that seen in SOD1-A4V-linked ALS.

**Future Directions:** A recent explosion in data pertaining to the genetics and pathology of ALS has allowed for a rethinking about the pathophysiology of ALS and multiple opportunities for designing rational therapies. Insights into functional pathways like RNA processing, ubiquitin-proteasome system and autophagy should provide new biologic targets for ALS. At the same time, new strategies for large-scale analysis of the human genome, like whole exome sequencing, will provide many new causative genes and functional pathways allowing for better genetic screening, testing, and counseling based on better phenotype-genotype correlation. Future studies should focus on identifying environmental risk factors and modeling familial ALS in animal models.

**BIBLIOGRAPHY:**

1. Brooks BR, Miller RG, Swash M, Munsat TL for the World Federation of Neurology Research Group on Motor Neuron Diseases. El Escorial revisited: Revised criteria for the diagnosis of amyotrophic lateral sclerosis. *Amyotroph Lateral Scler Other Motor Neuron Disord.* 2000;1:293-299.

2. Talbot K, Ansorge O. Recent advances in the genetics of amyotrophic lateral sclerosis and frontotemporal dementia: common pathways in neurodegenerative disease. *Hum Mol Genet.* 2006;15(spec no 2):R182-R187.

3. Brooks BR. El Escorial World Federation of Neurology criteria for the diagnosis of amyotrophic lateral sclerosis. *J Neurol Sci.* 1994;124(suppl):96-107.

4. Brooks BR. Clinical epidemiology of amyotrophic lateral sclerosis. *Neurol Clin.* 1996;14:399-420.

5. Wokke JH. Diseases that masquerade as motor neuron disease. *Lancet.* 1996;347:1347-1348.

6. Lacomblez L, Bensimon G, Leigh PN, Guillet P, Meininger V. Dose-ranging study of riluzole in amyotrophic lateral sclerosis. *Lancet.* 1996;374:1425-1431.

7. Bensimon G, Lacomblez L, Meininger V. A controlled trial of riluzole in amyotrophic lateral sclerosis. *N Engl J Med.* 1994;330:585-591.

8. Ajroud-Driss S, Saeed M, Khan H, et al. Riluzole metabolism and CYP1A1/2 polymorphisms in patients with ALS. *Amyotroph Lateral Scler.* 2007;8:305-309.

9. Moss AH, Casey P, Stocking CB, Roos RP, Brooks BR, Siegler M. Home ventilation for amyotrophic lateral sclerosis patients: outcomes, costs, and patient, family and physician attitudes. *Neurology.* 1993;43:438-443.

10. Allen J, Hall M, Wallery S, et al. Gastrostomy tube placement by endoscopy versus radiologic methods in patients with ALS: a retrospective review of complications and outcomes. *Neurology.* 2012;78 (meeting abstracts 1):P01.101

11. Fecto F, Siddique T. Making connections: pathology and genetics link amyotrophic lateral sclerosis with frontotemporal lobe dementia. *J Mol Neurosci.* 2011;45(3):663-675.

12. Appel SH, Rowland LP. Amyotrophic lateral sclerosis, frontotemporal lobar dementia, and p62: a functional convergence? *Neurology.* Oct 9 2012;79(15):1526-1527.

## Supplementary Information

**OMIM REFERENCES:**

[1] Amyotrophic Lateral Sclerosis 1; ALS1 (#105400)

[2] Frontotemporal Dementia and/or Amyotrophic Lateral Sclerosis; FTDALS (#105550)

[3] Amyotrophic Lateral Sclerosis 15, With or Without Frontotemporal Dementia; ALS15 (#300857)

**Alternative Names:**

- Lou Gehrig Disease
- Upper and Lower Motor Neuron Disease
- Motor neuron disease
- Charcot Disease

**Key Words:** ALS, amyotrophic lateral sclerosis, Lou Gehrig disease, motor neuron disease, genetics, diagnosis, treatment, mechanism

# 131 Myotonic Dystrophy Type 1

Nicholas E. Johnson and Richard T. Moxley III

## KEY POINTS

- *Disease summary:*
  - Myotonic dystrophy type 1 is a multisystemic disease with variable clinical manifestations.
  - Muscle weakness typically involves the face, long finger flexors, intrinsic hand muscles, and foot dorsiflexors.
  - Myotonia (impaired muscle relaxation) may be elicited with grip or percussion of the muscle. Myotonia is not present in infants or very young children with other features of myotonic dystrophy.
  - Early-onset cataract (age <50) is often present and may be the only disease feature in mildly affected individuals.
  - Severe cases of myotonic dystrophy type 1 may result in onset of symptoms at birth, known as congenital myotonic dystrophy. Features associated include hypotonia, respiratory failure, feeding difficulties, clubfoot, and cognitive delay.
  - Myotonic dystrophy type 1 affects the heart, smooth muscle, gastrointestinal (GI) system, endocrine system, central nervous system (CNS) in addition to the core features, as delineated in Table 131-1.

- *Hereditary basis:*
  - Myotonic dystrophy type 1 is an autosomal dominant condition due to an unstable CTG repeat expansion in the 3'untranslated region of the *DMPK* gene on chromosome 19q13.3. It has complete penetrance but disease manifestations are subject to anticipation. As such, subsequent generations have earlier onset of more severe symptoms due to greater expansion of the trinucleotide repeat length.

- *Differential diagnosis:*
  - Myotonic dystrophy type 2 may present similarly in adults, though the weakness is typically more proximal. Isolated myotonia without weakness can also occur in nondystrophic myotonias (myotonia congentia). Congenital myopathies, spinal muscular atrophy, and Pompe disease are all considerations in the evaluation of a congenital myotonic dystrophy patient.

## Diagnostic Criteria and Clinical Characteristics

***Diagnostic Criteria:*** Myotonic dystrophy type 1 has the most varied presentation of any muscular dystrophy. However, certain features are highly associated with myotonic dystrophy type 1:

- Early-onset cataracts (age <50)
- Muscle weakness, especially long finger flexors
- Myotonia
- Affected family member

***Clinical Characteristics:*** Myotonic dystrophy type 1 is characterized by weakness, myotonia, and early-onset cataracts. Many of the disease manifestations in Table 131-1 are commonly associated with the disease. It is typical for individuals within an affected kindred to have a variety of manifestations affecting different systems.

Congenital myotonic dystrophy typically occurs only from affected mothers with myotonic dystrophy type 1 and presents with hypotonia, generalized weakness, feeding difficulties, clubfoot deformity, respiratory failure requiring ventilation, or reduced fetal movement. Patients may require prolonged (>1 month) ventilation, in which case there is a 25% mortality rate in the first year. As these children grow older, they often have cognitive symptoms ranging from mild learning difficulties to severe mental retardation. Typical features of adult-onset myotonic dystrophy subsequently develop in the second and third decades.

## Screening and Counseling

***Screening:*** See Fig. 131-1 for screening of adult-onset myotonic dystrophy type 1 and Fig. 131-2 for screening of congenital myotonic dystrophy type 1.

***Counseling:*** Myotonic dystrophy type 1 is an autosomal dominant disorder with nearly 100% penetrance. Due to anticipation with unstable expansion in the CTG repeat length in the germ line, subsequent generations often become more severely affected and at an earlier age. There is typically instability of the CTG repeat length within the somatic germ line. This results in varying CTG repeat lengths in different cell lineages. As a result, patients experience greater disease burden in specific target tissues. This contributes to phenotypic variability within a family. Use of in vitro fertilization with prior genetic screening is an option for those individuals seeking children. During pregnancy, spontaneous abortion, hydramnios, prolonged first stage of labor, retained placenta, and preterm labor have all been complications associated with myotonic dystrophy.

## Management and Treatment

Current treatment of myotonic dystrophy relies on symptomatic and preventive multidisciplinary approaches. Early involvement of physical therapy, occupational therapy, and speech therapy as well as school assistance can be helpful in the management of the behavioral and cognitive abnormalities associated with the condition.

Mobility and ambulation may be addressed with the use of gait training and assistive devices to compensate for distal leg weakness. These assistive devices may range from ankle-foot orthoses to wheelchair depending on the severity and distribution of the weakness. In congenital myotonic dystrophy, foot deformities or scoliosis may benefit from bracing or surgery depending on severity. Symptomatic myotonia may benefit from the use of mexiletine, an antimyotonia-antiarrhythmic lidocaine derivative shown to be safe and effective. Dosages of 150 mg tid and 200 mg tid are effective in

*Table 131-1 System Involvement*

| System | Manifestation | Prevalence |
|---|---|---|
| Musculoskeletal | Weakness of the facial muscles, long finger flexors, intrinsic hand muscles, and foot dorsiflexors. Less commonly proximal upper extremity weakness. | Very common to have finger flexor weakness |
| Cardiac | Progressive heart block, prolonged QRS and PR interval, other cardiac conduction abnormalities. | Increased rate of sudden death |
| Gastrointestinal | Dysphagia, gastric regurgitation, constipation, diarrhea | Common symptoms |
| Pulmonary | Excessive daytime sleepiness and obstructive sleep apnea. Individuals may experience debilitating fatigue, frequent bouts of pneumonia, and respiratory failure after certain types of anesthesia. | Very common to have excessive daytime sleepiness |
| Endocrine | Insulin resistance, testicular atrophy, hyperlipidemia, thyroid dysfunction, and gonadal failure. | 67% of individuals have abnormal HbA$_{1c}$ |
| Central nervous system | May be mild with impairment of executive function, visuospatial processing, depression, and avoidant personality disorders. More severely affected individuals may have global cognitive delay. | Common to have difficulty thinking |
| Vision and hearing | Cataracts may be initial or only finding of myotonic dystrophy type 1. Sensorineural hearing loss may develop. | Very common to have cataracts |

reducing grip myotonia without evidence of prolongation of the PR interval, QTc, or QRS duration.

Patients require serial ECG monitoring given the life-threatening cardiac arrhythmias or progressive cardiac conduction block associated with this condition. Prompt placement of a pacemaker is life saving. Ongoing consultation with a cardiologist familiar with myotonic dystrophy is helpful in the monitoring patients.

Patients may also develop respiratory or diaphragmatic failure. They require serial supine and sitting forced vital capacity measurements.

When warranted, the use of biphasic positive airway pressure (BiPAP) is necessary for symptomatic relief of respiratory insufficiency. Myotonic dystrophy patients may also have obstructive sleep apnea as well as nocturnal hypoventilation. Patients with congenital myotonic dystrophy may require ventilation and feeding tubes depending on the severity of the disease. If suspected, a screening polysomnogram in a patient with excessive daytime sleepiness is warranted. Patients can benefit from nocturnal continuous positive airway pressure (CPAP) use. Excessive daytime

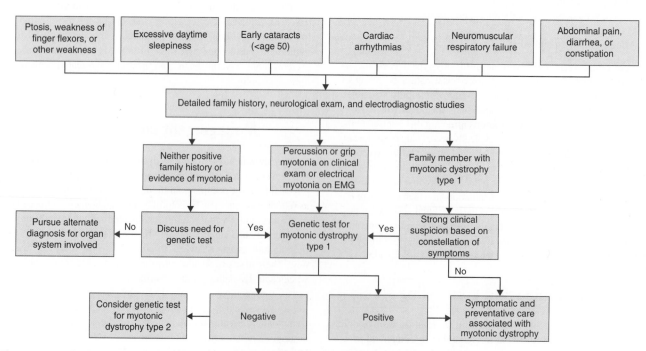

*Figure 131-1* Algorithm for Evaluation of Patient With Suspected Adult-Onset Myotonic Dystrophy Type 1.

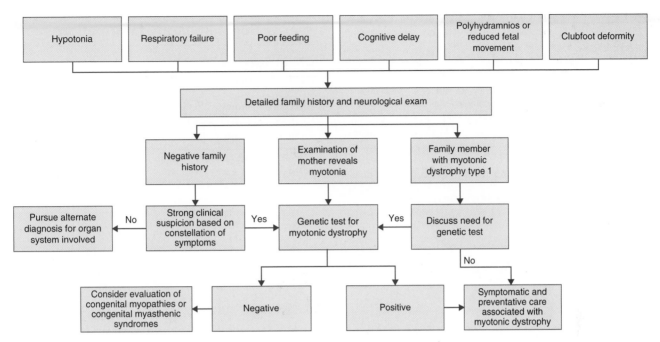

***Figure 131-2*** Algorithm for Evaluation of Patient With Suspected Congenital Myotonic Dystrophy.

sleepiness is common and may be related to a combination of obstructive sleep apnea and central hypoventilation. In this scenario, a trial of a stimulant such as modafinil in conjunction with CPAP use may be beneficial. Serial monitoring with slit-lamp examination with prompt surgical referral for symptomatic cataracts improves vision.

Patients may also have hearing loss. They will benefit from audiometric evaluations and hearing aids as appropriate.

Endocrine dysfunction including hypogonadism and insulin resistance is common. Patients should be periodically assessed for testosterone deficiency, insulin resistance, hyperlipidemia, and thyroid abnormalities with appropriate replacement.

Gastrointestinal dysmotility and gallbladder disease are also common. Patients with diarrhea may benefit from dietary adjustment with small, low-fat meals. Patients with abdominal pain or alternating diarrhea and constipation may benefit from a trial of antimyotonia therapy.

Particular caution should be given with anesthesia use. Patients may be sensitive to sedating medications and may have a paradoxical reaction to muscle depolarizing agents. These patients are at risk for cardiac arrhythmias during anesthesia and may need a prolonged ventilator wean following general anesthesia.

## Molecular Genetics and Molecular Mechanism

***Syndrome/Gene/Locus:*** DM1/dystrophia myotonica-protein kinase (*DMPK*)/19q13.3

*DMPK* is a serine or threonine kinase whose function is unclear. The normal gene for this protein has $[CTG]_n$ repeat length that ranges from 5 to 37 in the 3' UTR. Unstable expansion of this trinucleotide repeat in the germ line results in symptoms. The degree of expansion of the CTG repeat in leukocyte DNA correlates with

symptoms, with mildly affected individuals typically having 50 to 200 repeats, moderately affected individuals having 300 to 1000 repeats, and congenital onset often associated with greater than 1500 repeats. The expansion of this trinucleotide results in a hairpin formation in the RNA on the mutant allele and it accumulates in the nucleus. The accumulation sequesters nuclear regulatory proteins and alters the normal splicing of the pre-mRNA. This misregulation causes a splicopathy affecting the synthesis of a number of proteins. This includes the adult skeletal muscle chloride channel, the absence of which results in myotonia, as well as synthesis of the insulin receptor. Therefore, the expansion of the 3'UTR of the *DMPK* gene results in a toxic gain of function at the RNA level.

***Genetic Testing:*** Detection of the expanded CTG repeat in the *DMPK* gene by leukocyte DNA testing is widely available. Genetic testing may not be necessary for individuals with a clear phenotype and first-degree relative with a positive genetic test.

**BIBLIOGRAPHY:**

1. Harper PS. *Myotonic Dystrophy*. 3rd ed. London, UK: W.B. Saunders; 2001.

2. Fu YH, Pizzuti A, Fenwick RG Jr, et al. An unstable triplet repeat in a gene related to myotonic muscular dystrophy. *Science*. Mar 6 1992;255(5049):1256-1258.

3. Brook JD, McCurrach ME, Harley HG, et al. Molecular basis of myotonic dystrophy: expansion of a trinucleotide (CTG) repeat at the 3' end of a transcript encoding a protein kinase family member. *Cell*. Feb 21 1992;68(4):799-808.

4. Mahadevan M, Tsilfidis C, Sabourin L, et al. Myotonic dystrophy mutation: an unstable CTG repeat in the 3' untranslated region of the gene. *Science*. Mar 6 1992;255(5049):1253-1255.

5. Day JW, Ricker K, Jacobsen JF, et al. Myotonic dystrophy type 2: molecular, diagnostic and clinical spectrum. *Neurology*. Feb 25 2003;60(4):657-664.

6. Groh WJ, Groh MR, Saha C, et al. Electrocardiographic abnormalities and sudden death in myotonic dystrophy type 1. *N Engl J Med*. Jun 19 2008;358(25):2688-2697.

7. Heatwole CR, Miller J, Martens B, Moxley RT 3rd. Laboratory abnormalities in ambulatory patients with myotonic dystrophy type 1. *Arch Neurol*. Aug 2006;63(8):1149-1153.

8. Meola G, Sansone V. Cerebral involvement in myotonic dystrophies. *Muscle Nerve*. Sep 2007;36(3):294-306.

9. Logigian EL, Martens WB, Moxley RT 4th, et al. Mexiletine is an effective antimyotonia treatment in myotonic dystrophy type 1. *Neurology*. May 4 2010;74(18):1441-1448.

10. Campbell C, Sherlock R, Jacob P, Blayney M. Congenital myotonic dystrophy: assisted ventilation duration and outcome. *Pediatrics*. Apr 2004;113(4):811-816.

11. Wheeler TM, Sobczak K, Lueck JD, et al. Reversal of RNA dominance by displacement of protein sequestered on triplet repeat RNA. *Science*. Jul 17 2009;325(5938):336-339.

## Supplementary Information

**OMIM REFERENCE:**

[1] Myotonic Dystrophy 1 (DM1); DMPK (#160900)

**Alternative Names:**
- Dystrophia Myotonica 1
- Steinert Disease

**Key Words:** Myotonic dystrophy type 1, congenital myotonic dystrophy

# 132 Charcot-Marie-Tooth Disease

Philip M. Boone, Wojciech Wiszniewski, and James R. Lupski

## KEY POINTS

- *Disease summary:*
  - Charcot-Marie-Tooth disease (CMT), the broadest and most common disease class among the hereditary motor and sensory neuropathies (HMSNs), is a slowly progressive neurologic disease caused by dysfunction of the peripheral nerves with secondary muscle wasting, weakness, and sensory loss in a distal distribution. It is a distal symmetric polyneuropathy (DSP). DSP evidence-based medicine practice guidelines for laboratory and genetic testing have been established.
  - The disease is extremely heterogeneous both clinically and genetically (Table 132-1).
  - Electrophysiologic studies enable a distinction between the two major forms: (i) demyelinating (CMT1), with symmetrically slowed nerve conduction velocity (NCV); and (ii) axonal (CMT2), which is associated with normal nerve conduction velocity (NCV) but reduced compound muscle action potentials.

- *Hereditary basis:*
  - CMT can be observed as an autosomal dominant, autosomal recessive, or X-linked trait, predominately depending on the locus or gene involved. Many sporadic cases occur as a result of new mutation.
  - Thirty-six different genetic loci have been linked to CMT; for 30 of these loci, specific genes have been identified.
  - CMT subtypes are assigned broad designations based on nerve pathology and inheritance pattern: CMT1 = dominant, demyelinating; CMT4 = recessive, demyelinating; CMT2 = axonal; dominant, intermediate CMT (CMTDI) = dominant, mixed demyelinating and axonal; recessive, intermediate CMT (CMTRI) = recessive, mixed demyelinating and axonal; CMTX = X-linked. Within each class, specific designations are assigned for each separate gene or locus involved.
  - The most prevalent form of CMT disease, CMT1A, is caused in the vast majority of cases by copy-number gain of the *PMP22* gene and results from the CMT1A duplication and a gene dosage effect.
  - A deletion reciprocal to the CMT1A duplication results in hereditary neuropathy with liability to pressure palsies (HNPP), a milder condition characterized by recurrent episodes of nerve palsies at sites of compression.

- *Differential diagnosis:*
  - Acquired neuropathies associated with chronic disorders, including diabetes mellitus, vitamin deficiencies, and chronic infections (eg, HIV), paraneoplastic neuropathy, and iatrogenic causes (ie, side effect of chemotherapy; note that vincristine can cause a severe and sometimes lethal neuropathy in patients with CMT).
  - Other hereditary disorders with a neuropathic component, including other HMSNs, hereditary sensory and autonomic neuropathies (HSANs), distal hereditary motor neuropathy, etc.
  - Other conditions, such as myopathies, muscular dystrophy, amyotrophic lateral sclerosis (ALS), mitochondrial disorders, and many others.

## Diagnostic Criteria and Clinical Characteristics

***Diagnostic Criteria:*** Electrophysiologic studies: Symmetrically slowed NCVs of less than 38 m/s (normal value >45 m/s) indicates demyelinating CMT (CMT1; ~60%-70% of patients), while normal or slightly slowed NCVs with reduced compound muscle action potentials are features of axonal CMT (CMT2; ~20%-40% of patients).

Histopathologic evaluation of the sural nerve: Segmental demyelination and remyelination (onion bulb formation) in CMT1; normal myelin but reduced number of nerve fibers in CMT2.

***Clinical characteristics:*** CMT disease: Peripheral muscle weakness in lower and upper extremities, foot deformities, hammer toes, steppage gait, claw hand, hypo- or areflexia, sensory loss. Subtypes which have been studied appear to be highly penetrant. Age of symptom onset is variable, but usually occurs in the first or second decade of life. Most individuals with CMT1 walk without significant disability past middle age and a few (<5%) become wheelchair dependent.

HNPP: Nerve palsies following nerve compression. Focal thickening of myelin sheath (tomacula) on pathologic examination. Penetrance is unknown.

## Screening and Counseling

***Screening:*** CMT has an incidence of approximately 1 in 2500 individuals, making it a relatively commonly encountered illness among specialists. Thus, in a patient with symmetric lower motor and sensory neuron disease, particularly when inherited, CMT should be included in the differential diagnosis and genetic testing considered.

***Diagnostic Algorithm:*** Clinical features may point to a diagnosis of a particular CMT subtype. However, the following (or similar) algorithm may also be helpful. More complex, but sophisticated, algorithms are presented in (Bird, 2010; Saporta et al., 2011; Wiszniewski et al. 2013; and others).

☞SINGLE-GENE AND PANEL TEST APPROACH:

1. Positive family history → Obtain nerve conduction studies
   i. Demyelinating: test for the most commonly mutated genes based on inheritance pattern (AD = *PMP22* duplication, then *MPZ*, *PMP22* point mutations; AR = *GDAP1*, *PRX*, *SH3TC2*; XLD = *GJB1*).
   ii. Axonal: test for the most commonly mutated genes based on inheritance pattern (AD = *MFN2*, *MPZ*; AR = *GDAP1*; XLD = *GJB1*).

*Table 132-1* **Genetic Differential Diagnosis**

| Syndrome | OMIM ID | Gene Symbol | Inheritance[a] | Unique Associated Findings |
|---|---|---|---|---|
| CMT1A | #118220 | *PMP22* | AD | |
| CMT1B | #118200 | *MPZ* | AD | |
| CMT1C | #601098 | *LITAF (SIMPLE)* | AD | |
| CMT1D | #607678 | *EGR2* | AD | |
| CMT1E | #118300 | *PMP22* | AD | Sensorineural deafness |
| CMT1F | #607734 | *NEFL* | AD, AR | Early onset |
| CMT2A | #609260 | *MFN2* | AD, AR | |
| CMT2B | #600882 | *RAB7A* | AD | Notable sensory loss |
| CMT2B1 | #605588 | *LMNA* | AR | |
| CMT2B2 | #605589 | *MED25* | AR | |
| CMT2C | #606071 | *TRPV4* | AD | Vocal cord paresis, respiratory involvement |
| CMT2D | #601472 | *GARS* | AD | Involvement of hands more severe than of feet |
| CMT2E | #607684 | *NEFL* | AD | |
| CMT2F | #606595 | *HSPB1* | AD | |
| CMT2G | %608591 | Unknown gene at 12q12-q13 | AD | |
| CMT2H | 607731 | *GDAP1* | AR | |
| CMT2I | #607677 | *MPZ* | AD | |
| CMT2J | #607736 | *MPZ* | AD | Adie tonic pupil, deafness, marked sensory impairment |
| CMT2K | #607831 | *GDAP1* | AD, AR | |
| CMT2L | #608673 | *HSPB8* | AD | |
| CMT2N | #613287 | *AARS* | AD | |
| CMT2O | #614228 | *DYNC1H1* | AD | |
| CMT2P | #614436 | *LRSAM1* | AD, AR | |
| CMT4A | #214400 | *GDAP1* | AR | |
| CMT4B1 | #601382 | *MTMR2* | AR | Focally folded myelin sheaths (pathology) |
| CMT4B2 | #604563 | *SBF2 (MTMR13)* | AR | Juvenile glaucoma |
| CMT4C | #601596 | *SH3TC2* | AR | Spine deformities |
| CMT4D | #601455 | *NDRG1* | AR | Deafness, intra-axonal curvilinear profiles (pathology) |
| CMT4E | #607678 | *EGR2* | AR | Cranial nerve involvement, respiratory compromise |
| CMT4F | #145900 | *PRX* | AR | Focally folded myelin sheaths (pathology); loss of septate-like junctions and transverse bands and detachment of terminal paranodal myelin loops from axon (pathology) |
| CMT4G | %605285 | Unknown gene at 10q23 | AR | |
| CMT4H | #609311 | *FGD4* | AR | |
| CMT4J | #611228 | *FIG4* | AR | Rapidly progressive; severe motor involvement |
| CMTDIA | %606483 | Unknown gene at 10q24.1-q25.1 | AD | |
| CMTDIB (CMT2M) | #606482 | *DNM2* | AD | |
| CMTDIC | #608323 | *YARS* | AD | |

*(Continued)*

*Table 132-1  Genetic Differential Diagnosis (Continued)*

| Syndrome | OMIM ID | Gene Symbol | Inheritance[a] | Unique Associated Findings |
|---|---|---|---|---|
| CMTDID | #607791 | *MPZ* | AD | Focally folded myelin sheaths (pathology), bulbar and pupillary involvement, pronounced sensory involvement, intermittent symptoms |
| CMTRIA | #608340 | *GDAP1* | AR | |
| CMTRIB | #613641 | *KARS* | AR | |
| Charcot-Marie-Tooth disease, autosomal recessive, with vocal cord paresis | #607706 | *GDAP1* | AR | Vocal cord paralysis |
| Charcot-Marie-Tooth disease with glomerulopathy | #614455 | *INF2* | AD | Focal segmental glomerulosclerosis (FSGS) |
| CMTX1 | #302800 | *GJB1* (*CX32*) | XLD | Intermediate CMT; focal demyelination in CNS, deafness |
| CMTX2 | %302801 | Unknown gene at Xp22.2 | XLR | Intellectual disability |
| CMTX3 | %302802 | Unknown gene at Xq26 | XLR | Spasticity, pyramidal signs |
| CMTX4 | #310490 | Unknown gene at Xq24-q26.1 (locus denoted *NAMSD*) | XLR | Deafness, intellectual disability |
| CMTX5 | #311070 | *PRPS1* | XLR | Deafness, optic neuropathy |

[a]AD, autosomal dominant; AR, autosomal recessive; XLD, X-linked dominant; XLR, X-linked recessive.

Gene names: *PMP22*, peripheral myelin protein 22; *MPZ*, myelin protein zero; *LITAF*, lipopolysaccharide-induced TNF factor; *SIMPLE*, small integral membrane protein of lysosome or late endosome; *EGR2*, early growth response 2; *NEFL*, neurofilament, light polypeptide; *MFN2*, mitofusin 2; *RAB7A*, RAB7A, member RAS oncogene family; *LMNA*, lamin A/C; *MED25*, mediator complex subunit 25; *TRPV4*, transient receptor potential cation channel, subfamily V, member 4; *GARS*, glycyl-tRNA synthetase; *HSPB1*, heat shock 27kDa protein B1; *GDAP1*, ganglioside-induced differentiation-associated protein 1; *HSPB8*, heat shock 22kDa protein 8; *AARS*, alanyl-tRNA synthetase; *DYNC1H1*, dynein, cytoplasmic 1, heavy chain 1; *LRSAM1*, leucine-rich repeat and sterile alpha motif containing 1; *MTMR2*, myotubularin related protein 2; *SBF2*, SET binding factor 2; *MTMR13*, myotubularin related 13; *SH3TC2*, SH3 domain and tetratricopeptide repeats 2; *NDRG1*, N-myc downstream regulated 1; *PRX*, periaxin; *FGD4*, FYVE, RhoGEF, and PH domain containing 4; *FIG4*, FIG4 homolog, SAC1 lipid phosphatase domain containing (*Saccharomyces cerevisiae*); *DNM2*, dynamin 2; *KARS*, lysyl-tRNA synthetase; *YARS*, tyrosyl-tRNA synthetase; *INF2*, inverted formin FH2 and WH2 domain containing; *GJB1*, gap junction protein, beta 1, 32kDa; *CX32*, connexin 32; *NAMSD*, neuropathy, axonal, motor sensory with deafness and mental retardation (Cowchock syndrome); *PRPS1*, phosphoribosyl pyrophosphate synthetase 1.

2. Sporadic disease → Obtain nerve conduction studies
   i. CMT likely (ie, *de novo* mutation): test as earlier for positive family history.
   ii. Unclear → Sural nerve biopsy
      a. If not diagnostic of another (ie, non-CMT) condition, test as earlier for positive family history.

☞EXOME AND WHOLE GENOME SEQUENCING: Exome sequencing (ES) and whole genome sequencing (WGS), techniques that allow mutations in any gene within the genome to be identified, can be considered in lieu of panel testing after ruling out the CMT1A duplication and/or other often-mutated genes (eg, *GJB1*) (Lupski, et al., 2010; Montenegro, et al., 2011). Before ordering ES or WGS, the clinician should balance the time and cost involved with that of a traditional gene-by-gene or panel approach.

*Counseling:* CMT and related, inherited neuropathies display various forms of Mendelian inheritance (autosomal dominant, autosomal recessive, and X-linked dominant). New mutations are not infrequent; thus, absence of family history excludes neither a genetic etiology nor genetic testing.

Clinical symptoms of CMT usually begin in the first or second decades of life. Nonetheless, the disease can range from a severe, infantile-onset condition to a mild disease presenting in adulthood, such variability being possible even within one family (Lupski, et al. 2001). The penetrance of some CMT subtypes (eg, CMT1A) is known to be high; for the rest it is unknown.

☞GENOTYPE-PHENOTYPE CORRELATION: The broad CMT phenotype is characterized by genetic heterogeneity (mutations in multiple different genes may cause the same phenotype). Individual loci exhibit allelic affinity (different phenotypes can be due to mutations in the same gene). Even the inheritance pattern may vary between different kinds of mutations in the same gene.

## Management and Treatment

*Preventive Treatment:* Physical and occupational therapy to maintain function of muscles and joints, physical exercises, orthotic devices and assistive equipment, surgical interventions (hands and feet).

*Table 132-2* **Molecular Genetic Testing**

| | Gene | Testing Modality | Mutation Type | Detection Rate[a,b] (Saporta, et al. 2011; Wiszniewski, et al. In press) |
|---|---|---|---|---|
| **PMP22** | *PMP22* | Sequencing | SNV, indels | 2.5% of dominant CMT1; <2% of CMT1; 1%-4% of all CMT |
| | | MLPA | CNV | CMT1A duplication = 76%-90% of sporadic CMT1; ~80% of dominant CMT1; 54%-81% of CMT1; 25%-59% of all CMT; 3% of unassignable CMT |
| | | FISH | Large CNV | Tests for the CMT1A duplication can also detect the HNPP deletion, present in >90% of patients with symptoms of HNPP and ~6% of patients classified as CMT by Saporta, et al. 2011. |
| **Commonly mutated genes** | *GDAP1* | Sequencing | SNV, indels | ~5% of CMT2; most common cause (up to 25%) of AR CMT; <1% of all CMT |
| | *GJB1 (CX32)* | Sequencing | SNV, indels | 5%-19% of CMT1; 3%-57% of CMT2; 18% of unassignable CMT; 12% of X-linked CMT; second most common cause (~10%) of all CMT after *PMP22* duplication |
| | | MLPA | CNV | |
| | *MFN2* | Sequencing | SNV, indels | Most common cause (~20%) of CMT2; ~3% of all CMT |
| | | MLPA | CNV | |
| | *MPZ* | Sequencing | SNV, indels | 5% of dominant CMT1; 2%-7% of CMT1; 2%-40% of unassignable CMT; ~5% of all CMT |
| | | MLPA | CNV | |
| | *SH3TC2* | Sequencing | SNV, indels | 10%-26% of CMT4; <1% of all CMT |
| | | MLPA | CNV | |
| **Less commonly mutated genes** | *AARS* | Sequencing | SNV, indels | |
| | *EGR2* | Sequencing | SNV, indels | <1% of CMT1; <1% of all CMT |
| | *FGD4* | Sequencing | SNV, indels | |
| | *FIG4* | Sequencing | SNV, indels | |
| | *GARS* | Sequencing | SNV, indels | ~3% of CMT2; <1% of all CMT |
| | | MLPA | CNV | |
| | *HSPB1* | Sequencing | SNV, indels | |
| | | MLPA | CNV | |
| | *HSPB8* | Sequencing | SNV, indels | |
| | | MLPA | CNV | |
| | *LITAF (SIMPLE)* | Sequencing | SNV, indels | <2% of CMT1; <1% of all CMT |
| | *LMNA* | Sequencing | SNV, indels | <2% of all CMT |
| | | MLPA | CNV | |
| | *MED25* | Sequencing | SNV, indels | |
| | *MTMR2* | Sequencing | SNV, indels | <2% of all CMT |
| | *NDRG1* | Sequencing | SNV, indels | |
| | *NEFL* | Sequencing | SNV, indels | ~4% of CMT2; <1% of all CMT |
| | *PRPS1* | Sequencing | SNV, indels | |
| | | MLPA | CNV | |
| | *PRX* | Sequencing | SNV, indels | <1% of all CMT |
| | *RAB7A* | Sequencing | SNV, indels | |
| | *SBF2 (MTMR13)* | Sequencing | SNV, indels | |
| | *TRPV4* | Sequencing | SNV, indels | |

*(Continued)*

*Table 132-2* **Molecular Genetic Testing (Continued)**

| | Gene | Testing Modality | Mutation Type | Detection Rate[a,b] (Saporta, et al. 2011; Wiszniewski, et al. In press) |
|---|---|---|---|---|
| **Genomic Tests** | Many | Genome-wide aCGH, exon-targeted aCGH | CNV | |
| | All | Exome sequencing | Point mutations, indels | |

[a]CMT1 in this column refers to demyelinating CMT, and CMT2 to axonal CMT, regardless of inheritance pattern.

[b]The listed percentages likely differ in various ethnic populations.

SNV, single nucleotide variants; MLPA, multiplex ligation-dependent probe amplification; CNV, copy-number variation; FISH, fluorescence in situ hybridization; aCGH, array-based comparative genomic hybridization.

*Symptomatic Treatment:* Chronic pain, especially to lower back and legs (NSAIDs); neuropathic pain (gabapentin, topiramate, amitriptyline); tremor (beta-blockers, primidone); avoidance of neurotoxic medications and alcohol.

# Molecular Genetics and Molecular Mechanism

### Syndrome/Gene/Locus:

CMT1A/peripheral myelin protein 22 (*PMP22*)/17p12

CMT1B/myelin protein zero (*MPZ*)/1q22

CMT1C/lipopolysaccharide-induced TNF factor (*LITAF/ SIMPLE*)/16p13.13

CMT1D/early growth response 2 (*EGR2*)/10q21.3

CMT1E/peripheral myelin protein 22 (*PMP22*)/17p12

CMT1F/neurofilament, light polypeptide (*NEFL*)/8p21.2

CMT2A/mitofusin 2 (*MFN2*)/1p36.22

CMT2B/RAB7A, member RAS oncogene family (*RAB7A*)/3q21

CMT2B1/lamin A/C (*LMNA*)/1q22

CMT2B2/mediator complex subunit 25 (*MED25*)/19q13.3

CMT2C/transient receptor potential cation channel, subfamily V, member 4 (*TRPV4*)/12q24.11

CMT2D/glycyl-tRNA synthetase (*GARS*)/7p15

CMT2E/neurofilament, light polypeptide (*NEFL*)/8p21.2

CMT2F/heat shock 27kDa protein B1 (*HSPB1*)/7q11.23

CMT2G/unknown gene/12q12-q13

CMT2H/ganglioside-induced differentiation-associated protein 1 (*GDAP1*)/8q21.11

CMT2I/myelin protein zero (*MPZ*)/1q22

CMT2J/myelin protein zero (*MPZ*)/1q22

CMT2K/ganglioside-induced differentiation-associated protein 1 (*GDAP1*)/8q21.11

CMT2L/heat shock 22kDa protein 8 (*HSPB8*)/12q24.23

CMT2N/alanyl-tRNA synthetase (*AARS*)/16q22.1

CMT2O/dynein, cytoplasmic 1, heavy chain 1 (*DYNC1H1*)/14q32.31

CMT2P/leucine-rich repeat and sterile alpha motif containing 1 (*LRSAM1*)/9q34.13

CMT4A/ganglioside-induced differentiation-associated protein 1 (*GDAP1*)/8q21.11

CMT4B1/myotubularin related protein 2 (*MTMR2*)/11q21

CMT4B2/SET binding factor 2 (*SBF2/MTMR13*)/11p15.4

CMT4C/SH3 domain and tetratricopeptide repeats 2 (*SH3TC2*)/5q32

CMT4D/N-myc downstream regulated 1 (*NDRG1*)/8q24.22

CMT4E/early growth response 2 (*EGR2*)/10q21.3

CMT4F/periaxin (*PRX*)/19q13.2

CMT4G/unknown gene/10q23

CMT4H/FYVE, RhoGEF and PH domain containing 4 (*FGD4*)/12p11.21

CMT4J/FIG4 homolog, SAC1 lipid phosphatase domain containing (*S cerevisiae*) (*FIG4*)/6q21

CMTDIA/unknown gene/10q24.1-q25.1

CMTDIB/dynamin 2 (*DNM2*)/19p13.2

CMTDIC/tyrosyl-tRNA synthetase (*YARS*)/1p35.1

CMTDID/myelin protein zero (*MPZ*)/1q22

CMTRIA/ganglioside-induced differentiation-associated protein 1 (*GDAP1*)/8q21.11

CMTRIB/lysyl-tRNA synthetase (*KARS*)/16q23.1

Charcot-Marie-Tooth disease, autosomal recessive, with vocal cord paresis/ganglioside-induced differentiation-associated protein 1 (*GDAP1*)/8q21.11

Charcot-Marie-Tooth disease with glomerulopathy/inverted formin, FH2 and WH2 domain containing (*INF2*)/14q32.33

CMTX1/gap junction protein, beta 1, 32kDa (*GJB1/CX32*)/Xq13.1

CMTX2/unknown gene/Xp22.2

CMTX3/unknown gene/Xq26

CMTX4/unknown gene/Xq24-q26.1 (locus denoted *NAMSD*)

CMTX5/phosphoribosyl pyrophosphate synthetase 1 (*PRPS1*)/Xq22.3

CMT genes, most generally, encode proteins that are involved in the development, function, and/or preservation of peripheral motor and sensory nerves. The specific roles of each, however, are quite diverse: (1) myelination/myelin membrane proteins (PMP22, MPZ); (2) radial transport through the myelin sheath (GJB1); (3) axonal transport (NEFL); (4) transcription (EGR2, MED25); (5) signaling (PRX, MTMR2, MTMR13, NDRG1, FGD4); (6) mitochondrial function (GDAP1, MFN2); (7) endosome function or endocytic recycling (RAB7A, SH3TC2, FIG4); (8) chaperones (HSPB8, HSPB1); (9) protein synthesis (GARS, KARS, AARS, YARS); (10) nucleotide synthesis (PRPS1); (11) actin filament turnover (INF2); (12) vesicle and organelle motility along microtubules (DYNC1H1); (13) other functions (LMNA, DNM2, TRPV4, LRSAM1), and (14) unknown function (LITAF).

***Genetic Testing:*** The CMT1A duplication (and HNPP deletion) is easily detected with fluorescence *in situ* hybridization (FISH), array-based comparative genomic hybridization (aCGH), or multiplex ligation-dependent probe amplification (MLPA). Commercial sequencing is available for 24 CMT genes (Table 132-2). These tests can detect simple nucleotide variants (SNVs), but not small deletion or duplication mutations affecting these genes, necessitating MLPA or another method to detect DNA copy-number variations (CNVs), if desired. Genes may be tested one at a time, or a panel test may be ordered to assess multiple genes (eg, those sharing the same inheritance pattern) at once. Array CGH and exome or genome sequencing test for mutations (CNVs and SNVs, respectively) in multiple genes, or even in all genes.

See the Diagnostic Algorithm section for comments on the utility of testing and a testing algorithm.

## Bibliography:

1. Bird TD. Charcot-Marie-Tooth hereditary neuropathy overview. In: Pagon RA, Bird TD, Dolan CR, et al., eds. *GeneReviews* [Internet]. Seattle, WA: University of Washington; 2010.

2. England JD, Gronseth GS, Franklin G, et al. Practice parameter: evaluation of distal symmetric polyneuropathy: role of autonomic testing, nerve biopsy, and skin biopsy (an evidence-based review). Report of the American Academy of Neurology, American Association of Neuromuscular and Electrodiagnostic Medicine, and American Academy of Physical Medicine and Rehabilitation. *Neurology.* 2009;72:177-184.

3. England JD, Gronseth GS, Franklin G, et al. Practice parameter: evaluation of distal symmetric polyneuropathy: role of laboratory and genetic testing (an evidence-based review). Report of the American Academy of Neurology, American Association of Neuromuscular and Electrodiagnostic Medicine, and American Academy of Physical Medicine and Rehabilitation. *Neurology.* 2009;72:185-192.

4. GeneTests. http://www.ncbi.nlm.nih.gov/sites/GeneTests/?db= GeneTests. University of Washington. Accessed January 21, 2012.

5. Inoue K, Khajavi M, Ohyama T, et al. Molecular mechanism for distinct neurological phenotypes conveyed by allelic truncating mutations. *Nat Genet.* 2004;36:361-369.

6. Lupski JR, Garcia CA. Charcot-Marie-Tooth peripheral neuropathies and related disorders. In: Scriver CR, Beaudet AR, Sly D, Valle D, eds. *The Metabolic and Molecular Bases of Inherited Disease.* McGraw-Hill, New York;2001:5759-5788.

7. Lupski JR, Reid JG, Gonzaga-Jauregui C, et al. Whole-genome sequencing in a patient with Charcot-Marie-Tooth neuropathy. *N Engl J Med.* 2010;362:1181-1191.

8. Montenegro G, Powell E, Huang J, et al. Exome sequencing allows for rapid gene identification in a Charcot-Marie-Tooth family. *Ann Neurol.* 2011;69:464-470.

9. Online Mendelian Inheritance in Man (OMIM). http://www. omim.org. Johns Hopkins University. Accessed February 1, 2012.

10. Saporta AS, Sottile SL, Miller LJ, Feely SM, Siskind CE, Shy ME. Charcot-Marie-Tooth disease subtypes and genetic testing strategies. *Ann Neurol.* 2011;69:22-33.

11. Skre H. Genetic and clinical aspects of Charcot-Marie-Tooth's disease. *Clin Genet.* 1974;6:98-118.

12. Szigeti K, Lupski JR. Charcot-Marie-Tooth disease. *Eur J Hum Genet.* 2009;17:703-710.

13. Weedon MN, Hastings R, Caswell R, et al. Exome sequencing identifies a *DYNC1H1* mutation in a large pedigree with dominant axonal Charcot-Marie-Tooth disease. *Am J Hum Genet.* 2011;89:308-312.

14. Wiszniewski W, Szigeti K, Lupski JR. Hereditary motor and sensory neuropathies. In: Rimoin DL, Connor JM, Pyeritz RE, Korf BR, eds. *Emery and Rimoin's Principles and Practice of Medical Genetics.* Elsevier, Ltd., Philadelphia;2013:Ch.126, 1-24.

## Supplementary Information

**Alternative Names:**
- Hereditary Motor and Sensory Neuropathy
- Distal Symmetric Polyneuropathy

***Related Neuropathies:***
- Dejerine-Sottas Neuropathy
- Roussy-Lévy Syndrome
- Congenital Hypomyelinating Neuropathy

***Key Words:*** Peripheral neuropathy, slow NCV, lower motor neuron disease

# 133 Genetic Prion Disease

James Mastrianni

## KEY POINTS

- *Disease summary:*
  - Rare neurodegenerative diseases typically associated with rapidly progressive dementia and ataxia.
  - *Disease subtypes*—Sporadic (s) and familial (f) forms of Creutzfeldt-Jakob disease (sCJD and fCJD) and fatal insomnia (sFI and fFI). Gerstmann-Sträussler-Scheinker disease (GSS) is always genetic. Rarer forms caused by exposure to prions, include variant CJD (vCJD) and kuru. A new phenotype, labeled Variably Protease-Sensitive Prionopathy, has recently been recognized in a small number of patients.
  - *Transmissible properties*—Prions are misfolded isoforms of prion protein (PrP) that can interact with and convert normal prion protein (PrP$^C$) to the misfolded pathogenic isoform (PrP$^{Sc}$). Nervous tissues from affected patients with any subtype of prion disease can potentially transfer disease to healthy individuals, if directly introduced.
  - *Diagnostic tests*—For sCJD, brain magnetic resonance imaging (MRI) diffusion-weighted imaging (DWI) sequences often show hyperintensity of the cortical ribbon or basal ganglia, and electroencephalography (EEG) may demonstrate periodic sharp waves complexes of approximately 1 per second. Cerebrospinal fluid (CSF) may show elevation of 14-3-3 and/or extremely elevated tau protein. In FI, positron emission tomography (PET) scan of brain shows a hypometabolic thalamus. Genetic testing assists with diagnosis of familial forms of prion disease.
- *Hereditary basis:*
  - About 10% to 15% of all cases result from an autosomal dominant mutation of the PrP gene (*PRNP*). Homozygosity at the common polymorphic codon 129 of *PRNP* is more common in cases of sCJD and vCJD. Codon 129 genotype may influence the phenotype of some genetic prion diseases. No other genes are directly causal.
- *Differential diagnosis:*
  - Other neurodegenerative conditions, including Alzheimer disease, Huntington disease, frontotemporal lobar dementias, spinocerebellar ataxia, and dementia with Lewy bodies, among others. CNS viral and bacterial infections, paraneoplastic syndromes, Hashimoto encephalopathy, and Whipple disease are important considerations in the workup.

## Diagnostic Criteria and Clinical Characteristics

World Health Organization (WHO) criteria exists only for sporadic (s) CJD, which includes the following

**Probable sCJD**

**Rapidly progressive dementia *and* at least two of the following**

 i. Myoclonus
 ii. Visual or cerebellar signs
 iii. Pyramidal or extrapyramidal signs
 iv. Akinetic mutism

**And a positive result from at least one of the following**

a. Periodic EEG
b. Positive CSF 14-3-3 (*or significantly elevated tau protein >1200 pg/mL) in patients with disease under 2 years duration
c. MRI of brain with high-signal abnormalities in basal ganglia (*or cortical ribbon) by DWI or fluid attenuated inversion recovery (FLAIR)

**And the absence of**

- Routine investigations indicating an alternative diagnosis (*indicate author's modification of the WHO—levels may be greater than 3000 pg/mL)

**Possible sCJD**

**Progressive dementia and at least two of the following features**

 i. Myoclonus
 ii. Visual or cerebellar signs
 iii. Pyramidal or extrapyramidal signs
 iv. Akinetic mutism

And, the absence of a positive result [or unavailability of results] for any of the three tests described for probable CJD (a-c, earlier)
And, duration of illness less than 2 years
And, without routine investigations indicating an alternative diagnosis

**Definite**

Histopathologic presence of spongiform degeneration (vacuolation) and gliosis, and/or western blot presence of protease-resistant PrP. Note, this is the histopathology for CJD, not for other prion subtypes (see later).

*Clinical Characteristics:* Common core features include progressive dementia, ataxia, and myoclonus, although any neurologic or psychiatric feature can be seen, depending on the brain region affected by disease. There are four major subtypes of prion disease, outlined below. Kuru, a historic prion disease linked to cannibalistic rituals in New Guinea is not included. Although clinical features overlap considerably, the predominant presenting clinical feature is often used to distinguish between subtypes, although they are ultimately defined by their distinct histopathologies. Sporadic forms of disease generally present at a later age and progress faster than genetic forms. The four subtypes include

☞CREUTZFELDT-JAKOB DISEASE: Onset of progressive dementia, followed by ataxia, and myoclonus. Age at onset typically greater than or equal to 55 years for sporadic (s) cases (average 68 years) and less than or equal to 55 for familial (f) cases, but exceptions exist. Death typically occurs within 4 to 6 months (~90% <1 year) from the onset of sCJD and 1 to 3 years from the onset of fCJD. MRI and EEG findings appear to be more common in sCJD than fCJD. Histopathology demonstrates spongiform degeneration diffusely distributed throughout the cortex and deep

---

nuclei of the brain. Western blots reveal protease-resistant pathogenic prion protein (PrP^Sc).

☞**VARIANT CJD:** Onset typically with psychiatric symptoms, especially apathy and depression, followed by painful sensations (dysesthesias) in the distal extremities, then dementia, ataxia, and myoclonus. Teens and young adults more commonly affected (average onset ~28 years). Progression to death is slightly greater than 1 year from disease onset. MRI (proton density weighting or DWI) often shows hyperintensities in the pulvinar region of the thalamus. EEG and CSF are often normal. Histopathology includes PrP amyloid plaques surrounded by a halo of spongiform degeneration, described as "florid" plaques. This disease occurs only from exposure to prions (contaminated beef) originating from bovine spongiform encephalopathy (BSE), or "mad cow disease." Highest number of cases are from the United Kingdom. Occurrence has declined markedly since the first reports in 1995 to 1996. Three cases reported in the United States appear to have been exposed prior to emigration from the United Kingdom and Saudi Arabia.

☞**GERSTMANN-STRÄUSSLER-SCHEINKER DISEASE:** Ataxia of gait is the most common presentation, but cognitive or behavioral symptoms predominate in some. Most cases also include abnormalities in muscle tone and strength. Onset is generally 30s to 50s, and progression is relatively slow (5-7 years). Imaging, CSF, and EEG studies are generally nondiagnostic. All reported cases of GSS have been linked to a genetic alteration in *PRNP*. Histopathology is distinct from other subtypes and demonstrates diffusely distributed PrP amyloid plaques, especially within the cerebellum, and minimal spongiform degeneration.

☞**FATAL INSOMNIA:** Classically presents with progressive insomnia, autonomic dysfunction (alteration in blood pressure, lacrimation, sweating, etc), followed by other typical features of prion disease, including ataxia and myoclonus. Insomnia may be mild or not apparent at onset. A sleep study demonstrates total reduction in sleep time. PET of the brain shows selective hypometabolism within the thalamus. Sporadic (SFI) and familial (FFI) forms of FI are known. The polymorphic codon 129 is a key determinant of the FI phenotype. FFI is caused by a single base-pair change (Asp178Asn) in allelic phase with Met coding of the polymorphic codon 129, while the same Asp178Asn mutation coupled with Val coding at codon 129 produces a more typical fCJD phenotype. Histopathology demonstrates neuronal loss and gliosis in brain stem and thalamic nuclei, with minimal spongiform change.

☞**VARIABLY PROTEASE SENSITIVE PRIONOPATHY:** In this recently described subtype, common clinical features appear to include aphasia, ataxia, parkinsonian signs, or frontal lobe-like features, including impulsivity, euphoria, or apathy. Onset ranges from 48 to 81 years and duration is 2 to 6 years. It is distinguished from CJD primarily by the overall reduced protease-resistance of PrP^Sc isolated from the brain and the presence of punctate and target-like PrP amyloid deposits with moderate spongiform degeneration in histological sections. Diagnostic tests, such as EEG, MRI, and CSF studies are most often negative.

### *Evaluation of [a] patient with suspected prion disease:*

1. The WHO criteria for CJD, outlined under Diagnostic Criteria are used as a guideline for diagnosis.
2. Phenotypes described in Clinical Characteristics provide additional features of clinical presentation. Earliest symptoms help to define the subtype. Initial symptoms may be vague and consideration of prion disease is often delayed until obvious progression of disease.
3. Detailed family history—The presence of one or more documented cases of prion disease or unexplained deaths under age 55, raise suspicion for genetic prion disease and warrant genetic analysis of *PRNP*. A known mutation is nearly confirmatory, but a thorough evaluation is necessary to rule out another process that may masquerade as prion disease, despite the presence of the genetic defect.
4. Core diagnostic studies include
   - MRI—DWI of the brain is particularly useful, as it commonly shows hyperintensities of the cortical ribbon and/or basal ganglia (caudate and putamen) in sCJD, however, this finding is less common and not well documented in familial prion disease.
   - EEG—Periodic sharp wave complexes at a frequency of 0.5 to 2 per second in approximately 65% of sCJD cases, but less common or absent in other subtypes.
   - CSF—Mild increase in total protein (~10% above normal), high level of tau protein (>1200 pg/mL). 14-3-3 protein is also typically elevated, but false positives in association with herpes encephalitis, acute stroke, and other neurologic conditions that result in rapid neuron death. Normal cell count and glucose levels.

Other conditions confused with prion disease include other neurodegenerative diseases, such as dementia with Lewy bodies, Huntington disease, Alzheimer disease, spinocerebellar ataxias (SCA), frontotemporal lobar dementias (FTLD), including inclusion body myopathy with Paget disease of bone and/or FTD, CHMP2B-related FTD, and GRN-related FTD, in addition to autoimmune causes, such as Hashimoto encephalopathy, limbic encephalitis, and other paraneoplastic syndromes, heavy metal toxicity, vasculopathies, and CNS viral infections, among other conditions. Therefore, the workup is broad and, in addition to the usual dementia panel that includes complete blood count (CBC), a basic medical panel, vitamin $B_{12}$, folate, and thyroid function assessment, laboratory studies should also include antithyroglobulin and antithyroperoxidase antibodies, copper and ceruloplasmin, heavy metal screen, SPEP and UPEP, a paraneoplastic panel, including anti-Ma, anti-Ta, anti-GAD65, and anti-NMDA antibodies, in addition to a screen for inflammatory and connective tissue diseases (ESR, CRP, ANA, dsDNA, SS-A, SS-B, ANCA, etc). In addition to the proteins noted earlier, CSF analysis should rule out a CNS inflammatory and infectious disease, including polymerase chain reaction (PCR) for *Trophermyma.whippleii*.

## Screening and Counseling

***Screening:*** Genetic screening of asymptomatic individuals is not performed, unless directly requested by at-risk family members, and after genetic and psychiatric counseling. Screening of *PRNP* for mutations known to cause familial prion disease can be performed in symptomatic individuals with or without a family history of prion disease. In the presence of a family history, with a known mutation of *PRNP*, screening for individual mutations can be performed. However, complete genetic sequencing of the coding segment of *PRNP* is necessary to rule out genetic prion disease in patients without an obvious family history, or in those for whom the mutation is not known. Novel mutations continue to be identified, underscoring the importance of complete sequence analysis. See Table 133-1 for a summary of *PRNP* mutations associated with

*Table 133-1* **Summary of PRNP Mutations Associated With Genetic Prion Disease**

| Phenotype | Octapeptide Repeat Insertions (OPRI)[a] | Single Base-Pair Mutations |
|---|---|---|
| CJD | 1, 2, 4, and 5, (±7) OPRI more often associated with CJD histopathology, but highly variable | 178, 180, 183, 196, 200, 203, 208, 210, 211, 232, 238 |
| GSS | 8 or 9 OPRI most commonly associated with GSS histopathology[b] | 102, 105, 117, 131, 145[c], 160[c], 163[c], 198, 202, 212, 217, 226[c], 227[c] |
| FFI | None | D178N allelic with 129M |

[a]Normal PrP contains five repeat segments of approximately eight amino acids (Pro-[His/Gln]-Gly-Gly-Gly-(-/Trp)-Gly-Gln), between residues 51 and 91. Insertions of 1 to 9 repeat segments cause familial prion disease.

[b]GSS histopathology most consistent with 8 or 9 OPRI, but also reported in cases with less repeats.

A Huntington disease like-1 (HDL1) presentation has been associated with an 8-OPRI in a very limited number of cases. Pathology is GSS-like.

[c]Truncation mutations generate foreshortened PrP that lacks glycosylphosphatidylinisotol (GPI) anchor.

genetic prion disease and Table 133-2, for a detailed list of single base-pair alterations.

### Additional Genetic Aspects:

☞**POLYMORPHIC CODON 129:** Homozygosity (129MM or 129VV) is significantly more common (>80%) in patients affected with sCJD than controls (~50%). Codon 129 genotype also affects the phenotype of sCJD; 129MM is most often associated with rapidly progressive dementia, whereas 129VV or 129MV cases most often present with ataxia at onset and a slightly slower disease course. In some cases of genetic prion disease, homozygosity of codon 129 enhances disease onset and/or rate of disease progression. Codon 129 testing is not a useful genetic screen for sCJD, since the homozygous state is common in the normal population. All primary cases of vCJD caused by exposure to bovine spongiform encephalopathy are 129MM.

☞**GLU219LYS:** Primarily found in the Japanese population and associated with protection from sCJD. However, it has been detected in allelic phase with an autosomal dominant mutation, without obvious protection.

☞**GLY127VAL:** It is found in a specific population in New Guinea, where kuru was prevalent. It is thought to be protective.

☞**TRUNCATION MUTATIONS:** These occur at codons 145, 160, 163, 226, and 227. All promote a GSS phenotype, presumably by secretion of PrP, as a result of loss of the C-terminal GPI-anchor attachment site.

### Counseling:
Inheritance is autosomal dominant with nearly 100% penetrance. Some mutations have variable penetrance that appears to be age related, such as the *Val180Ile* mutation, which is commonly late onset. Family history is often negative in these cases, as at-risk mutation carriers may not reach the age of disease onset. The *Glu200Lys* mutation manifests from middle life (40s and 50s) to late life (up to the 80s), resulting in a scenario in which children of healthy parents develop CJD.

☞**GENOTYPE-PHENOTYPE CORRELATION:** Several mutations of *PRNP* are linked to, or strongly associated with, a specific clinical subtype, especially the histopathologic profile (Table 133-1 and 133-2), and the pattern of protease-resistant PrP^Sc fragments. The clinical features of disease are generally, but not strictly, associated with specific subtypes. The prominent clinical finding at onset, order of appearance of clinical features, and rate of progression, assist in characterizing phenotypes.

## Management and Treatment

There are no established pharmacologic agents for prion disease. Therapy is aimed at controlling symptoms; seizures are treated with general antiepileptic agents such as phenytoin or carbamazepine, myoclonus is managed with low doses of clonazepam, severe psychiatric symptoms, including hallucinations and/or delusions are best managed with atypical antipsychotics (eg, quetiapine or olanzapine). Evaluation by a social worker is mandatory to assist the family in planning. Life-sustaining procedures, such as feeding tubes and ventilatory support, should be discussed and decisions should be made about resuscitation in advance. Once the diagnosis is clearly established and the patient approaches the end of life, a palliative care consult and arrangement for hospice should be made.

## Molecular Genetics and Molecular Mechanism

☞**BASIC FUNCTION OF PRNP:** *PRNP* is positioned on the short arm of chromosome 20. A single exon encodes the 253 amino acid PrP. Differential splicing does not appear to occur. An

| Gene Name | Gene Symbol | Chromosomal Locus | Protein Name and Synonyms |
|---|---|---|---|
| Prion protein gene | *PRNP* | 20pter-p12 | Prion protein, PrP, PrP^C, PrP^Sc, CD230, CJD, GSS, prion, PrP27-30 |

*Table 133-2* **Selected PRNP Mutations and Histopathologic Phenotypes**

| Codon | Change | Codon 129 | Phenotype |
|-------|--------|-----------|-----------|
| 102 | Pro → Leu | Met or Val | GSS |
| 105 | Pro → Leu | Val | GSS |
| 105 | Pro → Thr | Val | GSS |
| 105 | Pro → Ser | Val | Atypical GSS |
| 114 | Gly → Val | Met | CJD |
| 117 | Ala → Val | Val | GSS |
| 129 | Met or Val | | Polymorphism |
| 131 | Gly → Val | Met | Atypical GSS |
| 133 | Ala → Val | Met | Atypical GSS |
| 145 | Tyr → Stop | Met | PrP-CAA |
| 148 | Arg → His | Met | CJD |
| 160 | Gln → Stop | Met | GSS |
| 163 | Tyr → Stop | | GSS |
| 171 | Asn → Ser | Val | Polymorphism |
| 178 | Asp → Asn | Val | CJD |
| 178 | Asp → Asn | Met | FFI |
| 180 | Val → Ile | Met | CJD |
| 183 | Thr → Ala | Met | CJD |
| 187 | His → Arg | Val | Atypical[a] |
| 168 | Thr → Lys | ? | CJD |
| 196 | Glu → Lys | Met | CJD |
| 198 | Phe → Ser | Val | GSS w/ NFTs |
| 200 | Glu → Lys | Met/Val | CJD |
| 202 | Asp → Asn | Val | GSS |
| 203 | Val → Ile | Met | CJD |
| 208 | Arg → His | Met | CJD |
| 210 | Val → Ile | Met | CJD |
| 211 | Glu → Gln | Met | CJD |
| 212 | Gln → Pro | Val | GSS |
| 217 | Gln → Arg | Val | GSS w/ NFTs |
| 219 | Glu → Lys | Met | Polymorphism |
| 226 | Tyr → Stop | Val | PrP-CAA |
| 227 | Gln → Stop | Val | GSS |
| 232 | Met → Arg | Met | CJD |
| 238 | Pro → Ser | Met | CJD |

[a]Either early psychiatric symptoms or dementia preceding ataxia with curly PrP deposits.

NFTs, neurofibrillary tangles; CAA, cerebral amyloid angiopathy.

amino-terminal 22 amino acid signal peptide, that directs translocation of PrP into the lumen of the endoplasmic reticulum, is post-translationally cleaved, as is a 23 residue signal sequence on the carboxy terminus prior to addition of a glycoinositol phospholipid (GPI) anchor. Two asparagine-linked glycosylation sites lie within a loop region of the protein created by a disulfide bond. PrP follows the secretory pathway to its destination on the outer leaflet of the plasma membrane. *PRNP* expression is regulated during development and constitutive in the adult. The highest levels of expression are within neurons, but lower levels of PrP are detected in other peripheral tissues including lung, heart, kidney, pancreas, testis, white blood cells, and platelets. Peripheral and central anterograde neuronal transport of PrP$^C$ has also been reported.

The primary function of the nonpathogenic isoform of PrP (PrP$^C$) is unknown, however; evidence exists that PrP may carry out one of several functions including the formation, function, and maintenance of synapses, cell signaling, neuritogenesis, and neuroprotection, copper binding and cellular delivery of copper (via the octapeptide repeat segments); antioxidant activity; cellular adhesion, and; a possible role in immune modulation. PrP knockout mice do not exhibit developmental or behavioral abnormalities, suggesting redundancy of function, although altered synaptic dysfunction within the hippocampus has been reported by some, but not others. More recently, adult PrP knockout mice have been reported to display spatial memory deficits and impaired peripheral nerve myelin maintenance. In recent years, a role for PrP in Alzheimer disease has been suggested, although the data have met with controversy, and the role of PrP appears to be at multiple levels. Initially, PrP$^C$ was reported to play a protective role by suppression of β-secretase, a key enzyme involved in the processing of amyloid precursor protein (APP) that leads to the generation of β-amyloid. In subsequent work by others, PrP$^C$ was suggested to act as a receptor to toxic β-amyloid oligomers, although several subsequent studies have not been able to reproduce that work. In addition to these roles, PrP$^C$ has also been suggested to enhance the generation of extracellular β-amyloid plaques. More studies are needed to clarify this complex relationship between PrP and Alzheimer disease.

***Genetic Testing:*** Not commercially available, but some centers are known to provide testing on a research basis (The National Prion Surveillance Center at Case Western Reserve University, or the Prion Laboratory at the University of Chicago, are two examples).

☞**INDICATIONS FOR TESTING:**

• **Establishing the diagnosis of genetic prion disease**. For the proband or patient with clinical features and diagnostic studies that support the diagnosis of prion disease, genetic testing can provide additional support for the diagnosis if a disease-associated mutation of *PRNP* is detected.

• **Predictive testing for at-risk asymptomatic adult family members**. This requires prior identification of a disease-associated mutation in the family. Genetic counseling and psychiatric consultation should be pursued prior to testing.

• **Prenatal diagnosis and preimplantation genetic diagnosis**. This requires prior identification of an at-risk family member who carries a disease-associated mutation.

**BIBLIOGRAPHY:**

1. Aguzzi A, Calella AM. Prions: protein aggregation and infectious diseases. *Physiol Rev*. 2009;89:1105-1152.

2. Brown K, Mastrianni JA. The prion diseases. *J Geriatr Psychiatry Neurol*. 2010;23:277-298.

3. Heath CA, Cooper SA, Murray K, et al. Diagnosing variant Creutzfeldt-Jakob disease: a retrospective analysis of the first 150 cases in the UK. *J Neurol Neurosurg Psychiatry*. 2011;82:646-651.

4. Isaacs JD, Jackson GS, Altmann DM. The role of the cellular prion protein in the immune system. *Clin Exp Immunol*. 2006;146:1-8.

5. Kovacs GG, Puopolo M, Ladogana A, et al. Genetic prion disease: the EUROCJD experience. *Hum Genet*. 2005;118:166-174.

6. Mastrianni JA. The genetics of prion diseases. *Genet Med*. 2010;12:187-195.

7. Montagna P, Gambetti P, Cortelli P, Lugaresi E. Familial and sporadic fatal insomnia. *Lancet Neurol*. 2003;2:167-176.

8. Prusiner SB. Prions (Les Prix Nobel Lecture). In: Frängsmyr T, ed. *Les Prix Nobel*. Stockholm, Sweden: Almqvist & Wiksell International; 1998:268-323.

9. Sanchez-Juan P, Green A, Ladogana A, et al. CSF tests in the differential diagnosis of Creutzfeldt-Jakob disease. *Neurology*. 2006;67:637-643.

10. Solforosi L, Criado JR, McGavern DB, et al. Cross-linking cellular prion protein triggers neuronal apoptosis in vivo. *Science*. 2004;303:1514-1516.

11. Will RG, Ironside JW, Zeidler M, et al. A new variant of Creutzfeldt-Jakob disease in the UK. *Lancet*. 1996;347:921-925.

## Supplementary Information

**OMIM References:**

[1] PRNP (#176640)

[2] Creutzfeldt-Jakob disease; CJD (#123400)

[3] Gerstmann-Sträussler disease; GSD (#137440)

[4] Huntington disease like-1; HDL1 (#603218)

[5] Insomnia, fatal familial; FFI (#600072)

*Key Words:* Prion disease, Creutzfeldt-Jakob disease, Gerstmann-Sträussler-Scheinker disease, fatal familial insomnia

# 134 The Hereditary Spastic Paraplegias

John K. Fink

## KEY POINTS

- *Disease summary:*
  - The hereditary spastic paraplegias (HSPs) are genetically heterogeneous disorders in which progressive difficulty walking due to spastic weakness of both legs is the predominant neurologic syndrome.
  - HSP clinical syndromes may be limited to difficulty walking due to lower extremity spastic weakness ("uncomplicated HSP") or may include other neurologic or systemic disturbances ("complicated HSP").
  - There may be wide variability in age-of-symptom onset, rate of worsening, degree of disability, and presence (and severity) of additional of neurologic involvement both within and between different genetic types of HSP.
  - Neuropathologic analyses of uncomplicated HSP generally reveals degeneration of corticospinal tract axons that is maximal in the thoracic spinal cord; degeneration of *fasciculus gracilis* fibers that is maximal in the cervicomedullary region; and a degree of demyelination that is considered to be secondary to axon degeneration.
  - Proteins encoded by *HSP* genes have diverse functions including mitochondrial function, axon transport, microtubule processing, protein folding and chaperone, endoplasmic reticulum morphology, and myelin structure.
- *Hereditary basis:*
  - More than 50 genetic types of HSP have been described (Table 134-1). Autosomal dominant, autosomal recessive, X-linked forms of HSP are each genetically heterogeneous. In addition, HSP due to *ATP6* gene mitochondrial gene mutation (and therefore, with maternally inherited HSP) has been recently described.
- *Differential diagnosis:*
  - Many different conditions have overlapping signs and symptoms. The differential diagnosis should include structural abnormalities of the brain and spinal cord, leukodystrophies, inflammatory disorders, metabolic disturbances, and infection.

## Diagnostic Criteria and Clinical Characteristics

### Diagnostic Criteria for Hereditary Spastic Paraplegia:

☞CLINICAL FEATURES: (1) typical clinical course (either nonprogressive [when symptoms begin in infancy] or insidiously progressive [when symptoms begin after infancy]); (2) typical clinical signs (~ symmetric lower extremity spasticity and weakness, often associated with urinary urgency and subtly diminished distal vibration sensation); and (3) careful exclusion of alternate disorders (see Differential Diagnosis, Table 134-2).

☞FAMILY HISTORY IS VARIABLE: The occurrence of similarly affected family members is helpful (but not mandatory) in supporting a clinical diagnosis of HSP. Family history may be entirely absent owing to X-linked or autosomal recessive inheritance, de novo mutation, incomplete genetic penetrance, or variable (including late) age-of-symptom onset.

☞GENETIC TESTING: *HSP* gene sequencing results must be interpreted in light of the clinical context. Identifying a mutation known to be associated with HSP is helpful in confirming a clinical diagnosis in subjects with clinical signs and symptoms of HSP (and for whom alternate diagnoses have been excluded). Conversely, the occurrence of previously unreported *HSP* gene mutations must be interpreted with caution, particularly in subjects with variant clinical syndromes.

*Clinical Characteristics:* *Clinical course:* nonprogressive, insidiously progressive, may reach functional plateau. The primary symptoms of uncomplicated HSP are impaired gait due to lower extremity weakness, increased tone (spasticity), and slowness of movement, frequently accompanied by urinary urgency and mild balance impairment. The course may be either nonprogressive and resemble spastic diplegic cerebral palsy (a common feature of SPG3A HSP); or may be insidiously progressive over many years. Subacute progression over weeks or months is not typical of HSP and suggests alternate disorders. After many years of worsening, it is not uncommon for gait impairment to reach an apparent clinical plateau after which the rate of functional worsening is consistent with effects of age and consequences of limited exertion.

*Neurologic examination* of subjects with "uncomplicated" forms of HSP demonstrates increased tone in the lower extremities (particularly hamstrings, quadriceps, adductors, and gastrocnemius-soleus muscles), weakness (particularly iliopsoas, hamstrings, and tibialis anterior muscles), lower extremity hyper-reflexia that is often, but not always accompanied by extensor plantar responses, and often a mild decrease in distal vibration sensation. Intelligence, cranial nerves, speech, swallowing, and upper extremity strength, tone, and dexterity are normal in uncomplicated HSP. Relative degrees of lower extremity weakness (none to severe) and spasticity (mild to severe) may be variable between individuals.

*Syndrome-specific features of "complicated HSP":* Many genetic types of HSP are sometimes (or usually) associated with additional clinical features. These include ataxia (eg, SPG7 due to paraplegin mutation), mental retardation and thin corpus callosum (eg, SPG11 due to spatacsin mutation), and distal muscle wasting (such as SPG20/spartin mutation, SPG 17/BSCL2 mutation, and SPG 39/NTE mutation).

## Screening and Counseling:

*Screening:* As with other disabling neurologic disorders for which there is no specific treatment, genetic screening of children and adults at risk of inheriting HSP is not recommended.

*Counseling:* The HSPs exhibit broad significant phenotypic variability, genetic penetrance that is age dependent and relatively high (70%-90%) but often incomplete, occasional de novo mutations,

Table 134-1 Genetic Types of HSP (updated from Fink JK, 2011)

| Spastic Gait (SPG) Locus | OMIM Number | Protein (genetic locus if protein is unknown) | Clinical Syndrome |
|---|---|---|---|
| Autosomal dominant HSP | | | |
| SPG3A | 182600 | Atlastin | Uncomplicated HSP: symptoms usually begin in childhood (and may be nonprogressive); symptoms may also begin in adolescence or adulthood and worsen insidiously. Genetic nonpenetrance reported. *De novo* mutation reported presenting as spastic diplegic cerebral palsy. |
| SPG4 | 128601 | Spastin | Uncomplicated HSP, symptom onset in infancy through senescence, single most common cause of autosomal dominant HSP (~40%); some subjects have late-onset cognitive impairment. |
| SPG6 | 600363 | Not imprinted in Prader-Willi/Angelman 1 (NIPA1) | Uncomplicated HSP: prototypical late-adolescent, early-adult onset, slowly progressive uncomplicated HSP |
| SPG8 | 603563 | KIAA0196/ strumpellin | Uncomplicated HSP |
| SPG9 | 601162 | (10q23.3-q24.2) | Complicated: spastic paraplegia associated with cataracts, gastroesophageal reflux, and motor neuronopathy |
| SPG10 | 604187 | Kinesin heavy chain (KIF5A) | Uncomplicated HSP or complicated by distal muscle atrophy |
| SPG12 | 604805 | Reticulon 2 (RTN2) | Uncomplicated HSP |
| SPG13 | 605280 | Chaperonin 60 (heat shock protein 60, HSP60) | Uncomplicated HSP: adolescent and adult onset |
| SPG17 | 270685 | BSCL2/seipin | Complicated: spastic paraplegia associated with amyotrophy of hand muscles (Silver Syndrome) |
| SPG19 | 607152 | (9q33-q34) | Uncomplicated HSP |
| SPG29 | 609727 | (1p31.1-21.1) | Complicated: spastic paraplegia associated with hearing impairment; persistent vomiting due to hiatal hernia inherited |
| SPG31 | 610250 | Receptor expression enhancing protein 1 (REEP1) | Uncomplicated HSP or occasionally associated with peripheral neuropathy |
| SPG33 | 610244 | ZFYVE27/protrudin | Uncomplicated HSP |
| SPG36 | 613096 | (12q23-24) | Onset age 14 to 28 years, associated with motor sensory neuropathy |
| SPG37 | 611945 | (8p21.1-q13.3) | Uncomplicated HSP |
| SPG38 | 612335 | (4p16-p15) | One family, 5 affected subjects, onset age 16-21 years. Subjects had atrophy of intrinsic hand muscles (severe in one subject at age 58) |
| SPG40 | (No OMIM #) | (Locus unknown) | Uncomplicated spastic paraplegia, onset after age 35, known autosomal dominant HSP loci excluded |
| SPG41 | 613364 | (11p14.1-p11.2) | Single Chinese family with adolescent onset, spastic paraplegia associated with mild weakness of intrinsic hand muscles |
| SPG42 | 612539 | Acetyl CoA transporter (SLC33A1) | Uncomplicated spastic paraplegia reported in single kindred, onset age 4-40 years, possibly one instance of incomplete penetrance |
| Autosomal recessive HSP | | | |
| SPG5 | 270800 | CYP7B1 | Uncomplicated or complicated by axonal neuropathy, distal or generalized muscle atrophy, and white matter abnormalities on MRI |

(Continued)

*Table 134-1  Genetic Types of HSP (updated from Fink JK, 2011)  (Continued)*

| Spastic Gait (SPG) Locus | OMIM Number | Protein (genetic locus if protein is unknown) | Clinical Syndrome |
|---|---|---|---|
| SPG7 | 607259 | Paraplegin | Uncomplicated or complicated: variably associated with mitochondrial abnormalities on skeletal muscle biopsy and dysarthria, dysphagia, optic disc pallor, axonal neuropathy, and evidence of "vascular lesions", cerebellar atrophy, or cerebral atrophy on cranial MRI |
| SPG11 | 604360 | Spatacsin (KIAA1840) | Uncomplicated or complicated: spastic paraplegia variably associated with thin corpus callosum, mental retardation, upper extremity weakness, dysarthria, and nystagmus; may have "Kjellin syndrome": childhood onset, progressive spastic paraplegia accompanied by pigmentary retinopathy, mental retardation, dysarthria, dementia, and distal muscle atrophy; juvenile, slowly progressive ALS reported in subjects with SPG11 HSP; 50% of autosomal recessive HSP is considered to be SPG11 |
| SPG14 | 605229 | (3q27-28) | Single consanguineous Italian family, 3 affected subjects, onset age ~30 years; complicated spastic paraplegia with mental retardation and distal motor neuropathy (sural nerve biopsy was normal) |
| SPG15 | 270700 | Spastizin/ZFYVE26 | Complicated: spastic paraplegia variably associated with pigmented maculopathy, distal amyotrophy, dysarthria, mental retardation, and further intellectual deterioration (Kjellin syndrome). |
| SPG18 | 611225 | ERLIN2 | Three families described. One with childhood-onset intellectual and motor disability and contractures; one with and spastic paraplegia complicated by mental retardation and thin corpus callosum; one with spastic paraplegia, mental retardation, and epilepsy |
| SPG20 | 275900 | Spartin | Complicated: spastic paraplegia associated with distal muscle wasting (Troyer syndrome) |
| SPG21 | 248900 | Maspardin | Complicated: spastic paraplegia associated with dementia, cerebellar and extrapyramidal signs, thin corpus callosum, and white matter abnormalities (Mast syndrome) |
| SPG23 | 270750 | (1q24-q32) | Complicated: childhood-onset HSP associated with skin pigment abnormality (vitiligo), premature graying, characteristic facies; Lison syndrome |
| SPG24 | 607584 | (13q14) | Complicated: childhood-onset HSP variably complicated by spastic dysarthria and pseudobulbar signs |
| SPG25 | 608220 | (6q23-q24.1) | Consanguineous Italian family, four subjects with adult (30-46 year)-onset back and neck pain related to disk herniation and spastic paraplegia; surgical correction of disk herniation ameliorated pain and reduced spastic paraplegia. Peripheral neuropathy also present. |
| SPG26 | 609195 | (12p11.1–12q14) | Single consanguineous Bedouin family with five affected subjects. Complicated: childhood onset (between 7 and 8 years), progressive spastic paraparesis with dysarthria and distal amyotrophy in both upper and lower limbs, nerve conduction studies were normal; mild intellectual impairment, normal brain MRI. |
| SPG27 | 609041 | (10q22.1-q24.1) | Complicated or uncomplicated HSP. Two families described. In one family (7 affected subjects) uncomplicated spastic paraplegia began between ages 25 and 45 years. In the second family (three subjects described) the disorder began in childhood and included spastic paraplegia, ataxia, dysarthria, mental retardation, sensorimotor polyneuropathy, facial dysmorphism, and short stature. |

*(Continued)*

**Table 134-1** *Genetic Types of HSP (updated from Fink JK, 2011)* *(Continued)*

| Spastic Gait (SPG) Locus | OMIM Number | Protein (genetic locus if protein is unknown) | Clinical Syndrome |
|---|---|---|---|
| SPG28 | 609340 | (14q21.3-q22.3) | Uncomplicated: childhood-onset progressive spastic gait |
| SPG29 | 609727 | (14q) | Uncomplicated HSP, childhood onset |
| SPG30 | 610357 | (2q37.3) | Complicated: spastic paraplegia, distal wasting, saccadic ocular pursuit, peripheral neuropathy, mild cerebellar signs |
| SPG32 | 611252 | (14q12-q21) | Mild mental retardation, brainstem dysraphia, clinically asymptomatic cerebellar atrophy |
| SPG35 | 612319 | Fatty acid 2-hydroxylase (FA2H) | Childhood onset (6-11 years), spastic paraplegia with extrapyramidal features, progressive dysarthria, dementia, seizures. Brain white matter abnormalities and brain iron accumulation; an Omani and a Pakistani kindred reported. |
| SPG39 | 612020 | Neuropathy target esterase (NTE) | Complicated: spastic paraplegia associated with wasting of distal upper and lower extremity muscles |
| SPG43 | (No OMIM #) | C19orf12 | Two sisters from Mali, symptom onset 7 and 12 years, progressive spastic paraplegia with atrophy of intrinsic hand muscles and dysarthria (one sister) |
| SPG44 | 613206 | Gap junction protein GJA12/GJC2, also known as connexin47 (Cx47) | Allelic with "Pelizaeus-Merzbacher-like disease" (PMLD, early-onset dysmyelinating disorder with nystagmus, psychomotor delay, progressive spasticity, ataxia). GJA/GJC2 mutation I33M causes a milder phenotype: late-onset (first and second decades), cognitive impairment, slowly progressive, spastic paraplegia, dysarthria, and upper extremity involvement. MRI and MR spectroscopy imaging consistent with a hypomyelinating leukoencephalopathy |
| SPG45 | 613162 | (10q24.3-q25.1) | Single consanguineous kindred from Turkey, five subjects described: affected subjects had mental retardation, infantile onset lower extremity spasticity and contractures, one subject with optic atrophy, two subjects with pendular nystagmus; MRI in one subject was normal. |
| SPG46 | 614409 | (9p21.2-q21.12) | Dementia, congenital cataract, ataxia, thin corpus callosum |
| SPG47 | See 603513 | AP4B1 | Two affected siblings from consanguineous Arabic family with early childhood onset slowly progressive spastic paraparesis, mental retardation, and seizures; one subject had ventriculomegaly; the other subject had thin corpus callosum and periventricular white matter abnormalities |
| SPG48 | 613647 | KIAA0415 | Analysis of *KIAA0415* gene in 166 unrelated spastic paraplegia subjects (38 recessive, 64 dominant, 64 "apparently sporadic") and control subjects revealed homozygous mutation in two siblings with late onset (6th decade) uncomplicated spastic paraplegia; and heterozygous mutation in one subject with apparently sporadic spastic paraplegia. |
| "SPOAN" syndrome | 609541 | (11q23) | Complicated: spastic paraplegia, optic atrophy, neuropathy (SPOAN) |
| No SPG designation | 256840 | Epsilon subunit of the cytosolic chaperonin-containing t-complex peptide-1 (Cct5) | Complicated spastic paraplegia associated with mutilating sensory neuropathy. |
| X-linked HSP | | | |
| SPG1 | 303350 | L1 cell adhesion molecule (L1CAM) | Complicated: associated with mental retardation, and variably, hydrocephalus, aphasia, and adducted thumbs |
| SPG2 | 312920 | Proteolipid protein | Complicated: variably associated with MRI evidence of CNS white matter abnormality; may have peripheral neuropathy |

*(Continued)*

**Table 134-1** *Genetic Types of HSP (updated from Fink JK, 2011)* *(Continued)*

| Spastic Gait (SPG) Locus | OMIM Number | Protein (genetic locus if protein is unknown) | Clinical Syndrome |
|---|---|---|---|
| SPG16 | 300266 | (Xq11.2-q23) | Uncomplicated or complicated: associated with motor aphasia, reduced vision, nystagmus, mild mental retardation, and dysfunction of the bowel and bladder |
| SPG22 | 300523 | Monocarboxylate transport 8 (MCT8) | Complicated (Allan-Herndon-Dudley syndrome): congenital onset, neck muscle hypotonia in infancy, mental retardation, dysarthria, ataxia, spastic paraplegia, abnormal facies |
| SPG34 | 300750 | (Xq24-25) | Uncomplicated, onset 12 to 25 years |
| Maternal (mitochondrial) inheritance HSP | | | |
| No SPG designation | (No OMIM #) | Mitochondrial *ATP6* gene | Adult onset, progressive spastic paraplegia, mild-to-severe symptoms, variably associated with axonal neuropathy, late-onset dementia, cardiomyopathy |

and occasionally, apparent genetic anticipation (in SPG3A and SPG4 HSP).

Significant phenotypic variability between genetic types of HSP (as well as within a given genetic type and even between affected individuals in the same family) may include wide differences in age-of-symptom onset (eg, childhood vs senescence), degree of severity (subtle hyper-reflexia vs disabling paraplegia), and the occurrence and severity of "complicating" features. For example, individuals with SPG7 HSP may or may not exhibit ataxia; those with SPG11 HSP may or may not exhibit cognitive impairment; and those with SPG10 may or may not exhibit distal muscle wasting.

Caution must be exercised in predicting whether the disorder will be early or late onset, cause mild or severe symptoms, or be associated with additional neurologic symptoms. A cautious, "wait and see" approach is recommended. Without genetic test results

indicating a particular type of HSP, caution must be exercised in estimating disease recurrence in progeny of subjects from families in which the disorder affects only siblings (because the disorder could be autosomal recessive or autosomal dominant with incomplete genetic penetrance). Phenotypes of only a few types of HSP (eg, SPG3A, SPG4, SPG7, and SPG11) have been well elaborated through descriptions of many subjects. Caution must be used in providing genetic counseling and prognosis for subjects for whom the genetic type is unknown, and for subjects with genetic types for which only limited clinical descriptions are available. Genetic counseling of subjects with SPG7 HSP must recognize that some *SPG7* mutations may cause either autosomal recessive or autosomal dominant HSP.

☞GENOTYPE-PHENOTYPE CORRELATION: Very little is known about genotype-phenotype correlation for most *HSP*

**Table 134-2** *Differential Diagnosis of Hereditary Spastic Paraplegia (adapted from)*

| Category | Examples (not inclusive) |
|---|---|
| Structural abnormalities of the brain or spinal cord | Tethered cord syndrome, spinal cord compression, parasagittal mass |
| Leukodystrophy | $B_{12}$ deficiency, adrenomyeloneuropathy, late-onset Krabbe disease, metachromatic leukodystrophy, Pelizeaus-Merzbacher disease, mitochondrial disorder |
| Inflammatory disorders | Paraneoplastic disorders, transverse myelitis, multiple sclerosis |
| Other motor neuron disorders | Amyotrophic lateral sclerosis, primary lateral sclerosis |
| Other neurodegenerative disorders | Mitochondrial disorder, spinocerebellar ataxia type 3 (Machado-Joseph disease), Friedreich ataxia, familial Alzheimer disease due to amyloid precursor protein or presenilin 1 or 2 gene mutation, Charlevoix-Saguenay (autosomal recessive, spastic ataxia) |
| Metabolic disturbance | Dopa-responsive dystonia, homocysteine remethylation defects (due to methylene tetrahydrofolate reductase [MTHFR] deficiency and cobalamin C disease), urea cycle defects (in particular, arginase deficiency and hyperornithinemia-hyperammonemia-homocitrullinuria), biotinidase deficiency, phenylketonuria |
| | Nonketotic hyperglycinemia, cerebral folate deficiency, homocarnosinosis, cerebrotendinous xanthomatosis, Sjögren-Larsson syndrome, polyglucosan body disease, nucleoside phosphorylase deficiency |
| Infection | Human immunodeficiency virus (HIV AIDS) |
| | Tropical spastic paraplegia (also known as human T-cell leukemia virus 1 [HTLV1]-associated myelopathy) |

gene mutations. Although some genetic types are usually associated with uncomplicated syndromes (eg, SPG3A or SPG4) and others typically associated with complicated syndromes (eg, SPG7 and SPG11), it is not uncommon for both complicated and uncomplicated syndromes to occur in a given genetic type of HSP. Indeed, sometimes complicating features (such as mental retardation or ataxia) may be present in one but not all affected subjects in a given family.

## Management and Treatment

Presently, there are no treatments that stop, reverse, or prevent nerve degeneration in HSP. For some subjects, reducing muscle spasticity may improve gait and reduce discomfort. Oral or intrathecal Lioresal or oral dantrolene or tizanidine and selective injection of botulinum toxin (Botox) may be helpful in this regard. Antispasticity medications provide greatest functional gait improvement in subjects with significant spasticity but only mild degrees of weakness. Conversely, excessive reduction of muscle spasticity in subjects with significant lower extremity weakness may worsen gait. Urinary urgency may be reduced with medications including oxybutynin.

Ankle-foot orthotic devices and gait-phase dependent, transcutaneous peroneal nerve stimulation may be useful in reducing toe-dragging. A daily regimen of physical therapy including stretching under the guidance of trained physical therapist or personnel trainer is generally recommended to maintain and improve cardiovascular conditioning, improve range of motion, maintain and increase lower extremity strength, and improve balance.

## Molecular Genetics and Molecular Mechanisms

Functional diversity of the encoded proteins of 28 discovered *HSP* genes implicates the following cellular and molecular processes in HSP pathogenesis: (1) disturbance in axon transport (eg, SPG10/KIF5A and possibly SPG4/Spastin), (2) disturbance in the development of endoplasmic reticulum morphology (eg, SPG3A/atlastin, SPG4/spastin, SPG12/reticulon 2, and SPG31/REEP1, all of which interact), (3) abnormal mitochondrial function (eg, SPG13/chaperonin 60/heat shock protein 60, SPG7/paraplegin, and mitochondrial ATP6), (4) primary myelin abnormality (eg, SPG2/proteolipid protein and SPG42/connexin 47), (5) protein degradation (eg, SPG18/ERLIN2) and misfolding leading to endoplasmic reticulum-stress response (SPG6/NIPA1, SPG8, SGP17/BSCL2, seipin, and "mutilating sensory neuropathy with spastic paraplegia" due to *CcT5* mutation), and (6) disturbance in corticospinal tract and other neurodevelopment (eg, SPG1/L1 cell adhesion molecule and SPG22/thyroid transporter MCT8).

*Genetic Testing:* Analysis of the subset of *HSP* genes for which clinical analysis is presently available (SPG2/PLP, SPG3A/atlastin, SPG4/spastin, SPG6/NIPA1, SPG7/paraplegin, SPG8/KIAA0196 [strumpellin], SPG11/spatacsin, SPG17/BSCL2, SPG31/REEP1) can identify mutations in approximately 75% of subjects with autosomal dominant HSP and approximately 20% of subjects with autosomal recessive HSP. Mutations in autosomal dominant or autosomal recessive HSP genes are identified in approximately 10% to 20% of subjects with no previous family history.

**BIBLIOGRAPHY:**

1. Fink JK. Hereditary spastic paraplegia. In: Rimoin D, Connor JM, Pyeritz RE, Korf BR, eds. 6th ed. Philadelphia, PA: Churchill Livingstone Elsevier; 2011.

2. Sedel F, Fontaine B, Saudubray JM, Lyon-Caen O. Hereditary spastic paraparesis in adults associated with inborn errors of metabolism: a diagnostic approach. *J Inherit Metab Dis.* 2007;30(6):855-864.

3. Durr A, Davoine C-S, Paternotte C, et al. Phenotype of autosomal dominant spastic paraplegia linked to chromosome 2. *Brain.* 1996;119:1487-1496.

4. Reddy PL, Seltzer WK, Grewal RP. Possible anticipation in hereditary spastic paraplegia type 4 (SPG4). *Can J Neurol Sci.* 2007;34(2):208-210.

5. Nielsen JE, Koefoed P, Abell K, et al. CAG repeat expansion in autosomal dominant pure spastic paraplegia linked to chromosome 2p21-p24. *Hum Mol Genet.* 1997;6:1811-1816.

6. Raskind WH, Pericak-Vance MA, Lennon F, Wolff J, Lipe HP, Bird TD. Familial spastic paraparesis: evaluation of locus heterogeneity, anticipation, and haplotype mapping of the SPG4 locus on the short arm of chromosome 2. *Am J Med Genet.* 1997; 74:26-36.

7. Burger J, Metzke H, Paternotte C, Schilling F, Hazan J, Reis A. Autosomal dominant spastic paraplegia with anticipation maps to a 4-cM interval on chromosome 2p21-p24 in a large German family. *Hum Genet.* 1996;98:371-375.

8. Raskind WH, Pericak-Vance MA, Lennon F, Wolff J, Lipe HP, Bird TD. Familial spastic paraparesis: evaluation of locus heterogeneity, anticipation and haplotype mapping of the SPG4 locus on the short arm of chromosome 2. *Am J Hum Genet.* 1997;74:26-36.

9. Xia CH, Roberts EA, Her LS, et al. Abnormal neurofilament transport caused by targeted disruption of neuronal kinesin heavy chain K1F5A. *J Cell Biol.* 2003;161:55-66.

10. Kasher PR, De Vos KJ, Wharton SB, et al. Direct evidence for axonal transport defects in a novel mouse model of mutant spastin-induced hereditary spastic paraplegia (HSP) and human HSP patients. *J Neurochem.* 2009;110(1):34-44.

11. Hansen JJ, Durr A, Cournu-Rebeix I, et al. Hereditary spastic paraplegia SPG13 is associated with a mutation in the gene encoding the mitochondrial chaperonin Hsp60. *Am J Hum Genet.* 2002;70:1328-1332.

12. Atorino L, Silvestri L, Koppen M, et al. Loss of m-AAA protease in mitochondria causes complex I deficiency and increased sensitivity to oxidative stress in hereditary spastic paraplegia. *J Cell Biol.* 2003;163:777-787.

13. Ferreirinha F, Quattrini A, Pirozzi M, et al. Axonal degeneration in paraplegin-deficient mice is associated with abnormal mitochondria and impairment of axonal transport. *J Clin Invest.* 2004;113:231-242.

14. Wilkinson PA, Crosby AH, Turner C, et al. A clinical and genetic study of SPG5A linked autosomal recessive hereditary spastic paraplegia. *Neurology.* 2003;61:235-238.

15. Casari G, Fusco M, Ciarmatori S, et al. Spastic paraplegia and OXPHOS impairment caused by mutations in paraplegin, a nuclear-encoded mitochondrial metalloprotease. *Cell.* 1998; 93:973-983.

16. Alazami AM, Adly N, Al DH, Alkuraya FS. A nullimorphic ERLIN2 mutation defines a complicated Hereditary Spastic Paraplegia locus (SPG18). *Neurogenetics.* Nov 2011;12(4):333-336.

17. Zhao J, Matthies DS, Botzolakis EJ, Macdonald RL, Blakely RD, Hedera P. Hereditary spastic paraplegia-associated mutations in the NIPA1 gene and its Caenorhabditis elegans homolog trigger

neural degeneration in vitro and in vivo through a gain-of-function mechanism. *J Neurosci.* 2008;28:13938-13951.

18. Clemen CS, Tangavelou K, Strucksberg KH, et al. Strumpellin is a novel valosin-containing protein binding partner linking hereditary spastic paraplegia to protein aggregation diseases. *Brain.* 2010;133(10):2920-2941.

19. Ito D, Suzuki N. Seipinopathy: a novel endoplasmic reticulum stress-associated disease. *Brain.* 2009;132(pt 1):8-15.

20. Ito D, Suzuki N. [Seipin/BSCL2-related motor neuron disease: seipinopathy is a novel conformational disease associated with endoplasmic reticulum stress]. *Rinsho Shinkeigaku.* 2007;47(6): 329-335.

21. Ito D, Fujisawa T, Iida H, Suzuki N. Characterization of seipin/BSCL2, a protein associated with spastic paraplegia 17. *Neurobiol Dis.* 2008;31(2):266-277.

22. Bouhouche A, Benomar A, Bouslam N, Chkili T, Yahyaoui M. Mutation in the epsilon subunit of the cytosolic chaperonin-containing t-complex peptide-1 (Cct5) gene causes autosomal recessive mutilating sensory neuropathy with spastic paraplegia. *J Med Genet.* 2006;43(5):441-443.

**ACKNOWLEDGEMENT:**
We gratefully acknowledge the support of the National Institutes of Health (R01 NS069700), Department of Veterans Affairs (Merit Review Award), the Spastic Paraplegia Foundation, the Geriatric Research Education and Clinical Center, Ann Arbor Veterans Affairs Medical Center, the generous support from the Katzman Family Fund, and the participation of subjects with hereditary spastic paraplegia and their family members.

## Supplementary Information

**Alternative Names:**
- Hereditary Spastic Paraparesis
- Familial Spastic Paraparesis
- Strumpell-Lorrain syndrome

*Key Words:* Spastic paraplegia, myelopathy, axon degeneration, motor neuron disease

# 135 Dystrophinopathies

Huma Q. Rana, Amy Yang, and Lakshmi Mehta

## KEY POINTS

- *Disease summary:*
  - The term dystrophinopathy encompasses three interrelated diseases: Duchenne muscular dystrophy (DMD), Becker muscular dystrophy (BMD), and DMD-associated dilated cardiomyopathy.
  - DMD has an incidence of approximately 1:4000 live male births and presents in early childhood with progressive proximal muscle weakness leading to loss of ambulation and, cardiomyopathy in the second decade with death in the third decade due to cardiorespiratory compromise. BMD causes later onset of muscle weakness with cardiomyopathy being the most common cause of death in the fourth to fifth decades. DMD-associated dilated cardiomyopathy is common in both phenotypes and may also be present in female carriers of *DMD* mutations.
  - Dystrophinopathies result from mutations in the *DMD* gene on Xp21.2 causing a reduced or deficient amount of dystrophin, a membrane-bound protein expressed in skeletal, cardiac, smooth muscle, and neurons. The type of mutation determines the amount of residual protein and the phenotype.

- *Hereditary basis:*
  - Deletions, duplications, insertions, and point mutations in the *DMD* gene, on Xp21.2, cause the dystrophinopathies.
  - Inheritance is X-linked and there is complete penetrance in males who inherit the mutation.
  - Manifestations in female heterozygotes including muscle weakness, myalgias, and cardiomyopathy, are usually due to skewed X-inactivation. In rare circumstances, females can have classic DMD or BMD. In these individuals a structural abnormality of the X chromosome should be ruled out.
  - One-third of mutations are *de novo*, and are not inherited.

- *Differential diagnosis:*
  - When considering the diagnosis of muscular dystrophy, the differential should include facioscapulohumeral muscular dystrophy, limb-girdle muscular dystrophy, Emery-Dreifuss muscular dystrophy, and dilated cardiomyopathy (Table 135-1).

## Diagnostic Criteria and Clinical Characteristics

### Diagnostic Criteria for Dystrophinopathies:
**Diagnostic evaluation should include the following**
- Three-generation pedigree to identify affected or at-risk family members
- Physical examination with particular attention paid to gait, ability to run and jump, proximal muscle weakness, calf hypertrophy, and Gower sign. Fasciculations are absent.
- Creatine kinase level
  - Elevated to greater than 10× normal in DMD
  - Elevated to greater than 5× normal in BMD
  - Increased in DMD-associated dilated cardiomyopathy
- DNA testing for deletion, duplication, or mutation of *DMD*. If no mutation identified, muscle biopsy with evaluation of histology and immunostaining for dystrophin

### Clinical Spectrum of Dystrophinopathies:
☞**Duchenne Muscular Dystrophy:** Symmetric muscle weakness worse in proximal muscles, calf hypertrophy, symptom onset less than 5 years of age, Gower sign, intellectual disability, loss of ambulation or wheelchair dependence by 13 years of age without treatment, dilated cardiomyopathy by age 18.

☞**Becker Muscular Dystrophy:** Symmetric muscle weakness as above but with milder, later onset; can present with muscle cramping with exercise, distal muscle hypertrophy; isolated quadriceps weakness; no cognitive impairment; loss of ambulation or wheelchair dependence after 16 years of age; preservation of neck flexor muscles; variable age of onset of dilated cardiomyopathy from mid-20s to mid-40s.

☞**Intermediate Phenotype:** Loss of ambulation or wheelchair dependence between 13 and 16 years of age.

☞**Female Heterozygotes of DMD Mutations:** Wide phenotypic variability ranging from asymptomatic to significant muscle disease. Up to 20% are thought to develop dilated cardiomyopathy.

☞**DMD-Associated Dilated Cardiomyopathy:** No or subclinical skeletal muscle involvement; dilated cardiomyopathy; may present with congestive heart failure, arrhythmias, or thromboembolic disease; age of onset later in women than men.

☞**Contiguous Gene Deletion Syndromes:** Xp21 deletions that include the *DMD* gene.

*Proximal deletion:* DMD with McLeod syndrome, chronic granulomatous disease, and/or retinitis pigmentosa.

*Distal deletion:* DMD with adrenal hypoplasia congenita and glycerol kinase deficiency.

## Screening and Counseling

### Screening:
See Fig. 135-1 for diagnostic screening.

☞**Carrier Screening:** No population wide carrier or newborn screening is currently recommended. Women who are at risk for being carriers of DMD mutations can be offered targeted mutation analysis if the familial mutation is known. If unknown, DMD deletion/duplication analysis and sequencing may be offered.

### Genetic Counseling:
Dystrophinopathies follow X-linked recessive inheritance and are fully penetrant in males, causing the Duchenne, Becker, or cardiomyopathy phenotypes. A *DMD* mutation may be inherited from a carrier mother, may arise spontaneously as a new

*Table 135-1 Genetic Differential Diagnosis*

| Syndrome | Genes/Loci | Associated Features |
|---|---|---|
| Facioscapulohumeral muscular dystrophy | Deletion of tandem repeats termed D4Z4 on 4q35 | Autosomal dominant inheritance; distal muscle involvement: scapular winging, facial weakness, foot drop, normal-to-elevated creatine kinase |
| Limb-girdle muscular dystrophy | Extensive locus heterogeneity | Recessive and dominant forms exist; progressive proximal muscle weakness with predominant shoulder and hip involvement, elevated creatine kinase |
| Emery-Dreifuss muscular dystrophy | *EMD* *FHL1* *LMNA* | X-linked, dominant and recessive forms exist with phenotypic heterogeneity. Contractures of elbows, Achilles tendons, spine, followed by muscular weakness and then cardiac conduction abnormalities and DCM; onset often before 20 years; normal-to-elevated creatine kinase |
| Dilated Cardiomyopathy (DCM) | Extensive locus heterogeneity | X-linked, dominant and recessive forms exist; left ventricular enlargement and systolic dysfunction |

mutation, or may be inherited because of mosaicism in the mother. The mother of a male proband has a two-thirds chance of being a carrier, one-third of mutations are *de novo*. Males with Duchenne muscular dystrophy are unlikely to reproduce. Males with Becker or DMD-associated DCM will pass on their X chromosome to their daughters who will be obligate carriers; none of their sons will be affected. Female carriers have a 50% chance of passing on the X chromosome with the *DMD* mutation, and a 50% chance of passing on the normal X chromosome. If the mother of a proband tests negative for a causative mutation, there is an empiric 15% to 20% chance that she may be mosaic for the mutation in germ cells (gonadal mosaicism) or somatic cells.

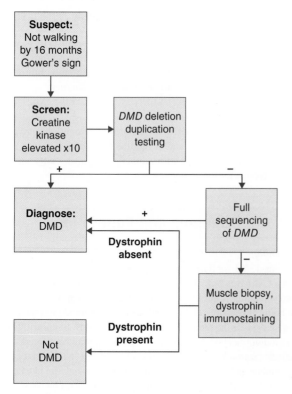

*Figure 135-1* Screening and Diagnosis of DMD.

Prenatal diagnosis for carriers of *DMD* mutations is available by chorionic villus sampling at 10 to 12 weeks gestation or amniocentesis at 16 weeks gestation, if the causative mutation in the family is known. Mothers of affected sons, who test negative, should be offered prenatal testing given the chance of gonadal or somatic mosaicism. Preimplantation genetic diagnosis may be an option if the causative mutation is known.

In families where the causative mutation is undetectable by molecular testing and where the diagnosis has been established by other means, linkage analysis using DNA from informative relatives may provide a means of obtaining prenatal diagnosis or diagnosis of carriers.

☞**GENOTYPE-PHENOTYPE CORRELATION:** The type of *DMD* mutation correlates with phenotype of the dystrophinopathy.

- Larger deletions tend to be more severe and predict a DMD phenotype.
- Mutations that alter the reading frame of the gene (out of frame) tend to predict a DMD phenotype, with an accuracy rate of 91% to 92%. Approximately 9% of mutations, especially duplications, do not obey the reading-frame rule.
- Deletions involving the cysteine-rich domain or a significant portion of the N-terminal actin binding domain are associated with a DMD phenotype.
- Deletions within the central rod domain cause a mild phenotype of muscle cramps and fatigue.
- Mutations or deletions that affect the muscle promoter, muscle exon 1, the hinge region, or select exons within the central rod domain cause dilated cardiomyopathy. Deletions within the muscle promoter or exon 1 cause lack of dystrophin in the heart muscle. The skeletal muscle is spared by activating the distal promoters normally active in the brain and Purkinje cells.
- Contiguous gene deletions—Larger deletions can involve genes proximal (5') or distal (3') to the *DMD* gene, causing contiguous gene deletion syndromes. At the proximal end, deletions involving the *XK, CYBB, RPGR,* and *OTC* genes can cause McLeod syndrome, chronic granulomatosis, cone-rod dystrophy, and ornithine transcarbamylase deficiency, respectively. Distally, deletions encompassing the *GK* and *NR0B1* genes manifest with glycerol kinase deficiency and adrenal hypoplasia, respectively.

## Management and Treatment

**Monitoring:**

- Developmental evaluation at diagnosis or as needed
- Cardiology evaluation including ECG and echocardiogram
  - At diagnosis
  - Ages 6 to 10: every 2 years
  - Age 10 and after: annual
  - BMD: every 2 years, beginning at age 10
  - Female carriers: baseline in late adolescence or early adulthood. Starting 25 to 30 years, every 5 years
- Cardiorespiratory evaluations prior to any surgery
- Bone health
  - Measure calcium, phosphorus, alkaline phosphatase, 25-OHD biannually
  - DEXA scan baseline at 3 years or start of steroid therapy. Repeat annually in high-risk patients
- Pulmonary
  - Pulmonary function tests at age 9 to 10 years (prior to loss of ambulation)
  - Twice yearly after age 12 years or if wheelchair bound, vital capacity less than 80%
- Orthopedic: monitor for scoliosis and contractures

**Management:** Management is largely supportive. However, concerted efforts have been made to provide standardized guidelines for care, by collaborators such as the TREAT-NMD EU network in Europe and the CDC (Centers for Disease Control) and MDA (Muscular Dystrophy Association) in the United States. Early and accurate diagnosis facilitates interventions and supportive care as well as genetic counseling for the family. Treatment should be through multidisciplinary clinics with appropriate expertise and significant commitment from families is necessary.

☞**CORTICOSTEROID THERAPY:** The only measure shown to slow progression of muscle weakness and delay loss of ambulation. Mechanism of action is unclear but includes anti-inflammatory or immunosuppressive effects. Prednisone at 0.75 mg/kg/d daily or deflazacort at 0.9 mg/kg/d has been shown to provide the best risk-benefit profile. Primary goals are to preserve ambulation and reduce cardiorespiratory and orthopedic complications. Steroid therapy is best initiated at the "plateau" phase of motor function, which often occurs at 4 to 6 years of age. However, steroids used even after loss of ambulation may have benefit in delaying cardiorespiratory decline. Numerous studies have evaluated dosing versus side effects. Lower doses of prednisone at 0.35 mg/kg/d (necessitated by weight gain or older age) have also been shown to have benefit, though effects are less robust. The following side effects of steroid therapy require regular monitoring: weight gain, hypertension, behavioral changes, glucose intolerance, gastroesophageal reflux disease (GERD), and gastrointestinal effects, bone involvement.

☞**CARDIAC CARE FOR DCM:** Early after load reduction therapy may improve myocardial function. There is no general consensus on when to initiate therapy, but several centers recommend starting angiotensin-converting enzyme (ACE) inhibitors at 5 to 10 years of age, or when echocardiogram suggests subclinical deterioration. Addition of beta-blockers is suggested when progressive echocardiographic deterioration occurs.

☞**PHYSICAL THERAPY:** Regular exercise and physical therapy promotes mobility and prevents contractures. Assistive and adaptive devices are needed to maintain mobility.

☞**VACCINE PROPHYLAXIS:** Routine vaccinations should be completed prior to initiation of steroid therapy. Pneumococcal and influenza vaccines should be taken annually.

☞**NUTRITION:** Balanced diet with adequate vitamin D and calcium intake.

☞**MANAGEMENT OF ADVANCED DISEASE:** Focus is on cardiopulmonary care, nutritional support, use of assisted ventilation as needed, and treatment of congestive heart failure.

☞**PSYCHOSOCIAL SUPPORT:** For patients, caretakers, and family considerations include advanced directives and end-of-life care planning. Palliative care consultation may be helpful.

**Clinical Trials:** DMD has been a major target for development of therapeutic strategies for genetic muscular dystrophies. Despite multiple clinical trials, there is as yet no effective molecular therapy.

☞**GENE AND CELL THERAPY:** Challenges remain the large size of the dystrophin gene, the large mass of target tissue, the lack of efficient gene vectors, and immunologic responses to cell grafts. Other molecular strategies include

*Rescue agents* targeted to nonsense mutations or deletions: antisense oligonucleotides to induce exon skipping.

*Read through* of stop codons: phase 2 human trials of PTC124 did not achieve sufficient clinical significance.

*Substitution of other proteins:* upregulation of utrophin, use of membrane stabilizers such as biglycan, block polymer P188.

*Enhancement of regeneration*—IGF1, myostatin inhibitors.

Information is available on the status of various clinical trials at www.clinicaltrials.gov.

## Molecular Genetics and Molecular Mechanism

**Syndrome/Gene/Locus:** DMD, BMD, DMD-associated DCM/ *DMD*/Xp21.2

The *DMD* gene is the largest known human gene and spans over 2.2 Mb in size, coding an mRNA with over 79 exons. It has at least four promoters, with many resultant isoforms. Due to its size, the mutation rate is higher in the *DMD* gene than average. More than 5000 different mutations have been described to date, most of which are listed in the Leiden Duchenne Muscular Dystrophy Mutation Database (www.dmd.nl). The full-sized dystrophin protein (427kD) has various distinct domains: the N-terminal actin-binding domain, 4 hinge regions, 24 spectrin-like units that form the central rod domain, a cysteine-rich domain, and a C-terminal domain. The N-terminal interacts with the intracellular actin, and the cysteine-rich domain binds to membrane proteins which interact with the extracellular matrix. Thus, dystrophin acts as a critical bridge between the intra- and extracellular architectures of the tissue in which it is expressed.

Over 60% of mutations are deletions that involve one or more exons. Duplications account for approximately 10% of mutations. Point mutations (small deletion, insertions, single nucleotide changes, and splice-site mutations) account for the rest (~30%), most of which result in frameshifts or stop codon. Rare missense mutations have been described. Deletions and duplications have a predilection for specific "hot spots." Approximately two-thirds of deletions involve exons 45 to 52. A minor hotspot for deletions occurs at exons 3 to 19. Duplications tend to occur toward the 5' end, with the majority involving exons 2 to 11.

***Genetic Testing:*** To establish the diagnosis, deletion or duplication analysis of *DMD* should be performed first. If a mutation is not identified, then gene sequencing can be pursued. If a mutation is still not identified with these two steps, then muscle biopsy and dystrophin immunostaining may confirm the diagnosis (Fig. 135-1). Deletions or duplications within the *DMD* gene can be identified on SNP or oligonucleotide based chromosomal microarray analysis, and may be an unexpected finding when the testing is being performed for other reasons. In such cases, molecular confirmation and genetic counseling is recommended.

## BIBLIOGRAPHY:

1. Aartsma-Rus A, Van Deutekom JCT, Fokkema IF, Van Ommen G-JB, Den Dunnen JT. Entries in the Leiden Duchenne muscular dystrophy mutation database: an overview of mutation types and paradoxical cases that confirm the reading-frame rule. *Muscle Nerve.* 2006;34(2):135-144.

2. Beggs AH, Hoffman EP, Snyder JR, et al. Exploring the molecular basis for variability among patients with Becker muscular dystrophy: dystrophin gene and protein studies. *Am J Hum Genet.* 1991;49(1):54-67.

3. Bushby K, Finkel R, Birnkrant DJ, et al. Diagnosis and management of Duchenne muscular dystrophy, part 1: diagnosis, and pharmacological and psychosocial management. *Lancet Neurol.* Jan 2010;9(1):77-93.

4. Bushby K, Finkel R, Birnkrant DJ, et al. Diagnosis and management of Duchenne muscular dystrophy, part 2: implementation of multidisciplinary care. *Lancet Neurol.* Feb 2010;9(2):177-189.

5. Darras BT, Miller DT, Urion DK. Dystrophinopathies. Sep 5 2000 [Updated Nov 23 2011]. In: Pagon RA, Bird TD, Dolan CR, et al., eds. GeneReviews™ [Internet]. Seattle, WA: University of Washington, Seattle; 1993.

6. Diegoli M, Grasso M, Favalli V, et al. Diagnostic work-up and risk stratification in X-linked dilated cardiomyopathies caused by dystrophin defects. *J Am Coll Cardiol.* 2011;58(9):925-934.

7. Flanigan KM, Dunn DM, von Niederhausern A, et al. Mutational spectrum of DMD mutations in dystrophinopathy patients: application of modern diagnostic techniques to a large cohort. *Hum Mutat.* 2009;30(12):1657-1666.

8. Guglieri M, Bushby K. Molecular treatments in Duchenne muscular dystrophy. *Curr Opin Pharmacol.* 2010;10:331-337.

9. Koenig M, Beggs AH, Moyer M, et al. The molecular basis for Duchenne versus Becker muscular dystrophy: correlation of severity with type of deletion. *Am J Hum Genet.* 1989;45(4):498-506.

10. Muntoni F, Melis MA, Ganau A, Dubowitz V. Transcription of the dystrophin gene in normal tissues and in skeletal muscle of a family with X-linked dilated cardiomyopathy. *Am J Hum Genet.* 1995;56(1):151-157.

11. Muntoni F, Torelli S, Ferlini A. Dystrophin and mutations: one gene, several proteins, multiple phenotypes. *Lancet Neurol.* 2003;2(12):731-740.

12. Partridge TA. Impending therapies for Duchenne muscular dystrophy. *Curr Opin Neurol.* 2011;24:415-422.

13. Sejerson T, Bushby K. Standards of care for Duchenne muscular dystrophy: brief treat-NMD recommendation. In: Espinos C, ed. *Inherited Neuromuscular Diseases, Advances in Experimental Medicine and Biology.* 2009;652:13-21.

14. White SJ, den Dunnen JT. Copy number variation in the genome; the human DMD gene as an example. *Cytogenet Genome Res.* 2006;115(3-4):240-246.

## Supplementary Information

### OMIM REFERENCES:

[1] DMD; DMD (#30037, 310200)

[2] BMD; DMD (#300376)

[3] DCM; DMD (#302045)

### Alternative Names:

- Duchenne Muscular Dystrophy
- Becker Muscular Dystrophy
- Dystrophinopathies
- X-linked Dilated Cardiomyopathy

## 136 **Depression**

Matthew Morris and Uma Rao

### KEY POINTS

- *Disease summary:*
  - Major depressive disorder (MDD) is a common and debilitating mood disorder associated with high morbidity and mortality.
  - It is estimated that 10% to 20% of the general population will experience clinical depression during the lifetime; rates differ by age (0.3%-2.5% for children, 10%-20% for adolescents and adults), gender (with women having about twice the risk compared to men), and ethnicity (with higher rates in non-Hispanic Whites).
  - MDD is characterized by both clinical and etiologic heterogeneity, involving a complex interplay among genetic, biologic, personality, cognitive, interpersonal, and environmental factors.

- *Differential diagnosis:*
  - Unipolar depression must be distinguished from bipolar disorder, bereavement, and mood disorders due to general medical conditions, substance use, or toxin exposure.

- *Monogenic forms:*
  - No single gene cause of MDD is known to exist.

- *Family history:*
  - There is a two- to threefold increased risk for the illness among first-degree relatives of probands with MDD. Family history of MDD is also associated with early age of onset and recurrence.

- *Twin studies:*
  - Heritability estimates for MDD based on monozygotic versus dizygotic twin concordance differences exhibit a modest heritable contribution of 37%, with a greater estimated contribution of 42% for women versus 29% for men. Evidence suggests that 31% to 42% of variance in liability to depression can be explained by additive genetic effects, 58% to 67% by individual specific environmental effects, and 0% to 5% by shared environmental effects.

- *Environmental factors:*
  - Strong evidence supports a link between stressful life events and the onset and maintenance of depression in both children and adults. Childhood trauma is associated with increased risk for early-onset depression and alterations in the hypothalamic-pituitary-adrenal (HPA) axis that are characteristic of depression.

- *Genome-wide associations:*
  - No studies have identified specific genetic variants that achieved genome-wide significance. Such studies require large-scale samples, with several thousand cases to study main effects and several tens of thousands of cases to investigate gene × gene or gene × environment interactions. Such large-scale samples have not been recruited into genome-wide association studies (GWASs) of MDD.

- *Pharmacogenomics:*
  - Although evidence suggests that genes implicated in pharmacokinetics or pharmacodynamics of antidepressant medications may predict response, replication of findings has been hampered by heterogeneity among samples across studies and because treatment outcome is likely determined by a combination of genetic variants exerting only modest unique effects.

## Diagnostic Criteria and Clinical Characteristics

***Diagnostic Criteria for Unipolar Major Depressive Disorder:***
Diagnostic evaluation should include five or more of the following symptoms, including depressed mood and/or anhedonia, present for at least two consecutive weeks and causing clinically significant distress or impairment in important areas of functioning (eg, social, occupational, self-care):

- Depressed mood: either subjective report (eg, feeling sad or empty) or observation made by others (eg, appears tearful); present most of the day, nearly every day. Note: can be irritable mood in children and adolescents.
- Anhedonia: either subjective report or observation made by others of markedly diminished interest or pleasure in most activities; present most of the day, nearly every day.
- Weight or appetite change: significant weight loss (not due to dieting) or weight gain (eg, change >5% of body weight in 1 month) and/or significant change in appetite (increase or

decrease) present almost daily. Note: can be a failure to make expected weight gain in children.

- Sleep disturbance: insomnia or hypersomnia; present nearly every day.
- Psychomotor disturbance: observation made by others of psychomotor retardation or agitation; present nearly every day.
- Fatigue: loss of energy or fatigue; present nearly every day.
- Worthlessness or guilt: feelings of worthlessness and/or excessive or inappropriate guilt; present nearly every day.
- Concentration or indecision: subjective report or observation made by others of difficulty thinking or concentrating and/or indecisiveness; present nearly every day.
- Suicide: recurrent morbid ideation or recurrent suicidal ideation with or without a specific plan or a suicide attempt.

### Clinical Characteristics:

Course

- Depression falls on a continuum of severity ranging from sad mood to diagnosable depressive disorders.
- MDD is highly recurrent (over 80% of depressed individuals experience more than one episode) and often chronic (up to 25% of individuals with MDD have a protracted episode).
- Median duration of MDD ranges from 19 to 22 weeks across multiple episodes in adults, and mean duration ranges from 26 to 36 weeks in children and adolescents.
- **Remission** is defined as a relatively brief period of symptom improvement after the onset of a major depressive episode (MDE) for at least 3 consecutive weeks but not longer than 4 months; the neurobiology of the MDE is assumed to be active; a return to the MDE before recovery is termed a **relapse**.
- **Recovery** is defined as a period of symptom improvement lasting at least 4 months after the onset of an MDE; the neurobiology of the MDE is assumed to be resolved; the development of an MDE after recovery is termed a **recurrence**.
- Seasonal affective disorder is a course specifier indicating that depressive episodes occur at a particular time of the year, for at least 2 years, with no episodes occurring during non-seasonal periods.

Age at onset

- Earlier age of onset for the first MDE is associated with increased risk for recurrence.

Sex differences

- Prevalence rates of MDD are approximately twice as high in females; sex differences emerge after puberty.

Subtypes

- Atypical depression is characterized by weight gain, appetite increase, and hypersomnia.
- Melancholic depression includes pervasive anhedonia or lack of mood reactivity and at least three of the following symptoms: distinct quality of mood, mood worse in the morning, terminal insomnia, psychomotor disturbance, significant anorexia or weight loss, and excessive guilt.

Sleep

- Electroencephalographic (EEG) sleep abnormalities characterize 40% to 60% of outpatients and up to 90% of inpatients

with an MDE. Persistence of these abnormalities into remission is associated with increased risk for relapse or recurrence.

## Screening and Counseling

*Screening:* There is only limited evidence from family studies for the role of genetic factors in antidepressant medication response.
*Counseling:* Lifetime risk for MDD in first-degree relatives of probands with MDD is two- to threefold compared to the risk in never-depressed individuals.

☞INHERITANCE, PENETRANCE: The mode of inheritance is complex. Replicated risk conferring gene variants exert a modest effect size that appears to contribute to overt phenotype expression in the context of a highly intricate concert of interrelated epigenetic and epistatic modifiers.

☞GENOTYPE-PHENOTYPE CORRELATION: The genotype-phenotype correlation is poor because of the clinical phenotype of MDD is broad. Moreover, other disorders (eg, bipolar disorder, anxiety disorders, internalizing personality traits) share some phenotypic aspects with MDD. As these partially overlapping phenotypes are likely polygenic in origin, a single small-effect gene could contribute in a modular fashion to more than one categorical phenotype, depending on individual constellations of interactive epigenetic and epistatic modifiers.

## Management and Treatment

☞PHARMACOTHERAPY: Pharmacotherapy is considered the standard of treatment for severe depression. Nevertheless, full remission following the administration of a single antidepressant drug is observed in only 30% of patients. Currently available antidepressant drugs target the monoaminergic system either by selectively or nonselectively blocking one of the three monoamine transporters (dopamine, norepinephrine, and/or serotonin). Tricyclic antidepressants (TCAs) mainly target the serotonergic system. The TCAs also have an affinity to a series of neurotransmitter transporters and receptors outside the monoaminergic system (eg, cholinergic and histaminergic systems), resulting in significant side effects. Monoamine oxidase inhibitors (MAOIs) increase monoamine levels by preventing their breakdown through blockade of the MAO. More recently, a number of antidepressant classes with a more selective profile and less side effects have been developed, such as the selective serotonin reuptake inhibitors (SSRIs), serotonin-norepinephrine reuptake inhibitors (SNRIs), norepinephrine-dopamine reuptake inhibitors (NDRIs), and norepinephrine reuptake inhibitors (NRIs).

☞PSYCHOTHERAPY: Cognitive behavior therapy (CBT), behavior therapy (BT), and interpersonal psychotherapy (IPT) are considered specific and efficacious psychosocial interventions for MDD; brief dynamic therapy (BDT) and emotion-focused therapy (EFT) are considered possibly efficacious. For the prevention of relapse or recurrence following treatment termination, CBT is considered efficacious and specific, mindfulness-based cognitive therapy (MBCT) is considered efficacious, and BDT and EFT are considered possibly efficacious. Combined psychotherapy and medication is superior to pharmacotherapy alone for preventing depressive relapses and recurrence. Depression prevention programs have demonstrated positive, though modest and short-lived, effects.

*Table 136-1 Pharmacogenetic Considerations in Unipolar Depression*

| Gene | Potential Medications | Variants | Association With Favorable Treatment Outcome |
|------|----------------------|----------|---------------------------------------------|
| SCLC6A4 (serotonin transporter) | Various AD drugs (specifically SSRIs) | 5-HTTLPR, Int2 VNTR STin2, rs25531 | 5-HTTLPR L allele |
| HTR1A (serotonin receptor 1A) | Various AD drugs | 1019 C/G (rs6295) 272 Gly/Asp (rs6295) | Possibly 1019 GG allele |
| HTR2A (serotonin receptor 2A) | Various AD drugs | 102 T/C rs6313) 1420 C/T (rs6306) 1438 A/G (rs6311) Various SNPs | Possibly 1438 GG allele Possibly 1420 C allele Possibly rs7997012 AA Possibly rs17288723 CC |
| HTR6 (serotonin receptor 6) | Various AD drugs | 256 C/T | Possibly 256 CT |
| FKBP5 (FK506-binding protein 5) | Various AD drugs | Various SNPs (rs1360780, rs3800373, rs4713916) | rs1360780 T allele rs3800373 C allele rs4713916 A allele |
| GRIK4 (glutamate receptor, ionotropic, kainite 4) | Various AD drugs | Various SNPS | rs 1954787 CC rs12800734 GG |
| COMT (catechol-O-methyltransferase) | Various AD drugs | 158 Val/Met (rs4680) various SNPs | rs4680 Val allele Possibly rs4680 Met allele rs165599 GG, rs165774 GG, rs174696 CC |
| BDNF (brain-derived neurotrophic factor) | Various AD drugs | 66 Val/Met (rs6265) various SNPs | Possibly Met allele Possibly rs908867 AA |
| TPH1 (tryptophan hydroxylase 1) | Various AD drugs | 218A/C (rs180052) various SNPs | Possibly 218 C allele, -7180 TG, -7065 TC, -5806 TG |
| TPH2 (tryptophan hydroxylase 2) | Various AD drugs | Various SNPs | Possibly rs10897346 C allele rs1487278 |
| GNB3 (G-protein beta 3) | Various AD drugs ECT | 825 C/T (rs5443) | Possibly 825 T allele |
| CRHR1 (corticotropin-releasing hormone receptor 1) | | | |
| MAOA (monoamine oxidase A) | Various AD drugs | VNTR Various SNPs 941 T/G (rs1799835) | No association detected |
| DTNBP1 (dysbindin) | Various AD drugs | Various SNPs | Possibly rs2005976 A allele |
| SCL6A2 (norepinephrine transporter) | Various AD drugs | 182 C/T (rs2242446) 1287 G/A (rs5569) Various SNPs | 182 T allele 1287 GG rs36029, rs1532701 |
| NR3C1 (glucocorticoid receptor) | Various AD drugs | ER22/23EK (rs6189/rs6190) N363S (rs6195) Bcl1 | Possibly ER22/23EK carriers rs852977, rs10482633, rs10052957 |
| PDE1A, PDE11A (cyclic nucleotide phosphodiesterases) | Various AD drugs | Various SNPs rs1549870, 1880916 | Possibly rs30585 GG, rs992185 AG |
| ACE (angiotensin-converting enzyme) | Various AD drugs ECT | ACE I/D | Possibly ACE D allele |

AD, antidepressant; SNP, single-nucleotide polymorphism; ECT, electroconvulsive therapy.

☞**ELECTROCONVULSIVE THERAPY:** Although electroconvulsive therapy (ECT) is considered efficacious for the treatment of severe MDD, particularly with psychotic symptoms, relapse rates are high following initial remission.

☞**ALTERNATIVE APPROACHES FOR TREATMENT-RESISTANT DEPRESSION:** Ablative procedures (anterior cingulotomy, anterior capsulotomy, subcaudate tractotomy, limbic leucotomy) lead to improvement in one-third to two-thirds of patients with treatment-resistant depression. Preliminary studies suggest that deep brain stimulation shows promise for individuals with treatment-resistance depression.

☞**PHARMACOGENETICS:** Recently, a number of pharmacogenetic studies on antidepressant drugs have been published. A summary of these studies indicates several strong candidate genes involved in the pharmacokinetic as well as pharmacodynamics of these drugs. However, the lack of standardized study design including diagnostic criteria, medications, outcome criteria, genetic coverage, and ethnic or racial background makes comparison across studies difficult. A summary of the candidate genes involved in antidepressant response is illustrated in Table 136-1.

*Genetic Testing:* A microarray test (AmpliChip CYP450 Test, Roche Diagnostics, Basel, Switzerland) is available to genotype variants in the cytochrome P450 (CYP450) system. CYP450 (particularly CYP2D6 and CYP2C19) plays a major role in the oxidative metabolism of various antidepressant drugs. This microarray test will allow the classification of metabolizer status (eg, poor metabolizer, extensive metabolizer) with a high degree of accuracy, thereby aiding in estimation of the risk of adverse effects and response profile, especially for TCAs and MAOIs which have a narrow dose or response window. For SSRIs, the most commonly used antidepressant drugs, no clear dose-response relationship has been established and to date no threshold toxic concentrations have been established. Therefore, metabolizer status-dependent dose adjustments might not be clinically relevant for these drugs.

*Future Directions:* Given the complex nature of unipolar depression, larger and more refined studies, both at the phenotypic as well as genetic level will be needed to move the field forward. Such markers could include clinical characteristics such as anxiety symptoms, environmental exposure, neuroimaging paradigms, endocrine studies, immune parameters, and peripheral blood mRNA expression to better understand the pathophysiology of unipolar depression and guide personalized treatments.

**BIBLIOGRAPHY:**

1. American Psychiatric Association. *Diagnostic and Statistical Manual of Mental Disorders.* 4th ed. Washington, DC; 2000.

2. Sullivan PF, Neale MC, Kendler KS. Genetic epidemiology of major depression: review and meta-analysis. *Am J Psychiatry.* 2000;157:1552-1562.

3. Kessler RC, Berglund P, Demler O, Jin R, Merikangas KR, Walters EE. Lifetime prevalence and age-of-onset distributions of DSM-IV disorders in the National Comorbidity Survey Replication. *Arch Gen Psychiatry.* 2005;62:593-602.

4. Solomon DA, Keller MB, Leon AC, et al. Recovery from major depression: a 10-year prospective follow-up across multiple episodes. *Arch Gen Psychiatry.* 1997;54:1001-1006.

5. Kendler KS, Karkowski LM. Prescott CA. Causal relationship between stressful life events and the onset of major depression. *Am J Psychiatry.* 1999;156:837-841.

6. Lohoff FW. Overview of the genetics of major depressive disorder. *Curr Psychiatry Rep.* 2010;12:539-546.

7. Anderson IM. Meta-analytical studies on new antidepressants. *Br Med Bull.* 2001;57:161-178.

8. Horstmann S, Binder EB. Pharmacogenomics of antidepressant drugs. *Pharmacol Ther.*2009;124:57-73.

**ACKNOLWEDGEMENTS:**

Matthew C. Morris was supported in part by an RCTR/MeTRC grant (U54 RR026140/MD007593), and an independent grant (R01 MH068391) from the National Institutes of Health. Uma Rao was supported in part by the grants from the National Institutes of Health (R01 DA017805, R01 MH068391, G12 RR003032/MD007586, UL1 RR024975/TR000445 and U54 RR026140/MD007593), and by the Endowed Chair in Brain and Behavior Research at Meharry Medical College.

## Supplementary Information

*Key Words:* Depression, environment, genetic, pharmacogenomics, phenotype

# 137 Bipolar Mood Disorder

Neera Ghaziuddin and Melvin McInnis

## KEY POINTS

- *Disease summary:*
  - Bipolar mood disorder (BP) is characterized by severe disturbances of mood that may include depression, mania or hypomania, or irritability. Manias are pathologically energized states with misguided volition and behavior in a mood state of intoxicating euphoria (or irritability) and depression. Depression consists of pathologically compromised energy and volition with a slowing of bodily functions, most prominently cognition and concentration. The disturbed mood may appear during distinct periods or as a more sustained disturbance. The underlying pathophysiology of the disorder is an interaction between multiple interacting genetic loci and environmental factors which trigger the disease.

- *Differential diagnosis:*
  - Depression with or without psychotic features, schizophrenia, personality disorder, substance or alcohol abuse, attention deficit hyperactivity disorder (ADHD), and anxiety disorders. Some medical disorders (hyperthyroidism, treatment with steroids among others) may mimic BP.

- *Monogenic forms:*
  - No single gene form of BP has been identified.

- *Family history:*
  - Positive family history of both unipolar and bipolar depression is noted in first-degree relatives and risk of any mood disorder increases as the number of close relatives increases. History of past diagnosis of ADHD is common possibly because of the overlapping symptoms between the two disorders. Increased history of consanguinity among parents of BP patients has been reported.

- *Twin studies:*
  - Concordance rate for monozygotic twins is reported to be in the range of 70% and the dizygote concordance in the range of 20%. This clearly supports the genetic basis of bipolar disorder. Based on this and additional genetic research the heritability has been estimated to be 85%.

- *Environmental factors:*
  - Environmental factors may include history of trauma and abuse (physical and sexual abuse), substance abuse disorders, temperamental factors, and the postpartum period. Different environmental factors may affect the onset and the recurrence of the disorder.

- *Genome-wide associations:*
  - There are no genes with risk variants that currently have clinical relevance for the actively managed patient with bipolar disorder. Genome-wide association studies (GWASs) have identified several risk genes and a number of them have been replicated in independent studies in BP. These include *ANK3* which regulates voltage-gated sodium channels, *CACNA1C* (a voltage-gated calcium channel gene), and *SYNE1* involved in neurogenesis and synaptic clustering. The calcium channel pathway evidence was confirmed and a new locus at ODZ4 was identified.

- *Pharmacogenomics:*
  - There are no laboratory or other tests that are recommended as standard of care for the assessment and management of bipolar disorder. The efforts in pharmacogenetics have identified several variants in genes that code for enzymes that commonly metabolize psychotropic medications. These include variants in genes that code for the enzymes CYP2D6, CYP2C19, and CYP3A4. However, the clinical relevance beyond good clinical knowledge of the patient and pharmacologic treatment remains to be determined.

## Diagnostic Criteria and Clinical Characteristics

***Diagnosing BP:*** The *Diagnostic and Statistical Manual IV* (DSM IV) describes four different forms of BP disorder: BP I, BP II, BP NOS, and cyclothymia. Essential criterion for BP I is the presence of at least one manic or one mixed episode. For BP II, one depressive episode and one hypomanic episode are required and for BP NOS the number or the duration of symptoms are insufficient to diagnose either BP I or BP II. Cyclothymia is a milder form of the illness, characterized by shifting back and forth between mild depression and hypomania for a 2-year period; however, the symptoms are not severe enough to meet the criteria for other forms of BP.

A thorough psychiatric and medical history is necessary for making accurate diagnosis. Standardized diagnostic interviews (SDIs) may be used in some instances.

There is no laboratory or psychologic test available for diagnosing these disorders. However, because of relatively high rates of comorbidity with psychiatric and medical disorders and because some general medical conditions may mimic BP, any patient experiencing the first episode of BP should receive a battery of laboratory tests (CBC with differential count, metabolic panel including electrolytes, thyroid function tests, liver function tests, and urine analysis and toxicology). Additional tests may be based on abnormal findings.

Contributing factors may include general medical conditions, medications with known association with mood disturbance, and alcohol and drug misuse. However, the symptoms of BP should not be directly related to these factors, to give an independent diagnosis of BP.

Psychosocial stress is commonly associated with the first episode and may be associated with recurrences. Symptoms may be incorrectly attributed as a reaction to stress, however, stressful events are best viewed as a precipitating or maintaining factors.

Brain imaging may be completed in some cases, especially when there is concern that space occupying lesions may be contributing to the pathology.

**Absence of the following criteria is necessary:**

- The symptoms of BP should not be accounted for by, or superimposed on schizophrenia, schizoaffective disorder, schizophreniform disorder, psychosis NOS, or delusional disorder.
- Symptoms should not be solely accounted for by a comorbid general medical disorder, medications with known mood effects and alcohol or illicit drugs. If the symptoms are related to one or more of these factors, the final diagnosis of BP should be deferred.

*Clinical Characteristics:* The central symptoms of BP are intermittent or chronic mood disturbance. Mood disturbance may include depression, elevated mood, and/or irritability presenting in different combinations. Additional symptoms include uncharacteristic changes in behavior, thought and speech, and rest-activity cycles. Cognitive deficits are not considered central to the illness. The symptoms may be cyclical with periods of complete or near-complete remission. BP is often missed in patients who may appear to be primarily depressed. Therefore, careful evaluation for BP is essential even in patients who present with symptoms of depression.

Increased energy and activity level are frequently noted; however, productivity may vary depending on the severity of symptoms. Impaired attention, distractibility, and task completion are common symptoms. Patients may report subjective experience of rapid thinking which may be apparent in speech. Common abnormalities of speech are pressured speech (excessive speed of speech), tangential speech, or loosening of associations (difficulty in maintaining clear boundaries between ideas). Speech abnormalities in more severe forms of illness may include punning, rhyming, and incoherence. Incoherent speech or "word salad" may present in the most severe forms of the illness. Psychotic symptoms (grandiosity, paranoia, hallucinations, and delusions) are common and in fact experienced by more than a half of all patients with BP.

Sleep disturbance is common and may include reduced total sleep time, prolonged periods of a complete lack of sleep, and frequent awakenings. Periods of insomnia may be associated with reduced need for sleep and followed by prolonged periods of sleep.

☞**BP Comorbid with Other Psychiatric Disorders:** Approximately, three-quarters of patients with BP suffer from one or more comorbid psychiatric disorders, such as, anxiety disorders (among the commonest), ADHD, personality, and eating disorders.

Substance abuse disorders are commonly reported, although the direction of this association is unclear. Both men and women with BP suffer from high rates of alcohol and other substance abuse disorders.

☞**BP and Comorbid Medical Disorders:** Medical disorders that are more common than expected by chance include migraine headaches, multiple sclerosis, and asthma. Comorbid medical conditions that are likely to be associated with the treatment

of BP, and not with the illness per se, include type 2 diabetes mellitus, hypothyroidism, polycystic ovarian disease, diabetes insipidus, renal failure, and skin rashes.

## Screening and Counseling

*Screening:* There are no specific screening approaches or tests for bipolar disorder. Typically, a parent is concerned over a child within the family unit and is interested to learn if they can be screened. The family members are advised that several comorbid features are not uncommon in bipolar disorder and are to be watched for (eg, anxiety and substance abuse) as they may be associated with earlier onset and a more problematic course of disease. If any concerns are expressed the family should have the person evaluated.

*Counseling:* The counseling of psychiatric disorders is challenging, as there is little to evaluate the biologic risk factors beyond the fact that there is an observed increased risk in family members of affected probands. The risk to the family member appears to increase with the perceived increasing severity of disease (the familial risk is greater in schizoaffective disorder compared to bipolar disorder) and when both parents (or two or more family members) are affected. The perceived burden of the illness is generally personal; an individual with a life experience of growing up in a family wherein bipolar disorder was present and poorly managed is likely to have a far greater negative perspective of the disorder than one with a neutral experience. Counseling related to genetic risk is notoriously difficult in the presence of observational clinic data. This is coupled with the variability in reports of the epidemiology of mood disorders. In families with high risk for mood disorder, there are many illnesses that segregate among the family; the presence of a bipolar family member predicts that up to 5% of first-degree relatives will have bipolar disorder (fivefold the accepted population risk) and 25% will have a mood disorder during their lifetime.

## Molecular Genetics and Molecular Mechanism

Early medications used to treat BP were found to bind to the bioamine receptors highlighting a potential biologic etiology of the illnesses. It is clear that susceptibility genes are being identified, albeit each with negligible effects, meaning that any one gene variant in the current knowledge status will by itself have essentially no effect on the disorder. Genes that influence stress and tissue growth factors are also strongly implicated. The genes and the internal and external environments are likely to work in an additive manner that may be specific in many respects to the individual. Many genetic variants with small effects at variable time periods may prove to be rather difficult to elucidate. It may be that the individual serving as their own control will be the most pragmatic approach to the study of molecular mechanisms, how the individual changes over time and the patterns of change in biologic parameters may identify insights to mechanisms.

## Management and Treatment

Early diagnosis and treatment of BP cannot be emphasized enough; early diagnosis and treatment are shown to ameliorate poor prognosis, improve long-term outcome, and prevent functional decline.

Patient groups that pose special treatment challenges include prepubertal children because of the difficulty with accurate diagnosis and definitions, patients with high rates of comorbid psychiatric and medical disorders, and those who display prominent risk-taking behaviors and thereby mislabeled as "personality disorders" or "temperamental problems" (adolescents and young adults in particular). There are additional challenges associated with substantial side effects of medications used in the treatment of BP. Special needs of women around childbirth include adjusting the dose of medications (or discontinuation) which may be necessary during periods of critical fetal development, restarting treatment during the second or the third trimester of pregnancy, changes in medication regimen if lactation is desired, and close monitoring for relapse, particularly during the high-risk postpartum period.

Although, the majority of patients with BP achieve good symptom control, a small but significant number are deemed as treatment resistant.

☞**MOOD STABILIZERS:** Majority of the patients are likely to benefit from one or a combination of mood stabilizers. Lithium is a commonly employed and an effective mood stabilizing agent. It has a narrow therapeutic window, requiring careful monitoring of side effects. Side effects may be minor such as nausea, changes in appetite, increased thirst, and weight gain. More serious side effects may include lithium toxicity which may result in vomiting, diarrhea, ataxia, seizures, changes in level of consciousness, and even death.

Cardiovascular complications including conduction defects and nephrogenic diabetes insipidus are rare complications.

A number of anticonvulsants such as valproate and carbamazepine can also be effective mood stabilizers.

☞**ANTIPSYCHOTIC AGENTS:** Second-generation antipsychotic agents are commonly used in the treatment of BP. Commonly employed agents are risperidone, quetiapine, olanzapine, aripiprazole, and ziprasidone among others. These agents are found to be useful in the management of acute mania and for the treatment of depressive symptoms associated with BP, although, the role of these agents for maintenance treatment has not been demonstrated.

☞**ANTIDEPRESSANTS:** Patients with BP are known to spend more time in depressed than in manic or hypomanic states. Therefore, treatment of depression is critical for optimum management of the disorder. Medications used for treatment of depression may include selective serotonin reuptake inhibitors (SSRIs), although close supervision and concurrent treatment with mood stabilizers is recommended because of the risk of inducing mania or hypomania, lithium, for its antidepressant and antisuicide properties, antiepileptic mood stabilizers (valproate, lamotrigine), and second-generation antipsychotics (quetiapine or olanzapine in particular).

☞**SLEEP AGENTS:** Many patients with BP suffer from chronic sleep problems, needing pharmacologic sleep aids across the age groups. Agents used may include benzodiazepines and nonbenzodiazepines on a short-term basis.

☞**ANTIANXIETY AGENTS:** Several agents have been used; however, there are no large trials specifically focused on the treatment of anxiety. Mood stabilizers and antipsychotic agents are commonly used, with modest evidence that divalproex may be the agent of choice in the treatment of anxiety.

☞**PSYCHOTHERAPY:** Although, pharmacotherapy remains the cornerstone treatment for the effective management of the illness, several other forms of therapy are also employed.

*Chronobiologic therapy:* This form of therapy regulates exposure to environmental stimuli, which are known to influence biologic or circadian rhythms. *Interpersonal and social rhythm therapy:* This form of therapy is based on the principles of interpersonal therapy and behavioral techniques to help patient regularize their daily routines, diminish interpersonal problems, and to adhere to medication regimens.

☞**NONPHARMACOLOGIC TREATMENTS:** Electroconvulsive therapy, repetitive transcranial brain stimulation (rTMS), and deep brain stimulation (DBS) are all being studied in patients who fail to respond to conventional treatments. The best data are probably available for electroconvulsive therapy (ECT) for the treatment of resistant cases, mixed-mood states, or when the disorder is associated with catatonia. DBS may benefit some patients whose depression fails to respond to conventional treatments, while promising preliminary data exist about the role of rTMS in selected patients with BP.

**Future Directions:** The future of medical research is dependent on the ongoing participation of individuals with the specific illness under study. While this is a straightforward and obvious statement, it is not clear that this is an accepted approach. Longitudinal studies are essential that maintain the engagement of patients over extended periods of time to monitor course of illness, outcomes, and response to interventions. The strategy of building an "onion" of data surrounding each individual will provide for an integrative approach that searches and characterizes relationships between biologic and clinical data from the individual in an etiologic and correlative analysis. However, there is inadequate commitment at an administrative level at the NIH to support ongoing longitudinal assessment and maintenance of study subjects. The example of the Framingham study represents the study design that is essential for the understanding of psychiatric diseases: ongoing follow-up of patients with the disorders with extensive collateral study using multidisciplinary methods that can be subsequently integrated.

**BIBLIOGRAPHY:**

1. Faraone SV, Tsuang MT, Tsuang DW, eds. Genetics of mental disorders: what practioners and students need to know. New York: Guildford Press; 2001.

2. Mansour H, Klei L, Wood J, et al. Consanguinity associated with increased risk for bipolar I disorder in Egypt. *Am J Med Genet B Neuropsychiatr Genet.* 2009;150B: 879-885.

3. McGuffin P, Rijsdijk F, Andrew M, Sham P, Katz R, Cardno A. The heritability of bipolar affective disorder and the genetic relationship to unipolar depression. *Arch Gen Psychiatry.* 2003;60:497-502.

4. Romero S, Birmaher B, Axelson D, et al. Prevalence and correlates of physical and sexual abuse in children and adolescents with bipolar disorder. *J Affect Disord.* 2009;112:144-150.

5. Ferreira MAR, O'Donovan MC, Meng YA, et al. Collaborative genome-wide association analysis supports a role for ANK3 and CACNA1C in bipolar disorder. *Nat Genet.* 2008;40:1056-1058.

6. Sklar P. Large-scale genome-wide association analysis of bipolar disorder identifies a new susceptibility locus near ODZ4. *Nat Genet.* 2011;43:977-983.

7. Steimer W. Pharmacogenetics and psychoactive drug therapy: ready for the patient? *Ther Drug Monit.* 2010;32:381-386.

8. APA. American Psychiatric Association. *Diagnostic and Statistical Manual of Mental Disorders.* 4th ed. Washington, DC: APPI; 1994.

9. Goodwin FK, Jamison KR, eds. *Manic Depressive Illness: Bipolar Disorders and Recurrent Depression.* 2nd ed. New York, NY: Oxford University Press; 2007.

10. Nurnberger J Jr., Guroff JJ, Hamovit J, Berrettini W, Gershon E. A family study of rapid-cycling bipolar illness. *J Affect Disord.* 1988;15:87-91.

11. Martinowich K, Schloesser RJ, Manji HK. Bipolar disorder: from genes to behavior pathways. *J Clin Invest.* 2009;119: 726-736.

12. Carter CJ. Multiple genes and factors associated with bipolar disorder converge on growth factor and stress activated kinase pathways controlling translation initiation: implications for oligo-dendrocyte viability. *Neurochem Int.* 2007;50:461-490.

13. Dallaspezia S, Benedetti F. Chronobiological therapy for mood disorders. *Expert Rev Neurother.* 2011;11:961-970.

14. Frank E, Swartz HA, Kupfer DJ. Interpersonal and social rhythm therapy: managing the chaos of bipolar disorder. *Biol Psychiatry.* 2000;48:593-604.

15. Levy D, Brink S. A change of heart. FDR's death shows how much we've learned about the heart. *US News World Rep.* 2005;138:54-57.

## Supplementary Information

***Key Words:*** Bipolar, depression, mania, comorbid, susceptibility, mood stabilizers

# 138 Schizophrenia

Pamela Sklar

## KEY POINTS

- *Disease summary:*
  - Schizophrenia (SCZ) is a severe, chronic psychiatric syndrome that is a complex genetic disorder involving the interactions of multiple genetic and nongenetic factors.
  - Clinical diagnosis is based on abnormalities in multiple domains including positive symptom domain, negative symptoms, cognition, and mood symptoms. No blood or neuroimaging tests are pathognomic.
  - Presentation is generally in adolescence or early adulthood but a premorbid prodrome is often apparent earlier suggesting a neurodevelopmental trajectory.
  - The course is most often chronic with significant impairments in social and work functioning.
  - Neuroimaging finds decreased activation in task-induced magnetic resonance imaging (MRI) paradigms in several brain regions including the dorsolateral prefrontal cortex and anterior cingulate. Diffusion tensor imaging has also identified white matter tract abnormalities.

- *Differential diagnosis:*
  - Major differential is with other psychotic disorders (bipolar disorder [BD], schizoaffective disorder, delusional disorder, and depression with psychotic features). Other significant differential includes (1) psychotic disorder due to medical conditions (eg, epilepsy, dementia, brain tumor, infections, and metabolic abnormalities), (2) substance use (eg, drugs of abuse, medications, toxins), and (3) brief or SCZ spectrum syndromes.

- *Monogenic forms:*
  - There are no agreed upon monogenic forms, no single gene has been demonstrated to cause SCZ.

- *Family history:*
  - Strongest risk for SCZ is a positive family history. Affected first-degree relatives confer a relative risk of 5% to 16%. A recent large-scale study shows that first-degree relatives are also at increased risk of BD (3.7%).

- *Twin studies:*
  - Monozygotic twins have 0.9 concordance rate, dizygotic twins have 0.5, with an estimated heritability of approximately 0.8.

- *Nonfamilial genetics:*
  - Advanced paternal age is associated with elevated relative risk (two- to threefold). De novo single-nucleotide polymorphism (SNP) and copy-number variants (CNV) rates are increased in SCZ.

- *Environmental factors:*
  - Multiple environmental factors have been associated with modest increased risk including obstetrical complications, prenatal infections, socioeconomic status, immigration status, urban living, maternal starvation, head injury, and cannabis use.

- *Genome-wide associations:*
  - Significant genome-wide associations exist for both CNVs and SNPs. Large CNVs are associated with larger risk, but produce pleiotropic phenotypes (ie, not specific for SCZ). Testing for CNVs or SNPs is not yet clinically validated for diagnosis or treatment selection.

- *Pharmacogenomics:*
  - Most antipsychotic medication is metabolized by the cytochrome P450 (CYP) system. Clinical efficacy of CYP testing has not been established.

## Diagnostic Criteria and Clinical Characteristics

***Diagnostic Criteria for SCZ:*** The clinical diagnostic criteria for SCZ are described in the *Diagnostic and Statistical Manual of Mental Disorders Fourth Edition Text Revision* (DSM-IV TR) and the *International Classification of Diseases*, 10th edition (ICD-10). DSM-IV TR is primarily used in the United States and ICD-10 in Europe. There is good agreement between the two systems.

- DSM1V criteria: (1) Two or more *characteristic symptoms* of delusions, hallucinations, disorganized speech, disorganized or catatonic behavior, or negative symptoms (only one if delusions are bizarre, or hallucinations with multiple voices or running commentary), (2) significant *functional decline* in work, self-care, or interpersonal relations, (3) *duration* of 6 months with 1 month of active symptoms, (4) *exclusions* include schizoaffective disorder, mood disorder with psychotic features, substance, general medical conditions, and autism spectrum disorders unless prominent active delusions and hallucinations. There are five subtypes: paranoid, disorganized, catatonic, undifferentiated, and residual.

- ICD-10 criteria: (1) *Active-phase symptoms* include one of either thought abnormalities (echo, insertion, withdrawal, or broadcasting), delusions of control or passivity, hallucinations of running commentary or conversing voices, culturally inappropriate delusions or two of either other hallucinations with delusions, thought disorder, catatonia, or negative symptoms, (2) significant *functional decline* not required, (3) *duration* of 1 month of active symptoms, (4) exclusions include psychosis during mood symptoms, alcohol or substance use, or organic brain diseases. There are seven subtypes: paranoid, hebephrenic, catatonic, undifferentiated, residual, simple, postschizophrenic depression.

**Diagnostic evaluation should include the following:**

- Clinical evaluation of patient that includes review of current and past symptoms, and duration and effect on the patient's functioning. In addition, a standard general medical review and physical examination are indicated including weight, height, and body mass index (BMI).

- Exclusion of medical conditions and substance intoxication that may cause psychotic symptoms via standard laboratory chemistries such as complete blood count (CBC), electrolytes, blood urea nitrogen (BUN)/creatinine, calcium and phosphorus, thyroid-stimulating hormone (TSH), liver function tests (LFTs), HIV screening, syphilis testing, vitamin $B_{12}$ and folate, and urine drug screen. Further testing should be based on level of clinical suspicion from history and physical particularly if presentation has atypical features.

- Imaging studies such as MRI and computed tomography (CT) are not generally recommended as yield is expected to be low unless there is additional clinical suspicion or atypical features.

### Clinical Characteristics:

☞**INITIAL PRESENTATION:** The initial presentation can take several forms. Often onset is acute with symptoms beginning over a short period of time that brings the patient to medical attention and hospitalization. Symptoms may evolve more slowly over a "prodromal" period of several years in which symptoms such as suspiciousness, depression, sleep problems, and decreased functioning may be noted, ultimately culminating in acute symptoms. Retrospective and premorbid studies show that cognitive deficits in intellectual, language, and behavioral measure may be present in childhood suggesting a neurodevelopmental etiology.

☞**ACUTE (POSITIVE) SYMPTOMS:** The characteristic acute symptoms are hallucinations and delusions. Hallucinations are false perceptions that can occur in any sensory modality, but most commonly are auditory. Typical examples include hearing a variety of sounds or hearing third person voices commenting negatively on the patient. Command hallucinations may direct a patient to perform specific potentially dangerous activities. Delusions are fixed, false beliefs that are not culturally appropriate. Typical examples include beliefs that the patient is being persecuted, or that random events have special meaning known only to the patient.

☞**NEGATIVE SYMPTOMS:** These are those symptoms that most negatively affect societal functioning and quality including lack of motivation (avolition), flat or blunted affect, poverty of speech (alogia), inability to experience pleasure (anhedonia), and associality. Negative symptoms are less responsive to antipsychotic treatment.

☞**COGNITIVE SYMPTOMS:** Deficits in a variety of areas that are independent of positive or negative symptoms have been characterized and include abnormalities in processing speed, attention or vigilance, working memory, verbal learning and memory, visual learning and memory, reasoning and problem solving, and verbal comprehension.

☞**COMORBIDITY:** A number of psychiatric syndromes are often comorbid, including depression and substance abuse. Lifetime suicide risk is approximately 5%. An elevated mortality rate from all causes is observed. There is a markedly elevated risk of cardiovascular disease.

## Screening and Counseling

***Screening:*** Genetic testing is not currently offered for SCZ. Genetic testing of DNA variants for diagnosis, reproductive choices, or treatment decisions is not yet validated and thus not recommended. Some clinicians advocate for pharmacogenetic testing of *CYP2D6* as a guide to antipsychotic dosing, however, there is controversy regarding its clinical utility. Surveys of treating clinicians and family members have indicated strong interest in providing and receiving genetic information and these recommendations may change in the future.

***Counseling:*** Traditional elements of genetic counseling apply. Familial clustering is observed, but the relatively low incidence, modest first-degree relative recurrence risk, late onset, and small modern family size can make familial cases difficult to discriminate from sporadic cases. There are no clear Mendelian forms of schizophrenia. General estimates of first-degree relative recurrence risks are 5% to 16%. Two recent large-scale population-based studies demonstrated recurrence risks for many family constellations for schizophrenia (first-degree, 8.2-10.7; second-degree, 2.5-3.8; third-degree, 2.3) as well as sibling recurrence risks of 3.7 for BD.

## Management and Treatment

***Management:*** The mainstay of treatment is antipsychotic medication. These have been shown to improve overall symptoms and decrease relapse risk. A variety of psychosocial interventions have been shown be effective including social skills training, psychoeducation, cognitive behavior therapy, and cognitive remediation.

☞**ANTIPSYCHOTICS:** Introduced in 1960s, first-generation antipsychotics (FGA), also referred to as typical antipsychotics, such as chlorpromazine and haloperidol, are potent dopamine receptor type 2 antagonists. The blockade is also thought to explain the observed nontherapeutic extrapyramidal side effects and prolactin elevation. In contrast, a second-generation antipsychotic (SGA) medications were developed that have been termed "atypical antipsychotics" and have reduced extrapyramidal side effects. In general, FGAs and SGAs do not differ in efficacy for positive symptoms, but have differing side effect profiles with FGAs having higher rates of extrapyramidal symptoms and tardive dyskinesia, and SGAs having increased weight gain and metabolic syndrome.

Management is divided into acute phase and maintenance phase. Acute phase, first-episode treatment may occur in the inpatient or outpatient setting, focuses on stabilization, diagnostic workup, and initiation of antipsychotic treatment. The majority of treatment guidelines suggest beginning treatment with an SGA (but not clozapine). Maintenance phase treatment focuses on preventing relapse with pharmacologic adherence and psychosocial therapy as well as monitoring and prevention of antipsychotic-related side effects including tardive dyskinesia and metabolic syndrome. Two antipsychotics, ziprasidone and aripiprazole have been shown to produce less weight gain in maintenance of schizophrenia and may be considered. Other medications are often used as adjuncts. These include antidepressants, anticonvulsants, and lithium to address affective symptoms and benzodiazepines for anxiety and agitation.

**Table 138-1 Pharmacogenetic Considerations in SCZ**

| Gene | Associated Medications | Goal of Testing | Variants | Effect |
|------|------------------------|-----------------|----------|--------|
| CYP2D6 | Most antipsychotics (eg, [a]aripiprazole, clozapine, iloperidone, perphenazine, risperidone, thioridazine) | Dose adjustment—not generally recommended for clinical practice | Multiple alleles: 4 common alleles (*3,*4,*5, and *6) account for the majority of poor metabolizers | Loss of function |
| CYP1A2 | Chlorpromazine, perphenazine, thioridazine, clozapine, olanzapine | Not available | Multiple alleles | Enzyme induction or inhibition |
| CYP3A4 | Haloperidol, quetiapine, ziprasidone | Not available | Multiple alleles | Decreased activity |

[a]Contains FDA-approved package labeling regarding *CYP2D6* metabolism.

Treatment refractory schizophrenia is defined as significant psychosis despite having been treated with adequate dosing of two or more antipsychotics. Treatment with clozapine is recommended at that point which requires monitoring of white blood cell and absolute neutrophil counts because of the risk of agranulocytosis.

☞MEDICAL MONITORING: Recent meta-analysis confirms that there is a high rate of metabolic syndrome averaging 32.5% associated with use of SGAs. This has been particularly noted with clozapine and olanzapine. Monitoring of baseline medical history and family history should be obtained at baseline. Weight/waist-hip ratio/BMI, blood pressure, fasting glucose, fasting lipids, and lifestyle is recommended at baseline, following drug treatment and annually.

☞PHARMACOGENETICS: This is an active area of research, however, at present there are no FDA-approved tests for clinical efficacy or side effect prediction.

Efficacy studies have focused on cytochrome P450 metabolism and a series of dopaminergic, serotonergic, and glutamatergic candidate genes (Table 138-1). Multiple functional variants in *CYP2D6* result in different enzyme activity leading to poor metabolizers, intermediate metabolizers, extensive metabolizers, and ultrarapid metabolizers. These phenotypes have not been associated with clinical efficacy and are not routinely used in practice.

Adverse effects studies have focused on tardive dyskinesia, extrapyramidal symptoms, antipsychotic-induced weight gain and metabolic syndrome, and clozapine-induced agranulocytosis. There are as yet no studies that have been consistently replicated, and have sufficient specificity and sensitivity to be used clinically.

# Molecular Genetics and Molecular Mechanism

Almost 100 years of family, twin and epidemiologic studies demonstrate conclusively that SCZ is heritable. Family studies consistently show increased recurrence risks to family members that vary directly with the closeness of the relationship and twin studies show increased monozygotic versus dizygotic concordance rates.

Increased risks of related phenotypes such as BD and major depressive disorder are also observed. In spite of this, traditional linkage analysis has not identified consistent genome-wide significant loci for positional cloning despite meta-analysis of over 3000 families. Thus, we can safely conclude that most cases of SCZ are not caused by a single or small number of genes containing variants of high penetrance, as is often observed in Mendelian disease. Many hundreds of candidate genes emerging from biologic theories, or from putative linkage peaks, have been tested for association to SCZ. Generally the evidence has been inconsistent and/or inconclusive, but can be found collated by the Schizophrenia Research Forum (http://www.szgene.org/).

Over the last few years, genome-wide association studies (GWASs) have discovered associations of common SNP and rare CNVs with SCZ. Common SNPs meeting genome-wide criteria for association have been identified. Like other common complex genetic diseases, the relative risks conferred by each locus and the combined overall proportion of heritability explained is small. At present there are approximately 11 loci (replicated, genome-wide significant loci are in Table 138-2a). The biologic impact of individual SNPs on disease pathology is not yet known. However, two lines of evidence suggest that the associations are not random. First, SCZ risk alleles are enriched for expression quantitative trait loci (eQTLs) in adult human brain samples. Second, replication studies indicate a significant excess of additional alleles have signal in the same direction as the original effect that can be detected as significant as sample sizes increase. Of note, intensively studied prior candidate genes such as *DISC1, DTNBP1, NRG1,* and *COMT* do not figure among the top ranks either individually or in bulk in GWAS.

A substantial proportion of risk comes from common variants of weakly associated (ie, not individually genome-wide significant) alleles. As a group, these alleles have been shown to account for approximately 25% to 30% of the variance in liability to SCZ. Furthermore, the polygenic alleles that characterize SCZ are also significantly enriched in BD. This coupled with the observation that several of the genome-wide significant SCZ risk alleles are also associated with BD indicate the need to re-examine the validity of disease distinctions that have previously been based entirely on clinical observation.

*Table 138-2a* **Disease-Associated Susceptibility Variants by GWAS**

| Candidate Gene (Chromosome Location) | Associated Variant | Relative Risk | Frequency of Risk Allele | Putative Functional Significance[a] | Associated Disease Phenotype |
|---|---|---|---|---|---|
| *MIR137* (1p21.3) | rs1625579 | 1.12 | 0.8 | - | SCZ |
| *SDCCAG8* (1q43) | rs6703335 | 1.09 | NA | - | SCZ |
| *VRK2* (2p15.1) | rs2312147 | 1.09 | 0.61 | - | SCZ |
| *ITIH3-ITIH4* (3p21.1) | rs2239547 | 1.11 | 0.74 | - | SCZ alone[b] and combined with BD |
| Extended MHC region (6p21.3-22-1) | Many | 1.13-1.36 | 0.78-0.92 | - | SCZ |
| *ANK3* (10q21.2) | rs10994359 | 1.22 | 0.69 | - | SCZ and BD combined only[c] |
| *CNNM2* (10q24.32) | rs7914558 | 1.08 | 0.59 | - | SCZ |
| *NRGN* (11q24.2) | rs12807809 | 1.12 | 0.83 | - | SCZ |
| *CACNA1C* (12p13.33) | rs4765905 | 1.09 | 0.35 | - | SCZ alone and combined with BD |
| *TCF4* (18q21.2) | rs9960767 | 1.2 | 0.056 | - | SCZ |
| *CCDC68* (18q21.2) | rs12966547 | 1.09 | 0.58 | - | SCZ |

[a]Functional effects of SNP variants have not been determined. In most cases SNPs are in LD with additional potentially functional variants.
[b]Genome-wide significance achieved for schizophrenia tested as a single phenotype.
[c]SCZ and BD analyzed together as a single phenotype.

*Table 138-2b* **Disease-Associated Copy-Number Variants**

| Locus (Chromosome Location Mb hg18) | Type of CNV | Relative Risk | Number of Genes (approximate) | Rate in SCZ Cases/ Rate in Controls | SCZ (Other Potentially Associated Disease Phenotypes)[b] |
|---|---|---|---|---|---|
| 1q21.1 (144.9-146.3) | Deletion | 9.2[a] | 12 | 0.18/0.02 | SCZ (ID, epilepsy, ASD) |
| 2p16.3 (*NRXN1*) | Exonic deletions | 7.5-8.97[a] | 1 | | SCZ (ID, epilepsy, ASD, ADHD) |
| 3q29 (197.4-198.8) | Deletion | 49.5[a] | 21 | 0.097/0.002 | SCZ (ID, ASD, BD) |
| 7q36.3 (158.4-158.8) | Duplication | 3.2[b] | 2 (*VIPR2*) | 0.19/0.06 | SCZ (ASD) |
| 15q11.2 (20.2-20.8) | Deletion | 2.2[a] | 8 | 0.57/0.27 | SCZ (ID, epilepsy) |
| 15q13.3 (28.7-30.3) | Deletion | 8.3[a] | 8 | 0.19/0.023 | SCZ (ID, epilepsy, ASD) |
| 16p13.1 (15.0-16.2) | Duplication | 2.1[a] | 8 | 0.28/0.13 | SCZ (ID, ADHD) |
| 16p11.2 (29.5-30.2) | Duplication | 9.8[a] | 26 | 0.3/0.031 | SCZ (ID, epilepsy, ASD, ADHD, BD) |
| 17p12 (14.0-15.4) | Deletion | 5.9[a] | 5 | 0.16/0.026 | SCZ (hereditary neuropathy with pressure palsies) |
| 17q12 (31.8-33.3) | Deletion | 18.4[a] | 17 | 0.06/0.0003 | SCZ (ID, ASD) |
| 22q11.2 (17.4-19.8) | Deletion | 44-infinity[a] | 30 | 0.31/0 | SCZ (LD, ASD) |

[a]Based on Grozeva D, et al. 2012 which included enhanced control population.
[b]Based on Grozeva D, et al. 2012.
ASD, autism spectrum disorder; ID, intellectual disability or developmental disability; BD, bipolar disorder.

*Table 138-2c* **De novo Variants Observed in Sequencing Studies**

| Reference | Samples | Controls | Genes or Regions Sequenced | Rate of Exonic SCZ de novo SNVs | Rate of Exonic Control de novo SNVs | Number of SCZ de novo Mutations | Number of Control de novo Mutations | Ms/Ns |
|---|---|---|---|---|---|---|---|---|
| Awadalla et al., 2010 | 143 SCZ probands | 185 | 401 synapse-expressed genes[a] | NA | NA | 8 | 1 | 2/2 |
| Xu et al., 2011 | 53 SCZ proband/ parent trios | 22 | Exome | 0.64 | 0.32 | 40 | 7 | 32/0 |
| Girard et al., 2011 | 14 SCZ proband/ parent trios | - | Exome | 1.88 | NA | 15 | NA | 11/4 |

[a]Only 39 genes found to have de novo variants in cases were sequenced in the controls.

Ms, missense; Ns, nonsense.

Rare CNVs have been associated with increased SCZ risk in several ways. First, rates of large (>100 kb), rare (<1%) CNVs are elevated in SCZ cases versus controls. Second, rates of de novo CNVs are elevated (although postulated to be enriched in sporadic cases, this has not been confirmed). Third, large-scale GWAS has identified specific locations in the genome that are recurrent sites of CNVs (Table 138-2b). These CNVs are often large, contain multiple genes, and confer larger relative risks (1.94 to >26) than the individual SNP loci. Furthermore, they often are observed in multiple additional disease phenotypes including most commonly autism spectrum disorder (ASD), learning disability (LD), and epilepsy. Hundreds of genes are contained within the frequently deleted or duplicated in CNVs. These genes are enriched in neuronal functions particularly those that are involved in synaptic activity and neurodevelopmental processes. Additional support for proteins-enriched synaptic signaling has been found in recent work on de novo CNVs.

Advanced paternal age is associated with increased risk of schizophrenia (age 45-49, relative risk =1.24; > 50 = 1.79) suggesting a role for de novo mutations. Deep sequencing of coding regions of candidate genes and whole exomes find that there may be an increased rate of de novo single-nucleotide variants, however the current studies are small and somewhat inconsistent (Table 138-2c). The exome studies did not observe multiple de novo mutations in any specific gene implying that there are not a small number of genes with large effect sizes attributable to rare de novo mutation and furthermore, that many of the observed mutations will not be pathogenic. Of note, mutations in *SHANK3* and *NRXN1*, previously implicated in CNV studies, were found in a candidate gene analysis.

The overall genetic architecture of SCZ remains unclear. However, the data is now strong that very many genes contribute to overall risk of developing the disease and that the allele spectrum will include rare and common variation. These data together suggest a threshold liability model and are consistent with both the elevated monozygotic concordance rates, as well as the observed high rates of sporadic cases, both of which are predicted for genetic diseases with prevalence in 1% range.

**Genetic Testing:** Currently clinical genetic testing is not available for SCZ.

**Future Directions:** Recent genomic studies have added significant information regarding loci conferring increased risk for SCZ particularly in the area of rare, large structural variation. In addition, GWAS have identified common variants at specific loci with consistent but modest effect sizes, as well as a polygenic signal implicating many genes in SCZ risk. Areas of extensive current research include (1) the role of de novo and inherited rare variation (eg, single nucleotide and indel), (2) exploration of phenotype-genotype correlations, and (3) exploration of genetic and environmental interactions.

Since available data support a highly complex genetic etiology for SCZ generally, rather than the existence of multiple homogeneous subsets of SCZ, strategies integrating across diverse types of data including DNA, RNA, and the epigenome will be needed to understand the pathways involved in SCZ pathogenesis. Extension of the current findings into large samples will be required to confidently apply these results to diagnostic testing, drug development, and to minimize drug side effects. However, the rapid pace of current advances gives us confidence that ultimately understanding the genetics of SCZ will enrich our understanding of basic cellular biology of the brain, as well as disease-specific neurobiology.

**BIBLIOGRAPHY:**

1. *Diagnostic and Statistical Manual of Mental Disorders, Fourth Edition Text Revision* (DSM-IV-TR). American Psychiatric Association; WHO ICD website. http://www.who.int/classifications/icd/en/.

2. Lichtenstein P, Björk C, Hultman CM, Scolnick E, Sklar P. Sullivan PF. Recurrence risks for schizophrenia in a Swedish national cohort. *Psychol Med.* Oct 2006;36(10):1417-1425.

3. Lichtenstein P, Yip BH, Björk C, Pawitan Y, Cannon TD, Sullivan PF, Hultman CM. Common genetic determinants of schizophrenia and bipolar disorder in Swedish families: a population-based study. *Lancet.* Jan 17 2009;373(9659):234-239.

4. Finn CT, Smoller JW. Genetic counseling in psychiatry. *Harv Rev Psychiatry.* 2006;14(2):109-121.

5. Grozeva D, Conrad DF, Barnes CP, et al. WTCCC. De novo CNV analysis implicates specific abnormalities of postsynaptic signalling complexes in the pathogenesis of schizophrenia. *Mol Psychiatry.* Feb 2012;17(2):142-153.

6. Malhotra D, Sebat J. CNVs: harbingers of a rare variant revolution in psychiatric genetics. *Cell.* Mar 16 2012;148(6):1223-1241.

7. Schizophrenia Psychiatric Genome-Wide Association Study (GWAS) Consortium. Genome-wide association study identifies five new schizophrenia loci. *Nat Genet.* Sep 18 2011;43(10):969-976.

8. Hamshere ML, Walters JT, Smith R, et al. The Schizophrenia Psychiatric Genome-wide Association Study Consortium (PGC), Wellcome Trust Case Control Consortium+ (WTCCC+), Wellcome Trust Case Control Consortium 2 (WTCCC2), Morris D, Gill M, Holmans P, Craddock N, Corvin A, Owen MJ, O'Donovan MC. Genome-wide significant associations in schizophrenia to ITIH3/4, CACNA1C and SDCCAG8, and extensive replication of associations reported by the Schizophrenia PGC. *Mol Psychiatry.* Jun 2013;18(6):738.

9. Lee SH, DeCandia TR, Ripke S, Yang J. Schizophrenia Psychiatric Genome-Wide Association Study Consortium (PGC-SCZ); International Schizophrenia Consortium (ISC); Molecular Genetics of Schizophrenia Collaboration (MGS), Sullivan PF, Goddard ME, Keller MC, Visscher PM, Wray NR. Estimating the proportion of variation in susceptibility to schizophrenia captured by common SNPs. *Nat Genet.* Feb 19 2012;44(3):247-250.

10. Xu B, Roos JL, Dexheimer P, et al. Exome sequencing supports a de novo mutational paradigm for schizophrenia. *Nat Genet.* Aug 7 2011;43(9):864-868.

11. Girard SL, Gauthier J, Noreau A, et al. Increased exonic de novo mutation rate in individuals with schizophrenia. *Nat Genet.* Jul 10 2011;43(9):860-863.

12. Fleeman N, McLeod C, Bagust A, et al. The clinical effectiveness and cost-effectiveness of testing for cytochrome P450 polymorphisms in patients with schizophrenia treated with antipsychotics: a systematic review and economic evaluation. *Health Technol Assess.* Jan 2010;14(3):1-157.

13. Visscher PM, Goddard ME, Derks EM, Wray NR. Evidence-based psychiatric genetics, AKA the false dichotomy between common and rare variant hypotheses. *Mol Psychiatry.* May 2012;17(5):474-485.

14. Tandon R, Nasrallah HA, Keshavan MS. Schizophrenia, "just the facts" 5. Treatment and prevention. Past, present, and future. *Schizophr Res.* Sep 2010;122(1-3):1-23.

15. Grozeva D, Conrad DF, Barnes CP, et al. Independent estimation of the frequency of rare CNVs in the UK population confirms their role in schizophrenia. *Schizophr Res.* 2012;135(1-3):1-7. Epub 2011 Nov 29.

16. Awadalla P, Gauthier J, Myers RA, et al. Direct measure of the de novo mutation rate in autism and schizophrenia cohorts. *Am J Hum Genet.* 2010 Sep 10;87(3):316-24.

## Supplementary Information

**OMIM REFERENCES:** Selection from >200 OMIM entries

[1] Schizophrenia; SCZD (#181500) Structural variant loci

[2] Schizophrenia; SCZD4 (#600850)

[3] Schizophrenia; SCZD13 (#613025)

[4] Schizophrenia; Chromosome 1q21.1 Deletion Syndrome (#612474)

[5] Schizophrenia; NRXN1 (#600565)

[6] Schizophrenia; Chromosome 17q12 Deletion Syndrome (#614527)

[7] Schizophrenia; Chromosome 3q29 Deletion Syndrome (#609425)

### Alternative Names:

- Dementia Praecox
- Schizoaffective Disorder
- Frequently Used But Incorrect Colloquial Names—Multiple Personality Disorder, Split Personality

***Key Words:*** Polygene, deletion, CNV, psychosis

# 139 Genetics of Drug Addiction

Noura S. Abul-Husn and Eric J. Nestler

## KEY POINTS

- *Disease summary:*
  - Drug addiction (termed as substance dependence or drug dependence by DSM-IV) is a complex neurobiologic disease characterized by genetic, psychosocial, and environmental factors.
  - Drug addiction is considered to be a maladaptive pattern of drug use that leads to clinically significant impairment or distress.
  - Addictive drugs are characterized by their ability to produce, after acute exposure, euphoria, a positive emotional state that motivates users to take the drug repeatedly. Addictive drugs include alcohol, nicotine, marijuana, opiates (eg, heroin, OxyContin), stimulants (cocaine, amphetamine, methamphetamine), psychotomimetics (eg, phencyclidine [PCP]), 3,4-methylenedioxymethamphetamine [MDMA or "ecstasy"]), etc.
- *Differential diagnosis:*
  - *Drug abuse:* In comparison with drug addiction, this is a milder disorder, in which the individual chooses to use a drug in spite of illegal, unsafe consequences, or inappropriateness of the drugging experience. This differs from drug addiction, which is characterized by impaired control over drug use.
  - *Physical or physiologic dependence:* This is an adaptive physiologic state that occurs with regular or prolonged drug use, and results in a characteristic withdrawal syndrome (characterized by a range of physical or psychological symptoms) when drug intake is terminated. Physical or physiologic dependence can exist in the absence of drug addiction.
  - *Tolerance:* This describes the diminished response that occurs with repeated drug use, such that larger doses of the drug are required to achieve the same effect. Tolerance can exist in the absence of drug addiction.
  - *Sensitization:* This is the opposite of tolerance, where repeated exposure to a constant dose of a drug elicits greater responses. Repeated exposure to a given drug can simultaneously produce tolerance and sensitization to its varying effects.
  - *Pseudoaddiction*: This represents patient behaviors that may occur when pain is not being adequately treated. Such patients may exhibit "drug seeking" behaviors or resort to taking illegal drugs. In contrast to true addiction, pseudoaddiction stops once the patient's pain is effectively controlled.
- *Monogenic forms:*
  - Genetic studies have failed to support single-gene models for the inheritance of addiction vulnerability. Addiction is a complex disorder that receives contributions from allelic variations in multiple genes.
- *Family history:*
  - Drug addiction vulnerability is familial. Indeed, genetic factors contribute to 40% to 60% of the overall vulnerability to drug addiction, while environmental factors provide the remainder.
- *Twin studies:*
  - Twin studies have shown a higher concordance rate for monozygotic twins in tobacco, alcohol, and other drug addictions. Twin data support the idea that much of the genetic vulnerability to the abuse of different addictive substances is shared. Although some elements of addiction vulnerability may be specific to particular substances, most genetic influences are common to different addictive substances.
- *Environmental factors:*
  - Environmental factors that contribute to addiction vulnerability have been identified in a number of epidemiologic studies. Shared and unique environmental factors contribute significantly to the risk for lifetime drug addiction, accounting for 28% to 38% of the phenotypic variance. Nonetheless, some individuals avoid addiction even in environments rich in addictive drugs. Moreover, none of these environmental influences is specific, as each is associated with increased risk for a range of neuropsychiatric disorders as well as with, in most cases, a normal outcome.
- *Pharmacogenomics:*
  - Despite the progress made in the prevention and treatment of drug addiction, available pharmacologic therapies are only effective in a fraction of addicted patients. The wide individual variation in therapeutic response has prompted a growing interest in the role that inherited factors play in the efficacy of various pharmacotherapies (Table 139-1).
- *Genome-wide associations:*
  - Genes that affect addiction vulnerability have recently begun to emerge from large family and population studies (Table 139-2). However, all of the genes identified thus far only represent a small fraction of the overall genetic risk for addiction.

## Diagnostic Criteria and Clinical Characteristics

***Diagnostic Criteria for Drug Addiction:*** According to DSM-IV criteria, drug dependence is diagnosed by three or more of the following, occurring at any time during the same 12-month period:

1. Tolerance—defined by either of the following
   a. A need for markedly increased amounts of the substance to achieve intoxication or the desired effect *or*
   b. Markedly diminished effect with the continued use of the same amount of the substance
2. Withdrawal—as manifested by either of the following
   a. The characteristic withdrawal syndrome for the substance *or*

*Table 139-1 **Pharmacogenetic Considerations in Drug Addiction***

| Gene | Associated Medications | Goal of Testing | Variants | Purported Effect |
|------|------------------------|-----------------|----------|------------------|
| *OPRM1* | Nicotine replacement therapy | Efficacy | Asn40Asp allele | Predicts a better response to nicotine-replacement therapy in nicotine addiction |
| *OPRM1* | Naltrexone | Efficacy | Asn40Asp allele | Predicts a better response to naltrexone treatment of alcohol addiction |
| *DRD4* | Olanzapine | Efficacy | L allele of a VNTR | Predicts a better response to olanzapine in alcohol addiction |
| *GRIK1* | Topiramate | Efficacy | rs2832407 in intron 9 | Predicts adverse events from treatment with topiramate in alcohol addiction |

b. The same (or closely related) substance is taken to relieve or avoid withdrawal symptoms

3. The substance is often taken in larger amounts or over a longer period than intended.
4. There is a persistent desire or unsuccessful efforts to cut down or control substance use.
5. A great deal of time is spent in activities necessary to obtain the substance, use the substance, or recover from its effects.
6. Important social, occupational, or recreational activities are given up or reduced because of substance use.
7. Substance use is continued despite knowledge of having a persistent physical or psychological problem that is likely to have been caused or exacerbated by the substance.

*Clinical Characteristics:*

☞**ACUTE INTOXICATION:** Addictive drugs affect multiple biologic systems, and their use can result in effects ranging from mild euphoria to psychotic episodes, respiratory or cardiovascular distress, accidental injury, or death. Signs and symptoms of drug use vary depending on the type and amount of drug used. Some examples are listed below:

*Alcohol*: Alcohol is a central nervous system (CNS) depressant. Its effects range from mildly impaired co-ordination and euphoria, marked ataxia, nausea or vomiting, and memory lapse, to severe respiratory failure, coma, and death.

*Nicotine*: Nicotine is a CNS stimulant characterized by euphoria, increased attention, and mild analgesia. Initial exposures can induce nausea, but this shows tolerance with repeated administration.

*Marijuana*: Marijuana generally causes mild euphoria, analgesia, and increased appetite. Other effects include impaired perception and motor skills, decreased short-term memory, anxiety, paranoia, and mild hallucinations.

*Opiates*: Opiates are commonly used clinically for their strong analgesic properties. Opiate overdose is characterized by respiratory depression, pinpoint pupils, decreased level of consciousness, or coma.

*Stimulants:* Stimulants such as cocaine, amphetamine, and methamphetamine cause hyperactivity and euphoria. They can also lead to fatal arrhythmias, seizures, or stroke and, after chronic administration, may induce paranoia.

*Psychotomimetics:* Phencyclidine (PCP) and related drugs (eg, ketamine) induce hallucinations and delusions as well as nausea or vomiting, seizures, coma, and death (often from accidental injury or suicide). Its sedative effects can interact with other CNS depressants, such as alcohol and benzodiazepines, leading to coma or accidental overdose.

☞**WITHDRAWAL:** Withdrawal symptoms occur upon the sudden discontinuation of a drug (or administration of an antagonist), and also vary depending on the drug involved. Withdrawal symptoms are typically opposite to the initial effects of a drug. Alcohol withdrawal can vary from mild symptoms such as sleep disturbances and anxiety, to severe and life-threatening symptoms, including hallucinations, seizures, delirium, and death. Opioid withdrawal ("cold turkey") can result in irritability, pain, nausea, and vomiting. Stimulant withdrawal can result in irritability, sleep disturbances, and depression.

☞**RELAPSE:** Repeated drug use can permanently affect the brain's reward circuitry to promote addiction by causing drug craving in response to environmental cues, stress, or the drug itself. For this reason, drug addicts are considered to be at lifelong risk for relapse.

☞**PERIPHERAL TOXICITY OF TOBACCO USE:** Chronic tobacco use contributes to respiratory and cardiovascular diseases, including myocardial infarction, stroke, chronic obstructive pulmonary disease (COPD), and cancer (particularly lung cancer, as well as cancers of the larynx and mouth). The contribution of nicotine per se to these sequelae remains uncertain.

☞**COMORBIDITIES:** There is a high rate of comorbidity between drug addiction and other psychiatric illnesses, including depression, bipolar disorder, anxiety, and schizophrenia. For example, individuals diagnosed with mood or anxiety disorders are twice as likely to suffer also from drug abuse or dependence, and vice versa.

## Screening and Counseling

*Screening:* Although numerous genes have been implicated in drug addiction risk, no screens are used clinically. The best characterized genetic contribution to addiction concerns mutations in enzymes that degrade alcohol (see later under "Molecular Genetics"); however, this is not used for routine screening. Another gene implicated in addiction risk is referred to as the *DRD2 TaqI* polymorphism; *DRD2* expresses the D2 dopamine receptor. Individuals with the A1 allele of this polymorphism are reported to show increased risk for alcohol and other drug addictions, but many groups have questioned the validity of this association.

*Table 139-2 Drug Addiction-Associated Susceptibility Variants*

| Candidate Gene (Chromosome Location) | Associated Variant [effect on protein] (assayed by Affymetrix/ Illumina) | Frequency of Risk Allele | Putative Functional Significance | Associated Disease Phenotype |
|---|---|---|---|---|
| ADH1B (4q22) | ADH1B*2 [nonsynonymous amino acid substitution R47H] | Common in Asian and Ashkenazi Jewish populations | Alcohol dehydrogenase with higher catalytic activity | Four- to fivefold reduction in alcohol addiction vulnerability |
| | ADH1B*3 [nonsynonymous amino acid substitution R369C] | Common in African-American and Native American populations | | Negative family history of alcohol addiction in African Americans. Absence of alcohol addiction in Native Americans. |
| ADH1C (4q22) | ADH1C*1 [nonsynonymous amino acid substitution I349V] | Common in Asians | | Decreased alcohol addiction vulnerability |
| ALDH2 (12q24.2) | ALDH2*2 [nonsynonymous amino acid substitution Q487K] | Common in Asians (~40%), rare in non-Asians | Inactive aldehyde dehydrogenase | Five to ninefold reduction in alcohol addiction vulnerability. Near-zero rate of alcohol addiction in homozygotes. |
| SLC6A4 (5-HTT) (17q11.1-q12) | 5-HTTLPR short S allele [lowers 5-HTT transcriptional activity] | 40% of European Americans | Decreased levels of serotonin transporter | ? Association with alcohol addiction—variable findings |
| CHRNA3 (15q24) | (rs1051730, rs6495308, rs1051730) | | α3 nicotinic acetylcholine receptor | Nicotine addiction |
| CHRNA5 (15q24-q25) | [nonsynonymous amino acid substitution D398N] (rs16969968) | 37%-43% in European and Middle Eastern populations. Uncommon in others. | α5 nicotinic acetylcholine receptor | Habitual smoking (20 cigarettes/d × 6 months or more) |
| GABRA1 (5q34-q35) | A15G AvaII restriction fragment length polymorphism (RFLP) | | GABA$_A$ receptor (α-1 subunit) | Alcohol addiction |
| GABRA2 (4p13-p12) | A 3-SNP haplotype: rs279871, rs279845, and rs279836 | 48.5% in families with many alcoholics | GABA$_A$ receptor (α-2 subunit) | Alcohol addiction |
| GABRA6 (5q31.1-q35) | T1519C AlwNI RFLP | | GABA$_A$ receptor (α-6 subunit) | Alcohol addiction |
| CHRM2 | (rs1824024, rs2061174, rs324650) | | Muscarinic cholinergic receptor | Alcohol addiction |
| | (rs324650) | | | Nicotine addiction |
| COMT (22q11.2) | Low activity L allele [nonsynonymous amino acid substitution V158M] | 25% Caucasians are homozygous for L allele | Catechol-O-methyltransferase with reduced activity and thermal instability | Alcohol addiction— variable findings |
| OPRM1 (6q24-q25) | Asp40 allele [nonsynonymous amino acid substitution N40D] | 2% in African Americans, 49% in Japanese | Altered function of the mu opioid receptor | Alcohol and other addictions—variable findings |

*Counseling:* Given the important role of environment in determining addiction vulnerability, genetic testing alone is unlikely to predict whether or not an individual will become an addict. However, genetic screening and counseling can serve to identify individuals at risk (eg, adolescents with a strong family history of alcoholism) and help to prevent drug addiction in these patients. Thus, genetic screening and counseling may eventually become incorporated into standard medical practice.

## Management and Treatment

*Management:* When the diagnosis of drug addiction is made, acute and long-term treatment is necessary. The most common treatment for drug addiction is drug-free outpatient counseling. Inpatient acute hospitalization is reserved for the most severely impaired patients, for example, with complicated withdrawal and/or medical or psychiatric comorbidities. Long-term residential treatment settings are also an option.

*Therapeutics:* Medications are an important element of treatment for some drug addictions. Medications can be used to reduce drug use as well as to prevent relapse once an initial remission is secured.

Pharmacotherapy is most useful when combined with counseling and other behavioral therapies. However, even when used optimally, only a fraction of patients benefit from existing medications.

- *Opioid addiction:* Methadone, a synthetic opiate and opioid receptor agonist, and buprenorphine, a semisynthetic opiate and opioid receptor partial agonist, are effective in helping patients addicted to heroin or other opiates. Naltrexone, an opioid receptor antagonist, is also used in the treatment of opiate addiction.
- *Alcohol addiction:* Disulfiram, an acetaldehyde dehydrogenase blocker, is used in the treatment of alcohol addiction. Disulfiram interrupts the metabolism of alcohol by preventing the breakdown of its metabolite acetaldehyde to acetic acid; this produces a severe and negative reaction to alcohol intake due to the accumulation of acetaldehyde. Naltrexone is effective in the treatment of alcohol addiction, and has been shown to reduce the frequency and severity of relapse. Acamprosate (which acts at N-methyl-D-aspartate [NMDA] and γ-aminobutyric acid [GABA] receptors) and topiramate (an anticonvulsant drug) are also used to treat alcohol addiction, though their mechanisms of action are less clear.
- *Nicotine addiction:* Nicotine replacement products, such as patches, gums, or lozenges, are commonly used as aides for smoking cessation. Also, oral medications such as varenicline (a partial agonist at nicotinic acetylcholine receptors), and bupropion (an antidepressant medication) have proven to be effective in the treatment of nicotine addiction.

☞**PHARMACOGENETICS:** Despite recent advances in pharmacogenetics, these have only just begun to influence the field of drug addiction. Of greatest clinical relevance are studies involving variants of the mu opioid receptor (OPRM1) in the treatment of drug addiction. Over 300 OPRM1 genetic variants have been identified; of these, the Asn40Asp SNP (resulting from an A118G transition) has been most extensively studied for its association with addiction. Though Asn40Asp does not appear to affect drug addiction vulnerability, it has been shown to moderate treatment response in several studies. In smokers on short-term nicotine replacement therapy, Asp40 carriers had a higher rate of abstinence compared to Asn40/

Asn40 homozygotes. In alcoholics prescribed naltrexone, Asp40 carriers had significantly lower rates of relapse, increased percent days abstinence, and decreased percent heavy drinking days compared to Asn40/Asn40 homozygotes.

However, other studies have not supported the association of OPRM1 Asn40Asp polymorphism with naltrexone treatment response; thus, further research is needed to accurately define this association.

Other studies of alcohol addiction have shown modest effects of different receptor variants in predicting treatment response as well as adverse effects (Table 139-1) [recently reviewed in ref. 8]. In the case of the D4 dopamine receptor (DRD4), a 7-repeat (long or L) allele of a 48-basepair variable number of tandem repeats (*VNTR*) polymorphism in exon III was shown to moderate the effects of the antipsychotic medication olanzapine on alcohol and drinking behavior. However, as this was demonstrated in a small study focusing on self-reported craving for alcohol, further research is needed to verify this effect. A variation in GRIK1, which encodes a subunit of the kainate receptor (GluR5) that selectively binds topiramate, was found to moderate adverse effects associated with topiramate treatment. These findings also need to be replicated as they have important clinical implications for the use of topiramate in the treatment of alcohol addiction.

## Molecular Genetics and Molecular Mechanisms

Though drug addiction is known to be highly heritable, the specific genes involved in addiction vulnerability remain largely unknown. To date, the most established genetic contribution to addiction is the protective effect of mutations in alcohol-metabolizing enzymes on alcohol addiction vulnerability. Mutations that increase alcohol dehydrogenase (ADH) activity and decrease aldehyde dehydrogenase (ALDH) activity are additive and promote the accumulation of acetaldehyde following alcohol intake. This produces intoxication at lower doses as well as an unpleasant flushing reaction, similar to the effects produced by disulfiram. These variants are common among individuals of East Asian descent, and individuals expressing these variants rarely abuse alcohol.

Other genes have recently been implicated in addiction vulnerability (Table 139-2) [reviewed in refs. 6,9,10]. The most established susceptibility loci are regions on chromosomes 4 and 5 containing GABA$_A$ receptor gene clusters linked to alcohol addiction, and the nicotinic acetylcholine receptor gene cluster on chromosome 15 associated with nicotine and alcohol addiction. Other addiction susceptibility loci include variants in catechol-*O*-methyl transferase COMT, the mu opioid receptor, and the serotonin transporter, although further work is needed to validate these findings.

*Genetic Testing:* Thus far, there is no established role for genetic testing in the diagnosis, prevention, or treatment of drug addiction.

*Future Directions:* Though many genes have been identified as contributing to drug addiction vulnerability, most of the genetic findings appear to be of small effect and will require replication to confirm the reported associations. To date, most studies of addiction genetics have focused on genes encoding proteins within the neurobiologic systems that are involved in the responses of drugs of abuse or are altered by exposure to drugs of abuse. Larger genome-wide scans are needed to further our understanding of molecular genetics and pharmacogenomics in the field of drug addiction.

An area of great potential clinical relevance is the ability to predict treatment responses in addicted patients. Advances in this area could eventually make it possible to match patients with specific treatments that are more likely to be successful.

Finally, despite their significant role, genetic factors are not the sole contributors to the development of addiction. Further studies are needed to understand the complex interplay between genetic and environmental factors in drug addiction, as well as a potential role for epigenetic mechanisms, in order to improve the development of pharmacologic and behavioral therapies for the prevention and treatment of drug addiction.

## BIBLIOGRAPHY:

1. Prescott CA, Kendler KS. Genetic and environmental contributions to alcohol abuse and dependence in a population-based sample of male twins. *Am J Psychiatry*. 1999;156:34-40.

2. Tsuang MT, Bar JL, Harley RM, Lyons MJ. The Harvard Twin Study of Substance Abuse: what we have learned. *Harv Rev Psychiatry*. 2001;9:267-279.

3. Kendler KS, Thornton LM, Pedersen NL. Tobacco consumption in Swedish twins reared apart and reared together. *Arch Gen Psychiatry*. 2000;57:886-892.

4. Tsuang MT, Lyons MJ, Meyer JM, et al. Co-occurrence of abuse of different drugs in men: the role of drug-specific and shared vulnerabilities. *Arch Gen Psychiatry*. 1998;55:967-972.

5. Noble EP. The DRD2 gene in psychiatric and neurological disorders and its phenotypes. *Pharmacogenomics*. 2000;1:309-333.

6. Khokhar JY, Ferguson CS, Zhu AZ, Tyndale RF. Pharmacogenetics of drug dependence: role of gene variations in susceptibility and treatment. *Annu Rev Pharmacol Toxicol*. 2010;50:39-61.

7. Lerman C, Wileyto EP, Patterson F, et al. The functional mu opioid receptor (OPRM1) Asn40Asp variant predicts short-term response to nicotine replacement therapy in a clinical trial. *Pharmacogenomics J*. 2004;4:184-192.

8. Kranzler HR, Edenberg HJ. Pharmacogenetics of alcohol and alcohol dependence treatment. *Curr Pharm Des*. 2010;16:2141-2148.

9. Dick DM, Bierut LJ. The genetics of alcohol dependence. *Curr Psychiatry Rep*. 2006;8:151-157.

10. Kreek MJ, Nielsen DA, LaForge KS. Genes associated with addiction: alcoholism, opiate, and cocaine addiction. *Neuromolecular Med*. 2004;5:85-108.

11. Renthal W, Nestler EJ. Epigenetic mechanisms in drug addiction. *Trends Mol Med*. 2008;14:341-350.

## Supplementary Information

### OMIM REFERENCES:

[1] Alcohol Dependence: ADH1B (#103780)

[2] Alcohol Dependence: ADH1C (#103730)

[3] Tobacco Addiction, Susceptibility to (#188890)

[4] Tobacco addiction, Susceptibility to: SLC6A4 (#126455).

**Alternative Names:**
- Drug Dependence
- Substance Dependence

***Key Words:*** Abuse, alcohol, dependence, nicotine, opiate, smoking

# 140 Nicotine Dependence

Ming D. Li, Thomas J. Payne, and Caryn Lerman

## KEY POINTS

- *Disease summary:*
  - Nicotine dependence (ND) is a complex psychiatric disorder determined by both genetics and environment, as well as gene-gene and gene-environment interactions.
  - About 20% of US adults use tobacco (primarily cigarettes); 70% of smokers want to quit, but only 4% to 7% are successful on a long-term basis without assistance.
  - Tobacco use is the leading preventable cause of morbidity and death in the United States.
  - It is the most common cause of cancer-related deaths in many countries, including cancers of the lung, larynx, esophagus, oral tissues, and bladder.
  - Tobacco use is also a leading cause of coronary artery disease, myocardial infarction, peripheral vascular disease, stroke, and chronic obstructive pulmonary disease (COPD).
  - Tobacco use is directly responsible for more than 443,000 premature deaths annually in the United States, with direct and indirect healthcare costs exceeding $193 billion.
  - Extensive research documents the relation between tobacco use and psychiatric conditions, particularly depression, anxiety disorders, substance abuse, and schizophrenia. Nicotine-dependent individuals appear more likely to develop depressive and anxiety disorders, and quitting partially reduces that risk. Tobacco users with psychiatric disorders are less likely to quit and are at risk for a substantially shortened life spans. Tobacco use prevalence rates for those with psychotic, depressive, or anxiety disorders or for those who are alcohol dependent is much higher than for the general population. In addition, nicotine alters the metabolism of many medications, including psychotropics, requiring close monitoring and dosage adjustment.
- *Monogenic forms:*
  - No single-gene cause of ND is known.
- *Family history:*
  - Initiation of smoking is two to four times more likely for adolescents whose parents and siblings smoke.
- *Twin studies:*
  - Monozygotic twins have a significantly higher concordance rate for ND than dizygotic twins. For example, one study revealed the concordance rate for ND in monozygotic twins to be 72% versus 28% for dizygotic twins.
- *Environmental factors:*
  - Many factors such as peers, friends, and family members who smoke, low socioeconomic status, or stressful environments are implicated as environmental triggers for ND.
- *Association studies:*
  - Many studies, including candidate gene-based association and genome-wide association (GWA) studies, have been conducted. Genetic variants associated with ND provide insight into the etiology of ND; however, testing for single-nucleotide polymorphisms (SNPs) is not yet clinically validated to diagnose or guide the management of ND.
- *Pharmacogenomics:*
  - There are reproducible and clinically significant associations of a phenotypic biomarker of nicotine metabolism rate (and CYP2A6 enzyme activity) with smoking cessation and response to nicotine replacement therapies. Although there is promising evidence for a role in smoking cessation for SNPs in the nicotinic receptor subunit genes β2, α5, and α3, effects are small and not consistently replicated.

## Diagnostic Criteria and Clinical Characteristics

***Diagnostic Criteria for ND:*** DSM-IV diagnosis of ND requires an individual to meet at least three of the following criteria during a 12-month period:

- Tolerance: the need for a markedly increased amount of nicotine to produce the desired effect or a diminished effect with continued use of the same amount of nicotine.
- Withdrawal, as manifested by either the characteristic syndrome, or use of nicotine or related substance to relieve or avoid withdrawal symptoms (ie, depressed mood, insomnia, irritability, anxiety, concentration difficulties, restlessness, decreased heart rate, and increased appetite or weight gain).
- Nicotine is used in larger amounts or over a longer period than intended.
- The individual has a persistent desire or makes unsuccessful attempts to cut down on use of tobacco.
- A great deal of time is spent in obtaining or using the substance.
- Reduced important social, occupational, or recreational activities because of tobacco use.
- Use of tobacco continues despite recurrent physical or psychological problems caused or exacerbated by tobacco; for example, continuing to smoke despite diagnoses such as hypertension, heart disease, cancer, bronchitis, and chronic obstructive lung disease.

The DSM-IV criteria for ND have been criticized for a variety of reasons. Primary among these is that a diagnosis of ND does not assess the degree of dependence. Thus, other instruments have been used as a supplement or replacement. The Fagerström Test for Nicotine Dependence (FTND) is one of the most commonly used questionnaires to characterize the degree to which the patient is physically dependent on cigarette smoking (Table 140-1).

Another option for measuring ND is the Wisconsin Inventory for Smoking Dependence Motives (WISDM), which provides greater information regarding various domains of smoking motivation. This is a relatively new scale with accumulating evidence suggesting its utility. Other scales are used less frequently and tend to be restricted to research applications.

Given the problems identified with the DSM-IV diagnostic criteria, substantial revisions are planned for the DSM-V edition. These proposed criteria call for (a) a total of 11 possible symptoms: the seven DSM-IV dependence criteria, three nicotine abuse criteria, and one new craving item; (b) reducing the number of required symptoms from three to two; and (c) establishing a severity indicator (ie, two or three symptoms for moderate, four or more symptoms for severe ND). However, only limited direct research has evaluated the viability of these new criteria to date.

*Clinical Characteristics:* Patterns of tobacco use vary considerably. Individuals may consume tobacco sporadically or on a daily basis, from small to relatively large amounts, and use a single versus multiple forms. The degree to which an individual's pattern of use is elicited by exposure to tobacco stimuli (eg, others smoking, distressing circumstances) is variable, as is the type, intensity, and duration of the particular withdrawal symptoms experienced. The general characteristics of the tobacco-using population are changing, with higher prevalence rates now evident among those of lower socioeconomic status and educational attainment and those with psychiatric diagnoses or symptoms. Overall, the risk of relapse postcessation generally is high, particularly for those who quit without professional assistance, or among certain subgroups (eg, pregnant women who smoke). Patients who have used tobacco products for an extended period often present with signs of compromised health, generally related to the length of smoking history. Depressive or anxiety symptoms or both are relatively common, but the clinician should be aware that the suicide rate for smokers is substantially higher than for the general population; the risk for former smokers falls in between.

## Screening and Counseling

*Screening:* No clear evidence to support genetic testing for ND or ability to quit smoking exists, and such tests have not yet been validated clinically. Although a number of SNPs in various candidate genes have been associated with ND or smoking cessation, only a few of them have been replicated in multiple independent samples, and most of these findings await further replication. So far, the most convincing example consists of variants in the nicotinic receptor subunit *CHRNA5/A3/B4* gene cluster on chromosome 15; a risk variant rs1051730 in this cluster has been used to predict the potential genetic risk for ND in individuals of European origin. However, the SNPs that have been studied account for a very small proportion of the variance (eg, <3%), and thus, predictive clinical validity would be low.

*Counseling:* Although there is substantial evidence for the involvement of genetic factors in ND and smoking cessation, no major Mendelian genes or variants have been identified. Familial clustering is common but not universal. Nevertheless, many variants have been implicated in ND and its treatment. Further validation is greatly needed in order to use this genetic information clinically.

## Management and Treatment

Healthcare-based interventions for tobacco dependence that include both counseling and pharmacologic evidence-based components comprise the most effective treatment approach. In general,

**Table 140-1** *Fagerström Test for Nicotine Dependence*

| Question | Selections | Score |
| --- | --- | --- |
| 1. How many cigarettes a day do you usually smoke? | ◦ 1-10 | 0 |
| | ◦ 11-20 | 1 |
| | ◦ 21-30 | 2 |
| | ◦ 31 or more | 3 |
| 2. How soon after you wake up do you smoke your first cigarette? | ◦ Within 5 minutes | 3 |
| | ◦ 6-30 minutes | 2 |
| | ◦ 31-60 minutes | 1 |
| | ◦ More than 60 minutes | 0 |
| 3. Do you smoke more frequently during the first 2 hours of the day than during the rest of the day? | ◦ Yes | 1 |
| | ◦ No | 0 |
| 4. Which cigarette would you hate the most to give up? | ◦ The first cigarette in the morning | 1 |
| | ◦ Any other cigarette | 0 |
| 5. Do you find it difficult to refrain from smoking in places where it is forbidden, such as church, at the movies, etc? | ◦ Yes | 1 |
| | ◦ No | 0 |
| 6. Do you still smoke even when you are so ill that you are in bed most of the day? | ◦ Yes | 1 |
| | ◦ No | 0 |
| **TOTAL** | | 0-10 |

interventions that incorporate higher levels of effort or resources increase the likelihood of success. With respect to counseling, this includes longer treatment times or more sessions, as well as input from providers from a variety of fields. When considering medications, recent evidence indicates higher dosing (as appropriate), some combination regimens, longer duration of therapy, and initiating prior to quit date (for nicotine replacement, similar to accepted protocols for other medications) generally are associated with higher quit rates.

***Psychosocial Interventions:*** Counseling for ND greatly improves long-term success. Although the particulars of how the intervention is delivered can take many forms, evidence suggests emphasis on two factors is the key: practical skills or problem solving, and intratreatment support. The delivery of services can vary with respect to intensity and modality. Intensity refers to the amount of time or number and spacing of sessions; the depth to which issues are dealt with, and level of patient participation are likely correlated features. Modality concerns the manner in which treatment is delivered. The following provides a brief overview of current options.

☞**Brief Interventions in the Primary Care Setting:** Primary care physicians and their staff operate in an environment that offers many advantages regarding the delivery of a standardized, brief intervention. The use of health information by experts to motivate patients, along with the capacity to counsel and provide prescription medications, is a highly effective combination. The major barriers are the perception of limited time to deliver these services, as well as inadequate reimbursement.

Brief interventions were developed in light of the usual operations in the outpatient clinic. They require little cost and/or staff time, with interventions as short as 3 minutes substantially increasing cessation rates. One widely employed option is the **"5A's"** method, which involves the following: (a) **Asking** about tobacco status at each visit; (b) **Advising** all tobacco users to quit; (c) **Assessing** the patient's willingness to quit; (d) **Assisting** the patient in quitting; and (e) **Arranging** for follow-up contact. Finally, if the intervention is unsuccessful or the provider believes a more potent intervention is necessary, patients can be provided with referrals to more intensive counseling programs.

☞**Specialty Tobacco Clinic Interventions:** This treatment option represents the highest end of the intensity dimension. Such programs are generally delivered by individuals who have received Tobacco Treatment Specialist training to conduct a multisession, face-to-face program (group or individual based) that addresses numerous issues related to achieving cessation. These programs often employ aggressive pharmacotherapy and more sophisticated counseling techniques and provide extended follow-up services.

☞**Quitlines:** Telephone-based services have the advantages of broad reach and somewhat more sophisticated counseling services, as well as easy access and relative anonymity. Pharmacotherapy options tend to be more limited, relying on patients working with their own physicians for complex options, and thus are not as tailored or closely monitored as Specialty Clinic options. Overall, they may be considered of moderate intensity, and represent a good option for many patients.

☞**Other Options:** Recently, other delivery modalities have emerged, including web-based and cellular telephone text-based options. Although available data are limited, early findings suggest the utility of these treatments.

***Therapeutics:*** National guidelines recommend that pharmacologic therapy be considered for all smokers attempting to quit unless it is medically contraindicated. Food and Drug Administration (FDA)-approved pharmacologic interventions for smoking cessation include nicotine replacement therapies (NRTs), bupropion hydrochloride, and varenicline tartrate, all of which enjoy extensive support for their effectiveness. Behavioral counseling is an important adjunct to any pharmacologic intervention for smoking cessation.

Nicotine replacement therapies deliver nicotine to ease withdrawal and craving while allowing the smoker to break the behavioral habits associated with tobacco use. Withdrawal symptoms are experienced by many when attempting to quit, and can reduce the likelihood of achieving and maintaining abstinence. There are five FDA-approved nicotine replacement options. Nicotine polacrilex gum and lozenges are available in 2-mg and 4-mg doses and are sold without a prescription. Patients must be instructed to use properly (eg, "chew and park" routine for the gum; avoid ingesting anything that alters the oral pH). The primary advantage is the ability to adjust administration as needed for changing circumstances. Nicotine transdermal patches (also over the counter) have the advantage of a delivery system that maintains steady nicotine concentrations over the course of the day. Both the nicotine nasal spray and the inhaler require a prescription. All NRTs may produce side effects, although these can often be reduced or eliminated with proper use tailored to the individual. The usual duration of use is approximately 3 months, although evidence is accumulating for improved long-term abstinence with longer periods of use.

Bupropion hydrochloride (Zyban) is an atypical antidepressant with noradrenergic and dopaminergic effects. Mechanisms of action include inhibition of dopamine reuptake in the nucleus accumbens, as well as nicotine antagonism in the ventral tegmental area. The recommended and maximum dose for smoking cessation is 300 mg per day, usually given as 150 mg twice daily. Dosing should begin at 150 mg a day, given daily for the first 3 to 7 days, followed by an increase to the recommended 300 mg a day, as tolerated. Therapy is typically begun 1 to 2 weeks before the patient's determined smoking quit date. Treatment should continue for at least the recommended 12 weeks.

Varenicline tartrate (Chantix) was approved by the FDA in 2006 for the treatment of ND. This medication appears to function as a partial agonist that binds with high affinity to the neuronal nicotinic acetylcholine receptor. Nicotine stimulation of this particular receptor, with which varenicline binds with high specificity, is associated with significant mesolimbic dopamine release which serves to reinforce nicotine ingestion. The high affinity with which varenicline binds to this receptor in conjunction with its long half-life reduces nicotine's capacity to stimulate the receptor, thereby reducing the reinforcing properties of nicotine ingestion, while providing sufficient stimulation to counter withdrawal symptoms. Dosing is uptitrated from 0.5 mg per day to 2 mg per day over the first week; 3 to 6 months of use is recommended.

## Molecular Genetics and Molecular Mechanism

Almost all approaches to human genetic studies have been used to search for susceptibility genomic regions and genes for ND, including genome-wide linkage analysis and candidate gene-based or GWA studies (Table 140-2). Although there is great variability in

**Table 140-2 Representative Susceptibility Variants for ND**

| Candidate Gene (symbol; chromosome location) | dbSNP ID; alleles [effect on protein] | Biologic Systems and Function | Associated Smoking Behavior |
|---|---|---|---|
| Catechol-O-methyltransferase (COMT; 22q11.21) | rs4680; G/A (V108M) | Met allele with lower enzyme activity may enhance dopamine signaling | Individuals with low-activity Met allele had lower dependence and higher quit rates |
| Dopamine receptor 1 (DRD1; 5q35.1) | rs686; A/G (3'-UTR) | Mediates dopamine effects; regulates RNA expression | Smoking quantity |
| Dopamine receptor 3 (DRD3; 3q13.3) | rs6280; C/T (G9S) | Mediates dopamine effects | Associated with CPD |
| Enzyme cytochrome P450 (CYP2A6; 19q13) | rs4105144; T/C (neighboring region) | | Associated with CPD |
| Nicotinic receptor β3 & α6 subunits (CHRNB3/CHRNA6; 8p11) | rs6474412; C/T (neighboring region) | | Associated with CPD and ND |
| Nicotinic receptor α4 subunit (CHRNA4; 20q13.33) | rs2236196; A/G (3-UTR) | Regulated RNA expression | Associated with CPD and smoking cessation |
| Nicotinic receptor α3 subunit (CHRNA3; 15q25.1) | rs1051730; G/A (exon 5) | Cause no amino acid change | Associated with CPD and heavy smoking |
| Nicotinic receptor α5 subunit (CHRNA5; 15q25.1) | rs1696968; A/G (D398N) | Regulates receptor-binding affinity | Associated with smoking quantity and heavy smoking |
| Taster receptor, type 2, member 38 (TAS2R38; 7q34) | rs713598 (C/G)-rs1726866 (C/T)-rs10246939 (C/T) P49A-A262V-V296I | Regulates taste status | Taster haplotype (PAV) is protective and nontaster haplotype (AVI) is risk for ND |

the detected linkage peaks among studies, primarily because of the small sample sizes, differences in measures of smoking behavior, and in ethnic backgrounds and environmental factors, regions on chromosomes 9, 10, 11, and 17 have been detected consistently by the greatest number of studies.

Genetic association studies investigate the association of a phenotype of interest with variants in genes implied in linkage analysis or those with strong biologic plausibility. The majority of these studies focused on genetic variants in the following three groups.

**Dopamine and other relevant neurotransmitter systems:** The majority of investigated genes are involved in the dopamine system, most often *DRD2*. Although many studies of the DRD2 *Taq*1A polymorphism reported an association with smoking behavior, a substantial number have failed to find one. Moreover, the functional significance of the DRD2 *Taq*1A polymorphism remains unclear, although evidence for an association with DRD2 receptor density has been reported. The *Taq*1A polymorphism apparently alters an amino acid residue in a protein kinase gene (*ANKK1*) near the *DRD2* locus. A modest number of studies have examined other dopamine receptor genes (eg, *DRD1*, *DRD3*, *DRD4*, and *DRD5*), the dopamine transporter (*DAT*), and genes involved in dopamine synthesis and metabolism, which include tyrosine hydroxylase (TH), dopamine beta hydroxylase (DBH), DOPA decarboxylase (*DDC*), and catechol-O-methyl transferase (*COMT*). There also have been studies of the GABAergic system. Subunit 2 of the GABAB

receptor (*GABAB2*) and GABAA receptor-associated protein gene (*GABARAP*) are significantly associated with ND. More recently, two independent high-density GWA studies implicated the neurexin gene family, including neurexins 1 and 3, in ND and polysubstance addiction. These findings strongly indicate that the GABAergic system is important in ND and other substance addictions.

**Nicotinic receptor subunit genes:** Several *nAChR* subunit genes have been examined. Whereas there is no evidence for an association of SNPs in *CHRNB2*, three recent studies provided evidence for the role of *CHRNA4*. A smaller study in schizophrenic smokers suggests that *CHRNA7* is associated with smoking status, although the relevance of this finding to the general population is unknown. Variants in *CHRNB1* and *CHRM1* are also associated with ND. Recently, several large-scale GWA and candidate gene-based association studies provided evidence for the association of variants in the *CHRNA5/A3/B4* cluster with ND and related phenotypes, as well as with lung cancer. Moreover, a significant association of *CHRNB3* with ND was found in a GWA study.

**Nicotine metabolism genes:** One of the most investigated genes of this family is *CYP2A6*, which encodes the enzyme cytochrome P450 CYP2A6. In humans, about 70% to 80% of nicotine is converted to cotinine by this liver enzyme. Approximately 33% to 40% of cotinine is converted to its primary metabolite, 3'-hydroxycotinine (3HC), also by *CYP2A6*. Variants in *CYP2A6* have been associated with several smoking-related phenotypes. Smokers with reduced or null activity *CYP2A6* alleles (CYP2A6*9, CYP2A6*12, CYP2A6*2, or CYP2A6*4) smoke fewer cigarettes and tend to be less nicotine dependent and more likely to quit than smokers with normal enzyme activity (CYP2A6*1) or increased enzyme activity (CYP2A6*1B). Several smoking cessation studies have reproducibly indicated that the nicotine metabolism rate predicts quitting success. Given the large number of *CYP2A6* alleles, as well as the influence of environmental factors on nicotine metabolism, a phenotypic biomarker of *CYP2A6* activity (3HC/cotinine) appears to be a more robust predictor of cessation than genotype. Interestingly, a recent GWA study revealed an association of reduced smoking quantity with rs4105144 SNP, which is in linkage disequilibrium with the *CYP2A6*2* reduced-activity allele.

**Future Directions:** The recent and current genetic studies of ND have already provided a wealth of new knowledge regarding the etiology of ND and its treatment. Insights into the molecular mechanisms underlying the etiology of ND and other smoking-related behaviors should provide new biologic targets for the treatment of ND. Although none of the susceptibility variants has provided a definitive genetic screening tool for the diagnosis of ND and its treatment, many susceptibility variants have been suggested. For example, although the SNP rs1051730 in the *CHRNA5/A3/B4* cluster has been suggested as predicting the risk of developing ND, the accuracy of that prediction remains to be explored; data on non-European smokers are particularly needed. Similarly, variation in the nicotine metabolism rate has been found to be a useful marker for treatment outcome and response to pharmacotherapy, but these findings were based on trials with relatively small samples. Thus, large-scale clinical studies correlating ND and response to treatment with genotype are needed, which may provide important new options for the prevention, treatment, and population screening for ND. Finally, pharmacogenetic research may facilitate the identification of individuals most susceptible to ND and those who may maximally benefit from certain medications.

**BIBLIOGRAPHY:**

1. Fagerstrom KO. Measuring degree of physical dependence to tobacco smoking with reference to individualization of treatment. *Addict Behav.* 1978;3:235-241.

2. Li MD. Identifying susceptibility loci for nicotine dependence: 2008 update based on recent genome-wide linkage analyses. *Hum Genet.* 2008;123:119-131.

3. Li MD, Cheng R, Ma JZ, Swan GE. A meta-analysis of estimated genetic and environmental effects on smoking behavior in male and female adult twins. *Addiction.* 2003;98:23-31.

4. Thorgeirsson TE, Gudbjartsson DF, Surakka I, et al. Sequence variants at CHRNB3-CHRNA6 and CYP2A6 affect smoking behavior. *Nat Genet.* 2010;42:448-453.

5. Tobacco and Genetics Consortium (TAG). Genome-wide meta-analyses identify multiple loci associated with smoking behavior. *Nat Genet.* 2010;42:441-447.

6. Lerman C, Jepson C, Wileyto EP, et al. Genetic variation in nicotine metabolism predicts the efficacy of extended-duration transdermal nicotine therapy. *Clin Pharmacol Ther.* 2010;87:553-557.

7. Lerman CE, Schnoll RA, Munafo MR. Genetics and smoking cessation improving outcomes in smokers at risk. *Am J Prev Med.* 2007;33:S398-S405.

8. Heatherton TF, Kozlowski LT, Frecker RC, Fagerstrom KO. The Fagerstrom Test for Nicotine Dependence: a revision of the Fagerstrom Tolerance Questionnaire. *Br J Addict.* 1991;86:1119-1127.

9. Furberg H, Ostroff J, Lerman C, Sullivan PF. The public health utility of genome-wide association study results for smoking behavior. *Genome Med.* 2010;2:26.

10. Bierut LJ, Stitzel JA, Wang JC, et al. Variants in nicotinic receptors and risk for nicotine dependence. *Am J Psychiatry.* 2008;165:1163-1171.

11. Fiore MC, Jae'n CR, Baker TB, et al. Treating tobacco use and dependence: 2008 update U.S. Public Health Service Clinical Practice Guideline executive summary. *Respir Care.* 2008;53:1217-1222.

12. Morissette SB, Tull MT, Gulliver SB, Kamholz BW, Zimering RT. Anxiety, anxiety disorders, tobacco use, and nicotine: a critical review of interrelationships. *Psychol Bull.* 2007;133:245-272.

13. Piper ME, Smith SS, Schlam TR, et al. Psychiatric disorders in smokers seeking treatment for tobacco dependence: relations with tobacco dependence and cessation. *J Consul Clin Psychol.* 2010;78:13-23.

## Supplementary Information

### OMIM REFERENCES:

[1] Tobacco Addiction, Susceptibility to; *SLC6A3, GPR51, CYP2A6,* and *CHRNA4* (#188890)

[2] Smoking as a Quantitative Trait Locus 3; SQTL3 (#612052)

[3] Smoking as a Quantitative Trait Locus 1; SQTL1 (#611003)

### Alternative Names:

- Nicotine Dependence
- Tobacco Dependence
- Smoking Addiction

**Key Words:** Nicotine dependence, tobacco, genetics, pharmacogenetics

# 141 **Spondyloarthropathies**

Matthew Brown and Philip Robinson

## KEY POINTS

- *Disease summary:*
  - The spondyloarthropathies (SpA) are a group of disorders causing inflammatory arthritis that typically involve the sacroiliac joints of the pelvis and usually the spine, and in which inflammation occurs at the insertion point of tendons into bone (enthesitis). They also share genetic associations notably with HLA-B27. Ankylosing spondylitis (AS) is the archetypal spondyloarthropathy; other members of this group include reactive arthritis (ReA), psoriatic arthritis (PsA), arthritis of inflammatory bowel disease (IBD), enteropathic arthritis, and axial spondyloarthritis (axial SpA). Where only peripheral joints are involved, the condition is termed peripheral SpA.
  - The main symptom of SpA is inflammatory back pain (IBP). This is chronic back pain that improves with activity, worsens with rest, and can cause patients to wake with back pain at night.
  - Inflammation in the sacroiliac joints (sacroiliitis) is universal in axial SpA.
  - Inflammation occurs where tendons join to bone (enthesitis). Commonly affected sites include the Achilles tendon, plantar fascia, and costal joints in SpA.
  - Peripheral arthritis occurs in axial SpA and usually involves large joints such as the knee, often asymmetrically.
  - Ankylosis, or bony fusion, of the sacroiliac joints and spinal vertebrae are the pathognomic feature of AS and other SpA.
  - SpA-associated conditions include skin psoriasis, IBD, and iritis.

- *Differential diagnosis:*
  - The most common alternate diagnoses for chronic back pain are degenerative lumbar disc disease (spondylosis) or facet joint osteoarthritis, and lumbar disc prolapse or tear. Diffuse idiopathic skeletal hyperostosis (DISH) often resembles AS radiographically but usually does not cause marked symptoms. The differential diagnoses of sacroiliitis include DISH, osteitis condensans ilii, degenerative arthritis, and septic arthritis.

- *Monogenic forms:*
  - No monogenic forms of SpA exist.

- *Family history:*
  - There is often a family history of one or more of the following: spondyloarthropathy, iritis, psoriasis, or IBD.

- *Twin studies:*
  - Twin studies in AS have shown that the environmental contribution to disease etiology is small; the identical twin concordance rate for the disease is greater than or equal to 60%. There is concordance among related individuals for SpA depending on the type of SpA, HLA-B27 status, and genetic relationship to the affected person (see Screening and Counseling section).

- *Environmental factors:*
  - ReA is caused by an immune reaction to microbial infection. Microbial infections are also thought to underlie the development of other forms of SpA, but thus far no specific organism has been convincingly implicated. Cigarette smoking increases the severity of AS and may also increase the risk of developing the disease.

- *Genome-wide associations:*
  - There have been three genome-wide association studies (GWASs) to date, one of which studied only nonsynonymous single-nucleotide polymorphisms (SNPs). These studies and other more targeted association studies have described 13 non-MHC confirmed associations. Along with the long known HLA-B association the results include SNPs in IL23R, ERAP1, CARD9, IL12B, TBKBP1, TNFR1, PTGER4, RUNX3, intergenic loci (2p15, 21q22), IL1R2, ANTXR2, and KIF21B. Some of these SNPs have also been identified in other autoimmune diseases like psoriasis and IBD.

- *Pharmacogenomics:*
  - There is currently limited evidence for the role of pharmacogenomics in SpA.

# Diagnostic Criteria and Clinical Characteristics

## Diagnostic Criteria for Spondyloarthritis:

☞THE 1984 MODIFIED NEW YORK CRITERIA FOR ANKYLOSING SPONDYLITIS:
- Clinical criteria
  - IBP
  - Limitation in chest expansion
  - Limitation in the movement of the lumbar spine
- Radiographic criterion
  - Either bilateral grade 2 sacroiliitis or unilateral grade 3 sacroiliitis on plain film
- Diagnosis requires one clinical criterion and the radiographic criterion

☞THE ASSESSMENT OF SPONDYLOARTHRITIS SOCIETY (ASAS) CLASSIFICATION CRITERIA FOR AXIAL SPONDYLOARTHRITIS: Either

1. Sacroiliitis* on imaging plus one or more SpA feature**, or
2. HLA-B27 plus two or more SpA features**

*Sacroiliitis on imaging is defined as (a) acute (active) inflammation on magnetic resonance imaging (MRI) highly suggestive of sacroiliitis associated with SpA, or, (b) definitive radiographic sacroiliitis according to the modified New York criteria.

**SpA features are defined as 1. IBP, 2. arthritis, 3. enthesitis (heel), 4. uveitis, 5. dactylitis, 6. Psoriasis, 7. Crohn disease or ulcerative colitis, 8. good response to nonsteroidal anti-inflammatory drugs (NSAIDs), 9. family history for SpA, 10. HLA-B27, and 11. elevated C-reactive protein (CRP).

☞THE ASAS CLASSIFICATION CRITERIA FOR PERIPHERAL SPONDYLOARTHRITIS: Arthritis or enthesitis or dactylitis **plus**

1. Greater than or equal to one of psoriasis, IBD, preceding infection, HLA-B27, uveitis, sacroiliitis on imaging (radiographs or MRI)
2. Or, two of the remaining: arthritis, enthesitis, dactylitis, IBP in the past, positive family history for SpA

☞INFLAMMATORY BACK PAIN CRITERIA: Numerous sets of criteria have been published for IBP. The main features are

- Morning stiffness
- Improvement with exercise and not with rest
- Improvement with NSAIDs
- Immobility stiffness
- Alternating buttock pain
- Waking in the second half of the night with back pain

### Diagnostic evaluation should include
- History of IBP, peripheral arthritis, psoriasis, IBD, and iritis.
- Physical examination, especially focused on axial spine, peripheral joints, and the skin.
- Assessment of inflammatory markers included CRP and/or erythrocyte sedimentation rate (ESR).
- Plain radiographs of the pelvis and spine.
- HLA-B27 assessment.
- There is no place for testing autoantibodies-like antinuclear antibody (ANA) or rheumatoid factor in patients with chronic back pain unless there are features suggestive of a connective tissue disease or alternate diagnosis such as rheumatoid arthritis.

### Diagnostic evaluation may include
- MRI of the axial spine and sacroiliac joints
- Assessment and/or investigation of suspected comorbid conditions such as iritis, IBD, and psoriasis

## Clinical Characteristics:

☞ANKYLOSING SPONDYLITIS: AS is the prototypic spondyloarthritis and symptoms include IBP, peripheral enthesitis, limitation of spinal movements, and commonly a peripheral arthritis. Hip disease occurs in about 40% of AS cases, and peripheral arthritis in other joints in approximately 10% of patients; the knee is the most commonly affected, and the arthritis is usually asymmetric. Inflammation of the tendon insertions into bone (enthesitis) occurs in AS, commonly affecting the Achilles tendon, costal joints (leading to anterior chest pain), and plantar fascia of the feet. Associated conditions include iritis in approximately 40%, IBD in approximately 10%, and skin psoriasis in approximately 5%. Approximately 10% of AS patients will have clinically apparent IBD, and over 60% of SpA patients have microscopic bowel inflammation on ileocolonoscopy. Patients with AS progressively develop ankylosis of their spine and sacroiliac joints leading to a loss of movement. This loss of movement leads to a loss of function that limits activities of daily living and work. AS also commonly leads to osteoporosis, and in combination with a fused spine leads to an increased risk of spinal fracture in particular.

☞REACTIVE ARTHRITIS: ReA is usually caused by either enteric or sexually transmitted infection. *Chlamydia* and *Campylobacter* are the two classic etiologic organisms, but many have been described. The actual causative organism is commonly not identified in individual patients. ReA usually manifests as an inflammatory oligoarthritis of the lower limbs. The disease course is variable with approximately one-third having a short self-limiting course of less than 6 months, one-third having a more extended course of between 6 and 24 months, and approximately one-third developing a chronic spondyloarthritis indistinguishable from AS. Having the HLA-B27 allele increases the risk of ReA to become a chronic AS-like SpA.

☞ENTEROPATHIC SPONDYLOARTHRITIS: Enteropathic SpA has a variable clinical presentation; it can be a predominately axial arthritis, or it can involve both axial and peripheral joints. It occurs in association with both Crohn disease and ulcerative colitis. As with other SpA, enthesitis and iritis also commonly occur. Skin lesions such as pyoderma gangrenosum and erythema nodosum occur in a minority of patients with this SpA. There is not any consistent correlation between the activity of gut and joint disease.

☞PSORIATIC ARTHRITIS: PsA is predominately a peripheral arthritis, which is not in the scope of this chapter, but a significant minority of patients also have axial involvement. Those with psoriatic spondyloarthritis can commonly develop dactylitis which is commonly referred to as "sausage digits" and is a combined synovitis and tenosynovitis of isolated fingers and toes.

☞AXIAL SPONDYLOARTHRITIS: Axial SpA is a heterogenous group of conditions which in addition to having inflammatory spinal disease may have any of a combination of SpA features including axial and peripheral arthritis, dactylitis, iritis, enthesitis, psoriasis, and bowel inflammation. An unknown proportion of these patients develop definitive AS.

## Screening and Counseling:

*Screening:* Population screening is not yet performed for AS because the low disease prevalence makes screening inefficient and expensive per case identified and because of limited data regarding whether there is a benefit to patients from early diagnosis. These factors may change in future, as genetic screening is becoming more advanced and because clinical trials in early AS or axial SpA suggest very good responses to treatment.

*Counseling:* Detailed studies of the recurrence risk of AS are available. Important knowledge for counseling is that in European populations HLA-B27 is present in 7% to 10% of the population (higher is some populations like the Finnish at 14%), but only 1% to 5% of patients with HLA-B27 will develop AS. The parent-child recurrence risk and sibling AS recurrence risk are both 8%. This estimate is modified by the presence of the HLA-B27 allele, with those carrying the B27 allele at increased risk relative to those not carrying the allele. The monozygotic twin AS concordance rate is 63%, first-degree relatives 8.2%, second-degree relatives 1%, and third-degree relatives 0.7%.

## Management and Treatment

*Management:* Management of SpA is focused on education, physiotherapy, and medication. Education empowers patients and is a critical aspect of SpA management. In addition to patient education self-help groups and/or arthritis associations are valued by some patients. Exercise programs have been shown to improve flexibility and function in AS patients with supervised physiotherapy being better than home-based therapy. NSAIDs are a mainstay in the pharmacologic therapy of SpA. Tumor necrosis factor inhibitors (TNFi) are used in a large proportion of AS patients who fail to be adequately treated with NSAIDs alone.

Treatment of the complications and comorbidities of SpA is an integral part of care. This often involves other specialties including ophthalmology for treatment of iritis, gastroenterology for the care of IBD, and dermatology for the care of psoriasis. Patients with greater than 20 years history of AS should be screened for osteoporosis, noting that spinal BMD is typically artificially elevated due to ankylosis.

*Therapeutics:* NSAIDs are a core therapeutic in SpA. Both traditional nonselective NSAIDs and the COX-2 inhibitors are effective in AS and other SpA. To be effective they have to be taken at maximal dose on a regular basis. Proton pump inhibitors are often coprescribed to avoid gastrointestinal side effects. In older patients and those with cardiovascular risk factors a careful assessment of the risk-benefit ratio is required before prescribing NSAIDs due to the increased rate of myocardial infarction.

TNFi are widely used and highly effective for treating the inflammation of AS. They have no effect on the bone formation or ankylosis of AS. The currently indicated agents for AS include etanercept, adalimumab, golimumab, and infliximab. Current consensus is that they all have similar efficacy, although etanercept is not effective for IBD associated with AS. Patient preference and comorbidity usually drive the choice of specific agent used; for patients that are overweight, especially greater than 100 kg as the dose of etanercept, adalimumab, and golimumab is fixed, infliximab (the dose of which is adjusted according to weight) is preferred. Etanercept, adalimumab, and golimumab are subcutaneously administered at weekly, fortnightly, or monthly intervals respectively; infliximab is administered intravenously every 6 weeks after initial loading doses. Side effects include local injection site reactions, allergy and anaphylaxis, reactivation of latent tuberculosis, and an increased rate of serious infection. There is also an increased rate of both melanoma and nonmelanoma skin cancer with TNFi. In addition, they rarely cause autoimmune problems like drug-induced lupus. TNFi are also effective in reducing the frequency of iritis, and also improve bone density in AS.

Sulfasalazine (SSZ) is effective in peripheral but not axial arthritis associated with SpA. Methotrexate (MTX) may also be effective in peripheral SpA-associated arthritis. Oral corticosteroids can be used in severe treatment-resistant disease, but AS is more resistant to corticosteroids than seropositive arthritis, and the risk of osteoporosis needs to be considered. Intra-articular corticosteroid can be used in both peripheral and sacroiliac joints.

☞PHARMACOGENETICS: At this stage there is no role for genetic testing to predict treatment response or toxicity in medications used in AS. HLA-B27–negative patients respond less well to TNFi, but the difference with HLA-B27–positive cases is not so great as to be clinically useful.

## Molecular Genetics and Molecular Mechanism

Since the discovery of the association of HLA-B27 with AS in 1973 exhaustive efforts have gone into trying to determine how this molecule contributes to disease pathogenesis. There have been a number of theories to date and recent data has shed further light on the possible mechanism.

HLA-B27 is a class I major histocompatibility complex (MHC) molecule which presents mainly intracellular proteins on the cell surface. MHC class I molecules display the intracellular content of the cell to the immune system to detect intracellular infection or cancerous transformation.

The leading theory of how HLA-B27 predisposes to AS is through antigen presentation to CD8+ lymphocytes or killer immunoglobulin receptors, which also interact with class I MHC molecules. A further theory involves misfolding of HLA-B27. This may lead to accumulation of misfolded HLA-B27 in the endoplasmic reticulum, leading to an "unfolded protein response" (UPR), inducing endoplasmic reticulum stress, a cellular response that attempts to deal with the accumulated misfolded protein. This UPR can have significant effects on the cell including cell cycle arrest and has been shown to increased IL-23 production. Alternately, HLA-B27 is known to form self-dimers, leading to the presence of homodimers on the cell surface. These homodimers could lead to aberrant T-cell activation and a subsequent pathologic immune response. HLA-B27 may not be the causal association, it may tag another nearby causal variant, but recent GWAS results have made this possibility very unlikely. A further possibility is that there may be molecular mimicry between some exogenous antigen and an endogenous, likely enthesial antigen.

A number of other variants associated with AS have been discovered, they are detailed in Table 141-1. The associations with ERAP1 and IL23R explain the most heritability in AS after HLA-B. CARD9 is a significant association as it could support the theory of an environmental microbial trigger.

**Table 141-1 Spondyloarthritis-Associated Susceptibility Variants**

| Candidate Gene (Chromosome Location) | Associated Variant [effect on protein] | Relative Risk | Frequency of Risk Allele (HapMap-CEU) | Putative Functional Significance | Associated Disease Phenotype |
|---|---|---|---|---|---|
| HLA-B (6p21) | *B27 [tags HLA-B27] (rs4349859) | 40.8 [A] | 0.025 | Antigen presentation | AS |
| IL23R (1p31) | R381Q [nonsynonymous SNP] (rs11209026) | 1.20 [G] | 0.959 | Actions on IL-23R expressing cells | AS |
|  | [noncoding] rs11209032 | 1.20 [A] | 0.306 |  |  |
| ERAP1 (5q15) | K528R [nonsynonymous SNP] (rs30187) | 1.35 [T] | 0.300 | Peptide trimming prior to antigen presentation | HLA-B27–positive AS |
|  | D575N [nonsynonymous SNPs] (rs10050860) | 1.17 [C] | 0.743 |  |  |
| KIF21B (1q32) | Intronic (rs2297909) | 1.14 [G] | 0.658 | Unknown | AS |
| Gene desert (2p15) | Intergenic (rs10865331) | 1.32 [A] | 0.288 | Unknown | AS |
| Gene desert (21p22) | Intergenic (rs378108) | 1.23 [G] | 0.496 | Unknown | AS |
| RUNX3 (1p36) | Intergenic (rs11249215) | 1.19 [A] | 0.517 | Lymphocyte counts | AS |
| IL1R2 | Intergenic (rs2310173) | 1.18 [A] | 0.45 | Response to IL-1 | AS |
| IL12B (5q33) | Intergenic (rs6556416) | 1.18 [C] | 0.271 | Actions on IL-23R expressing cells | AS |
| LTBR-TNFRSF1A (12p13) | Intergenic (rs11616188) | 1.21 [A] | 0.433 | TNF receptor | AS |
| ANTXR2 (4q21) | Intronic (rs4389526) | 1.15 [A] | 0.55 | Unknown | AS |
| CARD9 (9p34) | Intergenic (rs10781500) | 1.18 [T] | 0.487 | Innate immune system activation | AS |
| PTGER4 (5p13) | Intergenic (rs10440635) | 1.13 [A] | 0.659 | Promoting IL-23 expression in response to physical stress at enthuses | AS |
| TBKBP1 (17p21) | Intergenic (rs8070463) | 1.13 [A] | 0.504 | TNF/NFKB pathway | AS |

SNP, single-nucleotide polymorphism; AS, ankylosing spondylitis; TNF, tumor necrosis factor; NFκB, nuclear factor kappa beta.
Intergenic means the polymorphism does not occur in an exonic region.

Endoplasmic reticulum aminopeptidase 1 (ERAP1) is a multifunctional aminopeptidase. Its physiologic function is to cleave peptides within the endoplasmic reticulum down to nine amino acids in length, prior to them being loaded onto MHC class I molecules such as HLA-B27, and being presented on the cell surface. Results from the recent Welcome Trust Case Control Consortium 2 and the Anglo-Australian-American Spondylitis Consortium (WTCCC2-TASC) GWAS demonstrate ERAP1 SNPs are only associated with HLA-B27–positive AS and this suggests that ERAP1 contributes to disease pathogenesis via the antigen presentation pathway. Similarly, ERAP1 is associated with HLA-Cw6–positive but not –negative psoriasis, suggesting that HLA-B27 and HLA-Cw6 operate by similar mechanisms to cause AS and psoriasis, respectively.

SNPs in IL23R have been associated with AS, psoriasis, and IBD. These SNPs are protective, and functional studies in healthy have demonstrated that the A allele is associated with reduced IL-17 production and STAT3 phosphorylation compared to the G allele. This leads to reduced T-helper 17 activation, a proinflammatory T-helper subset.

CARD9 is a mediator of signals from pattern recognition receptors that are triggered by evolutionarily conserved sequences on yeasts and other micro-organisms. The association of CARD9 with AS provides further clues to the involvement of microbes in the etiology of AS.

**Genetic Testing:** Genetic testing for HLA-B27 is widely available and routinely used in the assessment of SpA. HLA-B27 is present in 80% to 90% of AS patients, 14% to 80% of ReA patients depending on the source of the cohort, and 85% of enteropathic SpA patients. In interpreting this, it is important to remember that the HLA-B27 allele is present in 7% to 10% of European descent populations but only 1% to 5% of those HLA-B27 positive will develop AS.

Traditionally polymerase chain reaction (PCR) primer-based approaches have been used to test for B27, but more recently the WTCCC2-TASC group has described a SNP (rs4349859) which tags B27 with 98% sensitivity and 99% specificity. This SNP tags all the European HLA-B27 AS-associated subtypes, but does not tag Asian or African B27 subtypes associated with AS. This SNP could be used in the future to test B27 in European populations at reduced cost compared to the current PCR-based techniques.

☞**UTILITY OF TESTING:** Rudwaleit and colleagues published a decision tree on the diagnosis of axial SpA. They started with chronic low back pain patients (5% probability of SpA) and then assessed IBP and SpA features. In those with IBP and no SpA features, the pretest probability of axial SpA was 14%, and this rose to a probability of 59% if HLA-B27 was positive. In those with one to two SpA features, the pretest probability was 35% to 70%, and this rose to 80% to 90% with a positive HLA-B27. Therefore B27 testing provides some utility in a clinical setting, but must be combined with history, examination, and radiology findings in making the diagnosis of axial SpA. HLA-B27 testing is now formally included in the definition of axial SpA, which can be diagnosed in HLA-B27–positive individuals with two more clinical features of SpA, even in the absence of radiographic evidence of disease.

**Future Directions:** With the current GWAS data researchers are examining the ability of this information to be used for disease screening or prognosis prediction. In addition researchers are currently working on genetic predictors of radiologic progression in AS and these results may help elucidate mechanisms of ankylosis in AS which to date have eluded identification. In the future exome and whole genome sequencing approaches will be applied to the SpA for further genetic variant discovery. Interethnic studies can also be utilized to further examine genetic variants associated with the SpA.

Clinically, the current emphasis is on earlier diagnosis of AS, and trialling medications in early axial SpA in the hope that in this patient cohort effects on the natural history of the disease will be more easily obtained. New medications, such as IL-17 blockade are in trial, and show promise in SpA, as suggested by the genetic studies described earlier.

**BIBLIOGRAPHY:**

1. Brown MA. Genetics of ankylosing spondylitis. *Curr Opin Rheumatol*. 2010;22(2):126-132.
2. Brown MA, Kennedy LG, MacGregor AJ, et al. Susceptibility to ankylosing spondylitis in twins the role of genes, HLA, and the environment. *Arthritis Rheum*. 1997;40(10):1823-1828.
3. van der Linden S, Valkenburg HA, de Jongh BM, Cats A. The risk of developing ankylosing spondylitis in HLA-B27 positive individuals. *Arthritis Rheum*. 1984;27(3):241-249.
4. TASC, WTCCC2. Interaction between ERAP1 and HLA-B27 in ankylosing spondylitis implicates peptide handling in the mechanism for HLA-B27 in disease susceptibility. *Nat Genet*. 2011;43(8):761-767.
5. Brown MA. Progress in the genetics of ankylosing spondylitis. *Brief Funct Genomics*. Sep 2011;10(5):249-257.
6. Rudwaleit M, van der Heijde D, Landewé R, et al. The development of Assessment of SpondyloArthritis international Society classification criteria for axial spondyloarthritis (part II): validation and final selection. *Ann Rheum Dis*. 2009;68:777-783.
7. Rudwaleit M, van der Heijde D, Landewé R, et al. The Assessment of SpondyloArthritis international Society classification criteria for peripheral spondyloarthritis and for spondyloarthritis in general. *Ann Rheum Dis*. 2011;70:25-31.
8. van der Linden S, Valkenburg HA, Cats A. Evaluation of diagnostic criteria for ankylosing spondylitis. A proposal for modification of the New York criteria. *Arthritis Rheum*. 1984;27:361-368.
9. Seitz M, Wirthmuller U, Moller B, Villiger PM. The 308 tumour necrosis factor-alpha gene polymorphism predicts therapeutic response to TNF alpha-blockers in rheumatoid arthritis and spondyloarthritis patients. *Rheumatology*. 2007;46:93-96.
10. Davila L, Ranganathan P. Pharmacogenetics: implications for therapy in rheumatic diseases. *Nat Rev Rheum*. 2011;7(9):537-550.
11. Rudwaleit M, van der Heijde D, Khan M, Braun J, Sieper J. How to diagnose axial spondyloarthritis early. *Ann Rheum Dis*. 2004;63(5):535-543.

## Supplementary Information

**OMIM REFERENCES:**

[1] Spondyloarthropathy (#106300)

[2] HLA-B (+142830)

**Alternative Names:**

- Spondyloarthritis
- Enteropathic Arthritis
- Axial Spondyloarthritis
- Marie-Strumpell Disease
- Bechterew Syndrome

**Key Words:** Spondyloarthritis, spondyloarthropathies, ankylosing spondylitis, HLA-B27

# 142 Systemic Lupus Erythematosus

Ornella J. Rullo, Yun Deng, and Ornella J. Rullo

## KEY POINTS

- *Disease summary:*
  - Systemic lupus erythematosus (SLE) is a complex, autoimmune disease characterized by the presence of antibodies to nuclear components. An interplay of genetic and environmental factors contribute to the immunologic manifestations and disease pathogenesis, which can involve the skin, kidneys, hematologic system, nervous system, joints, mucosal and serosal membranes, and/or other organs.
  - Clinically, the disease spectrum is varied and affected individuals can experience periods of disease activity and remission.
  - Women are affected more frequently than men, with a reported ratio of up to 9:1, and diagnosis most often occurring in the third through fifth decades of life.
  - The diagnosis of SLE is clinical, and a typical presentation is often a young woman with constitutional, skin, and musculoskeletal complaints.
  - Organ involvement, such as kidney, central nervous system, or cardiopulmonary, can occur early in the disease course or at diagnosis, and can be severe and dominate the patient's disease course.

- *Differential diagnosis:*
  - Some important general considerations when evaluating an individual with potential SLE include drug-induced lupus, infection, malignancy, and other autoimmune conditions. Due to the number of possible clinical manifestations of SLE, it is beyond the scope of this review to fully summarize the differential diagnosis. However, if one organ manifestation dominates, then the differential will include related conditions. For example, in a patient presenting with seizures, considerations for diagnosis include new-onset epilepsy, metabolic abnormalities, drug toxicity or withdrawal, and hypoxia, among others.

- *Monogenic forms:*
  - Several rare mutations that lead to either a deficiency of classical complement components, or impaired DNA degradation, clearance, and/or antigen signaling have been identified in small numbers of patients with SLE or lupus-like manifestations. The genes include *C1Q* (1p36), *C1R/C1S* (12p13), *C4A&B* (6p21.3), *C2* (6p21.3), *TREX1* (3p21.31), *DNASE1* (16p13.3), *ACP5* (19p13), *SIAE* (11q24), and *DNASE1L3* (3p14.3).

- *Family history:*
  - Most individuals with SLE do not have an affected family member. However, a familial prevalence of up to 12% has been reported. In families with clusters of members with SLE, the inheritance pattern does not follow a classic single-gene Mendelian pattern.

- *Twin studies:*
  - The disease concordance rate is 2% to 5% for dizygotic twins and 24% to 58% for monozygotic twins. The rate of concordance in monozygotic twins supports the possibility that development of disease is multifactorial, which may include multiple genes, as well as environmental and hormonal factors.

- *Environmental factors:*
  - Several infections have been associated with the development of SLE, with the strongest evidence linked to Epstein-Barr virus; the correlation of disease flares in patients with SLE who develop viral infections supports this possibility. Environmental exposures or contaminants, such as trichloroethylene (an industrial solvent) and various pesticides have all been suggested in epidemiologic studies as possible triggers of SLE in susceptible individuals, but further study in this area is necessary. Plausible biologic evidence links SLE and other autoimmune diseases to silica exposure, which can occur due to diverse occupations such as farming, construction, mining, and manufacturing. High silica exposure has been associated with the development of SLE (odds ratio [OR] 4.6, 1.4-15.4). Additionally, a number of medications have been implicated in precipitating SLE, including hydrochlorothiazide, antihistamines, calcium channel blockers, terbinafine, and naproxen. Antitumor necrosis factor-alpha therapy and interferon-alpha therapy have been associated with antinuclear antibodies (ANA)—typically anti–double-stranded DNA (dsDNA) antibodies—and the development of lupus manifestations. Furthermore, hormone-induced SLE may occur in some clinical settings.

- *Genome-wide associations:*
  - In the vast majority of cases, SLE fits the common disease-common variant hypothesis, in which nonrare risk variants lead to a modest magnitude of risk (OR 1.1-2.5) and account for a portion of overall genetic susceptibility to disease. Genetic dissection of SLE utilizing the rapidly advancing technology applied in genome-wide association (GWA) studies have confirmed disease associations with previously established risk loci, and identified several novel risk loci. Up to 1 million single-nucleotide polymorphisms (SNPs) have been genotyped in each of six GWA studies, and in a series of large-scale replication studies of individuals of both European and Asian descent. Current understanding of SLE pathogenesis can group several of the identified genes into major immunologic pathways, such as defective clearance of immune complexes containing nuclear antigens (eg, *TREX1*, complement components, *ITGAM*, *FCGR*s); toll-like receptor activation with secretion of type I interferons (eg, *TLR*s, *IRF5*, *STAT4*, *IRAK1*); and amplification of the adaptive immune response

(eg, *PTPN22, BANK1, BLK, LYN, FCGR2B, TNFSF4*). Certain immunologic pathways are common to multiple autoimmune disorders, which likely explains that a growing number of SLE-susceptibility genes also predispose to conditions including rheumatoid arthritis, Crohn disease, psoriasis, type 1 diabetes, and systemic sclerosis.

- *Pharmacogenomics:*
  - Testing for *TPMT* (thiopurine methyltransferase) mutations can be utilized in clinical practice before initiation of a thiopurine drug such as azathioprine (Table 142-1). Defects in the *TPMT* gene can lead to increased levels of the pharmacologically active metabolite, with potential bone marrow toxicity.

## Diagnostic Criteria and Clinical Characteristics

***Diagnostic Criteria for SLE:*** The diagnosis of SLE can be readily made in a young woman who presents with hallmark features of the disease, such as fatigue, fevers, malar rash or photosensitivity, alopecia, oral or nasal ulcerations, and/or arthralgias or arthritis. Hypertension, pleuritic chest pain with friction rub, purpura, hepatosplenomegaly, and/or lymphadenopathy may also be present at the initial evaluation.

**Diagnostic evaluation should include**

- Laboratory testing: complete blood count, comprehensive metabolic panel, erythrocyte sedimentation rate or C-reactive protein, and urinalysis.
- Autoantibody testing: ANA titer, anti-dsDNA titer, antiribosomal binding protein antibody titers (including anti-Smith, antiribonucleoprotein [RNP], anti-SSA/Ro, anti-SSB/La), and antiphospholipid antibody titers. Over 90% of individuals with SLE demonstrate ANA positivity, therefore the absence of ANAs would weigh strongly against a diagnosis of SLE.
- Additional testing if indicated: protein and creatinine urine collection over 24 hours, Coombs antibody test, reticulocyte count, amylase or lipase, and lupus anticoagulant activity.

Organ involvement can be identified with evidence of nephritis or nephrosis, elevated liver enzymes, interstitial lung disease or pulmonary hypertension, cardiac valvular involvement, etc. Additional workup for the evaluation of specific organ involvement can include, when indicated

- Biopsy: skin or kidney
- Imaging: chest and/or joint radiographs, magnetic resonance imaging and/or angiography of the brain, computed tomography (CT) scan of the abdomen

- Other: electrocardiogram, echocardiogram, pulmonary function test, lumbar puncture, scan for pulmonary embolism

The American College of Rheumatology has developed a set of criteria that differentiate individuals with SLE from other autoimmune diseases for the purposes of inclusion in clinical trials. When 4 of 11 criteria are present, serially or simultaneously, the sensitivity and the specificity for the classification of SLE are each 96%; these criteria include malar rash, discoid rash, photosensitivity, oral ulcers, arthritis, serositis (pleuritis or pericarditis), renal disorder (proteinuria of 500 mg/d or cellular casts present), neurologic disorder (seizures or psychosis), hematologic disorder (hemolytic anemia, leucopenia, lymphopenia, or thrombocytopenia), immunologic disorders, and an abnormal ANA titer.

***Clinical Characteristics:*** Constitutional symptoms and/or specific organ symptoms can occur in the setting of an individual with SLE. A brief overview of major clinical characteristics at disease onset or at a time of increased disease activity is as follows:

*Constitutional:* Fatigue, malaise, and fever can occur.
*Mucocutaneous:* The most common skin lesion is the facial butterfly rash (sparing the nasolabial folds), with associated photosensitivity. Alopecia as well as oral and nasal ulcerations can be frequent. Discoid rash lesions (discrete plaques which tend to scar) are less common.
*Arthritis:* Arthritis is a common manifestation in SLE and is seen in over 60% of individuals. It tends to be symmetrical and nondeforming.
*Renal:* Renal involvement can develop in up to 75% of individuals diagnosed with SLE in the first or second decade of life, and usually complicates early stages of the disease. Adult-onset of SLE is associated with lower rates of renal involvement. There are a number of types of renal disease in SLE, which are typically differentiated by renal biopsy.
*Pulmonary:* Pleuritic chest pain is fairly common in SLE, with up to 50% involvement. Interstitial lung disease is

**Table 142-1 Pharmacogenetic Considerations in SLE**

| Gene | Associated Medications | Goal of Testing | Variants | Effect |
|---|---|---|---|---|
| *TPMT* (thiopurine methyltransferase) | Azathioprine | Safety Efficacy | *2 (G238C), *3A (G460A and A719G), *3B (G460A), and *3C (A719G) | Decreased enzymatic activity and the ability to detoxify azathioprine |
| *MTHFR* (5,10-methylene tetrahydrofolate reductase) | Methotrexate | Safety Efficacy | C677T A1298C | Decreased enzymatic activity, associated with greater susceptibility to methotrexate toxicity |

less commonly seen, but can lead to pulmonary hypertension when untreated. Acute pneumonitis, pulmonary hemorrhage, and shrinking lung syndrome are rarely seen complications.

*Hematologic:* The major hematologic manifestations of SLE are anemia, leukopenia, thrombocytopenia, and the antiphospholipid syndrome.

*Neuropsychiatric:* The frequency of neuropsychiatric manifestations in SLE has been estimated anywhere between 10% and 90%. Cognitive dysfunction can be frequent, whereas seizures and psychosis are quite less common, although they remain a significant cause of morbidity. Headaches, neuropathies, and psychiatric abnormalities can also complicate the disease course in SLE.

*Cardiovascular:* Pericarditis, noninfectious valvular (Libman-Sacks) endocarditis, and increased risk of coronary artery disease are cardiac risks of SLE. Thromboembolic disease, vasculitis, and the antiphospholipid syndrome are additional important considerations in the disease course.

*Gastrointestinal:* Peritonitis and rarely pancreatitis can occur in SLE.

## Screening and Counseling

**Screening:** There is no evidence supporting the routine screening of family members of individuals with SLE, in the absence of clinical signs or symptoms. The genetic testing of identified SLE susceptibility SNPs has not been validated in clinical studies in the general population or in relatives of patients with SLE. Because of the strong penetrance of C1q deficiency for development of immune deficiency and/or autoimmunity, some experts have advocated screening for the mutation identified in the index case among family members to identify C1q-deficient patients and carriers, and provide genetic counseling. This situation, however, is rare (SLE reported in less than 50 C1q deficiency cases worldwide), and often is offspring of consanguineous marriages.

**Counseling:** The incidence of SLE or lupus-like manifestation in individuals with a complete deficiency, due to a homozygous mutation, in one of the classical complement pathway genes ranges from 10% to 93%. There is an extremely high genetic risk for SLE and glomerulonephritis in C1q-deficient (93% penetrant) individuals. Individuals deficient in both *C4A* and *C4B* genes have a high risk to develop SLE or a lupus-like manifestation (75% penetrant). Despite the strong association between C1q deficiency and development of SLE at an extremely young age, the clinical presentation of hereditary C1q deficiency can be very diverse, with symptoms ranging from mild recurrent infections to severe bacterial meningitis, sepsis, glomerulonephritis, and/or angioedema or SLE-like skin involvement.

The general sibling risk ratio for the development of SLE is approximately 30. Additionally, there seems to be familial aggregation of autoimmune disease in general in some families with SLE. Sporadic cases of SLE do not present with different disease features overall compared with familial cases; however, familial aggregates tend to display similar disease characteristics as well as immunologic manifestations.

Importantly, several recent GWA studies have begun to investigate the genotype-phenotype relationship in SLE with some interesting reported associations, particularly in regards to the development of autoantibody production as well as renal disease. Ongoing research into this area may ultimately provide uniquely personalized care and recommendations.

## Management and Treatment

**Management:** The basic management of individuals with SLE includes avoidance of known triggers of disease, and maintaining good general health.

☞**SUN AVOIDANCE:** Sun avoidance should be recommended to all patients, as ultraviolet radiation can promote disease activity likely through the stimulation of proinflammatory cytokines and increased generation of apoptotic material in the skin that can act as autoantigens.

☞**VITAMIN D/CALCIUM SUPPLEMENTATION:** Due to the recommended sun avoidance in all people with SLE, the assessment of circulating vitamin D levels with appropriate supplementation should be routine. Additionally, the use of calcium supplementation should be considered, particularly in patients with SLE who have required glucocorticoid therapy and would therefore be at increased risk for osteoporosis.

☞**VACCINES:** Routine vaccinations should be encouraged in individuals with SLE, especially prior to initiation of immune suppression (if possible), including the annual influenza vaccine. However, any individual on therapy with immune-modulating agents, with the exception of perhaps hydroxychloroquine, should avoid live virus vaccines.

☞**DIET AND EXERCISE:** No specific dietary recommendations exist for individuals with SLE, although a healthy and varied diet is encouraged. Weight loss should be recommended in any overweight individuals with SLE. Exercise is recommended for general health maintenance and for prevention of loss of muscle mass and bone demineralization in individuals with active disease. Smoking cessation is recommended in all individuals with SLE.

**Therapeutics:** Medical therapy with immune-modulating agents is considered in many individuals with SLE. A mainstay of management of SLE includes the use of antimalarials, such as hydroxychloroquine, which can be used for skin and musculoskeletal complaints. Hydroxychloroquine has also been shown to reduce the rate of flares in individuals with stable SLE, therefore it is often continued while individuals are stable as well as in conjunction with other medications in individuals who are experiencing increased disease activity. Glucocorticoids are used in acute flares, with dosing ranges chosen based on type of organ involvement and whether the flare is organ or life threatening. Renal or central nervous system involvement typically necessitates prednisone doses of 1 to 2 mg/kg/d, or equivalent, or intermittent intravenous methylprednisolone doses, whereas skin or musculoskeletal flares can often be managed with oral prednisone doses of 15 mg per day or less. Specific organ involvement often necessitates the use of additional agents such as cyclophosphamide, mycophenolate mofetil, azathioprine or methotrexate, based on the presenting clinical situation. The efficacy of B-cell depletion therapy, such as with rituximab, remains controversial; however, the use of other novel targeted B-cell therapies, such as belimumab—the first FDA-approved treatment for SLE in over 50 years—shows promise.

# Molecular Genetics and Molecular Mechanism

Early epidemiologic and genetic studies, particularly in multiplex families, have long pointed toward an important genetic component to the development of SLE. Work over several decades utilizing methods such as linkage analysis and candidate gene association analysis confirmed several important genetic signals. The complex pathophysiology of SLE has been underscored by the many promising susceptibility candidates from nearly all aspects of the immune system. Our understanding of the genetic contribution to pathogenesis and progression of disease in SLE has been greatly advanced, however, by recent GWA studies in populations of European and Asian ancestries. The *HLA* genetic region is a good example. Both HLA class II and class III genes are significantly associated with susceptibility of SLE; the major role of class II molecules is the presentation of antigens to T cells, which can in turn stimulate B cells to produce antibodies. Identification of gene variants associated with abnormalities of apoptotic cell clearance and initiation of the autoimmune response include regulators of the complement components *CFHR3, CFHR1 C1Q, C3,* and *CR2*. Low levels of complement has long been recognized as a feature of SLE, and genetic variants that result in lower levels of complement components can contribute to risk for SLE.

Knowledge of the role of both the innate and adaptive immune system has been increased by GWA studies, which have provided convincing evidence for genetic association of these pathways in SLE pathophysiology. Immune complexes consisting of nucleic acid self-antigens are known to bind the pattern recognition receptors, TLR7 and TLR9. These receptors activate transcription factors leading to activation of the type I interferon pathway, an important early proinflammatory mechanism utilized as a response to viral infection. Overly abundant activation of this pathway leads to the persistent production of interferon-inducible, antiviral genes and has been implicated in SLE disease activity. Variants of genes within this pathway, including *IRF5/7, STAT4, TLR7/8, IRAK1, TYK2,* and *TNFAIP3*, have reached genome-wide significance and illustrate the importance of innate immunity in SLE pathophysiology. Additionally, SLE is characterized by a loss of tolerance at the level of the adaptive immune system, which leads ultimately to the formation of autoantibodies. GWA studies have identified multiple susceptibility genes involved in T- and B-cell signaling, such as *PTPN22, TNFSF4, NCF2, BLK, BANK1, LYN, ETS1, IKZF1,* and *IL10*; these findings highlight the importance of lymphocyte function and activation in SLE pathogenesis.

The loci (Table 142-2) were identified through GWAS, GWA meta-analysis studies, candidate gene studies, or replication papers, and include common variants (allelic frequency >5%) reaching genome-wide significance (*p* value ≤5*10^-8). Most genetic studies in SLE have been undertaken primarily in European-derived populations, and for that reason we list the frequency of the risk allele in Caucasians. In addition, we have listed rare variants that appear to be monogenic. The putative functional significance is based in most cases on what is known about the gene and its relationship to potential autoimmunity; the actual function of many gene variants and their gene products in relationship to the pathogenesis of SLE

*Table 142-2 SLE-Associated Susceptibility Variants*

| Candidate Gene (Chromosome Location) | Associated Variant [effect on protein] (dbSNP) | Odds Ratio of SLE | Frequency of Risk Allele | Putative Functional Significance | Associated Disease Phenotype |
|---|---|---|---|---|---|
| *PTPN22* (1p13.2) | C1988T [nonsynonymous amino acid substitution R620W] (rs2476601) | 1.4-2.4 | 0.14 | Reduced removal of autoreactive B cells | SLE in general |
| *C1Q* (1p36) | Homozygous mutations [deficiency] | >90% penetrant | 64 individuals | Reduced handling of apoptotic cell debris and immune complexes | Renal disorder; photosensitivity; neurologic disorder |
| | SNPs | 1.4-2.2 | 0.05-0.56 | | Renal disorder; photosensitivity |
| *FCGR2A* (1q23) | A550G [nonsynonymous amino acid substitution H131R] (rs1801274) | 1.3-1.4 | 0.43 | Reduced immune complex clearance | Renal disorder; APS, malar rash |
| *FCGR3A* (1q23) | T660G [nonsynonymous amino acid substitution F158V] (rs396991) | 1.2-1.5 | 0.3 | | Renal disorder |

*(Continued)*

*Table 142-2* **SLE-Associated Susceptibility Variants** *(Continued)*

| Candidate Gene (Chromosome Location) | Associated Variant [effect on protein] (dbSNP) | Odds Ratio of SLE | Frequency of Risk Allele | Putative Functional Significance | Associated Disease Phenotype |
|---|---|---|---|---|---|
| *FCGR2B* (1q23) | T822C [nonsynonymous amino acid substitution I232T] (rs1050501) | 1.3-2.5 | 0.18* | 232T risk allele reduces inhibitory activity of BCR signaling | *232T and risk of SLE susceptibility has been established mainly in patients of Asian descent |
| *FCGR3B* (1q23) | Low copy number | 1.7-2.3 | 0.04-0.05 | Influences clearance of immune complexes | Renal disorder |
| *TNFSF4* (1q25) | SNPs | 1.2-1.5 | 0.23-0.49 | Influences T-cell activation | Renal disorder |
| *NCF2* (1q25) | (rs10911363) | 1.23 | 0.37 | Increases B-cell differentiation | SLE in general |
| *IL10* (1q31-q32) | (rs3024505) | 1.2-1.3 | 0.09 | Downregulates immune responses | aCL-IgM, anti-Sm, anti-SSA antibodies: discoid rash; renal and neurologic disorders |
| *CFHR* (1q32) | Heterozygous and homozygous deletions | 1.5 | 0.04-0.33 | Regulation of alternative complement pathway | SLE in general |
| *IFIH1* (2q24) | G3058A [nonsynonymous amino acid substitution A946T] (rs19903760) | 1.17 | 0.37 | Increased sensing of dsRNA | SLE in general |
| *RASGRP3* (2p25-p24) | (rs13385731) | 1.2-1.4 | 0.08 | Lymphocyte activation | Malar rash; discoid rash; anti-ANA |
| *STAT4* (2q32) | (rs7574865) | 1.5-1.8 | 0.25 | Immune cell signal transduction | Early age at disease onset; renal disorder; Anti-dsDNA; APS |
| | (rs7582694) | 1.4 | 0.27 | | Anti-dsDNA |
| *PXK* (3p14.3) | (rs6445975) | 1.2-1.3 | 0.32 | Functions are not well characterized | Photosensitivity |
| *DNASE1L3* (3p14.3) | Autosomal recessive null mutation (decreased activity) | Identified rarely in patients of Arab descent (in offspring of consanguineous marriages) | 0.08 | Reduced clearance of apoptotic material | Antineutrophil cytoplasmic antibodies; renal disorder |
| *TREX1* (3p21.31) | Heterozygous mutations (decreased activity) | RR 25 | 0.03 | Removal of nucleic acids | SLE in general |
| | SNPs | 1.6-1.7 | 0.43-0.46 | | Neuropsychiatric SLE |
| *BANK1* (4q24) | SNPs | 1.2-1.4 | 0.65-0.70 | Attenuates B-cell proliferation and survival | SLE in general |

*(Continued)*

**Table 142-2 SLE-Associated Susceptibility Variants (Continued)**

| Candidate Gene (Chromosome Location) | Associated Variant [effect on protein] (dbSNP) | Odds Ratio of SLE | Frequency of Risk Allele | Putative Functional Significance | Associated Disease Phenotype |
|---|---|---|---|---|---|
| IL21 (4q26-q27) | SNPs | 1.1-1.6 | 0.36-0.70 | TH17 cell response | Hematologic disorder |
| TNIP1 (5q32-q33) | (rs10036748) | 1.3-1.4 | 0.46 | NFKB inhibition | Photosensitivity; vasculitis |
| HLA-DR2 & HLA-DR3 (6p21.3) | SNPs | 1.5-2.5 | 0.10-0.16 | Peptide presentation to CD4+ T cells | Anti-Ro/La, and anti-dsDNA antibodies |
| C4A & C4B (6p21.3) | Low copy number | 1.6-6.5 | 0.02-0.27 | Clearance of immune complex; propagating complement cascade | Arthritis |
| | Homozygous deficiency | >70% penetrant | 28 individuals | | Renal disorder |
| C2 (6p21.3) | Homozygous deficiency | 10%-20% penetrant | <0.01 | Early key regulator of complement cascade | Renal disorder |
| UHRF1BP1 (6p21) | A1595G [nonsynonymous amino acid substitution Q454R] (rs11755393) | 1.2-1.3 | 0.47 | Transcription and methylation factor | Immunologic disorder |
| PRDM1/ATG5 (6q21) | SNPs | 1.2-1.3 | 0.28-0.37 | Hyperproliferation of T cells (PRDM1)/formation of autophagosomes (ATG5) | SLE in general |
| TNFAIP3 (6q23) | SNPs | 1.7-2.5 | 0.03-0.21 | Restricts TNF and NFκB signals | Renal and hematologic disorders |
| IKZF1 (7p13-p11) | (rs2366293) | 1.2-1.4 | 0.13 | Perturbed TH1/TH2 balance | Malar rash; renal disorder |
| JAZF1 (7p15.2) | (rs849142) | 1.2 | 0.28 | Functions are not well characterized | SLE in general |
| IRF5 (7q32) | SNPs | 1.3-1.9 | 0.11-0.46 | Transcription factor that induces interferon-alpha and downstream gene production | Anti-dsDNA and anti-Ro antibodies |
| BLK (8p23) | SNPs | 1.2-1.6 | 0.25-0.35 | B-cell development | APS; anti-dsDNA antibodies |
| XKR6 (8p23.1) | SNPs | 1.2-1.3 | 0.46-0.50 | Functions are not well characterized | SLE in general |
| LYN (8q13) | SNPs | 1.2-1.3 | 0.78 | B-cell activation | Discoid rash, hematologic disorder |
| WDFY4 (10q11.2 LRCC18/WDFY4 (10q11.23) | G5524A [nonsynonymous amino acid substitution R1816Q] (rs7097397) | 1.2-1.3 | 0.4* | Functions are not well characterized | *1816R and risk of SLE susceptibility has been established mainly in patients of Asian descent |
| PDHX/CD44 (11p15) | SNPs | 1.2-1.4 | 0.43 | Lymphocyte activity (CD44) | Thrombocytopenia |

*(Continued)*

*Table 142-2 SLE-Associated Susceptibility Variants (Continued)*

| Candidate Gene (Chromosome Location) | Associated Variant [effect on protein] (dbSNP) | Odds Ratio of SLE | Frequency of Risk Allele | Putative Functional Significance | Associated Disease Phenotype |
|---|---|---|---|---|---|
| *PDHF1/IRF7* (11p15) | (rs4963128) | 1.3-2.0 | 0.31 | Transcription factor that induces interferon-alpha and downstream gene production (IRF7) | Anti-dsDNA and anti-Sm antibodies; immunologic disorder |
| | (rs702966) | 1.8 | 0.29 | | Anti-dsDNA antibodies |
| | A1684G [nonsynonymous amino acid substitution Q412R] (rs1131665) | 1.3-1.8 | 0.28 | | SLE in general |
| *ETS1* (11q23.3) | SNPs | 1.3-1.7 | 0.33-0.42 | B- and T-cell differentiation | Early age at disease onset |
| *C1R/C1S* (12p13) | Homozygous deficiency | 65% penetrant | 19 individuals | Early key regulators of complement cascade | Renal disorder |
| *SLC15A4* (12q24.32) | SNPs | 1.1-1.3 | 0.41 | NF$\kappa$B signaling pathway regulation | Discoid rash |
| *ITGAM* (16p11.2) | G328A [nonsynonymous amino acid substitution R77H] (rs1143679) | 1.3-2.1 | 0.09 | Leukocyte activation and migration; phagocytosis | Discoid rash; arthritis; renal, neurologic, Hematologic, and immunologic disorders |
| | (rs9888739) | 1.3-1.4 | 0.22 | | Anti-dsDNA antibodies; arthritis |
| *PRKCB* (16p11.2) | (rs16972959) | 1.2 | 0.16 | B-cell activation; apoptosis induction | SLE in general |
| *DNASE1* (16p13.3) | Heterozygous mutation with decreased activity | ND | 2 patients with SLE | Clearance of apoptotic debris | SLE in general |
| *IRF8* (16q24.1) | (rs2280381) | 1.16 | 0.3 | B-cell differentiation | SLE in general |
| *ACP5* (19p13) | Biallelic mutations with decreased activity | ND | 8 patients with SPENCD | Overactivation of IFN-alpha | ANA and anti-dsDNA antibodies; renal disorder; arthritis; thrombocytopenia |
| *C3* (19p13) | SNPs | 1.2-1.4 | 0.08-0.50 | Central complement component | Decreased serum C3 level |
| *TYK2* (19p13.2) | (rs280519) | 1.16 | 0.47 | Interaction with IFN receptor | SLE in general |
| *UBE2L3* (22q11.21) | (rs5754217) | 1.2-1.3 | 0.36 | Regulation of the TLR response | Anti-dsDNA antibodies |
| *TLR7/TLR8* (Xp22) | (rs3853839) | 1.2-2.3 | 0.38 | Bind nucleic acid-containing immune complexes; induce interferon-alpha response | Anti-RBP antibodies |

*Table 142-2* *SLE-Associated Susceptibility Variants (Continued)*

| Candidate Gene (Chromosome Location) | Associated Variant [effect on protein] (dbSNP) | Odds Ratio of SLE | Frequency of Risk Allele | Putative Functional Significance | Associated Disease Phenotype |
|---|---|---|---|---|---|
| *IRAK/MECP2* (Xq28) | SNPs | 1.1-1.6 | 0.14-0.25 | Suppression of TLR response (IRAK)/ regulation of methylation-sensitive genes (*MECP2*) | SLE in general |

ND, not determined; SPENCD, immuno-osseous dysplasia spondyloenchondrodysplasia

remains a work in progress. The associated disease phenotypes are based on observational data from genetic studies.

**Genetic Testing:** No role yet exists for genetic testing in the diagnosis of SLE.

**Future Directions:** SLE is a complex disorder, with many new genetic associations to consider in the evolving understanding of its pathogenesis. Though many gene associations have been identified, causal variants for SLE pathogenesis are largely not known. Next-generation sequencing techniques will continue to aid researchers in identifying functional genetic variants in autoimmunity. The majority of large-scale genetic studies in SLE have been undertaken in European-derived populations, and secondly in Asian populations; focusing on other genetic backgrounds, including African American and Hispanic American, will lead to greater understanding of common pathways to autoimmunity. Critical susceptibility genes shared among ethnic groups will be important in drug development for novel therapy. Currently, immune-modulating therapeutic strategies have serious side effects and vary in efficacy between individuals. Therapy for organ involvement could be more effective, and unnecessary treatment toxicities would be mitigated if genes known to influence disease and therapeutic delivery could be utilized in optimal selection of treatment and dosing. Ongoing work is attempting to explore how identified SLE susceptibility genes may contribute to pathology. The correlation of the individual's clinical course of disease with the specific genetic profile is underway: variation in the presentation of SLE could be explained and predicted by genetic factors. Thus, currently evolving information and technology has the potential to permit significant strides toward the goal of improved medical management in SLE, and ultimately preventative care in individuals at risk for SLE.

**BIBLIOGRAPHY:**

1. Gualtierotti R, Biggioggero M, Penatti AE, Meroni PL. Updating on the pathogenesis of systemic lupus erythematosus. *Autoimmun Rev.* 2010;10(1):3-7.
2. Costenbader KH, Gay S, Riquelme ME, Iaccarino L, Doria A. Genes, epigenetic regulation and environmental factors: which is the most relevant in developing autoimmune diseases? *Autoimmun Rev.* 2012;11(8):604-609.
3. Kelley JM, Edberg JC, Kimberly RP. Pathways: strategies for susceptibility genes in SLE. *Autoimmun Rev.* 2010;9(7):473-476.
4. Deng Y, Tsao BP. Genetic susceptibility to systemic lupus erythematosus in the genomic era. *Nat Rev Rheumatol.* 2010;6(12):683-692.
5. Truedsson L, Bengtsson AA, Sturfelt G. Complement deficiencies and systemic lupus erythematosus. *Autoimmunity.* 2001;40(8):560-566.
6. Yuan YJ, Luo XB, Shen N. Current advances in lupus genetic and genomic studies in Asia. *Lupus.* 2010;19(12):1374-1383.
7. Delgado-Vega AM, Alarcón-Riquelme ME, Kozyrev SV. Genetic associations in type I interferon related pathways with autoimmunity. *Arthritis Res Ther.* 2010;12(suppl 1):S2.
8. Kariuki SN, Franek BS, Kumar AA, et al. Trait-stratified genome-wide association study identifies novel and diverse genetic associations with serologic and cytokine phenotypes in systemic lupus erythematosus. *Arthritis Res Ther.* 2010;12(4):R151.
9. Yildirim-Toruner C, Diamond B. Current and novel therapeutics in the treatment of systemic lupus erythematosus. *J Allergy Clin Immunol.* 2011;127(2):303-312.
10. Sestak AL, Furnrohr BG, Harley JB, et al. The genetics of systemic lupus erythematosus and implications for targeted therapy. *Ann Rheum Dis.* 2011;70(suppl1):i37-i43.

## Supplementary Information

**OMIM REFERENCE:**

[1] Systemic Lupus Erythematosus; SLE: (#152700)

**Alternative Name:** None.

**Key Words:** Autoimmunity, antinuclear antibodies, anti–double-stranded DNA antibodies, lupus nephritis, immune complex deposition

# 143 Articular Chondrocalcinosis
Matthew Brown

## KEY POINTS

- *Disease summary:*
  - The diagnostic for calcium pyrophosphate dihydrate (CPPD) crystal deposition is given after the identification of CPPD crystals in synovial fluid (SF) or in tissue sections.
  - The terminology of CPPD-related diseases is still not uniform; the following definitions are the most commonly used:
    - Pseudogout—acute clinical syndrome of synovitis associated with CPPD deposition
    - Pyrophosphate arthropathy—structural abnormality of cartilage and bone associated with articular CPPD deposition
    - Chondrocalcinosis (CC)—radiographic observation of calcification of fibro and/or hyaline articular cartilage
  - CPPD deposition is the main cause of radiographic articular calcification of the knee, that is, CC. The deposition of other calcium salts, such as hydroxyapatite, can also be the cause of articular calcification.

- *Hereditary basis:*
  - CPPD deposition disease (CPDD) can occur as a familial monogenic disorder showing an autosomal dominant pattern of inheritance.

- *Differential diagnosis:*
  - Certain metabolic diseases predispose to CPDD deposition such as hemochromatosis, Gitelman syndrome, and hyperparathyroidism. It is possible to screen these disorders by laboratory hematologic testing and evaluate elevated serum calcium, decreased serum phosphate, elevated parathyroid hormone or parathormone, elevated alkaline phosphatase, and increased serum ferritin. However, it is important to refer that these disorders have strong genetic component themselves. In Table 143-1, it is possible to see how to perform a genetic differential diagnosis.

## Diagnostic Criteria and Clinical Characteristics

### Diagnostic Criteria:

**At least two of the following**

- **Demonstration of calcium pyrophosphate crystal deposition in tissue or SF by definitive means**.
- Identification of crystals showing weakly or no positive birefringence by compensated polarized light microscopy.
- Presence of typical radiographic calcifications.
- Acute arthritis, especially of knees or other large joints.
- Chronic arthritis, especially of knee, hip, carpus elbow, shoulder, or metacarpophalangeal (MCP) joint, especially if accompanied by acute exacerbation; the chronic arthritis shows the following features, which are helpful in differentiating it from osteoarthritis:
  - Uncommon sites: wrist, MCP joint, elbow, shoulder
  - Radiographic—or patellofemoral joint-space narrowing, especially if isolated
  - Subchondral cyst formation
  - Severity of degeneration—progressive, with subchondral bony collapse and fragmentation with formation of intra-articular radiodense bodies
  - Osteophyte formation—variable and inconsistent
  - Tendon calcifications, especially triceps, Achilles, obturators

### Categories
- Definite disease: I or IIa and IIb must be fulfilled
- Probable disease: IIa or IIb must be fulfilled
- Possible disease: IIIa or IIIb should alert the clinician to the possibility of underlying calcium pyrophosphate deposition

*Clinical Characteristics:* CPPD-CC is clinically heterogeneous, including

- An *asymptomatic* presentation, common in elderly people, affecting mainly the knee by the deposition of CPPD crystals in articular hyaline and fibrocartilage (CC)
- An acute form of CPPD arthropathy, known as *pseudogout,* typically monoarticular but sometimes subacute and/or polyarticular
- A chronic progressive CPPD arthropathy known as *pseudo-osteoarthritis,* affecting multiple joints with or without acute inflammatory reaction, usually bilateral and symmetrical
- *Pseudorheumatoid arthritis,* which is less common and characterized by bilateral and symmetrical polyarthritis, with low-grade inflammation lasting weeks or months
- A *miscellaneous* pattern mimicking ankylosing spondylitis, among other disorders
- A *tophaceous pseudogout* resulting from the deposition of calcium pyrophosphate crystals as large soft tissue masses

## Screening and Counseling

*Screening:* Aging is the most important risk factor for CC.

In patients with CPPD-CC onset less than 55 years other metabolic disorders should be screened (hemochromatosis, Gitelman syndrome, and hyperparathyroidism). It is also possible that, in these patients, a familial predisposition may exist. The only monogenic cause known for CPPD-CC is gain-of-function mutations in *ANKH*. Mutations in this gene are more likely in younger patients or in cases there is florid polyarticular CC. However, it has been recently suggested that cases of apparently sporadic chondrocalcinosis can also be caused by polymorphisms in *ANKH* gene.

*Table 143-1* **Genetic Differential Diagnosis**

| Syndrome | Gene Symbol | Associated Findings |
|---|---|---|
| Hemochromatosis | *HFE, TFR2, HJ, HAM, SLC40A1* | Group of phenotypically and genetically heterogeneous disorders characterized by iron overload. CPPD-CC has a well-known association with hemochromatosis affecting about 67% of the patients. |
| Gitelman syndrome | *SLC12A3* | Variant of Barter syndrome in which patients present hypokalemic alkalosis in conjunction with hypocalciuria and hypomagnesemia. CPPD-CC has been widely associated with this syndrome affecting a large majority of these patients. |
| Hypophosphatasia | *ALPL* | Heterogeneous biochemical and clinical features which include low levels of serum alkaline phosphatase, high levels of serum pyridoxal-5-prime-phosphate, early loss of teeth (odontohypophosphatasia), bowed legs, calcification of paraspinous ligaments, joint pains, and peri- and intra-articular calcifications of joints of the hands, feet, and knees and calcification of the anterior spinous ligament in the lumbar area. |
| Hyperparathyroidism | *MEN1, HPRT2, HRPT3* | This is the most common familial form of primary hyperparathyroidism. Primary chief cell hyperplasia is the main characteristic of this disorder. Many patients show hypercalcemia and radiologic changes characteristic of chondrocalcinosis. |
| Familial hypocalciuric hypercalcemia, type I | *CASR* | This was the first disorder described where renal tubular defect in calcium reabsorption is independent of parathormone. A ratio of renal calcium clearance to creatinine clearance below 0.01 suggests FHH1. The only complications attributable to the hypercalcemia are pancreatitis and chondrocalcinosis. Both the kidneys and the parathyroid glands seem insensitive to chronic hypercalcemia in this disease. |

Gene names: *HFE*, hemochromatosis; *TFR2*, transferrin receptor-2; *HJV*, hemojuvelin; *HAMP*, hepcidin antimicrobial peptide; *SLC40A1*, solute carrier family 40 member 1; *ALPL*, alkaline phosphatase; *MEN1*, menin; *HRPT2*, hyperparathyroidism 2; *HRPT3*, hyperparathyroidism 3; *CASR*, calcium sensing receptor.

CC is very common in elderly patients (>55 years). Hyperparathyroidism should be screened in all patients.

Osteoarthritis (OA) is a common finding in these patients as well. It is still not fully understood the relationship between OA and CC, but CC does not appear to be a risk factor for more rapid cartilage degradation.

**Counseling:** Although most cases of CPPD-CC are nonfamilial, there are many reports of kindreds with a familial form of this disorder, indicating a significant genetic impact in the disease. Two main different clinical phenotypes have been observed in all these kindreds. The first is characterized by the early onset, polyarticular involvement, and variable severity of arthropathy; the second is similar to that observed in sporadic disease cases and is characterized by late-onset oligoarticular CC with arthritis. The large majority of the investigated families have shown an autosomal dominant pattern of transmission. Each sibling has 50% chance of inheriting this disease.

The disease segregates equally on males and females and is thought to be highly penetrant. There is not a difference between clinical phenotypes shown by sporadic patients when compared with those with familial story. The phenotypic severity in CPPD-CC is variable and this is apparently associated with the specific mutation which is causing the disease.

## Management and Treatment

- Management of CPDD depends on the clinical manifestations observed (Table 143-2).

- Asymptomatic CPDD should not be treated. Other syndromes should be screened and treated accordingly.
- Pseudogout may be treated with joint aspiration and intra-articular corticosteroid injection, systemic corticosteroids, nonsteroidal anti-inflammatory drugs (NSAIDs) and colchicines. Pseudorheumatoid arthritis can be treated with corticosteroids.
- Methotrexate has been used in patients with severe disease and joint destruction.
- Anakinra has recently been reported to treat and prevent acute attacks of pseudogout in end-stage renal failure.
- Surgical excision of calcifications from the joint may be helpful but this has to be further investigated.

## Molecular Genetics and Molecular Mechanism

☞**CHONDROCALCINOSIS 1/UNKNOWN/8Q:** Two chromosomal regions have been linked to this disease. Genetic linkage between markers on human chromosome 8q and the disease in a large family from Maine with early-onset CPPD and severe degenerative OA [CCAL1, MIM 600668] was reported. The disease-causing gene has yet to be mapped but there is a strong possibility that this gene is primarily related with OA and that the CPPD deposition is secondary, enhanced by the degenerative changes in cartilage.

☞**CHONDROCALCINOSIS 2/ANKH/5P15.1:** Greater success has been experienced with a second form of autosomal

*Table 143-2* **Algorithm for Screening and Management of Patient With CPPD Chondrocalcinosis**

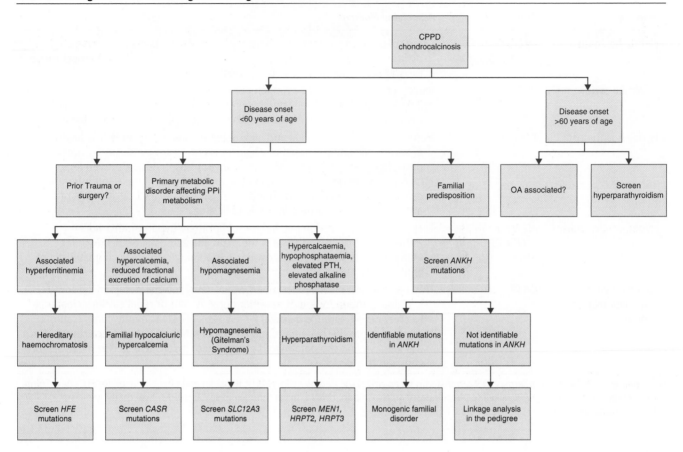

dominant CPPD deposition disease CCAL2 [CCAL2, MIM 118600] (Table 143-3). This condition was initially described and genetically localised in five English families with CPPD crystal deposition. Subsequently, in two CPPD-CC unrelated families, one from Argentina and the other from France, another zone in the same chromosome mapping just centromeric to the first, was further identified through recombination analysis. Linkage was well established to chromosome 5p where the responsible gene *ANKH* has been identified.

ANKH is a transmembrane protein that regulates the transport of PPi out of the cell for the extracellular matrix.

Mutations in *ANKH* have also been shown to cause another autosomal dominant condition characterised by hyperostosis and sclerosis of the skull, together with flaring and abnormal modelling of the metaphyses of long bones—Jackson craniometaphyseal dysplasia [CMD, MIM 123000].

***Genetic Testing:*** Genetic testing for familial forms of CPPD-CC is not clinically used and is not widely available. Identification of mutations associated with CPPD-CC is still not in the clinical genetic testing domain. Genetic testing for CMD where *ANKH* mutations are identified through direct sequencing is clinically available.

*Table 143-3* **ANKH Molecular Genetic Testing**

| Mutation Type | Modification | Amino Acid Change | Location |
|---|---|---|---|
| Regulatory | CGGG(G-A)ACTATG | Noncoding | 5' UTR, -4bp from initiation codon |
| Regulatory | CCCA(C-T)GGCG | Noncoding | 5'UTR, -11bp from initiation codon |
| Missense | CCG-ACG | Pro-Thr | Codon 5 |
| Missense | CCG-CTG | Pro-Leu | Codon 5 |
| Missense | ATG-ACG | Met-Thr | Codon 48 |
| Missense | GGG-AGG | Gly-Arg | Codon 389 |
| Small deletion | GAGgagAAT | Glu deletion | Codon 490 |

The utility of testing, for the moment, is limited in terms of clinical practice since there is still no appropriate treatment for this disorder based on the genetic information. On the contrary, the utility of genetic testing for investigational purposes is enormous for it will allow the development of knowledge in this area of expertise and will surely lead to the development of new drugs with pharmacologic treating potential.

## BIBLIOGRAPHY:

1. Ryan LM. Calcium pyrophosphate dehydrate crystal deposition. In: Weyand CM, Wortman R, Klippel JH, eds. *Primer of Rheumatic Diseases.* 11th ed. Atlanta, GA: Arthritis Foundation; 1997:226-229.

2. Richete P, Bardin T, Doherty M. An update on the epidemiology of calcium pyrophosphate dihydrate crystal deposition disease. *Rheumatology.* 2009;48(7):711-715.

3. Zhang Y, Johnson K, Russell RG, et al. Association of sporadic chondrocalcinosis with a 4-basepair G-to-A transition in the 5'-untranslated region of ANKH that promotes enhanced expression of ANKH protein and excess generation of extracellular inorganic pyrophosphate. *Arthritis Rheum.* 2005;52(4):1110-1117.

4. Williams CJ, Zhang Y, Timms A, et al. Autosomal dominant familial calcium pyrophosphate dihydrate deposition disease is caused by mutation in the transmembrane protein ANKH. *Am J Hum Genet.* 2002;71(4):985-991.

5. Ea HK, Liote F. Calcium pyrophosphate dehydrate and basic calcium phosphate crystal-induced arthropathies: update on pathogenesis, clinical features and therapy. *Curr Rheumatol Rep.* 2004;6(3):221-227.

6. Announ N, Palmer G, Guerne PA, Gabay C. Anakinra is a possible alternative in the treatment and prevention of acute attacks of pseudogout in end-stage renal failure. *Joint Bone Spine.* Jul 2009;76(4):424-426.

7. Baldwin CT, Farrer LA, Adair R, Dharmavaram R, Jimenez S, Anderson L. Linkage of early-onset osteoarthritis and chondrocalcinosis to human chromosome 8q. *Am J Hum Genet.* 1995;56:692-697.

8. Hughes AE, McGibbon D, Woodward E, Dixey J, Doherty M. Localisation of a gene for chondrocalcinosis to chromosome 5p. *Hum Mol Genet.* 1995;4(7):1225-1228.

9. Andrew LJ, Brancolini V, de la Pena LS, et al. Refinement of the chromosome 5p locus for familial calcium pyrophosphate dihydrate deposition disease. *Am J Hum Genet.* 1999;64(1):136-145.

10. Pendleton A, Johnson MD, Hughes A, et al. Mutations in ANKH cause chondrocalcinosis. *Am J Hum Genet.* 2002;71(4):933-940.

11. Gurley KA, Reimer RJ, Kingsley DM. Biochemical and genetic analysis of ANK in arthritis and bone disease. *Am J Hum Genet.* 2006;79(6):1017-1029.

12. Nurnberg P, Thiele H, Chandler D, et al. Heterozygous mutations in ANKH, the human ortholog of the mouse progressive ankylosis gene, result in craniometaphyseal dysplasia. *Nat Genet.* 2001;28:37-41.

13. Human Genetic Mutation Database: www.hgmd.cf.ac.uk

## Supplementary Information

### OMIM REFERENCES:

[1] Chondrocalcinosis 2; ANKH (#118600)

[2] Chondrocalcinosis 1; (%600668)

[3] Gitelman Syndrome; (#263800)

[4] Hyperparathyroidism; (#145000)

[5] Hypophosphatasia, Adult; (#146300)

[6] Hypocalciuric Hypercalcemia, Familial, Type I; (#145980)

[7] Bartter Syndrome, Type III; (# 607364)

### Alternative Names:
- Familial Articular Chondrocalcinosis
- Calciumgout
- Calcium Pyrophosphate Arthropathy
- Calcium Pyrophosphate Dehydrate Deposition Disease

*Key Words:* Chondrocalcinosis, pseudogout, osteoarthritis, *ANKH*, arthritis, carpal tunnel, crystal deposition, pyrophosphate, epidemiology, ankylosis, hemochromatosis, hypomagnesemia, hypercalcemia, hyperparathyroidism, Gitelman syndrome, hypophosphatasia

## 144 Cystic Diseases of the Kidney, Polycystic Kidney Disease

Maria V. Irazabal and Vicente Torres

### KEY POINTS

- *Disease summary:*
  - Cystic diseases of the kidney are a heterogeneous group of hereditary, developmental, or acquired disorders that have in common the presence of renal cysts.
  - A renal cyst is a fluid-filled cavity lined by epithelial cells that derives primarily from the renal tubules, loosing its connection with their origin tubule once developed.
  - Polycystic kidney disease (PKD) is a group of monogenic disorders that result in renal cyst development, being autosomal dominant polycystic kidney disease (ADPKD) and autosomal recessive polycystic kidney disease (ARPKD) the most common forms.
  - ADPKD, caused by mutation in *PKD1* or *PKD2*, is generally a late-onset multisystem disorder characterized predominantly by bilateral renal cysts and variable extra renal manifestations (extrarenal cysts, cardiac valvular defects, arterial aneurysms, colonic diverticulosis, abdominal wall hernias)
  - ARPKD, most commonly affecting newborns and young children, is caused by mutation in *PKHD1* and is characterized by enlarged echogenic kidneys and congenital hepatic fibrosis.

- *Hereditary basis:*
  - ADPKD is the most frequent inherited renal disorder (1 in 400-1000) and follows an autosomal dominant inheritance pattern with complete penetrance and high intrafamilial variability.
  - ARPKD follows an autosomal recessive inheritance with an incidence of approximately 1:20.000; the frequency of heterozygosity is approximately 1:70.

- *Differential diagnosis:*
  - Cystic diseases in the differential diagnosis of ADPKD: ARPKD, other systemic diseases associated with renal cysts such as tuberous sclerosis complex (TSC), von Hippel-Lindau disease (VHL), and orofacial digital syndrome type 1 (OFDS), acquired renal cystic disease (ARCD) in patients with end-stage renal disease (ESRD), medullary sponge kidney, and simple cysts (Table 144-1).
  - Cystic diseases in the differential diagnosis of ARPKD: early-manifesting ADPKD, a group of inherited pleiotropic disorders causing polycystic kidneys (nephronophthisis [NPHP], Joubert syndrome and related disorders [JSRD], Meckel syndrome [MKS], Bardet-Biedl syndrome [BBS]), glomerulocystic kidney disease, and diffuse cystic dysplasia.

## Diagnostic Criteria and Clinical Characteristics

### Diagnostic Criteria for ADPKD:

**At least one of the following when there is a family history of ADPKD**

- Unified diagnostic criteria based on ultrasound findings in individuals at risk for ADPKD
  - Three or more (unilateral or bilateral) renal cysts if between 15 and 39 years and genotype unknown
  - Two or more cysts per kidney if between 40 and 59 years
  - Four or more cysts per kidney if patient is more than or equal to 60 years
- No established diagnostic criteria exist based on computed tomography (CT) or magnetic resonance imaging (MRI). Ultrasound criteria could reasonably be applied to CT or MRI if restricted to cysts measuring greater than or equal to 1 cm in diameter (MRI and contrast-enhanced CT are more sensitive than ultrasound to detect smaller cysts).
- Identification of a known *PKD1* or *PKD2* mutation by sequence analysis or genetic diagnosis based on linkage analysis.

**In the absence of a family history of ADPKD**

- More than 10 cysts per kidney in the absence of manifestations, suggestive of a different renal cystic disease (presumptive diagnosis)
- Identification of a *PKD1* or *PKD2* mutation by sequence analysis

### Diagnostic Criteria for ARPKD:

**At least two of the following**

- Kidney involvement
  - Infants or early childhood: bilateral renal enlargement with loss of corticomedullary differentiation
  - Older patients: precalyceal tubular ectasia or bilateral renal cysts

*Table 144-1 Genetic Differential Diagnosis*

| Disease | Gene Symbol | Associated Findings | |
|---------|-------------|---------------------|---|
| ADPKD | *PKD1* | ~85% of cases of ADPKD; more aggressive disease. Average onset of ESRD 54.3 years. | Bilateral macrocysts (from all parts of the nephron), liver cysts, intracranial aneurysms, cardiac valve abnormalities, abdominal wall hernias. |
| | *PKD2* | ~15% of cases of ADPKD; milder disease with fewer cysts. Average onset of ERSD 74 years. | |
| ARPKD | *PKHD1* | More frequent in newborns/young children<br>Bilateral microcysts (fusiform dilations of the collecting tubules)<br>Bile duct proliferation and ectasia with congenital hepatic fibrosis (CHF) | |
| TSC | *TSC1, TSC2* | Renal angiomyolipomas, facial angiofibromas, nontraumatic ungual or periungual fibromas, hypomelanotic macules, shagreen patch, retinal nodular hamartomas, cortical tubers, subependymal giant cell astrocytoma, cardiac rhabdomyoma, multiple renal cysts, "confetti" skin lesions | |
| VHL | *VHL* | Hemangioblastomas of the brain, spinal cord, and retina; renal cysts and renal cell carcinoma; pheochromocytoma; and endolymphatic sac tumors | |
| OFDS | *OFD1* | Malformations of the face, oral cavity, and digits; CNS abnormalities; renal cysts, glomerulocystic kidney. | |
| NPHP | *NPHP2* | ESRD 1-3 years, tubulointerstitial nephritis with cortical microcysts; Senior-Loken syndrome (retinitis pigmentosa), situs inversus and ventricular septal defect, hypertension, hepatic fibrosis | |
| | *NPHP1, 3-11* | ESRD 5-25 years. First symptoms: polyuria and polydipsia; late symptoms: related to the progressive renal insufficiency (nausea, anorexia, weakness). Small cysts in the medulla; Senior-Loken syndrome. | |
| JSRD | *JBTS1-JBTS10* | Hypo/dysplasia of the cerebellar vermis "molar tooth sign," developmental delay, retinal dystrophy, nephronophthisis, hepatic fibrosis, and polydactyly. | |
| MKS | *MKS1, MKS3* | Renal cystic dysplasia, central nervous system defects (typically occipital encephalocele), polydactyly, and biliary dysgenesis. | |
| BBS | *BBS1-BBS14* | Obesity, polydactyly, pigmentary retinopathy, learning disabilities, various degrees of cognitive impairment, hypogonadism, renal cystic dysplasia. | |

Gene names: *PKD1*, polycystic kidney disease 1; *PKD2*, polycystic kidney disease 2; *PKHD1*, polycystic kidney and hepatic disease 1; *TSC1*, tuberous sclerosis complex 1; *TSC2*, tuberous sclerosis complex 2; *VHL*, von Hippel-Lindau tumor suppressor; *OFD1*, orofacial digital 1; *NPHP1-11*, nephronophthisis 1-11; *JBTS1-JBTS10*, Joubert syndrome 1-10; *MKS1*, Meckel syndrome 1; *MKS3*, Meckel syndrome 3; *BBS1-BBS14*, Bardet-Biedl syndrome 1-14.

- Evidence of ductal plate malformation
  - Diagnosis of congenital hepatic fibrosis (CHF) on liver biopsy *or*
  - Radiologic findings consistent with intrahepatic bile duct dilatation
- Detection of *PKHD1* mutation by direct sequencing
- Definite diagnosis of ARPKD, CHF, or Caroli disease in a sibling

**And the absence of**
- Renal cysts in both parents demonstrated by ultrasound (US)
- Manifestations suggesting a different renal cystic disease in the child

***Clinical Characteristics:*** ADPKD is characterized by the progressive, bilateral development, and enlargement of renal cysts, frequently resulting in ESRD. The typical presenting symptoms include hypertension, flank pain, hematuria, and less frequently urinary tract infections and nephrolithiasis. The most common extrarenal manifestations are hepatic cysts, followed by cysts in other organs (seminal vesicles, arachnoid). The most important noncystic manifestations include intracranial (ICA) and other arterial aneurysms.

In ARPKD, the severity of the renal and hepatic manifestations is inversely correlated and depends on the age at diagnosis. In the perinatal period, the disease often presents with greatly enlarged echogenic kidneys and minimal hepatic fibrosis. Severe renal impairment in utero leads to oligohydramnios and subsequent pulmonary hypoplasia. Infants usually manifests with renal and hepatic involvement. Patients often develop ESRD and/or portal hypertension. Older children or adolescents usually present with hepatic involvement with portal hypertension and less severe renal involvement.

## Screening and Counseling

*Screening:* In patients over the age of 18 years, with family history of ADPKD, abdominal US remain the main screening method and should be the initial evaluation. Abdominal CT and MRI are useful in the differential diagnosis and to establish a prognosis. Genetic testing should be considered when imaging findings are equivocal. Although gene-based diagnosis is not necessary in most of the patients, it is particularly helpful for obtaining a definitive diagnosis in a young person who is a potential living-related donor.

Molecular genetic testing is usually not necessary to confirm the diagnosis of ARPKD when clinical diagnostic criteria are met; sequence analysis or mutation scanning can establish the diagnosis in most of the other cases.

In an index case, the relative likelihood of these disorders can be predicted based on (a) age at diagnosis, and (b) kidney characteristics. Clinical features of ADPKD most frequently begin between the third and fifth decade of life, but cysts may be detectable in childhood and in utero. ARPKD typically presents in utero or during the neonatal period, but can also be diagnosed in childhood or even adolescents or young adults (Table 144-2).

In addition, diagnosis based on relative likelihood is outlined in Table 144-3.

*Counseling:* ADPKD is inherited as an autosomal dominant trait with complete penetrance. Each child of an affected parent has 50% risk of inheriting the disease. The majority of the patients have an affected parent, but in 5% to 10% of the patients no family history can be found, suggesting a high spontaneous mutation rate. Presymptomatic screening should be offered to all first-degree relatives of an affected individual; however, proper information about the advantages and disadvantages of being screened should be given prior testing.

ARPKD is inherited as an autosomal recessive trait, and therefore, may occur in siblings but not in parents. Each sibling of an affected patient has a 25% chance of inheriting both disease-causing alleles and thus being affected. Penetrance is 100%, although considerable phenotypic variability may be observed.

Due to the poor prognosis of early manifestations of ARPKD, molecular diagnostics for prenatal testing and preimplantation genetic diagnosis have been used. On the other hand, molecular testing for prenatal or preimplantation diagnosis of ADPKD is not usually requested as the disease generally first manifests in adults.

☞GENOTYPE-PHENOTYPE CORRELATION: Mutations on *PKD1* are associated with a more severe disease and a higher number of cysts, with earlier diagnosis, a higher incidence of hypertension and hematuria and ESRD occurring on average 20 years earlier (54.3 vs 74 years). Both PKD1 and PKD2 can be associated with severe polycystic liver disease (PLD) and vascular abnormalities.

In ARPKD, a clear genotype or phenotype correlation has been described, where patients with two truncating mutations are associated with the most severe phenotype (neonatal death). On the other hand, patients with two missense changes or a missense and a truncating change present with a moderate phenotype.

## Management and Treatment

Current therapy in PKD is directed toward reducing the morbidity and mortality from the renal and extrarenal complications: blood pressure control, pain management, prompt treatment of infections and other disease complications, and management of ESRD.

Advances in the understanding of the genetics of ADPKD and mechanisms of cyst development and growth have facilitated the development of clinical trials and identification of promising drugs (tolvaptan, octreotide, lanreotide). Angiotensin-converting enzyme inhibitors (ACEi) and angiotensin II receptor blockers (ARB) may be superior to other antihypertensive medications because of the role of the renin angiotensin system in the pathogenesis of hypertension in ADPKD. Pain should be treated with simple analgesia, but surgical management (cyst decompression, denervation) may be required. Kidney transplant is the treatment of choice for ESRD; complications after transplant are no greater than in the general population. MR angiography is the gold standard screening method for ICA and should be limited to those patients with a family history of aneurismal rupture, previous aneurysm rupture, or preparation for major elective surgeries.

The results of Consortium for Radiologic Imaging for the Study of Polycystic Kidney disease (CRISP) have shown that the rate of renal growth is a good predictor of functional decline and justify the use of kidney and cyst volume as markers of disease progression.

The initial management of ARPKD affected neonates should be oriented toward stabilization of the respiratory function. If the neonate presents with oliguria or anuria, peritoneal dialysis may be required. Hypertension is managed with ACEi or ARB. Children that present with portal hypertension may require a portacaval shunt. Renal transplantation may be necessary in a large number of patients and is the preferred choice for ESRD in children.

## Molecular Genetics and Molecular Mechanism

*Disease/Gene/Locus:*

ADPKD/polycystic kidney disease 1 (*PKD1*)/16p13.3
ADPKD/polycystic kidney disease 2 (*PKD2*)/4q21
ARPKD/polycystic kidney and hepatic disease 1 (*PKHD1*)/6q21.1-12

The PKD1 and PKD2 proteins, polycystin-1 (PC1 ~460 KDa) and polycystin-2 (PC2, ~110 KDa) belong to a subfamily (TRPP) of transient receptor potential (TRP) channels. PC1, with a large extracellular N-terminal region, 11 transmembrane regions, and a short intracellular C-terminal region, has the structure of a receptor or adhesion molecule and may function as a receptor involved in cell-cell and/or cell-matrix interaction. PC2, with a short N-terminal cytoplasmic region, 6 transmembrane domains, and a short C-terminal portion, functions as a $Ca^{2+}$-permeable channel. Both proteins interact through their cytoplasmic region and transmit fluid flow–mediated mechanosensation, which is detected by the primary cilium of renal epithelium. Disruption of normal polycystin function by mutations predispose to cyst formation through loss of mechanical cues in tubular epithelial cells that regulate tissue morphogenesis.

Fibrocystin (~447 KDa), the protein encoded by *PKHD1*, is an integral membrane protein with a large extracellular region, a single transmembrane domain, and a short cytoplasmic tail. The extracellular region contains 12 TIG/IPT domains (immunoglobulin-like fold shared by plexins and transcription factors). Fibrocystin is

**Table 144-2 Algorithm for Diagnostic Evaluation of Patient With Renal Cysts**

Kidney cysts
- Adults
  - Syndromic presentation
    - Renal cysts + Renal angiomyolipomas; facial angiofibromas; shagreen patch; cortical tubers; "confetti" skin lesions → **TSC**
    - Renal cysts + Hemangioblastoma; Renal Cell Carcinoma; pheochromocytoma → **VHL**
    - Renal cysts + Female w/ malformations of the face, oral cavity, and digits; CNS abnormalities → **OFDS**
  - No Family History of PKD
    - ESRD → **Acquired Renal Cystic Disease (ARCD)**
    - Precalyceal tubular ectasia; renal cysts in medulla → **Medullary Sponge Kidney (MSK)**
    - Few unilateral/bilateral renal cysts → **Simple Cysts**
    - Bilateral renal cysts, many cysts, often liver cysts → **Unrecognized or de novo ADPKD**
  - Family History of PKD
    - Bilateral renal cysts, many cysts, ESRD in an affected family member ≤ 50 y.o. → **PKD1**
    - Bilateral renal cysts, fewer cysts, sufficient renal function in an affected family member ≥ 70 y.o. → **PKD2**
  - Family History of ESRD, gout
    - ESRD 50–70 y.o. → **MCKD1**
    - ESRD 30–50 y.o. → **MCKD2** Uromodulin
- Children
  - Family History of PKD
    - Infantile presentation of markedly enlarged echogenic kidneys, one of the parents with renal cysts → **PKD1 >> PKD2; PKD1/TSC2 contiguous gene syndrome**
  - Absence of renal cysts in both parents demonstrated by US
    - Bilateral microcysts + CHF → **ARPKD**
  - Syndromic presentation
    - Renal cystic dysplasia, central nervous system defects; polydactyly and biliary dysgenesis. → **MKS** *MKS1, MKS3, NPHP3, CEP290, RPGRIP1L, CC2D2A, TMEM216/ MKS2*
    - Hypo/dysplasia of the cerebellar vermis "molar tooth sign", developmental delay, nephronophthisis, hepatic fibrosis → **Joubert Syndrome** *AHI1, NPHP1, CEP290, MKS3, RPGRIP1L, ARL13B, CC2D2A*
    - Renal cystic dysplasia + Obesity, polydactyly, pigmentary retinopathy, learning disabilities. → **BBS 1–14**
    - Renal cysts, fibrosis ± Senior-Loken syndrome (retinitis pigmentosa) → **NPHP**
      - ESRD 1–3 y.o; normal or enlarged kidneys with cysts; situs inversus; hepatic fibrosis. → **NHPH2**
      - ESRD 5–25 y.o.; small kidneys with medullary cysts → **NHPH1,3-11**

*Table 144-3* **Genes Associated With Different Presentations**

| Presentation | PKD1 | PKD2 | PKHD1 |
|---|---|---|---|
| Bilateral renal cysts, many cysts, ESRD in an affected family member ≤ 50 years<br>Adults | 1 | 2 | 3 |
| Bilateral renal cysts, fewer cysts, sufficient renal function in an affected family member ≥70 years<br>Adults | 2 | 1 | 3 |
| Infantile presentation of markedly enlarged echogenic kidneys, unaffected parents<br>Children | 2 | 3 | 1 |
| Infantile presentation of markedly enlarged echogenic kidneys, one of the parents with cystic kidneys<br>Children | 1 | 2 | 3 |
| Cystic kidneys and manifestations of portal hypertension in an adolescent or young adult | 2 | 3 | 1 |

Scale 1 to 3, 1 most likely and 3 least likely.

*Table 144-4* **Molecular Genetic Testing**

| Gene | Testing Modality | Mutation Type | Detection Rate |
|---|---|---|---|
| PKD1 | Sequence analysis | Sequence variants | ~88% |
| PKD2 | Sequence analysis/mutation scanning | Sequence variants | ~92% |
|  | Linkage analysis | N/A | N/A |
|  | Deletion/duplication analysis | Partial or whole gene deletions | <1% |
| PKHD1 | Mutation scanning | Sequence variants | 57%-75% two mutations, 18%-39% one mutation, and 2%-8% no mutations |
|  | Sequence analysis |  | Unknown |
|  | Linkage analysis | N/A | N/A |
|  | Deletion/duplication analysis | Partial or whole gene deletions | Unknown |
|  | Targeted mutation analysis | Panel of mutations | [a] |

[a]Panels of mutations specific to different population groups are offered by some laboratories listed in the *GeneTests Laboratory Directory*.

expressed in the primary cilia of renal and bile duct epithelial cells. The precise function of fibrocystin is still unknown, but may mediate its activity through PC2, and is believed to have a role in collecting-duct and biliary differentiation.

***Genetic Testing:*** Testing for *PKD1*, *PKD2*, and *PKHD1* mutations is clinically available (Table 144-4). The decision on which gene to test and testing modality should be based on clinical presentation, family history, the availability and willingness of family members to be tested and a previous identification of the disease-causing mutation in the family.

## BIBLIOGRAPHY:

1. Pei Y, Obaji J, Dupuis A, et al. Unified criteria for ultrasonographic diagnosis of ADPKD. *J Am Soc Nephrol*. 2009;20:205-212.

2. Pirson Y, Chauveau D, Torres V. Management of cerebral aneurysms in autosomal dominant polycystic kidney disease. *J Am Soc Nephrol*. 2002;13:269-276.

3. MacDermot KD, Saggar-Malik AK, Economides DL, Jeffery S. Prenatal diagnosis of autosomal dominant polycystic kidney disease (PKD1) presenting in utero and prognosis for very early onset disease. *J Med Genet*. 1998;35:13-16.

4. Zerres K, Senderek J, Rudnik-Schöneborn S, et al. New options for prenatal diagnosis in autosomal recessive polycystic kidney disease by mutation analysis of the PKHD1 gene. *Clin Genet*. 2004;66:53-57.

5. Hateboer N, v Dijk MA, Bogdanova N, et al. Comparison of phenotypes of polycystic kidney disease types 1 and 2. European PKD1-PKD2 Study Group. *Lancet*. 1999;353:103-107.

6. Rossetti S, Chauveau D, Kubly V, et al. Association of mutation position in polycystic kidney disease 1 (PKD1) gene and development of a vascular phenotype. *Lancet*. 2003a;361:2196-2201.

7. Rossetti S, Torra R, Coto E, et al. A complete mutation screen of PKHD1 in autosomal-recessive polycystic kidney disease (ARPKD) pedigrees. *Kidney Int*. 2003b;64:391-403.

8.  Bergmann C, Senderek J, Sedlacek B, et al. Spectrum of mutations in the gene for autosomal recessive polycystic kidney disease (ARPKD/PKHD1). *J Am Soc Nephrol.* 2003;14:76-89.

9.  Koulen P, Cai Y, Geng L, et al. Polycystin-2 is an intracellular calcium release channel. *Nat Cell Biol.* 2002;4:191-197.

10. Nauli SM, Alenghat FJ, Luo Y, et al. Polycystins 1 and 2 mediate mechanosensation in the primary cilium of kidney cells. *Nat Genet.* 2003;33:129-137.

11. Igarashi P, Somlo S. Genetics and pathogenesis of polycystic kidney disease. *J Am Soc Nephrol.* 2002;13:2384-2398.

12. Rossetti S, Consugar MB, Chapman AB, et al. Comprehensive molecular diagnostics in autosomal dominant polycystic kidney disease. *J Am Soc Nephrol.* 2007;18:2143-2160.

13. Consugar MB, Wong WC, Lundquist PA, et al. Characterization of large rearrangements associated in autosomal dominant polycystic kidney disease and the PKD1/TSC2 contiguous gene syndrome. *Kidney Int.* 2008;74:1468-1479.

14. Sharp AM, Messiaen LM, Page G, et al. Comprehensive genomic analysis of PKHD1 mutations in ARPKD cohorts. *J Med Genet.* 2005;42:336-349.

15. Bergmann C, Senderek J, Schneider F, et al. PKHD1 mutations in families requesting prenatal diagnosis for autosomal recessive polycystic kidney disease (ARPKD). *Hum Mutat.* 2004;23:487-495.

16. Bergmann C, Senderek J, Windelen E, et al. Clinical consequences of PKHD1 mutations in 164 patients with autosomal-recessive polycystic kidney disease (ARPKD). *Kidney Int.* 2005;67:829-848.

## Supplementary Information

**OMIM References:**

[1] Polycystic Kidneys (#173900)

[2] Polycystic Kidney Disease 1; PKD1 (#601313)

[3] PKD2 Gene; PKD2 (#173910)

[4] Polycystic Kidney Disease, Autosomal Recessive; ARPKD (#263200)

[5] PKHD1 Gene; PKHD1 (#606702)

[6] von Hippel-Lindau; VHL (#193300)

**Alternative Names:**

- Polycystic Kidney Disease
- Polycystic Renal Disease
- Autosomal Dominant Polycystic Kidney Disease
- Cysts—Kidneys
- Kidney—Polycystic

*Key Words:* Renal cysts, polycystic kidney disease (PKD), autosomal dominant polycystic kidney disease (ADPKD), polycystic kidney disease 1 (PKD1), polycystin-1 (PC1), polycystic kidney disease 2 (PKD2), polycystin-2 (PC2), autosomal recessive polycystic kidney disease (ARPKD), polycystic kidney and hepatic disease 1 (PKHD1), fibrocystin, end-stage renal disease (ESRD), congenital hepatic fibrosis (CHF), ultrasound (US), genetic testing

# 145 Nephrolithiasis

John A. Sayer

## KEY POINTS

- *Disease summary:*
  - Nephrolithiasis is the pathologic process of stone (calculus) formation within the renal tract. The resulting renal calculi are composed of calcium salts, uric acid, cystine, and other insoluble complexes.
- *Hereditary basis:*
  - Nephrolithiasis may occur either as part of the phenotype of rare single gene disorders or as an "idiopathic" renal stone-forming disease with a polygenic inheritance.
  - The genetic basis of single gene disorders includes autosomal recessive, autosomal dominant, and X-linked disorders. Each of these single gene disorders usually leads to a significant metabolic risk factor for nephrolithiasis.
  - Idiopathic renal stone formation is caused by an interplay of environmental, dietary, and genetic factors. Twin studies demonstrate a significant contribution of genetic factors in stone formation, whilst the recent rise in stone formation in Westernized societies is likely to be secondary to nongenetic factors such as diet and obesity.
  - Hypercalciuria is the most commonly found metabolic risk factor in "idiopathic" stone formers. There are many candidate genes for "idiopathic" hypercalciuric stone formers but the genetic basis remains elusive since hypercalciuria is a quantitative trait and may be polygenic.
  - The genetic basis of other metabolic risk factors such as hyperuricosuria, hyperoxaluria, and hypocitraturia is beginning to be understood as molecular transporters of various solutes are cloned and characterized.
- *Differential diagnosis:*
  - Nephrolithiasis may be part of a more generalized calcification of the kidney termed nephrocalcinosis. It may be part of multisystem disorders and congenital abnormalities of the kidney or urinary tract (CAKUT). Nephrolithiasis may be a complicating feature of autosomal dominant polycystic kidney disease and medullary sponge kidney due to architectural and metabolic abnormalities associated with these conditions.
  - It is useful to distinguish between calcium-containing and noncalcium-containing stones (eg, urate, cystine), as this will determine the best imaging modality for diagnosis and follow-up.

## Diagnostic Criteria and Clinical Characteristics

*Diagnostic Criteria:* Nephrolithiasis is derived from the Greek words nephros and lithos meaning kidney stone. Urolithiasis is defined as a condition giving rise to a stone within the urinary tract (including kidneys, ureters, and bladder). Nephrocalcinosis is calcification of the kidney which can be microscopic or macroscopic.

The diagnosis of nephrolithiasis is made clinically by presenting features that may include loin pain, spasms of pain radiating to the groin (renal colic), hematuria (visible and nonvisible), urinary frequency, urgency, and dysuria. The diagnosis is confirmed using imaging of the stone (radiologic or ultrasound studies), serum and urine biochemistry, and, once the stone is passed or removed, by physical and chemical examination of the stone morphology and composition.

Urinary tract infection may present concurrently with a renal stone. Stones may be a complication of other anatomic abnormalities of the kidneys, including autosomal dominant polycystic kidney disease. Nephrolithiasis, strictly speaking, is a symptom rather than a diagnosis and an underlying cause must be sought in all cases.

*Clinical Characteristics:* Stones may vary in size from microscopic crystals forming within the urine and within renal tissues to huge "staghorn" calculi that completed fill or replace the renal pelvis. The majority of renal stones are composed of calcium oxalate (60%) or calcium phosphate (20%) and are therefore radio-opaque. Uric acid (~10%), struvite (~8%), and cystine (~2%) are rarer but can all give rise to Staghorn calculi. Stones may present acutely as an episode of renal colic or an obstructed urinary system, necessitating urgent decompression. Nephrocalcinosis and some forms of renal stone disease (eg, 2,8-dihydroxyadenine [DHA] stones) are more insidious and may present with chronic kidney disease or end-stage renal failure rather than renal colic. It is important to note that hypercalciuria or crystalluria per se may be a cause of invisible (microscopic) hematuria.

## Screening and Counseling

*Screening:* A diagnostic algorithm approach to all patients with nephrolithiasis will aid the identification of a metabolic diagnosis in idiopathic stone formers. Establishing such a diagnosis allows both metabolic and molecular screening of family members at risk of inherited renal stone disorders. No clear evidence of benefit from screening of family members exists for idiopathic stone diseases whilst monogenic disorders may be screened according to the specific diagnosis.

*Counseling:* For known monogenic diseases, genetic counseling and advice should be given, according to the Mendelian pattern of the disease. Examples of X-linked forms of nephrolithiasis include Dent disease. Autosomal dominant forms of nephrolithiasis include forms of distal renal tubular acidosis and an example of an autosomal recessive disorder would be primary hyperoxaluria.

Family clustering is common with idiopathic hypercalciuric renal stones, with around half of patients with this diagnosis having a family history of kidney stones. The inheritance pattern is likely to be polygenic, given that hypercalciuria is a phenotype which is

*Table 145-1* **Monogenic Causes of Nephrolithiasis Associated With Hypercalciuria**

| Monogenic Cause | OMIM | Gene Symbol/Name | Associated Features |
|---|---|---|---|
| Hypophosphatemic nephrolithiasis/osteoporosis 1 (NPHLOP1) | 182309 | SLC34A1/sodium phosphate cotransporter | Phosphate wasting, osteoporosis, hypercalciuria, nephrolithiasis |
| Hereditary hypophosphatemic rickets with hypercalciuria (HHRH) | 241530 | SLC34A3/sodium phosphate cotransporter | Phosphate wasting, hypercalciuria, nephrolithiasis |
| Dent disease | 300009 | CLCN5/chloride/proton exchanger | Hypercalciuria, hyperphosphaturia, low molecular weight proteinuria, rickets nephrocalcinosis, nephrolithiasis |
| Lowe oculocerebrorenal syndrome | 309000 | OCRL/phosphatidylinositol 4,5-bisphosphate 5 phosphatase | Hypercalciuria, aminoaciduria, hyperphosphaturia nephrocalcinosis, nephrolithiasis |
| Renal hypomagnesemia 3 | 248250 | CLDN16/claudin 16 | Hypercalciuria, renal magnesium wasting, nephrocalcinosis, nephrolithiasis |
| Renal hypomagnesemia 5 | 248190 | CLDN19 | Hypercalciuria, renal magnesium wasting, nephrocalcinosis, nephrolithiaisis, ocular involvement |
| Bartter syndrome type 1 | 601678 | Sodium-potassium chloride cotransporter | Hypercalciuria, nephrocalcinosis |
| Bartter syndrome type 2 | 241200 | Renal outer medullary potassium channel | Hypercalciuria, nephrocalcinosis |
| Bartter syndrome type 3 | 607364 | Chloride channel | Hypercalciuria |
| Bartter syndrome type 4 | 602522 | Barttin | Congenital deafness |
| Bartter syndrome type 5 | 601199 | Calcium-sensing receptor | Hypercalciuria |
| Autosomal dominant hypocalcemia | 146200 | CASR/calcium-sensing receptor | Hypercalciuria, nephrolithiasis |
| Distal renal tubular acidosis with deafness | 267300 | ATP6V1B1/V-ATPase, beta subunit | Nephrocalcinosis, hypercalciuria, nephrolithiasis |
| Distal renal tubular acidosis | 602722 | ATP6V0A4/V-ATPase, alpha subunit | Nephrocalcinosis, hypercalciuria |
| Distal renal tubular acidosis | 179800 | SLC4A1/anion exchanger | Nephrocalcinosis, nephrolithiasis |
| Distal renal tubular acidosis | 259730 | CAII/carbonic anhydrase II | Nephrocalcinosis, nephrolithiasis, osteopetrosis, brain calcifications |
| Beckwith-Wiedemann syndrome | 130650 | Genes within the 11p15.5 region including KIP2, CDKN1C, H19, and LIT1. | Exomphalos, macroglossia, and gigantism Hypercalciuria, nephrocalcinosis, renal stones |
| MEN1 syndrome with hyperparathyroidism | 131100 | MEN1/menin | Hyperparathyroidism, hypercalciuria, nephrocalcinosis, and nephrolithiasis |
| Hyperparathyroidism type 2 | 145001 | HRPT2/parafibromin | Hyperparathyroidism, jaw tumors, hypercalciuria, nephrolithiasis |
| Metaphyseal chondrodysplasia Jansen type | 156400 | PTHR1/parathyroid hormone receptor 1 | Hypercalciuria, hyperphosphaturia, nephrolithiasis |

a continuous variable and the fact that the molecular genetic identification of monogenic causes of hypercalciuria has not proven to be the sole cause of many idiopathic hypercalciuric stone formers (Tables 145-1 and 145-2).

## Management and Treatment

Aside from the emergency urology or radiology referral for acute renal colic and obstructive nephropathy, the accurate diagnosis of the underlying metabolic defect in a stone former

(Table 145-3) allows the appropriate medical management to be given (Table 145-4), the aim of which is to prevent recurrent stone episodes from occurring.

## Molecular Genetics and Molecular Mechanism

☞IDIOPATHIC HYPERCALCIURIC STONE FORMERS: Hypercalciuria is the commonest metabolic abnormality found in stone formers. Increased urinary calcium concentration may be

*Table 145-2* **Monogenic Causes of Nephrolithiasis (Without Hypercalciuria)**

| Monogenic Cause | OMIM | Gene Symbol/Name | Associated Features |
|---|---|---|---|
| Hyperoxaluria type 1 (HP1) | 259900 | *AGXT*/alanine-glyoxylate aminotransferase | Calcium oxalate stone formation |
| Hyperoxaluria type 2 (HP2) | 260000 | *GRHPR*/glyoxylate reductase/hydroxypyruvate reductase | Calcium oxalate stone formation |
| Hyperoxaluria type 3 (HP3) | 613616 | *HOGA1*/4-hydroxy-2-oxoglutarate aldolase 1 | Calcium oxalate stone formation |
| Cystinuria | 220100 | *SLC3A1*/amino acid transporter *SLC7A9* subunit | Cystine stones, dibasic aminoaciduria |
| 2,8-dihydroxyadenine urolithiasis | 102600 | *APRT*/adenine phosphoribosyl transferase | Urolithiasis |
| Xanthinuria | 278300 | *XDH*/xanthine dehydrogenase | Hypouricemia, xanthine stones |

*Table 145-3* **Algorithm for Diagnosis and Investigation of the Patient With Nephrolithiasis**

| | |
|---|---|
| Review risk factors for renal stones | Family history of renal stones or of end-stage renal failure, previous documented UTI, renal tract abnormalities, low fluid intake, multiple or previous stones, type 2 diabetes mellitus, obesity, dietary factors and use of vitamin supplements, bowel surgery/gastrointestinal disorders including inflammatory bowel conditions, medications which may potentiate stone formation (eg, loop diuretics) |
| Baseline investigations | Serum creatinine, serum bicarbonate, serum calcium, serum urate, serum PTH. Spot urine for calcium/creatinine ratio, spot urine for cystine, spot urine for pH. Urine for culture to exclude infection |
| If single stone, no risk factors and normal baseline investigations | General advice (fluid intake, dietary) and discharge |
| If risk factors/abnormal serum or urine biochemistry or urine pH, investigate further | 24-hour urine collections for calcium, oxalate, citrate, and urate. If spot urine suggestive, 24-hour urine for cystine quantification. Early morning urine for pH. Urine microscopy for crystalluria. |
| Diagnosis of underlying metabolic disorder (allows appropriate preventative measures to be undertaken) | Hypercalciuria, hyperoxaluria, hyperuricosuria, cystinuria, hypocitraturia. If early morning urine pH >5.5 consider renal tubular acidosis. If urine pH persistently acidic consider uric acid stones. Hexagonal crystals seen with urine microscopy indicate cystinuria. Distinctive brownish crystals seen with urine microscopy suggest 2,8-dihydroxyadenine (DHA) stones |

*Table 145-4* **Management and Treatment of the Patient With Nephrolithiasis**

| Risk Factor | Dietary Intervention | Pharmacologic Intervention |
|---|---|---|
| Low urine volume | Drink >2 L per day | |
| Hypercalciuria | Salt restriction, protein moderation, high potassium diet | Thiazide diuretic and/or amiloride Potassium citrate |
| Hypocitraturia | Protein moderation | Potassium citrate |
| Hyperoxaluria | Oxalate restriction, sodium restriction | Pyridoxine (for primary hyperoxaluria) |
| Hyperuricosuria | Purine restriction | Allopurinol |
| Low urine pH | Animal protein restriction | Potassium citrate |
| High early morning urine pH | | Sodium bicarbonate, potassium citrate |
| Urinary tract infection | | Antibiotics according to sensitivities |
| Cystinuria | Drink >3 L per day, sodium restriction | Potassium citrate, D-penicillamine, Beta-mercaptopropionyl glycine (tiopronin), captopril |

explained by various contributing and interacting mechanisms. Firstly, increased gastrointestinal calcium resorption may give rise to increased serum calcium and leading to increased urinary calcium. Secondly, there may be defects in the ability of the renal tubules to regulate calcium reabsorption. Thirdly, an increased bony resorption of calcium into the circulation leading to hypercalciuria may occur. Clearly, both environmental (such as diet) and genetic factors (such as solute transporters) may influence all these mechanisms.

The genetic factors underlying hypercalciuria remain elusive. Epidemiologic data suggest that many patients with idiopathic hypercalciuria have a family history of stones. Efforts to identify loci to determine heritability have been frustrated by the fact that urinary calcium excretion is quantitative. Statistical modeling was undertaken by Loredo-Osti et al. following analysis of stones in 221 French-Canadian families with at least two affected individuals with calcium stones. Computer programs predicted the best inheritance fit with a model of single gene codominant model or a mixed codominant or polygenic model. Both models gave a heritability score of 58%, suggesting a genetic tendency to underlying renal stone formation. Twin studies have also confirmed this strong heritability of hypercalciuria. Two large studies have used monozygotic and dizygotic twins to compare inheritance rates of kidney stones; the St. Thomas UK Adult Twin Registry examined 1747 adult female twin pairs and showed that the heritability of hypercalciuria was 52%, with a higher correlation for calcium excretion in monozygotic twins compared to dizygotic twins. The VET Registry also showed the rate of kidney stones was greater in monozygotic twins (32.4%) than dizygotic twins (17.3%). Based on this, a genetic predisposition is likely to account for the tendency to form stones and genes determine over 50% of the urinary calcium excretion rate.

Hypercalciuria may also occur in a range of monogenic disorders but so far polymorphisms in genes underlying these rarer diseases have not been able to account for the majority of patients with idiopathic hypercalciuria. A few molecular candidates have been identified using linkage and genome-wide association approaches (Table 145-5). Three families with a severe phenotype of absorptive hypercalciuria were used in a genome-wide search for linkage. A highly significant LOD score of 3.3 was shown in a single locus on chromosome 1 and sequence variants in the human soluble adenylate cyclase gene (*sAC*), a divalent cation, and bicarbonate sensor, were identified. The functional significance of these sequence variants has yet to be determined.

Polymorphisms in *CASR* have been described in patients with kidney stones and those with hyperparathyroidism. Indeed, the *CASR* polymorphism (R990G) exists in hypercalciuric (nonstone forming) females, with evidence from in vitro studies that this polymorphism had an "activating" effect on the CASR, thus promoting hypercalciuria. Heterozygous and homozygous carriers of the R990G allele had a significant increase in calcium excretion in comparison with women homozygous for the 990R allele. The R990G allele occurred in 15% of hypercalciuric females studied (compared to only 3% of the normocalciuric control population).

There have been several genetic studies that have pointed to the *VDR* gene as being implicated in hypercalciuric nephrolithiasis. The *VDR* is within a genetic locus for hypercalciuria identified in families from northern India. *VDR* polymorphisms may define bone mineral density and calcium homeostasis, producing a "resorptive" type of hypercalciuria.

Claudin-16 is a tight junction protein and mutations in the gene encoding it, *CLDN16*, give rise to a syndrome of familial hypomagnesemia with hypercalciuria and nephrocalcinosis, leading to renal failure. The defect is in the TAL of the loop of Henle, where paracellular calcium and magnesium resorption occurs. Heterozygous *CLDN16* mutations may give rise to a much milder phenotype and delay renal impairment. The contribution of such functional polymorphisms to idiopathic hypercalciuria has not been investigated.

Polymorphisms in a distal nephron calcium channel, TRPV6, have also been associated with absorptive hypercalciuria in humans. A related epithelial calcium channel, TRPV5 and the regulating serine-threonine kinase WNK4, are also implicated in idiopathic hypercalciuria. Mutations in *WNK4* lead to familial hyperkalemic hypertension (FHH) and affected patients carrying the *Q565E* mutation exhibit marked hypercalciuria.

☞**DEFECTS OF PHOSPHATE RESORPTION OR RENAL PHOSPHATE WASTING:** Various molecules and transporters regulate proximal tubular phosphate transport and mutations leading to a risk of nephrolithiasis have been identified in a number of disorders (Table 145-6).

### Other Monogenic Forms of Renal Stone Disease:

☞**HYPEROXALURIA TYPE I/AGXT/2Q36-Q37 AND HYPEROXALURIA TYPE II:** Hyperoxaluria is detected as the underlying metabolic abnormality in 10% to 20% of stone formers. The distinction between a primary genetic cause or metabolic syndrome of overproduction of oxalate and other idiopathic causes of hyperoxaluria should be made. In the autosomal recessive primary hyperoxaluria conditions (type I and II) an accumulation of oxalate

*Table 145-5 Candidate Genes for Idiopathic Hypercalciuria*

| Candidate Gene | Function | Features/Associated Variant |
|---|---|---|
| sAC | Divalent cation and bicarbonate sensor | Absorptive hypercalciuria |
| CASR | Calcium-sensing receptor in kidney and parathyroid gland | Hyperparathyroidism |
| VDR | Vitamin D receptor | Reduced bone mineral density |
| CLDN16 | Tight junction protein | Heterozygous carriers may be hypercalciuric with renal stones |
| TRPV6 | Epithelial calcium channel | Absorptive hypercalciuria |
| WNK4 | Regulator of sodium chloride cotransporter | Hypertension, hyperkalemia, hypercalciuria |

**Table 145-6** *Genes Underlying Renal Phosphate Transport*

| Disorder Leading to Hyperphosphaturia | Gene Implicated | Locus | Function | Features Associated Variant |
|---|---|---|---|---|
| Hypophosphatemic nephrolithiasis/osteoporosis 1 (NPHLOP1) | SLC34A1 | 17q25.1 | Sodium-dependant phosphate transporter Npt2a | Phosphate wasting, osteoporosis, hypercalciuria, nephrolithiasis |
| Hypophosphatemic nephrolithiasis/osteoporosis 2 | SLC9A3R1 | 17q25.1 | Regulator of sodium-dependant phosphate transporter Npt2a | Phosphate wasting, decreased bone mineral density, nephrolithiasis |
| Hereditary hypophosphatemic rickets with hypercalciuria (HHRH) | SLC34A3 | 9q34 | Sodium-dependant phosphate transporter Npt2c | Phosphate wasting, hypercalciuria, nephrolithiasis |

occurs in the kidney, resulting in renal failure. The biochemical defect in type I hyperoxaluria is a decreased or absent AGXT activity leading to the inability to transaminate glyoxylate. The accumulated glyoxylate is oxidized to oxalate, which precipitates in various tissues as calcium oxalate. Pyridoxine is a coenzyme of AGXT. Type I hyperoxaluria is characterized by an increased level of urinary glycolate. In type II hyperoxaluria is caused by mutations in the glyoxylate reductase or hydroxypyruvate reductase gene (*GRHPR*) affecting another pathway of glyoxylate metabolism. Here there is hyperoxaluria and increased urinary excretion of L-glyceric acid.

☞**CYSTINURIA TYPE I/SLC3A1/2P16.3 AND CYSTINURIA TYPE II/SLC7A9/19Q13.11:** Cystine stones account for 1% to 2% of kidney stones. Stones may occur in young children or not until adulthood, with a median age of onset of around 12 years of age. Defects in a cystine or dibasic amino acid transporter (and its subunit) underlie this disorder giving rise to excessively high urinary cystine levels, which precipitate to form stones. Two genes are known, *SLC3A1* and *SLC7A9*, but it is noteworthy that in around 25% of cystinuria patients, mutations may not be found in these genes, implicating other unknown gene defects. Other genetic defects may also give rise to cystinuria including the hypotonia-cystinuria syndrome (OMIM 606407) and the 2p21 deletion syndrome, which are contiguous gene deletion syndromes that include SLC3A1.

SLC3A1 encodes a heavy chain subunit (rBAT) that forms a heterodimer with the gene product of SLC7A9 to facilitate proximal tubular (and small intestine) transport of cystine and dibasic amino acids. rBAT facilitates transport of the dimmer to the brush border membrane. Mutations in the gene affect heterodimer formation and trafficking.

☞**RENAL HYPOURICEMIA TYPE I/SLC22A12/ 11Q13 AND RENAL HYPOURICEMIA TYPE II/SLC2A9/4P16-P15.3:** Hyperuricosuria is detected in 2% to 8% of patients with nephrolithiasis. Medical causes underlying hyperuricosuria include myeloproliferative disorders, chronic diarrheal states, insulin resistance, and monogenic metabolic disorders, such as Lesch-Nyhan syndrome. Defects in renal excretion (hypouricemia) of uric acid may cause urate stones, with these stones forming preferentially in acidic urine. Molecular identifies of urate transporters now include the human urate transporter 1 (hURAT1, alias SLC22A12) and homozygous loss of function mutations have been found in subjects with idiopathic renal hypouricemia and nephrolithiasis. URAT1 encodes

a proximal tubule urate transporter and mutations lead to a raised fractional excretion of urate which predispose to calculi formation. As well as renal stone disease, mutations may also lead to exercise-induced renal failure. Recently another renal urate transporter SLC2A9 has been identified as a genetic cause of hypouricemia, and represents a novel candidate gene for uric acid stone formation as a result of increased excretion of uric acid. Genome-wide association studies have implicated a number of additional loci involved in urate regulation and transport and these represent candidate genes for uric acid stone formation.

☞**2,8-DIHYDROXYADENINE STONES/APRT/16Q24.3:** This autosomal recessive inherited form of renal stones is secondary to adenine phosphoribosyltransferase (APRT) deficiency. Excess adenine is oxidized to 2,8-DHA by the enzyme xanthine oxidase. The clinical phenotype may vary from no calculi, to "gravel" calculi, and Staghorn calculi. Like uric acid stones, 2,8-DHA stones are radiolucent. The diagnosis may be made using routine urine microscopy where urinary sediment shows spherical brownish crystals that have a birefringent and pseudo-Maltese cross appearance under polarized light. A simple treatment based on allopurinol (a xanthine oxidase inhibitor) administration, high-fluid intake, and a low-purine diet can reverse or halt renal damage and avoid renal failure.

☞**XANTHINURIA TYPE I/XHL/2P23-22:** Xanthinuria is an autosomal recessive disorder characterized by a urinary excess of xanthine, leading to the formation of xanthine stones. Uric acid levels are low in both urine and serum. Type I xanthinuria is secondary to an isolated deficiency of xanthine dehydrogenase whilst in type II there is a deficiency in both xanthine dehydrogenase and aldehyde oxidase, although the molecular basis of this disease is not known.

## Genetic Testing

DNA sequence analysis is clinically available for hyperoxaluria (see UK Genetics Testing Network). The genotyping of patients with hyperoxaluria is clinically relevant as responsiveness to pyridoxine and progression to end-stage renal failure may be predicted.

Genetic testing is available for other monogenic stone-forming disorders including forms of hypophosphatemic nephrolithiasis, cystinuria, renal hypouricemia, 2,8-dihydroxyadenine urolithiasis, and xanthinuria type 1.

**BIBLIOGRAPHY:**

1. Cochat P, Liutkus A, Fargue S, Basmaison O, Ranchin B, Rolland MO. Primary hyperoxaluria type 1: still challenging! *Pediatr Nephrol.* 2006;21:1075-1081.

2. Devuyst O, Pirson Y. Genetics of hypercalciuric stone forming diseases. *Kidney Int.* 2007;72:1065-1072.

3. Gambaro G, Vezzoli G, Casari G, Rampoldi L, D'Angelo A, Borghi L. Genetics of hypercalciuria and calcium nephrolithiasis: from the rare monogenic to the common polygenic forms. *Am J Kidney Dis.* 2004;44:963-986.

4. Goodyer P. The molecular basis of cystinuria. *Nephron Exp Nephrol.* 2004;98:e45-e49.

5. Karim Z, Gerard B, Bakouh N, et al. NHERF1 mutations and responsiveness of renal parathyroid hormone. *N Engl J Med.* 2008;359:1128-1135.

6. Loredo-Osti JC, Roslin NM, Tessier J, Fujiwara TM, Morgan K, Bonnardeaux A. Segregation of urine calcium excretion in families ascertained for nephrolithiasis: evidence for a major gene. *Kidney Int.* 2005;68:966-971.

7. Moe OW. Kidney stones: pathophysiology and medical management. *Lancet.* 2006;367:333-344.

8. Moe OW, Bonny O. Genetic hypercalciuria. *J Am Soc Nephrol.* 2005;16:729-745.

9. Pak CY, Poindexter JR, Adams-Huet B, Pearle MS. Predictive value of kidney stone composition in the detection of metabolic abnormalities. *Am J Med.* 2003;115:26-32.

10. Sayer JA. The genetics of nephrolithiasis. *Nephron Exp Nephrol.* 2008;110:e37-e43.

11. Sayer JA, Carr G, Simmons NL. Nephrocalcinosis: molecular insights into calcium precipitation within the kidney. *Clin Sci (Lond).* 2004;106:549-561.

12. Suzuki Y, Pasch A, Bonny O, Mohaupt MG, Hediger MA, Frey FJ. Gain-of-function haplotype in the epithelial calcium channel TRPV6 is a risk factor for renal calcium stone formation. *Hum Mol Genet.* 2008;17:1613-1618.

13. Vezzoli G, Tanini A, Ferrucci L, et al. Influence of calcium-sensing receptor gene on urinary calcium excretion in stone-forming patients. *J Am Soc Nephrol.* 2002;13:2517-2523.

## Supplementary Information

**Alternative Names:**
- Urolithiasis
- Renal Stones
- Calculi
- Nephrolithiasis

*Key Words:* Hypercalciuria, hyperoxaluria, hypouricemia, hypocitraturia, cystinuria, xanthinuria, dihydroxyadenine

# 146 Alport Syndrome

Varun Chawla and Martin Pollak

## KEY POINTS

- *Disease summary:*
  - Alport syndrome is a hereditary glomerular disease caused by mutations in the genes encoding type IV collagen. It is often associated with hearing loss and ocular abnormalities.
  - The most common form of inheritance is X-linked. Classically the affected males present with asymptomatic hematuria in the first decade of life. With advancing age they develop proteinuria, renal insufficiency, and hypertension. They typically progress to end-stage renal disease (ESRD). Males without hematuria in the first decade of life are unlikely to be affected.
- *Hereditary basis:*
  - The most common mode of transmission of Alport syndrome is X-linked and a small percentage is autosomal recessive.
- *Differential diagnosis:*
  - It is important to distinguish Alport syndrome from other causes of hematuria. These include other glomerulonephritides (IgA nephropathy, MPGN, PSGN), tubulointerstitial diseases (acute pyelonephritis, sickle cell anemia), urinary tract (structural anomalies, hypercalciuria), and vascular anomalies (nut cracker syndrome).
  - The evaluation includes a thorough history including family history, physical examination, evaluation of the urinary sediments (to ascertain if glomerular hematuria), urine and blood studies, renal ultrasound, audiometry, and ophthalmologic examination. Evaluation of urine sediment of family members may aid in the diagnosis. Once the family history, laboratory evaluation, audiometry, and ophthalmologic examination point toward Alport syndrome, skin and renal biopsy can confirm the diagnoses. Genetic testing when available may be the test of choice.

## Diagnostic Criteria and Clinical Characteristics

**Diagnostic Criteria:** The suspicion for Alport syndrome is high if the proband and other family members meet at least three of the following:

1. Positive family history of macro- or microscopic hematuria or chronic renal failure
2. Electron microscopic evidence of AS on renal biopsy
3. Characteristic ophthalmic signs (anterior lenticonus and macular flecks)
4. Sensorineural deafness

These criteria strongly suggest Alport syndrome, for a firm diagnosis genetic testing may be required.

**Clinical Characteristics:** Clinical features of a typical male with X-linked Alport syndrome include persistent hematuria with progression to ESRD, hearing loss, and ocular abnormalities (Table 146-1). Isolated persistent hematuria is the key finding of Alport syndrome. Males without hematuria in the first decade of life are highly unlikely to have Alport syndrome. Proteinuria, hypertension, and renal insufficiency develop with advancing age with finally progression to ESRD. Sensorineural hearing loss starts in childhood with initially hearing loss to higher frequencies. This progresses to other frequencies including conversational range. Ocular abnormalities include anterior lenticonus (conical protrusion on the anterior aspect of the lens due to thinning of the lens capsule), corneal changes (posterior polymorphous dystrophy and recurrent corneal erosion), and retinal changes (bilateral white or yellow granulations in the retina surrounding the foveal area). A small percentage of patients and carriers have leiomyomas within the respiratory, gastrointestinal, and female reproductive tracts.

## Screening and Counseling

**Screening:** Given the low prevalence of Alport syndrome in the population, there is no data to suggest screening members of the general population for Alport syndrome. Relatives of the index case should be offered screening for Alport syndrome. Determining the at-risk individuals would depend on the mode of inheritance. In case of a male proband with X-linked Alport syndrome (XLAS), at-risk relatives are the mother, siblings, and the daughters (obligate carriers). In autosomal recessive Alport syndrome (ARAS) screening should be offered to parents, siblings, and children (who may be obligate carriers. Screening tests include urinalysis for hematuria and proteinuria, serum creatinine, and blood pressure monitoring).

**Counseling:** The most common mode of transmission of Alport syndrome is X-linked (XLAS). A small percentage is autosomal recessive. In XLAS, fathers can never transmit the disease-causing mutation to their sons; they will necessarily transmit the disease-causing variant to their daughters. The chance of mother transmitting the disease-causing mutation is 50%. If the male inherits the gene defect, he will be affected. If a daughter inherits the gene defect, the phenotypic expression can vary considerably.

The reason for variable phenotype in females is X-inactivation (lyonization), a process by which one of the two copies of the X chromosomes in female mammals is inactivated. As a result, approximately one-half of their cells will express the mutant gene and the remaining cells express the normal gene leading to a variable phenotype. Prenatal testing is available for XLAS.

☞GENOTYPE-PHENOTYPE CORRELATION: XLAS is clinically and genetically heterogeneous. There is a high number of mutations in the *COL4A5* gene with associated phenotypic variability. In a study with 681 male participants from 175 families, the age of onset of ESRD varied for different genetic mutations. The median time was longest for missense mutations (37 years) as

*Table 146-1  System Involvement*

| System | Manifestation | Incidence 1-3 |
|---|---|---|
| Renal | Hematuria | XLAS males 100%<br>XLAS heterozygous females ~90%<br>Males and females with ARAS 100% |
| | Proteinuria, hypertension, and renal insufficiency | XLAS males—all ARAS males and females—all with advancing age |
| | Progression to ESRD | XLAS Males—60% by 30 years, 90% by 40 years<br>XLAS heterozygous females—12% by 40 years, 40% by 80 years<br>ARAS males and females all by 20 to 30 years |
| Auditory system | Sensorineural hearing loss | XLAS males 80% by 15 years<br>XLAS heterozygous females 20% by 15 years |
| Vision | Anterior lenticonus—conical protrusion on the anterior aspect of the lens due to thinning of the lens capsule is pathognomonic of Alport syndrome. Retinal changes include white or yellow granulations around the fovea. In the cornea, changes that can be seen include posterior polymorphous dystrophy and recurrent corneal erosions. | XLAS males 30% to 40% |

XLAS, X-linked Alport syndrome; ARAS, autosomal recessive Alport syndrome; ESRD, end-stage renal disease.

compared with splice-site mutations (28 years), truncating mutations (25) years, large deletions (22 years), and small deletion mutations (22 years). Ocular changes also varied with the mutation type, with more changes in those with large deletion, splice-site, and truncating mutations compared with missense and small deletion mutations. Similarly, missense mutations were associated with a lower incidence of hearing impairment.

## Management and Treatment

There is no specific treatment for Alport syndrome. Once patients reach ESRD either dialysis or transplantation can be performed. Recurrence of the disease does not occur in the transplant (since the donor glomerular basement membrane [GBM] is normal). A low percentage of transplanted males do develop de novo anti-GBM antibody disease. Patients with reduced kidney function should receive the same management for the complications of chronic kidney disease of other etiologies. If significant proteinuria is present, treatment with angiotensin-converting enzyme inhibitors or angiotensin receptor blockers should be considered.

## Molecular Genetics and Molecular Mechanism

***Syndrome/Gene/Locus/Protein:*** XLAS/*COL4A5*/Xq22.3/collagen alpha-5(IV) chain

Type IV collagen is comprised of three alpha chains coiled around each other to form a triple helix. There are six different alpha chains that have been identified, encoded by separate genes: *COL4A1* and *COL4A2* (at 13q34), *COL4A3* and *COL4A4* (at 2q35-37), and *COL4A5* and *COL4A6* (at chromosome X). In the basement membrane of immature nephrons, the collagen trimer is alpha 1, alpha 1, alpha 2; this is replaced with alpha 3, alpha 4, alpha 5 as the nephron matures. The organ of Corti basement membrane and lens capsule also have alpha 3, alpha 4, alpha 5 type IV collagen. In XLAS, there is a mutation of *COL4A5* which leads to absent or defective alpha 5 chain. This impairs the congregation of the alpha 3, alpha 4, alpha 5 triple helix thus leading to an abnormal basement membrane.

***Genetic Testing:*** Molecular genetic testing is slowly becoming the diagnostic test of choice (see Table 146-2). As the rate of progression of the disease is dependent on the type of mutation, it may help

*Table 146-2  Molecular Genetic Testing*

| Gene | Testing Modality | Mutation Type | Detection Rate |
|---|---|---|---|
| COL4A5 | Targeted mutation analysis | c.4692G>A, c.4946T>G, c.5030G>A (most common mutations in US) | 100% for the three mutations |
| | Sequence analysis | Sequence variants | 80% |
| | Deletion/duplication analysis | multiexonic deletions or duplications | 10% |
| COL4A3/A4 | Sequence analysis | Sequence variants | 100% |
| | Deletion/duplication analysis | Multiexonic deletions or duplications | Unknown |

provide more prognostic information than a renal or skin biopsy. The availability of testing can be obtained at http://www.ncbi.nlm.nih.gov/sites/GeneTests/lab/clinical_disease_id/2306?db=genetests

## BIBLIOGRAPHY:

1. Kashtan CE. Collagen IV-Related Nephropathies (Alport Syndrome and Thin Basement Membrane Nephropathy). 1993.

2. Jais JP, Knebelmann B, Giatras I, et al. X-linked Alport syndrome: natural history and genotype-phenotype correlations in girls and women belonging to 195 families: a "European Community Alport Syndrome Concerted Action" study. *J Am Soc Nephrol.* 2003;14(10):2603-2610.

3. Jais JP, Knebelmann B, Giatras I, et al. X-linked Alport syndrome: natural history in 195 families and genotype-phenotype correlations in males. *J Am Soc Nephrol.* 2000;11(4):649-657.

4. Hanson H, Storey H, Pagan J, Flinter F. The value of clinical criteria in identifying patients with X-linked Alport syndrome. *Clin J Am Soc Nephrol.* 2011;6(1):198-203.

5. Bekheirnia MR, Reed B, Gregory MC, et al. Genotype-phenotype correlation in X-linked Alport syndrome. *J Am Soc Nephrol.* 2010;21(5):876-883.

6. Kashtan CE, Butkowski RJ, Kleppel MM, First MR, Michael AF. Posttransplant anti-glomerular basement membrane nephritis in related males with Alport syndrome. *J Lab Clin Med.* 1990;116(4):508-515.

7. Gubler MC. Inherited diseases of the glomerular basement membrane. *Nat Clin Pract Nephrol.* 2008;4(1):24-37.

8. Tryggvason K, Zhou J, Hostikka SL, Shows TB. Molecular genetics of Alport syndrome. *Kidney Int.* 1993;43(1):38-44.

9. Inoue Y, Nishio H, Shirakawa T, et al. Detection of mutations in the COL4A5 gene in over 90% of male patients with X-linked Alport's syndrome by RT-PCR and direct sequencing. *Am J Kidney Dis.* 1999;34(5):854-862.

10. Boye E, Mollet G, Forestier L, et al. Determination of the genomic structure of the COL4A4 gene and of novel mutations causing autosomal recessive Alport syndrome. *Am J Hum Genet.* 1998;63(5):1329-1340.

11. Proesmans W, Knockaert H, Trouet D. Enalapril in paediatric patients with Alport syndrome: 2 years' experience. *Eur J Pediatr.* 2000;159(6):430-433.

## Supplementary Information

### OMIM REFERENCES:

[1] X-linked Alport Syndrome (#301050)

[2] Autosomal Recessive Alport Syndrome (#203780)

[3] Alport Syndrome With Diffuse Leiomyomatosis (#308940)

***Key Words:*** Hereditary nephritis, a hereditary glomerular disease, hematuria, collagen type IV, sensorineural hearing loss, renal failure, anterior lenticonus, collagen trimer

# 147 Age-related Cataract

Alan Shiels and J. Fielding Hejtmancik

## KEY POINTS

- *Disease summary:*
  - Age-related cataract is a complex disorder of the ocular lens involving environmental and genetic risk factors. In addition to decreased visual acuity, early symptoms include myopic shift, astigmatism, monocular diplopia, glare, color shift, and reductions in contrast-sensitivity, light transmission, and visual field. Despite surgical treatment, age-related cataract remains a universally important cause of progressive low vision and blindness.
  - Clinical presentations are morphologically described as nuclear cataract, cortical cataract, posterior subcapsular cataract (PSC), or mixed cataract.
  - Age-at-onset is usually within the sixth to eighth decades; however, in some populations, onset may occur as early as the third to fourth decades (eg, India).

- *Differential diagnosis:*
  - Presenile cataract may present in the second to fifth decades and can be associated with genetic or metabolic disorders, including myotonic dystrophy-associated cataract, hereditary hyperferritinemia cataract syndrome (HHCS), adult i blood group phenotype, female carriers of X-linked forms of cataract (eg, Nance Horan "cataract-dental" syndrome [NHS]; Lowe oculocerebrorenal syndrome [OCRL]), oil droplet cataract and diabetic cataract. Other adult-onset forms of cataract may result from local ocular disease (eg, uveitis, retinal dystrophy or degeneration, glaucoma, ocular tumors), certain drugs (eg, chronic corticosteroid regimens), radiation exposure, electrocution, metal ion deposits (eg, siderotic cataract), and trauma.

- *Monogenic forms:*
  - Many Mendelian forms of cataract are known. Most present with an early onset, ranging from birth or infancy (congenital or infantile) through the second decade (juvenile) either in association with other ocular and/or systemic abnormalities, or as an isolated lens phenotype often with autosomal dominant inheritance. Mutations in genes encoding crystallins and gap-junction (or connexin) proteins account for approximately 70% of autosomal dominant cataract.

- *Family history:*
  - A positive family history has been indicated as a risk factor for cortical cataract, nuclear cataract, and mixed nuclear and cortical cataract but has not been replicated for PSC.

- *Twin studies:*
  - Heritability estimates for cortical cataract lie in the range of 53% to 58% mostly due to dominant genetic effects, and those for nuclear cataract are approximately 48% due to additive effects.

- *Environmental factors:*
  - Cortical cataract and PSC are associated with UV-B exposure, diabetes, alcohol consumption, and topical or oral steroid use. Nuclear cataract is strongly linked with tobacco smoking. Other risk factors include female gender, myopia, metabolic syndrome, severe dehydration or diarrhea and malnutrition.

- *Genome-wide associations:*
  - The strongest genetic association is obtained at the *EPHA2* locus on chromosome 1p36 with cortical cataract in Caucasian and Chinese populations and with cortical cataract and PSC in Southern India (Table 147-1). An unidentified locus on chromosome 6p12-q12 has been associated with cortical cataract in Caucasians. Genetic testing for single-nucleotide polymorphisms (SNPs) is not clinically validated for diagnosis.

- *Pharmacogenomics:*
  - No clinically valid testing is available. Protective effects of statins and nutritional supplements including daily multivitamins, antioxidants, and n-3 fatty acids, remain controversial.

Table 147-1 **Summary of Gene Variants Associated With Age-Related Cataract***

| Cytogenetic Locus | Physical Locus (Mbp) | Gene | Exon/Intron | DNA Change | Coding Change | Origin | Cataract Phenotype |
|---|---|---|---|---|---|---|---|
| 1p36 | 16,450,832 - 16,482,582, complement | EPHA2 | 5'-region | rs477558 (G/A >1Mb) | | China | Age-related cortical |
| 1p36 | | EPHA2 | Ex3 | rs6678616 (c.573G>A) | p.L191L | Australia, UK, USA | Age-related cortical |
| 1p36 | | EPHA2 | IVS3 | rs6603867 | | Australia, UK, USA | Age-related cortical |
| 1p36 | | EPHA2 | IVS3 | rs3768293 | | Australia, UK, USA | Age-related cortical |
| 1p36 | | EPHA2 | Ex13 | rs116506614 (c.2162G>A) | p.R721Q | USA | Age-related cortical |
| 1p36 | | EPHA2 | Ex17 | rs3754334 (c.2874C>T) | p.I958I | Australia, UK, USA | Age-related cortical |
| 1p36 | | EPHA2 | 3'-region | rs7543472 (T/C), rs11260867 (C/G) | | Italy | Age-related cortical, cortical and/or nuclear |
| 1p36 | | EPHA2 | 3'-region | rs7543472 (T/C), rs11260867 (C/G) | | India | Age-related cortical and posterior sub-capsular |
| 1p36 | | EPHA2 | 3'-region | rs7548209 (G/C) | | Australia, UK, USA | Age-related cortical |
| 1p36 | | EPHA2 | 3'-region | rs7548209 (G/C) | | China | Age-related cortical |
| 1q21.1 | 147,374,946 - 147,381,395 | GJA8 | IVS1 | rs9437983 (A/G), rs1495960 (G/T) | | China | Age-related nuclear |
| 1q21.1 | | GJA8 | Ex2 | c.823G>A | p.V275I | China | Age-related cortical |
| 9p13 | 34,646,635 - 34,650,573 | GALT | Ex9 | rs111033773 (c.855G>T) | p.K285N | Slovenia | Idiopathic, presenile |
| 10q23.31 | 91,190,051 - 91,295,313, complement | SLC16A12 | Ex3 | rs3740030 (c.49T>G) | p.W17G | Swiss | Age related |
| 10q23.31 | | SLC16A12 | Ex3 | c.77A>G | p.E26G | Swiss | Age related |
| 12q13 | 56,843,286 - 56,848,435, complement | MIP | 5'-region | rs2269348 (c.-84T>C) | | China | Age related |
| 12q13 | | MIP | 5'-UTR | rs117788190 (c.-4T>C) | | China | Age related |
| 12q13 | | MIP | Ex1 | rs74641138 (c.319G>A) | p.V107I | China | Age related |
| 13q11-q12 | 20,712,395 - 20,735,183, complement | GJA3 | IVS1 | c.-39C>G (IVS1-22C>G) | | China | Age-related nuclear |

| Location | Gene | Exon | Nucleotide change | Protein change | Country | Phenotype |
| --- | --- | --- | --- | --- | --- | --- |
| 13q11-q12 | GJA3 | Ex2 | c.415G>A | p.V139M | China | Age-related cortical |
| 16q21 67,197,288 - 67,203,848 | HSF4 | Ex4 | c.182A>G | p.Q61R | China | Age-related cortical |
| 17q24 73,754,018 - 73,761,280, complement | GALK1 | Ex4 | rs80084721 (c.593C>T) | p.A198V | Japan | Age-related (Asian) |
| 19q13.33 49,468,566 - 49,470,136 | FTL | 5'-IRE | c.-415C>A | | Italy | Bilateral (50 years of age) |
| 19q13.4 51,883,163 - 51,891,210, complement | LIM2 | Ex2 | rs142517355 (c.57G>A) | p.L19L | China | Age-related cortical |
| 19q13.4 | LIM2 | Ex2 | c.67A>C | p.M23L | China | Age-related cortical |
| 21q22.3 44,589,141 - 44,592,913 | CRYAA | Ex1 | rs872331C/T (c.6G>A) | p.D2D | India | Age-related nuclear, cortical, mixed |
| 21q22.3 | CRYAA | Ex2 | c.213C>A | p.F71L | India | Age-related nuclear, mixed |

*Genomic coordinates are based on human reference sequence GRCh37 (Feb 2009, hg19)

## Diagnostic Criteria and Clinical Characteristics

***Diagnostic Criteria for Age-Related Cataract:*** Diagnostic evaluation should include digital slit-lamp examination of the lens and visual acuity testing (eg, Snellen or Early Treatment Diabetic Retinopathy Study [EDTRS] charts).

***Clinical Characteristics:*** Clinical classification of age-related cataract is largely based on the location, size, shape, density, and color of opacities when visualized in the lens with a slit lamp. Defined by lens location, three pure subtypes may be distinguished (see Fig. 147-1).

- Nuclear cataract affects the central core of the lens. In addition to aging-induced light scattering (nuclear white scatter) it is often associated with pigment accumulation (nuclear brunescence) ranging in color from amber through brown to black ("cataracta nigra"). Prevalent in white populations and indigenous populations from Africa, India, and Southern China.
- Cortical cataract usually appears as wedge-shaped or spoke-like opacities, affecting the outer cortex of the lens particularly in the lower nasal quadrant that is most impacted by solar radiation. Prevalent in Icelandic, African-American, and most East Asian populations.
- PSC, which usually appears as a granular deposit or plaque-like opacity, is confined to the back of the lens, lying just beneath the capsule or basement membrane that envelopes the lens mass.

Although PSC is prevalent in India, it represents the least prevalent type in other populations studied. PSC is frequently observed in neurofibromatosis type 2 (NF2) and chronic corticosteroid regimens.

Pure subtypes of age-related cataract can be further graded for severity according to their size, density, or color by evaluation of lens photographs taken with a slit-lamp digital camera. In practice, however, age-related opacities often occur in combination (ie, mixed nuclear and cortical with or without posterior subcapsular) and may eventually progress to total opacification of the lens. Left untreated, hypermature or Morgagnian cataract can result from liquefaction and resorption of the lens.

## Screening and Counseling

***Screening:*** Comprehensive dilated eye examination and slit-lamp grading of lens opacities. Young or adult females presenting with either faint Y-sutural opacities or cortical dot-like and subcapsular plaque-like opacities may indicate obligate carrier status of X-linked NHS or OCRL, respectively. Genetic testing for myotonic dystrophy type-1 (DM1) or type-2 (DM2) may detect asymptomatic or very mild cases of myotonia presenting with cortical iridescent opacities and/or posterior cortical opacities. No genetic testing for cataract-associated variants is clinically validated. Laboratory tests

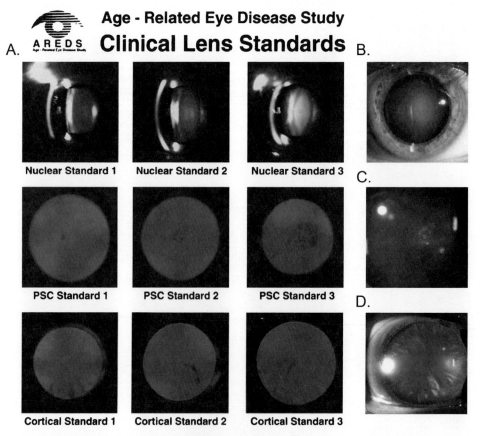

**Age - Related Eye Disease Study**
A. A.R.E.D.S. **Clinical Lens Standards** B.

Nuclear Standard 1  Nuclear Standard 2  Nuclear Standard 3  C.

PSC Standard 1  PSC Standard 2  PSC Standard 3  D.

Cortical Standard 1  Cortical Standard 2  Cortical Standard 3

***Figure 147-1*** Three Main Types of Age-Related Cataract. (*A*) The Age-Related Eye Disease Study (AREDS) System for Classifying Cataract From Photographs. (*B*) Nuclear Cataract. (*C*) Posterior Subcapsular Cataract. (*D*) Cortical Cataract.
Used with permission from Dr. M. Datiles III and the National Eye Institute AREDS.

for serum ferritin (FTL) levels, I/i blood group (GCNT2), red cell galactokinase-1 (GALK1) activity, and acetylated hemoglobin (HbA$_{1c}$) levels may detect undiagnosed cases of cataract associated with HHCS, adult i blood group phenotype, GALK1 deficiency, and uncontrolled diabetes mellitus, respectively.

***Counseling:*** Sibling and twin studies have provided statistical evidence for familial aggregation of cortical and/or nuclear, but probably not posterior subcapsular, forms of age-related cataract. Heritability estimates range from 14% to 36% for nuclear cataract, 24% to 58% for cortical cataract, and 4% for PSC, after adjustment for likely shared environmental factors. Suspected cases of "syndromic" cataract should undergo appropriate genetic counseling for the relevant genetic disorder. Patients should be advised about the benefits of reduced ocular exposure to UV-B radiation and cessation of cigarette smoking. However, the protective benefits of nutritional supplements remain inconclusive. Patients with diabetes mellitus or long-term users of oral or inhaled corticosteroids should be informed of their increased risk of cataract formation. Cataract surgery is the only accepted treatment to enhance vision for reading, driving, and to prevent falls. Patients with coexisting ocular disease (eg, age-related macular degeneration) should be informed about the increased risk of a poor visual outcome following cataract surgery.

## Management and Treatment

***Surgery:*** The primary indication for cataract surgery is impaired visual function for which surgical removal provides a reasonable likelihood of improved vision. Extracapsular cataract extraction (ECCE) with ultrasonic phacoemulsification or femtosecond laser fragmentation, followed by posterior-chamber intraocular lens (IOL) implantation is standard of care. Intracapsular cataract extraction (ICCE) and anterior-chamber IOLs may be indicated for difficult or complicated cases (eg, partly dislocated lenses, ruptured or degraded posterior capsule). Presurgical counseling should include discussion of the surgical process (eg, type of anesthesia, intraoperative visual sensations), IOL options (eg, multifocal, accommodating, aspheric, toric), and postoperative recovery (eg, follow-up visits, eye-drop use), sight-threatening complications, and expected visual outcomes. The most common late postsurgical complication is posterior capsule opacification (PCO, or secondary cataract) that occurs in about 25% of eyes and requires Nd-YAG laser capsulotomy. Other complications (<2% of eyes) include endophthalmitis, uveitis, increased risk of aphakic glaucoma and retinal detachment, and residual refractive error.

## Molecular Genetics and Molecular Mechanism

Heritability estimates for age-related cataract range from 35% to 48% for nuclear cataract, and 24% to 58% for cortical cataract. By contrast with Mendelian forms of congenital or early onset cataract, relatively few genes have been unambiguously associated with risk of age-related cataract. However, sequence variants in several genes underlying inherited cataract are emerging as candidates for age-related cataract (Table 147-1).

The "Osaka" variant (rs80084721) of the gene for galacto-kinase-1 (*GALK1*), which catalyzes the first step in galactose metabolism to glucose, has been detected at increased frequency (~7%) in a Japanese cohort with age-related cataract. This heterozygous protein-coding variant involves an amino acid substitution (p.Ala198Val) that results in reduced stability of the variant enzyme and mild galactokinase deficiency equivalent to about 20% of normal levels. The Osaka variant was also present in Koreans (frequency 2.8%) but had a lower incidence in Chinese, and was not detected in blacks and whites from the United States or in a North Italian cohort with age-related cataract. These observations suggest that the genetic contribution to age-related cataract might vary in different populations. Interestingly, severe homozygous mutations in the *GALK1* gene are usually associated with classic autosomal recessive galactokinase-1 deficiency and isolated congenital cataracts as a result of galactitol accumulation in the lens. These findings show that different variations in the *GALK1* gene can contribute to both congenital and age-related forms of cataract; a principle that is also borne out by an increased incidence of presenile cataract in individuals (age range 20-55 years) heterozygous for *GALK1* deficiency.

Association of cortical cataract with variations in the gene for Eph-receptor type-A2 (*EPHA2*), have been replicated in Caucasian, Chinese, and Indian populations. Mutations in *EPHA2* have been linked with autosomal dominant and recessive forms of familial cataract, and mice lacking Epha2 have been reported to develop cataract with a penetrance of approximately 80%. However, the precise role of *EPHA2* in lens biology remains unclear.

In addition, variants in certain other genes linked with inherited congenital or early onset cataract have been reported to be associated with age-related cataract. These include the genes for alpha-crystallin (*CRYAA*), lens intrinsic membrane proteins (*MIP, LIM2*), gap-junction or connexin proteins (*GJA3, GJA8*), a heat shock transcription factor (*HSF4*), and a solute carrier protein (*SLC16A12*). Further, variants of several other genes involved in diverse biologic functions have been tentatively implicated in age-related cataract including those mediating antioxidant metabolism (*GSTM1, GSTT1*), DNA repair (*ERCC2*), folate metabolism (*MTHFR*), kinesin motor transport (*KLC1*), estrogen metabolism, and systemic inflammation. Further replication and validation studies of these genes, coupled with functional expression studies of the variant proteins, will be required to substantiate their role in age-related cataractogenesis. However, it is likely that all of the currently implicated genes will account for a relatively small percentage of the genetic risk for age-related cataract.

***Future Directions:*** Family-based linkage studies and case-control association studies in different populations will continue to identify, test, and validate candidate genes for inherited and age-related forms of cataract. In addition, the advent of next-generation sequencing techniques capable of deciphering genetic variation in large numbers of individuals will provide powerful insights regarding the molecular genetic basis of age-related cataract including gene-gene and gene-environment interactions. Ultimately, a genomic understanding of cataract, combined with improved phenotyping of animal models, may translate into nonsurgical means to treat, delay, or even prevent cataract onset.

**BIBLIOGRAPHY:**

1. Asbell PA, Dualan I, Mindel J, et al. Age-related cataract. *Lancet.* 2005;365:599-609.

2.  Shiels A, Bennett TM, Hejtmancik JF. *Cat-Map*: putting cataract on the map. *Mol Vis*. 2010;16:2007-2015.

3.  Congdon N, Browman KW, Lai H, et al. Nuclear cataract shows significant familial aggregation in an older population after adjustment for possible shared environmental factors. *Ophthalmology*. 2005;112:73-77.

4.  Sanfilippo PG, Hewitt AW, Hammond CJ, et al. The heritability of ocular traits. *Surv Ophthalmol*. 2010;55:561-583.

5.  Iyengar SK, Klein BE, Klein R, et al. Identification of a major locus for age-related cortical cataract on chromosome 6p12-q12 in the Beaver Dam Eye Study. *Proc Natl Acad Sci USA*. 2004;101:14485-14490.

6.  Sperduto RD, Clemons TE, Lindblad AS, et al. Cataract classification using serial examinations in the age-related eye disease study: age-related eye disease study report no. 24. *Am J Ophthalmol*. 2008;145:504-508.

7.  Wussuki-Lior O, Abu-Horwitz A, Netzer I, et al. Hematologic biomarkers in childhood cataracts. *Mol Vis*. 2011;17:1011-1015.

8.  Okano Y, Asada M, Fujimoto A, et al. A genetic factor for age-related cataract: identification and characterization of a novel galactokinase variant, "Osaka," in Asians. *Am J Hum Genet*. 2001;68:1036-1042.

9.  Shiels A, Bennett TM, Knopf HL, et al. The EPHA2 gene is associated with cataracts linked to chromosome 1p. *Mol Vis*. 2008;14:2042-2055.

10. Jun G, Guo H, Klein BE, et al. EPHA2 is associated with age-related cortical cataract in mice and humans. *PLoS Genet*. 2009;5:e1000584.

11. Tan W, Hou S, Jiang Z, et al. Association of *EPHA2* polymorphisms and age-related cataract in a Han Chinese population. *Mol Vis*. 2011;17:1553-1558.

12. Sundaresan P, Ravindran RD, Vashist P, et al. EPHA2 polymorphismsandage-related cataract in India. *PloSOne*. 2012;7:e33001.

## Supplementary Information

**OMIM REFERENCES:**

[1] Cataract, Age-Related Cortical, 1; ARCC1 (%609026)

[2] Cataract, Age-Related Cortical, 2; ARCC2 (#116600)

[3] Cataract, Age-Related Nuclear (#601371)

**Alternative Names:**
- Senile Cataract(s)
- Nuclear Sclerosis

*Key Words:* Candidate genes, cataract, cortical, ephrin receptor, galactokinase-1, lens, nuclear, posterior subcapsular, presenile

*Websites:*
1.  World Health organization (WHO): http://www.who.int/en/
2.  National Eye Institute (NEI) of the United States: http://www.nei.nih.gov/
3.  Prevent Blindness America: http://www.preventblindness.org/

# 148 Primary Open Angle Glaucoma

Janey L. Wiggs

## KEY POINTS

- *Disease summary:*
  - Primary open angle glaucoma (POAG) is a genetically and clinically complex disease with multiple genetic risk factors and environmental exposure influencing disease susceptibility.
  - POAG is defined by progressive degeneration of the optic nerve. Elevation of intraocular pressure (IOP) is a risk factor for optic nerve degeneration, however, approximately 30% of POAG patients have optic nerve degeneration despite IOPs in the normal range (called normal-pressure glaucoma or NPG, also normal-tension glaucoma or NTG).
  - Ocular traits other than IOP also contribute to POAG risk including the thickness of the central cornea, the size of the optic nerve (optic nerve area), and the size of the optic nerve "cup" relative to the overall size of the nerve (optic nerve cup-to-disc-ratio, CDR).
- *Differential diagnosis:*
  - Exfoliation glaucoma, pigment dispersion glaucoma, developmental glaucoma, angle-closure glaucoma
- *Monogenic forms:*
  - Autosomal dominant juvenile-onset primary open-angle glaucoma caused by mutations in the *MYOC* gene.
- *Family history:*
  - Siblings and first-degree relatives have a 7 to 10 times increased risk of developing POAG overall.
- *Twin studies:*
  - Monozygotic twins have an increased risk of disease when compared to dizygotic twins.
- *Environmental factors:*
  - Postmenopausal hormone use and body mass index (BMI) have been suggested as environmental risk factors for POAG.
- *Genome-wide associations:*
  - Genome-wide association studies (GWAS) have identified five genes or loci for POAG: *CDKN2BAS* (POAG and NPG), *CAV1/CAV2* (POAG), *TMCO1* (POAG), *SIX1/SIX6* (POAG), and 8q22 (NPG). GWAS for ocular quantitative traits relevant to POAG have also yielded results: *CDKN2BAS* (CDR), *SIX1/SIX6* (CDR), *ATOH7* (optic nerve area), and a number of genes or loci for central corneal thickness (CCT), a trait that is a risk factor for the disease. Disease-associated genetic variants (single-nucleotide polymorphisms [SNPs]) have provided insight into disease pathogenesis; testing for SNPs is not yet clinically validated to diagnose or guide management of POAG.
- *Pharmacogenomics:*
  - Testing for common variants has not yet been shown to influence management of POAG.

## Diagnostic Criteria and Clinical Characteristics

### Diagnostic Criteria for POAG:

**Diagnostic evaluation should include the following (Fig. 148-1 algorithm):**

- Clinical examination of the ocular anterior segment (cornea, trabecular meshwork, iris, lens) using the slit lamp
- Evaluation of the optic nerve by fundoscopy and other imaging modalities (optic nerve photography, laser scanning imaging [HRT], ocular computed tomography [OCT])
- Visual field evaluation
- Measurement of IOP
- Measurement of CCT

**And the absence of**

- Narrow angles (angle-closure glaucoma)
- Exfoliation material (pseudoexfoliation syndrome)
- Increased pigment in the trabecular meshwork (pigment dispersion syndrome)
- Absence of transillumination defects in the iris (pigment dispersion syndrome)
- Developmental abnormalities of the anterior segment (developmental glaucoma)

A patient potentially at risk for glaucoma is identified through general eye care screening because of elevated IOP (>21 mm Hg), asymmetry of the optic nerve CDR, or a family history of disease. The patient undergoes further clinical examination of the ocular anterior segment (slit-lamp examination). For some types of glaucoma, specific anatomic abnormalities will establish a diagnosis other than POAG. If the ocular anterior segment is anatomically normal then the patient undergoes optic nerve imaging and visual field testing. If detects are not detected the patient is considered a glaucoma suspect and is re-evaluated on an annual basis. If visual field and/or optic nerve defects are identified the patient is given a diagnosis of POAG. After IOP and CCT testing, if the patient has high IOP and disease onset was at 20 years old or younger they are given the diagnosis of juvenile open-angle glaucoma (JOAG) and are referred for *MYOC* gene testing. If the patient has high IOP and is between 20 and 50 years of age at disease onset and also has a family history of disease, referral for *MYOC* gene testing is indicated. All patients with *MYOC* mutations and/or a family history of glaucoma are referred for genetic counseling. Patients older than 50 years of age at time of disease onset are less likely to have

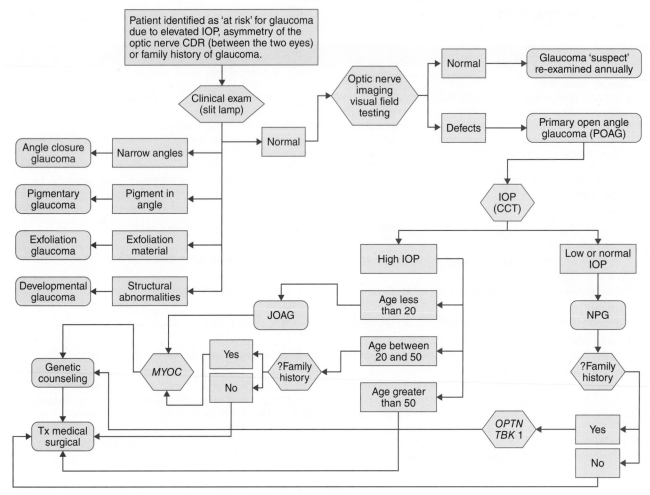

**Figure 148-1** Algorithm for Diagnostic Evaluation of Patient at Risk for Glaucoma.

*MYOC* mutations. All patients with POAG are treated with medications and possibly surgery to lower the IOP. For POAG patients with low IOP (≤21 mm Hg), they are given the diagnosis of NPG and if there is a family history of NPG they are referred for *OPTN* and *TBK1* gene testing. All patients with gene mutations and/or a family history are referred for genetic counseling. All patients with NPG are treated with medications and possibly surgery to lower IOP.

### Clinical Characteristics:

**Adult-Onset POAG:** Glaucoma causes progressive painless degeneration of the optic nerve. If left untreated, the optic nerve damage results in irreversible and complete blindness. The disease onset is typically in the sixth and seventh decades, although individuals may be affected by age 40 and patients carrying mutations in *MYOC* develop an early-onset form of the disease during the first and second decades of life. Loss of vision typically begins in the peripheral visual fields where it may not be noticed by the patient. Gradually the peripheral visual field defects progress to involve the high acuity central visual fields. In POAG, elevation of IOP precedes the damage to the optic nerve and IOP screening can identify individuals at early disease stages when treatment is most effective. IOP measurement should be accompanied by measurement of the CCT because the corneal thickness can influence the IOP measurement, and studies suggest that low CCT (<530 nm)

is an independent risk factor for POAG. High IOP is typically greater than 21 mm Hg while "normal" IOP is less than or equal to 21 mm Hg. In the NPG form of POAG, without elevated IOP, patients may initially present for treatment at advanced stages of the disease with severe optic nerve damage.

**Early-Onset (Juvenile) POAG:** Patients that develop POAG as children (juvenile-onset POAG also known as JOAG with onset between the ages of 3 and 20) typically have very high IOP (>25 mm Hg) and rapidly progressive optic nerve disease. Children who are carriers of *MYOC* mutations frequently require surgery to control the IOP.

## Screening and Counseling

**Screening:** Screening for IOP elevation can be effective for patients at risk for the high-pressure form of POAG. Screening for mutations in *MYOC* can be useful for patients with onset of disease before the age of 20, or with a history of affected family members with onset of disease before age 50. The only effective screening test for NPG is yearly visual field testing and imaging of the optic nerve.

**Counseling:** First-degree relatives of patients carrying a *MYOC* mutation have a 50% chance of developing the early-onset form of POAG. This form of the disease is highly penetrant except for individuals with several specific mutations known to be associated with milder disease including *GLN368X*, the most common *MYOC* mutation. For patients developing POAG after age 50, there is also significant heritability with an overall risk for a primary family member increasing to 7 to 10 times that of the general population. For NPG rare monogenic forms exist due to one mutation in *OPTN* (E50K) and a duplication of *TBK1*. First-degree relatives of affected individuals carrying these mutations have up to a 50% chance of developing the disease; however, the penetrance of these mutations is not well understood.

☞GENOTYPE-PHENOTYPE CORRELATION: Most mutations in *MYOC* cause severe early-onset glaucoma (before age 20), however several, especially THR377MET and GLN368X are associated with later disease onset (between 20 and 50). Genotype-phenotype correlations for other glaucoma-associated genes are not yet known.

## Management and Treatment

*Management:* Ideally, effective treatment for glaucoma would include neuroprotection and/or repair of the optic nerve, however such therapies are not yet available. Current disease management in glaucoma patients is directed toward normalization of the IOP. Although not curative, reduction of IOP can slow the rate of disease progression, even in patients with NPG. IOP-lowering therapy is most effective at early stages of the disease, making strategies for screening, early detection, and diagnosis important.

*Therapeutics:* A number of different medications, delivered topically to the eye, are commonly used to reduce IOP. The IOP level is determined by the rate of production of intraocular fluid (aqueous humor) by the ciliary body and the rate of fluid removal by the trabecular meshwork or other pathways. Prostaglandin analogues increase the flow of fluid from the eye while all the other commonly used medications reduce formation of the aqueous humor (beta-blockers, carbonic anhydrase inhibitors, and alpha agonists).

Use of topical medication is the first-line therapy for glaucoma. Beta-blocker and prostaglandin "nonresponders" have been clinically described, however the underlying responsible genetic factors are not yet known.

If medications fail to adequately reduce IOP then surgery can be used to create an alternative exit route for the intraocular fluid. Surgical procedures include laser therapies to open the trabecular outflow pathways, incision procedures such as trabeculectomy to create an alternative path for fluid flow and implantation of tubes and other devices to facilitate the flow of fluid from the eye.

☞PHARMACOGENETICS: Pharmacogenetics has not yet been incorporated into the clinical management of glaucoma patients. Future work identifying genetic variants influencing therapeutic responses will be of interest in this regard.

## Molecular Genetics and Molecular Mechanism

☞JOAG: *MYOC* missense mutations account for approximately 35% of cases of juvenile-onset (prior to age 20) POAG (Table 148-1). The majority of *MYOC* disease-associated mutations are located in the olfactomedin domain encoded by the third exon. *MYOC* mutations are probably gain of function, as null mice and humans with complete deletion of the gene do not develop glaucoma. Myocilin is expressed in the trabecular meshwork outflow pathways as well as other ocular tissues and structures. The role of myocilin in IOP elevation is not completely known however in vitro studies have shown that myocilin mutants are misfolded and detergent resistant. Myocilin mutations may be secretion-incompetent and accumulate in the endoplasmic reticulum (ER) inducing ER stress. Recent studies using a transgenic mouse have indicated that compounds that relieve ER stress can also reduce the mutation-associated elevation of IOP. Several other loci for JOAG have been mapped to 9q21, 20q13, and 15q, however additional causative genes have not yet been identified.

*Table 148-1 Disease-Associated Susceptibility Variants*

| Candidate Gene (Chromosome Location) | Associated Variant [minor allele] | Relative Risk | Frequency of Risk Allele | Putative Functional Significance | Associated Disease Phenotype |
|---|---|---|---|---|---|
| *CDKN2BAS* (9p21) | rs4977756[A] | 1.5 (OR) | 0.69 | Not known | POAG |
| *CDKN2BAS* (9p21) | rs2157719:G | 0.58 (OR) | 0.30 | Not known | NPG |
| *CAV1/CAV2* (7q35) | rs4236601[A] | 1.36 (OR) | 0.29 | Not known | POAG |
| *TMCO1* (1q24) | rs4656461[G] | 1.68 (OR) | 0.17 | Not known | POAG |
| *SIX1/SIX6* (14q23) | rs10483727[A] | 1.32 (OR) | 0.46 | Not known | POAG CDR |
| 8q22 | rs284489:G | 0.62 (OR) | 0.30 | DNaseI hypersensitivity site | NPG |
| *MYOC* | Many different missense alleles located in the third exon. One common nonsense allele (GLN368X) | High | Rare | Gain of function | Early-onset POAG JOAG |
| *OPTN* | E50K (protein) | High | Rare | Probable loss of function | NPG |
| *TBK1* (12q14) | Gene duplication | High | Rare | Not known | NPG |

☞**NPG:** Two gene mutations are rare causes of familial NPG: the E50K missense change in *OPTN* (optineurin) and a duplication of the *TBK1* (TANK-binding kinase 1) on chromosome 12q14. Both products of these genes participate in TNF-alpha signaling. The E50K mutation is found in approximately 1% of NPG cases, while the *TBK1* duplication has been described in two families so far. Other common polymorphisms in *OPTN* have been inconsistently associated with disease. A recent genome-wide association study (GWAS) that included NPG subgroup analysis identified common SNPs associated with NPG in the *CDKN2BAS* gene region and in a regulatory region on chromosome 8q22. The role of these variants in development of optic nerve disease is not yet understood.

☞**POAG:** Mutations in *MYOC* account for approximately 4% of cases of POAG, especially those cases with onset between ages of 20 and 50 and with a family history of the disease. In particular, two *MYOC* mutations, *GLN368X* and *Thr377Met* result in adult-onset POAG. Recent (GWAS) have identified five genes that may contribute to disease development: *CAV1/CAV2* encoding caveolin 1 and caveolin 2; *CDKN2BAS* which codes for a long antisense RNA (ANRIL) that regulates expression of a number of genes including *CDKN2A* and *CDKN2B*; *TMCO1*, coding for a coiled-coiled domain protein; *SIX1/SIX6*, coding for developmentally regulated sine oculis 1 and 6 proteins that participate in development of the optic nerve; and a regulatory region on 8q22 that may target several genes in the region. Two other genes, *WDR36* and *NTF4*, may contribute to POAG pathogenesis, however their association has not been consistently reported.

**Genetic Testing:** Several laboratories offer genetic testing for glaucoma including the Carver Laboratory (University of Iowa) (https://www.carverlab.org) and the eyeGENE network (http://www.nei.nih.gov/resources/eyegene.asp). Individuals diagnosed with glaucoma at age 20 or younger should be tested for mutations in *MYOC* if the IOP is high (>21 mm Hg) or *OPTN* and *TBK1* if the IOP is low (<21 mm Hg). Patients with onset of disease between the ages of 20 and 50 should also be tested for mutations in *MYOC* if they have a family history of disease and their pressure is high or *OPTN* and *TBK1* if they have a family history of NPG and their pressure is low (Fig. 148-1). Patients with disease onset after age 50 are not likely to have mutations in these genes. Genes currently known to be associated with adult-onset POAG (ie, age of onset after age 40) do not have sufficient sensitivity and specificity to warrant gene-based testing. For patients with a family history of glaucoma genetic counseling can be helpful. Patients with mutations in *MYOC*, *OPTN*, or *TBK1* will also benefit from genetic counseling which may prompt testing of appropriate family members. Individuals who are carriers of mutations in these genes can be targeted for increased surveillance and aggressive therapy.

**Future Directions:** Although GWAS have successfully identified genes that are associated with POAG, these studies also suggest that larger datasets will be required to fully delineate the genetic architecture of POAG. Additionally, well-phenotyped cohorts will facilitate subset analyses that may be more likely to reveal important genes for this clinically and genetically heterogeneous disease. Larger datasets will also make gene-gene and gene-environment analyses possible. Ultimately the discovery of a comprehensive set of genes predisposing to POAG will facilitate efficient and useful genetic screening for POAG. Correlations between genes and specific disease features as well as response to therapy will help establish diagnostic and prognostic outcomes for patients leading to an effective personalized approach for glaucoma treatment.

**BIBLIOGRAPHY:**

1. Burdon KP, Macgregor S, Hewitt AW, et al. Genome-wide association study identifies susceptibility loci for open angle glaucoma at TMCO1 and CDKN2B-AS1. *Nat Genet.* 2011;43:574-578.

2. Fan BJ, Wiggs JL. Glaucoma: genes, phenotypes, and new directions for therapy. *J Clin Invest.* 2010;120:3064-3072.

3. Fingert JH, Robin AL, Stone JL, et al. Copy number variations on chromosome 12q14 in patients with normal tension glaucoma. *Hum Mol Genet.* 2011;20:2482-2494.

4. Kwon YH, Fingert JH, Kuehn MH, Alward WL. Primary open-angle glaucoma. *N Engl J Med.* 2009;360:1113-1124.

5. Nagabhushana A, Bansal M, Swarup G. Optineurin is required for CYLD-dependent inhibition of TNFα-induced NF-κB activation. *PLoS One.* 2011;6:e17477.

6. Thorleifsson G, Walters GB, Hewitt AW, et al. Common variants near CAV1 and CAV2 are associated with primary open-angle glaucoma. *Nat Genet.* 2010;42:906-909.

7. Wiggs JL, Yaspan BL, Hauser MA, et al. Common variants at 9p21 and 8q22 are associated with increased susceptibility to optic nerve degeneration in glaucoma. *PLoS Genet.* 2012;8:e1002654.

8. Zode GS, Bugge KE, Mohan K, et al. Topical ocular sodium 4-phenylbutyrate rescues glaucoma in a myocilin mouse model of primary open-angle glaucoma. *Invest Ophthalmol Vis Sci.* 2012;53(3):1557-1565.

## Supplementary Information

**OMIM REFERENCES:**

[1] Primary Open-Angle Glaucoma; (#137760)

[2] Juvenile Open-Angle Glaucoma; MYOC (#601652)

[3] Normal-Tension Glaucoma; (#606657)

[4] Optineurin; OPTN (#602432)

**Alternative Names:**
- Normal-Pressure Glaucoma (NPG)
- Juvenile Open-Angle Glaucoma (JOAG)
- Primary Open-Angle Glaucoma (POAG)

**Key Words:** Optic nerve, intra ocular pressure, visual field, blindness

# 149 Age-Related Macular Degeneration

Scott E. Brodie

## KEY POINTS

- *Disease summary:*
  - The "macula" is the central portion of the retina, where the greatest density of cone photoreceptors provides clear central vision. With increasing age, the macula is susceptible to disruption of the normal cellular architecture.
  - In the early stages, toxic metabolic waste products, especially metabolites of the retinal photopigments, accumulate in the retinal pigment epithelial cells immediately beneath the retinal photoreceptors. Accumulations of photoreceptor debris overwhelm the cellular transport mechanisms and form extracellular deposits known as "drusen" between the retinal pigment epithelium and the underlying basement membrane. While small, isolated drusen are essentially innocuous, larger, coalescent drusen indicate a high risk of atrophic breakdown of the retinal pigment epithelium and the underlying capillary bed, the choriocapillaris. This often takes the form of sharply demarcated atrophic patches, referred to as "geographic atrophy" or "dry" macular degeneration. The overlying retinal photoreceptors cease to function, resulting in central scotomas and loss of visual acuity. In some cases, the underlying vascular bed reacts to the atrophic process by the elaboration of vascular membranes which proliferate under the retinal pigment epithelium, or between the retinal pigment epithelium and the retina. These neovascular membranes are prone to extravasation into the extracellular space, causing macular edema, as well as subretinal hemorrhage, again leading to loss of central vision. This "wet" or "exudative" macular degeneration is much less frequent than "dry" macular degeneration, but accounts for most cases of severe visual loss from macular disease.
  - Age-related macular degeneration (AMD) (or macular degeneration, for short) is a leading cause of acquired blindness in developed countries, accounting for 54% of legal blindness in the United States.
  - There is a strong racial predilection: prevalence among adults age 45 to 85 is 5.4% among Caucasians, 4.6% among ethnic Chinese, 4.3% among Hispanics, 2.4% among African Americans. The prevalence increases rapidly in all ethnic groups after age 80.
- *Differential diagnosis:*
  - Geographic atrophy: hereditary macular dystrophies (Stargardt disease, retinitis pigmentosa, cone and cone-rod dystrophy, central areolar pigment epithelial dystrophy), congenital retinal abnormalities (coloboma, Leber congenital amaurosis), traumatic injuries, retinal drug toxicity.
  - Exudative maculopathy: diabetic retinopathy with macular edema, central serous chorioretinopathy, juvenile retinoschisis, myopic retinal degeneration, Best vitelliform dystrophy, serpiginous choroiditis, familial exudative vitreoretinopathy, epiretinal membranes with macular pucker.
  - Diagnosis is based on ophthalmoscopic appearance, then confirmed by fluorescein angiography to identify subretinal neovascularization, and optical coherence tomography imaging (OCT) to confirm and measure macular edema.
- *Monogenic forms:*
  - No single-gene cause of age-related macular degeneration is known. Candidate genes which may contribute to risk for AMD include *APOE* (apolipoprotein E—found in drusen, affects lipid transport), and genes for several Mendelian disorders somewhat akin to AMD: *ABCA4*—Stargardt disease; *TIMP3*—Sorsby fundus dystrophy; *VMD2*—Best vitelliform dystrophy; *Fibulin*-3—Malattia leventinese, *RDS-peripherin*—pattern dystrophies; *A4917G*—a mitochondrial DNA polymorphism; *TLR4*—toll-like receptor 4.
- *Family history:*
  - Comparison of prevalence of AMD between parents and children is difficult, as information about parents is frequently unavailable by the time their children are old enough to be at significant risk for AMD. After controlling for race and other known risk factors for AMD, the odds ratio (OR) for AMD in the siblings of patients with AMD compared with siblings of unaffected probands is between 3.6 and 10.3, depending on the stage of disease.
- *Twin studies:*
  - Concordance for AMD in twin studies has ranged from 90% to 100% in monozygotic twins, compared with about 40% in dizygotic twins.
- *Environmental factors:*
  - Smoking increases the risk of AMD 3.5-fold. Dietary supplementation with antioxidant vitamins and zinc is weakly protective against AMD in patients at high risk.
- *Genome-wide association studies:*
  - Linkage signals have been demonstrated to 1q25-31 (*CFH*) and 10q26 (*ARMS2/HTRA1*). Association signals have been confirmed to *ABCA4*, *CFI*, *C2-CFB*, and *C3*.
  - The locus associated with AMD at or near 1q31 is the gene for complement factor H (CFH). Unfavorable single-nucleotide polymorphisms (SNPs) at this locus and other complement factor loci are associated with ORs for development of AMD of 2.0 to 4.0.
  - Two genes at 10q26, *LOC387715* (of unknown function), and *HTRA1* have been associated with AMD. Variations in alleles of these two loci account for as much as 63% of the variation in risk for AMD, with ORs in combination as great as 57.6.
- *Pharmacogenomics:*
  - Data are very preliminary. Specific SNPs of *CFH* and *LOC387715* have been associated with small variations in the degree of protection against AMD by nutritional supplements, and frequency of injections of antivascular endothelial growth factor (anti-VEGF) treatments (see later).

## Diagnostic Criteria and Clinical Characteristics

The diagnosis of AMD is based on ophthalmoscopic findings and clinical imaging.

Findings of dry AMD include

- Clumping and irregularity of the macular pigment epithelium
- Drusen
- Geographic atrophy of the macular pigment epithelium
- Abnormal transmission of "choroidal flush" during early phases of fluorescein angiography ("window defects")

Findings of wet AMD include

- Macular edema
- Turbid or cloudy subretinal fluid
- Subretinal hemorrhage
- Progressive intensification and spreading of subretinal fluorescence during late phases of fluorescein angiography

Drusen, atrophy of the retinal pigment epithelium, subretinal neovascularization, and macular edema can be visualized with OCT.

## Screening and Counseling

**Screening:** Patients at risk for AMD should receive routine eye examinations every 1 to 2 years. If macular pigment irregularities or drusen are noted, patients should regularly use an "Amsler grid" (a small square of graph paper) to check for distortion of central vision ("metamorphopsia").

Dilated fundus examination should be performed whenever metamorphopsia or reduction in visual acuity is noted. Fluorescein angiography and/or OCT imaging should be performed if subretinal neovascularization is suspected.

**Counseling:** Antioxidant vitamins and zinc diet supplements (the "AREDS" formula) may be recommended for patients at high risk for AMD. (NB: The Vitamin A component of the AREDS supplement formula is not recommended for smokers, as it carries an increased risk of lung cancer. Alternative supplements which omit the vitamin A are available for these patients, though the degree of protection against AMD is reduced.)

Patients at increased risk for AMD should continue regular dilated fundus examinations, and frequently check for metamorphopsia with the Amsler grid.

☞GENOTYPE-PHENOTYPE CORRELATION: Genotype testing for AMD is not currently routine clinical practice. Testing for CFH mutations may soon become helpful in identifying and advising patients at risk.

## Management and Treatment

**Management:**
- There is no known treatment for dry AMD.
- Historically, wet AMD has been treated by ablation of subretinal neovascular membranes with thermal laser or photodynamic therapy (PDT—intravenous infusion of a sensitizing agent followed by irradiation of the retina with ultraviolet light to generate free radicals which selectively destroy neovascular tissue).
- Ablation treatments slow the rate of visual deterioration due to wet AMD, but do not arrest or reverse progression.
- Ablation treatment has largely been supplanted by intravitreal injection of drugs directed against VEGF, a tissue factor elaborated by ischemic retinal tissue which increases vascular permeability, and stimulates growth of neovascular tissue.
- The first anti-VEGF drug, pegaptanib sodium (Macugen) was shown to slow the impairment of vision due to wet AMD. Subsequent anti-VEGF drugs ranibizumab (Lucentis) and bevacizumab (Avastin—used off label for AMD) have been shown to reverse loss of visual acuity in a substantial fraction of patients, and to improve or stabilize visual acuity in a significant majority of patients with wet AMD.

**Therapeutics:** Anti-VEGF drugs are presently administered by intravitreal injection. The FDA-approved regimen for ranibizumab is for injections to be repeated on a monthly basis, indefinitely. Alternative regimens, based on monthly monitoring for recurrence of macular edema or loss of visual acuity, with injections repeated on an as-needed basis, have achieved visual results almost as good as regular monthly injections.

- Bevacizumab (Avastin), a monoclonal antibody directed against VEGF (from which the ranibizumab molecule was derived) has been used extensively on an off-label basis with visual results and safety comparable to ranibizumab, at much lower cost.

☞PHARMACOGENETICS: See Table 149-1.

*Table 149-1 Pharmacogenetic Considerations in AMD*

| Gene | Associated Medications | Goal of Testing | Variants | Effect |
|------|------------------------|-----------------|----------|--------|
| *CFH* | Bevacizumab | | CC (vs TT or TC) | Better visual acuity |
| *LOC3087715* | Bevacizumab | | TT (vs GG or GT) | Better visual acuity (not statistically significant) |
| *CFH* | AREDS supplement formula | | TT (vs CC) | Nonrisk TT phenotype associated with proportionally greater risk reduction |

*Table 149-2 Disease-Associated Susceptibility Variants*

| Candidate Gene (Chromosome Location) | Associated Variant [effect on protein] (assayed by affymetrix/illumina) | Relative Risk | Putative Functional Significance |
|---|---|---|---|
| CFH (1q32) | SNP Y402H | Heterozygous: 2.4 Homozygous: 6.2 | Hyperactivity of complement pathway |
| C2 | | 2 | |
| CFB | | 2.8 | |
| C3 | | Heterozygous: 1.85 Homozygous: 4.08 | |
| C3 and ARMS2 | | 57.6 | |
| CFI | | 1.4 | |
| LOC387715 | | Heterozygous: 2.5 Homozygous: 7.3 | |

## Molecular Genetics and Molecular Mechanism

See Table 149-2.

**Genetic Testing:** Clinical testing is not routinely available and the utility of testing is unproven.

**Future Directions:** Elucidate the mechanism of action of the complement cascade in the pathogenesis of wet AMD, in order to understand the role of mutations in the determination of risk, and, ultimately, to develop immunomodulatory agents for the prevention and treatment of AMD.

### BIBLIOGRAPHY:

1. Katta S, Kaur I, Chakrabarti S. The molecular genetic basis of age-related macular degeneration: an overview. *J Genet.* 2009;88:425-449.

2. Montezuma SR, Sobrin L, Seddon JM. Review of genetics in age related macular degeneration. *Semin Ophthalmol.* 2007;22:229-240. Review.

3. Klein RJ, Zeiss C, Chew EY, et al. Complement factor H polymorphism in age-related macular degeneration. *Science.* 2005;308:385-389.

4. Edwards AO, Ritter R 3rd, Abel KJ, Manning A, Panhuysen C, Farrer LA. Complement factor H polymorphism and age-related macular degeneration. *Science.* 2005;308:421-424.

5. Haines JL, Hauser MA, Schmidt S, et al. Complement factor H variant increases the risk of age-related macular degeneration. *Science.* 2005;308:419-421.

6. Seddon JM, Reynolds R, Maller J, Fagerness JA, Daly MJ, Rosner B. Prediction model for prevalence and incidence of advanced age-related macular degeneration based on genetic, demographic, and environmental variables. *Invest Ophthalmol Vis Sci.* 2009;50:2044-2053.

7. Zhang K, Kniazeva M, Hutchinson A, Han M, Dean M, Allikmets R. The ABCR gene in recessive and dominant Stargardt diseases: a genetic pathway in macular degeneration. *Genomics.* 1999;60:234-237.

8. Zhou J, Kim SR, Westlund BS, Sparrow JR. Complement activation by bisretinoid constituents of RPE lipofuscin. *Invest Ophthalmol Vis Sci.* 2009;50:1392-1399.

9. Age-Related Eye Disease Study Research Group. A randomized, placebo-controlled, clinical trial of high-dose supplementation with vitamins C and E, beta carotene, and zinc for age-related macular degeneration and vision loss: AREDS report no. 8. *Arch Ophthalmol.* 2001;119:1417-1436.

10. Klein ML, Francis PJ, Rosner B, et al. CFH and LOC387715/ARMS2 genotypes and treatment with antioxidants and zinc for age-related macular degeneration. *Ophthalmology.* 2008;115:1019-1025.

11. Rosenfeld PJ, Brown DM, Heier JS, et al. Ranibizumab for neovascular age-related macular degeneration. *N Engl J Med.* 2006;355:1419-1431.

12. Rich RM, Rosenfeld PJ, Puliafito CA, et al. Short-term safety and efficacy of intravitreal bevacizumab (Avastin) for neovascular age-related macular degeneration. *Retina.* 2006;26:495-511.

## Supplementary Information

### OMIM REFERENCES:

[1] Macular Degeneration, Age-Related, 7; ARMD7 (#610149)

[2] LOC387715 Gene; (+611313)

[3] Macular Degeneration, Age-Related, 4; ARMD4 (#610698)

# 150 Retinitis Pigmentosa

Fowzan S. Alkuraya

## KEY POINTS

- *Disease summary:*
  - Retinitis pigmentosa (RP) is the commonest "monogenic" form of photoreceptor degeneration affecting 1 in 3000 individuals.
  - Age of onset varies from early childhood to adulthood.
  - Patients typically present with night blindness and display a characteristic fundus appearance and constricted visual field (tunnel vision). Legal blindness eventually ensues.
  - A significant minority of RP patients have evidence of other system involvement, the recognition of which can facilitate specific syndromic diagnosis which has important consequences on the management, molecular diagnosis, and genetic counseling.

- *Hereditary basis:*
  - RP is one of the most genetically heterogeneous disorders in man. Mutations in any of approximately 50 genes can cause the disease typically in a Mendelian fashion. These mutations account for three quarters of RP cases with the remaining quarter assumed to be caused by mutations in yet unidentified genes.
  - Autosomal dominant (sometimes with reduced penetrance) and X-linked inheritance (mostly males but sometimes in females with variable severity) are seen each in about 30% and 15% of the cases, respectively, with the remaining 50% likely to be autosomal recessive. This distribution is not simply a reflection of the frequency of the respective loci but rather of the mutation frequency and population characteristics, for example, founder effect and level of consanguinity.

- *Differential diagnosis:*
  - The significant overlap between the different forms of retinal degeneration means that a patient may have less than classical RP phenotype or even a phenotype typical of a clinically distinct form of retinal degeneration and yet have mutation of a known RP gene. These other forms of retinal degeneration include cone or cone-rod dystrophy and macular dystrophy.
  - Leber congenital amaurosis (LCA) was previously viewed as a distinct clinical entity in which blindness is observed during infancy but many RP genes are also mutated in LCA patients so LCA can be viewed as a variant of RP with an extremely early onset.
  - Although RP is typically a rod disease, cones are inevitably lost as the disease progresses, so it is also referred to as rod-cone dystrophy. In cone and cone-rod dystrophies, there is preferential predilection to cones.
  - Macular dystrophies are a special form of cone dystrophy that is limited in distribution to the macula.
  - Many syndromes feature pigmentary retinal changes consistent with RP. In fact, some of the genes known to be mutated in these syndromes can be mutated in patients with isolated RP. For example, BBS3 and BBS9 are linked to Bardet-Biedl syndrome (BBS) which is characterized by RP, obesity, polydactyly, renal malformation, and hypogenitalism, but were also found to be mutated in patients with nonsyndromic RP. Other syndromes known to manifest with RP or RP-like lesions include Usher syndrome, Cohen syndrome, Cockayne syndrome, Refsum syndrome, neuronal ceroid lipofuscinosis, and abetalipoproteinemia.

## Diagnostic Criteria and Clinical Characteristics

***Diagnostic Criteria:*** The diagnosis of RP is based on characteristic history and fundus findings. Patients present with night blindness typically in early to late childhood. Physical examination will reveal constricted visual field and the fundus typically displays the classical triad of bone spicule pigmentation, attenuation of arterioles, and optic disc pallor. In early stages, electroretinographic (ERG) findings would show more severe deterioration in scotopic vision (rods) than photopic vision (cones) but as the disease progresses a severely diminished ERG recording in both test conditions is typical.

RP or RP-like lesions (including LCA picture) can be part of various syndromes which, based on the author's experience, can be missed unless the patient is evaluated by a clinical geneticist or an ophthalmologist who is experienced in the recognition of syndromic RP diagnoses.

Clinical evaluation of a patient with RP should include the following:

- Growth parameters: Microcephaly is a primary feature of Cohen syndrome whereas obesity is characteristic of BBS. Obesity is also seen in Alstrom syndrome but this syndrome typically manifests in cone-rod dystrophy rather than RP. Cachectic dwarfism is commonly seen in Cockayne syndrome. This author is aware of a novel form of RP with short stature that maps to a novel locus (unpublished).
- Facial features: Prominent upper incisors and a grimacing smile are features of Cohen syndrome whereas sunken eyes with cachectic appearance should point to Cockayne syndrome. Subtle facial dysmorphism can accompany BBS, mainly in the form of round facies.
- Skeletal features: Polydactyly is very common in BBS; history of removed extra digits should always be sought and the examiner should thoroughly search for tiny postaxial skin appendages that may be the only manifestation of polydactyly. Even in the

absence of polydactyly, brachydactyly (short digits) can be seen, so the digits should be closely inspected.

- Neurologic features: Developmental delay and intellectual disability should serve as a warning sign that RP is probably syndromic in nature. It is important to note that intellectual disability is not a consistent feature of BBS, so its absence does not rule this diagnosis out. In addition to BBS, Cohen syndrome and Cockayne syndromes are also characterized by developmental delay. Ataxia with impaired proprioception is characteristic of the Posterior Column Ataxia and RP syndrome but may also be seen in abetalipoproteinemia. Impaired hearing is a telltale sign of Usher syndrome. Although Refsum disease can rarely masquerade as Usher syndrome (unpublished), it is typically associated with more sensorimotor neuropathy. Hypertonia in the context of neurodegeneration and RP should alert to the diagnosis of neuronal ceroid lipofuscinosis (NCL).

## Screening and Counseling

*Screening:* History of difficulty seeing in dim light conditions is an effective screening tool. When the onset is early in childhood, it is necessary to rely on parental observation although this is not always accurate. Early retinal changes may not be easy to recognize unless assessed by an experienced retina specialist (they could be missed by a pediatric ophthalmologist) but ERG can be diagnostic even at early stages so it can serve as a presymptomatic screening tool in the setting of positive family history. ERG can also be helpful to identify female carriers of X-linked forms of RP which can be very helpful for counseling. Early recognition of the disease is important particularly for young children whose parents may not be aware of the recurrence risk.

*Counseling:* Genetic counseling can be straightforward when pedigrees are highly informative. Recurrence risk in the case of autosomal recessive RP is 25%, parents are obligate carriers and healthy siblings are at 67% risk of being carriers. In autosomal dominant RP the recurrence risk is up to 50% because reduced penetrance needs to be considered. In typical X-linked pedigrees, the obligate carrier female has 50% risk of having an affected son and 50% risk of having a "carrier" daughter. Caution is required when counseling these families about the potential visual involvement of carrier females.

Atypical pedigrees are not infrequently encountered and can pose significant counseling challenges. For instance, sporadic occurrence of RP with no family history could be the result of a de novo dominant or autosomal recessive mutation and these have very different recurrence risk both to the parents of the index as well as his/her offspring. The remarkable genetic and allelic heterogeneity of RP makes it unusually difficult for a counseling session to be based on actual knowledge of the mutation but recent developments in molecular diagnostics promise to change this trend (see later). Almost all syndromic RP diagnoses are autosomal recessive in nature which underscores the importance of recognizing them clinically to facilitate testing and counseling. Despite the increasingly recognized role of genes linked to syndromic RP in the pathogenesis of nonsyndromic RP, little is known about how to counsel in these scenarios. For instance, a family has recently been published where the index has nonsyndromic RP caused by *BBS9*

mutation whereas her two sisters, who are similarly homozygous for the same mutation, have the full blown BBS phenotype.

## Management and Treatment

Recognition of syndromic RP diagnoses is important for the proper management of syndrome-specific complications, for example, renal evaluation in BBS, neutrophil count determination in Cohen, avoidance of sun exposure in Cockayne, and administration of lipid-soluble vitamins in abetalipoproteinemia. For nonsyndromic RP, many therapies have been tried in the past but nothing has been convincingly shown to alter the disease course. Nonspecific ciliary neurotrophic factor (CNTF) has shown mixed results in slowing the disease progression. More recently, gene therapy has shown great promise but the gene-specific nature of this treatment modality and the requirement for surviving photoreceptors are among the main obstacles that hamper its widespread use. A recent breakthrough in slowing the decline of RP regardless of the underlying mutation involves the genetic modification of cones that became light insensitive as part of the natural history of RP to respond to light by bypassing the rhodopsin-mediated phototransduction pathway. Recent advances in stem cell-based therapies will probably translate into clinical trials within the few coming years.

Finally, retinal prostheses (electronic chip retina implants) have witnessed steady improvement over the years but significant technical hurdles need to be overcome to fully realize the potential of artificial vision. It is not uncommon for patients with end-stage RP to seek unproven therapies out of desperation so it is critical that they be warned against experimenting with unproven and unregulated therapies which may indeed worsen their retina function or even render them ineligible for future promising treatment modalities.

## Molecular Genetics and Molecular Mechanism

*Gene/Locus/Basic Gene Function:* Because the list of genes that are known to be mutated in RP is constantly changing with the discovery of more RP genes, the reader is encouraged to consult RETNET database for the most up-to-date list.

A comprehensive review of every RP gene is beyond the scope of this chapter but a few highlights are worth making in the context of the molecular pathogenesis of RP. The connecting cilium which plays a critical role in the delivery of proteins and membranes from the inner to the outer segment of photoreceptors also appears to confer high degree of vulnerability to their survival, the largest group of RP genes being implicated in the structure and/ or function of the cilia. Genes involved in phototransduction and retinal metabolism represent a second major group. What is less understood are genes that appear to have more generic functions and how they result is an eye-specific phenotype; this is particularly true for genes involved in splicing. Considering the extremely diverse nature of the gene products that are linked to RP pathogenesis, a theme emerges wherein photoreceptors in general and rods specifically are among the most vulnerable cells in the body and that their highly specialized physiology comes at the expense of very limited tolerance to any perturbation in their cellular homeostasis. The secondary loss of cones in the natural history of RP is a poorly understood phenomenon but one that leads to the most morbid symptoms of advanced RP.

***Genetic Testing:*** The following factors have traditionally complicated mutation analysis in patients with RP:

- Remarkable degree of genetic and allelic heterogeneity means that not only is there a prohibitive number of genes to be tested but they often need to be sequenced in full. This translates to hundreds to sequencing reactions per patient which until recently was impractical. Although homozygosity mapping can be an effective tool in reducing the number of candidate genes to be sequenced, its utility in RP diagnostics in outbred populations is unknown.
- With very few exceptions, the clinical phenotype of RP patient does not predict the underlying genotype, so testing algorithms analogous to those devised for other genetically heterogeneous conditions are not feasible.
- Not infrequently, pedigree analysis is not informative enough to suggest a particular inheritance pattern and even when it does there are many genes that display different modes of inheritance.
- Despite the recent momentum in discovering novel RP genes, all the genes discovered combined only account for 75% of the cases and it seems unlikely that any of the yet-to-be-discovered genes will account for a sizable proportion of cases.

Establishing a molecular diagnosis is essential for accurate genetic counseling and for the implementation of preventive services such as cascade, premarital and preconception carrier testing, and preimplantation and prenatal genetic diagnosis. In addition, recent advances in gene therapy have increased the demand on establishing molecular diagnosis to determine potential eligibility.

Until recently, chip-based solutions offered the only alternative to sequencing of hundreds of amplicons representing the coding segments of tens of RP genes. These chips were either designed to detect known mutations (targeted mutation analysis) or to sequence polymerase chain reaction (PCR)-generated amplicons (resequencing chips). The former has the obvious limitation of not being able to detect novel mutations while the latter is hampered by the requirement to generate hundreds of amplicons which puts to question the throughput of this method. However, recent advances in sequencing technology have now made it possible for the first time to sequence the entire genome at an ever decreasing cost. A more attractive alternative to whole genome sequencing is exome sequencing since most disease-causing Mendelian mutations are in the exons or flanking intronic sequences. Exome sequencing will reveal the causative mutation in one of the known RP or LCA genes in about 75% of patients with family history suggestive of autosomal recessive inheritance (Alkuraya, 2013). Interestingly, this technique also has a high yield in patients with no family history, although this is based on a consanguineous population where sporadic patients are likely to represent autosomal recessive cases so caution is advised in extrapolating these results to outbred populations.

## BIBLIOGRAPHY:

1. Daiger SP, Bowne SJ, Sullivan LS. Perspective on genes and mutations causing retinitis pigmentosa. *Arch Ophthalmol.* 2007;125:151-158.
2. Abu Safieh L, Aldahmesh MA, Shamseldin H, et al. Clinical and molecular characterisation of Bardet-Biedl syndrome in consanguineous populations: the power of homozygosity mapping. *J Med Genet.* 2010;47:236-241.
3. Ho AC. *Retina: Color Atlas and Synopsis of Clinical Ophthalmology.* McGraw-Hill, Medical Pub Division; 2003.
4. Aldahmesh MA, Al-Hassnan ZN, Aldosari M, et al. Neuronal ceroid lipofuscinosis caused by MFSD8 mutations: a common theme emerging. *Neurogenetics.* 2009;10:307-311.
5. Talcott KE, Ratnam K, Sundquist SM, et al. Longitudinal study of cone photoreceptors during retinal degeneration and in response to ciliary neurotrophic factor treatment. *Invest Ophthalmol Vis Sci.* 2011;52:2219-2226.
6. Busskamp V, Duebel J, Balya D, et al. Genetic reactivation of cone photoreceptors restores visual responses in retinitis pigmentosa. *Science.* 2010;329:413-417.
7. Weiland JD, Cho AK, Humayun MS. Retinal prostheses: current clinical results and future needs. *Ophthalmology.* 2011;118:2227-2237.
8. Wright AF, Chakarova CF, Abd El-Aziz MM, et al. Photoreceptor degeneration: genetic and mechanistic dissection of a complex trait. *Nat Rev Genet.* 2010;11:273-284.
9. Aldahmesh MA, Safieh LA, Alkuraya H, et al. Molecular characterization of retinitis pigmentosa in Saudi Arabia. *Mol Vis.* 2009;15:2464-2469.
10. Alkuraya FS. Homozygosity mapping: one more tool in the clinical geneticist's toolbox. *Genet Med.* 2010;12:236-239.
11. Berger W, Kloeckener-Gruissem B, Neidhardt J. The molecular basis of human retinal and vitreoretinal diseases. *Prog Retin Eye Res.* 2010;29:335-375.
12. Booij JC, Bakker A, Kulumbetova J, et al. Simultaneous mutation detection in 90 retinal disease genes in multiple patients using a custom-designed 300-kb retinal resequencing chip. *Ophthalmology.* 2011;118:160-7 e1-e3.
13. Vallespin E, Cantalapiedra D, Riveiro-Alvarez R, et al. Mutation screening of 299 Spanish families with retinal dystrophies by Leber congenital amaurosis genotyping microarray. *Invest Ophthalmol Vis Sci.* 2007;48:5653-5661.
14. Abu-Safieh L, Alrashed M, Alkuraya H, et al. Autozygome-guided exome sequencing in retinal dystrophy patients reveals pathogenetic mutations and novel candidate disease genes. *Genome Res.* 2013;23(2):236-247.

# 151 Nonsyndromic Sensorineural Hearing Loss

## KEY POINTS

- *Disease summary:*
  - Hearing loss (HL) is the most common sensory deficit in humans, occurring in 1 in 500 births and affecting 278 million people worldwide.
  - Conductive HL (CHL) is characterized by abnormalities of the external and/or middle ear, while sensorineural hearing loss (SNHL) is caused by malfunction of the inner ear, and mixed HL is a combination of both CHL and SNHL.
  - Nonsyndromic HL (NSHL) is not associated with any abnormalities of the external ear or any other organs and comprises the majority (70%) of hereditary HL (Fig. 151-1).

- *Hereditary basis:*
  - Most cases of NSHL have a genetic etiology.
  - NSHL is genetically heterogeneous with 64 genes currently implicated in the disorder (Table 151-1).
  - Mutations in the gene encoding the gap junction protein connexin 26 (*GJB2*) are the most common genetic cause of NSHL, occurring in an estimated 25% of autosomal recessive cases in the US population.

- *Differential diagnosis:*
  - Environmental causes of hearing impairment (acquired HL) account for approximately 30% of NSHL in developed countries
    - Acquired HL in children may be caused by
      - Prenatal infections from TORCH organisms (*Toxoplasmosis, Rubella, Cytomegalovirus* [CMV], and *Herpes*) with infection comprising the majority of environmental HL in children
      - Postnatal infections, particularly bacterial meningitis caused by *Neisseria meningitides, Haemophilus influenzae,* or *Streptococcus pneumoniae*
    - Acquired HL in adults is most often due to environmental noise exposure, though there is evidence for gene-environment interactions in "age-related" HL.
  - Syndromic hearing impairment is characterized by hearing loss and abnormal findings of at least one other organ system. There are more than 400 genetic syndromes that include hearing impairment and only the most common are briefly outlined here.
    - Autosomal dominant syndromic hearing impairment
      - Waardenburg syndrome: variable SNHL, pigmentary abnormalities including white forelock, and heterochromia iridis
      - Branchiootorenal syndrome (BOR syndrome): CHL, SNHL, or mixed HL, branchial cleft cysts, malformations of the external ear, and renal anomalies
      - Stickler syndrome: progressive SNHL, cleft palate, and spondyloepiphyseal dysplasia leading to arthritis
    - Autosomal recessive syndromic hearing impairment
      - Usher syndrome (USH): the most common cause of deaf-blindness is characterized by congenital SNHL, retinitis pigmentosa, and vestibular dysfunction. There are three types of USH differentiated by hearing and vestibular phenotypes:
        - USH type I: severe-to-profound SNHL, vestibular deficits
        - USH type II: mild-to-severe SNHL, normal vestibular function
        - USH type III: progressive SNHL and progressive loss of vestibular function
      - Pendred syndrome: severe-to-profound SNHL and euthyroid goiter associated with an abnormality of the bony labyrinth on CT examination (Mondini dysplasia or enlarged vestibular aqueduct [EVA])
      - Jervell and Lange-Nielsen syndrome: congenital deafness and prolongation of the QT interval leading to syncopal episodes
    - X-linked syndromic impairment
      - Alport syndrome: progressive SNHL and progressive glomerulonephritis which can lead to end-stage renal disease along with variable ophthalmologic findings (eg, anterior lenticonus)

- NSHL is distinguished by a lack of visible abnormalities of the external ear or other organ systems, however, it can be associated with abnormalities of the middle and/or inner ear (Table 151-1). NSHL is categorized by mode of inheritance and the different gene loci are designated DFN (for DeaFNess) and then given a letter according to inheritance pattern.
- Autosomal dominant NSHL (DFNA): generally progressive and moderate to severe. Significant genotype-phenotype correlations exist (eg, *WFS1*, DFNA6/14, causes low-frequency SNHL).
- Autosomal recessive NSHL (DFNB): generally congenital severe to profound, with exceptions (eg, *TECTA*, DFNB21, causes moderate NSHL).
- X-linked NSHL (DFNX): there are two identified X-linked NSHL genes with variable phenotypes.
- Mitochondrial NSHL: mutations in two mitochondrial genes cause NSHL by a mechanism that is not understood and some cases (eg, *MT-RNR1* mutations) susceptibility to developing deafness is conferred by aminoglycoside administration.

## Diagnostic Criteria and Clinical Characteristics

### Diagnostic Criteria for Inherited NSHL:
- Presence of
  - Bilateral, typically symmetrical hearing loss
  - Family history of hearing loss often elicited (notable exception—autosomal recessive)
- Absence of
  - Unilateral hearing loss
  - Syndromic features
  - Aminoglycoside antibiotic treatment
  - Prenatal infections associated with hearing loss
  - Significant noise exposure

### Clinical Characteristics:
*Onset:* congenital (from birth), prelingual (prior to speech development), or postlingual (after speech development)

*Severity:* mild (26-40 dB hearing threshold), moderate (41-55 dB), moderately severe (56-70 dB), severe (71-90 dB), or profound (>90 dB)

*Frequency:* low frequency (<500 Hz), mid frequency (501-2000 Hz), or high frequency (>2000 Hz)

*Progression:* progressive (deteriorates over time) or stable

*Inner ear malformations:* common malformations include Mondini dysplasia and EVA associated with DFNB4 hearing loss and perilymphatic gusher associated with DFNX3 hearing loss

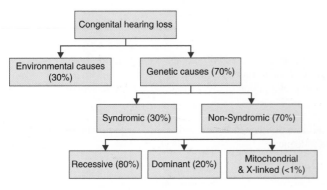

*Figure 151-1* Causes of Congenital NSHL.

*Inheritance pattern:* autosomal recessive (ARNSHL, DFNB), autosomal dominant (ADNSHL, DFNA), X-linked (DFNX), or mitochondrial

## Screening and Counseling

***Screening:*** It is clear that genetic testing provides important information to families including recurrence chance, prognosis (ie, progression and severity), and treatment options. Patients presenting with apparent NSHL according to the criteria outlined earlier should be referred for genetic testing. If inner ear malformations are detected they can be used to direct genetic screening. For example, presence of EVA is indicative for screening of the *SLC26A4* (DFNB4) gene.

In all cases of ARNSHL, screening of *GJB2/GJB6* (DFNB1 locus) should be completed first or as part of a comprehensive genetic screen, as mutations in this gene account for up to 50% of ARNSHL in many outbred world populations. If mutations in *GJB2* are excluded, selecting the next gene to screen is difficult due to the large number of known deafness genes (Table 151-1) and, in most cases, lack of distinguishing features. Fortunately, screening platforms based on new sequencing technologies that simultaneously target hundreds of known deafness-causing mutations, a subset of the commonly mutated NSHL genes, or all known NSHL genes have been developed to streamline genetic testing for NSHL. The important features of these tests are summarized in Table 151-2. If all-inclusive platforms are used, there is no for sequential screening strategies (for example, there is no need to screen *GJB2* first in cases of ARNSHL).

There is no single gene that accounts for the majority of ADNSHL cases. However, there are clear genotype-phenotype correlations that can be used to direct screening. A computer software tool is now publicly available that can predict the likely *ADNSHL* gene from a patient audiogram (AudioGene). AudioGene was developed using several thousand audiograms from genetically diagnosed patients to prioritize genes for screening in families with idiopathic ADNSHL. This phenotypic analysis will support the new high throughput genetic screening methods described earlier.

***Counseling:*** There are special considerations in counseling individuals with hearing loss. Deaf (small "d") is a colloquial term that implies severe-to-profound hearing loss by audiometry, whereas Deaf culture (capital "D") refers to members of the Deaf community in the United States who are deaf and use American Sign Language for communication. The Deaf community has a culture

*Table 151-1* **Genes Associated With NSHL**

| Gene | Deafness Locus | Full Name | OMIM # | Phenotype |
|------|----------------|-----------|--------|-----------|
| **Autosomal Recessive NSHL Genes**[a] | | | | |
| BSND | DFNB73 | Barttin | 606412 | Prelingual, severe |
| CDH23 | DFNB12 | Cadherin-related 23 | 601386 | Prelingual, relatively stable |
| CLDN14 | DFNB29 | Claudin 14 | 605608 | Prelingual, profound |
| COL11A2 | DFNB53/DFNA13 | Collagen, type XI, alpha 2 | 609706 | Postlingual (second decade), mid frequency |
| ESPN | DFNB36 | Espin | 609006 | Prelingual, vestibular areflexia |
| ESSRB | DFNB35 | Estrogen-related receptor beta | 608565 | Prelingual, profound |
| GIPC3 | DFNB15/DFNB95 | GAIP C-terminus interacting protein 3 | 601869 | Prelingual, mid-high frequency |
| GJB2 | DFNB1/DFNA3 | Gap junction protein, beta 2 | 220290 | Prelingual, relatively stable, all frequencies or high frequency |
| GJB3 | DFNA2 | Gap junction protein, beta 3 | 600101 | Details not available |
| GJB6 | DFNB1/DFNA3 | Gap junction protein, beta 6 | 220290 | Details not available |
| GPSM2 | DFNB82 | G-protein signaling modulator 2 | 613557 | Prelingual, stable, profound |
| GRXCR1 | DFNB25 | Glutaredoxin cysteine-rich 1 | 613285 | Prelingual, severe to profound |
| HGF | DFNB39 | Hepatocyte growth factor | 608265 | Prelingual, severe to profound |
| ILDR1 | DFNB42 | Ig-like domain-containing receptor 1 | 609646 | Prelingual, mid-to-high frequency |
| LHFPL5 | DFNB66/67 | Lipoma HMGIC fusion partner-like 5 | 610212 | Prelingual, severe to profound |
| LOXHD1 | DFNB77 | Lipoxygenase homology domain-containing 1 | 613079 | Prelingual, mid-to-high frequency, progressive |
| LRTOMT | DFNB63 | Leucine-rich transmembrane OMT | 611451 | Prelingual, profound |
| MARVELD2 | DFNB49 | MARVEL domain-containing 2 | 610153 | Prelingual, moderate to profound |
| MSRB3 | DFNB74 | Methionine sulfoxide reductase B3 | 613719 | Prelingual, profound |
| MYO3A | DFNB30 | Myosin IIIA | 607101 | Progressive, affects high then mid frequencies |
| MYO6 | DFNB37/DFNA22 | Myosin VI | 607821 | Prelingual or postlingual high frequency |
| MYO7A | DFNB2/DFNA11 | Myosin VIIA | 600060 | Prelingual or postlingual (first decade) |
| MYO15A | DFNB3 | Myosin XVA | 600316 | Prelingual, stable, severe to profound |
| OTOA | DFNB22 | Otoancorin | 607039 | Prelingual, moderate to severe |
| OTOF | DFNB9 | Otoferlin | 601071 | Prelingual, stable |
| PCDH15 | DFNB23 | Protocadherin-related 15 | 609533 | Prelingual, severe to profound |
| PJVK | DFNB59 | Pejvakin | 610220 | Prelingual, severe-to-profound, auditory neuropathy |
| PTPRQ | DFNB84 | Protein-tyrosine phosphatase receptor | 613391 | Prelingual, severe to profound |
| RDX | DFNB24 | Radixin | 611022 | Prelingual, profound |
| SERPIN | DFNB91 | Serpin peptidase inhibitor, clade B, member 6 | 173321 | Postlingual, moderate to severe, progressive |
| SLC26A4 | DFNB4 | Solute carrier family 26, member 4 | 600792 | Prelingual or postlingual, stable or progressive, EVA |
| SLC26A5 | DFNB61 | Solute carrier family 26, member 5 | 604943 | Prelingual, severe to profound |
| STRC | DFNB16 | Stereocilin | 603720 | Prelingual, stable, primarily high frequencies |
| TECTA | DFNB21/DFNA8/DFNA12 | Tectorin alpha | 603629 | Prelingual, moderate, mid frequency |
| TMC1 | DFNB7/DFNB11/DFNA36 | Transmembrane channel-like 1 | 600974 | Prelingual, stable |

*(Continued)*

**Table 151-1** *Genes Associated With NSHL (Continued)*

| Gene | Deafness Locus | Full Name | OMIM # | Phenotype |
|---|---|---|---|---|
| *TMIE* | DFNB6 | Transmembrane inner ear | 600971 | Prelingual, stable |
| *TMPRSS3* | DFNB8/DFNB10 | Transmembrane protease, serine 3 | 601072 | Prelingual or postlingual, stable or progressive |
| *TPRN* | DFNB79 | Taperin | 613307 | Prelingual, severe to profound |
| *TRIOBP* | DFNB28 | TRIO and F-actin binding protein | 609823 | Prelingual, severe to profound |
| *USH1C* | DFNB18 | Usher syndrome 1C homolog | 602092 | Prelingual, stable |
| *WHRN* | DFNB31 | Whirlin | 607084 | Prelingual, profound |
| | | **Subtotal** | | **38 genes** |
| **Autosomal Dominant NSHL Genes**[a] | | | | |
| *ACTG1* | DFNA20/26 | Actin, gamma 1 | 604717 | Postlingual, high frequency |
| *CCDC50* | DFNA44 | Coiled-coil domain containing 50 | 607453 | Postlingual, moderate, all frequencies |
| *CEACAM16* | DFNA4 | Carcinoembryonic antigen-related cell adhesion molecule 16 | - | Postlingual, moderate |
| *COCH* | DFNA9 | Coagulation factor C homolog, cochlin | 601369 | Postlingual (second decade), high frequency |
| *CRYM* | - | Crystallin, mu | 123740 | Postlingual high frequency |
| *DFNA5* | DFNA5 | Deafness, autosomal dominant 5 | 600994 | Postlingual (first decade), high frequency |
| *DIAPH1* | DFNA1 | Diaphanous homolog 1 | 124900 | Postlingual (first decade), low frequency |
| *DSPP* | DFNA39 | Dentin sialophosphoprotein | 605594 | Postlingual, high frequency |
| *EYA4* | DFNA10 | Eyes absent homolog 4 | 601316 | Postlingual (third/fourth decade), mid-high frequency |
| *GRHL2* | DFNA28 | Grainyhead-like 2 | 608641 | Postlingual, mid-high frequency |
| *KCNQ4* | DFNA2 | Potassium voltage-gated channel | 600101 | Postlingual (second decade), high frequency |
| *MYH14* | DFNA4 | Myosin, heavy chain 14, nonmuscle | 600652 | Postlingual, mid-to-high frequency |
| *MIRN96* | DFNA50 | MicroRNA 96 | 611606 | Postlingual, mild to profound, progressive |
| *MYH9* | DFNA17 | Myosin, heavy chain 9, nonmuscle | 603622 | Postlingual high frequency |
| *MYO1A* | DFNA48 | Myosin IA | 607841 | Postlingual |
| *POU4F3* | DFNA15 | POU class 4 homeobox 3 | 602459 | Postlingual high frequency |
| *SLC17A3* | DFNA25 | Solute carrier family 17, member 3 | 605583 | Postlingual high frequency |
| *TJP2* | DFNA51 | Tight junction protein 2 | 613558 | Postlingual high frequency |
| *WFS1* | DFNA6/DFNA14 | Wolfram syndrome 1 (wolframin) | 600965 | Prelingual, low frequency |
| | | **Subtotal** | | **17 genes** |
| **X-Linked NSHL Genes** | | | | |
| *POU3F4* | DFNX3 | POU-domain class 3 transcription factor 4 | 300030 | Prelingual, associated with EVA |
| *PRPS1* | DFNX2 | Phosphoribosylpyrophosphate synthetase 1 | 304400 | Prelingual, severe |
| | | **Subtotal** | | **2 genes** |
| **Mitochondrial NSHL Genes** | | | | |
| *MT-RNR1* | - | Mitochondrially encoded 12S RNA | 500008 | Aminoglycoside-induced HL |
| *MT-TS1* | - | Mitochondrially encoded tRNA ser 1 | 590080 | |
| | | **Subtotal** | | **2 genes** |
| | | **Grand Total** | | **59 genes** |

[a]Genes that cause both ARNSHL and ADNSHL are included under ARNSHL.

*Table 151-2  Newly Developed High-Throughput Genetic Tests for NSHL*

| Test Name | Location of Development | DNA Sequencing Technology | Screened | Advantages/ Disadvantages | Reference |
|---|---|---|---|---|---|
| HHLAPEM[a] | Stanford University | Single basepair primer extension | 198 deafness mutations | Inexpensive/only screens 198 mutations, not direct sequencing | Rodriguez-Paris et al. *PLOS One*. 2010 |
| OtoChip | Harvard University | Resequencing microarray | 13 deafness genes | Inexpensive/only examines 13 of 64 known deafness genes | Kothiyal et al. *BMC Biotechnol*. 2010 |
| OtoSCOPE | University of Iowa | Sequence capture followed by massively parallel sequencing | 59 deafness genes | Screens all known deafness genes, uses direct sequencing/more expensive | Shearer et al. *PNAS*. 2010 Shearer et al. *J Med Genet*. 2013 |

[a]Hereditary hearing loss arrayed primer extension microarray.

that is characterized by unique social and societal attributes, as are other cultures.

The deaf do *not* consider themselves to be hearing "impaired" nor do they feel that they have a hearing "loss." Instead, they consider themselves deaf. Their deafness is viewed as a distinguishing characteristic and not considered a pathology that needs to be treated or cured. However, there are individuals with deafness or in the Deaf community who seek information on medical, educational, and social services and possibly management and treatment. Clinicians should remain sensitive to these cultural differences.

Recurrence chance depends on mode of inheritance. Phenotypic characteristics of NSHL are largely gene or mutation dependent (Table 151-1). Progression can range from rapidly progressive to stable, and severity from mild to profound.

When counseling individuals with autosomal dominant hearing loss, family history may appear to be negative due to failure to diagnose hearing loss, failure to recognize environmental contributions, late-onset hearing loss, reduced penetrance, or de novo mutations.

## Management and Treatment

Management of NSHL is best performed by a team that includes an otolaryngologist, audiologist, clinical geneticist, and pediatrician. In some cases the services of an educator of the Deaf, neurologist, and ophthalmologist may be required. Sequential audiograms are the key for documenting stability or progression of hearing loss, unless the genetic causes has been established and audioprofile data are available (for example, through AudioGene).

Auditory deprivation through the age of 2 years is associated with poor reading performance, poor communication skills, and poor speech production; therefore early intervention is paramount. Furthermore, it has been shown that although decreased cognitive skills and performance in mathematics and reading are associated with deafness, these deficiencies are not linked inextricably to deafness and can be significantly improved by habilitation options such as hearing aids or cochlear implants.

Due to the varying deafness phenotypes, it is important to determine the best mode of treatment. Treatment options include hearing aids, vibrotactile devices, or cochlear implantation. It is important to note that although educational intervention is in itself important it is insufficient to remediate deficiencies without medical interventions.

## Molecular Genetics and Molecular Mechanism

Due to the extreme genetic heterogeneity of NSHL, it is outside the scope of this chapter to review the molecular mechanisms of all known NSHL genes (Table 151-1). NSHL can be caused by mutations in genes encoding ion channels, cytoskeletal proteins, and transcription factors, and other protein types, and this underlies the complexity of the human auditory system. There are many excellent reviews on this subject for interested readers. ***Genetic Testing:*** Due to the genetic heterogeneity of NSHL, gene sequencing approaches are preferred to mutation detection approaches. There are numerous molecular genetic laboratories that offer genetic testing for deafness. In all cases, clinical testing laboratories should be CLIA certified and JACO approved to ensure high-quality testing. Readers are referred to the GeneTests website (http://www.genetests.org) for an up-to-date list of laboratories that offer genetic testing for NSHL.

**BIBLIOGRAPHY:**

1. Putcha GV, Bejjani BA, Bleoo S, et al. A multicenter study of the frequency and distribution of GJB2 and GJB6 mutations in a large north american cohort. *Genet Med*. 2007;9:413-426.

2. Huyghe JR, Van Laer L, Hendrickx JJ, et al. Genome-wide SNP-based linkage scan identifies a locus on 8q24 for an age-related hearing impairment trait. *Am J Hum Genet*. 2008;83: 401-407.

3. Konings A, Van Laer L, Van Camp G. Genetic studies on noise-induced hearing loss: a review. *Ear Hear*. 2009;30:151-159.

4. Hilgert N, Smith RJ, Van Camp G. Forty-six genes causing nonsyndromic hearing impairment: which ones should be analyzed in DNA diagnostics? *Mutat Res*. 2009;681:189-196.

5. Rodriguez-Paris J, Pique L, Colen T, Roberson J, Gardner P, Schrijver I. Genotyping with a 198 mutation arrayed primer extension array for hereditary hearing loss: assessment of its diagnostic value for medical practice. *PLoS One*. 2010;5:e11804.

6. Kothiyal P, Cox S, Ebert J, et al. High-throughput detection of mutations responsible for childhood hearing loss using resequencing microarrays. *BMC Biotechnol*. 2010;10:10.

7. Shearer AE, Deluca AP, Hildebrand MS, et al. Comprehensive genetic testing for hereditary hearing loss using massively parallel sequencing. *Proc Natl Acad Sci USA*. 2010;107:21104-21109.

8. Hildebrand MS, DeLuca AP, Taylor KR, et al. A contemporary review of AudioGene audioprofiling: a machine-based candidate gene prediction tool for autosomal dominant nonsyndromic hearing loss. *Laryngoscope*. 2009;119:2211-2215.

9. Dror AA, Avraham KB. Hearing impairment: a panoply of genes and functions. *Neuron*. 2010;68:293-308.

10. Petit C, Richardson GP. Linking genes underlying deafness to hair-bundle development and function. *Nat Neurosci*. 2009;12:703-710.

11. Hilgert N, Smith RJH, Van Camp G. Forty-six genes causing nonsyndromic hearing impairment: which should be analyzed in DNA diagnostics? *Mut Res Revs*. 2009;681:189-196.

12. Hilgert N, Smith RJH, Van Camp G. Function and expression pattern of nonsyndromic deafness genes. *Cur Mole Med*. 2009;9:546-564.

13. Shearer AE, Black-Ziegelbein EA, Hildebrand MS, et al. Advancing genetic testing for deafness with genomic technology. *J Med Genet*. 2013;Jun 26[Epub ahead of print].

## Supplementary Information

**OMIM Reference:**

[1] Included in Table 151-1.

**Alternative Name:** None

**Key Words:** Hearing loss, hearing impairment, deafness, nonsyndromic hearing loss

# 152 Syndromic Hearing Loss

Amy L. Hernandez and Heidi Rehm

## KEY POINTS

- *Disease summary:*
  - Usher syndrome is characterized by sensorineural hearing loss and retinitis pigmentosa (RP) with or without vestibular dysfunction.
  - Pendred syndrome is characterized by nonsyndromic hearing loss with enlarged vestibular aqueducts (EVA) and/or Mondini dysplasia (incomplete partition or common cavity malformation of the inner ear) in combination with euthyroid goiter or thyroid dysfunction. DFNB4 hearing loss is characterized by the same features of Pendred syndrome without thyroid abnormalities.

- *Hereditary basis:*
  - Usher syndrome is inherited in an autosomal recessive manner.
  - Pendred syndrome or DFNB4 hearing loss is inherited in an autosomal recessive manner. However, there are rare reports of possible digenic inheritance involving the *FOXI1* and *KCNJ10* genes.

- *Differential diagnosis:*
  - Usher syndrome
    - Nonsyndromic hearing loss or nonsyndromic RP
    - Deafness-dystonia-optic neuronopathy (DDON)
    - Mitochondrial disorders
    - Diabetic neuropathy
    - Viral infections
    - Alstrom syndrome
    - Bardet-Biedl syndrome
  - *Pendred syndrome*
    - Branchiootorenal syndrome (BOR)
    - Brachiooto syndrome (BO)
    - Waardenburg syndrome
    - Deafness associated with the recessive form of distal renal tubular acidosis

## Diagnostic Criteria and Clinical Characteristics

***Diagnostic Criteria:*** A clinical diagnosis of Usher syndrome can be made based on the following features:

- Sensorineural hearing loss with typical presentations as follows
  - Congenital severe to profound for type 1
  - Congenital moderate-to-severe sloping for type 2
  - Variable age of onset and severity for type 3, often progressive
- RP
- Vestibular dysfunction for type 1, which may also occur in type 3
- Family history suggestive of autosomal recessive inheritance (though many cases are singletons)
- Absence of other physical abnormalities such as dystonia/ataxia (DDON), obesity/cardiomyopathy/insulin resistance (Alstrom syndrome), obesity/postaxial polydactyly/cognitive impairment/genital abnormalities/renal abnormalities (Bardet-Biedl syndrome), or features suggestive of a mitochondrial disorder.

A genetic diagnosis of Usher syndrome can also be made based on the presence of two pathogenic variants in a gene that has been associated with Usher syndrome (Table 152-1). However, some pathogenic variants in *USH1C*, *CDH23*, *PCDH15*, and *DFNB31* have also been associated with recessive nonsyndromic hearing loss. This is further addressed under the section on genetic counseling.

A clinical diagnosis of Pendred syndrome and DFNB4 hearing loss can be made based on the following features:

- Sensorineural hearing loss that is typically congenital.
- Bilateral enlarged vestibular aqueducts with or without incomplete partition (Mondini deformity). Goiter, hypothyroidism, or abnormal perchlorate discharge test result (this feature is absent in DFNB4).
- Family history suggestive of autosomal recessive inheritance (though many cases are singletons).

A genetic diagnosis of Pendred syndrome or DFNB4 hearing loss can be made based on the presence of two pathogenic variants in the *SLC26A4* gene (Table 152-1). These mutations in combination with a goiter or an abnormal perchlorate discharge test would confirm a diagnosis of Pendred syndrome.

***Clinical Characteristics:***

☞USHER SYNDROME: Usher syndrome is one of the most common types of autosomal recessive syndromic hearing loss and is the most common genetic cause of combined deafness and blindness. Its prevalence is at least 4/100,000, with an estimated carrier frequency of 1/70. Recent data suggest that 10% of hearing loss cases, negative for *GJB2* mutations, will develop Usher syndrome.

Usher syndrome is subdivided into three clinical types depending on the severity and onset of hearing impairment and RP, as well as the presence of vestibular dysfunction (Table 152-2). Types 1 and 2 are equally frequent in the general population, while type 3 is considerably less common in the general population although

*Table 152-1* **Genetic Differential Diagnosis**

| Syndrome | Gene Symbol | Associated Findings |
|---|---|---|
| Pendred syndrome | SLC26A4 | Sensorineural hearing loss, EVA, Mondini dysplasia, thyroid dysfunction |
| DFNB4 | SLC26A4[a] | Sensorineural hearing loss, EVA, Mondini dysplasia |
| Usher syndrome type 1B | MYO7A[b] | Congenital severe-to-profound sensorineural hearing loss with RP and vestibular dysfunction |
| Usher syndrome type 1C | USH1C[a] | |
| Usher syndrome type 1D | CDH23[a,b] | |
| Usher syndrome type 1F | PCDH15[a] | |
| Usher syndrome type 1G | USH1G | |
| Usher syndrome type 2A | USH2A[b] | Congenital mild-to-severe sensorineural hearing loss with RP and intact vestibular response |
| Usher syndrome type 2C | GPR98 | |
| Usher syndrome type 2D | DFNB31[a] | |
| Usher syndrome type 3A | CLRN1 | Progressive mild-to-profound sensorineural hearing loss with RP and variable impairment of vestibular response |

[a]Gene has also been associated to nonsyndromic hearing loss.
[b]Atypical presentations have been reported.
Gene and protein names: *SLC26A4*, pendrin; *MYO7A*, myosin VIIA; *USH1C*, Usher syndrome type-1C protein-binding protein 1; *CDH23*, cadherin-23; *PCDH15*, protocadherin-15; *USH1G*, Usher syndrome type-1G protein; *USH2A*, usherin; *GPR98*, G protein-coupled receptor 98; *DFNB31*, whirlin; *CLRN1*, clarin-1.

it has a higher prevalence in the Finnish and Ashkenazi Jewish populations.

RP, a type of retinal dystrophy, is a group of hereditary retinal diseases in which there is degeneration of the rod and cone photoreceptors. RP can occur as an isolated condition or be part of at least 30 different syndromes. Usher syndrome is the most common syndromic form of RP, accounting for 10% to 20% of all individuals with RP. RP is a highly variable disorder with respect to age of onset, severity, and progression. Individuals often present with difficulties with dark adaptation and night blindness followed by reduction in peripheral (tunnel vision) then central vision loss.

The vestibular problems associated with Usher syndrome often present as delayed walking (>18 months), especially in Usher syndrome type 1. The presence of vestibular dysfunction in an individual with significant hearing loss increases the possibility for Usher syndrome.

*Table 152-2* **Clinical Features of Usher Syndrome**

| | Bilateral Hearing Loss | Vestibular System | Retinitis Pigmentosa |
|---|---|---|---|
| Type 1 | Congenital severe to profound | Impaired | Onset prepuberty |
| Type 2 | Congenital mild-to-severe sloping | Normal | Onset in teens—early 20s |
| Type 3 | Variable severity, progressive later onset | Variable, often progressive balance problems | Variable age of onset |

Usher syndrome type 1 is the most severe form of the condition and is characterized by congenital, bilateral, profound sensorineural hearing loss, vestibular dysfunction, and the onset of RP in childhood. Individuals with Usher Syndrome type 2 also have congenital hearing loss (usually milder and worse in the higher frequencies), but vestibular problems are typically absent. In type 2, RP presents later, typically in teens—early 20s. The hearing loss associated with Usher syndrome type 3 may not be present at birth. Vestibular dysfunction may or may not be present, and RP usually develops later than it does in types 1 and 2.

There are atypical forms of Usher syndrome and overlap between the three types, which can make it difficult to make a clinical distinction between the three different types. In addition, *CDH23*, *DFNB31*, *PCDH15*, and *USH1C* have also been associated with recessive nonsyndromic hearing loss and USH2A can also cause nonsyndromic RP.

☞**PENDRED SYNDROME:** The incidence of Pendred syndrome is 7.5/100,000, which accounts for approximately 5% to 10% of childhood-onset hereditary hearing loss. Hearing loss associated with Pendred syndrome or DFNB4 is typically bilateral severe-to-profound sensorineural hearing loss that can be progressive or fluctuating. In some cases progression can be associated with head injury, infection, and delayed secondary hydrops. The most common abnormalities are enlarged vestibular aqueduct and incomplete partition (Mondini deformity).

The presence of thyroid abnormalities is what distinguishes Pendred syndrome from DFNB4 hearing loss. The thyroid abnormalities associated with Pendred syndrome are caused by a partial defect in iodine organification. The euthyroid goiter typical of Pendred syndrome presents in late childhood or early adulthood. Approximately 10% will also develop hypothyroidism. An abnormal perchlorate discharge test can be diagnostic, though this type of test is not widely available and can be difficult to establish a normal range. Vestibular problems can also been seen in individuals with Pendred syndrome.

## Screening and Counseling

*Screening:* In addition, diagnosis based on relative likelihood as outlined in Table 152-3.
*Counseling:* Usher syndrome and Pendred syndrome are inherited in an autosomal recessive manner. The penetrance is 100% but expressivity can vary. Some patients with *SLC26A4* mutations will develop Pendred syndrome and others develop only

**Table 152-3 *Genes Associated With Different Presentations***

| Presentation | Gene 1 | Gene 2 | Gene 3 | Gene 4 | Gene 5 |
|---|---|---|---|---|---|
| Usher syndrome type 1 | *MYO7A* (39%-55%) | *CDH23* (19%-35%) | *PCDH15* (10%-20%) | *USH1C* (6%-7%) | *USH1G* (7%) |
| Usher syndrome type 2 | *USH2A* (80%) | *GPR98* (15%) | *DFNB31* (5%) | *PDZD7* (rare/ digenic/modifier) | |
| Usher syndrome type 3 | *CLRN1* (100%) | | | | |
| Pendred syndrome | *SLC26A4* (~100%) | *FOXI1* (rare/ digenic?) | *KCNJ10* (rare/ digenic?) | | |
| DFNB4 hearing loss | *SLC26A4* (100%) | | | | |

Percentages describe the relative distribution of identified mutations.

hearing loss. Some individuals with two pathogenic variants in *CDH23*, *DFNB31*, *PCDH15*, and *USH1C* will only have recessive nonsyndromic hearing loss and not develop RP and some individuals with mutations in *USH2A* will only develop RP. For some genes, such as *CDH23*, presentation is based on the severity of mutations with biallelic truncating leading to a syndromic presentation and having at least one copy of the gene containing a missense variant that leaves the protein with partial function allows for a nonsyndromic presentation with vision and vestibular function preserved. For other genes such as *DFNB31*, the location of the mutations seems to dictate phenotype. With CDH23 and PCDH15 only certain missense mutations have been associated with nonsyndromic hearing loss. Therefore, for CDH23 and PCDH15, a predicted development of RP should only be made if both alleles have truncating mutations or missense variants previously associated with Usher syndrome and for DFNB31, only if the mutations reside in the gene region associated with Usher syndrome. USH1C contains seven alternatively spliced exons that are not expressed in the retina and mutations in these exons have only been associated with nonsyndromic hearing loss. However, mutations outside of these alternatively spliced exons have been associated both with Usher syndrome and nonsyndromic hearing loss. Therefore, prediction of nonsyndromic hearing loss should only be made if both mutations are located in the alternatively spliced exons.

## Management and Treatment

***Usher Syndrome:*** The hearing loss in Usher syndrome should be managed according to severity with hearing aids or cochlear implants. Learning oral communication instead of, or in combination with, manual communication can greatly benefit individuals with Usher syndrome as their vision will become impaired creating difficulty in the use of manual communication. For those with profound deafness, bilateral cochlear implantation should be considered to allow for better sound localization when vision is impaired.

Individuals with Usher syndrome should have their vision monitored by an ophthalmologist. There are different tests to monitor retinal function which include an electroretinogram (ERG) and dark adaptive thresholds. The ERG can be used to diagnose RP and can be used to track the progressive retinal degeneration and associated vision loss. ERGs measure electrical responses of the retina, including rod and cone photoreceptors. There are currently no approved treatments for RP. However, there is some data to suggest that safe levels of vitamin A supplements and/or wearing sunglasses may slow

progression of the vision loss. There are also a number of clinical trials enrolling patients for a variety of treatment approaches.

Vestibular function can be assessed and monitored with many different tools including assessing for delayed motor milestones, video-oculography (VOG), computerized rotary chair (CRC), computerized dynamic posturography (CDP), and vestibular-evoked myogenic potentials (VEMPs).

***Pendred syndrome:*** After an initial evaluation by otolaryngology and genetics, patients with *SLC26A4* mutations should have semi-annual or annual evaluations by an audiologist and endocrinologist. Hearing loss is typically treated with hearing aids, cochlear implantation, and other standard approaches to managing sensorineural hearing loss. Repeat audiometry should be every 3 to 6 months if hearing loss is progressive. Surveillance for goiter should include volumetric baseline measurement of the thyroid by ultrasonography with periodic (every 2-3 years) reassessment. If hypothyroidism develops it can be treated with thyroid hormone supplementation.

## Molecular Genetics and Molecular Mechanism

***Syndrome/Gene/Locus:***

Pendred syndrome/solute carrier family 26, member 4 (*SLC26A4*)/7q31

*SLC26A4* encodes the 780-amino acid (86-kd) protein, pendrin, which functions as a chloride, iodide, bicarbonate, and formate transporter. The protein is expressed in the endolymphatic sac and duct epithelium, on the apical membrane of transitional calls in the saccule, utricle, and ampulla and in many different cell types of the cochlea where it is thought to help condition endolymph pH and maintain ionic balance in the endolymphatic fluid. Pendrin is also expressed in the apical membrane of the thyroid follicular cells where it may play a role in mediating apical iodide efflux into the endolymph. Pendrin is also expressed in kidney, airways, mammary gland, testis, placenta, endometrium, and liver.

Usher syndrome type 1B/myosin VIIA (*MYO7A*)/11q13.5

Usher syndrome type 1C/Usher syndrome 1C (autosomal recessive, severe) (*USH1C*)/11p15.1

Usher syndrome ype 1D/cadherin-related23 (*CDH23*)/10q21-q22

Usher syndrome type 1F/protocadherin-related 15 (*PCDH15*)/ 10q21-q22

Usher syndrome type 1G/Usher syndrome 1G (autosomal recessive) (*USH1G*)/17q24-q25

**Table 152-4 Molecular Genetic Testing**

| Gene | Missense | Truncating[a] | Partial or Full gene Deletion/Duplication | Regulatory |
|------|----------|------------|-------------------------------------------|------------|
| SLC26A4 | Pendred, DFNB4 | Pendred, DFNB4 | Pendred | Pendred |
| MYO7A | Usher, AR NSHL, AD NSHL | Usher | Usher (deletion) | |
| USH1C | Usher, AR NSHL | Usher, AR NSHL | Usher (deletion) | |
| CDH23 | Usher, AR NSHL | Usher | Usher (deletion) | |
| PCDH15 | Usher, AR NSHL | Usher | Usher (deletion/duplication) | |
| USH1G | Usher | Usher | | |
| USH2A | Usher, AR RP | Usher, AR RP | Usher (deletion) | |
| GPR98 | Usher | Usher | Usher (deletion) | |
| DFNB31 | Usher, AR NSHL | Usher, AR NSHL | | |
| CLRN1 | Usher | Usher | | |

[a]Truncating mutations include splice-site mutations, nonsense mutations, and frameshift mutations.

AR NSHL, autosomal recessive nonsyndromic hearing loss; AD NSHL, autosomal dominant nonsyndromic hearing loss; AR RP, autosomal recessive retinitis pigmentosa.

Usher syndrome type 2A/Usher syndrome 2A (autosomal recessive, mild) (*USH2A*)/1q41

Usher syndrome type 2C/G protein-coupled receptor 98 (*GPR98*)/5q14.3

Usher syndrome type 2D/deafness, autosomal recessive 31 (*DFNB31*)/9q32-q34

Usher syndrome type 3A/clarin 1 (*CLRN1*)/3q21-q25

Most of the Usher proteins are large proteins expressed in the inner hair cells of the cochlea and photoreceptor cells of the retina. These proteins interact to form a network of proteins that are involved in maintaining the structure and function of the inner hair cell stereocilia as well as functioning in the photoreceptor cells. Specifically many of the proteins are expressed in the connecting cillium of the photoreceptor cells.

**Genetic Testing:** Testing for *SLC26A4* is available (GeneTests) and includes DNA sequencing of the coding regions and splice junctions of the gene. Pathogenic mutations in the *SLC26A4* gene were identified in 30% (14/47) of sporadic cases and 82% (9/11) of hereditary cases of hearing loss with EVA. However, only 9/23 (three simplex, six multiplex) had mutations detected on both alleles. Therefore, some mutations probably reside outside these coding regions or are not detectable by typical molecular approaches. At least one large deletion has been reported in *SLC26A4*, which would not be detectable by DNA sequencing, but would be detectable by deletion or duplication test methodologies (Table 152-4). *FOXI1* and *KCNJ10* have been suggested to be rare causes Pendred syndrome or DFNB4 when mutations in those genes are seen in double heterozygosity with a *SLC26A4* mutation; however, these studies have not been replicated.

Current testing for Usher syndrome includes DNA sequencing of all nine identified genes (*MYO7A, USH1C, CDH23, PCDH15, USH1G, USH2A, GPR98, DFNB31,* and *CLRN1*) either through individual gene tests or as a panel of all nine genes (GeneTests). In addition to point mutations detectable by sequencing, deletions and duplications have also been described for most of the Usher genes and deletion/duplication testing is now available for all nine genes (Table 152-4). Genotyping tests are also available for individuals of certain ancestral backgrounds known to have founder mutations: Arg245X in *PCDH15* and Asn48Lys in *CLRN1* for the Ashkenazi Jewish population, 216G>A in *USH1C* and 4338_4339delCT in *USH2A* for the Acadian or French Canadian population and Tyr176X in *CLRN1* for the Finnish population.

**BIBLIOGRAPHY:**

1. Azaiez H, Yang T, Prasad S, et al. Genotype-phenotype correlations for SLC26A4-related deafness. *Hum Genet.* 2007;122:451-457.
2. Boughman JA, Vernon M, Shaver KA. Usher syndrome: definition and estimate of prevalence from two high-risk populations. *J Chronic Dis.* 1983;36:595-603.
3. Rosenberg T, Haim M, Hauch AM, Parving A. The prevalence of Usher syndrome and other retinal dystrophy-hearing impairment associations. *Clin Genet.* 1997;51:314-321.
4. Kimberling WJ, Hildebrand MS, Shearer AE, et al. Frequency of Usher syndrome in two pediatric populations: implications for genetic screening of deaf and hard of hearing children. *Genet Med.* 2010;12:512-516.
5. Pakarinen L, Karjalainen S, Simola KO, Laippala P, Kaitalo H. Usher's syndrome type 3 in Finland. *Laryngoscope.* Jun 1995;105(6):613-617.
6. Ness SL, Ben-Yosef T, Bar-Lev A, et al. Genetic homogeneity and phenotypic variability among Ashkenazi Jews with Usher syndrome type III. *J Med Genet.* Oct 2003;40(10):767-772.
7. Hartong DT, Berson EL, Dryja TP. Retinitis pigmentosa. *Lancet.* Nov 18 2006;368(9549):1795-1809.
8. Teschner M, Neuburger J, Gockeln R, Lenarz T, Lesinski-Schiedat A. "Minimized rotational vestibular testing" as a screening procedure detecting vestibular areflexy in deaf children: screening cochlear implant candidates for Usher syndrome type I. *Eur Arch Otorhinolaryngol.* 2008;265:759-763.
9. Cohen M, Bitner-Glindzicz M, Luxon L. The changing face of Usher syndrome: clinical implications. *Int J Audiol.* 2007;46:82-93.
10. Fraser GR. Association of congenital deafness with goitre (Pendred's syndrome) a study of 207 families. *Ann Hum Genet.* 1965;28:201-249.
11. Park HJ, Shaukat S, Liu XZ, et al. Origins and frequencies of SLC26A4 (PDS) mutations in east and south Asians: global implications for the epidemiology of deafness. *J Med Genet.* 2003;40:242-248.
12. Luxon LM, Cohen M, Coffey RA, et al. Neuro-otological findings in Pendred syndrome. *Int J Audiol.* 2003;42:82-88.

13. Ito T, Choi BY, King KA, et al. SLC26A4 genotypes and phenotypes associated with enlargement of the vestibular aqueduct. *Cell Physiol Biochem*. 2011;28:545-552.

14. Pryor SP, Madeo AC, Reynolds JC, et al. SLC26A4/PDS genotype-phenotype correlation in hearing loss with enlargement of the vestibular aqueduct (EVA): evidence that Pendred syndrome and non-syndromic EVA are distinct clinical and genetic entities. *J Med Genet*. 2005;42:159-165.

15. Alasti F, Van Camp G, Smith RJH (Updated 12/22/2011). Pendred syndrome/DFNB4. In: GeneReviews at GeneTests: Medical Genetics Information Resource (database online). University of Washington, Seattle. 1997-2011. http://www.genetests.org. Accessed August, 2012.

16. Schultz JM, Bhatti R, Madeo AC, et al. Allelic hierarchy of CDH23 mutations causing non-syndromic deafness DFNB12 or Usher syndrome USH1D in compound heterozygotes. *J Med Genet*. 2011;48:767-775.

17. Ebermann I, Scholl HP, Charbel Issa P, Becirovic E, Lamprecht J, Jurklies B, Millán JM, Aller E, Mitter D, Bolz H. A novel gene for Usher syndrome type 2: mutations in the long isoform of whirlin are associated with retinitis pigmentosa and sensorineural hearing loss. *Hum Genet*. 2007;121(2):203-211.

18. Ahmed ZM, Riazuddin S, Aye S, et al. Gene structure and mutant alleles of PCDH15: nonsyndromic deafness DFNB23 and type 1 Usher syndrome. *Hum Genet*. 2008;124:215-223.

19. Ouyang XM, Xia XJ, Verpy E, et al. Mutations in the alternatively spliced exons of USH1C cause non-syndromic recessive deafness. *Hum Genet*. 2002;111:26-30.

20. Berson EL, Rosner B, Sandberg MA, et al. A randomized trial of vitamin A and vitamin E supplementation for retinitis pigmentosa. *Arch Ophthalmol*. 1993;111:761-772.

21. Peng YW, Zallocchi M, Wang WM, Delimont D, Cosgrove D. Moderate light-induced degeneration of rod photoreceptors with delayed transducin translocation in shaker1 mice. *Invest Ophthalmol Vis Sci*. 2011;52(9):6421-6427.

22. Valente LM. Assessment techniques for vestibular evaluation in pediatric patients. *Otolaryngol Clin North Am*. 2011;44:273-290.

23. Alasti F, Van Camp G, Smith RJH. Pendred Syndrome/DFNB4. *GeneReviews*. 1998 Sep 28 [Updated 2012 Dec 20].

24. Choi BY, Muskett J, King KA, et al. Hereditary hearing loss with thyroid abnormalities. *Adv Otorhinolaryngol*. 2011;70:43-49.

25. Dossena S, Nofziger C, Tamma G, et al. Molecular and functional characterization of human pendrin and its allelic variants. *Cell Physiol Biochem*. 2011;28:451-466.

26. Reiners J, Nagel-Wolfrum K, Jürgens K, Märker T, Wolfrum U. Molecular basis of human Usher syndrome: deciphering the meshes of the Usher protein network provides insights into the pathomechanisms of the Usher disease. *Exp Eye Res*. 2006;83:97-119.

27. Campbell C, Cucci RA, Prasad S, Green GE, Edeal JB, Galer CE, Karniski LP, Sheffield VC, Smith RJ. Pendred syndrome, DFNB4, and PDS/SLC26A4 identification of eight novel mutations and possible genotype-phenotype correlations. *Hum Mutat*. 2001;17(5):403-411.

28. Pera A, Villamar M, Viñuela A, et al. A mutational analysis of the SLC26A4 gene in Spanish hearing-impaired families provides new insights into the genetic causes of Pendred syndrome and DFNB4 hearing loss. *Eur J Hum Genet*. 2008;16:888-896.

29. Yang T, Gurrola JG, Wu H, et al. Mutations of KCNJ10 together with mutations of SLC26A4 cause digenic nonsyndromic hearing loss associated with enlarged vestibular aqueduct syndrome. *Am J Hum Genet*. 2009;84:651-657.

30. Yang T, Vidarsson H, Rodrigo-Blomqvist S, Rosengren SS, Enerback S, Smith RJ. Transcriptional control of SLC26A4 is involved in Pendred syndrome and nonsyndromic enlargement of vestibular aqueduct (DFNB4). *Am J Hum Genet*. 2007;80:1055-1063.

31. Aller E, Jaijo T, García-García G, et al. Identification of large rearrangements of the PCDH15 gene by combined MLPA and a CGH: large duplications are responsible for Usher syndrome. *Invest Ophthalmol Vis Sci*. 2010;51:5480-5485.

32. Hilgert N, Kahrizi K, Dieltjens N, et al. A large deletion in GPR98 causes type IIC Usher syndrome in male and female members of an Iranian family. *J Med Genet*. 2009;46:272-276.

33. Le Guédard S, Faugère V, Malcolm S, Claustres M, Roux AF. Large genomic rearrangements within the PCDH15 gene are a significant cause of USH1F syndrome. *Mol Vis*. 26 2007;13:102-107.

34. Bitner-Glindzicz M, Lindley KJ, Rutland P, et al. A recessive contiguous gene deletion causing infantile hyperinsulinism, enteropathy and deafness identifies the Usher type 1C gene. *Nat Genet*. 2000;26:56-60.

35. Aleman TS, Duncan JL, Bieber ML, et al. Macular pigment and lutein supplementation in retinitis pigmentosa and Usher syndrome. *Invest Ophthalmol Vis Sci*. 2001;42:1873-1881.

36. GeneTests: Medical Genetics Information Resource (database online). Copyright, University of Washington, Seattle. 1993-2011. http://www.genetests.org. Accessed August, 2011.

## Supplementary Information

**OMIM References:**

[1] Pendred Syndrome; SLC26A4 (#274600)

[2] Usher Syndrome Type 1B; MYO7A (#276900)

[3] Usher Syndrome Type 1C; USH1C (#276904)

[4] Usher Syndrome Type 1D; CDH23 (#601067)

[5] Usher Syndrome Type 1F; PCDH15 (#602083)

[6] Usher Syndrome Type 1G; USH1G (#606943)

[7] Usher Syndrome Type 2A; USH2A (#276901)

[8] Usher Syndrome Type 2C; GPR98 (#605472)

[9] Usher Syndrome Type 2D; DFNB31 (#611383)

[10] Usher Syndrome Type 3A; CLRN1 (#276902)

**Alternative Names:**

- Usher Syndrome
  - Retinitis Pigmentosa and Congenital Deafness
- Pendred Syndrome
  - Deafness With Goiter
  - Goiter-Deafness Syndrome
  - Thyroid Dyshormonogenesis 2B; TDH2B
  - Thyroid Hormonogenesis, Genetic Defect in, 2B
  - Hypothyroidism, Congenital, due to Dyshormonogenesis, 2B
  - SLC26A4-Related Pendred Syndrome
  - Enlarged Vestibular Aqueduct and Goiter
- DFNB4; Deafness, Autosomal Recessive 4
  - Enlarged Vestibular Aqueduct; EVA
  - Deafness, Autosomal Recessive 4; DFNB4
  - Neurosensory Nonsyndromic Recessive Deafness 4; NSRD4
  - Dilated Vestibular Aqueduct; DVA
  - DFNB4 Nonsyndromic Hearing Impairment and EVA

*Key Words:* Sensorineural hearing loss, hearing loss, retinitis pigmentosa, enlarged vestibular aqueduct, dilated vestibular aqueduct, Mondini dysplasia, temporal bone, goiter, night blindness

# 153 Waardenburg Syndrome

Seema Jamal and Jeffrey M. Milunksy

## KEY POINTS

- *Disease summary:*
  - Waardenburg syndrome types 1 to 4 are a group of auditory-pigmentary syndromes that comprise sensorineural hearing loss (due to the absence of melanocytes in the stria vascularis of the cochlea), and hypomelanosis of the eyes, hair, and/or skin.
  - Since Waardenburg syndrome types 1 to 4 are disorders related to neural crest cells and their derivatives, they are considered to be neurocristopathies.

- *Hereditary basis:*
  - Waardenburg syndrome is one of the most common syndromic causes of hearing loss and accounts for approximately 2% to 5% of all congenital sensorineural hearing loss.
  - Waardenburg syndrome demonstrates both inter- and intrafamilial variable expressivity, as well as locus and allelic heterogeneity.
  - Waardenburg syndrome type 1 (WS1), Waardenburg syndrome type 2 (WS2), and Waardenburg syndrome type 3 (WS3) are transmitted in an autosomal dominant manner, while Waardenburg syndrome type 4 (WS4) is inherited either as an autosomal recessive condition, with mutations within the endothelin-3 (*EDN3*) or endothelin-B receptor (*EDNRB*) genes, or as an autosomal dominant condition with heterozygous mutations within the SRY-related HMG-box 10 (*SOX10*) gene.

- *Differential diagnosis:*
  - Well over 400 genetic syndromes that include hearing loss have been described. While nonsyndromic hearing loss accounts for the vast majority of hearing loss, syndromic hearing impairment is thought to account for up to 30% of prelingual deafness.
  - Piebaldism [MIM 172800] is an autosomal dominant condition that has a clinical phenotype similar to that of Waardenburg syndrome. A white forelock is commonly seen along with absent pigmentation of the medial forehead, eyebrows, chest, abdomen, and limbs. A characteristic feature is hyperpigmented borders surrounding the hypopigmented areas. In contrast to Waardenburg syndrome, hearing loss is not characteristic of this syndrome.
  - Tietze syndrome [MIM 103500] is an autosomal dominant condition characterized by congenital hearing loss and uniform hypopigmentation. Tietze syndrome is allelic to WS2 with heterozygous mutations within the *MITF* gene described in affected individuals. In contrast to WS2, the Tietze phenotype does not include heterochromia.
  - Craniofacial-deafness-hand syndrome [MIM 122880] is an autosomal dominant condition with characteristic facial features, profound sensorineural hearing loss, and radiologic abnormalities of the maxilla, nasal bones, and hands. This condition is also allelic to WS1 and WS3 with a heterozygous mutation within the *PAX3* gene described in an affected individual.

## Diagnostic Criteria and Clinical Characteristics

**Diagnostic Criteria for Waardenburg Syndrome Type 1 (as proposed by the Waardenburg Consortium):**

**An individual must have two major criteria *or* one major and two minor criteria:**

Major criteria
- Congenital sensorineural hearing loss
- Hair hypopigmentation
  - White forelock
  - White hairs within eyebrow, eyelashes
- Pigmentation abnormality of the iris
  - Complete heterochromia iridum (irides of different color)
  - Partial or segmental heterochromia (two different colors in same iris, typically brown and blue)
  - Hypoplastic blue irides, or brilliant blue (sapphire) irides
- Dystopia canthorum: W index >1.95*
- First-degree relative (parent, sibling, or offspring) with WS1 as defined by the above criteria

Minor criteria
- Skin hypopigmentation (congenital leukoderma)
- Synophrys or medial eyebrow flare
- Broad high nasal root, prominent columella
- Hypoplasia of the alae nasi
- Premature graying of the hair (before age 30 years)

*W index: The measurements necessary to calculate the W index (in mm) are as follows: inner canthal distance (a), interpupillary distance (b), and outer canthal distance (c).

Calculate $X = (2a - 0.2119c + 3.909)/c$
Calculate $Y = (2a - 0.2479b + 3.909)/b$
Calculate $W = X + Y + a/b$
An abnormal W index result is greater than 1.95.

**Diagnostic Criteria for Waardenburg Syndrome Type 2:**
**An individual must have two criteria:**
- Congenital sensorineural hearing loss
- Hair hypopigmentation
  - White forelock
  - White hairs within eyebrow, eyelashes
- Pigmentation abnormality of the iris
  - Complete heterochromia iridum (irides of different color)
  - Partial or segmental heterochromia (two different colors in same iris, typically brown and blue)
  - Hypoplastic blue irides, or brilliant blue (sapphire) irides

- First-degree relative (parent, sibling, or offspring) with WS2 as defined by the above criteria

**And the absence of**
- Dystopia canthorum: Thus, W-index should be less than 1.95.

### Diagnostic Criteria for Waardenburg Syndrome Type 3:
**An individual must have the presence of**
- WS1 features (+ dystopia canthorum)

And
- Skeletal abnormalities
  - Axial or limb anomalies
    - Hypoplasia of the musculoskeletal system
    - Flexion contractures of the fingers
    - Fusion of the carpal bones
    - Syndactyly

### Diagnostic Criteria for Waardenburg Syndrome Type 4:
**An individual must have the presence of**
- Waardenburg syndrome features (+/− dystopia canthorum)

And
- Intestinal dysfunction: often presents as chronic unremitting constipation
  - Hirschsprung disease
    - Total colonic aganglionosis: includes the entire large intestine
    - Long segment colonic aganglionosis: proximal to the sigmoid colon
    - Short segment colonic aganglionosis: restricted to the rectosigmoid colon
  - Chronic intestinal pseudo-obstruction*

*Chronic intestinal pseudo-obstruction is defined as repetitive episodes or continuous symptoms of bowel obstruction, in the absence of a mechanical occluding lesion.

**Clinical Characteristics:** Refer to Table 153-1.

☞**Waardenburg Syndrome Type 1:** Dystopia canthorum is observed in virtually all individuals with WS1. The hearing loss observed in 60% of patients with WS1 is typically congenital, sensorineural, nonprogressive, and unilateral or bilateral. Most often the hearing loss is bilateral and profound (>100 dB). The majority of individuals with WS1 have either a classic white forelock (observed in ~45% of affected individuals) or premature graying of the scalp hair. The classic white forelock and congenital leukoderma are more common in WS1 than WS2. While the classic forelock is most commonly in the midline, the patch of white hair may also be elsewhere. Other associated features occurring rarely include cleft lip and/or palate and spina bifida.

☞**Waardenburg Syndrome Type 2:** The main distinguishing feature between WS2 and WS1 is the absence of dystopia canthorum. Hearing loss and heterochromia iridum are the two most characteristic features of WS2. Both features are more common in WS2 than WS1.

☞**Waardenburg Syndrome Type 3:** WS3 is an allelic disorder to WS1 caused by mutations in the *PAX3* gene. Skeletal malformations in WS3 range from minimal contractures of the fingers with or without syndactyly to hypoplasia of the upper limbs and/or pectoral girdle. Other skeletal abnormalities observed in affected individuals include hypoplastic or absent terminal phalanges of the toes.

☞**Waardenburg Syndrome Type 4:** Intestinal dysfunction is a feature unique to this type of Waardenburg syndrome.

**Table 153-1  System Involvement**

| Clinical Findings | Percent of Affected Individuals | |
| --- | --- | --- |
| | WS1 | WS2 |
| Sensorineural hearing loss | 47%-58% | 77%-80% |
| White forelock | 43%-48% | 16%-23% |
| Complete heterochromia irides | 15%-31% | 42%-54% |
| Partial heterochromia irides | 4% | 27% |
| Hypoplastic blue eyes | 15%-18% | 3%-23% |
| Dystopia canthorum | ~100% | 0% |
| Leukoderma | 22%-36% | 5%-12% |
| Medial eyebrow flare | 63%-73% | 7%-12% |
| Broad/high nasal root | 52%-100% | 0%-14% |
| Early graying | 23%-38% | 14%-30% |

(Liu et al. 1995) (Pardono et al. 2003) (Tamayo et al. 2008) (Read et al. 1997)

Precise percentage of clinical findings within WS3 and WS4 is not yet known. Skeletal abnormalities are characteristic of WS3, and intestinal dysfunction is characteristic of WS4.

All forms of Hirschsprung disease have been described in individuals with WS4, with total colonic aganglionosis being the most prevalent. Symptoms of short segment Hirschsprung disease include chronic constipation, malabsorption, and enterocolitis. Long-segment Hirschsprung disease presents with intestinal obstruction findings such as bilious vomiting, abdominal distention, inability to feed orally in the first few days of life, and delayed meconium passage. Neurologic symptoms including peripheral demyelinating neuropathy and central neuropathy are typically only observed in affected individuals with terminal *SOX10* mutations. In addition, the penetrance of Hirschsprung disease is close to 100% in individuals with *SOX10* mutations, whereas it is not as prevalent in individuals with *EDN3* or *ENDRB* mutations. Other dysautonomic features including asialia, alacrima, and reduced sweating may also be observed in affected individuals with *SOX10* mutations.

## Screening and Counseling

**Screening:** An algorithm for the diagnostic evaluation of a patient suspected of having Waardenburg syndrome is outlined in Fig. 153-1.

**Counseling:** WS1, WS2, WS3, and WS4 when associated with *SOX10* gene mutations are transmitted in an autosomal dominant fashion. Each child of an affected parent has a 50% chance of inheriting the condition. WS4, when associated with *EDN3* or *EDNRB* gene mutations, is inherited in an autosomal recessive fashion. Siblings of an affected individual have a two-thirds chance of being a carrier. Parents of an affected child are obligate carriers and have a 25% recurrence risk in each pregnancy of having an affected child. *EDN3* or *EDNRB* carrier individuals may be asymptomatic or have some features of WS4 including Hirschsprung disease. Prenatal diagnosis is clinically available for pregnancies at increased risk. Testing can determine whether a fetus has inherited a familial mutation, however it cannot determine the clinical manifestations or their severity.

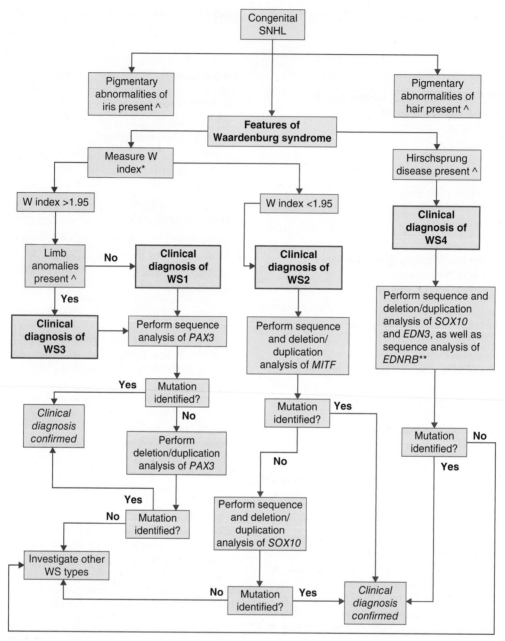

***Figure 153-1*** Algorithm for Diagnostic Evaluation of a Patient With Waardenburg Syndrome.

SNHL, sensorineural hearing loss.

*W index: The measurements necessary to calculate the W index (in mm) are as follows: inner canthal distance (a), interpupillary distance (b), and outer canthal distance (c).

Calculate $X = (2a - 0.2119c + 3.909)/c$; calculate $Y = (2a - 0.2479b + 3.909)/b$; calculate $W = X + Y + a/b$

^Consult Diagnostic Criteria and Clinical Characteristics for further details.

**If neurologic symptoms present, perform sequence and deletion analysis of *SOX10*. If negative, then proceed to *EDNRB*, *EDN3* analysis. If <u>no</u> neurologic symptoms present, perform sequence analysis of *EDNRB*, and *EDN3*. If negative, then proceed to *SOX10* analysis.

Given that the *PAX3* gene is expressed in the neural crest, folic acid supplementation in pregnancy is recommended for women at increased risk of having a child with WS1 due to the possible increased risk of neural tube defects in association with WS1.

Although the majority of individuals with WS1 have an affected parent, a minority of individuals do not have and are presumed to have a de novo mutation. In situations of apparent de novo mutations, germline mosaicism in an unaffected parent needs to be considered. Additionally, possible nonmedical explanations including nonpaternity or maternity (eg, with assisted reproduction) or undisclosed adoption could also be explored.

WS1 is thought to have penetrance close to 100%. However, due to variable expressivity, it is not uncommon for a parent of an affected individual to escape diagnosis due to a milder phenotypic expression. Penetrance for the other WS types has not been determined.

☞**Genotype-Phenotype Correlation:** Genotype-phenotype correlations in the *PAX3* gene are not well established, aside for the Asn47His (N47H) mutation in WS3, and the Asn47Lys (N47K) mutation described in craniofacial-deafness-hand Syndrome. Homozygosity for the Tyr90His (Y90H) *PAX3* mutation has been described in an individual with WS3. Both parents were confirmed to be heterozygous for the mutation and had evidence of dystopia canthorum, while only the father had a white forelock. It was proposed that heterozygous inheritance of the *Y90H* mutation causes WS1, while homozygosity leads to a more severe phenotype as seen in patients with WS3. There appears to be no appreciable difference in severity between partial and whole *PAX3* gene deletions and other mutations described within the *PAX3* gene.

Somatic *PAX3* mutations have been observed in alveolar rhabdomyosarcoma. Specifically, a recurring acquired chromosomal translocation t(2;13)(q35;q14) creates a novel fusion gene whereby the 5' region of the *PAX3* gene including the first seven exons is juxtaposed to the 3' region of the *FKHR* gene including the last two exons. This fusion gene creates a gain-of-function mechanism that results in alveolar rhabdomyosarcoma. Individuals with alveolar rhabdomyosarcoma resulting from this mechanism do not have Waardenburg syndrome.

Mutations within the *MITF* gene are causative of WS2 and Tietze syndrome. A recurring in-frame 3-bp deletion (ΔR217) has been described as causative of Tietze syndrome, and the missense Asn210Lys (*N210K*) mutation has also been described in a seven-generation family with Tietze syndrome.

Mutations within the *SOX10* gene are causative of WS4 and WS2 syndromes. Some individuals with *SOX10* mutations present with neurologic features, either peripheral demyelinating neuropathy, central neuropathy or both, which leads to a syndrome called PCWH: peripheral demyelinating neuropathy, central dysmyelinating leukodystrophy, Waardenburg syndrome, and Hirschsprung disease. Truncating mutations located in the first coding exons (exons 3 and 4) activate the nonsense-mediated mRNA decay (NMD) pathway, leading to haploinsufficiency and the classic form of WS4. Truncating mutations located in the last coding exon (exon 5) escape NMD, leading to translation of an abnormal SOX10 protein with a dominant negative effect and thus resulting in the more severe PCWH phenotype. Deletions of single and multiple exons, as well as the entire gene have been described in individuals with WS2 and WS4.

Homozygous or compound heterozygous mutations within the *EDN3* gene are causative of WS4, while heterozygous mutations have been observed in individuals with isolated Hirschsprung disease. The *EDN3* gene is a susceptibility gene for Hirschsprung disease with mutations within this gene accounting for approximately 5% of all Hirschsprung disease. Haddad syndrome (congenital central hypoventilation syndrome [MIM 209880] with Hirschsprung disease) has been described in one patient with a 1bp insertion within exon 4 of the *EDN3* gene.

Homozygous or compound heterozygous mutations within the *EDNRB* gene are causative of WS4, while heterozygous mutations have also been observed in individuals with isolated Hirschsprung disease. The *EDNRB* gene is also a susceptibility gene for Hirschsprung disease, and mutations within this gene accounts for approximately 7% of all Hirschsprung disease. In 1995, Gross et al. described a consanguineous Kurdish family of five siblings with albinism, black locks, cell migration disorder of the neurocytes of the gut, and deafness, demonstrating autosomal recessive inheritance. This syndrome was named ABCD [MIM 600501]. In 2002, Verheij et al. examined the initial proband of this family, and discovered that homozygosity for the Arg201Term (*R201X*) mutation within the *EDNRB* gene was causative of ABCD. It was proposed by the authors that ABCD syndrome is not a separate entity, but rather an expression of WS4.

## Management and Treatment

Evaluations following an initial or suspected diagnosis of Waardenburg syndrome should include a thorough clinical and family history, an audiology assessment, and physical examination to assess facial features, calculating the W index, examining the skin and hair for hypopigmentation, and to assess for upper limb anomalies. For individuals suspected of having WS4, an abdominal x-ray, barium enema, anorectal manometry, and rectal biopsy may be required.

As the hearing loss in Waardenburg syndrome is most often nonprogressive, repeating audiograms is typically not necessary. As profound hearing loss is typical for Waardenburg syndrome, amplification is typically of limited benefit. Cochlear implantation is a well-established method of auditory rehabilitation for children with severe-profound sensorineural hearing loss. Children with Waardenburg syndrome benefit from cochlear implantation to an extent that is comparable to the general population of implanted children. Some individuals with Waardenburg syndrome have abnormalities of the bony architecture of the inner ear, including hypoplasia of the cochlea and internal acoustic canal, and absence of the posterior semicircular canal. Additionally, a poorly developed vestibule, and short, stubby semicircular canals have also been described. Therefore, a high-resolution computed tomography (CT) of the temporal bone in the workup of a patient with Waardenburg syndrome to determine candidacy for cochlear implantation may be considered.

For individuals with Hirschsprung disease, treatment includes surgical resection of the aganglionic bowel.

## Molecular Genetics and Molecular Mechanism

**Syndrome/Gene/Locus:**

WS1/paired box 3 (*PAX3*)/2q36.1
WS2/microphthalmia-associated transcription factor (*MITF*)/3p14.1
   Other WS2 loci: SRY-related HMG-box 10 (*SOX10*)/22q13.1
      Unknown gene/1p21-p13.3
      Unknown gene/8p23
WS3/paired box 3 (*PAX3*)/2q36.1
WS4/SRY-related HMG-box 10 (*SOX10*)/22q13
   Other WS4 loci: endothelin 3 (*EDN3*)/20q13.32
      Endothelin 3 receptor type B (*EDNRB*)/13q22.3

**Gene Function:** The *PAX3* gene is comprised of ten exons, with the paired box DNA-binding domain housed within exons 2 to 4, and the homeobox DNA-binding domain within exons 5 to 6. The C-terminal region contains a proline-, serine- and threonine-rich transactivation domain. The *PAX3* gene is a member of the paired box (PAX) family of transcription factors which are known to play critical roles during fetal development.

The *MITF* gene is comprised of twelve exons, and the first four exons (exon 1A, exon 1H, exon 1B, exon 1M) are isoform specific exons with alternative promotors. These alternatively spliced transcript variants play a critical role in the differentiation of various cell types as neural crest-derived melanocytes, mast cells, osteoclasts, and optic cup-derived retinal pigment epithelium. The remaining eight exons, 2 to 9, are common to all isoforms.

The *SOX10* gene is comprised of five exons, while only exons 3 to 5 encode the SOX10 protein. The *SOX10* gene encodes a member of the SOX (SRY-related HMG-box) family of transcription factors involved in the regulation of embryonic development and in the determination of the cell fate. The encoded protein acts as a nucleocytoplasmic shuttle protein and is important for neural crest and peripheral nervous system development. The *SOX10* gene contains an HMG domain and a transactivation domain. Similar to other HMG proteins, SOX10 binds its target DNA sequences via its HMG domain. Mutations in the HMG box disrupt SOX10 structure and compromise its binding to DNA. Similar to the *PAX3* gene, the C-terminal region of the *SOX10* gene contains a proline-, serine- and glutamine-rich transactivation domain. Deletion of this region abolishes the ability of SOX10 to induce promoter activity of its target genes in vitro.

The *EDN3* gene is comprised of five exons. The protein encoded by the *EDN3* gene is a member of the endothelin family, which are vasoactive peptides involved in a variety of biologic functions. The EDN3 protein is a ligand for endothelin receptor type B (EDNRB). The interaction of EDN3 with EDNRB is essential for development of neural crest-derived cell lineages, such as melanocytes and enteric neurons.

The *EDNRB* gene is comprised of seven exons and six introns. Each intron occurs near the border of the putative transmembrane domain in the coding region.

**Genetic Testing:** DNA sequence analysis is clinically available for the *PAX3*, *MITF*, *SOX10*, *EDNRB*, and *EDN3* genes. Deletion or duplication analysis via multiplex ligation-dependent probe amplification (MLPA) is also clinically available for the *PAX3*, *MITF*, *SOX10*, and *EDN3* genes (see GeneTests: http://www.genetests.org/).

More than 110 mutations spread throughout the *PAX3* gene have been reported (http://www.hgmd.cf.ac.uk/docs/login.html. Accessed August 27, 2013) as causative of WS1. Missense mutations within the *PAX3* gene have also been reported as causative of WS3. The majority of these mutations are nucleotide substitutions resulting in missense mutations, usually in the regions encoding the paired box or homeobox-binding domains. Thirty-six mutations spread throughout the *MITF* gene have been reported (http://www.hgmd.cf.ac.uk/docs/login.html. Accessed August 27, 2013). More than 80 predominantly nonsense and frameshift mutations spread throughout the *SOX10* gene have been reported (http://www.hgmd.cf.ac.uk/docs/login.html. Accessed August 27, 2013) to be causative of WS4 or a more severe phenotype: peripheral demyelinating neuropathy, central dysmyelinating leukodystrophy, Waardenburg syndrome, Hirschsprung disease (PCWH). Deletions and point mutations within the *SOX10* gene have been reported as causative of WS2. Nineteen mutations spread throughout the *EDN3* gene have been reported (http://www.hgmd.cf.ac.uk/docs/login. html. Accessed August 27, 2013) to be causative of WS4 or isolated Hirschsprung disease. More than 50 mutations spread throughout the *EDNRB* gene have been reported http://www.hgmd.cf.ac.uk/docs/login.html. Accessed August 27, 2013) to be causative of WS4 or isolated Hirschsprung disease.

The decision about which gene to test first is often based on overall incidence of mutations. For detection rates, please refer to Table 153-2.

**Table 153-2 *Molecular Genetic Testing***

| Gene | Testing Modality | Mutation Type | Detection Rate | |
|------|-----------------|---------------|----------------|---|
| *PAX3* | Sequence analysis | Missense, nonsense, splice site, small deletions, small insertions | WS1/WS3 | >90% |
| | Deletion/duplication analysis | Partial/whole exon deletions, entire gene deletions | WS1/WS3 | ~6% |
| *MITF* | Sequence analysis | Missense, nonsense, splice site, small deletions | | ~10%-20% |
| | Deletion/duplication analysis | | | Unknown |
| *SOX10* | Sequence analysis | Missense, nonsense, small deletions, small insertions | WS2 | Unknown |
| | | | WS4 | ~40%-50% |
| | Deletion/duplication analysis | Partial/whole exon deletions, entire gene deletions | WS2 | ~15% |
| | | | WS4 | ~5% |
| *EDN3* | Sequence analysis | Missense, nonsense, small insertions | | ~20%-30% |
| | Deletion/duplication analysis | a | | |
| *EDNRB* | Sequence analysis | Missense, nonsense, splice site, small deletions, small insertions | | |

(Bondurand et al. 2007) (Milunsky et al. 2007) (HGMD)

[a]No gross deletions or duplications have been described. However, clinical testing is available.

**BIBLIOGRAPHY:**

1. Toriello H, Reardon W, Gorlin RJ. *Hereditary Hearing Loss and Its Syndromes.* Oxford University Press Inc., New York; 2004.

2. Pingault V, Guiochon-Mantel A, Bondurand N, et al. Peripheral neuropathy with hypomyelination, chronic intestinal pseudo-obstruction and deafness: a developmental "neural crest syndrome" related to a SOX10 mutation. *Ann Neurol.* 2000;48(4):671-676.

3. Farrer L, Grundfast KM, Amos J, et al. Waardenburg syndrome (WS) type I is caused by defects at multiple loci, one of which is near ALPP on chromosome 2: first Report of the WS Consortium. *Am J Hum* Genet. 1992;50:902-913.

4. Hoth C, Milunsky A, Lipsky N, Sheffer R, Clarren SK, Baldwin CT. Mutations in the paired domain of the human PAX3 gene cause Klein-Waardenburg syndrome (WS-III) as well as Waardenburg syndrome type I (WS-1). *Am J Hum Genet.* 1993;52:455-462.

5. Goodman R, Yahav Y, Frand M, Barzilay Z, Nissan E, Hertz M. A new white forelock (poliosis) syndrome with multiple congenital malformation in two sibs. *Clin Genet.* 1980;17(6):437-442.

6. Read AP, Newton VE. Waardenburg syndrome. *J Med Genet.* 1997; 34:656-665.

7. Asher JH Jr, Sommer A, Morell R, Friedman TB. Missense mutation in the paired domain of PAX3 causes craniofacial-deafness-hand syndrome. *Hum Mutat.* 1996;7(1):30-35.

8. Wollnick B, Tukel T, Uyguner O, et al. Homozygous and heterozygous inheritance of PAX3 mutations causes different types of Waardenburg syndrome. *Am J Med Genet.* 2003;122A:42-45.

9. Wang W, Fang WH, Krupinski J, Kumar S, Slevin M, Kumar P. Pax genes in embryogenesis and oncogenesis. *J Cell Mol Med.* 2008;12:2281-2294.

10. Tassabehji M. Newton VE, Liu XZ, et al. The mutational spectrum in Waardenburg syndrome. *Hum Mol Genet.* 1995;11:2131-2137.

11. Smith S, Kelley PM, Kenyon JB, Hoover D. Tietz syndrome (hypopigmentation/deafness) caused by mutation of MITF. *J Med Genet.* 2000;37:446-448.

12. Bondurand N, Dastot-Le Moal F, Stanchina L, et al. Deletions at the SOX10 gene locus cause Waardenburg syndrome types 2 and 4. *Am J Hum Genet.* 2007;81:1169-1185.

13. Bolk S, Angrist M, Xie J, et al. Endothelin-3 frameshift mutation in congenital central hypoventilation syndrome. *Nat Genet.* 1996;13(4):395-396.

14. Gross A, Kunze J, Maier RF, Stoltenburg-Didinger G, Grimmer I, Obladen M. Autosomal-recessive neural crest syndrome with albinism, black lock, cell migration disorder of the neurocytes of the gut, and deafness: ABCD syndrome. *Am J Med Genet.* 1995;56(3):322-326.

15. Verheij J, Kunze J, Osinga J, van Essen AJ, Hofstra RM. ABCD syndrome is caused by a homozygous mutation in the EDNRB gene. *Am J Med Genet.* 2002;108:223-225.

16. Migirov L, Henkin Y, Hildesheimer M, Muchnik C, Kronenberg J. Cochlear implantation in Waardenburg's syndrome. *Acta Otolaryngol.* 2005;125:713-717.

17. Oysu C, Oysu A, Aslan I, Tinaz M. Temporal bone imaging findings in Waardenburg's syndrome. *Int J Pediatr Otorhinolaryngol.* 2001;58:215-221.

18. Schweitzer VG, Clack TD. Waardenburg's syndrome: a case report with CT scanning and cochleovestibular evaluation. *Int J Pediatr Otorhinolaryngol.* 1984;7(3):311-322.

19. Udono T, Yasumoto K, Takeda K, et al. Structural organization of the human microphthalmia-associated transcription factor gene containing four alternative promotors. *Biochim Biophys Acta.* 2000;1491(1-3):205-219.

20. Pingault V, Bondurand N, Kuhlbrodt K, et al. SOX10 mutations in patients with Waardenburg-Hirschsprung disease. *Nat Genet.* 1998;18:171-173.

21. Mollaaghababa R, Pavan WJ. The importance of having your SOX on: role on SOX10 in the development of neural crest-derived melanocytes and glia. *Oncogene.* 2003;22:3024-3034.

22. Bondurand N, Pingault V, Goerich DE, et al. Interaction among SOX10, PAX3 and MITF, three genes altered in Waardenburg syndrome. *Hum Mol Genet.* 2000;9(13):1907-1917.

23. HGMD (database online). Copyright, Cardiff University, Cardiff. 2013. http://www.hgmd.cf.ac.uk/ac/index.php. Accessed August 27, 2013.

24. Iso M, Fukami M, Horikawa R, Azuma N, Kawashiro N, Ogata T. SOX10 mutation in Waardenburg syndrome type II. *Am J Med Genet.* 2008;146A:2162-2163.

25. Milunsky JM, Maher TA, Ito M, Milunsky A. The value of MLPA in Waardenburg syndrome. *Genet Test.* 2007;11(2):179-182.

26. Milunsky JM. (Updated August 4, 2009). Waardenburg syndrome type I. In: *GeneReviews* at GeneTests: Medical Genetics Information Resource (database online). Copyright, University of Washington, Seattle. 1997-2009. http://www.genetests.org. Accessed August 27, 2009.

27. Shah N, Dalal SJ, Desai MP, Sheth PN, Joshi NC, Ambani LM. White forelock, pigmentary disorder of irides, and long segment Hirschsprung disease: possible variant of Waardenburg syndrome. *J Pediatr.* 1981;99(3):432-435.

28. Liu XZ, Newton VE, Read AP. Waardenburg syndrome type II: phenotypic findings and diagnostic criteria. *Am J Med Genet.* 1995;55(1):95-100.

29. Pardono E, van Bever Y, van den Ende J, et al. Waardenburg syndrome: clinical differentiation between types I and II. *Am J Med Genet.* 2003;117A(3):223-35.

30. Tamayo ML, Gelvez N, Rodriguez M, et al. Screening program for Waardenburg syndrome in Colombia: clinical definition and phenotypic variability. *Am J Med Genet.* 2008;146A(8):1026-31.

## Supplementary Information

**OMIM REFERENCES:**

[1] Waardenburg Syndrome, Type 1; PAX3 (#193500)

[2] Waardenburg Syndrome, Type 2A; MITF (#193510)

[3] Waardenburg Syndrome, Type 2E; SOX10 (#611584)

[4] Waardenburg Syndrome, Type 3; PAX3 (#148820)

[5] Waardenburg Syndrome, Type 4; EDNRB (#131244), EDN3 (#131242), SOX10 (#602229)

**Alternative Names:**

• Waardenburg Syndrome Type 3: Klein-Waardenburg Syndrome
• Waardenburg Syndrome Type 4: Shah-Waardenburg Syndrome

*Key Words:* Waardenburg syndrome, sensorineural hearing loss, heterochromia, Hirschsprung disease, dystopia canthorum, white forelock, upper limb abnormalities, broad nasal root, early graying, colonic aganglionosis, cochlear implant, neurologic symptoms, hypopigmentation, leukoderma

# 154 Vestibular Schwannoma and Neurofibromatosis 2

Fabio P. Nunes and Scott R. Plotkin

## KEY POINTS

- *Disease summary:*
  - Vestibular schwannomas (formerly known as acoustic neuromas) are benign tumors arising from the vestibular branch of the VIII cranial nerve. Vestibular schwannomas (VS) are usually isolated tumors, but can occur as part of neurofibromatosis 2 tumor suppressor syndrome (NF2).
  - The most common presenting symptom of VS is unilateral hearing loss, often noticed when using the phone. Tinnitus, imbalance, and facial nerve dysfunction can also occur.
  - NF2 is a hereditary condition associated with presence of bilateral vestibular schwannomas (BVS), schwannomas of other cranial and peripheral nerves, meningiomas, gliomas (spinal ependymomas), and posterior subcapsular cataracts (Table 154-1).
  - The National Institutes of Health (NIH) diagnostic criteria for NF2 requires presence of BVS, or a first-degree family member with NF2 plus unilateral VS or two other NF2-associated features as detailed in Table 154-2. The modified diagnostic criteria were expanded to include patients with presumed NF2 who not yet meet NIH diagnostic criteria.
  - Average age of onset of NF2 is usually in the early 20s. Earlier age of onset is associated with heavier tumor burden and more severe disease.
  - About 25% to 30% of founders with bilateral VS are found to be mosaic for mutation in the *NF2* gene.
  - The likelihood of meeting criteria for NF2 after being diagnosed with a unilateral VS is inversely proportional to the age at diagnosis of the VS (Table 154-3).

- *Hereditary basis:*
  - Sporadic VS are not associated with higher recurrence rates in family members, although patients with NF2 may present with unilateral VS, prior to developing other tumors.
  - NF2 is an autosomal dominant condition, which gives an affected individual a 50% risk of passing the condition to their children.
  - NF2 is fully penetrant, meaning that individuals inheriting the mutated *NF2* gene will develop symptoms in 100% of the cases.

- *Monogenic forms:*
  - NF2 is caused by mutations in the *NF2* gene on chromosome 22.
  - The *NF2* gene codes for a cytoskeleton protein named merlin, and is involved in cell growth regulation.
  - NF2 is a classic tumor suppressor syndrome, requiring both copies of the *NF2* gene to be inactivated in the cell for tumor formation. In patients with NF2, the first *NF2* inactivation event is either inherited or occurs early in embryogenesis and is present in all cells of the body. The second inactivating event occurs in somatic cells and leads to formation of schwannomas, meningiomas, and ependymomas, depending on the type of cell involved.
  - Loss of *NF2* has been associated with sporadic VS formation. In sporadic tumors, both *NF2* inactivating events occur at the cellular level, with no *NF2* mutations found in nontumor tissues.

- *Family history:*
  - Children of patients with nonmosaic NF2 have a 50:50 risk of inheriting the disease. Siblings of patients with NF2 who have clinically unaffected parents are at a higher risk of developing NF2 than the general population due to the risk of low-level gonadal mosaicism in one of the parents. In practice, we find the risk of gonadal mosaicism to be small in unaffected parents of NF2 patients.

- *Environmental factors:*
  - There are no specific environmental factors associated with NF2 or VS formation. Although cell phone use has been suggested to be associated with an increased risk for brain tumor formation, no definitive research to date has found an association between VS and cell phone use. For patients with NF2, excessive use of radiation for diagnostic or therapeutic purposes should be avoided based on the theoretical risk of inducing tumor formation in patients with a tumor suppressor syndrome. Magnetic resonance imaging (MRI) scans are preferred to computed tomographic (CT) scans or x-rays when imaging is needed, particularly in children.

- *Differential diagnosis:*
  - Schwannomatosis (multiple central and peripheral schwannomas without VS, intradermal schwannomas, or any other NF2-associated tumors); multiple meningioma syndrome (two or more intracranial meningiomas without other clinical stigmata of NF2).

*Table 154-1 System Involvement in NF2*

| System | Manifestation | Incidence |
|---|---|---|
| Nervous system | Bilateral vestibular schwannomas | Almost 100% |
| | Schwannomas of other cranial nerves | 25% |
| | Intracranial meningiomas | 50% |
| | Gliomas (mostly spinal ependymomas) | 33%-53% |
| | Cutaneous schwannomas (peripheral nerves) | 68% |
| | Spinal tumors (spinal meningiomas and schwannomas) | 55% |
| | Peripheral neuropathy (probably underestimate) | 3%-5% |
| Eye | Posterior subcapsular cataracts (lenticular opacities) | 70%-80% |
| | Epiretinal membranes | 25% |

# Diagnostic Criteria and Clinical Characteristics

### Diagnostic Criteria:

**Clinical Characteristics:** Sporadic VS are relatively common benign tumors accounting for about 8% of all intracranial tumors. Initial symptoms of sporadic VS and NF2-associated VS are indistinguishable, and usually associated with eighth cranial nerve dysfunction in adults, including hearing loss, tinnitus, and imbalance. Progressive tumor growth can lead to complete deafness, brainstem compression, and death. In order to identify small VS, MRI of the brain should include gadolinium and internal auditory canal (IAC) protocol (3-mm thick cuts with no skip). This imaging method has been shown to better assess tumor size for treatment and to identify any small contralateral VS.

BVS are the hallmark of NF2, with virtually all patients developing bilateral eighth cranial nerve tumors during their life. The average age of symptom onset in NF2 is the early 20s, but patients can become symptomatic as early as the first and as late as the seventh decades. Earlier age of onset of symptoms is associated with disease severity and heavier tumor burden. Interestingly, hearing loss from VS in NF2 patients does not correlate with tumor size. In children, presenting symptoms are less likely to be associated with VS, and more likely to result from other cranial or peripheral nerve tumors.

Half of all NF2 patients will develop one or more intracranial meningiomas during their lifetime. Symptoms from these benign tumors arise from compression of adjacent brain parenchyma, with seizures as the most common presenting symptom. Meningiomas are a major cause of morbidity and mortality in NF2 patients, with the large tumor burden making it impossible to perform surgical resection in all tumors.

Up to 90% of NF2 patients have at least one spinal tumor. Extramedullary tumors (meningiomas and schwannomas) are more often symptomatic, while intramedullary tumors (ependymomas) are often clinically silent, not causing significant problems.

Posterior subcapsular ("juvenile") cataracts are the only nontumorous diagnostic criterion for NF2, found in over 70% of patients, but other retinal manifestations can also occur, including epiretinal membranes and hamartomas. The natural history of NF2 is of progressive decline in hearing, balance, and sometimes vision. With the associated intracranial and spinal tumor burden and the need for repeated surgical procedures, NF2 leads to significant morbidity. The life expectancy and quality of life in NF2 patients are related to the severity of the disease. Factors associated with increased risk

*Table 154-2 Manchester Modified Diagnostic Criteria for NF2*

- Bilateral vestibular schwannomas, or
- A first degree family relative with NF2, and unilateral vestibular schwannoma or any two of:
  - Meningiomas
  - Schwannomas
  - Gliomas
  - Neurofibroma
  - Posterior subcapsular lenticular opacities, or
- Unilateral vestibular schwannoma and any two of:
  - Meningioma
  - Schwannoma
  - Glioma
  - Neurofibroma
  - Posterior subcapsular lenticular opacities, or
- Multiple meningiomas (two or more) and unilateral vestibular schwannoma or any two of:
  - Schwannoma
  - Glioma
  - Neurofibroma
  - Cataract

Adapted from Baser ME, Friedman JM, Wallace AJ, et al. *Neurology.* 2002;59:1759-1765.

*Table 154-3 Likelihood of Meeting Diagnostic Criteria for NF2 After Diagnosis of Unilateral VS*

| Decade of Unilateral VS Diagnosis | Percentage of Patients That Will Meet NF2 Diagnostic Criteria in Their Lifetime. |
|---|---|
| 10-19 | 1% |
| 20-29 | 0.45% |
| 30-39 | 0.15% |
| 40-49 | 0.06% |
| 50-59 | 0.03% |

Reproduced with permission from DGR Evans, RT Ramsden, C Gokhale, N Bowers, SM Huson, A Wallace. Should NF2 mutation screening be undertaken in patients with an apparently isolated vestibular schwannoma? in *Clinical Genetics*. John Wiley and Sons, 2007.

of mortality in NF2 patients include age at diagnosis, intracranial meningioma status, type of constitutional *NF2* mutation (ie, truncating mutations), and type of treatment center.

## Screening and Counseling

*Screening:* There are no specific screening recommendations for NF2 or sporadic VS.

*Counseling:* Individuals with NF2 have a 50:50 chance of passing the mutated gene to their offspring. There is no anticipation phenomenon in NF2, with a strong intrafamilial homogeneity in phenotypes. However, founders (the first individual diagnosed with NF2 in a family) can sometimes have a milder clinical course when compared to their offspring due to undetected somatic mosaicism. Somatic mosaicism has been reported in 25% to 30% of founders.

Genotype-phenotype studies in NF2 have shown that truncating mutations (nonsense and frameshift mutations), which lead to premature termination of the NF2 protein, are associated with a more severe phenotype. Missense mutations and large deletions (encompassing the entire *NF2* gene) are associated with a milder phenotype, whereas splice-site mutations can present with either clinical course. Interestingly, in neurofibromatosis type 1 (NF1), large deletions of the gene *NF1* are associated with severe phenotypes. It is unclear why in NF2 large deletions cause a mild phenotype, but it is possible that loss of both copies of the *NF2* gene caused by loss of heterozygosity (LOH) in tumors from patients with large deletions as germline events are lethal at a cellular level and do not lead to tumor formation.

For NF2 patients interested in having children, preimplantation genetic diagnosis (PGD) and prenatal testing are available if the family mutation is known. In cases where the *NF2* mutation cannot be identified, testing can be performed using a combination of linkage analysis and LOH analysis of tumors for identification of the mutated allele. These techniques should be used with caution, particularly if founders are included in the analysis due to the risk of mosaicism. Caution should also be exercised if the mutation identified in the affected family member has never been reported before, or is an atypical event, such as a missense mutation or a splice-site mutation outside of the consensus sequence, as these may not represent the true causative event.

## Management and Treatment

Treatment of sporadic VS is primarily surgical. Three surgical techniques can be used, including middle fossa, translabyrinthine, and retrosigmoid approaches. Surgeries in higher-volume hospitals and high-volume surgeons provide superior short-term outcomes. Postsurgical hearing loss or facial nerve dysfunction is important complication that affects quality of life. As VS are slow-growing tumors, the option of watchful waiting can be adopted for small tumors, and for patients in which the surgical option includes higher risks due to advanced age or comorbidities. Tumor size, hearing function, and facial nerve function prior to surgery are important indicators of successful hearing preservation after VS resection. Interestingly, small tumor size and intact hearing function have also been associated with symptom-free watchful

waiting in patients with sporadic VS. For example, in a study of sporadic VS in patients with intact hearing function at diagnosis, 69% of patients maintained good hearing function after 10 years of clinical monitoring.

Timing for surgical intervention in NF2-associated VS is complicated. With the potential for bilateral hearing loss and blindness during the course of the disease, hearing preservation whenever possible is paramount. Surgical outcomes in NF2 patients are also worse than sporadic tumors, with approximately 66% of patients with tumors smaller than 1.5 cm having preserved hearing function after surgery in a highly specialized neuro-otologic center. Worse surgical prognosis may reflect different histologic patterns of NF2 tumors, which are more likely to be multilobulated and to encompass fascicles of the VII and VIII cranial nerve (rather than displacing nerve fascicles as in sporadic VS).

Intracranial meningiomas usually have an indolent course, with years to decades between diagnosis and development of symptoms. Treatment is also surgical for the majority of symptomatic tumors, with complete resection of meningiomas possible for small tumors, easily accessible sites, and tumors not causing significant compression of adjacent structures. Skull base meningiomas represent a significant clinical challenge due to the lack of good options for resection and compression of lower cranial nerves. Decision on the timing of intervention is dictated by worsening neurologic symptoms, tumor growth, or development of surrounding edema on imaging studies.

Spinal tumors in NF2 can be divided between intramedullary (ependymomas) and extramedullary tumors (schwannomas, meningiomas). Intramedullary tumors are usually found incidentally on imaging studies, with the cervical spine as a site of predilection for these tumors. Surgery is not usually needed, with less than 15% of intramedullary tumors requiring surgery due to worsening symptoms. Extramedullary tumors tend to be more aggressive, requiring resection in almost 60% of patients with tumors due to worsening symptoms.

Surveillance of affected patients includes yearly brain MRIs with an IAC protocol and audiology that includes testing for pure-tone thresholds and word recognition scores. Yearly spinal imaging may be considered based on previous knowledge about presence of spinal tumors or symptomatology. For asymptomatic at-risk relatives who cannot receive presymptomatic molecular diagnosis, brain imaging with an IAC protocol should be performed every 1 to 3 years starting at 10 to 12 years of age until at least the fourth decade.

Surgical resection of all tumors in NF2 patients is neither possible nor warranted. The large tumor burden caused by intracranial meningiomas, VS, and other cranial nerve schwannomas can lead to increased intracranial pressure and brainstem compression, while multiple surgical procedures can lead to debilitating neurologic sequelae. Treatment options are limited for tumors that recur despite surgical resection or that are not amenable to surgery. Radiation therapy has been used as an alternative in sporadic VS with approximately 60% of patients retaining hearing function after the procedure, but no long-term (ie, decades of follow-up) studies have been published. Chemotherapy for VS is also an area of active research. Recently, bevacizumab (Avastin), an antivascular endothelial growth factor (anti-VEGF) antibody, has been shown to improve hearing function and lead to VS shrinkage in 10 NF2 patients, but further research is needed to confirm these findings. Developments on the molecular biology of NF2 should create new avenues for therapies.

*Table 154-4 Molecular Genetic Testing*

| Gene | Testing Modality | Mutation Type | Detection Rate |
|------|------------------|---------------|----------------|
| NF2 | Mutation scanning with SSCP or sequence analysis | Sequence variants, small deletions/insertions | 65%-75% |
| | Deletion/duplication testing | Partial or whole gene deletions | 10%-15% |
| | Linkage analysis | N/A | N/A |
| | LOH analysis of tumors | N/A | N/A |

## Molecular Genetics and Molecular Mechanism

The *NF2* gene was cloned in 1993 by two independent groups, with the NF2 protein named merlin (moesin, ezrin, radixin-like protein) by one group, due to its similarities to other members of the 4.1 protein family, while the second group named it schwannomin for its role in schwannoma formation.

The *NF2* gene has 17 exons with the last two exons being alternatively spliced. Disease-causing mutations can be found throughout the gene from exons 1 to 15, with no deleterious mutations ever reported on the alternatively spliced exons 16 and 17. Two recent meta-analyses compiling 12 years of *NF2* research showed that two-thirds of mutations detected by sequencing in NF2 patients are truncating in nature (nonsense or frameshift), with exons 2, 6, 8, 11, and 15 as warm-spots, accounting for almost half of all mutations. Approximately 25% of the mutations were splice-site events, while only 9% were missense mutations. In patients in whom sequence analysis of the *NF2* gene does not yield any mutations, intragenic and whole gene deletions have been reported, accounting for approximately 15% of all cases, with chromosomal rearrangements being rarely reported.

*NF2* is the only gene associated with sporadic VS formation, with mutations found in 76% to 86% of schwannomas studied (including VS and other cranial or peripheral schwannomas). Recently, *INI1* or *SMARCB1* gene located proximal to *NF2* on chromosome 22 was identified as the molecular event involved in schwannomatosis. Patients with schwannomatosis develop two or more schwannomas, without VS or any other clinical stigmata of NF2. The molecular biology of schwannomatosis is very peculiar as *INI1* or *SMARCB1* mutations seem to lead to instability of the *NF2* gene, with each one of the schwannomas from schwannomatosis patients developing a different (usually truncating) *NF2* gene mutation. No germline *NF2* mutations can be identified in schwannomatosis patients. The exact mechanism for the interaction between *NF2* and *INI1* or *SMARCB1* is still unclear.

NF2 is a cytoskeletal protein with multiple inter- and intraprotein interactions, including cytoskeletal actin and multiple cell signaling and growth regulatory factors, including hepatocyte growth factor-regulated tyrosine kinase, synthenin, and schwannomin-interacting protein 1. The precise mechanism of tumor formation in NF2 patients is not entirely known. NF2 seems to be inactivated by phosphorylated Pak1, and in a feedforward mechanism, inactive NF2 is unable to suppress Rac/cdc42. Activated Rac/cdc42 perpetuates Pak1 phosphorylation. New research suggests that NF2 also interacts with the MAPK-PI3K-Akt-mTOR cellular pathway for its tumor suppressor function, but the exact site of interaction has not yet been identified. Recently, two papers described new roles for NF2, one regulating epidermal growth factor receptor (EGFR) expression on the cytoskeleton membrane, showing that upon cell-cell contact NF2 leads to negative regulation of EGFR by restraining EGFR into a membrane compartment from which it cannot signal. The second article showed that the closed conformation of NF2 can be found in the nucleus, binding to E3 ubiquitin ligase CRL4$^{DCAF1}$ and suppressing its activity.

***Genetic Testing:*** Since the cloning of the *NF2* gene, mutation analysis for patients has been commercially available. For patients with confirmed diagnosis by clinical criteria, mutation analysis does not add to clinical care. Mutation analysis is indicated in cases where somatic mosaicism is suspected, or patients are willing to undergo testing for presymptomatic diagnosis of at-risk relatives or PGD. In patients whom the diagnosis is not certain, imaging surveillance is recommended. Although genotype-phenotype correlations in NF2 exist, no specific recommendation for patient care based on the mutation found has been established.

Mutation scanning using single-strand conformational polymorphism (SSCP) for exons 1 through 15 or exon sequencing has been the standard techniques for mutational analysis of the *NF2* gene with a detection rate of 65% to 75% of patients meeting diagnostic criteria (Table 154-4). Deletion testing with multiplex ligation-dependent probe amplification (MLPA) is able to detect an additional 10% to 15% of patients with partial or whole gene deletions. When the causative mutation is not identified in a family, combination of linkage analysis for the *NF2* gene and LOH analysis of resected tumors can help identify the affected allele in a family for presymptomatic, prenatal, or PGD diagnosis.

**BIBLIOGRAPHY:**

1. Li W, You L, Cooper J, et al. Merlin/NF2 suppresses tumorigenesis by inhibiting the E3 ubiquitin ligase CRL4(DCAF1) in the nucleus. *Cell.* 2010;140:477-490.
2. Curto M, Cole BK, Lallemand D, Liu CH, McClatchey AI. Contact-dependent inhibition of EGFR signaling by Nf2/Merlin. *J Cell Biol.* 2007;177:893-903.
3. Ahronowitz I, Xin W, Kiely R, Sims K, MacCollin M, Nunes FP. Mutational spectrum of the NF2 gene: a meta-analysis of 12 years of research and diagnostic laboratory findings. *Hum Mutat.* 2007;28:1-12.
4. Nunes F, MacCollin M. Neurofibromatosis 2 in the pediatric population. *J Child Neurol.* 2003;18:718-724.
5. Baser ME. Contributors to the International NF2 Mutation Database. The distribution of constitutional and somatic mutations in the neurofibromatosis 2 gene. *Hum Mutat.* 2006;27:297-306.

6. Patronas NJ, Courcoutsakis N, Bromley CM, Katzman GL, Mac-Collin M, Parry DM. Intramedullary and spinal canal tumors in patients with neurofibromatosis 2: MR imaging findings and correlation with genotype. *Radiology*. 2001;218:434-442.

7. Evans DG, Ramsden RT, Gokhale C, Bowers N, Huson SM, Wallace A. Should NF2 mutation screening be undertaken in patients with an apparently isolated vestibular schwannoma? *Clin Genet*. 2007;71:354-358.

8. Gutmann DH, Aylsworth A, Carey JC, et al. The diagnostic evaluation and multidisciplinary management of neurofibromatosis 1 and neurofibromatosis 2. *JAMA*. 1997;278:51-57.

9. Plotkin SR, Stemmer-Rachamimov AO, Barker FG 2nd, et al. Hearing improvement after bevacizumab in patients with neurofibromatosis type 2. *N Engl J Med*. 2009;361:358-367.

10. Stangerup SE, Thomsen J, Tos M, Cayé-Thomasen P. Long-term hearing preservation in vestibular schwannoma. *Otol Neurotol*. 2010;31:271-275.

11. Barker FG 2nd, Carter BS, Ojemann RG, Jyung RW, Poe DS, McKenna MJ. Surgical excision of acoustic neuroma: patient outcome and provider caseload. *Laryngoscope*. 2003;113:1332-1343.

12. Baser ME, Friedman JM, Wallace AJ, Ramsden RT, Joe H, Evans DG. Evaluation of clinical diagnostic criteria for neurofibromatosis 2. *Neurology*. 2002;59:1759-1765.

## Supplementary Information

### OMIM REFERENCE:

[1] Neurofibromatosis, Type II; NF2 (#101000)

### Alternative Names:
- Central Type Neurofibromatosis
- Bilateral Acoustic Schwannomas
- Acoustic Neuromas

*Key Words:* Vestibular schwannomas, neurofibromatosis, NF2, schwannomatosis, multiple meningiomas

## 155 Achondroplasia

Bryn D. Webb, Julie E. Hoover-Fong, and Ethylin Wang Jabs

### KEY POINTS

- *Disease summary:*
  - Achondroplasia is the most common form of inherited short stature.
  - Incidence is approximately 1 in 15,000 to 1 in 40,000 live births.
  - Clinical features include rhizomelic disproportionate short stature, macrocephaly, midface hypoplasia, trident hand conformation with brachydactyly, lordosis, genu varum, and normal cognitive development.
  - Neurologic complications occur with cervicomedullary cord compression, spinal stenosis, and kyphosis. Potential respiratory complications include central sleep apnea due to cervicomedullary cord compression, and mechanical sleep apnea due to midface hypoplasia and relatively large adenotonsillar tissue compounded by hypotonia.

- *Hereditary basis:*
  - Achondroplasia is inherited in an autosomal dominant fashion and has 100% penetrance.
  - Approximately 99% of patients with achondroplasia have a point mutation (G changed to an A or G changed to a C) at nucleotide 1138 in the gene fibroblast growth factor receptor 3 (*FGFR3*) located at chromosome 4p16.3. This nucleotide change (G>A or G>C) results in a Gly380Arg amino acid substitution.
  - Approximately 80% of patients with achondroplasia are born to parents of average height without *FGFR3* mutations. De novo mutations have been associated with advanced paternal age.

- *Differential diagnosis:*
  - Achondroplasia can be distinguished from other forms of disproportionate short stature including hypochondroplasia (OMIM 146000) and severe achondroplasia with developmental delay and acanthosis nigricans (SADDAN), both caused by different *FGFR3* mutations. Thanatophoric dysplasia I (OMIM 187600) and thanatophoric dysplasia II (OMIM 187601) are also caused by mutations in *FGFR3*, but are easily differentiated from achondroplasia by their more severe pulmonary phenotype and lethality.

## Diagnostic Criteria and Clinical Characteristics

**Diagnostic Criteria:** Clinical features of achondroplasia include
- Rhizomelic (proximal limb) short stature
- Macrocephaly with frontal bossing
- Midface hypoplasia
- Trident hands
- Genu varum (bow legs)
- Limitation of elbow extension

Distinctive radiographic features include

- Hypolucency at proximal femora
- Interpedicular narrowing of the lumbar vertebrae
- Broad metaphyses and shortened tubular bones

Clinical features are often apparent at birth and radiographic features are diagnostic at any time. For patients with a suspected clinical diagnosis, molecular testing can be performed to confirm the diagnosis.

**Clinical Characteristics:** Achondroplasia is characterized by disproportionate short stature with rhizomelic shortening (shortening of the proximal segments of the limbs), macrocephaly, prominent forehead, and depressed nasal bridge. Hands are noted to have a trident configuration due to fingers of roughly the same length. The average adult height is 131 cm for males and 124 cm for females. Most individuals with achondroplasia have normal intelligence and lifespan.

Skeletal abnormalities in patients with achondroplasia include lumbar lordosis, kyphosis, limited elbow extension, limited hip extension, and tibial bowing. Tibial bowing results from the relative overgrowth of the fibula when compared to the tibia.

The most serious complication of achondroplasia is cervicomedullary cord compression, which may cause sudden death in infants. In adults, neurologic complications include claudication and lumbosacral spinal stenosis. Claudication is rarely seen prior to adolescence and symptoms include tingling, numbness, and weakness that are transient and generally occur with exercise. Claudication is relieved with rest and with maneuvers aimed to increase the volume of the lumbosacral canal, such as the "achondroplasia squat" (squatting with a straight back against a wall). In contrast to claudication, symptoms from lumbosacral spinal stenosis are persistent and are often due to bony compression of the spinal cord. The average age of onset of symptoms is 38 years. Symptoms include persistent weakness, persistent sensory deficits,

*Table 155-1* **System Involvement**

| System | Manifestation | Incidence (if available) |
|---|---|---|
| Skeletal | Lumbar lordosis | 80% of children |
| | Persistent kyphosis | 10% |
| | Tibial bowing, genu varus | 90%, 42% of adult patients |
| | Limited elbow extension | 70% |
| | Posterior dislocation of the radial head | |
| Neurologic | Lumbar spine stenosis (L1-L4) | 37%-89% |
| | Cervicomedullary spinal cord compression | |
| | Hydrocephalus | |
| | Claudication | 80% by the sixth decade of life |
| Dental | Teeth crowding | |
| Respiratory | Obstructive sleep apnea | >16% |
| ENT | Chronic otitis media | At least 25% of children |
| | Conductive hearing loss | 38% of adults |
| Gynecologic | Menorrhagia | |
| | Fibroids | |
| Metabolic | Obesity | |

hyperreflexia, bladder or bowel incontinence. Lumbosacral spinal stenosis is treated with decompressive surgery.

Other symptoms, other than neurologic and skeletal, may be involved as well. Dental problems include class III malocclusion, cross-bite, and teeth crowding. Respiratory symptoms may arise due to a small chest or upper airway obstruction. Obstructive sleep apnea is common. Patients with achondroplasia often have numerous middle ear infections as children due to shortened eustachian tubes. Chronic ear infections can lead to conductive hearing loss, which affects as many as 40% of adults with achondroplasia. There may also be an increased incidence of fibroids and menorrhagia in female patients with achondroplasia. Obesity is also common and a major cause of increased morbidity due to worsening of joint problems and an increase in heart disease-related deaths seen in patients with achondroplasia (Table 155-1).

### Screening and Counseling

**Screening:** Clinical features of achondroplasia are often apparent at birth, though up to 20% may not be diagnosed until into the first year of life. Clinical suspicion may lead to confirmatory molecular testing (Table 155-2).

**Counseling:** For unaffected parents who have had a child with achondroplasia, there is a 0.02% recurrence risk due to possible gonadal mosaicism.

Persons with achondroplasia who have children with average stature partners have a 50% risk of each child having achondroplasia due to autosomal dominant inheritance. Couples with both parents affected with achondroplasia have a 25% chance of the conceptus being unaffected, a 50% chance of the conceptus having classical achondroplasia (heterozygous mutation), and a 25% chance of the conceptus having a homozygous mutation, a lethal condition. For couples with achondroplasia, preimplantation genetic diagnosis, chorionic villus sampling (CVS), or amniocentesis may be performed.

During pregnancy, achondroplasia may be suspected in the third trimester when prenatal ultrasound shows long bone shortening; however, this finding is not specific for the disorder. The diagnosis of achondroplasia may be confirmed by molecular testing with fetal material obtained from either CVS or amniocentesis. Cesarean section delivery is needed for pregnant women with achondroplasia and may be needed for average stature women carrying a fetus with achondroplasia due to cephalopelvic disproportion.

## Management and Treatment

Primary care physicians should plot growth parameters, including length or height, weight, and head circumference at every visit.

*Table 155-2* **Molecular Genetic Testing**

| Gene | Testing Modality | Mutation Type | Detection Rate |
|---|---|---|---|
| FGFR3 | Targeted mutation analysis | c.1138G>A substitution | ~98% |
| FGFR3 | Targeted mutation analysis | c.1138G>C substitution | ~1% |

Weight for age charts and body mass index (BMI) charts are available for children with achondroplasia and should be utilized. Obesity is common and measures to control it including diet and exercise are started in early childhood and maintained into adulthood.

The short limbs of achondroplasia have been treated with limb lengthening, growth hormone (GH) therapy, or both. Limbs are usually lengthened surgically by callotasis (callus distraction). Multiple studies have shown limited increase in average final height with the use of GH in achondroplasia patients. Limitations of elbow and hip extension and lumbar hyperlordosis rarely interfere with activities of daily living (ADLs) and generally do not require aggressive treatment. However, adaptive equipment may be needed for ADLs (eg, toileting, reaching) if back range of motion is compromised after surgical spinal fusion. Genu varus is extremely common in achondroplasia, but only 10% to 22% of patients with this deformity require tibial osteotomies for comprised function or excessive pain.

Physicians should monitor for signs of spinal stenosis and nerve compression by performing a detailed neurologic examination with deep tendon reflexes, tone, and sensation, as well as computed tomography (CT), magnetic resonance imaging (MRI), somatosensory-evoked potentials, and polysomnography in some cases every 3 to 5 years when adult patients reach midlife. Claudication symptoms can be minimized with weight loss and exercises aimed to reduce hyperlordosis. Decompressive surgery is the treatment of choice for lumbosacral spinal stenosis. Restenosis is common and patients often require repeated surgeries.

Physicians should continue to screen for symptoms of obstructive sleep apnea at routine visits. If screening is positive, patients should be referred for sleep studies. Treatment may include adenotonsillectomy, weight loss, and nasal-mask continuous positive airway pressure (CPAP).

Adult patients with achondroplasia should continue to be assessed for orthodontic problems. Approximately 50% of patients have orthodontic issues related to crowding.

Patients may have difficulties in social adjustment with families, peers, and employment and may seek advice from social awareness programs and support groups, such as the Little People of America (www.lpaonline.org).

## Molecular Genetics and Molecular Mechanism

*FGFR3* encodes one of four closely related fibroblast growth factor receptors. These receptors are composed of an extracellular ligand-binding domain consisting of three immunoglobulin subdomains, a transmembrane domain, and a split intracelullar tyrosine kinase domain. The binding of fibroblast growth factor (FGF) ligands causes dimerization of FGF receptors with activation of intracellular tyrosine kinase domains. This activation leads to autophosphorylation and phosphorylated tyrosine residues serve as docking sites for adaptor proteins and effector molecules. Activation of FGFR3 results in inhibition of proliferation and terminal differentiation of growth plate chondrocytes. The G380R mutation is located at a critical region in the tyrosine kinase domain and results in constitutive activation of FGFR3, and thus achondroplasia results from a gain-of-function mutation.

***Genetic Testing:*** Currently many laboratories offer targeted mutation analysis, sequence analysis of select exons, and analyses of the entire coding region. Targeted mutation analysis is most commonly performed and identifies the c.1138G>A and c.1138G>C substitutions (both resulting in the Gly380Arg amino acid substitution), which account for the majority of cases of achondroplasia. Other rare mutations include c.1125G>T (Gly375Cys), c.1037G>A (Gly346Glu), c.742C>T (Arg248Cys), and c.1620C>G (Asn540Lys).

### BIBLIOGRAPHY:

1. Richette P, Bardin T, Stheneur C. Achondroplasia: from genotype to phenotype. *Joint Bone Spine*. 2008;75:125-130.
2. Pauli, RM. The natural histories of bone dysplasias in adults—vignettes, fables and just-so stories. *Am J Med Genet (Semin Med Genet)*. 2007;145C:309-321.
3. Hunter AG, Bankier A, Rogers JG, et al. Medical complications of achondroplasia: a multicentre patient review. *J Med Genet*. 1998;35:705-712.
4. Horton WA, Hall JG, Hecht JT. Achondroplasia. *Lancet*. 2007;370:162-172.
5. Wynn J, King TM, Gambello MJ, et al. Mortality in achondroplasia study: a 42-year follow-up. *Am J Med Genet*. 2007;143:2502-2511.
6. Shirley ED, Ain MC. Achondroplasia: manifestations and treatment. *J Am Acad Orthop Surg*. 2009;17:231-241.
7. Mettler G, Fraser FC. Recurrence risk for sibs of children with "sporadic" achondroplasia. *Am J Med Genet*. 2000;90:250-251.
8. Trotter TL, Hall JG. Health supervision for children with achondroplasia. *Pediatrics*. 2005;116:771-783.
9. Hoover-Fong JE, McGready J, Schulze KJ, et al. Weight for age charts for children with achondroplasia. *Am J Med Genet*. 2007;143:2227-2235.
10. Hoover-Fong JE, Schulze KJ, McGready J, et al. Age-appropriate body mass index in children with achondroplasia: interpretation in relation to indexes of height. *Am J Clin Nutr*. 2008;88:364-371.
11. Hecht JT, Hood OJ, Schwartz RJ, et al. Obesity in achondroplasia. *Am J Med Genet*. 1988;31:597-602.
12. Haga N. Management of disabilities associated with achondroplasia. *J Orthop Sci*. 2004;9:103-107.

## Supplementary Information

### OMIM REFERENCES:

[1] Achondroplasia (#100800)

[2] Fibroblast growth factor receptor 3 (FGFR3) (*134934)

### Alternative Name:

- Rhizomelic Dwarfism

***Key Words:*** Short stature, dwarfism, FGFR3

# 156 Malignant Hyperthermia

Henrik Rueffert and Henry Rosenberg

- *Disease summary:*
  - Malignant hyperthermia (MH) is a pharmacogenetic disorder of skeletal muscle that is triggered by potent halogenated volatile anesthetics and depolarizing muscle relaxants and in rare case by strenuous exercise and/or heat exposure, too.
  - Susceptible individuals have an inherited abnormality of muscle metabolism that is compensated under everyday life conditions (no clinical symptoms). However, patients with central core disease (CCD) who are at risk for MH may display muscle weakness.
  - Upon exposure to triggering agents muscle cell metabolism is massively accelerated with potentially fatal consequences. The resulting hypermetabolic syndrome is characterized by typical clinical signs such as tachycardia, hypercapnia, acidosis, muscle rigidity, and breakdown as well as hyperthermia.
  - The underlying abnormality relates to an uncontrolled release of calcium from the sarcoplasmic reticulum (SR) resulting in elevation of intracellular calcium. This in turn leads to activation of muscle contractile elements, and elevated anaerobic and aerobic metabolism.
  - The ryanodine receptor subtype 1 (RYR1; fast calcium-releasing channel) is considered to play a key role in the pathogenesis of MH. It controls the calcium release from the SR into the cytoplasm in normal skeletal muscle cells.
  - The response of the RYR1 to MH triggering substances is functionally affected in MH patients. This results in an uncontrolled calcium release via the SR membrane.
  - Early recognition of MH and its immediate treatment is essential for the patient's survival. Besides symptomatic therapy dantrolene sodium is the only effective and specific treatment drug for MH (RYR1 antagonist).
  - MH susceptibility may reliably be detected by standardized in vitro contracture testing of biopsied skeletal muscle. Upon exposure to compounds such as halothane, caffeine, ryanodine, and other calcium release agents, marked contracture of the muscle is noted.
  - DNA analysis can be used in up to 30% of MH families, mainly for the screening of family members that carry a MH-associated mutation in the *RYR1* gene.
  - A patient advocacy organization exists in the United States, Malignant Hyperthermia Association of the United States (MHAUS) (www.mhaus.org). A registry of patients with MH in North America is sponsored by MHAUS.
  - In Europe, the European MH Group (www.emhg.org) sponsors meetings and research into the syndrome.
- *Hereditary basis:*
  - The disposition to MH is inherited in humans in an autosomal dominant fashion with variable penetrance and expressivity.
  - The majority of MH cases (>70%) is linked to the ryanodine receptor 1 gene (*RYR1*) located on chromosome 19q13.1 (MHS-1). Another gene locus is the *DHPR* gene. Other gene loci (MHS 2-6) are of minor importance.
  - There is a considerable allelic heterogeneity in the *RYR1* gene with over 200 mutations which were detected in MH patients. About 30 *RYR1* mutations were proven causal for MH.
- *Differential diagnosis:*
  - Malignant neuroleptic syndrome, sepsis, serotonergic syndrome, heat stroke, thyroid crisis, drug intoxication (ecstasy, cocaine), hyperkalemic cardiac arrest during anesthesia in patients with occult myopathy
  - Iatrogenic: rapid uptake of carbon dioxide incident to laparoscopic surgery, overheating, hypoventilation, anesthesia machine malfunction
  - Neuromuscular disorders
    - CCD: causal relationship to MH (same gene locus)
    - Multiminicore disease (MmD): MmD patients with mutations in the *RYR1* gene (minority)
  - Other: for example muscle dystrophies (Duchenne, Becker), myotonias

## Diagnostic Criteria and Clinical Characteristics

***Diagnostic Criteria:*** To make an accurate diagnosis can be difficult because clinical signs associated with MH are not unique. Each sign allows a number of differential diagnoses, so the provider must be able to recognize a pattern of signs.

In the presence of potent volatile anesthetics and/or succinylcholine

*Early signs:*
- Tachycardia, arrhythmia, hypertension or hypotension
- Masseter spasm, generalized muscle rigidity
- Tachypnea (if breathing spontaneously), raised end-tidal $CO_2$
- Mixed acidosis
- Cyanosis, skin mottling

*Later signs*
- Hyperkalemia
- Rapid increase of core body temperature (up to >40°C)

*Table 156-1  System Involvement*

| System | Manifestation | Incidence |
|---|---|---|
| Skeletal muscle | Masseter spasm, general muscle rigidity | up to 80% |
| | Rhabdomyolysis, myoglobinemia myoglobinuria | ~50% |
| Cardiovascular | Tachycardia, arrhythmia | up to 80% |
| | Severe hyper or hypotension, cardiac arrest | <1% |
| (Hyper) metabolism | Hypercapnea,[a] hyperthermia,[b] acidosis[c] | ~80%,[a] ~30%,[b] ~70%[c] |
| Electrolytes | Hyperkalemia (secondary to acidosis and muscle breakdown) | ~30% |
| Renal | Acute renal failure (secondary to myoglobinuria) | <5% |
| Respiratory | Hyperventilation; respiratory acidosis | ~50% |
| Hematologic | Disseminated intravascular coagulation syndrome | <1% |

- Muscle breakdown: creatinine kinase (CK) elevation, myoglobinemia, myoglobinuria
- Disseminated intravascular coagulation particularly with marked hyperthermia
- Cardiac arrest, multiorgan failure

A clinical grading scale may retrospectively help determine the likelihood that the incident was really attributable to MH. However, this scoring system depends on the manifestation of the clinical signs in the grading scale. Multiple organ systems may be affected, see Table 156-1.

### Clinical Characteristics:

- Onset of signs of MH is variable and may occur on induction, during maintenance of anesthesia, and within 1 hour of termination of anesthesia.
- There are different clinical courses of MH: fulminant crisis, delayed onset with only a few clinical signs, postoperative rhabdomyolysis.
- Most MH susceptibles will manifest jaw and peripheral muscle rigidity with succinylcholine. Muscle rigidity may be present, but less common, in the absence of succinylcholine.
- Muscle rigidity is not relieved by nondepolarizing muscle relaxants or benzodiazepines.
- There is marked variability in the progression of the signs of MH.
- Hyperthermia exceeding 40°C may occur within 20 to 30 minutes of onset.
- HyperCKemia with or without myoglobinuria is characteristic. The peak CK levels occur between 14 and 20 hours of onset.
- Once a MH crisis is suspected, trigger agents must be immediately stopped, hyperventilation begun along with active cooling if hyperthermia is present.
- Dantrolene sodium, IV at a dose of 2.5 mg/kg reverses the signs of MH, although in some cases up to 10 mg/kg or more are needed.

## Screening and Counseling

### Screening:

- A personal or family history of MH, unexplained anesthetic death, history of myopathy should arise suspicion of MH.

- There is no reliable laboratory test for preclinical screening for MH.
- Each suspected case of MH should be referred to a MH center for further investigation (muscle biopsy and in vitro caffeine/halothane contracture test, DNA testing) in order to confirm or to exclude the clinical diagnosis.
- Confirmed MH cases (MH susceptible diagnosis in the caffeine/halothane test) may be considered for DNA testing and screened for MH-associated mutations in the *RYR1* gene.
- If a MH-associated mutation is present in the index patient all relatives should be tested for the familial *RYR1* mutation. CLIA certified testing laboratories are listed on the web site of MHAUS.
- For diagnostic work up, see Fig. 156-1.

### Counseling:

☞INHERITANCE, PENETRANCE: MH is transmitted in an autosomal dominant pattern; hence 50% of first-degree relatives of an index person are at risk to develop the syndrome and that the susceptibility to MH does not skip generations. However, not every predisposed person develops the syndrome on exposure to trigger agents and the severity of clinical signs may vary.

The genetic prevalence of MH (frequency of MH-associated mutations in the normal population) is estimated at 1 in approximately 3000, whilst the clinical incidence is between one in 50,000 and 100,000 surgical procedures involving general anesthesia.

☞GENOTYPE-PHENOTYPE CORRELATION: Most mutations in the *RYR1* gene are concordant with pathologic findings in the in vitro caffeine/halothane test, in particular the 30 MH-causal *RYR1* mutations.

Severity of presentation is not related to specific mutations. Frequency of specific mutations varies among different ethnic groups. Most mutations are private.

## Management and Treatment

### Treatment:
Treatment of a MH crisis is based on three fundamental measures that have to begin immediately after making a diagnosis:

1. Stop exposure to trigger agents.
2. Administer dantrolene sodium IV at a dose of 2.5 mg/kg. Continue dosing until resolution of signs.

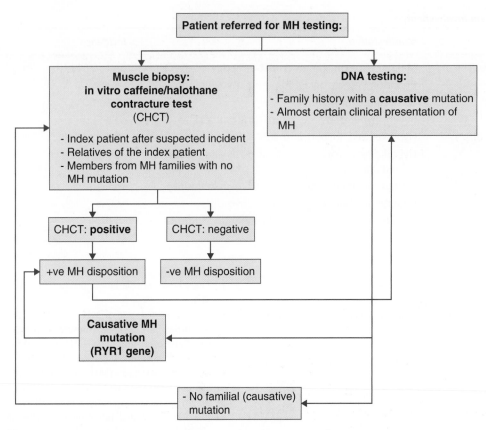

***Figure 156-1*** Algorithm for Screening and Management of Patient With Malignant Hyperthermia.

3. Continue dantrolene at 1 to 2 mg/kg for at least 36 hours after resolution of signs since recrudescence occurs in 25% of patients.
4. Symptomatic therapy (cooling, buffering, dialysis, etc).

**Anesthesia in patient susceptible to MH**
- Safe are trigger-free anesthesia (total intravenous), local anesthesia, regional anesthesia.
- Use of standardized monitoring: ECG, blood pressure, capnometry, pulse oximetry, continuous measurement of core body temperature.

## Molecular Genetics and Molecular Mechanism

***Syndrome/Gene/Locus:***

Malignant hyperthermia susceptibility-1/RYR1/19q13.1
Malignant hyperthermia susceptibility-2/MHS2/17q11.2-q24
Malignant hyperthermia susceptibility-3/MHS3/7q21-q22
Malignant hyperthermia susceptibility-4/MHS4/3q13.1
Malignant hyperthermia susceptibility-5/CACNA1S/1q32
Malignant hyperthermia susceptibility-6/MHS6/5p

***Description of Basic Gene Functions:*** The underlying mechanism for the immense activation of cellular and systemic metabolism is an abnormal calcium homeostasis in the muscle fibers during the MH event. The ryanodine receptor 1, which is located in the membrane

of the SR and is activated by the voltage-dependent dihydropyridine receptor (DHPR), is normally responsible for the controlled calcium release from the SR into the cytoplasm. Calcium acts as a cofactor for ATP-generating processes (actin-myosin interactions, glycolysis, glycogenolysis). RYR1s seem to play the key role in the pathogenesis of MH by generating an increased and sustained transmembranal calcium release. This is based on functionally altered gating properties and on higher sensitivity and affinity to agonists (caffeine, chloro-m-cresol, ryanodine). The uncontrolled release of calcium induces an excessive ATP turnover in the cells resulting in typical signs of a MH crisis.

In line with the disturbance of intracellular calcium homeostasis, genetic linkage studies identified the gene encoding the ryanodine receptor of the skeletal muscles on chromosome 19q13.1 as the primary locus of MH susceptibility (MHS-1 locus) in humans. Additional five MH loci (MHS 2-6) have been suggested as being responsible for MH susceptibility but appear to be of minor importance. With the exception of MHS-5 locus (*CACNA1S* gene, encoding the α1 subunit of the dihydropyridine receptor) neither putative candidate genes nor MH-associated mutations have been identified in these loci as yet.

To date, more than 200 different missense mutations (predominately heterozygous point mutations) have been identified in the *RYR1* gene. The majority of *RYR1* mutations are clustered in three regions of the gene: MH region 1 close to the N-terminus (amino acid 35-614), MH region 2 in the central protein segment (2163-2458), and MH region 3 in the C-terminus, which encodes the pore

*Table 156-2 Molecular Genetic Testing*

| Gene | Testing Modality | Mutation Type | Detection Rate |
|---|---|---|---|
| *RYR1* | MH-index patient: analysis of the entire gene: direct sequencing | Point mutations; in few exceptional cases: deletions, insertions | >70% |
| | Family members: (in families with a causal MH mutation) Sequence analysis of selected exons (sequencing, DHPLC, restriction enzyme analysis, MLPA) | Point mutation | 50% |
| *CACNA1S* | MH-index patient: analysis of selected exon | Point mutation | <0.5% |

region and is often associated with the CCD phenotype, too. However, MH mutations have also been found across the entire region of the gene.

More than 30 *RYR1* mutations have also been proved clearly causative for MH by functional analyses in sufficient homologous and heterologous cell systems. Accentuated release of calcium is shown on exposure to agonists such as caffeine when the mutant allele is inserted into the cell's DNA. In addition, knock-in genetically engineered mice incorporating one or more causal mutations demonstrate typical MH signs.

When screening the entire coding region of a clearly positive diagnosed MH patient (MH susceptible phenotype confirmed by the CHCT), for example by direct sequencing, a detection rate of *RYR1* mutations of more than 70% can be reached.

### Genetic Testing:

☞**CLINICAL AVAILABILITY OF TESTING:** Genetic testing is available in two CLIA-approved laboratories in the United States, in about 10 MH centers in Europe as well as in a few laboratories in Australia and New Zealand and South America.

☞**UTILITY OF TESTING:** The identification of an accepted causative mutation permits a positive MH diagnosis ("MH susceptible") without further confirmation by the muscle test. The European MH group has published a list of accepted causative *RYR1* mutations (www.emhg.org) that is periodically updated. The genetics group of North America has also developed a consensus panel of *RYR1* mutations for genetic testing and suggested using molecular genetic analysis whenever possible and appropriate.

Genetic testing is predominately valuable in families that carry a causal *MH* mutation because the family members can be screened fast and less invasive by means of a blood investigation. However, the absence of the familial mutation the MH-negative diagnosis must be confirmed by the CHCT (due to possible allelic heterogeneity in *RYR1*).

Genetic testing is also of value where a death has occurred and tissue is not available for in vitro muscle biopsy contracture testing. In future, it can also be a promising option for prenatal diagnosis in MH families. See also Table 156-2.

### BIBLIOGRAPHY:

1. Larach MG, Localio AR, Allen GC, et al. A clinical grading scale to predict malignant hyperthermia susceptibility. *Anesthesiology*. 1994;80:771-779.
2. Rosenberg H, Davis M, James D, Pollock N, Stowell K. Malignant hyperthermia. *Orphanet J Rare Dis*. 2007;2:21.
3. Litman RS, Rosenberg H. Malignant hyperthermia: update on susceptibility testing. *JAMA*. 2005;293(23):2918-2924.
4. MacLennan DH, Duff C, Zorzato F, et al. Ryanodine receptor gene is a candidate for predisposition to malignant hyperthermia. *Nature*. 1990;343(6258):559.
5. Rosero EB, Adesanya AO, Timaran CH, Joshi GP. Trends and outcomes of malignant hyperthermia in the United States, 2000 to 2005. *Anesthesiology*. 2009;110(10):89-94.
6. Carpenter D, Ringrose C, Leo V, et al. The role of CACNA1S in predisposition to malignant hyperthermia. *BMC Med Genet*. 2009;10:104.
7. Sambuughin N, Holley H, Muldoon, et al. Screening of the entire ryanodine receptor type 1 coding region for sequence variants associated with malignant hyperthermia susceptibility in the North American population. *Anesthesiology*. 2005;102:515-521.
8. Levano S, Vukcevic M, Singer M, et al. Increasing the number of diagnostic mutations in malignant hyperthermia. *Hum Mutat*. 2009;30(4):590-598.
9. Robinson RL, Anetseder MJ, Brancadoro V, et al. Recent advances in the diagnosis of malignant hyperthermia susceptibility: how confident can we be of genetic testing? *Eur J Hum Genet*. 2003;11(4):342-348.
10. Nathan A, Ganesh A, Godinez RI, Nicolson SC, Greeley WJ. Hyperkalemic cardiac arrest after cardiopulmonary bypass in a child with unsuspected Duchenne muscular dystrophy. *Anesth Analg*. 2005;100(3):672-674.
11. Rosenberg H, Rueffert H. Clinical utility gene card for: malignant hyperthermia. *Eur J Hum Genet*. Jun 2011;19(6).

## Supplementary Information

### OMIM REFERENCES:

[1] Malignant Hyperthermia; RYR1 (#180901)

[2] Malignant Hyperthermia; CACNA1S (#114208)

[3] Malignant Hyperthermia (Disease) (#145600)

### Alternative Names:
- Malignant Hyperpyrexia
- Hyperthermia of Anesthesia
- MHS (MH Susceptible)
- King-Denborough Syndrome

*Key Words:* Malignant hyperthermia, ryanodine receptor, anesthetic death

# 157 Noonan Syndrome and Related Disorders

Constance Weismann and Bruce D. Gelb

## KEY POINTS

- *Disease summary:*
  - Noonan syndrome is the "prototype" of a spectrum of clinical entities that during the last few years was found to be caused by mutations in various genes along the RAS-MAPK pathway. This pathway is well known for its role in cancer. There is a strong correlation between the clinical phenotype and the genetic defect, which so far is unique to this disease entity.
  - *Features:* congenital heart disease (especially pulmonary stenosis), hypertrophic cardiomyopathy, facial dysmorphia, webbed neck, lymphedema, short stature, mild developmental delay, delayed onset of puberty, cryptorchidism, male infertility, bleeding disorders, malignancies, malrotation, hepatosplenomegaly, renal anomalies, ophthalmologic and dermatologic problems to a variable degree
  - *Incidence:* 1:1000-1:2500
  - *Disease genes: PTPN11* (41%), *SOS1* (11%), *RAF1* (5%), *BRAF* (1%), *KRAS* (1%), *NRAS* (<1%), *SHOC2* (2%)
- *Hereditary basis:*
  - Autosomal dominant, de novo mutation; complete penetrance, variable phenotype
- *Differential diagnosis:*
  - *Noonan syndrome with multiple lentigines:* formerly known as LEOPARD syndrome with major features including lentigines, echocardiogram (ECG) conduction anomalies, ocular hypertelorism, pulmonary stenosis, abnormal genitalia, retardation of growth, and sensorineural deafness, same cardiac defects as Noonan syndrome, but higher prevalence of hypertrophic cardiomyopathy
  - *Cardiofaciocutaneous syndrome:* more severe variant of Noonan syndrome with more coarse facial features, hyperkeratotic skin, curly hair and sparse eyebrows and eyelashes, severe developmental delay, hypotonia, seizures, structural brain anomalies
  - *Costello syndrome:* more severe variant of Noonan syndrome with prenatal overgrowth and postnatal growth delay, more coarse facial features, benign cutaneous papillomata, and 15% childhood incidence of solid tumors (rhabdomyosarcoma, neuroblastoma, bladder carcinoma)
  - *Neurofibromatosis-Noonan syndrome:* features of both neurofibromatosis type 1 and Noonan syndrome
  - *Legius syndrome:* axillary freckling, café-au-lait spots, macrocephaly, and facial dysmorphism resembling Noonan syndrome

## Diagnostic Criteria and Clinical Characteristics

**Diagnostic Criteria:**
- Diagnosis is made by clinical examination.
- Van der Burgt et al. developed a scoring system to aid in the clinical diagnosis of Noonan syndrome (Table 157-1):
  - Typical facial features *plus* one major or two minor criteria
  - Suggestive facial features *plus* two major or three minor criteria

**Clinical Characteristics:** Noonan syndrome (OMIM 163950) was first described by Jacqueline Noonan in 1968. She noticed a recurring pattern of defects in patients with pulmonary stenosis, dysmorphic facial features with hypertelorism, ptosis and low-set ears, webbed neck, and chest deformities. Several male patients also had cryptorchidism. Because the phenotype resembled that of Turner syndrome, it was previously called "male Turner syndrome." Noonan syndrome is inherited in an autosomal dominant pattern or caused by spontaneous mutations of genes along the RAS-MAPK pathway, most commonly *PTPN11*. Noonan syndrome is the most common syndrome associated with congenital heart disease with an estimated incidence of 1 in 1000 to 2500 live births. One study demonstrated 1% prevalence among patients with congenital heart disease which again has an incidence of approximately 1% of all live births.

Since Noonan syndrome was first described a number of other cardiac and noncardiac features have been identified (Table 157-2). Cardiac involvement is reported in 80% to 90% of patients with Noonan syndrome. While hypertrophic cardiomyopathy and valvar pulmonary stenosis are the most well-known defects in Noonan syndrome, other forms of congenital heart disease occur not uncommonly. The largest study included 136 Noonan syndrome patients with heart disease and showed the following defects: pulmonary stenosis (39%), partial atrioventricular canal defect (15%), hypertrophic cardiomyopathy (10%), aortic coarctation (9%), atrial septal defect (8%), anomalies of the mitral valve (6%), and tetralogy of Fallot (4%). While echocardiography of newborns will detect congenital heart disease, hypertrophic cardiomyopathy may develop during infancy or later in life. Thus periodic cardiology follow-up is recommended for all Noonan syndrome patients throughout life.

Noncardiac clinical manifestations can be categorized into the following organ systems: dysmorphism, skeletal/growth, gastrointestinal, genitourinary, hematologic/oncologic, neurologic/developmental, lymphatic, and ectodermal.

Facial features include hypertelorism, downslanting palpebral fissures with high-arched eyebrows, epicanthal folds, ptosis, low-set and/or posteriorly rotated ears, a full upper lip, depressed nasal root with a wide nasal base, and a high forehead. Webbing of the

*Table 157-1  Diagnostic Criteria*

| Feature | Major | Minor |
|---|---|---|
| Cardiac | Pulmonary stenosis, hypertrophic obstructive cardio-myopathy, and/or typical ECG changes | Other cardiac defect |
| Height | <3rd percentile | <10th percentile |
| Chest wall | Pectus carinatum/excavatum | Broad thorax |
| Family history | First-degree relative with confirmed NS | First-degree relative with possible NS |
| Other | Mental retardation, cryptorchidism, and lymphatic dysplasia | Mental retardation, cryptorchidism, or lymphatic dysplasia |

*Table 157-2  System Involvement*

| System | Manifestation | Incidence |
|---|---|---|
| Cardiovascular | Pulmonary stenosis (39%), partial atrioventricular canal defect (15%), hyper-trophic cardiomyopathy (10%), aortic coarctation (9%), atrial septal defect (8%), anomalies of the mitral valve (6%) and tetralogy of Fallot (4%). ECG anomalies include wide QRS complex, negative pattern in left precordial leads, left axis deviation, giant Q waves | 80%-90% |
| Facial | Hypertelorism, downslanting palpebral fissures with high-arched eyebrows, epicanthal folds, ptosis, low-set and/or posteriorly rotated ears, a full upper lip, depressed nasal root with a wide nasal base, high forehead. Phenotype often mild in adults | 100% |
| Neck | Short and/or webbed neck | 23% |
| Growth | Normal prenatal growth, postnatal growth delay involving height and weight (50%) but not cranial growth, feeding problems during infancy (76%), mean adult height 162.5 cm in males and 152.7 cm in females (<third percentile) | 50% |
| Skeletal | Pectuscarinatus superiorly and pectus excavatum inferiorly most common; thoracic scoliosis (10%), talipes equinovarus, joint contractures, radioulnar synostosis, and cervical spine fusion less common | 95% |
| Neurological | Hypotonia, mild-to-moderate developmental delays (20% require special education), attention deficit disorder, Chiari malformation | 20% |
| Gastrointestinal | Splenomegaly, hepatosplenomegaly, malrotation (rare), choledochal cyst (rare) | 50% |
| Renal | Pyeloureteric stenosis with or without hydronephrosis | 10% |
| Genital | Cryptorchidism, male infertility, delayed onset of puberty by 2 years | 70% |
| Hematologic | Moderate-severe bleeding diathesis, may resolve with age | 25% |
| Oncologic | Juvenile myelomonocytic leukemia (JMML) and acute lymphoblastic leukemia (ALL) although still rare. Spontaneous resolution of JMML common unlike in nonsyndromic patients. Hepatosplenomegaly of unknown origin may be due to subclinical myelodysplasia | <10% |
| Lymphatic | Neonatal lymphedema, lymphangiectasia of lungs (chylothorax) or gastroin-testinal tract (protein-losing enteropathy), peripheral lymphedema | <20% |
| Ophthalmologic | Strabismus, refractive errors, amblyopia, and nystagmus, visuomotor integration | 95% |
| ENT | Conductive hearing loss | 40% |
| Dermatologic | Extra prominence on the pads of all fingers and toes most common (67%), less common are curly and thick (29%) or sparse hair (11%), follicular kera-tosis (14%), café-au-lait spots, multiple lentigines (>100 in 3%) | >70% |
| Dental | High-arched palate most common, less frequent dental malocclusion (50%-67%), articulation difficulties (72%), micrognathia (33%-43%) | 55%-100% |

neck occurs in only 23% of cases. In adults, facial dysmorphism is often mild and may pose diagnostic difficulties. While a child's face may appear coarse and myopathic with prominent eyes and a short neck, the face becomes more triangular with less prominent eyes and a more normal-looking neck during adolescence.

Birth length and weight are typically normal, but postnatal growth delay involving height and weight affects about 50%. Cranial growth is spared. Feeding problems occur in 76% of patients during infancy, requiring tube feeding in 24%. In most patients, feeding difficulties resolve by around age 18 months. Onset of puberty and bone maturity is delayed by approximately 2 years. Mean adult height is 162.5 cm in males and 152.7 cm in females, which are below the third percentile. Noonan syndrome-specific growth data and charts are available, (http://www.norditropin-us.com/hcp/resources.asp). Abnormal growth hormone (GH) secretion and decreased sensitivity to GH have been described in Noonan syndrome. While the effect on adult height is not as strong as in idiopathic GH deficiency, GH treatment of Noonan syndrome patients still significantly improves final compared to predicted adult height (10.9 cm for males, 9.2 cm for females). Duration of prepubertal GH therapy was an important predictor of growth. In children with hypertrophic cardiomyopathy, however, and those carrying certain *RAF1* mutations, GH therapy should not be initiated due to its known effect on cardiac muscle mass.

Skeletal features include pectus carinatum superiorly and pectus excavatum inferiorly in 95% of the patients. Thoracic scoliosis, talipes equinovarus, joint contractures, radioulnar synostosis, and cervical spine fusion are less common.

The only gastrointestinal anomalies described are unexplained (hepato) splenomegaly (50%) which may be due to subclinical myelodysplasia, and rarely malrotation. Regarding the genitourinary system, cryptorchidism occurs in 70% of males and infertility may be associated with it. Renal anomalies, primarily pyeloureteric stenosis with or without hydronephrosis, occur in 10% of patients.

Mild-to-moderate bleeding diathesis is a common problem in Noonan syndrome. Mildly abnormal bleeding (ie, easy bruising with raised bruises >5 cm in diameter occurring over the whole body after minor trauma) is reported in 34% of the patients. Moderately abnormal bleeding (ie, major bruising after surgery or postoperative bleeding lasting >24 h) occurs in 21%. However, severe hemorrhage requiring an emergent blood transfusion happens in only 3%. The etiology is variable and may be a combination of clotting factor or platelet deficiencies, and/or abnormal platelet function. These reports are in concordance with abnormalities found in the intrinsic coagulation cascade in 50% of Noonan syndrome patients. Hematologic evaluation prior to major surgical procedures is generally recommended.

Noonan syndrome patients are at increased risk for juvenile myelomonocytic leukemia (JMML, OMIM 607785) and acute lymphoblastic leukemia (ALL), although only occurring in 1% to 2% of children. While JMML in the general population has a very poor prognosis, cases of spontaneous regression have been described in Noonan syndrome. Lifetime risk of other cancers does not appear to be increased.

Mild developmental delay and learning problems affect about one-third of Noonan syndrome patients. Individuals with *SOS1* mutations have generally better neurocognitive outcome, while those with *KRAS* mutations fare poorly. Some motor delay can be attributed to the hypotonia that is often observed during infancy. There is also an increased incidence of attention deficit hyperactivity disorder (ADHD), and impaired emotion recognition in adult with Noonan syndrome. Seizure disorders are rare.

Noonan syndrome is associated with lymphatic dysplasia in about 20% of cases. This may present as hydrops in the fetus, peripheral lymphedema in the young infant that often resolves in the first few years of life due to delayed lymphatic development and maturation, or as peripheral lymphedema in the adolescents or adults. Other lymphatic problems in Noonan syndrome include chylous pleural effusions, chylothorax, pulmonary lymphangiectasis, intestinal lymphangiectasia, hypoplastic leg lymphatics, anomalous lymphatic vessels in the thoracic cage and aplasia or absence of the thoracic duct, hypoplastic inguinal and iliac lymphatic vessels, and testicular lymphangiectasis. Management of these conditions can be difficult and patients should be referred to lymphedema specialists.

Visual problems are highly prevalent among Noonan syndrome patients. They include strabismus, refractive errors, amblyopia, and nystagmus. More recently abnormal visuomotor integration was identified in 30% of the patients. Hearing loss has been described in about 40% of patients. Dental anomalies are high-arched palate, malocclusion, articulation difficulties, and micrognathia.

## Screening and Counseling

***Screening:***

☞**PRENATAL SCREENING:** Cystic hygroma, increased nuchal translucency, polyhydramnios, and rarely hydrops fetalis may occur in fetuses with Noonan syndrome. Prenatal and even preconception testing is available for cases where a parent is affected and a mutation is known. In fetuses with cystic hygroma and normal karyotype, 16% carry *PTPN11* mutations (Table 157-3).

***Counseling:***

☞**INHERITANCE, PENETRANCE:** The mode of inheritance is autosomal dominant with complete penetrance but the phenotype can be variable. An affected parent is present in 30% to 75% of the cases. An affected parent may be identified following the diagnosis of a more severely affected child. The recurrence risk for future pregnancies is 50% if a parent is affected. If careful evaluation of both parents shows no evidence of Noonan syndrome, the recurrence risk approaches the risk for the general population which is presumed to be 1:1000-1:2500 plus the theoretical possibility of gonadal mosaicism for Noonan syndrome in one of the parents, which is rare.

☞**GENOTYPE-PHENOTYPE CORRELATION:** For Noonan syndrome, there are genotype-phenotype associations that depend on which of the seven known disease genes is mutated and, less frequently, which particular mutation is present. To some extent, this enables one to predict the likely genotype based on the patient's phenotype. More importantly, a known genotype can guide further screening and management; for example, an infant with a known *RAF1* mutation who has a normal echocardiogram should have close cardiology follow-up because she is likely to develop hypertrophic cardiomyopathy.

## Management and Treatment

Recommendations for screening and management of patients with Noonan syndrome are provided in Table 157-3.

**Table 157-3** *Algorithm for Screening and Management of Patients With Noonan Syndrome*

| Clinical Specialty Issue | Recommendations |
|---|---|
| Cardiovascular | • Pediatric cardiology referral at diagnosis<br>• If initial evaluation is normal, periodic ECGs every 3-5 years *through adolescence* for hypertrophic cardiomyopathy<br>• Avoid using aspirin if possible because of bleeding tendency |
| Growth and endocrine | • Assess and plot growth on growth chart three times a year for the first 3 years of life, and yearly thereafter<br>• Refer to pediatric endocrinology around 8 to 10 years of age or earlier if growth delay present for possible growth hormone treatment<br>• Children with delayed-onset of puberty (no breast development in girls by age 13 years, no testicular enlargement in boys by age 14 years) should be referred to a pediatric endocrinologist |
| Renal and genitourinary | • Kidney ultrasound at diagnosis<br>• Orchiopexy should be performed for cryptorchidism by 1 year of age |
| Gastrointestinal | • Pediatric gastroenterology/nutrition consult for feeding difficulties if indicated |
| Hematologic | • Coagulation workup prior to surgery or otherwise electively during early childhood<br>• Splenomegaly: CBC with differential count |
| Neurological, cognitive, and behavioral | • Developmental screening annually<br>• Complete neuropsychologic testing if screening abnormal<br>• Early intervention programs beginning in infancy if delays noted<br>• Speech therapy, physical therapy (PT), and occupational therapy (OT) if delays in speech, gross motor or fine motor skills, respectively<br>• Individualized education plan for school age children<br>• Electroencephalography (EEG) and referral to neurology if seizures suspected |
| Ophthalmologic | • Detailed examination at diagnosis<br>• Follow-up as indicated or every 2 years if initial evaluation normal |
| Otologic | • Hearing test at diagnosis, thereafter annually throughout early childhood<br>• Aggressive management of ear infections to minimize hearing loss |
| Orthopedic | • Annual examination of chest and back<br>• Orthopedics referral as indicated |
| Dental | • Referral to dentist between age 1 and 2 years with yearly visits thereafter |

# Molecular Genetics and Molecular Mechanism

## Syndrome/Gene/Locus:

☞DESCRIPTION OF BASIC GENE FUNCTIONS: There are seven Noonan syndrome disease genes that have been identified to date. They have in common that they encode proteins relevant for signal transduction through the RAS-MAPK pathway. Most Noonan syndrome-related mutations have gain-of-function effects. Prior to discovering its role in the development of Noonan syndrome and related disorders, this signaling pathway's relevance for human disease was primarily for acquired gain of function for various cancers. Mutations in the seven known disease genes account for approximately 60% of Noonan syndrome cases, implying the existence of additional disease genes (Table 157-4).

*PTPN11* was the first Noonan syndrome disease gene identified and mutations are found in 41% of cases. It was identified through a positional candidacy approach in 2001. *PTPN11* (OMIM 176876) encodes SHP2, a widely expressed cytoplasmic Src homology 2 (SH2) domain-containing protein tyrosine phosphatase. SHP2 plays important roles during development and regulates cell migration, proliferation, survival, and differentiation. It primarily occupies a positive role

in RAS-MAPK signaling. SHP2 has two N-terminal SH2 domains (N-SH2 and C-SH2) and a catalytic domain (PTP) C-terminal domain. The protein has a molecular switching mechanism involving interactions between amino acid residues in the N-SH2 and catalytic domains such that the SHP2 has active and inactive conformations. Nearly all *PTPN11* mutations found in Noonan syndrome are missense defects, most altering amino residues relevant for SHP2's molecular switch and lead to constitutive or prolonged activity. Among patients with Noonan syndrome due to *PTPN11* mutations, there is a relatively higher prevalence of pulmonary stenosis, whereas hypertrophic cardiomyopathy and severe developmental delay are less common. *PTPN11* mutations also account for nearly 90% of cases of Noonan syndrome with multiple lentigines. The amino acid substitutions for Noonan syndrome and Noonan syndrome with multiple lentigines are essentially mutually exclusive. While strictly gain of function in Noonan syndrome, there are discrepant data for the two most common Noonan syndromes with multiple lentigines mutations: biochemically, they are phosphatase deficient while they have gain-of-function effects on development in fruit fly models. This partially explains the enigma of how loss- and gain-of-function mutations in the same gene lead to similar phenotypes.

Children with Noonan syndrome are predisposed to malignancies, including JMML, a clonal myeloproliferative disorder of

*Table 157-4 Molecular Genetic Testing*

| Gene | Disease | Testing Modality | Mutation Type | Detection Rate |
|------|---------|------------------|---------------|----------------|
| *PTPN11* | Noonan syndrome, LEOPARD syndrome | Sequencing | Missense mutation, duplication (rare) | 41% 85% |
| *SOS1* | Noonan syndrome | Sequencing | Missense mutation | 11% |
| *KRAS* | Noonan syndrome, CFC syndrome, Costello syndrome | Sequencing | Missense mutation | 1% 8% 10% |
| *NRAS* | Noonan syndrome | Sequencing | Missense mutation | <1% |
| *RAF1* | Noonan syndrome, LEOPARD syndrome | Sequencing | Missense mutation | 5% 3% |
| *BRAF* | Noonan and LEOPARD syndrome CFC syndrome | Sequencing | Missense mutation | 1% 35% |
| *SHOC2* | Noonan syndrome with loose anagen hair | Sequencing | Missense mutation | 2% |
| *HRAS* | Costello syndrome | Sequencing | Missense mutation | 90% |
| *MEK1/2* | CFC syndrome | Sequencing | Missense mutation | 10% |

childhood. JMML is characterized by hypersensitivity of myeloid progenitor colony growth in response to GM-CSF, which is due to an inability to downregulate RAS function. A germline mutation, *Thr73Ile*, that is not very common among Noonan syndrome patients without leukemia, is the most common mutation found in patients with JMML and Noonan syndrome. In children with nonsyndromic JMML, somatic *PTPN11* mutations are identified in one-third and there is nearly mutual exclusivity between those inherited through the germline that cause Noonan syndrome and the somatic mutations causing nonsyndromic JMML. Further, SHP2 mutants associated with malignancies tend to be more activating on a biochemical level than observed with the Noonan syndrome-associated mutant proteins.

Taking these data together, it is now believed that SHP2 mutants associated with NS have relatively milder gain-of-function effects in that they are able to perturb development but not activating enough to induce leukemia. The somatic *PTPN11* mutations observed in isolated JMML and other hematologic malignancies are associated with higher gain of function, and presumably would be embryonically lethal if occurring as germline mutations. The subgroup of Noonan syndrome patients with JMML carry distinct *PTPN11* mutations which have an effect that is in between the prior two groups. This might explain why patients with Noonan syndrome and JMML have a relatively good prognosis.

The second most commonly mutated gene causing Noonan syndrome is *SOS1*, which encodes a RAS-specific guanine nucleotide exchange factor that is important for RAS activation. *SOS1* mutations are missense and are found in 11% of Noonan syndrome patients. Noonan syndrome-causing *SOS1* mutations cluster in regions implicated in the maintenance of *SOS1* autoinhibition, and, therefore, have gain-of-function effects on RAS-MAPK signaling. The phenotype associated with *SOS1* defects is significant for a high prevalence of ectodermal abnormalities (keratosis pilaris/hyperkeratotic skin, sparse eyebrows) but normal cognitive development and growth. Unlike *PTPN11*, *SOS1* mutations do not appear to play a role in the development of malignancies.

Based on the link between the functions of SHP2 and RAS, two groups independently used a candidate gene approach to discover that *KRAS* mutations can cause Noonan syndrome. *KRAS* missense mutations account for 1% of Noonan syndrome cases. They act by impairing the switch between the active and inactive conformation leading to an exaggerated response of KRAS to growth factor stimulation. The phenotype of patients carrying these mutations generally is relatively severe. JMML and craniosynostosis have been described as well. Sometimes the phenotype is difficult to distinguish from cardiofaciocutaneous syndrome. Not surprisingly, *KRAS* mutations have also been identified in individuals with the latter syndrome. Of note, Noonan syndrome-causing *KRAS* mutations are distinct from the somatic mutations found in human cancers.

Other members of the RAS family of GTPases are *HRAS* and *NRAS*. Missense mutations in *HRAS* cause Costello syndrome, which is a severe variant of Noonan syndrome with a strong potential for developing cancer. *HRAS* mutations are found in almost all patients with Costello syndrome, and vice versa, the absence of an *HRAS* mutation essentially excludes the diagnosis. *HRAS* mutations are missense, and mainly affect two residues, that is, Gly and Gly. These are the two residues commonly mutated in human cancers, although the prevalence of the specific amino acid substitutions differs between Costello syndrome and cancer. The functional effect again is gain of function. Two *NRAS* missense mutations, *T50I* and *G60E*, have been found in a total of four patients with Noonan syndrome. No genotype-phenotype correlation has been established for this genetic form of Noonan syndrome yet.

Downstream of RAS are the RAF family of serine-threonine kinases which include ARAF, BRAF, and RAF1 (also known as CRAF). RAF proteins phosphorylate and activate the dual-specificity kinases, MEK1 and MEK2, which in turn promote the activation of ERK1 and ERK2. While BRAF has stronger kinase activity, RAF1 is unique in that it has kinase-independent functions. Missense mutations of *RAF1* are found in 5% of patients with Noonan syndrome and 2% to 3% of cases of Noonan syndrome with multiple lentigines. Mutations cluster in three regions: an N-terminal negative regulatory domain, the activation segment, and the C-terminal domain. While in vitro data show that the former and latter groups of mutations cause an increased activation of ERK, mutations in the activation segment do not. Interestingly, the clinical phenotype correlates with these findings in that patients carrying mutations in the N-terminal and C-terminal regions almost all have hypertrophic cardiomyopathy whereas patients carrying mutations in the activation segment rarely develop hypertrophic cardiomyopathy. Also, Noonan syndrome patients with *RAF1* mutations have a predisposition to hyperpigmented cutaneous lesions, that is, multiple nevi, lentigines, and/or café-au-lait spots, which are detectable in one-third of the group. There is no apparent increased risk of developing malignancies in patients with germline *RAF1* mutations. In general, somatic *RAF1* mutations are rare in human cancer when compared to *BRAF* mutations. Further, inherited mutations causing Noonan syndrome affect different residues than somatic mutations seen in cancer.

While missense mutations in ***BRAF*** are known to be a common cause of CFC syndrome (35%), they were recently identified in 1% of Noonan and Noonan syndrome with multiple lentigines patients as well. Of note, Noonan syndrome-associated mutations do not overlap with those occurring in CFC syndrome. In vitro data shows that CFC syndrome mutations are more activating than Noonan or Noonan syndrome with multiple lentigines-causing mutations, suggesting a genotype-phenotype correlation. There was a recent case report on a CFC patient carrying a 93-kb deletion that included the entire CR1 domain of BRAF, which is the first time that a large intragenic deletion has been shown to cause a Noonan syndrome-related phenotype. Clinically, Noonan syndrome patients carrying *BRAF* mutations have more severe cognitive deficits and a higher prevalence of neonatal growth failure and feeding difficulties, hypotonia, multiple nevi, and lentigines. Normal intelligence does not exclude this genotype. Germline *BRAF* mutations differ from those commonly found in human cancer, and they are less activating *in vitro*. This goes along with the observation that there is no increased risk of developing cancer in these patients.

A distinct N-terminal missense mutation in ***SHOC2*** was identified in a subgroup of Noonan syndrome patients termed Noonan syndrome with loose anagen hair. SHOC2 is a scaffolding protein that links RAS to downstream signal transducers. The *S2G SHOC2* mutation causing Noonan syndrome introduces an N-myristoylation site, resulting in aberrant targeting of SHOC2 to the plasma membrane and impairing translocation to the nucleus upon growth factor stimulation. This mutation is found in approximately 2% of Noonan syndrome patients. Clinically, these patients commonly have hair anomalies including easily pluckable, sparse, thin, slow-growing hair, reduced growth often with proven growth hormone deficiency, more severe cognitive deficits, hyperactive behavior that tends to improve with age, a hypernasal voice, and darkly pigmented skin with eczema or ichthyosis. Among cardiac anomalies, dysplastic mitral valves and septal defects are unusually common for Noonan syndrome.

Taken together, the understanding of Noonan syndrome and related disorders has changed fundamentally over the last 8 years. While originally presumed to be separate diseases it is now clear that they all have in common the dysregulation of the RAS-MAPK pathway. Mutations in identified disease genes account for approximately 60% of affected individuals with Noonan syndrome, indicating that other disease genes responsible for this disorder remain to be identified. There is a strong genotype-phenotype correlation with respect to the individual disease genes, but also regarding different alleles of the same disease gene. Knowledge of the affected gene in the individual patient is important for prognostication and counseling, and may guide further surveillance and treatment.

### Genetic Testing:

☞**CLINICAL AVAILABILITY OF TESTING:** Genetic testing for *PTPN11, SOS1, HRAS, KRAS, NRAS, RAF1, BRAF, MEK1/2, and SHOC2* is commercially available. For up-to-date contact information, visit http://www.genetests.org.

☞**UTILITY OF TESTING:** Genetic testing plays a large role in the prognostication and counseling of Noonan syndrome patients and their families since the genotype often predicts the phenotype that may evolve over time. For example, infants with *KRAS* mutations are likely to exhibit more severe cognitive deficits and thus early intervention should be initiated. Another example would be patients with certain *RAF1* mutations who are likely to develop hypertrophic cardiomyopathy and therefore need close cardiology follow-up. For infants, in whom differentiating Noonan syndrome from its related disorders can be very challenging; gene testing may enable earlier and more precise diagnosis.

### BIBLIOGRAPHY:

1. Allanson JE. Noonan syndrome. *Am J Med Genet C Semin Med Genet.* 2007;145C:274-279.

2. Van der Burgt I, Berends E, Lommen E, van Beersum S, Hamel B, Mariman E. Clinical and molecular studies in a large Dutch family with Noonan syndrome. *Am J Med Genet.* 1994;53:187-191.

3. Sharland M, Burch M, McKenna WM, Paton MA. A clinical study of Noonan syndrome. *Arch Dis Child.* 1992;67:178-183.

4. Witt DR, Keena BA, Hall JG, Allanson JE. Growth curves for height in Noonan syndrome. *Clin Genet.* 1986;30:150-153.

6. Tartaglia M, Mehler EL, Goldberg R, et al. Mutations in *PTPN11*, encoding the protein tyrosine phosphatase SHP-2, cause Noonan syndrome. *Nat Genet.* 2001;29:465-468.

7. Tartaglia M, Niemeyer CM, Fragale A, et al. Somatic mutations in PTPN11 in juvenile myelomonocytic leukemia, myelodysplastic syndromes and acute myeloid leukemia. *Nat Genet.* 2003;34: 148-150.

8. Tartaglia M, Pennacchio LA, Zhao C, et al. Gain-of-function *SOS1* mutations cause a distinctive form of Noonan syndrome. *Nat Genet.* 2007;39:75-79.

9. Carta C, Pantaleoni F, Bocchinfuso G, et al. Germline missense mutations affecting KRAS isoform B are associated with a severe Noonan syndrome phenotype. *Am J Hum Genet.* 2006;79:129-135.

10. Schubert S, Zenker M, Rowe SL, et al. Germline KRAS mutations cause Noonan syndrome. *Nat Genet.* 2006;38:331-336.

11. Aoki Y, Niihori T, Kawame H, et al. Germline mutations in HRAS proto-oncogene cause Costello syndrome. *Nat Genet.* 2005;37:1038-1034.

12. Cirstea IC, Kutsche K, Dvorsky R, et al. A restricted spectrum of *NRAS* mutations causes Noonan syndrome. *Nat Genet.* 2010;42:27-29.

13. Pandit B, Sarkozy A, Pennacchio LA, et al. Gain-of-function RAF1 mutations cause Noonan and LEOPARD syndromes with hypertrophic cardiomyopathy. *Nat Genet.* 2007;39:1007-1012.

14. Yu S, Graf WD. BRAF gene deletion broadens the clinical spectrum of neuro-cardio-facila-cutaneous syndromes. *J Child Neurol.* Dec 2011;26:1593-1596.

15. Cordeddu V, Di Schiavi E, Pennacchio LA, et al. Mutation of SHOC2 promotes aberrant protein N-myristoylation and causes Noonan-like syndrome with loose anagen hair. *Nat Genet.* 2009;41:1022-1026.

## Supplementary Information

**OMIM References:**

[1] Noonan Syndrome (#163950)

[2] Noonan Syndrome With Multiple Lentigines (#151100)

[3] Costello Syndrome (#218040)

[4] CFC Syndrome (#115150)

[5] Neurofibromatosis-Noonan Syndrome (#601321)

[6] Noonan-Like Syndrome With Loose Anagen Hair (#607721)

[7] PTPN11(#176876)

[8] SOS1(#182530)

[9] RAF1(#164760)

[10] BRAF(#164757)

[11] KRAS(#190070)

[12] NRAS(#164790)

[13] HRAS(#190020)

[14] SHOC2(#602775)

[15] MEK1(#176872)

[16] MEK2(#601263)

**Alternative Name:**

• Male Turner Syndrome

*Keywords:* Noonan syndrome, Noonan-like syndrome with loose anagen hair, LEOPARD syndrome, Noonan syndrome with multiple lentigines, Costello syndrome, CFC syndrome, Neurofibromatosis-Noonan syndrome, Turner syndrome, PTPN11, SOS1, RAF1, BRAF, KRAS, NRAS, HRAS, SHOC2, MEK1, MEK2, developmental delay, mental retardation, growth short stature, lentigines, congenital heart defect, pulmonary stenosis, hypertrophic cardiomyopathy, leukemia, JMML

# 158 Hereditary Hemorrhagic Telangiectasia

Reed E. Pyeritz

## KEY POINTS

- *Disease summary:*
  - Hereditary hemorrhagic telangiectasia (HHT) is a disorder of vascular development that results in direct communication between arteries and veins.
  - Multiple organs are affected and the development of clinical features is age dependent. Telangiectases in the nose cause epistaxis severe enough to cause chronic anemia. Vascular anomalies in the brain and spinal column cause stroke or seizures. Pulmonary arteriovenous malformations (PAVMs) cause hypoxemia and high-output cardiac failure because of shunting and provide a conduit for clots and bacteria to cause embolic stroke and cerebral abscess. Hepatic AVMs cause high-output cardiac failure and cirrhosis. A late finding is gastrointestinal (GI) telangiectases that cause chronic blood loss.
  - While today mortality is only modestly increased, the clinical features cause considerable morbidity and diminished quality of life.
- *Hereditary basis:*
  - HHT is an autosomal dominant condition of considerable variability found in all populations. Reproduction is little affected so sporadic cases are uncommon. Most cases (>80%) are due to mutations in either *ENG* or *ACVRL1*, the products of which function as cell surface receptors in the TGF-β/BMP signaling pathway. Mutations in *SMAD4* cause HHT combined with juvenile polyposis. Some families show linkage to none of these loci.
- *Differential diagnosis:*
  - A number of syndromes include cutaneous or sclera telangiectases (ataxia telangiectasia, CREST syndrome, chronic liver disease, hereditary benign telangiectasia, pregnancy) but not the visceral vascular anomalies.
  - An isolated PAVM can occur in the absence of other features of HHT.
  - Vascular dysplasias can accumulate in GI mucosa with age and cause chronic blood loss.

## Diagnostic Criteria and Clinical Characteristics

**Diagnostic Criteria for HHT:** The Curacao criteria have been expanded to include molecular genetic testing. In the absence of a mutation, three of the following four criteria are required to diagnose HHT:

- Epistaxis
- Visceral AVMs
- Mucocutaneous telangiectases
- A family history of documented HHT

Having two of these criteria qualify for possible HHT.

Having a pathogenic mutation in *ENG*, *ACVRL1*, or *SMAD4* known to cause HHT in either the patient's family of another individual with documented HHT qualifies for a diagnosis of HHT.

**Clinical Characteristics:** Patients present with recurrent epistaxis, anemia, cutaneous telangiectases, dyspnea due to hypoxemia or heart failure, liver failure, embolic or hemorrhagic stroke, or cerebral abscess.

## Screening and Counseling

**Screening:** When HHT is suspected, such as in a relative of a person with documented HHT or in a person with one of the Curacao criteria, a protocol for establishing or discarding the diagnosis of HHT is as follows:

- In a family in which the pathogenic mutation is known, DNA testing is the most effective and most economic method of screening.

- Brain magnetic resonance imaging (MRI) to detect cerebral vascular anomalies and occult stroke(s) and cerebral abscess.
- Contrast echocardiogram to detect elevated pulmonary artery pressure or delayed passage (4-8 cardiac cycles) of contrast from the right ventricle into the left atrium. Immediate passage of contrast suggests a cardiac septal defect, especially a patent foramen ovale, and no information about the integrity of the pulmonary capillary circulation can be inferred. In either case of contrast in the left atrium, a high-resolution computed tomographic angiogram (CTA) of the lungs is needed to determine whether a pulmonary AVM (PAVM) is present, how many, where, and the size of the feeding artery(ies).
- Typically, the chest CT also visualizes much of the liver, so information about the presence of hepatic AVMs is also obtained. But if a chest CT is not needed, then screening of the liver is generally not needed for diagnostic purposes.
- Upper and lower endoscopy of the GI tract can detect mucosal telangiectases; while the presence of such lesion may be useful for satisfying the Curacao criterion of visceral AVMs, such testing is generally not used for screening purposes.

**Counseling:**

☞INHERITANCE AND PENETRANCE: HHT is an autosomal dominant syndrome with age dependency and variable expression. True nonpenetrance is uncommon. Males and females are equally frequently and severely affected.

Presymptomatic testing can be performed based on a familial mutation. This is important to reassure those unaffected relatives who can then be spared clinical screening. If the familial mutation is not known or if a person is mutation-positive, then the individual should undergo the clinical screening protocol detailed earlier.

Women with HHT of childbearing age should have their clinical status evaluated carefully before undertaking a pregnancy. PAVMs should be treated and anemia corrected.

☞**Genotype-Phenotype Correlation:** Mutations in *ACVRL1* may cause primary pulmonary hypertension, HHT, or a combination. Mutations in *SMAD4* cause juvenile polyposis and HHT. There is little consistent difference among patients with HHT who have mutations in *ENG* or *ACVRL1*.

## Management and Treatment

☞**Epistaxis:** Conservative measures such as intranasal emollients and humidification of indoor air can help minimize bleeding in many patients. Patients who have persistent bleeding that interferes with daily activities or causes transfusion-dependent anemia should be evaluated by a rhinologist with experience with HHT. Laser coagulation of bleeding telangiectases can stem hemorrhage, at least for a time. Septal dermoplasty, using the patient's skin, can provide longer-term relief, but eventually telangiectases appear on the surface of the skin. Some patients have benefited from off-label use of thalidomide or bevacizumab (Avastin), but controlled trials are just beginning.

☞**PAVMs:** Lesions with a feeding artery of greater than 1 mm should be considered for occlusion using a coil that incites a thrombus. A PAVM with a large feeding artery, or a complex AVM, may require occlusion with an Amplatzer device. Occlusion of multiple lesions can be accomplished in one outpatient procedure. Occlusion of peripheral PAVMs may result in transient pleuritis. Imaging of occluded PAVMs should be performed by CTA after 6 months to ensure persistent occlusion. Lesions too small to treat should be imaged periodically (every 3-5 years) by CTA because expansion can occur.

☞**Hepatic Vascular Lesions:** Several types of abnormal vascular connections can occur, including hepatic artery to hepatic vein, hepatic artery to portal vein, hemangiomas, and diffuse telangiectases. The clinical syndrome depends on the type of abnormal connection and the size of the shunt. Hepatocyte dysfunction should be treated by standard approaches. Often a picture of multinodular cirrhosis, resembling hepatoma, develops; liver biopsy should be avoided because of the risk of severe bleeding. Liver transplant can be used for end-stage disease. Some patients have benefited from off-label use of thalidomide or bevacizumab (Avastin), but controlled trials are just beginning.

☞**Gastrointestinal Bleeding:** Blood loss from the GI tract before middle age is uncommon. Thereafter occult and chronic blood loss can occur. Testing stool for heme is not helpful since most patients regularly swallow blood from epistaxis. Upper and lower endoscopy can be used to detect telangiectases and to exclude an ulcer or a tumor, but ablation of telangiectases is rarely helpful because of their number and tendency to emerge persistently. Similarly, push enterostomy and capsule endoscopy can detect mucosal lesions but rarely visualize a lesion bleeding so actively that surgical therapy would be warranted.

☞**Mucocutaneous Telangiectases:** Lesions in the mouth occasionally bleed and can be treated with laser cautery. Lesions on the face bleed recurrently from shaving and can also be cauterized. Otherwise, lesions are primarily of cosmetic concern.

☞**Cerebrovascular Anomalies:** Anyone suspected of HHT should undergo noncontrast MRI imaging. Neurosurgical or neurovascular consultation should be sought for any patient with an aneurysm, hemangioma, or AVM detected. Similarly, a cerebral abscess should prompt neurosurgical and infectious disease consultation, and a search for a PAVM.

☞**Anemia:** The hemoglobin should be checked periodically in any patient with HHT, frequently with active epistaxis or known anemia. Iron deficiency is common, particularly in premenopausal women. Aggressive iron replacement, first orally and if ineffective or not tolerated, intravenously, should be undertaken. If the hemoglobin cannot be maintained greater than 9 to 10 g/dL, then transfusions of packed red cells are necessary. Transfusion dependency should prompt consideration of aggressive treatment of epistaxis or GI bleeding as described earlier.

## Molecular Genetics and Molecular Mechanism

*Genes/Loci:*

Endoglin/*ENG*/9q34.1

Activin A receptor, type II-like 1/*ACVRL1*/12q11-q14

Mothers against decapentaplegic, *Drosophila* homolog of, 4/*SMAD4*/18q21.1

HHT3/5q31.3-q32

HHT4/7p14

The three known genes encode proteins that are involved in TGF-β and BMP signaling. Virtually all of the other components of canonical signaling through these pathways have been screened for mutations in probands that have no detectable mutations in the three known genes, to no avail. A proband with classic HHT has an 87% chance of having a mutation detected in one of the three known genes.

HHT is a disorder primarily of endothelial cell dysfunction and the manifestations can begin in the embryo. Some infants are born with severe manifestations, such as large PAVMs or cerebral AVMs. In the majority of patients features emerge during childhood or adolescence. Whether this represents the development of new vascular anomalies during growth, or the expansion of embryologic lesions, remains unclear.

Molecular pathogenesis is an area of active investigation, and may uncover targets amenable to potential therapies. Currently, off-label treatments with agents that interfere with angiogenesis (thalidomide, bevacizumab) have helped some patients with severe epistaxis, bleeding from the GI tract, and hepatic failure from vascular shunts. However, not all patients benefit and the potential adverse effects of some agents can be severe.

*Genetic Testing:* DNA sequencing and deletion or duplication analyses of *ENG*, *ACVRL1*, and *SMAD4* are available from number of laboratories in North America and around the world (see Gene Tests    http://www.ncbi.nlm.nih.gov/sites/GeneTests/lab/disease/hht?db=genetests&search_param=contains). Except for the patient who has GI polyps, for whom *SMAD4* testing should be conducted first, then *ENG* and *ACVRL1* are analyzed. About 87% of probands with classic HHT will have a mutation detected.

**Bibliography:**

1. Bernhardt BA, Zayac C, Trerotola SO, Asch DA, Pyeritz RE. Cost savings through molecular diagnosis for hereditary hemorrhagic telangiectasia. *Genet Med.* 2012;14:604-610.

2. Faughnan ME, Palda VA, Garcia-Tsao G, et al. International guidelines for the diagnosis and management of hereditary hemorrhagic telangiectasia. *J Med Genet*. 2011:48:73-87.

3. Gallione CJ, Repetto GM, Legius E, et al. A combined syndrome of juvenile polyposis and hereditary haemorrhagic telangiectasia associated with mutations in MADH4 (SMAD4). *Lancet*. 2004;363:852-859.

4. Garcia-Tsao G, Korzenik JR, Young L, et al. Liver disease in patients with hereditary hemorrhagic telangiectasia. *N Engl J Med*. 2000;343:931-936.

5. Guttmacher A, et al. Hereditary hemorrhagic telangiectasia. In: Rimoin DL, Pyeritz RE, Korf BR, eds. *Emery and Rimoin's Essential Medical Genetics*. Oxford; Academic Press, 2013;184-191.

6. McDonald J, Pyeritz RE. (Updated Aug 2011.) Hereditary hemorrhagic telangiectasia. In: GeneReviewsatGeneTests: Medical Genetics Information Resource [database online]. Copyright, University of Washington, Seattle.1997-2011. http://www.genetests.org.

7. McDonald J, Bayrak-Toydemir P, Pyeritz RE. Hereditary hemorrhagic telangiectasia: an overview of diagnosis, management and pathogenesis. *Genet Med*. 2011;13:607-616.

8. McDonald J, Damjanovich K, Millson A, et al. Molecular diagnosis in hereditary hemorrhagic telangiectasia: findings in a series tested simultaneously by sequencing and deletion/duplication analysis. *Clin Genet*. 2011;79:335-344.

9. Shovlin CL, Guttmacher AE, Buscarini E, et al. Diagnostic criteria for hereditary hemorrhagic telangiectasia (Rendu-Osler-Weber syndrome). *Am J Med Genet*. 2000;91:66-67.

10. Trerotola SO, Pyeritz RE. PAVM embolization: an update. *AJR Am J Roentgenol*. 2010;195:837-845.

11. van Tuyl SA, Letteboer TG, Rogge-Wolf C, et al. Assessment of intestinal vascular malformations in patients with hereditary hemorrhagic teleangiectasia and anemia. *Eur J Gastroenterol Hepatol*. 2007;19:153-158.

## Supplementary Information

**OMIM Reference:**

[1] 187300; 600376; 175050; 601101; 610655

***Key Words:*** Epistaxis, anemia, arteriovenous malformation, GI bleeding, iron deficiency

# 159 Fragile X Syndrome and Related Conditions

Gretchen Schneider

## KEY POINTS

- *Disease summary:*
  - Fragile X syndrome is characterized by neurodevelopmental dysfunction including intellectual disability and behavioral problems, facial dysmorphism, and connective tissue findings. Clinical features may be subtle in childhood while developmental delays typically present at a young age. Manifestations in affected females tend to be milder than those seen in males.
  - Fragile X-associated late-onset tremor-ataxia syndrome (FXTAS) is a progressive neurodegenerative disorder that typically presents after age 50 and affects men more commonly than women.
  - Fragile X-associated premature ovarian insufficiency (FXPOI) can present as decreased ovarian reserve, decreased fertility, elevated follicle-stimulating hormone (FSH) levels, or premature ovarian failure (POF).
- *Hereditary basis:*
  - Fragile X syndrome, FXTAS, and FXPOI are caused by triplet repeat expansions in the *FMR1* gene on the X chromosome.
    - Greater than 99% of fragile X syndrome is associated with repeat sizes of greater than 200 (full mutation). Less than 1% is associated with other mutations that silence the *FMR1* gene.
    - FXTAS and FXPOI are associated with repeat sizes of 55 to 200 (premutation)
  - Females with a pre or full mutation have a 50% of passing an expansion mutation to their offspring.
    - Expansion of a premutation to a full mutation only occurs during female meiosis and depends on premutation size in carrier females.
  - Fragile X syndrome affects approximately 1/4000 males and 1/8000 females. The carrier frequency for *FMR1* premutations in females in the United States is estimated to be 1/382.
- *Differential diagnosis:*
  - Fragile X syndrome is the most common single gene cause of intellectual disability and autism. Therefore, it should be considered at the top of the differential diagnosis for males and females affected with either of the two.
  - Intellectual disability is seen as a part of many genetic syndromes, however, the presence of clinical features consistent with other conditions may help to rule out other diagnoses.
  - Genetic conditions that warrant consideration when a diagnosis of fragile X syndrome cannot be established include fragile XE syndrome, Sotos syndrome, and other chromosomal abnormalities.

## Diagnostic Criteria and Clinical Characteristics

**Fragile X Syndrome:** The clinical findings seen in individuals with fragile X syndrome are summarized in Table 159-1. Features tend to be milder in affected females than males, with 50% of females with a full mutation having normal intellect. Intellectual disability in males includes a spectrum of mild to severe with most falling in the moderate range with an IQ of 70 or lower. The facial features and connective tissue findings vary significantly and are often subtle or absent in young children. Macroorchidism, a hallmark feature of fragile X syndrome (not listed in Table 159-1), is not evident in boys until after puberty.

A definitive diagnosis of fragile X syndrome is made when an individual with any of the above clinical findings is found to have a silencing mutation in the *FMR1* gene.

☞**FXTAS:** FXTAS is an adult-onset progressive neurologic condition that typically presents after age 50. Men with *FMR1* premutations are at significantly higher risk than female carriers. Diagnostic criteria for FXTAS include both clinical and neuroimaging findings.

- Major criteria—intension tremor and cerebellar ataxia on clinical examination and white matter lesions of the middle cerebellar peduncles or brain stem on magnetic resonance imaging (MRI)
- Minor criteria—short-term memory deficits, defects in executive function, parkinsonism, white matter lesions in the cerebral white matter, generalized atrophy on MRI

Definite diagnosis of FXTAS is made in an individual with an *FMR1* premutation and one major clinical and one major imaging finding. A probable diagnosis of FXTAS requires the presence of two major clinical signs of one major imaging finding with one minor clinical sign. Additional neurologic findings associated with FXTAS can include cognitive decline, dementia, peripheral neuropathy, and muscle weakness. The majority of individuals with an *FMR1* premutation are of normal intelligence although learning disabilities in children and mental health issues in females with premutations have been reported.

☞**FXPOI:** Clinical findings are present in approximately 21% of women with an *FMR1* premutation and include elevated FSH levels, decreased ovarian reserve, educed fertility, and cessation of menses prior to 40. The risk of FXPOI increases with repeat sizes from 55 to 95 then stabilizes and then decreases with higher repeat number up until 200. Women with evidence of reports

**Table 159-1  Summary of Clinical Findings in Individuals With Fragile X Syndrome**

| Neurodevelopmental | Facial Features | Connective Tissue |
|---|---|---|
| Intellectual disability | Macrocephaly | Smooth skin |
| Autism | Large forehead | Hyperextensible joints |
| Attention deficit | Long face | Flat feet |
| Speech impairment | Enlarged ears | Mitral valve prolapse |
| Anxiety | Prominent chin | |
| Developmental delay | High-arched palate | |
| Hypotonia | Strabismus | |

**Table 159-2  Expansion of FMR1 Premutation**

| Maternal Repeats | Risk of Full Mutation in Offspring |
|---|---|
| 55-59 | 3.70% |
| 60-69 | 5.30% |
| 70-79 | 31.10% |
| 80-89 | 57.80% |
| 90-99 | 80.10% |
| >100 | 94%-100% |

have demonstrated the ability to conceive with FXPOI, but with a markedly reduced success rate from the general population.

## Screening and Counseling

**Screening:** Screening for mutations in the *FMR1* gene is indicated for

- Individuals with a family history of fragile X syndrome or intellectual disability of unknown etiology
- Individuals with a family history of FXTAS or FXPOI, or clinical findings suggestive of either diagnosis, especially if there are also individuals in the family with intellectual disability
- Individuals of either gender with developmental delay, intellectual disability, or autism
- Individuals with clinical findings suggestive of FXTAS or FXPOI

Screening of newborns for fragile X syndrome has been discussed but concerns about the identification of premutations in otherwise normal individuals and the lack of data on improved clinical outcome have impeded its adoption. A collaborative newborn screening pilot program for fragile X syndrome is ongoing, primarily looking at allele frequencies across a broad population. Population screening for *FMR1* mutations in women of childbearing age has also been discussed but is not universally agreed upon. A recent American College of Obstetricians and Gynecologists (ACOG) recommends testing for women who ask for it regardless of family history and a recent American Academy of Pediatrics (AAP) recommendation encourages ACOG and the American Society of Reproductive Medicine (ASRM) to endorse offering *FMR1* testing to all women of reproductive age, regardless of family history.

**Counseling:** Fragile X syndrome, FXTAS, and FXPOI are inherited in an X-linked semidominant fashion.

All males with a gene silencing *FMR1* mutation (usually a CGG repeat >200) will have signs and symptoms of fragile X syndrome. Rare individuals whose full mutations are unmethylated or individuals who are mosaic for either repeat size or methylation status may have a milder phenotype and higher cognitive function.

Approximately 50% of females with a full mutation will show physical and/or neurodevelopmental signs of fragile X syndrome, which are usually milder that those seen in affected males.

FXTAS displays age-related penetrance, with an overall incidence of 40% to 45% in males with a premutation over age 50 and a 75% of FXTAS in males age 80 or older. Estimated prevalence of FXTAS in females with a premutation is approximately 8% to 16%.

Approximately 21% of females with an *FMR1* premutation will develop FXPOI. Males with a full mutation typically have significant intellectual disability and are unlikely to reproduce. Females with a full mutation have a 50% chance of passing their mutation on to any offspring. Males who inherit a full mutation from their mother will have fragile X syndrome while females will have approximately a 50% chance of being affected, often with milder manifestations than their male counterparts.

Males with a premutation will pass their mutation on to all of their daughters and none of their sons. As premutations do not expand during male meiosis, daughters will all be premutation carriers, and be at increased risk for FXTAS, FXPOI as well as for having children with fragile X syndrome.

Females with a premutation have a 50% chance of passing on their mutation to any offspring. The likelihood of expansion from a pre to full mutation is dependent on the number of repeats (Table 159-2) as well as the number of interspersed AGG repeats within the CGG expansion which are known to cause stabilization.

Identification of a pre or full mutation in an individual has implications for other family members. Analysis of family history information can help determine other family members for which genetic counseling and testing is warranted.

## Management and Treatment

Newly diagnosed children with fragile X syndrome should have a complete developmental evaluation and behavioral assessment, physical examination to monitor for connective tissue irregularities, and/or hypotonia and screening for other findings that would potentially require treatment such as heart murmur, strabismus, and recurrent otitis. While no treatments are currently available for individuals with fragile X syndrome, early intervention, ongoing educational planning, and behavioral management can be very beneficial to affected individuals and their families.

Individuals diagnosed with FXTAS should be evaluated by neuroimaging and neurologic examination to delineate the extent of their symptoms. No treatment, other than supportive measures, is currently available.

For females with FXPOI, hormonal studies and ultrasound may be used to determine the extent of the ovarian insufficiency. Options for managing reduced fertility can be discussed with a reproductive endocrinologist.

*Table 159-3 FMR1 CGG Repeat Ranges*

| Normal | 5-44 |
|---|---|
| Intermediate | 45-54 |
| Premutation | 55-200 |
| Full mutation | >200 |

# Molecular Genetics and Molecular Mechanism

***Syndrome/Gene/Locus:*** Fragile X syndrome, FXTAS, FXPOI/ *FMR1*/Xq27.3

The *FMR1* gene has an area of CGG triplet repeats in the 5' untranslated region. Repeat sizes fall into one of four categories (Table 159-3). Alleles within the normal range are not expected to expand significantly, while there are some reports of alleles in the intermediate range expanding to a premutation. Premutation and full mutation alleles have distinct clinical phenotypes associated with them and premutation alleles can expand further to a full mutation. The risk of this expansion is dependent on the number of CGG repeats (Table 159-3) as well as the number of interspersed AGG repeats within the CGG expansion which are known to cause stabilization.

The protein product of the *FMR1* gene, fragile X mental retardation 1 protein (FMRP), is expressed in many tissues and is particularly important in the proper neuronal function. It functions as an RNA-binding protein that shuttles mRNA between the nucleus and cytoplasm. Full mutations result in hypermethylation of *FMR1* and silencing of the gene. Premutations result in overexpression of *FMR1*, leading to an overabundance of mRNA which is thought to be toxic.

***Genetic Testing:*** Molecular testing of the *FMR1* gene is clinically available and is useful in confirming a diagnosis of fragile X syndrome in an individual with suggestive clinical or neurodevelopmental findings. Testing is also valuable for at-risk family members in identifying other individuals with pre or full mutations.

Combined testing by polymerase chain reaction (PCR) and Southern blot analysis detects greater than 99% of *FMR1* mutations in all repeat size ranges and determines methylation status in those with full mutations.

Sequence analysis, duplication or deletion analysis, and fluorescence in situ hybridization (FISH) studies can be used to identify the less than 1% of gene silencing mutations in the *FMR1* gene.

**BIBLIOGRAPHY:**

1. Abrams L, Cronister A, Brown WT, et al. Newborn, carrier and childhood screening recommendations for fragile-X. *Pediatrics.* 2012;130:1-10.

2. American College of Obstetricians and Gynecologists Committee on Genetics. ACOG Opinion No. 469. Carrier screening for fragile-X syndrome. *Obstet Gynec.* 2010;116:1008-1010.

3. Coffey SM, Cook K, Tartaglia N, et al. Expanded clinical phenotype of women with the FMR1 premutation. *Am J Med Genet.* 2008;146A:1009-1016.

4. Cronister A, DiMaio M, Mahoney MJ, Donnenfeld AE, Hallam S. Fragile X syndrome carrier screening in the prenatal genetic counseling setting. *Genet Med.* 2005;7:246-250.

5. Finucane B, Abrams L, Cronister A, Archibold AD, Bennett RL, McConkie-Rosell A. Genetic counseling and testing for *FMR1* gene mutations: practice guidelines of the national society of genetic counselors. *J Genet Couns.* Dec 2012;21(6):752-760.

6. Grigsby J, Brega AG, Jacquemont S, et al. Impairment in the cognitive functioning of men with fragile X-associated tremor/ataxia syndrome (FXTAS). *J Neurol Sci.* 2006;248:227-233.

7. Hagerman RJ, Berry-Kravis E, Kaufmann WE, et al. Advances in the treatment of fragile X syndrome. *Pediatrics.* 2009;123:378-390.

8. Hagerman RJ, Hagerman PJ. The fragile X premutation: into the phenotypic fold. *Curr Opin Genet Dev.* 2002;12:278-283.

9. Jacquemont S, Hagerman RJ, Hagerman PJ, Leehey MA. Fragile-X syndrome and fragile X-associated tremor/ataxia syndrome: two faces of FMR1. *Lancet Neurol.* 2007;6:45-55.

10. Nolin SL, Brown WT, Glicksman A, et al. Expansion of the fragile X CGG repeat in females with premutations or intermediate alleles. *Am J Hum Gen.* 2003;72:454-464.

11. Sherman S, Pletcher BA, Driscoll DA. Fragile X syndrome: diagnostic and carrier testing. *Genet Med.* 2005;7:584-587.

# Supplementary Information

## OMIM REFERENCE:

[1] Fragile X Syndrome, FXTAS, FXPOI; FMR1 (#309550)

## Alternative Names:
- *FMR1*-Related Conditions
- Martin-Bell Syndrome

***Key Words:*** Autism, intellectual disability, developmental delay, hypotonia, mitral valve prolapse, macroorchidism, intension tremor, cerebellar ataxia, executive function disorder, premature ovarian failure, elevated FSH

# 160 Werner Syndrome

Dru F. Leistritz, George M. Martin, Junko Oshima

## KEY POINTS

- *Disease summary:*
  - Werner syndrome is an adult-onset genetic disorder characterized by features suggestive of accelerated aging ("segmental progeroid syndrome") and cancer predisposition.
  - Individuals with Werner syndrome appear to develop normally during the first decade of life. The first sign often recognized retrospectively is the lack of a growth spurt during the early teen years.
  - Early findings (usually observed in the 20s) include loss and graying of hair, hoarseness or high-pitched voice, and scleroderma-like skin changes, followed by bilateral ocular cataracts, type 2 diabetes mellitus, hypogonadism, skin ulcers (particularly of the ankles), and osteoporosis in the 30s.
  - Myocardial infarction and cancer are the most common causes of death, at about age 54 years.

- *Hereditary basis:*
  - Werner syndrome is caused by mutations in the *WRN* gene. The *WRN* gene encodes a helicase that unwinds DNA. Werner syndrome is inherited in an autosomal recessive manner.

- *Differential diagnosis:*
  - Atypical Werner syndrome refers to a small subset of individuals with a normal *WRN* gene sequence, normal WRN protein, and some signs and symptoms that sufficiently overlap with the Werner syndrome such that clinicians submit these cases to the International Registry. These individuals may give a history of comparatively early age of onset and a faster rate of progression than those with typical Werner syndrome. Among this group, 4 of 26 individuals so far investigated (15%) had novel heterozygous missense mutations in *LMNA*, which encodes the nuclear intermediate filament lamin A/C. These mutations are N-terminal to the canonical C-terminal mutations of the classical Hutchinson-Gilford progeria syndrome (HGPS) (see later).
  - Mandibuloacral dysplasia (MAD) is characterized by short stature; thin, hyperpigmented skin; partial alopecia, prominent eyes, beaked nose, tooth loss, small recessed chin, and short fingers. The *Arg527His* mutation in the C-terminal region of lamin A/C accounts for approximately 90% of the recessive MAD caused by *LMNA* mutations. A small subset of MAD is caused by mutations in the *ZMPSTE24* gene, whose gene product is involved in the processing of lamin A.
  - The HGPS or progeria of childhood, like Werner syndrome, affects multiple organs with presentations suggestive of accelerated aging. Newborns with HGPS usually appear normal, but profound failure to thrive occurs during the first year. Characteristic facies, partial alopecia progressing to total alopecia, loss of subcutaneous fat, stiffness of joints, bone changes, and abnormal tightness of the skin over the abdomen and upper thighs usually become apparent during the second to third year. Motor and mental development is normal. Individuals with HGPS develop severe atherosclerosis. Death usually occurs as a result of complications of cardiac or cerebrovascular disease generally between age 6 and 20 years. Average life span is approximately 13 years. About 90% of individuals with HGPS have the same p.Gly608Gly in exon 11 of the *LMNA* gene, a mutation that creates a cryptic splice site. Inheritance is autosomal dominant. All individuals with HGPS have a de novo mutation, although inheritance via a mosaic testicular mutation is a potential mechanism.
  - Early-onset type 2 diabetes with secondary complications of vascular disease and skin complications could mimic some features of Werner syndrome.
  - Though bilateral ocular cataracts (probably presenting as posterior subcapsular cataracts) are one of the most commonly observed features of Werner syndrome, the age of onset is typically in the second decade when graying of hair and skin findings would likely be present. Isolated juvenile cataracts are therefore not likely to be a feature of Werner syndrome. Myotonic dystrophy type 1 or myotonic dystrophy type 2 could be a consideration with young adult-onset cataracts; there may be muscle wasting, although other manifestations (myotonia, cardiac conduction abnormalities) are quite different and onset is usually in adulthood.
  - Scleroderma, mixed connective tissue disorders, and lipodystrophy may present skin features similar to those of Werner syndrome. Distal atrophy and skin ulcerations in the absence of other manifestations characteristic of Werner syndrome could raise the possibility of Charcot-Marie-Tooth disease or familial leg ulcers of juvenile onset.
  - Other cancer-prone syndromes, including Rothmund-Thomson syndrome (RTS), caused by mutations in a member of the same family of helicases, and Bloom syndrome, caused by mutations in a related helicase, (*BLM*) may be considered if cancer is the presenting symptom. However, RTS and Bloom syndrome are childhood-onset disorders. Werner syndrome cells do not exhibit the increased sister chromatid exchange typical of Bloom syndrome. Li-Fraumeni syndrome (caused by mutations in *TP53*) may present multiple cancers, including nonepithelial cancers similar to those observed in Werner syndrome, but juvenile-onset cataracts and other manifestations of Werner syndrome are not part of Li-Fraumeni syndrome.

## Diagnostic Criteria and Clinical Characteristics

### Diagnostic Criteria for Werner Syndrome:

Cardinal signs and symptoms (onset after age 10 years)
- Bilateral cataracts
- Characteristic skin (tight skin, atrophic skin, pigmentary alterations, ulceration, hyperkeratosis, regional subcutaneous atrophy)
- Characteristic facies, described as "bird-like" (ie, the nasal bridge appears pinched and subcutaneous tissue is diminished)
- Short stature
- Premature graying and/or thinning of scalp hair
- Parental consanguinity (third cousin or closer) or affected sibling

Further signs and symptoms
- Type 2 diabetes mellitus
- Hypogonadism (secondary sexual underdevelopment, diminished fertility, testicular or ovarian atrophy)
- Osteoporosis
- Radiographic evidence of osteosclerosis of distal phalanges of fingers and/or toes
- Soft tissue calcification
- Evidence of premature atherosclerosis (eg, history of myocardial infarction)
- Neoplasms, especially mesenchymal (eg, meningiomas, sarcomas), rare neoplasms (eg, unusual sites of melanomas and osteosarcomas, and multiple neoplasms)
- Abnormal voice (high pitched, squeaky, or hoarse)
- Flat feet

The International Registry of Werner syndrome uses the above findings to establish a "definite," "probable," or "possible" diagnosis pending molecular genetic confirmation:

- Definite diagnosis: all of the cardinal signs and two others
- Probable diagnosis: the first three cardinal signs and any two others
- Possible diagnosis: either cataracts or dermatologic alterations and any four others
- Exclusion of the diagnosis: onset of cardinal signs and further symptoms before age 10 years, except for short stature, which is typically caused by lack of the usual adolescent growth spurt

**Clinical Characteristics:** Werner syndrome is characterized clinically by the premature appearance of some (but not all) features associated with normative aging, and cancer predisposition.

Individuals with Werner syndrome develop normally until the end of the first decade. The first symptom, often recognized retrospectively, is the lack of a growth spurt during the early teen years. Symptoms typically start in the 20s. The youngest patient with a molecular confirmation of the diagnosis was of age 16 years. Initial findings include loss and graying of hair, hoarseness, and scleroderma-like skin changes, followed by bilateral ocular cataracts, type 2 diabetes mellitus, hypogonadism, skin ulcers, and osteoporosis in the 30s. Median age of diagnosis is 38 years. A characteristic facial appearance, termed "bird-like" because of the pinched appearance at the bridge of the nose, evolves during the third or fourth decade.

Affected individuals exhibit several forms of arteriosclerosis; the most serious form, coronary artery atherosclerosis, may lead to myocardial infarction which, together with cancer, is the most common cause of death. The most recent data on the mean age of death in individuals with Werner syndrome is 54 years, somewhat older than that reported in earlier studies.

The spectrum of cancers in individuals with Werner syndrome is unusual in that it includes a large number of sarcomas and very rare types of cancers, often in atypical locations. The most common cancers in Japanese individuals (for whom the most data exist) are soft tissue sarcomas, osteosarcomas, melanomas, and thyroid carcinomas. Acral lentiginous melanomas (most often observed on the feet and nasal mucosa) are particularly prevalent compared to levels observed the general population.

The osteoporosis of individuals with Werner syndrome is unusual in that it especially affects the long bones. In contrast, osteoporosis during normative aging preferentially involves the vertebral bodies, particularly in females. Characteristic osteolytic lesions of the distal joints of the fingers are observed on radiographs.

Deep, chronic ulcers around the ankles (Achilles tendons, medial malleolus, and lateral malleolus) are highly characteristic.

Controversy exists concerning the degree to which the brain is involved. While individuals with Werner syndrome may have central nervous system complications of arteriosclerosis, they do not appear to be unusually susceptible to Alzheimer disease. Cognitive changes are not typically observed. Diffuse changes observed on brain magnetic resonance imaging (MRI) in some individuals warrant further investigation in research studies.

Fertility appears to decline soon after sexual maturity. This decline in fertility is associated with testicular atrophy and a probable accelerated rate of loss of primordial follicles in the ovaries, although data are sparse. Early menopause is common in women as are multiple miscarriages, but successful pregnancies have also been reported. Men have fathered children, usually at younger ages.

### Genetic Counseling:

☞**COUNSELING:** Werner syndrome is inherited in an autosomal recessive manner. Parents of a proband are obligate heterozygotes for a disease-causing mutation and, therefore, carry one mutant allele. Although systematic clinical studies have not been reported, heterozygotes do not appear to be at increased risk for any Werner syndrome-specific symptoms, although additional research is needed on this subject.

The offspring of an individual with Werner syndrome are obligate heterozygotes for a disease-causing mutation. Due to the very low prevalence in the US population, the risk of Werner syndrome in the offspring of an affected individual is negligible unless the affected individual and his or her reproductive partner are consanguineous. In Japan, where heterozygotes may be as common as 1/150, the risk for Werner syndrome in an offspring is still less than 1/500.

☞**GENOTYPE-PHENOTYPE CORRELATIONS:** The chronologic order of the onset of signs and symptoms appears to be similar in all individuals with Werner syndrome regardless of the specific *WRN* mutations.

The specific cell type in which cancer develops may depend on the type of *WRN* mutation present. In individuals of Japanese descent, papillary carcinoma of the thyroid has been associated with an N-terminal mutation, whereas follicular carcinoma of the thyroid is more frequently observed with a C-terminal mutation. This finding clearly contradicts the original assumption that all WRN mutations that truncate nuclear localization signals act as null mutations. Further studies may reveal additional genotype-phenotype correlations.

## Management and Treatment

***Clinical Evaluation:*** To establish the extent of disease in an individual diagnosed with Werner syndrome, the following evaluations are recommended:

- Screen for type 2 diabetes mellitus by standard clinical assays
- Lipid profiles
- Physical examination for cancers common in Werner syndrome, (eg, thyroid nodules, skin tumors, meningiomas)
- Ophthalmologic examination for the detection of cataracts, including slit-lamp examination
- Skin examination for common findings, especially early ulcerations of the feet, with special attention to nail beds and soles of feet for lentiginous melanoma
- MRI if neurologic symptoms are present (eg, chronic headaches that could suggest a diagnosis of meningioma, a common neoplasm in Werner syndrome)
- Assessment of coping and psychologic fitness in light of prognosis

***Treatment of Manifestations:***
- Aggressive treatment of skin ulcers with standard or novel techniques.
- Control of type 2 diabetes mellitus.
- Use of cholesterol-lowering drugs if lipid profile is abnormal. Muscle atrophy is a potential complication of statins, however.
- Surgical treatment of ocular cataracts.
- Treatment of malignancies in a standard fashion.
- Prevention of secondary complications
  - Lifestyle counseling for smoking avoidance, regular exercise, and weight control to reduce atherosclerosis and cancer risk
  - Excellent skin care, trauma avoidance, and examination to treat problems early

***Surveillance:***
- Screening for type 2 diabetes mellitus at least annually
- Annual lipid profile
- Annual physical examination seeking malignancies common in Werner syndrome and other skin manifestations
- Annual ophthalmologic examination for cataracts
- Attention to signs of angina
- Agents or circumstances to avoid
  - Smoking and excess weight, which increase the risk of atherosclerosis and cancer
  - Trauma to the extremities

## Molecular Genetics and Molecular Mechanism

***WRN Gene Product:*** The *WRN* gene encodes a 1432 amino-acid multifunctional nuclear protein that has both helicase and exonuclease activities. The N-terminal region contains ATP-dependent 3'->5' exonuclease domains and the central region contains an ATP-dependent 3'->5' helicase, a member of the RecQ family of DNA helicases. The C-terminal region contains a nuclear localization signal. *WRN* maps to 8p12-p11.2.

Biochemical and cell biologic studies suggest that the WRN protein is involved in DNA repair and recombination, DNA replication, telomere maintenance, and transcription. The WRN protein preferentially unwinds or digests aberrant DNA structures accidentally generated during various DNA transactions. It participates in the regulation of DNA recombination and repair processes by unwinding or digesting intermediate DNA structures. Cells isolated from Werner syndrome patients exhibit accelerated replicative senescence. The S phase is prolonged and there is stochastic loss of telomere sequences. Genomic instability is a hallmark and is reflected in elevated point mutations and intragenic deletions as well as mosaicism for a variety of chromosomal translocations, inversions, and deletions. Hypersensitivity to certain genotoxic agents has been demonstrated. Mouse models of Werner syndrome show some features consistent with accelerated aging if there is experimentally induced attrition of the unusually long telomeres of laboratory strains.

***Genetic Testing:*** DNA sequencing of the *WRN* gene is available on a research basis (see www.wernersyndrome.org). Genomic sequencing of the *WRN* coding region detects mutations in both alleles in approximately 90% of affected individuals. Mutations may occur within the relatively large introns and regulatory regions; however, these are not routinely analyzed. Western blot analysis is also carried out for the detection of altered mobility and amounts of the WRN protein. In typical Werner syndrome patients there is an absence of WRN protein.

More than 70 different disease-causing *WRN* mutations have been identified, the majority consisting of stop codons, insertions, or deletions that result in a frameshift. Splicing donor or acceptor site mutations have been shown to result in skipped exons and frameshifts. A few cases of genomic rearrangements and missense mutations have also been reported. A homozygous double amino acid substitution that results in an unstable protein has been identified in an individual from Germany. The most common pathologic variant is c.1105C>T (pR369X), which accounts for 20% to 25% of mutations in the Caucasian and Japanese populations. A founder effect in the Japanese population is seen with the IVS 26-1G>C allele, which accounts for approximately 60% of mutations in this group.

**BIBLIOGRAPHY:**

1. Martin GM. Genetic syndromes in man with potential relevance to the pathobiology of aging. *Birth Defects Orig Artic Ser.* 1978;14(1):5-39.
2. Epstein CJ, Martin GM, Schultz AL, Motulsky AG. Werner's syndrome a review of its symptomatology, natural history, pathologic features, genetics and relationship to the natural aging process. *Medicine (Baltimore).* 1966;45(3):177-221.
3. Goto M. Hierarchical deterioration of body systems in Werner's syndrome: implications for normal ageing. *Mech Ageing Dev.* 1997;98(3):239-254.
4. Martin GM, Oshima J, Gray MD, Poot M. What geriatricians should know about the Werner syndrome. *J Am Geriatr Soc.* 1999;47(9):1136-1144.
5. Yu CE, Oshima J, Fu YH, et al. Positional cloning of the Werner's syndrome gene. *Science.* 1996;272(5259):258-262.
6. Chen L, Lee L, Kudlow BA, et al. LMNA mutations in atypical Werner's syndrome. *Lancet.* 2003;362(9382):440-445.

7. Broers JL, Ramaekers FC, Bonne G, Yaou RB, Hutchison CJ. Nuclear lamins: laminopathies and their role in premature ageing. *Physiol Rev.* 2006;86(3):967-1008.

8. Martin GM, Oshima J. Lessons from human progeroid syndromes. *Nature.* 2000;408(6809):263-266.

9. Singh DK, Ahn B, Bohr VA. Roles of RECQ helicases in recombination based DNA repair, genomic stability and aging. *Biogerontology.* 2009;10(3):235-252.

10. Huang S, Lee L, Hanson NB, et al. The spectrum of WRN mutations in Werner syndrome patients. *Hum Mutat.* 2006;27(6):558-567.

11. Goto M, Miller RW, Ishikawa Y, Sugano H. Excess of rare cancers in Werner syndrome (adult progeria). *Cancer Epidemiol Biomarkers Prev.* 1996;5(4):239-246.

12. Ishikawa Y, Sugano H, Matsumoto T, Furuichi Y, Miller RW, Goto M, Unusual features of thyroid carcinomas in Japanese patients with Werner syndrome and possible genotype-phenotype relations to cell type and race. *Cancer.* 1999;85(6):1345-1352.

13. Brosh RM Jr, Opresko PL, Bohr VA. Enzymatic mechanism of the WRN helicase/nuclease. *Methods Enzymol.* 2006;409: 52-85.

14. Friedrich K, Lee L, Leistritz DF, et al. WRN mutations in Werner syndrome patients: genomic rearrangements, unusual intronic mutations and ethnic-specific alterations. *Hum Genet.* 2010;128(1):103-111.

## Supplementary Information

**OMIM References:**

[1] Werner Syndrome; WRN (#277700)

[2] RECQL2—RecQ Protein-Like 2; RECQL2 (#604611)

**Alternative Names:**

- Progeria of Adults
- DNA Helicase, RecQ-Like, Type 3; RECQ3

***Key Words:*** Short stature, cataracts, beaked nose, atherosclerosis, osteoporosis, slender limbs, scleroderma-like skin, diabetes mellitus, hypogonadism, malignancy, progeroid syndrome, genomic instability syndrome

# 161 Prader-Willi and Angelman Syndromes: Examples of Genomic Imprinting

Merlin G. Butler

## KEY POINTS

- *Disease summary:*
  - Prader-Willi syndrome (PWS)
    - Characteristic face with a small upturned nose, narrow bifrontal diameter, thin upper lip with downturned corners of mouth, sticky saliva, and enamel hypoplasia.
    - Hypogonadism or hypogenitalism, hypopigmentation, hypotonia, poor suck and feeding difficulties, and growth hormone deficiency noted during infancy.
    - Short stature and small hands and feet noted during childhood without growth hormone treatment. Growth hormone therapy increases muscle mass, decreases fat mass, and improves strength in children.
    - Hyperphagia is noted in early childhood with subsequent obesity, if diet restriction and behavior modifications are unsuccessful addressing the eating issues.
    - Developmental delay noted during infancy with mental deficiency (average IQ = 65) and behavioral problems (skin picking, outbursts, obsessive-compulsive disorder) observed during childhood, adolescence, and adulthood.
    - Paternal 15q11-q13 deletion (in about 70% of cases), maternal uniparental disomy 15 (in 25%), and imprinting defects or other chromosome 15 abnormalities in the remaining subjects.
    - Genetic subtypes such as maternal disomy 15 and typical 15q11-q13 deletions (type I or type II) produce variation in clinical phenotype with compulsions, and self-injury being more common and adaptive and cognitive assessment scores reported lower in those with the type I deletion compared with maternal disomy 15 or type II deletions.
    - Adults with PWS are at increased risk of osteoporosis, sleep apnea, and psychosis. Increased pain threshold and impaired temperature sensitivity can delay the recognition of illnesses among PWS adults.
  - Angelman syndrome (AS)
    - Characteristic face with acquired microcephaly, a broad-appearing head, a prominent nose, large mouth with a protruding tongue and swallowing difficulties, widely spaced teeth, frequent drooling, and prognathism.
    - Seizures, abnormal electroencephalogram (EEG) (high-amplitude spikes and slow waves at 2 to 3 Hz noted anteriorly), severe developmental delay or intellectual disability, absent or nearly absent speech, inappropriate laughter, and sleep problems.
    - Unsteady wide-based gait with abnormal jerky arm movements, hypotonia with occasional hyper-reflexia, and abnormal head computed tomography (CT) scan (cerebral atrophy).
    - Maternal 15q11-q13 deletion (in about 70% of cases), paternal disomy 15 (about 5%), *UBE3A* gene mutations (about 10%), imprinting center defects (about 5%), and other chromosome 15 abnormalities in the remaining subjects.
    - Clinical differences correlate with genetic subtypes as seen in PWS with typical 15q11-13 deletions having more seizures (particularly in type I deletions), microcephaly, and hypopigmentation than in the other genetic subtypes.
    - Adults with AS typically retain the facial features, lack of speech and seizures (seizures may get worse with age), but are also at increased risk of obesity and decreased mobility due to ataxia, contractures, and scoliosis.
- *Hereditary basis:*
  - Prader-Willi and Angelman syndromes are genomic imprinting disorders due to alterations of an epigenetic phenomenon controlling methylation of CpG-rich regions of genes regulating gene allele expression based on the gender of the transmitting parent. This phenomenon evolved over 150 million years ago. Many imprinted gens are arranged in clusters or imprinted domain areas.
- *Differential diagnosis:*
  - Several disorders can strongly resemble PWS including Cohen, Bardet-Biedl, fragile X, and Alström syndromes. Cytogenetic abnormalities in similarly affected individuals include duplications of 3p25.3-p26.2 and Xq27.2-qter and deletions of chromosomes 1p36, 2q37.3, 6q16.2, 10q26, 11p12-p14, 16p11.2, 20q13.13-q13.32, and Xq26.3. In addition, genome-wide studies have identified at least 58 gene loci associated with an obesity phenotype (eg, *FTO, POMC, SH2B1, MC4R, TUB, BNDF*). Several of these genes are known to contribute to extreme childhood obesity and increased body mass index, waist circumference, or waist-to-hip ratio.
  - Differential diagnosis of AS includes Rett syndrome (*MECP2* gene defect) and Pitt-Hopkins syndrome which are both due to different genetic defects but have overlapping features. Other conditions with a similar clinical presentation to AS include Mowat-Wilson and Smith-Magenis syndromes. Due to the same-appearing chromosome 15q11-q13 deletion as seen in PWS, confusion in laboratory diagnosis between the two disorders is evident in prenatal diagnosis and during the neonatal period. Chromosome abnormalities in individuals with similar findings include the 22q13.3, 1p36, 17q21.3, and 2q23.1 deletions.

## Diagnostic Criteria and Clinical Characteristics

The first clinical diagnostic criteria in PWS was reported in 1993 and revised later in 2001. Diagnostic criteria were reported for both PWS and AS before comprehensive laboratory testing became available. Most health-related features in PWS relate to behaviors (hyperphagia, self-injury, outbursts) and associated obesity-related complications (Table 161-1). Most of the important health-related problems in AS are related to the nervous system including severe intellectual disabilities, lack of speech, hyperactivity, wide-based gait with unusual arm movements, and sleep disturbances (Table 161-2).

*Diagnostic Criteria:*

☞PRADER-WILLI SYNDROME (summarized by Holm et al., 1993 and Gunay-Aygun et al., 2001):

**Major criteria**

- Neonatal and infantile central hypotonia with poor suck and feeding problems
- Excessive or rapid weight gain (if food intake not limited) with hyperphagia or food foraging and obsession
- Characteristic facial features with dolichocephaly in infancy, narrow face or bifrontal diameter, almond-shaped eyes, small-appearing mouth with thin upper lip, down-turned corners of the mouth
- Hypogonadism and hypogenitalism (small penis and cryptorchidism in males)
- Global development delay (mild intellectual disability) and behavior problems (skin picking, temper tantrums)
- 15q11-q13 deletion, maternal disomy 15, or imprinting center defects

**Minor or associated criteria:**

- Decreased fetal movement
- Characteristic behavior problems—temper tantrums, violent outbursts, and obsessive-compulsive behavior
- Sleep disturbance or apnea
- Short stature for genetic background
- Unusual skill with jigsaw puzzles
- Hypopigmentation
- Small hands and feet
- Narrow hands with straight ulnar border
- Decreased vomiting
- Eye abnormalities (esotropia, myopia)

*Table 161-1  System Involvement in Prader-Willi Syndrome*

| System | Manifestation | Incidence (%) |
|---|---|---|
| Gestation | Reduced fetal activity | ~75 |
| | Breech presentation | ~25 |
| Early infancy | Developmental delay | 98 |
| | Hypotonia (weak muscle tone) | ~95 |
| | Feeding problems | ~95 |
| | Low birth weight | 30 |
| Brain function and behavior | Mental deficiency (for family background) | 97 |
| | Personality problems | ~40 |
| | Seizures | 20 |
| Growth | Obesity (childhood onset) | ~95 |
| | Short stature (if untreated with growth hormone) | ~75 |
| | Delayed bone age | 50 |
| Face | Narrow forehead | 75 |
| | Almond-shaped eyes | 75 |
| | Strabismus | 50 |
| | Early dental cavities/enamel hypoplasia | 40 |
| Sexual development | Hypogenitalism/hypogonadism (males and females) | 95 |
| | Cryptorchidism (males) | ~90 |
| | Menstruation (females) | ~40 |
| Skeletal | Small hands and feet | ~80 |
| | Scoliosis | ~40 |
| Other | Skin picking | ~80 |
| | Reduced glucose tolerance/diabetes mellitus | 20 |

Adapted from Butler, 1990. Butler MG. Prader-Willi Syndrome: obesity due to genomic imprinting. *Curr Genomics.* 2011;12:204-21.

*Table 161-2* **System Involvement in Angelman Syndrome**

| System | Manifestation | Incidence (%) |
|---|---|---|
| Brain Function & Behavior | Severe mental retardation | 100 |
| | Absent or limited speech | 100 |
| | Ataxia, wide-based unsteady gait, jerky unusual arm movements and position | 99 |
| | Abnormal EEG | ~90 |
| | Inappropriate laughter | ~90 |
| | Seizures | ~80 |
| | Hypotonia | ~60 |
| | Hyper-reflexia | ~60 |
| | Abnormal head CT scan | 35 |
| | Hypertonia | ~10 |
| Face | Macrostomia | 97 |
| | Prognathism | ~90 |
| | Maxillary hypoplasia | 80 |
| | Protruding or thrusting tongue with swallowing difficulties | ~80 |
| | Microcephaly | ~80 |
| | Brachycephaly | ~50 |
| Pigmentary | Pale blue eyes | ~90 |
| | Blond hair | 65 |
| | Hypopigmentation | ~40 |
| Other | Frequent drooling/excessive chewing | ~80 |
| | Sleep problems | ~80 |
| | Strabismus | ~40 |
| | Scoliosis | ~20 |
| | Childhood obesity | ~20 |

Adapted from Yamada and Volpe, Angelman's syndrome in infancy. Dev Med and Williams CA, Driscoll DJ, Dagli AI. Clinical and genetic aspects of Angelman syndrome. *Genet Med.* 2010;12:385-395.

- Thick, viscous saliva, dental anomalies
- Speech articulation defects
- Osteoporosis, scoliosis, kyphosis

☞ANGELMAN SYNDROME (summarized by Yamada and Volpe, 1990 and Williams et al., 2010):

**Major criteria**

- Severe developmental delay or intellectual disability
- Movement or balance disorder, tremulous, wide-based gait with uplifted, flexed arm position upon walking
- Frequent inappropriate laughter, easy excitability, hyperactivity
- Speech impairment (<10 words), receptive and nonverbal communication skills higher than verbal
- Early-onset seizures (usually <3 years of age) with abnormal EEG
- Characteristic facial findings including brachymicrocephaly, flat occiput, protruding tongue with thrusting and suck or swallowing difficulties, prognathia, wide-appearing mouth, wide-spaced teeth, and frequent drooling
- 15q11-q13 deletion, paternal disomy 15, *UBE3A* gene mutations, or imprinting defects

**Minor or associated criteria:**

- Feeding problems and/or truncal hypotonia during infancy
- Sensitivity to heat
- Abnormal sleep and awake patterns
- Hyperactive deep tendon reflexes
- Attraction or fascination with water
- Hypopigmentation

*Clinical Characteristics:*

☞PRADER-WILLI SYNDROME: PWS was first described in 1956 and recognized as a complex neurodevelopmental disorder with major features of infantile hypotonia, feeding difficulties due to a poor suck, decreased muscle mass and strength, developmental delay, temperature instability, hypogonadism or hypogenitalism, cryptorchidism in males, and growth hormone deficiency leading to short stature and small hands and feet. Reduced fetal activity, breech presentation, and nonterm delivery are also observed. As individuals with PWS enter early childhood (about 2-4 years of age), additional features appear including food-seeking behavior, leading to hyperphagia and obesity, if not controlled, mental deficiency and personality and behavioral problems (compulsions, outbursts, self-injury), a high pain threshold, enamel hypoplasia, sticky saliva, a characteristic face (a narrow forehead, strabismus, almond-shaped eyes, short upturned nose, downturned corners of the mouth, thin upper lip), and hypopigmentation.

Obesity is recognized as the most significant health problem in PWS, and without dietary intervention, adolescents may weigh 250 to 300 lb. Hyperphagia and obesity-related complications may include diabetes, hypertension, cardiopulmonary compromise, and orthopedic problems which impact on morbidity and mortality. Food stealing and hoarding can be problematic as well as consuming discarded or inedible food items. Eating-related fatalities do occur, including choking on gorged food and gastric necrosis and rupture.

Hypogonadism, a small penis, hypoplastic scrotum, and cryptorchidism are seen in 90% of PWS males while a hypoplastic labia majora and minora with a small clitoris are seen in most females. In males with palpable testes, the size is seldom greater than 6 mL in volume. The testes may descend spontaneously in males during childhood and puberty, but surgery is often required. Nearly all individuals with PWS require sex hormone replacement. Males are thought to be sterile although on rare occasions females with PWS have established pregnancies. Musculoskeletal problems including scoliosis are common in PWS and accompanied by kyphosis or lordosis. Hypotonia, decreased muscle mass, and obesity contribute to these problems. Bone density is also decreased. Scoliosis defined as a lateral spinal curvature of greater than 10 degrees should be followed closely particularly if the child is on growth hormone.

Individuals with PWS with the typical chromosome 15 deletion are hypopigmented and more homogeneous in their clinical presentation. Those with maternal disomy 15 have fewer typical facial features and are less likely to have certain behavioral findings such as skin picking, unusual skill with jigsaw puzzles, a high pain threshold and articulation problems seen in most PWS individuals with deletions. However, PWS individuals with maternal disomy 15 are often diagnosed later in life, which may reflect a milder phenotype. PWS individuals with the 15q11-q13 deletion have a greater number of compulsive symptoms than those with maternal disomy 15, but less likely to have autism or psychosis in adulthood.

Academic achievement is usually impaired in PWS and become more apparent after 6 years of age. About one-third of PWS children function in the low-normal range (70-100 IQ) and the remaining function in the mild-to-moderate range (50-70 IQ). Measures of intellectual function and academic achievement in PWS have shown that those with maternal disomy 15 have significantly higher verbal IQ scores than those with the typical deletion and have superior visual recognition memory. Further characterization of clinical differences in PWS subjects with type I or type II deletions have shown that those with type I deletions scored significantly worse in self-injurious and maladaptive behavior assessments and academic achievement scores compared with type II deletions. Obsessive-compulsive behavior and increased grooming were also more common in type I deletions along with other maladaptive behaviors. The presence or absence of specific genes can greatly influence the phenotypes observed in PWS. Type I deletion subjects are missing four extra genes, *TUBGCP5*, *CYFIP1*, *NIPA1*, and *NIPA2*, which are known to play a role in brain function (eg, *CYFIP1* gene product interacts with the fragile X syndrome protein [FMRP]). The four genes located between BP1 and BP2 apparently play a role in decreased cognition and behavioral impairment reported in subjects with the typical type I deletion in relationship with type II deletions.

☞**ANGELMAN SYNDROME:** AS, an entirely different clinical condition, was first reported in 1965 and characterized by severe mental deficiency, lack of speech, inappropriate laughter, unsteady wide-based gait with unusual jerky arm movements, an abnormal EEG with seizures, hypotonia with occasional hyper-reflexia, hypopigmentation, and a particular facial appearance (macrostomia, prognathism, wide-spaced teeth, a protruding tongue, a large-appearing nose, acquired microcephaly, and a broad-head shape).In addition, a fascination with water is reported thus close supervision is required around swimming pools, bathing, or other water-related activities. They also have a happy disposition and display laughter with smiling at inappropriate times but appear to be unrelated to happiness. Hand flapping, easy excitability, and hyperactivity with a short attention span are generally observed beginning in infancy with frequent placement of hands in the mouth with drooling. Absent-to-severe speech delay (<10 words) are noted in most individuals with severe motor delays and locomotion problems represented by severe jerkiness and ataxia. Receptive skills may be sufficient to understand simple commands but most use a form of sign language for communication. Sleep problems are common in both males and female with a decreased need to sleep. Delayed milestones are present in AS with sitting at about 2 years of age and abnormal forms of walking at about 3 to 5 years. Toe-walking with a stiff and robot-like wide-based gait is present with jerkiness, uplifted arms, and flexed elbows. About 10% of individuals with AS can never walk. Abnormal EEG findings such as very large amplitudes and slow activity at 2 to 3 Hz occur predominantly in the anterior range of the brain. The EEG patterns are specific and point strongly to the diagnosis of AS. Other major organ systems are generally not involved as individuals are reported to live into their 70s.

Clinical differences in AS also correlate with genetic subtypes as seen in PWS with the typical 15q11-q13 deletion having more seizures, microcephaly, and hypopigmentation than the other genetic subtypes. Those AS subjects with the larger type I deletion have more language impairment and autistic traits than those with the smaller type II deletion. Those with paternal disomy 15 have a milder phenotype and may not have seizures. Their head size may also be within normal range and have better development and language abilities, but yet perform at a severe-to-profound level. Those with paternal disomy 15 may also have fewer movement problems with milder ataxia. Those individuals with AS and *UBE3A* gene mutations or with imprinting defects are more likely to have clinical severity judged to be between those seen with the typical 15q11-q13 deletion or paternal disomy 15.

## Screening and Counseling

Both PWS and AS occur in about 1 in 20,000 deliveries and with the same-appearing de novo chromosome 15q11-q13 deletion seen in the majority of cases, but of different parental origin (ie, paternal deletion in PWS and maternal deletion in AS). The typical 15q11-q13 deletion occurs in about 70% of affected individuals (AS or PWS) and of two types (larger type I and smaller type II) due to the location of novel low copy DNA repeats clustered at or near two major proximal breakpoints (BP1 and BP2) and at a distal breakpoint (BP3) in the chromosome 15q11-q13 region (Fig. 161-1).

Maternal disomy 15 (both chromosome 15s from the mother) is the second most frequent finding in PWS and result from the

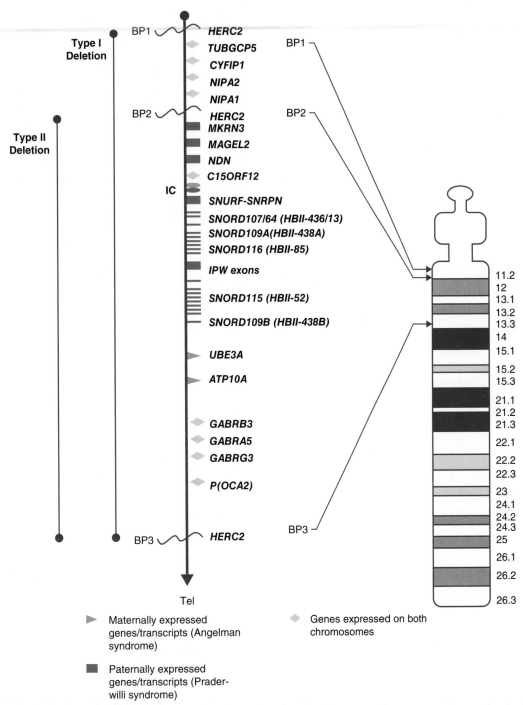

**Figure 161-1** Ideogram of Chromosome 15 Showing the Order of Protein-Coding and Noncoding Genes and Transcripts in the 15q11-q13 Region. The location of breakpoints BP1, BP2, and BP3 are shown for the typical type I and type II deletions. Tel, telomere; BP, breakpoint; IC, imprinting center.

fertilization by a normal sperm of an oocyte with two maternal chromosome 15s due to nondisjunction in meiosis. This leads to a zygote which is trisomic for chromosome 15 and not compatible with development, thus a relatively common cause of early miscarriage. Through a trisomy rescue event in the fetus, the pregnancy can be salvaged and not spontaneously aborted. This occurs by removal of the paternal chromosome 15 in a cell and a normal chromosome count results with two maternal chromosome 15s in the fetus producing PWS.

About 25% of PWS subjects have maternal disomy 15 while approximately 5% of AS subjects have paternal disomy 15 (both 15s from the father). Uniparental disomy 15 results from errors in meiosis leading to trisomy 15 rescue in a PWS pregnancy from trisomic 15 fetus due to two chromosome 15s from the mother and monosomy 15 rescue in AS due to paternal disomy 15 caused by fertilizing an egg missing a chromosome 15 by a normal sperm containing a single chromosome 15. This single chromosome 15 from the father becomes duplicated leading to a normal 46 chromosome count in the AS fetus. The remaining subjects with PWS have either defects of the imprinting center or other chromosome 15 abnormalities whereby AS is due to a disturbance of a single imprinted gene (*UBE3A*) which is maternally expressed. *UBE3A* mutations are found in about 10% of AS individuals with a recurrence risk of 50%. If a microdeletion of the imprinting center is present in the father in a PWS family, then the recurrence risk would be 50%. The recurrence risk is 1% for the typical 15q11-q13 deletions or uniparental disomy 15 in either PWS or AS families.

## Management and Treatment

There are established clinical indicators supporting genetic testing for PWS such as central hypotonia and a poor suck during the neonatal period in the absence of metabolic or structural brain abnormalities. At 2 to 6 years of age, the diagnosis of PWS should be considered when hypotonia, increased weight gain, and a history of poor suck and global developmental delay are present. At 6 to 12 years of age, a history of hypotonia with a poor suck and global developmental delay and excessive eating leading to central obesity are strong indicators for PWS genetic testing. At a later age (12 years through adulthood), cognitive impairment (usually mild) and excessive eating with central obesity along with hypothalamic hypogonadism and/or typical behavior problems including temper tantrums, skin picking, and compulsive features are sufficient to warrant genetic testing for PWS. Establishing the genetic subtype (deletion, maternal disomy 15, or an imprinting defect) is important for accurate and informative genetic counseling and in developing medical management and treatment plans to control obesity and behavioral problems (Table 161-3).

Food-seeking behavior often necessitates locking the refrigerator and food storage areas to prevent excessive eating, thus precluding independent living as adults. However, individuals with PWS can live into their 60s if obesity is controlled by caloric restriction and exercise. The typical diet in PWS consists of about 60% of caloric requirements for non-PWS individuals thus requiring strict mealtime regimes. Thirty minutes of exercise is also encouraged daily. Adequate protein is encouraged to conserve and increase lean body mass particularly during growth hormone treatment and diet restrictions. Growth hormone therapy will increase stature and muscle mass and decrease fat mass. In addition to restricted caloric intake, vitamin and calcium supplementation is generally required by age 2 years to prevent osteoporosis.

Sleep disorders and respiratory problems in PWS such as hypoventilation and oxygen desaturation are common in childhood and continue to adulthood. These findings should be closely monitored and treated before growth hormone treatment. Adolescents and adults often fall asleep during the day, particularly when inactive. Behavioral and psychiatric problems such as compulsions, outbursts, and self-injury often require medical treatment and behavioral management. Psychosis is evident in young adulthood

*Table 161-3 Molecular Genetic Testing for Prader-Willi and Angelman Syndromes*

| Test Modality | Purpose |
|---|---|
| DNA methylation of *SNRPN* gene with Southern blotting or PCR amplification | Confirm the diagnosis of PWS or AS by identifying characteristic methylation patterns (will not distinguish among the different genetic subtypes). |
| Fluorescence in situ hybridization (FISH) of 15q11-q13 probes | Identify the proximal 15q deletion in PWS and AS. |
| Chromosome microarray hybridization | Detect the 15q11-q13 deletion and determine the larger type I or smaller type II typical deletion in both PWS or AS. Specific chromosome microarrays with SNP probes are used to determine the hetero-, iso- or segmental isodisomy status of chromosome 15. |
| Methylation-specific multiplex ligation-dependent probe amplification (MS-MLPA) testing | Determine the methylation and deletion status using multiple specific DNA markers from the 15q11-q13 region in both PWS or AS. |
| DNA analysis of polymorphic markers within and outside of the 15q11-q13 region | Identify biparental inheritance (normal), maternal disomy 15 (in PWS), or paternal disomy 15 (in AS). |
| Real-time PCR quantitative or other research techniques (eg, quantitative microsphere hybridization, digital PCR) | Determine microdeletions or epimutations of the imprinting center in PWS or AS. |
| Pathogenic DNA sequence analysis | Changes identified in the *UBE3A* gene in a subset of individuals with AS. |

in about 10% of individuals with PWS. Based on population studies, the death rate is estimated at 3% per year.

A multidisciplinary approach is required for both PWS and AS with particular emphasis on early diagnosis and treatment specific for each disorder and required throughout life. Specifically, in PWS, genetic counseling, caloric restriction, exercise programs, and behavioral modification and growth hormone therapy are important to improve quality of life. Expertise in genetics, neurology, orthopedics, cognitive, communication, and syndrome-specific behavioral therapies are required in treating individuals with AS.

## Molecular Genetics and Molecular Mechanism

About 100 nonredundant genes or transcripts are recognized in the 15q11-q13 region and at least a dozen are imprinted and paternally expressed. These paternally expressed genes serve as candidates for causing PWS while two other imprinted genes (*UBE3A* and *ATP10A*) are maternally expressed. Disturbances of the *UBE3A* gene causes AS. The *UBE3A* gene produces a cellular ubiquitin ligase enzyme that targets damaged proteins for degradation or proteins no longer needed for normal function in cells including the brain. In addition, AS mice models with altered *UBE3A* gene function share characteristics seen in humans such as ataxia, motor dysfunction and learning, memory and sleep problems.

Several paternally expressed genes in the 15q11-q13 region include the bicistronic *SNURF-SNRPN* locus, *NDN*, *MKRN3*, *MAGEL2*, andmultiple copies of small untranslated nucleolar RNAs (snoRNAs or SNORDs) involved with processing specific RNA transcripts (eg, serotonin receptor 2C). These genes become candidates for causing PWS. For example, Necdin (*NDN*) impacts on axonal nerve growth while *MAGEL2* plays a role in circadian rhythm, behavior, and fertility. *MKRN3* encodes specific proteins (makorins) abundantly present in the brain. Genes in the region expressed on both chromosome 15s include three gamma-aminobutyric acid (GABA) neurotransmitter receptors (*GABRB3*, *GABRA5*, *GABRG3*), *HERC2*, and the *P(OCA2)* locus for oculocutaneous albinism type 2, along with four genes (*TUBGCP5*, *CYFIP1*, *NIPA1*, and *NIPA2*) located between breakpoints BP1 and BP2. An estimated 40% of brain neurons utilize GABA as an important inhibitory neurotransmitter. The promoter and first exon of the *SNURF-SNRPN* gene are components of the imprinting center, and when paternally disturbed, leads to loss of function of paternally expressed genes in this region under its control. A separate imprinting center located upstream to the PWS imprinting center controls the two imprinted maternally expressed genes (*UBE3A* and *ATP10A*) involved in AS. Several antisense transcripts produced in this region, including *UBE3A*, are paternally expressed thereby blocking expression of the paternal allele. Recent clinical reports of individuals presenting with features of PWS (eg, hyperphagia, obesity, learning/behavior problems) have shown small atypical deletions of the snoRNAs (ie, *SNORD116*, *SNORD115*) further supporting a role in PWS.

*Syndrome/Gene/Locus:* PWS appears to be a contiguous gene disorder with several imprinted paternally express genes in the 15q11-q13 region accounting for its phenotype with the snoRNAs (*SNORD116*, *SNORD115*) playing a significant role. In contrast, AS

is due to a single imprinted maternally expressed gene (*UBE3A*), a ubiquitin ligase enzyme that targets damaged protein in the brain for degradation.

*Genetic Testing:* DNA methylation testing is now the most sensitive assay for genetic confirmation of all forms of genetic lesions in PWS or AS based on differences in methylation patterns in both maternally or paternally inherited alleles in the 15q11-q13 region. This test was initially based on Southern blotting techniques but later, methylation-sensitive polymerase chain reaction (PCR) amplification and methylation-specific multiplex ligation-dependent probe amplification (MS-MLPA) simplified the testing (Fig. 161-2). However, this test will not differentiate among the separate molecular classes seen in either syndrome. Fluorescent insitu hybridization (FISH) using specific probes in the region (eg, *SNRPN*) and newer techniques are used to identify deletions such as chromosomal (DNA) microarrays, genotyping with DNA markers, or MS-MLPA.

DNA microarrays are used to identify copy number variants (CNV) in the 15q11-q13 region and single-nucleotide polymorphisms (SNPs) are used to establish the deletion size (type I, type II, or atypical) and uniparental disomy 15 status. MS-MLPA can be used to identify the methylation status as well as copy number assignment (deletions or duplications) (Fig. 161-3). Genotyping of DNA markers on chromosome 15 is required to identify biparental (or normal) inheritance of the chromosome 15s in the affected individuals with abnormal DNA methylation in order to identify uniparental disomy 15 (and its type) or imprinting center defects. If the mother is a carrier of a recessive allele for a genetic condition on one of her chromosome 15s (eg, Bloom syndrome), then the type of maternal disomy status (isodisomy or segmental disomy) could impact on the presence of this second genetic condition.

Once biparental inheritance is established and normal-appearing (nondeleted) chromosome 15s identified, then an imprinting center defect must be present either due to a microdeletion within the center or due to an error in the DNA methylation pattern (epimutation) impacting on the activity of imprinted genes in the region. Individuals with imprinting defects (microdeletion vs epimutation) will require specialized testing in a research laboratory to determine the specific type of imprinting defect.

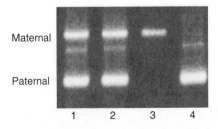

**Figure 161-2** Methylation-Specific Polymerase Chain Reaction (PCR) Analysis of the *SNRPN* Gene Promoter Showing DNA Methylation Patterns From Two Normal Controls (Lanes 1 and 2), an Individual With Prader-Willi Syndrome (lane 3) and an Individual With Angelman Syndrome (lane 4). The top band represents the PCR fragment generated from the mother and the bottom band from the father. Only the top (maternal) band is seen in Prader-Willi syndrome and only the bottom band is seen in Angelman syndrome while normal control individuals have both bands.

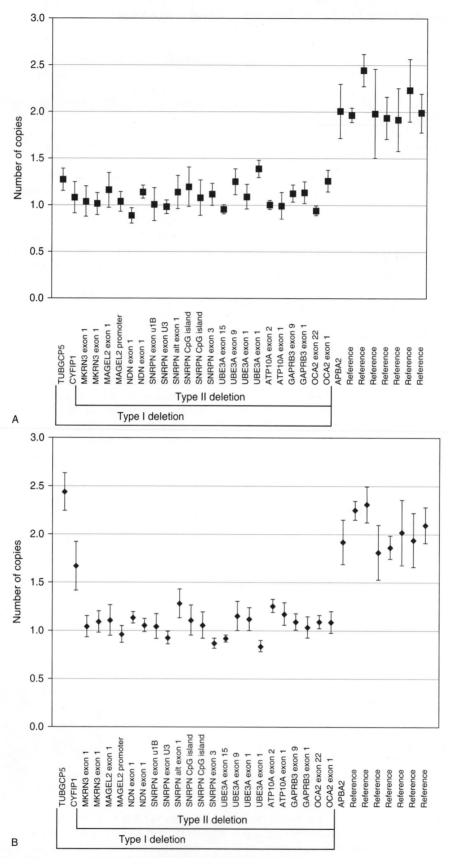

***Figure 161-3*** Scatter Plot of Mean Normalized Values With Standard Deviations for Probes Using Methylation-Specific Multiplex Ligation-Dependent Probe Amplification (MS-MLPA) to Determine the Deletion Status in both Prader-Willi or Angelman Syndromes. **(A)** Gene copy number of an individual with Prader-Willi syndrome and the typical type I deletion of the 15q11-q13 region extending from *TUBGCP5* to *OCA2* with other genes not deleted on chromosome 15 (eg, *APBA2*) or other chromosomes (copy number of 1.0 = deletion; copy number of 2.0 = nondeletion). **(B)** Gene copy number of an individual with Prader-Willi syndrome and the typical type II deletion extending from *MKRN3* to *OCA2* with other genes not deleted on chromosome 15 (eg, *APBA2*) or other chromosomes (copy number of 1.0 = deletion; copy number of 2.0 = nondeletion).

## BIBLIOGRAPHY:

1. Schrander-Stumpel CT, Sinnema M, van den Hout L, et al. Healthcare transition in persons with intellectual disabilities: general issues, the Maastricht model, and Prader-Willi syndrome. *Am J Med Genet C Sem Med Genet.* 2007;145C:241-247.

2. Smith JC. Angelman syndrome: evolution of the phenotype in adolescents and adults. *Dev Med Child Neurol.* 2001;43:476-480.

3. Angelman H. "Puppet children": a report on three cases. *Dev Med Child Neruol.* 1965;7:681.

4. Das R, Hampton DD, Jirtle RL. Imprinting evolution and human health. *Mamm Genome.* 2009;20:563-572.

5. Butler MG. Genomic imprinting disorders in humans: a minireview. *J Assist Reprod Genet.* 2009;26(9-10):477-486.

6. Butler MG. Prader-Willi Syndrome: obesity due to genomic imprinting. *Curr Genomics.* 2011;12:204-215.

7. Butler MG. Prader-Willi syndrome: current understanding of cause and diagnosis. *Am J Med Genet.* 1990;35:319-332.

8. Yamada KA, Volpe JJ. Angelman's syndrome in infancy. *Dev Med Child Neruol.* 1990;32:1005-1021.

9. Williams CA, Driscoll DJ, Dagli AI. Clinical and genetic aspects of Angelman syndrome. *Genet Med.* 2010;12:385-395.

10. Holm VA, Cassidy SB, Butler MG, et al. Prader-Willi syndrome: consensus diagnostic criteria. *Pediatrics.* 1993;91:398-402.

11. Gunay-Aygun M, Schwartz S, Heeger S, O'Riordan MA, Cassidy SB. The changing purpose of Prader-Willi syndrome clinical diagnostic criteria and proposed revised criteria. *Pediatrics.* 2001;108:E92.

12. Cassidy SB, Driscoll DJ. Prader-Willi syndrome. *Eur J Hum Genet.* 2009;17:3-13.

13. Goldstone AP, Holland AJ, Hauffa BP, Hokken-Koelega AC, Tauber M. Recommendations for the diagnosis and management of Prader-Willi syndrome. *J Clin Endocrinol Metab.* 2008;93:4183-4197.

14. Butler MG, Lee PDK, Whitman BY. In: Butler MG, Lee PDK, Whitman BY, eds. *Management of Prader-Willi Syndrome.* 3rd ed. New York, NY: Springer-Verlag; 2006.

15. Burnside RD, Pasion R, Mikhail FM, et al. Microdeletion/microduplication of proximal 15q11.2 between BP1 and BP2: a susceptible region for neurological dysfunction including developmental and language delay. *Hum Genet.* 2010;130:517-528.

## Supplementary Information

### OMIM REFERENCES:

[1] Prader-Willi Syndrome (#176270)

[2] Angelman Syndrome (#105830)

***Key Words:*** Prader-Willi syndrome, Angelman syndrome, genetic subtypes, clinical features, obesity, seizures, hypopigmentation, typical 15q11-q13 deletions, genomic imprinting, maternal disomy 15, paternal disomy 15, diagnostic criteria, imprinting center defects, *UBE3A* and *SNURF—SNRPN* genes, snoRNAs (SNORDs), chromosome breakpoints, BP1, BP2, BP3

# 162 Down Syndrome

David J. Harris and Fowzan S. Alkuraya

## KEY POINTS

- *Disease summary:*
  - Down syndrome (DS) is a chromosomal aneuploidy of chromosome 21 and represents the most frequently identified cause of intellectual disability, with a wide range of severity.
  - In addition to typical facial features, the phenotype includes skeletal, neurologic, gastrointestinal, endocrine, and hematologic components or risks. Anticipatory guidance is the key to the prevention and treatment of these complications.
  - DS is associated with increased mortality in childhood (usually due to congenital heart disease) and in adulthood (due to Alzheimer disease and premature aging, among other factors).
  - Prenatal screening for DS is widely practiced and has evolved from ultrasound-based approach to combined ultrasound and biochemical marker-based approach to DNA-based approach.
- *Hereditary basis:*
  - DS is usually caused by the sporadic de novo occurrence of a meiotic error involving chromosome 21 in the parent (usually the mother especially in the older age group), which is associated with a low recurrence risk.
  - A much higher recurrence risk is observed when the meiotic error is the result of a constitutional parental translocation (<5% of DS cases) or parental mosaicism (frequency unknown).
- *Differential diagnosis:*
  - Single palmar (Simian) crease, sandal gap, upslanting palpebral fissures, epicanthic folds, protruding tongue, and hypotonia are seen in the majority of DS but can also be seen in normal individuals and this explains why clinical diagnosis is only accurate in two-thirds of the cases in the neonatal period. Hypothyroidism may present with similar features. Other rare disorders, such as peroxisomal disorders and Menkes syndrome are possible alternatives in infants. Short stature and mental retardation occur in a number of disorders.

## Diagnostic Criteria and Clinical Characteristics

***Diagnostic Criteria for Down Syndrome:***

Common features
Epicanthic folds
Upslanting palpebral fissures
Protruding tongue
Single palmar creases
Hypotonia
Sandal gap (abnormally wide gap between the first and second toes)

In one study, the above six features were identified in 100% of trisomy DS and 90% of translocation DS but in 38% of those with mosaic DS. Any of these features in isolation can be seen in normal individuals and the presence of these features combined strongly predict DS but karyotypic testing is a must to both confirm the clinical suspicion and to determine the recurrence risk (see Counseling).

***Clinical Characteristics:*** The conspicuous profile of DS makes it highly unlikely that the diagnosis is first made in adulthood. A summary of the clinical features seen in adults with DS is summarized in Table 162-1. Individuals with mosaicism have variable expression of the clinical characteristics that is dependent on the proportion of trisomic cells.

## Screening and Counseling

***Screening:*** Screening for DS is usually done prenatally. In 2006, the American College of Obstetrics and Gynecology issued recommendations that all women regardless of their age should be offered noninvasive screening and the option for chorionic villous sampling (CVS) or amniocentesis. According to the new recommendations, "first-trimester screening using both nuchal translucency (NT) and a blood test is an effective screening test in the general population, and that women found to be at increased risk of having a baby with DS with first-trimester screening should be offered genetic counseling and the option of CVS or mid-trimester amniocentesis." Recently, isolation of circulating cell-free fetal DNA followed by next-generation sequencing has shown a remarkable degree of sensitivity and specificity and is currently offered clinically.

It is highly unusual that a DS patient will reach adulthood without being diagnosed but one should consider making the diagnosis in an adult patient with intellectual disability and typical facial features. More relevant to the issue of screening in adult DS patients is the screening for certain health conditions that occur at a higher frequency compared to the general population and these are detailed in Table 162-2 in which a guideline for anticipatory guidance is recommended. Several health issues deserve a special mention. Normal eyes are considered to be the exception in adults with DS so regular assessment for the development of cataract, keratoconus, and other visual problems is important. Just like in children, DS adults are more likely than others to have undiagnosed otitis media and failure to recognize and treat these infections can lead to a more severe mastoiditis so regular ENT assessment is recommended. Obesity, which is very common in DS adults, can result in hypoventilation and sleep apnea, so this needs to be considered in the regular assessment of these patients. Although Alzheimer disease is much more common in DS adults compared to the general population, a decrease in cognitive function should be investigated considering other possibilities including hypothyroidism which is

**Table 162-1** *Clinical Characteristics of Adult Patients With DS (based on 36 adults, adapted from van Allen et al. 1999)*

Visual concerns 79%
Congenital cataracts (2.6%)
Adult-onset cataracts (50%)
Blindness (21%)
Strabismus (36.8%)
Recurrent keratitis (21%)
Keratoconus (15.8%)
Refractive errors (34.2%)
Hearing concerns (44.7%)
Chronic otitis media (44.7%)
Hearing loss NI (25%)
Chronic mastoiditis (18.4%)
Mastoidectomy (15.8%)
Respiratory concerns (60.5%)
Pulmonary hypertension (7.9%)
Pneumonia (55.3%)
Asthma/bronchitis (7.9%)
Recurrent aspiration with chronic interstitial lung changes on x-ray (30%)
Cardiovascular concerns (57.9%)
CHD (15.8%)
Rheumatic heart disease (2.6%)
Arteriosclerotic heart disease (13.2%)
Cerebral vascular accidents (5.3%)
Gastrointestinal concerns (15.8%)
Hiatal hernia (7.9%)
Gastroesophageal reflux (18.4%)
Fundoplication for gastroesophageal reflux (2.6%)
Prolapsed rectum (7.9%)
Genitourinary concerns (31.6%)
Recurrent urinary tract infection (7.9%)
Bladder neck resection (10.5%)
Hydronephrosis (5.2%)
Renal failure (2.6%)
Musculoskeletal (5.3%)
Paraplegia due to compression fracture (5.3%)

very common in this patient population and should be screened for on an annual basis.

***Counseling:*** For families who have had an affected child, recurrence risk depends on the cytogenetic result. A woman who has a child with trisomy 21 has a risk of another affected child estimated at twice her age-specific risk. If the child has a translocation, the risk depends on the specifics of the translocation. A carrier of a homologous robertsonian 21;21 translocation can only have affected children (with the very rare exception of a trisomy rescue and resulting UPD 21 in the fetus). For a parent who is a carrier of nonhomologous robertsonian translocation (eg, 14;21), there is a theoretical DS risk of one-third because of unviable

**Table 162-2** *Healthcare Screening of Adults With Down Syndrome*

| Health assessment | Initial | Annual | Periodic | PRN |
|---|---|---|---|---|
| Central and peripheral nervous system | | | | |
| Neurological history and exam | X | X | | X |
| Cognitive skills assessment | X | X | q 5 y[†] | X |
| Behavioral assessment | X | X | | X |
| Seizure evaluation | X | X | | X |
| EEG | * | * | | X |
| Neurology consultation | ** | *,** | | X |
| Ear, nose, and throat (ENT) | | | | |
| History and exam | X | X | | X |
| ENT specialist consultation | ** | *,** | | ** |
| Visual system | | | | |
| History and exam | X | X | | X |
| Ophthalmology consultation | X | *,** | | ** |
| Auditory system | | | | |
| History and exam | X | X | | X |
| Hearing testing | X | * | q 3-5 y | X |
| Audiology consultation | ** | *,** | | ** |
| Pulmonary system | | | | |
| History and exam | X | X | | X |
| CXR | X | * | | X |
| Tuberculosis skin test | X | | q 5 y | |
| Specialist consultation | ** | *,** | | ** |
| Hematologic system | | | | |
| History and exam | X | X | | X |
| Complete blood count, differential, platelets | X | X | | X |
| Hematology consultation | ** | * | | ** |
| Cardiovascular system | | | | |
| History and exam | X | X | | X |
| CXR/ echocardiogram | X | * | | X |
| Lipid profile | X | * | | |
| Cardiology consultation | *,** | *,** | | ** |

(Continued)

*Table 162-2 Healthcare Screening of Adults With Down Syndrome (Continued)*

| Gastrointestinal system | | | | |
|---|---|---|---|---|
| History and exam | X | X | | X |
| Hepatitis screening/ immunization | X | | | |
| Specialist consultation | *,** | *,** | | ** |
| **Genitourinary system** | | | | |
| History and exam | X | X | | X |
| Sexual activity/ knowledge counseling | X | + | + | |
| Urinalysis, renal function tests | X | X | | X |
| Routine pelvic exam and PAP smear | X | + | + | |
| Specialty consultation | *,** | *,** | | ** |
| **Endocrine and autoimmune disorders** | | | | |
| History and exam | X | X | | X |
| Thyroid function tests | X | X | | X |
| Diet counseling | X | X | | |
| Specialty consultation | *,** | *,** | | ** |
| **Musculoskeletal system** | | | | |
| History and exam[a] | X | X | | X |
| Spine radiography/ odontoid views | X | X | | |
| Counsel regarding sports activities | X | X | | |
| Orthopedic consultation | *,** | *,** | | ** |

†q 5 y, every 5 years formal testing with specialist; X, evaluate focusing on concerns related to DS; *, evaluate based on clinical assessment and/or specialist's recommendation; **, obtain consultation if there is history of concerns, ongoing concerns, or suspected new concerns; +, screening frequency based on individual DS adults, their tolerance, and activities.

[a]Assess for osteoporosis.

offspring. However, in reality, the rate is between 10% and 15% with a carrier mother and even lower if the father is a carrier. A family with more than one affected child may have a mosaic parent with a normal phenotype. Adults with DS are typically sterile especially males but the few reported cases suggest a preponderance of normal karyotype in their offspring.

## Management and Treatment

Demographic information on the survival of individuals with DS is limited. The median age at death was 25 years in 1983, increasing to 49 in 1997. Death certificates list congenital heart disease, dementia, hypothyroidism, and leukemia more frequently than in the general population. Survival is continuing to improve, with better preservation of cognitive functioning. In a recent longitudinal study, the most important problems related to mortality were dementia, mobility restriction, visual impairment, and epilepsy.

Although most postmortem examination of the brains of individuals with DS show Alzheimer-like changes, not all are clinically demented. This difference may be a consequence of the difficulty of accurately identifying cognitive and other changes associated with dementia. Seizures, particularly of the myoclonic type, may also contribute to cognitive decline as well as problems of vision, hearing, and hypothyroidism. In a longitudinal study of 200 adults, 22 (11%) had subclinical hypothyroidism, 22 (10.5%) had definite hypothyroidism, and 6 (3%) were hyperthyroid at the start of the program. The results are complicated by mortality, but 80% of the group remained euthyroid. The hypothyroid state may be related to autoimmunity, and Hashimoto encephalopathy may occur. The risk of leukemia in DS is 1:150 and extends into adulthood. DS adults appear to be at reduced risk for most solid malignancies but at increased risk for lymphomas, extragonadal germ cell tumors, testicular germ cell tumors, and, a possible increase in retinoblastoma and pancreatic and bone tumors.

Primary healthcare of DS adults require familiarity with the health issues they are at risk for in addition to those relevant to the general population. Table 162-2 summarizes the recommendations for anticipatory guidance of DS patients based on van Allen et al, 1999.

## Molecular Genetics and Molecular Mechanism

### *Syndrome/Gene/Locus:*

Down Syndrome, Trisomy 21, Included/*DS*/21q22.3

The classical view of DS pathogenesis is that it results from perturbation of dosage-sensitive genes as a result of the triplication of greater than 300 genes that are present on the human chromosome 21. Linking specific genes on chromosome 21 to the various phenotypic manifestations of DS has been aided by the study of human patients with partial trisomy 21 and mouse models in which triplication of the syntenic region of human chromosome 21 is engineered. These studies challenge the notion of a DS "critical locus" and suggest that a wide array of genes on chromosome 21 are involved in the pathogenesis. Some of the best studied of these dosage-sensitive genes is APP-encoding amyloid beta A4 precursor protein because the increased dose of this gene has been experimentally shown to increase the deposition of amyloid beta, the main component of the amyloid plaques in Alzheimer disease brains although mouse studies suggest that this in itself is not sufficient to cause Alzheimer disease in DS brain. For an excellent review on the current knowledge of all candidate dosage-sensitive genes that are implicated in DS pathogenesis, please refer to Lana-Elola et al.

## Genetic Testing:

☞**PRENATAL DIAGNOSIS:** Standard cytogenetic analysis is widely available to identify trisomy 21. The extra chromosome material can also be identified in cells with fluorescent in situ hybridization (FISH), or by chromosomal microarray with either bacterial artificial chromosomes (BAC), oligonucleotide probes or single-nucleotide polymorphisms (SNPs).

## BIBLIOGRAPHY:

1. Sivakumar S, Larkins S. Accuracy of clinical diagnosis in Down's syndrome. *Arch Dis Child.* 2004;89:691.

2. Devlin L, Morrison PJ. Accuracy of the clinical diagnosis of Down syndrome. *Ulster Med J.* 2004;73:4-12.

3. Papavassiliou P, York TP, Gursoy N, Hill G, et al. The phenotype of persons having mosaicism for trisomy 21/Down syndrome reflects the percentage of trisomic cells present in different tissues. *Am J Med Genet A.* 2009;149A:573-583.

4. ACOG Practice Bulletin No. 77: screening for fetal chromosomal abnormalities. *Obstet Gynecol.* 2007;109:217-227.

5. Palomaki GE, Kloza EM, Lambert-Messerlian GM, et al. DNA sequencing of maternal plasma to detect Down syndrome: an international clinical validation study. *Genet Med.* 2011;13:913-920.

6. Palomaki GE, Deciu C, Kloza EM, et al. DNA sequencing of maternal plasma reliably identifies trisomy 18 and trisomy 13 as well as Down syndrome: an international collaborative study. *Genet Med.* 2012;14:296-305.

7. Harris DJ, Begleiter ML, Chamberlin J, Hankins L, Magenis RE. Parental trisomy 21 mosaicism. *Am J Hum Genet.* 1982;34:125-133.

8. Bovicelli L, Orsini LF, Rizzo N, Montacuti V, Bacchetta M. Reproduction in Down syndrome. *Obstet Gynecol.* 1982;59:S13-S17.

9. Yang Q, Rasmussen SA, Friedman JM. Mortality associated with Down's syndrome in the USA from 1983 to 1997: a population-based study. *Lancet.* 2002;359:1019-1025.

10. Coppus AM, Evenhuis HM, Verberne GJ, et al. Survival in elderly persons with Down syndrome. *J Am Geriatr Soc.* 2008;56:2311-2316.

11. Jensen KM, Davis MM. Health care in adults with Down syndrome: a longitudinal cohort study. *J Intellect Disabil Res.* 2012.

12. van Allen MI, Fung J, Jurenka SB. Health care concerns and guidelines for adults with Down syndrome. *Am J Med Genet.* 1999;89:100-110.

13. Jensen KM, Taylor LC, Davis MM. Primary care for adults with Down syndrome: adherence to preventive healthcare recommendations. *J Intellect Disabil Res.* 2013;57(5):409-421.

14. Salehi A, Delcroix JD, Belichenko PV, et al. Increased App expression in a mouse model of Down's syndrome disrupts NGF transport and causes cholinergic neuron degeneration. *Neuron.* 2006;51:29-42.

15. Lana-Elola E, Watson-Scales SD, Fisher EM, Tybulewicz VL. Down syndrome: searching for the genetic culprits. *Dis Model Mech.* 2011;4:586-595.

16. http://www.aafp.org/afp/2001/0915/p1031.html

## Supplementary Information

**OMIM REFERENCE:**

[1] Down Syndrome; DS (#190685)

**Alternative Name:**

• Trisomy 21

***Key Words:*** Down syndrome, trisomy, translocation, thyroid, retardation

# 163 Turner Syndrome

Carolyn A. Bondy

## KEY POINTS

- *Disease summary:*
  - Caused by complete or partial loss of the second sex chromosome (45,X karyotype).
  - The great majority of 45,X gestations end in fetal demise by end of first trimester.
  - Approximately 1/2500 live born females have Turner syndrome (TS).
  - Extreme short stature may be prevented by growth hormone RX during childhood.
  - Secondary sexual development and normal sexual functioning are achieved with estrogen replacement treatment.
  - The other features if diagnosed and remedied in a timely manner need not impair longevity or quality of life.
- *Hereditary basis:*
  - TS is a sporadic disorder occurring due to nondisjunction or fragmentation of sex chromosomes during gametogenesis or early embryonic development.
- *Differential diagnosis*
  - Noonan syndrome—the physical phenotype may mimic TS, with short stature and residual evidence fetal lymphedema (eg, neck webbing) and congenital heart disease (CHD). The karyotype of this autosomal dominant syndrome is normal, however.
  - Idiopathic short stature with constitutional delay of puberty—the karyotype in these children is also normal.

## Diagnostic Criteria and Clinical Characteristics

*Diagnostic Criteria for Turner Syndrome:* Criteria include short stature and at least one or other of the cardinal or major features listed below in a phenotypic female, confirmed with a 20-cell karyotype revealing loss of all or parts of one sex chromosome.

- Cardinal features (>90% of cases) include phenotypic female, short stature most evident by age 12, ovarian failure, absent pubertal development, infertility by age 12 to 20.
- Major features (~50% of cases) include CHD, sensorineural hearing loss by age 30 to 40 and thyroid autoimmune disease begins in childhood, peaking approximately at age 50.
- Minor features (≤30% of cases) include renal anomalies such as horseshoe kidney, hypertension—may begin in childhood, type 2 diabetes in adults aged 30 and up, lymphedema-neck webbing (a residual of fetal cystic hygroma; a few patients have persistent peripheral lymphedema).

## Screening and Counseling

*Screening:* In the setting of an abnormal fetal ultrasound (cystic hygroma, hydrops, cardiovascular defects) the finding of 45,X from chorionic villous or amniocentesis carries a grave prognosis in terms of fetal survival. However, this scenario is compatible with delivery of a viable newborn. In a contrasting situation, a sex chromosome anomaly is detected during routine prenatal screening; the degree of mosaicism detected prenatally is not generally predictive of the severity of the TS phenotype. Particularly if the fetal ultrasound is normal, there may be little clinical consequence of the prenatal karyotype, and chromosomes need to be re-evaluated in the newborn. In general, prenatally diagnosed girls tend to be less affected than those diagnosed postnatally.

*Counseling:* TS is a sporadic disorder but recurrence that has rarely been reported suggests that recurrence risk is probably increased after the first TS pregnancy and an estimate of 1.4% has been reported based on one small case series of 140 TS patients.

## Management and Treatment

*Practice Guidelines:*

☞INDICATIONS FOR KARYOTYPE: TS should be suspected in any female with short stature (determined based on parental heights), premature ovarian failure, and left-sided congenital heart defects (aortic coarctation, aortic valve disease, and hypoplastic left heart). Physical diagnosis in addition may find multiple pigmented nevi, high-arched palate, neck webbing, low posterior hairline, low-set or malrotated ears, micrognathia, short fourth metacarpals. The diagnosis of TS requires a genetic confirmation that is currently provided by a 20-cell karyotype on peripheral white blood cells (Fig. 163-1).

☞Y CHROMOSOME: If the karyotype contains Y-chromosome material, the patient has an increased risk of developing gonadoblastoma. The actual risk for a clinically significant (malignant or metastatic) tumor is not known; however, current recommendations suggest removal of the usually rudimentary gonads. If a patient with TS exhibits virilization, or if the karyotype contains a marker or ring chromosome that is suspicious for Y material, further genetic studies to identify Y-chromosome material are needed.

☞REQUIRED MEDICAL SCREENING UPON DIAGNOSIS:
- All patients with the diagnosis of TS need comprehensive cardiologic evaluation by an expert in CHD, since this feature poses great risk of morbidity and mortality. This evaluation must include cardiovascular magnetic resonance imaging (MRI), since transthoracic echo does not adequately visualize the aortic valve or aortic arch. The diameter of the aorta must be indexed to the patient size, since aortic aneurysm and dissection occur at significantly lower diameters in these small women.

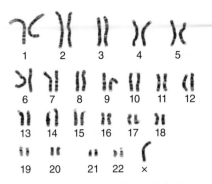

**Figure 163-1** Human Karyotype Containing Only One Sex Chromosome, Hall Mark of the Diagnosis of Turner Syndrome. These are G-banded metaphase chromosomes microphotographed and then sorted according to the size and centromere location, with the sex chromosomes always last.

- BP in all four extremities.
- Renal ultrasound.
- Hearing evaluation.
- Liver function tests (LFTs) and thyroid function tests (TFTs), celiac screen, lipids, HgA$_{1C}$.
- Age-appropriate pubertal development—need for estrogen replacement.
- Growth, educational, and psychosocial evaluations for pediatric patients.

☞**ONGOING MONITORING:**
- If cardiologic abnormality was detected, follow-up per cardiology specialist
- BP, liver and thyroid, lipids, HgA$_{1C}$ annually
- Age-appropriate evaluation of pubertal development and psychosexual adjustment
- Evaluation of ovarian hormone treatment for older girls and adults annually
- Celiac screen and audiology every 3 to 5 years
- Bone mineral density by dual-energy x-ray absorptiometry (DXA) at transition from pediatric to adult care and at age 40 to 50

☞**HEART DISEASE IN TS:** Heart disease is the major source of morbidity and premature mortality in TS. The problems include both congenital defects (aortic valve disease, aortic aneurysms and dissection, anomalous pulmonary veins) and premature atherosclerosis. Thus intensive cardiology evaluation by a unit familiar with these issues is essential. Cardiothoracic MR angiography is essential to visualize the entire aorta and pulmonary veins. This may be done at diagnosis for older girls and adults, and at the transition to adult care for pediatric cases.

☞**PREGNANCY IN TS:** Spontaneous pregnancy occurs in a very few women with TS, but in recent years many women with infertility due to this syndrome have sought assisted reproductive technology (ART) usually with donor oocytes to achieve pregnancy. However, several studies have reported a high rate of catastrophic aortic complications during late pregnancy in women with TS. Thus recent guidelines from the American Society for Reproduction suggest that TS is a relative contraindication to ART pregnancy, and requires comprehensive cardiovascular consultation prior to and follow-up during pregnancy.

*Treatment:* Girls are optimally treated by a pediatric endocrinologist, who will address issues of growth hormone treatment to enhance adult stature, monitor for spontaneous pubertal development (in ~15%), and initiate sexual development with low-dose estrogen as needed.

Adults with TS may be cared for by an internist or endocrinologist. Provision of suitable ovarian hormone replacement is essential to build and maintain adequate bone health. Estrogen doses may need to be higher in young women with TS than those typically used for postmenopausal patients. Oral contraceptives provide adequate estrogen and are well tolerated and adhered to in most cases. In young women with some contraindication for oral contraceptive (OC) (eg, smoking, clotting disorder) and in older women transdermal estradiol at 50 to 100 μg is preferred. In most cases we aim to taper and discontinue estrogen treatment by age 50. Hypothyroidism, hypertension, hyperlipidemia, osteoporosis, and type 2 diabetes are common and respond to standard treatment.

## Molecular Genetics and Molecular Mechanism

The most common genetic constitution in TS is 45,X (~50% of cases) due to complete loss of a sex chromosome in gametogenesis. The next most common genotype includes cell line mosaicism for 45,X/46,XX or 45,X/47,XXX or 45,X/46,XY (~20% of cases) which occurs as a result of nondisjunction during early embryonic development. The last important category includes sex chromosome fragmentation that results in loss of all or major portions of a sex chromosome short arm (Xpdel or Ypdel). This category includes iso and ring X or Y chromosomes containing short arm deletions; such karyotypes are often mosaic for 45,X cell lines due to loss of the abnormal chromosome during mitotic cell divisions.

*Genetic Testing:* Karyotype is the gold standard test in TS (Fig. 163-1). This test involves the preparation and staining of chromosomes from live dividing cells using standard culture techniques. Most patients with TS are diagnosed based on a karyotype prepared from blood lymphocytes. Karyotypes from cultured chorionic villous tissues or amniocytes are used to diagnose TS prenatally. Occasionally, suspicion of mosaicism for X monosomy will necessitate preparing additional karyotypes from skin-derived cultured fibroblasts. Fluorescent in situ hybridization (FISH) is used to characterize fragmentary 'ring' or 'marker' chromosomes, and for detecting aneuploidy on interphase nuclei. New diagnostic tests using single nucleotide polymorphism (SNP) genotyping arrays are currently undergoing evaluation for the diagnosis of TS.

**BIBLIOGRAPHY:**
1. Koeberl DD, McGillivray B, Sybert VP. Prenatal diagnosis of 45,X/46,XX mosaicism and 45,X: implications for postnatal outcome. *Am J Hum Genet.* 1995;57:661-666.
2. Gunther DF, Eugster E, Zagar AJ, Bryant CG, Davenport ML, Quigley CA. Ascertainment bias in Turner syndrome: new insights from girls who were diagnosed incidentally in prenatal life. *Pediatrics.* 2004;114:640-644.
3. Larizza D, Danesino C, Maraschio P, Caramagna C, Klersy C, Calcaterra V. Familial occurrence of Turner syndrome: casual event or increased risk? *J Pediatr Endocrinol Metab.* 2011;24:223-225.

4. Bondy C. Care of girls and women with Turner syndrome: a guideline of the Turner Syndrome Study Group. *J Clin Endocrinol Metab*. 2007;92:10-25.

5. Rivkees S, Hager K, Hosono S, et al. A highly sensitive, high-throughput assay for the detection of Turner syndrome. *J Clin Endocrinol Metab*. 2011;96:699-705.

6. Schoemaker M, Swerdlow A, Higgins C, Wright A, Jacobs P. Cancer incidence in women with Turner syndrome in Great Britain: a national cohort study. *Lancet Oncol*. 2008;9:239-246.

7. Sachdev V, Matura L, Sidenko S, et al. Aortic valve disease in Turner syndrome. *J Am Coll Cardiol*. 2008;51:1904-1909.

8. Bondy CA. Aortic dissection in Turner syndrome. *Curr Opin Cardiol*. 2008;23:519-526.

9. Stochholm K, Juul S, Juel K, Naeraa RW, Hojbjerg Gravholt C. Prevalence, incidence, diagnostic delay, and mortality in Turner syndrome. *J Clin Endocrinol Metab*. 2006;91:3897-3902.

10. Practice Committee of American Society For Reproductive Medicine. Increased maternal cardiovascular mortality associated with pregnancy in women with Turner syndrome. *Fertil Steril*. 2012;97:282-284.

11. Hjerrild BE, Mortensen KH, Gravholt CH. Turner syndrome and clinical treatment. *Br Med Bull*. 2008;86:77-93.

## Supplementary Information

***Key Words:*** Turner syndrome, gonadoblastoma, growth hormone, amenorrhea, mosaicism

# 164 Klinefelter Syndrome and Related Sex Chromosome Aneuploidies

Prasanth Surumpudi and Ronald Swerdloff

## KEY POINTS

- *Disease summary:*
  - Klinefelter syndrome is characterized by a sex chromosome aneuploidy in males. Affected males have an extra X chromosome. Males with other rare sex chromosome aneuploidy conditions have single or multiple extra X and/or Y chromosomes.
  - Klinefelter syndrome is the most common sex chromosome abnormality with incidence of 1 in 500 live male births to 1 in 700 live male births. Often the diagnosis of Klinefelter syndrome is made after the onset of puberty.
  - Classically, males with Klinefelter syndrome present with primary hypogonadism, small testes, azoospermia or severe oligospermia, gynecomastia, an increased arm-to-leg ratio, and learning (dyslexia) and executive skill difficulties. There is an increased risk of low bone density, cardiovascular disease, immunologic diseases, and psychiatric disorders.
  - Signs and symptoms are influenced by several factors including how many cells have an additional X chromosome, the number of X chromosomes, X-chromosome gene inactivation on the extra X chromosome(s), and the number of CAG repeats in the androgen receptor gene.

- *Hereditary basis:*
  - Klinefelter syndrome is a chromosomal disorder that occurs due to meiotic nondisjunction. There is a near-equal distribution of maternal and paternal meiotic nondisjunction events.
  - Parental age may be related to an increased risk of Klinefelter syndrome.
  - Mitotic nondisjunction can cause postfertilization and can result in individuals with mosaic forms of Klinefelter syndrome.

- *Differential diagnosis:*
  - Klinefelter syndrome involves many systems (Table 164-1). The severity and pattern differ among patients. The differential diagnostic characteristics depend on the symptom complex of the individual patient.
  - The differential diagnoses based on hypogonadism include other causes of primary hypogonadism, hypogonadotropic hypogonadism (eg, Kallmann syndrome), mutations in luteinizing hormone (LH) or follicle-stimulating hormone (FSH) receptor genes, microdeletions in specific regions of the Y chromosome, cryptorchidism, fragile X syndrome (see Chap. 159), defects in 3β-hydroxysteroid dehydrogenase, and 17α-hydroxylase enzymes.
  - The differential diagnosis for learning disorders includes other causes of dyslexia. The impairment of behavioral or executive dysfunctions and behavioral disorders provide another category of diagnostic consideration (eg, ADD/ADHD).

## Diagnostic Criteria and Clinical Characteristics

*Diagnostic Criteria:* Klinefelter syndrome and higher-order sex chromosome aneuploidies are diagnosed through karyotype analysis. Cytogenetic studies will reveal the presence of an extranumerary X chromosome. The classic karyotype for individuals with Klinefelter syndrome is 47,XXY. Individuals can have mosaic forms such as 47,XXY/46,XY, 48,XXXY/46,XY, and 48,XXXY/47,XXXY. It is very rare to find cases that are due to a structurally abnormal X in addition to a normal X and Y, such as 47,X,i(Xq)Y and 47,X,del(X)Y. Higher-order sex chromosome aneuploidies 48,XXYY, 48,XXXY, and 49,XXXXY have been classified in the past as variants of Klinefelter syndrome. These higher-order chromosomal aneuploidies may be alternatively considered as independent sex chromosomal aneuploidial syndromes.

Individuals with Klinefelter syndrome have decreased secondary sexual characteristics, testicular dysgenesis (eg, small testes), azoospermia or severe oligospermia, and gynecomastia. Laboratory values will reveal primary hypogonadism (high LH, high FSH, low inhibin B, and low total testosterone).

*Clinical Characteristics:* Classically affected men present with infertility due to azoospermia (most common) or oligospermia. Normal-to-moderately reduced Leydig cell function, small testes (typically 4-6 mL), decreased secondary sexual characteristics (eg, body hair), tall stature, broad hips, gynecomastia, psychologic and learning disabilities are all commonly observed. The phenotypic presentation can vary in individuals with Klinefelter syndrome. There is a spectrum of clinical characteristics, and a spectrum of childhood and adult capabilities. For systemic involvement, please see Table 164-1.

Individuals with mosaic forms such as 47,XXY/46,XY can have mild phenotypic presentations of Klinefelter syndrome. Individuals with more X chromosomes have more severe phenotypic presentations.

## Screening and Counseling

*Screening:* Children may present with learning and behavioral disorders. A workup is warranted in pubertal males who have not attained signs of secondary male characteristics. Karyotype analysis and hypogonadal workup (eg, testicular examination, LH, FSH, total testosterone, inhibin B) will help to guide the diagnosis (Fig. 164-1).

*Table 164-1 System Involvement*

| System | Manifestation | Incidence |
|---|---|---|
| GU and reproductive | Small testes | 95% |
| | Infertility, azoospermia | 95%-99% |
| | Decreased libido | 70% |
| | Erectile dysfunction | Similar rates to those in non-XXY in those with severe hypogonadism |
| Dermatology | Decreased facial hair | 60%-80% |
| | Decreased pubic hair | 30%-60% |
| | Gynecomastia | 38%-75% |
| Endocrine | Abdominal obesity | 50% |
| | Hypogonadism | 99%-100% |
| | Metabolic syndrome | 44% |
| | Decreased insulin sensitivity, type 2 diabetes | 10%-39% |
| Musculoskeletal | Tall stature | Common |
| | Osteopenia | 25%-40% |
| | Osteoporosis | 6%-15% |
| | Rheumatologic diseases (eg, lupus) | Uncommon but higher than non-XXY |
| Cardiovascular | Varicose veins; sometimes venous ulcers | Up to 40% |
| | Ischemic heart disease | Actual incidence unknown but similar to other hypogonadal states |
| | Anemia | Actual incidence unknown but similar to other hypogonadal states |
| Pulmonary | Diseases of the respiratory system | Actual incidence unknown but increased in XXY |
| | Deep vein thrombosis and pulmonary embolism | Actual incidence unknown but increased in XXY |
| Neurologic/psychiatric | Learning disorders, attention deficit disorder/attention deficit hyperactivity disorder | Some degree of dyslexia is near universal |
| | Depression, anxiety, psychosis | More frequent in KS subjects than XY males |
| | Epilepsy | More frequent in KS subjects than XY males |
| Malignancy | Malignant neoplasms (eg, mediastinal tumors, breast cancer) | Rare but increased in XXY |
| | Breast cancer | 20- to 30-fold higher than in XY males but less than in females |

| System | Manifestation | Relative Mortality |
|---|---|---|
| Endocrine | Endocrine, metabolic, and nutritional disorders | 1.8%-4.8% |
| | Decreased insulin sensitivity, type 2 diabetes | 1.6%-5.8% |
| Cardiovascular | Disorders of the circulatory system | 1.3%-1.41% |
| Pulmonary | Diseases of the respiratory system | 2.3%-2.97% |
| | Chronic lower respiratory disease/chronic obstructive airway disease | 2.1%-3.16% |
| Neuropsychiatric | Neuropsychiatric disorders | 2.62%-2.8% |
| | Depression, anxiety, psychosis | 1.45%-3.7% |
| Malignancy | Malignant neoplasms (eg, mediastinal tumors, breast cancer) | 1.1%-1.2% |

Adapted from Bojesen A, Gravholt CH. Morbidity and mortality in Klinefelter syndrome (47,XXY). *Acta Paediatr.* 2011;100(6):807-813. Review; and Swerdlow AJ, Higgins CD, Schoemaker MJ, Wright AF, Jacobs PA; United Kingdom Clinical Cytogenetics Group. Mortality in patients with Klinefelter syndrome in Britain: a cohort study. *J Clin Endocrinol Metab.* 2005;90(12):6516-6522.

The most common scenario is an adult male who has reported infertility and gynecomastia. Karyotype analysis and hypogonadal workup will be ordered as part of workup for infertility and gynecomastia. Screening should also be considered for males who want to conceive using reproductive technologies (eg, intracytoplasmic sperm injection [ICSI], in vitro fertilization [IVF]). Preimplantation genetic diagnostic testing (cytogenetic analysis of fetal cells obtained from chorionic villus sampling or amniocentesis) should be offered to individuals with Klinefelter syndrome, mosaic Klinefelter syndrome, or other higher-order sex chromosome aneuploidy. There

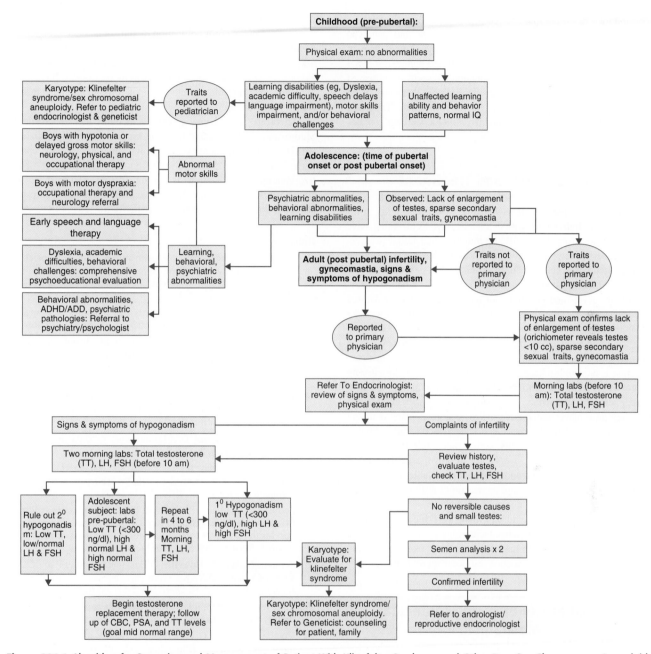

**Figure 164-1** Algorithm for Screening and Management of Patient With Klinefelter Syndrome and Other Rare Sex Chromosome Aneuploidy Conditions.

is an increased risk of sex chromosomal aneuploidies and autosomal aneuploidies in the offspring with sex chromosomal aneuploidies.

***Counseling:*** An essential aspect of the counseling is absolving the parents' unfounded sense of guilt. The recurrence risk for Klinefelter syndrome in a patient's siblings is not increased.

Extranumerary X chromosome arises from either meiosis stage I or stage II in maternal nondisjunction or meiosis I errors in paternal nondisjunction. An extranumerary X chromosome may also arise from postfertilization mitotic nondisjunction. The extra X chromosome may be of paternal or maternal origin and there appears to be a near-equal distribution of maternal and paternal meiotic nondisjunction. The nondisjunction does not follow an autosomal recessive or dominant pattern. There may be an increase of nondisjunction in paternal and maternal gametes of older parents. To date,

studies have not definitively demonstrated a significant phenotypic difference between the paternally and maternally derived cases of Klinefelter syndrome.

☞**GENOTYPE-PHENOTYPE CORRELATION:** The length of CAG repeats in the androgen receptor gene (on the X chromosome) appears to influence the responsiveness to testosterone. Individuals with large CAG repeats in the androgen receptor gene have more severe phenotypic presentations of the disease. Other gene(s) on the X chromosome that are responsible for the phenotypic presentation are still being elucidated.

Signs and symptoms are dependent on how many cells have an additional X chromosome(s). Individuals who have the mosaic form may have milder signs and symptoms, depending on the percentage of cells that harbor an extra X chromosome. There are more abnormalities in phenotype with each additional X or Y chromosome. Overall, the correlation between phenotype and genotype is better with higher-order sex chromosome aneuploidies than in classic Klinefelter syndrome. There are increased features of facial and skeletal malformations and psychomotor retardation observed in 48,XXXY and 49,XXXXY males. In addition, there can be an increased incidence of intrauterine growth retardation. There are more severe neurodevelopmental and psychologic features in males with 48,XXYY.

## Management and Treatment

*Testosterone Replacement Therapy, Gynecomastia, and Reproduction:* Individuals with Klinefelter syndrome often have adequate testosterone levels for the initiation and initial progression of puberty. However, they may not have adequate testosterone levels to attain maximal secondary sex characteristics. Testosterone replacement therapy can be initiated after the determination of low testosterone levels and symptoms of hypogonadism. In the United States, testosterone injections and testosterone gel preparations are the more common methods of testosterone administration. The goal of testosterone replacement therapy is to raise testosterone levels to the mid-normal range and minimize the symptoms of hypogonadism. The dose is adjusted to keep hematocrit less than 52%. Monitoring of prostate-specific antigen (PSA) is warranted in aging men with Klinefelter syndrome who are on testosterone replacement therapy. Testosterone replacement therapy helps to correct some deficient secondary sexual characteristics (such as decreased facial and pubic hair), low libido, sense of vitality, sexual function, self-image, and physical strength. However, it *does not* improve testicular size or fertility. The effects on mood and behavior are variable. Testosterone replacement therapy may prompt regression of mild gynecomastia; however, surgical intervention may be needed in more severe cases.

Men with Klinefelter syndrome may have biologic children with the assistance of reproductive technologies. Oligospermia and azoospermia individuals can have sperm isolated from epididymal sperm aspiration or microdissection testicular sperm extraction.

## Molecular Genetics and Molecular Mechanism

*Syndrome/Gene/Locus:* The extranumerary X chromosome may exert its effects through one or more mechanisms including (1) X-chromosome inactivation, (2) the influence of genes that escape X-chromosome inactivation, (3) the influence of genes from the long arm versus short arm of the X chromosome, (4) CAG repeats in the androgen receptor gene, (5) and DNA methylation of genes on the X-chromosome. The phenotype seen in Klinefelter syndrome may be due to either two active copies of X-linked genes, three active copies of X-Y homologous genes, or genes that have escaped X-chromosome gene inactivation. Currently, there is increased support that the Lyon law (inactivation of the supernumerary X genes) also occurs in males with Klinefelter syndrome. Genes that escape inactivation are often on the short arm of the X chromosome. It is unknown at present which genes that escape inactivation are important in Klinefelter syndrome. It is also unknown at present which combination of genes result in the variable phenotype of the Klinefelter syndrome. There may be

inappropriate transcription of genes (eg, excess gene products) on the X chromosome or modification of autosomal gene products.

*Genetic Testing:* The gold standard for diagnosing Klinefelter is a karyotype that demonstrates at least one extra X chromosome in a metaphase spread from cultured cells (peripheral blood lymphocytes, skin fibroblasts, cells obtained through amniocentesis or chorionic villus sampling).

There are several new screening methods that are available. Studies have demonstrated that fluorescence in situ hybridization (FISH) studies can identify sex chromosomal number and can be performed on sperm. Microarray technology (eg, array comparative genomic hybridization) is currently being used to detect sex chromosome gene abnormalities. Barr body detection (eg, in buccal cells) does not have adequate sensitivity for screening.

BIBLIOGRAPHY:

1. Aksglaede L, Skakkebaek NE, Almstrup K, Juul A. Clinical and biological parameters in 166 boys, adolescents and adults with nonmosaic Klinefelter syndrome: a Copenhagen experience. *Acta Paediatr.* 2011;100(6):793-806.
2. Bojesen A, Gravholt CH. Morbidity and mortality in Klinefelter syndrome (47,XXY). *Acta Paediatr.* 2011;100(6):807-813. Review.
3. Swerdlow AJ, Higgins CD, Schoemaker MJ, Wright AF, Jacobs PA. United Kingdom Clinical Cytogenetics Group. Mortality in patients with Klinefelter syndrome in Britain: a cohort study. *J Clin Endocrinol Metab.* 2005;90(12):6516-6522.
4. Dillon S, Aggarwal R, Harding JW, et al. Klinefelter syndrome (47,XXY) among men with systemic lupus erythematosus. *Acta Paediatr.* 2011;100(6):819-823.
5. Frühmesser A, Kotzot D. Chromosomal variants in Klinefelter syndrome. *Sex Dev.* 2011;5(3):109-123.
6. Herlihy AS, Halliday JL, Cock ML, McLachlan RI. The prevalence and diagnosis rates of Klinefelter syndrome: an Australian comparison. *Med J Aust.* 2011;194(1):24-28.
7. Scofield RH, Bruner GR, Namjou B, et al. Klinefelter syndrome (47,XXY) in male systemic lupus erythematosus patients: support for the notion of a gene-dose effect from the X chromosome. *Arthritis Rheum.* 2008;58(8):2511-2517.
8. Tartaglia N, Ayari N, Howell S, D'Epagnier C, Zeitler P. 48,XXYY, 48,XXXY and 49,XXXXY syndromes: not just variants of Klinefelter syndrome. *Acta Paediatr.* Jun 2011;100(6):851-860. Review.
9. Tüttelmann F, Gromoll J. Novel genetic aspects of Klinefelter syndrome. *Mol Hum Reprod.* Jun 2010;16(6):386-395. Review.
10. Vignozzi L, Corona G, Forti G, Jannini EA, Maggi M. Clinical and therapeutic aspects of Klinefelter syndrome: sexual function. *Mol Hum Reprod.* 2010;16(6):418-424. Review. PMID: 20348547.
11. Wikström AM, Dunkel L. Klinefelter syndrome. *Best Pract Res Clin Endocrinol Metab.* 2011;25(2):239-250. Review.

## Supplementary Information

**OMIM REFERENCE:**

[1] Condition: Klinefelter Syndrome

**Alternative Name:**
• Sex Chromosomal Aneuploidy

*Key Words:* Klinefelter syndrome, hypergonadotropic hypogonadism, primary testicular failure, sex chromosomal aneuploidy, infertility, childhood learning disorders

# 165 The 22q11.2 Deletion Syndrome

Donna M. McDonald-McGinn, Kristine Dickinson, Alice Bailey, and Elaine H. Zackai

## KEY POINTS

- *Disease summary:*
  - The 22q11.2 deletion (22q11.2DS) has been identified in the majority of patients with DiGeorge syndrome, velocardiofacial syndrome (VCFS), and conotruncal anomaly face syndrome, and in some individuals with autosomal dominant Opitz G/BBB syndrome and Cayler cardiofacial syndrome (asymmetric crying facies).
  - The most frequent significant clinical features in individuals with 22q11.2 deletion include the following: immunodeficiency, congenital heart disease, palatal defects, hypocalcemia, renal anomalies and dysphagia, and developmental disabilities.
  - 85% of individuals have the same large greater than 3 Mb hemizygous deletion (referred to as A-D) involving approximately 45 functional genes including *TBX1*, a member of the T-box transcription factor family of genes, known to play a crucial role in development.
  - Conversely, 15% of individuals have "nested" or atypical deletions which may or may not include *TBX1* as it resides between low copy repeat (LCR) blocks A-B.
  - Nested deletions may include A-B, A-C, B-C, B-D, C-D.
  - Phenotypic features in Individuals with deletions which do not include A-B/*TBX1* are similar to those with the full standard deletion suggesting either a downstream effect of *TBX1* and/or the importance of other downstream genes such as *CRKL1* located between C and D.
  - Variable expressivity may be due to stochastic, environmental, and/or genetic factors such as modifier genes or variations in the remaining allele of *TBX1*. See Table 165-1 for a summary of molecular genetic testing associated with 22q11.2 DS.
- *Hereditary basis:*
  - 22q11.2DS most often occurs as a de novo event.
  - Approximately 10% of cases are familial and affected individuals have a 50% recurrence risk.
  - Germline and somatic mosaicism has been observed so parental testing and prenatal monitoring is suggested.
  - Inter- and intrafamilial phenotypic variability is common including between identical twins.
- *Differential diagnosis:*
  - Structural anomalies found in association with 22q11.2DS can also be observed as an isolated finding in an otherwise normal individual.
  - Syndromes with overlapping features include Smith-Lemli-Opitz, Alagille, VATER, oculo-auriculo-vertebral spectrum or Goldenhar, and Kabuki.
  - Individuals with both unicoronal and bicoronal craniosynostosis in whom molecular causes for known craniosynostosis syndromes have been excluded are candidates for deletion studies.
  - Individuals suspected of having 22q11.2DS with negative fluorescence in situ hybridization (FISH) studies may have a smaller nested or atypical deletion within 22q11.2 which will require further study using multiplex ligation-dependent probe amplification (MLPA) or array technology; aneuploidy involving some other chromosomal region such as a cytogenetically detectable 10p13-10p14 deletion; a mutation in *TBX1*; or a mutation in *CHD7*, associated with CHARGE syndrome.
  - It is important to note that individuals with 22q11.2DS have presented with concomitant diagnoses such as those detailed in Table 165-2.

## Diagnostic Criteria and Clinical Characteristics

**Diagnostic Criteria:** Due to the enormous phenotypic variability, there are currently no established diagnostic criteria for 22q11.2DS. However, genetic testing is often prompted by one or more of the most common clinical features, but varies depending on the age of the patient.

- Conotruncal cardiac anomalies
- Palatal abnormalities/hypernasal speech/nasopharyngeal reflux
- Hypocalcemia
- Dysphagia, gastroesophageal reflux disease (GERD)
- Characteristic facial features
- Intellectual deficits, autism
- Behavioral problems, psychiatric illness

Identification in adolescents and adults frequently requires an enhanced index of suspicion; therefore adults may only come to attention following the diagnosis in their child. An individual lacking any apparent clinical features may go undiagnosed and unknowingly pass the deletion to his or her child. Non-Caucasians are more likely to remain undetected.

**Clinical Characteristics:** 22q11DS is the most common microdeletion syndrome in humans with wide inter- and intrafamilial phenotypic variability most frequently involving congenital cardiac anomalies, palatal differences, immune deficiency, hypoparathyroidism, renal abnormalities, dysphagia, and mild craniofacial differences. Behavioral problems and intellectual disabilities are common, including delays in acquisition of motor milestones and emergence of language, while a subset of individuals meet criteria for a psychiatric diagnosis such as autism, pervasive developmental disorder not otherwise specified (PDD-NOS), attention deficit hyperactivity disorder (ADHD), anxiety, obsessive-compulsive

*Table 165-1* **Molecular Genetic Testing**

| Gene | Testing Modality | Mutation Type | Detection Rate |
|---|---|---|---|
| Approximately 45 Functional genes | FISH | All deletions that include the clinically available probes, N25 and TUPLE | 85% A-D (remainder involves other deletions, some of which are detected by FISH) |
| | aCGH | Atypical, nested | No rate available |
| | genome-wide microarray | Atypical, nested | Highly accurate |
| | MLPA | Atypical, nested | |

*Table 165-2* **System Involvement**

| System | Manifestation | Incidence |
|---|---|---|
| Immunologic | Immunodeficiency (impaired T-cell production, humoral defects, IgA deficiency); chronic otitis media, sinusitis, upper airway bacterial infections, fungal infections; autoimmune disease (juvenile rheumatoid arthritis, vitiligo, autoimmune neutropenia, idiopathic thrombocytopenia, thyroid disease); allergies; malignancies (hepatoblastoma, leukemia, lymphoma) | 77% (Immunodeficiency) |
| Cardiovascular | Any congenital defect but most frequently conotruncal anomalies: tetralogy of Fallot, ventricular septal defect, interrupted aortic arch type B, truncus arteriosus; right aortic arch; vascular ring; atrial septal defect; dilated aortic root; arrhythmias | 75% (Structural defect) |
| Craniofacial (palatal and related) | Palatal anomalies (velopharyngeal incompetence, submucous cleft palate, bifid uvula, overt cleft palate, cleft lip, cleft lip and palate); microtia/anotia; craniosynostosis; short forehead/low anterior hairline; malar flatness; hooded eyelids, hypertelorism; thick, overfolded, crumpled helices, protuberant ears, attached lobes; prominent nasal root, bulbous nasal tip with hypoplastic alae nasi, nasal crease or groove with or without small nasal strawberry hemangioma; small mouth; asymmetric crying facies; micrognathia; dental enamel hypoplasia | 75% (Palatal anomaly) |
| Endocrine | Hypocalcemia, hypoparathyroidism; hypo- or hyperthyroidism; failure to thrive; short stature, growth hormone deficiency; diabetes | 50% (Hypocalcemia) |
| Musculoskeletal | Butterfly vertebrae; hemivertebrae; coronal clefts; rib anomalies; scoliosis; hypoplastic scapulae; cervical spine abnormalities; pre-/postaxial polydactyly of hands and feet; clubfoot; 2-3 toe syndactyly; cervical cord compression; tethered cord; craniosynostosis | 50% (Cervical spine anomalies) |
| Gastrointestinal | Dysphagia; gastroesophageal reflux; nasopharyngeal reflux; prominence of the cricopharyngeal muscle; abnormal cricopharyngeal closure; diverticulum; constipation; diaphragmatic hernia, intestinal malrotation/nonrotation, Hirschsprung disease, imperforate anus/anal stenosis, umbilical/inguinal hernia | 35% (Dysphagia) |
| ENT/audiology | Conductive, sensorineural, or mixed hearing loss; Mondini malformation of the cochlea; chronic otitis media; laryngeal web, T-E fistula, esophageal atresia; preauricular pits/tags, microtia/anotia | ~35% |
| Genitourinary | Renal abnormalities (single/multicystic/dysplastic/hypoplastic/absent kidney); hydronephrosis; vesicoureteral reflux, irregular bladder/bladder wall thickening; dysfunctional voiding; nephrocalcinosis; horseshoe kidney; duplicated collecting system; renal tubular acidosis; enuresis; hypospadias; cryptorchidism; primary amenorrhea; absent uterus | 31% (Renal anomalies) |

*(Continued)*

**Table 165-2** *System Involvement (Continued )*

| System | Manifestation | Incidence |
|---|---|---|
| Hematologic | Idiopathic thrombocytopenia, Bernard-Soulier; autoimmune neutropenia; leukemia; lymphoma | Platelet abnormalities (common) |
| Neuromuscular | Hypotonia in infancy; learning disabilities; psychosis (most frequently schizophrenia); hypocalcemic seizures; idiopathic seizures; asymmetric crying facies; ataxia; cerebellar atrophy; multicystic white matter lesions of unknown significance; perisylvian dysplasia; hypoplasia of the pituitary gland; polymicrogyria; cervical cord compression, neural tube defects; abdominal migraines; tethered cord | Hypotonia and learning disabilities **common;** Schizophrenia in ∼ 25%; specific neurologic manifestations **uncommon** |
| Respiratory | Symptoms result from associated factors such as congenital heart disease, asthma, laryngotracheoesophageal anomalies, GERD (aspiration pneumonia) | Common |
| Ophthalmologic | Posterior embryotoxon; tortuous retinal vessels; hooded eyelids; strabismus; ptosis; amblyopia; tilted optic nerves; astigmatism; myopia; hyperopia sclerocornea, coloboma, micro/anophthalmia | Varies |

disorder (OCD), depression, schizophrenia, and other psychotic disorders.

An additional subset of patients have less frequent but important associated features such as cardiac differences (vascular ring, dilated aortic root, arrhythmias), endocrine issues (growth hormone deficiency, hypo- or hyperthyroidism, diabetes), ENT differences (chronic otitis media, sensorineural or conductive hearing loss, cochlear abnormalities, laryngeal web, T-E fistula, esophageal atresia, preauricular pits or tags, microtia or anotia), gastrointestinal problems (diaphragmatic hernia, intestinal malrotation or nonrotation, Hirschsprung disease, imperforate anus, umbilical or inguinal hernia), genitourinary findings (hypospadias, cryptorchidism, absent uterus, dysfunctional voiding, nephrocalcinosis), hematologic or oncologic issues (idiopathic thrombocytopenia, Bernard-Soulier, autoimmune neutropenia, leukemia, lymphoma, hepatoblastoma), immune or autoimmune problems (IgA deficiency, juvenile rheumatoid arthritis, vitiligo), neurologic problems (unprovoked seizures, polymicrogyria, cerebellar abnormalities, cervical cord compression, neural tube defects, abdominal migraines), ophthalmologic findings (sclerocornea, coloboma, micro/anophthalmia, posterior embryotoxon, tortuous retinal vessels, ptosis), pulmonary (asthma, aspiration pneumonia), and skeletal anomalies (cervical/thoracic vertebral differences, tethered cord, polydactyly, craniosynostosis).

## Screening and Counseling

*Screening:* See Table 165-3 for management and screening guidelines.

*Counseling:* It is estimated that a 22q11.2 deletion occurs in 1 of every 2000 births at minimum. The majority of affected individuals (93%) acquire the deletion as a de novo event. This is due to the inherent structure of chromosome 22q11.2 where LCRs with high homology to each other make this region especially susceptible to rearrangements because of unequal meiotic crossovers and thus aberrant interchromosomal exchanges (nonallelic homologous recombination). These LCRs flank the common deletion and define the breakpoints. Parental studies

are encouraged in all families with an affected child in order to identify mildly affected parents and to rule out somatic and germline mosaicism, which have both been reported previously. An affected individual has a 50% chance of passing the deletion to his or her child. Although the pattern of inheritance is similar to that seen in an autosomal dominant disorder, as there are many genes involved in the 22q11.2 microdeletion syndrome, as opposed to a single gene, this is considered a contiguous deletion syndrome.

Genetic counseling is often difficult due to the wide inter- and intrafamilial variability of the deletion. Any number of the following abnormalities may or may not be present in an affected individual: cardiac disease, palatal involvement, immune deficiency and autoimmune disorders, hypoparathyroidism, neurologic involvement, speech and learning disabilities, and feeding and gastrointestinal problems.

## Molecular Genetics and Molecular Mechanism

*Syndrome/Gene/Locus:* The occurrence of 22q11.2 deletions is related to the genomic architecture of the chromosome 22q11.2 region. LCP sequences with high homology to each other make this region especially susceptible to rearrangements because of unequal meiotic crossovers and thus aberrant interchromosomal exchanges. These LCR sequences flank the common 22q11.2 deletions and define the common breakpoints. Breakpoints that are not flanked by LCRs, however, may involve other repeat elements and mechanisms that are yet to be defined.

*Genetic Testing:* The 22q11.2 deletion was originally identified using standard cytogenetic testing in a small number of individuals with DiGeorge syndrome. Subsequent laboratory advances utilizing FISH with probes such as N25 and TUPLE within the commonly deleted "DiGeorge critical region" followed, allowing for the identification of submicroscopic deletions. The pitfalls of FISH, that it is time consuming, relatively expensive, and limited to one target sequence within the DiGeorge critical region, have caused

*Table 165-3  Algorithm for Screening and Management of Patient With the 22q11.2 Deletion*

| | |
|---|---|
| Indications for screening | Conotruncal cardiac anomalies |
| | Variant cardiac defects in conjunction with another characteristic anomaly |
| | VPI, especially in conjunction with dysmorphic features and/or learning disability |
| | A combination of findings such as facial dysmorphia, hypocalcemia, T-cell abnormalities, skeletal abnormalities, and/or a nonverbal learning disability |
| | Detection of the deletion in a biologic child |
| Management of systems | **Cardiac:** immediate completion of a cardiovascular physical examination including echocardiogram, electrocardiogram, and chest x-ray; close attention to respiratory symptomatology |
| | **Palate:** immediate evaluation by a Cleft Palate Team; early surgical intervention as indicated |
| | **Immune**: completion of a full immunologic evaluation; protection from infection, pneumocystis prophylaxis, and prophylactic antibiotics as indicated; immunizations with inactivated viruses |
| | **Feeding:** evaluation for gastroesophageal reflux; intestinal malrotation; constipation; dysphagia; Hirschsprung disease; imperforate or anteriorly placed anus; introduction of a feeding tube as indicated |
| | **Growth:** testing for growth hormone deficiency; referral to diagnosis specific growth charts |
| | **Skeletal:** completion of cervical spine films; ongoing scoliosis screening; evaluation for butterfly or hemivertebrae; attention to extremities including polydactyly and leg pain; attention to skull shape to rule out craniosynostosis; and evaluation by an Orthopedist |
| | **Neurology:** close attention to possible neurologic symptoms such as idiopathic epilepsy and polymicrogyria |
| | **Neurodevelopment:** early developmental evaluation and therapeutic intervention; attainment of services such as OT, PT, and ST; attention to possible associated phenotypes such as ADHD, OCD, ODD, and psychosis |

newer techniques such as microarray comparative genomic hybridization (CGH), whole genome-wide array, and MLPA to be more frequently utilized both to screen for abnormalities in people with multiple congenital anomalies and/or developmental disabilities and to precisely define the deletion breakpoints in people with classic phenotypic features of the 22q11.2 deletion.

## BIBLIOGRAPHY:

1. Bassett A, McDonald-McGinn D, Devriendt K, et al. Practical guidelines for managing patients with 22q11.2 deletion syndrome. *J Pediatrics*. 2011;159:332-339.

2. McDonald-McGinn D, Kohut T, Zackai EH. Deletion 22q11.2 (velo-cardio-facial syndrome/DiGeorge syndrome). *Management of Genetic Syndromes*. 3rd ed. Hoboken: Wiley-Blackwell; 2005:263-284.

3. McDonald-McGinn D, Zackai EH. Genetic counseling. *Velo-Cardio-Facial Syndrome: A Model for Understanding Microdeletion Disorders*. 1st ed. Cambridge: Cambridge University Press. 2005:200-218.

4. McDonald-McGinn DM, Tonnesen MK, Lauger-Cahana A, et al. Phenotype of the 22q11.2 deletion in individuals identified through an affected relative: cast a wide FISHing net! *Genet Med*. 2001;3:23-29.

5. McDonald-McGinn DM, LaRossa D, Goldmuntz E, et al. The 22q11.2 deletion: screening, diagnostic workup, and outcome of results; report on 181 patients. *Genet Test*. 1997;1:99-108.

## Supplementary Information

### OMIM REFERENCE:

[1] DiGeorge Syndrome; DGCR (#188400/194230)

*Clinical Names Previously Associated With the Diagnosis:*
- DiGeorge Syndrome
- Velocardiofacial Syndrome
- Conotruncal Anomaly Face Syndrome
- Autosomal Dominant Opitz G/BBB Syndrome
- Cayler Cardiofacial Syndrome/Asymmetric Crying Facies

*Key Words:* 22q11.2 deletion, DiGeorge syndrome, velocardiofacial syndrome, CTAF, Opitz G/BBB, Cayler cardiofacial syndrome, CATCH 22, VPI, immunodeficiency, hypocalcemia, congenital heart disease, cleft palate

# 166 Mitochondrial Disorders in Adult Patients

Vijay Hegde and Katherine Sims

## KEY POINTS

- *Disease summary:*
  - Dysfunction of the electron transport chain (ETC) causes a group of multisystem disorders which can present in any age group. Mitochondrial disorders should be suspected in patients with diffuse involvement of several organ systems that does not conform to an established pattern of conventional disease, particularly in the presence of myopathy or neurologic symptoms.
  - The major clinical features of mitochondrial diseases include stroke or stroke-like events, dementia, seizures, myopathy, external ophthalmoplegia, pigmentary retinopathy, optic atrophy, hearing loss, cardiomyopathy, cardiac conduction abnormalities, hepatopathy, severe gastrointestinal (GI) dysmotility, autonomic dysfunction, and endocrinopathies.
  - Clinical features most specific to mitochondrial disorders include strokes that do not follow vascular territory, external ophthalmoplegia, unexplained lactic acidosis, and maternal inheritance pattern. The most common symptoms reported by patients include migraine, fatigue or exercise intolerance, heat intolerance, dyspnea, and GI dysmotility.
  - While many patients develop clusters of symptoms that fall into discrete clinical syndromes (Table 166-1), most affected individuals do not fit neatly into any particular syndromic category.
- *Hereditary basis:*
  - Mitochondrial disease can result from mutations of both nuclear and mitochondrial genes.
  - Nuclear mutations can be inherited in autosomal dominant, autosomal recessive, or X-linked patterns.
  - Mutations of the mitochondrial DNA (mtDNA) are inherited through the maternal lineage. Each cell carries multiple copies of the mitochondrial genome and deleterious mutations usually affect some but not all copies of the mitochondrial genome (heteroplasmy). The expression of mitochondrial disease due to mtDNA mutations depends on the relative proportions of normal and abnormal mtDNA.

## Diagnostic Criteria and Clinical Characteristics

***Diagnostic Criteria:*** When a patient presents with a classic mitochondrial syndrome, or with typical clinical features and a family history of maternal inheritance, molecular genetic testing often establishes the diagnosis of mtDNA-associated disease. A definite molecular genetic diagnosis, particularly in those with presumed nuclear DNA (nDNA) etiology, is difficult to establish in most patients. A variety of diagnostic criteria have been proposed and include the following:

- Clinical evidence of myopathy including proximal myopathy, cardiomyopathy, rhabdomyolysis, or abnormal electromyography (EMG).
- Clinical evidence of central nervous system (CNS) involvement including strokes, cortical blindness, seizures, developmental delay, or complex migraines.
- Progressive external ophthalmoplegia.
- Evidence of unexplained multisystem disease including loss of vision, hearing loss, GI dysmotility, autonomic dysfunction, endocrine disorders, nephropathy, or hepatic dysfunction.
- Elevated lactate or alanine levels in plasma or cerebrospinal fluid (CSF), or elevated lactate by magnetic resonance (MR) spectroscopy of the brain.
- MR imaging (MRI) evidence of metabolic strokes or Leigh disease.
- Muscle biopsy showing ragged red fibers, subsarcolemmal accumulation of mitochondria, or crystalline inclusions, abnormal COX or SDH histochemical staining or decreased ETC enzymatic activity.

***Clinical Characteristics:***

☞**NEUROLOGIC:** Patients with mitochondrial disease can develop a variety of neurologic symptoms including strokes, seizures, subacute neurodegeneration, multiple sclerosis (MS)-like illness, and migraines. Metabolic strokes do not follow typical vascular distribution. They usually involve the occipital and/or parietal lobes. These lesions are extremely epileptogenic and patients may present with focal status epilepticus. Leigh syndrome is characterized by focal, bilateral lesions consisting of areas of demyelination, gliosis, necrosis, spongiosis, or capillary proliferation. A MS-like illness has been described in women with Leber hereditary optic neuropathy (LHON). Migraines are one of the most common symptoms in mitochondrial patients.

☞**MUSCLE:** Weakness, pain, and cramping are common complaints and patients typically complain of fatigue with minimal exertion. After exercise, patients may have dyspnea and tachycardia out of proportion to the degree of work. The exercise intolerance is usually severe relative to muscle weakness. After a short rest, patients usually can resume their activity.

☞**CARDIAC:** There is a high prevalence of cardiovascular involvement in adults with mitochondrial diseases. Common ECG abnormalities include Wolff-Parkinson-White (WPW) syndrome and cardiac conduction defects. Cardiomyopathy has been described in a variety of mitochondrial diseases, the majority of which is of the hypertrophic type.

☞**OPHTHALMOLOGIC:** Ophthalmologic pathology is very common and includes retinopathy, optic atrophy, and external ophthalmoplegia. Retinal degeneration, specifically pigmentary retinopathy, is seen in both syndromic and nonsyndromic mitochondrial diseases. Optic nerve atrophy is classically associated with LHON. Progressive external ophthalmoplegia is seen in a variety of deletion and depletion syndromes.

*Table 166-1* **Syndromic Presentations**

| Syndrome | Gene Symbol | Clinical Phenotype |
|---|---|---|
| MELAS | *MT-TL1, MT-ND5, MTTQ, MTTH, MTTK, MTTS1, MTND1, MTND5, MTND6, MTTS2* | The cardinal feature of MELAS is recurrent stroke-like episodes with resultant transient hemiparesis, hemianopsia, or cortical blindness. Repeated stroke-like episodes lead to impairment of cognitive, motor, and visual abilities. Seizures, recurrent headaches, exercise intolerance, weakness, and sensorineural hearing loss are commonly seen. |
| MERRF | *MTTK, MTTL1, MTTH, MTTS1, MTTS2, MTTF, MTND5* | MERRF is characterized by myoclonic seizures, proximal myopathy, ataxia, and cognitive decline. Other common findings include cardiomyopathy, Wolff-Parkinson-White (WPW) syndrome, optic atrophy, hearing loss, and short stature. Multiple symmetrical lipomatosis (Madelung disease) has been described in some patients. |
| NARP | *MTATP6* | The cardinal features of NARP are sensory motor neuropathy, cerebellar ataxia, and retinitis pigmentosa. Other common findings include dementia, seizures, proximal muscle weakness, and hearing loss. Usually there is no histologic evidence of mitochondrial myopathy. |
| LHON | *MTND1, MTND4, MTND6* | LHON is characterized by bilateral painless visual loss and usually presents in young adults. Males are approximately four times more likely to be affected. Other features include cardiac arrhythmias, myopathy, peripheral neuropathy, dystonia and WPW syndrome. A minority of female LHON carriers develop clinical and neuroimaging features indistinguishable from multiple sclerosis. |
| MIDD | *MTTL1, MTTE, MTTK* | Hearing loss develops in early adulthood and frequently precedes the diagnosis of diabetes. Other features include basal ganglia calcification, cerebral or cerebellar atrophy, visual loss and night blindness, proximal myopathy, left ventricular hypertrophy, WPW syndrome, atrial fibrillation, and short stature. Patients may also develop end-stage renal disease which may precede the diagnosis of diabetes or deafness. Men are more commonly affected. |
| Progressive external ophthalmoplegia (PEO) | Multiple mtDNA deletions; nuclear: *POLG, C10orf2, SLC25A4, OPA1* | PEO is characterized by ptosis, paralysis of the extraocular muscles (ophthalmoplegia), and proximal limb weakness. Patients usually experience bilateral, symmetrical, progressive ptosis, followed by ophthalmoparesis. Additional symptoms are variable, and may include cataracts, hearing loss, sensory axonal neuropathy, ataxia, depression, hypogonadism, and parkinsonism. Both autosomal dominant and autosomal recessive inheritance can occur. |
| Kearns-Sayre syndrome | mtDNA deletion | Kearns-Sayre syndrome consists of ophthalmoparesis, pigmentary retinopathy and onset before 20 years. Other clinical features include sensorineural hearing loss, renal tubular acidosis, cardiac conduction blocks, cerebellar ataxia, proximal myopathy, and short stature. Patients often have multiple endocrinopathies including diabetes mellitus, hypoparathyroidism, and Addison disease. Cerebrospinal fluid (CSF), protein of greater than 100 mg/dL is frequently seen. |
| Sensory ataxic neuropathy, dysarthria, and ophthalmoparesis (SANDO) | POLG | An autosomal recessive systemic disorder resulting from mitochondrial DNA depletion which is characterized by adult onset of sensory ataxic neuropathy, dysarthria, and ophthalmoparesis. Other clinical features include myopathy, seizures, hearing loss, gastroparesis, cardiomyopathy, migraines, and depression. |
| MNGIE | *TYMP* | Clinical features include nausea, early satiety, episodic abdominal pain, diarrhea, gastroesophageal reflux, postprandial emesis, progressive gastrointestinal dysmotility, dysphagia, and progressive cachexia. Other features include ophthalmoparesis, hearing loss, peripheral neuropathy, and distal muscle weakness. |

☞GASTROINTESTINAL: Progressive GI dysmotility is very commonly seen in mitochondrial disease patients. Patients frequently complain of abdominal pain, bloating, early satiety, nausea, dysphagia, postprandial emesis, and diarrhea. Chronic GI dysmotility causes cachexia, and many patients require feeding tubes or parenteral nutrition.

☞HEARING: Bilateral sensorineural hearing loss occurs both in syndromic and nonsyndromic presentations. Some patients with mitochondrial disease have hearing loss as their initial presenting symptom. Nonsyndromic sudden hearing loss in mitochondrial patients can occur days to weeks after receiving aminoglycoside antibiotics. This type of hearing loss is exposure and not dose related.

### Diagnostic evaluation of patient with mitochondrial disease

- Supporting evidence for the diagnosis of mitochondrial disease can be obtained by measuring serum lactate and alanine CSF lactate, creatine phosphokinase (CPK), ammonia, plasma carnitine, and acyl carnitine profile, and urinary organic acids.
- Neurologic evaluation of mitochondrial disease may include lumbar puncture for CSF analysis and lactate level, an electroencephalogram (EEG) to evaluate for seizures, computed tomography (CT) scan to look for basal ganglia calcification, and brain MRI and MR spectroscopy to look for strokes and increased lactate levels, respectively.
- Muscle biopsy should be considered in all patients suspected of having mitochondrial disease. Significant findings on light microscopy include ragged red fibers and altered SDH and COX histochemical staining. Significant mitochondrial electron microscopic findings include subsarcolemmal accumulation, large dysmorphic mitochondria, and paracrystalline inclusions.
- Respiratory chain (ETC) enzyme activity can help differentiate between isolated defects in individual complexes from multicomplex deficiencies. This information will help determine target genes for molecular genetic testing.
- Molecular genetic testing may include mtDNA sequencing to look for mutations, southern hybridization to look for deletions or rearrangements, qPCR for mtDNA depletion, and sequencing of specific nuclear genes.

### Diagnostic algorithm

- If the patient presents with classic syndromic features or has a typical family history of maternal inheritance, the clinician should proceed directly with molecular genetic testing. See Table 166-2.
- When the clinical picture is highly suggestive but is not a typical syndromic presentation, further studies are recommended before proceeding to molecular testing. These may include lactate levels (plasma or CSF), plasma carnitine and acylcarnitine profile, organic acid profile, MRI and MR spectroscopy, and muscle biopsy for light microscopy, histochemistry, electron microscopy, and respiratory chain function studies.

## Screening and Counseling

*Screening:*
- Abnormal cardiopulmonary exercise-testing may identify patients with mitochondrial diseases. Common findings include

reduction of forced vital capacity (FVC), maximum minute ventilation, and maximal oxygen consumption (decreases VO$_2$ max).
- Plasma lactate can be increased in mitochondrial disease, particularly when metabolically stressed. Any patient with unexplained lactic acidosis should be evaluated for mitochondrial disease.

*Counseling:* mtDNA point mutations, deletions, or duplications can be sporadic or inherited through the maternal line. The father of a proband is not at risk while the mother could carry the mitochondrial mutation. The risk to the siblings depends on the genetic status of the mother. Disease penetrance and expressivity within the same family varies greatly due to heteroplasmy and threshold effects. mtDNA deletions generally occurs de novo and thus there is no significant risk to other family members.

Mutations of the nuclear DNA could occur de novo or be inherited in autosomal dominant, autosomal recessive, or X-linked patterns. Identification of dominant mutations is sometimes difficult due to varied penetrance and expressivity of these mutations, that is, one of the parents may carry the same mutation but may not have the disease symptoms.

## Management and Treatment

*Screening:*
- Cardiac conduction defects and cardiomyopathy are commonly seen in mitochondrial diseases. ECG and echocardiographic evaluation should be done to identify appropriate patients for pacemaker and automatic implantable cardioverter defibrillators (AICD) placement.
- As both hearing and vision are commonly affected, regular hearing and vision testing is important in early identification of dysfunction.
- Seizures should be treated and valproic acid should be avoided as it interferes with mitochondrial function.
- GI dysfunction is common and can lead to malnutrition and cachexia. Periodic nutritional assessment will help identify patients needing nutritional support such as percutaneous endoscopic gastrostomy (PEG) tube feeding and parenteral nutrition.
- Screening for endocrinopathies, particularly diabetes mellitus should be routinely done. Metformin should be avoided in these patients due to the risk of lactic acidosis.
- Respiratory muscle weakness and failure are known to occur in late-stage disease and regular spirometric evaluation will identify patients who would need respiratory support.
- Bulbar muscle weakness is seen in advanced stages and could cause sleep apnea and aspiration pneumonia. Sleep and swallowing studies should be considered in patients suspected with bulbar muscle weakness.

*Treatment:*
- The mainstay of management of mitochondrial disease consists of symptom management and avoidance of metabolic stresses by ensuring adequate rest, avoiding dehydration or prolonged fasting, and promptly treating infections.
- CoQ10 and its analogs (ubiquinone and idebenone) are currently in clinical trials for the treatment of mitochondrial disorders.
- L-arginine has shown promising results in the treatment and prevention of stroke-like episodes in patients with MELAS.

*Table 166-2* **Diagnostic Algorithm and Recommended Testing**

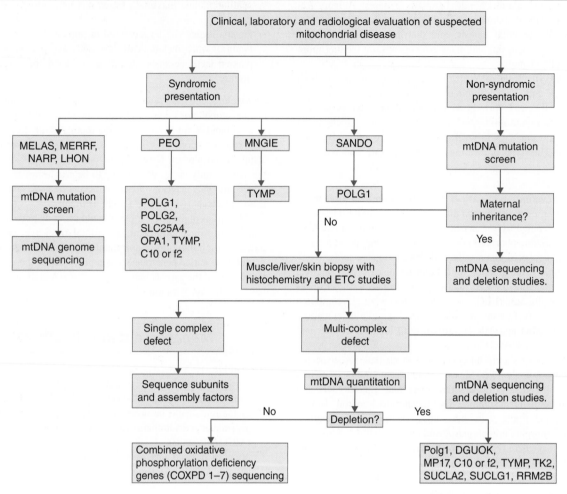

- Low aerobic conditioning exercise training can improve functional capacity in patients with mitochondrial myopathy.

*Management:*

- Patients with mitochondrial disease do not tolerate prolonged fasting. To avoid metabolic crisis an intravenous (IV) dextrose infusion should be initiated in any patient who may need to fast for a procedure. Lactated Ringer solution should be avoided as an IV fluid, as it contains lactic acid.
- Valproate should be avoided as it is a mitochondrial poison and can trigger a metabolic crisis.

# Molecular Genetics and Molecular Mechanism

The mitochondrial respiratory chain (ETC) consists of five enzyme complexes located on the inner mitochondrial membrane whose function is to produce ATP. Unique to the ETC, its component proteins are encoded by two genomes, nDNA and mtDNA. The nuclear genome encodes the majority of ETC subunits, assembly factors of the ETC, and genes involved in the maintenance and replication of the mitochondria and its genome. Mutations

of the subunits or assembly factors of the ETC result in isolated deficiency of a complex, while mutations in nucleotide transport and DNA repair mechanisms can result in multiunit dysfunction. Human mtDNA is a 16.6-kb circular, double-stranded molecule, which contains 37 genes: 2 rRNA genes, 22 tRNA genes, and 13 structural genes encoding subunits of the mitochondrial respiratory chain. Each cell contains hundreds or thousands of mtDNA copies, which at cell division distribute randomly among daughter cells. Deleterious mutations of mtDNA usually affect some but not all mtDNAs (heteroplasmy), and the clinical expression of a pathogenic mtDNA mutation is determined largely by the relative proportions of normal and mutant genomes in different tissues. Thus, a variety of molecular mechanisms are involved in mitochondrial respiratory chain disorders. While the cellular mechanism of toxicity is not known, energy deficiency is thought to play a major role.

*Genetic Testing:* It is often difficult to achieve a definite molecular diagnosis when the etiologic locus is in the nDNA. Many of the nuclear genes are yet to be identified and clinical testing is available for only a few genes. Testing of the mitochondrial genome can be done by testing for specific mutations, sequencing the entire mitochondrial genome, Southern blot to evaluate for deletions and duplication, and qPCR to assess for mtDNA depletion (http://www.ncbi.nlm.nih.gov/sites/GeneTests/lab/clinical_disease_id/ 2516?db=genetests).

## BIBLIOGRAPHY:

1. Finsterer J, Eichberger H. Phenotype variability in 130 adult patients with respiratory chain disorders. *J Inherit Metab Dis.* 2001;24(5):560-576.

2. Kovács GG, Jakab G. Neuropathology of white matter disease in Leber's hereditary optic neuropathy. *Brain.* 2005;128(pt 1):35-41.

3. Murphy R, Hattersley AT. Clinical features, diagnosis and management of maternally inherited diabetes and deafness (MIDD) associated with the 3243A>G mitochondrial point mutation. *Diabet Med.* 2008;25(4):383-399.

4. Walker UA, Byrne E. Respiratory chain encephalomyopathies: a diagnostic classification. *Eur Neurol.* 1996;36(5):260-267.

5. Bernier FP, Thorburn DR. Diagnostic criteria for respiratory chain disorders in adults and children. *Neurology.* 2002;59(9):1406-1411.

6. Morava E, Smeitink JA. Mitochondrial disease criteria: diagnostic applications in children. *Neurology.* 2006;67(10):1823-1826.

7. Parikh S. The neurologic manifestations of mitochondrial disease. *Dev Disabil Res Rev.* 2010;16(2):120-128.

8. Limongelli G, Elliott PM. Prevalence and natural history of heart disease in adults with primary mitochondrial respiratory chain disease. *Eur J Heart Fail.* 2010;12(2):114-121.

9. Chinnery PF, Griffiths TD. The spectrum of hearing loss due to mitochondrial DNA defects. *Brain.* 2000;123 (pt 1):82-92.

10. Clay AS, Brown KK. Mitochondrial disease: a pulmonary and critical-care medicine perspective. *Chest.* 2001;120(2):634-648.

11. Patrick F Chinnery. Mitochondrial Disorders Overview. GeneReviews—NCBI Bookshelf.

12. Cope land WC. Inherited mitochondrial diseases of DNA replication. *Annu Rev Med.* 2008;59:131-146.

## Supplementary Information

### OMIM REFERENCES:

[1] MELAS (#540000)

[2] MERR (#545000)

[3] NARP (#551500)

[4] LHON (#535000)

[5] PEO (#157640)

[6] Kearns-Sayre (#530000)

[7] MNGIE (#603041)

[8] MIDD (#520000)

[9] Leigh Syndrome (#256000)

[10] Complex I Deficiency (#252010)

[11] Complex II Deficiency (#252011)

[12] Complex III Deficiency (#124000)

[13] Complex IV Deficiency (#220110)

[14] Complex V Deficiency (#604273)

***Key Words:*** Lactic acidosis, cardiomyopathy, myopathy, retinopathy, ophthalmoplegia, WPW syndrome, stroke, myoclonus, optic atrophy, GI dysmotility, cachexia, autonomic neuropathy, deafness

# 167 Chromosomal Disorders in Adults

Leslie Manace-Brenman. Lisa Edelmann, and Ethylin Wang Jabs

## KEY POINTS

- *Disease summary:*
  - Cytogenetics is the study of chromosome structure, function, and disorders by combining cytology (the study of cells) with clinical genetics (the study of inherited variation). The normal diploid complement of chromosomes consists of 46 chromosomes: 22 pairs of numbered autosomal chromosomes and one pair of lettered sex chromosomes (X and Y) (Fig. 167-1). One haploid complement is composed of 23 chromosomes, inherited from the mother in the egg or the father in the sperm. A complete diploid set of 46 chromosomes is present in the zygote, and upon replication, they are present in every cell nucleus of the offspring. A normal chromosome complement (or karyotype) is designated as 46,XX for females and 46,XY for males. Chromosomes each have a short arm (p) and a long arm (q). Chromosome regions as well as gene locations are annotated as the chromosome number followed by "p" or "q" (for the short or long arm, respectively) followed by the band number (organized by the banding pattern chromosomes uniformly display on in vitro staining). During metaphase the region between the p and q arms is condensed and constricted and is designated the centromeric region where the spindle apparatus is attached. Some chromosomes such as chromosome 1, 6, 7, 11, 14, 15, 18, 19, and 20 contain regions that are differentially methylated, or "imprinted," based on the parent of origin; imprinted portions of chromosomes are transcriptionally silenced, meaning genes in those segments are not translated to protein. The term *chromosome disorder* refers to a clinical condition secondary to an abnormality in the quantity, content, and/or arrangement of the 23 pairs of chromosomes comprised of the nuclear genomic DNA.

- *Chromosomal abnormalities (see Table 167-1):*
  - *Aneuploidy*, alteration in the total number of chromosomes, such as trisomy and monosomy
  - *Euploidy*, a multiple of the normal number of chromosomes, 46 (eg, 69,XXX or 92,XXXX, which are embryonic lethal)
  - *Deletion*, loss of a portion of a chromosome (eg, DiGeorge or velocardiofacial syndrome due to deletion of 22q11.2, or chromosome 22, q arm region, band 11.2 [designated "one one point two"])
  - *Duplication*, gain of a portion of a chromosome (eg, Charcot-Marie-Tooth type 1 due to duplication of the *PMP22* gene in chromosome17p12)
  - *Insertion*, gain of a portion of a chromosome
  - *Pericentric inversion*, inversion of a portion of a chromosome including the centromeric region
  - *Paracentric inversion*, inversion of a portion of a chromosome arm not including the centromeric region
  - *Robertsonian translocation*, fusion of two acrocentric chromosomes 13, 14, 15, 21, or 22 (chromosomes with a very small p arm) with breakpoints at or near the centromere with loss of repeated DNA sequences from the short p arms that usually is without clinical consequence. A karyotype with a robertsonian translocation has a total of 45 chromosomes.
  - *Reciprocal translocation*, rearrangement of portions of two different chromosomes formed by the reciprocal exchange between portions from autosomal or sex chromosomes (Fig. 167-2)
  - *Isochromosome*, abnormal arrangement of chromosome arms with either fusion of two p arms separated by a centromere without a q arm or fusion of two q arms separated by a centromere without a p arm forming a chromosome
  - *Ring chromosome*, abnormal arrangement of a chromosome with breakage and fusion in the p arm and q arm to form a ring
  - *Uniparental disomy*, inheritance of both maternal and paternal copies of the same chromosome, instead of the normal inheritance of one maternal and one paternal chromosome forming a complementary pair. This may result in an abnormal phenotype or a particular syndrome if the chromosome involved is imprinted (eg, Prader-Willi syndrome due to maternal uniparental disomy of chromosome 15)
  - *Trinucleotide repeat* expans*ion*, a sequence of three nucleotides that may not cause symptoms in the "premutation or carrier" status, but may expand in number of repeats during gametogenesis and lead to disease in an offspring
  - *Other variant chromosomes*, telomeric fusions and complex rearrangements

- *Chromosome disorders*
  - These are either present from embryogenesis and are constitutionally present in the individual (germline) or develop over time as a result of DNA replication errors and dysfunctional DNA repair (somatic); the latter are important in cancer biology.
  - Constitutional chromosome abnormalities that may not be detected until adulthood are usually rearrangements in which no significant DNA material is lost or gained. These alterations are termed balanced, and usually do not result in phenotypic abnormality unless a gene is interrupted in the breakpoints of the rearrangement, or regulatory elements for a gene are disturbed (positional effect).
  - Cancer chromosomal abnormalities include hundreds of different mutations, many of which are recurrent aneuploidies and reciprocal translocations. Chromosome mutations that accumulate in cancer are acquired, somatic genetic changes that generally interrupt or activate oncogenic or tumor suppressor loci.
  - Certain translocations carry prognostic import for responsiveness to therapy, rate of recurrences, and survival, particularly in hematologic malignancies.
  - Certain chromosomes have fragile sites prone to an abnormal thin or stretched appearance when grown in folate-deficient media that may be correlated with clinical syndromes depending on the chromosome location. Common fragile sites that are inherited or of unknown clinical significance can be induced with aphidicolin or 5-azacytidine.

- Chromosome breakage syndromes demonstrate chromosome fragility and structural abnormalities on chromosome analysis and are often diagnosed in childhood due to heightened cancer disposition and immune malfunction.
- Mosaicism refers to the existence of more than one distinct chromosomal constitution within cells of one or multiple tissue types.
- All females are mosaic with two different cell types because one X chromosome (maternally or paternally derived) is actively transcribed and the other X is randomly inactivated (or lyonized) forming a Barr body. Inactivation is propagated along the inactive X chromosome by the expression of *Xist* RNA from the inactive X, followed by chromatin condensation and methylation.
- A chromosomal abnormality may be found as a tissue-limited mosaic line and result in mild or no features of the full chromosomal disorder (eg, trisomy 21 may be found in certain tissues and not others, resulting in a mild or no features of Down syndrome; or mosaicism for X chromosome rearrangements with interruption of genes in particular chromosome locations, or loci, resulting in the neurocutaneous syndrome, hypomelanosis of Ito).
- *Technology* to analyze chromosomes has evolved from gross examination of metaphase chromosomes (karyotype) at a resolution from about 5 Mb (million DNA base pairs) to a submicroscopic resolution of about 50 to 200 kb using fluorescently labeled probes for specific chromosome regions, fluorescent in situ hybridization (FISH), and whole genome dosage examination at a resolution of at least 10 kb using array comparative genomic hybridization (array CGH, or microarray). Array resolution depends on the density of probes (either single-nucleotide polymorphisms, SNPs, or stretches of DNA, known as oligonucleoties) tiled along the microarray chip.
- Microdeletions and microduplications comprise a set of well-characterized syndromes due to deletion or duplication of a chromosomal segment or region and thereby haploinsufficiency or triplosufficiency for the dosage-sensitive genes in that locus. Many are recurrent at a predictable rate in the population, and are caused by aberrant recombination between repeated sequences or nonallelic homologous recombination.
- Copy number variants (CNVs) are the most common type of structural variation in the human genome, representing regions of chromosomes that are deleted or duplicated. Some CNVs are de novo (arised during gametogenesis or embryogenesis and present newly in offspring) and may be associated with clinical significance, whereas others may be inherited usually with no phenotypic consequences.

- *Medical history:*
  - Chromosomal disorders that come to clinical attention in adults are often detected during workup for pubertal delay, reproductive problems, abnormalities in an offspring, or cancer
  - Primary amenorrhea in a female
  - Oligospermic or nonobstructive azoospermic infertility (failure to conceive regardless of age after 1 year of unprotected intercourse) in a male
  - Infertility in a female (failure to conceive regardless of age after 1 year of unprotected intercourse)
  - Recurrent miscarriage (three or more consecutive spontaneous abortions)
  - Chromosomal disorder detected in a child (usually on workup for multiple congenital anomalies and developmental delay)
  - Balanced translocation (with no DNA lost or gained) carriers are at risk to pass on an unbalanced derivative chromosome leading to an abnormal phenotype in an offspring inheriting what appears as grossly the same translocation (imbalance detected on karyotype or higher-resolution analysis, such as array CGH)
  - Hematologic malignancy, Wilms tumor

- *Family history:*
  - Recurrent miscarriage
  - Two or more first- (children, siblings, parents) or second-degree relatives (grandparents, aunts, uncles) with multiple congenital anomalies and mental retardation
  - Multiple cases of cancer at young ages of diagnosis and/or immunologic defects

- *Differential diagnosis:*
  - Other causes of delayed puberty include endocrine disorders.
  - Other causes of female infertility include endocrine disorders, gynecologic factors, metabolic diseases, infectious etiologies.
  - Other causes of male infertility include cystic fibrosis mutation.

- *Pharmacogenomics:*
  - Use of imatinib mesylate (Gleevec) for chronic myelogenous leukemia is based on the presence of the Philadelphia chromosome translocation (between chromosomes 9 and 22) and a hyperactive bcr-abl protein. The drug inhibits the chimeric protein in cancerous cells.

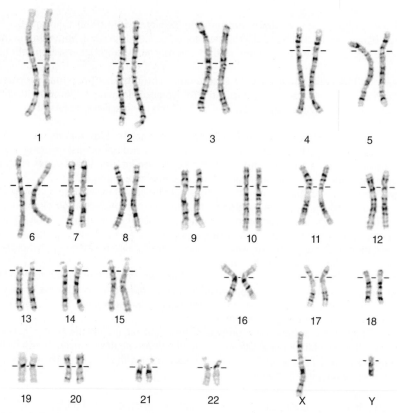

**Figure 167-1** Normal Male G-Banded Karyotype at 650 Band Resolution.

**Table 167-1** **Common Chromosome Disorders Frequency and Clinical Consequence**

| Chromosome Disorders | Abnormality | Population Frequency | Penetrance | Risk of Abnormal Offspring | Associated Phenotypes |
|---|---|---|---|---|---|
| Sex chromosome aneuploidy | Abnormal number of sex chromosomes | 1/1000 | Variable | Adult is often infertile | Delayed or absent puberty, hypogonadism, infertility |
| Balanced translocation | Reciprocal or robertsonian translocation | 1/500 | Variable | 1%-15% for affected offspring, empiric risk | Usually none; infertility, recurrent miscarriage, depending on chromosome breakpoints |
| 22q.11.2 microdeletion | Loss of a small segment of one chromosome arm | 1/2000 to 1/4000 | Complete penetrance with variable expressivity | 50% for affected offspring | Palatal abnormalities, congenital heart defect, immune deficiency, learning disability |
| Pericentric inversion | Rearrangement of chromosome material including the centromeric region | 1/150 to 1/800 | May be a benign population variant or a unique rearrangement | None | Usually of no clinical consequence or in some cases reproductive loss or infertility |
| Somatic t(9;22) | Balanced reciprocal translocation | 95% of chronic myeloid leukemia cases | Complete | None | Chronic myeloid leukemia, acute lymphoblastic leukemia |

Before translocation                After translocation

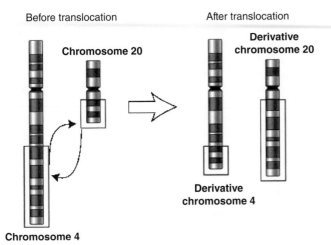

*Figure 167-2* Reciprocal, Balanced Translocation Diagram. National Genome Research Institute.

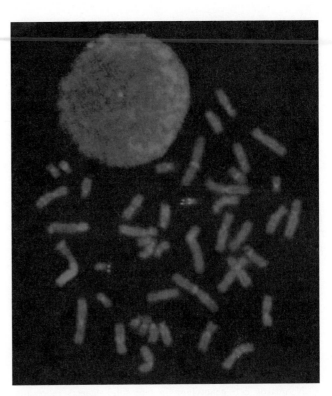

*Figure 167-3* 22q11.2 deletion FISH, loss of signal from one copy of chromosome 22

## Diagnostic Criteria and Clinical Characteristics

### Diagnostic Indications for Chromosome Analysis:

- Primary amenorrhea in females defined as the absence of menstrual bleeding
- Delayed puberty or hypogonadism in males
- Infertility defined as failure to conceive after 1 year of unprotected intercourse
- Recurrent miscarriage defined as three or more pregnancy losses
- Mental retardation in a male or female
- Congenital malformations including cardiac, cerebral, and renal anomalies, particularly in the setting of mental retardation
- Cancer subtyping and prognostic evaluation

### And the absence of

- Endocrine, gynecologic, or other etiology of primary amenorrhea or delayed puberty
- Gynecologic, metabolic, infectious, or other etiology in the cases of infertility

### Diagnostic Evaluation:

- High-resolution chromosome analysis generally for suspected aneuploidy or balanced rearrangement as in cases of recurrent miscarriages
- Array CGH analysis generally for cases of mental retardation and/or congenital malformations
  - Identification of CNV
  - Detection of microdeletions and microduplications
  - Cannot detect balanced rearrangements
- FISH analysis generally for rapid aneuploidy screening or targeted assay for a suspected syndrome as in the case of 22q11.2 deletion in DiGeorge or velocardiofacial syndrome (Fig. 167-3)
  - Detection of dosage abnormalities (deletions or duplications)
  - Identification of chromosomes involved in a rearrangement or derivative structure

### Clinical Findings:

- No clinical signs or symptoms may be found for some chromosome disorders outlined earlier such as in the case of balanced translocations and mosaicism.
- Normal phenotypes have been documented for maternal or paternal uniparental disomy (UPD) of chromosomes 13, 21, and 22.
- Sex chromosome disorders are the most common chromosomal abnormalities and generally present with learning disability, pubertal delay or absence, or infertility.
- Sex reversal and hermaphroditism in 46,XY is due to deletions or translocations involving the segment of the Y chromosome containing the sex-determining region Y (*SRY*) gene at Yp11.3, and in 46,XX males if there is translocation of the SRY-containing region to the X chromosome.
- Primary or secondary amenorrhea: 45,X (Turner syndrome), structural X aberrations, mosaicism with X abnormalities.
- Infertility in a female: 47,XXX, balanced autosomal rearrangement.
- Infertility in a male: sex chromosome disorder including 47,XXY, structural Y aberrations, Y-autosomal translocation, and robertsonian translocations especially der(13;14)(q10;q10).
- Aspermic males have the highest rate of chromosome disorder at 15%.
- Recurrent miscarriage (one parent carries a balanced translocation in 3%-30% of couples with a history of three or more spontaneous abortions)
- Family history of multiple cases of Down syndrome not associated with advanced maternal age
- Most familial Down syndrome is due to robertsonian translocation involving chromosomes 14 and 21, der(14;21)(q10;q10).

- Relatively common, recurrent interstitial microdeletion 22q11.2 deletion, or DiGeorge/velocardiofacial, syndrome may not cause major malformation and thus go unnoticed or incidentally detected on workup for learning disability or psychiatric disorder.
- Congenital defects including cardiac, cerebral, and renal malformation.
- Familial cancer syndrome in which a point mutation in the associated tumor suppressor gene or oncogene is not identified.
- In cancers, a chromosomal disruption of the tumor suppressor gene or oncogene by reciprocal translocation or other aberration acts as the "first hit," followed by somatic mutation of the other tumor suppressor gene or oncogene allele as the "second hit" allowing cancer development.
- Constitutional reciprocal translocations t(5;10)(q22;q25) and t(5;8)(q22;p23.1) (designating the chromosomes involved in the rearrangement, 5 and 10 in the former and 5 and 8 in the latter, and the breakpoints along the chromosome arms) have been detected that disrupt the *APC* gene at the 5q22 breakpoint causing familial adenomatous polyposis.
- Retinoblastoma is rarely caused by constitutional del(13)(q14) (interstitial deletion of the long arm of chromosome 13).
- Translocations involving the *VHL* locus on chromosome 3p25.3 lead to clear-cell renal carcinoma.
- Neoplastic cell genotyping in rare solid cancers (adenomatous polyposis, juvenile polyposis, Gorlin syndrome basal cell carcinoma, retinoblastoma, Wilms tumor) and hematologic malignancies.

## Screening and Counseling

### Screening:

- Approximately 1 in 500 people in the general population is a reciprocal translocation carrier, which may have arisen de novo in the individual, or be inherited and present in other members of the family.
- See section Diagnostic Indications for Chromosomal Analysis.

### Counseling:

☞INHERITANCE:

- Carriers for a microdeletion, duplication, or other chromosome dosage abnormalities have a 50% risk of passing the change on to offspring, unless the abnormality is found in a male and involves the X chromosome, for which a patient is at 100% risk for passing the altered chromosome X to 46,XX daughters and 0% to 46,XY sons.
- Unaffected, balanced reciprocal translocation carriers are at risk for abnormal offspring due to malsegregation of the translocated chromosomes during meiosis which leads to partial monosomy and partial trisomy.
- There are different risks for abnormal offspring in translocation carriers depending on sex and chromosomes involved (for those who carry a chromosome 21 robertsonian translocation, a female carrier is at 15% risk for a fetus with translocation trisomy 21, while a male carrier is at 1% risk, likely due to reduced viability of sperm with unbalanced quantity of chromosome 21).
- Aneuploidy may be due to parental germline nondisjunction of chromosomes during meiosis, or somatic nondisjunction and not in the germline (particularly in mosaic autosomal trisomies).

- Trisomy represents the most common abnormality encountered in spontaneous abortion.
- Vast majority of trisomies are maternal in origin as a result of meiosis I error during egg gametogenesis, and the risk increases exponentially with maternal age.
- Predisposition to nondisjunction is rarely a familial, inherited trait.
- Chromosome disorders found in tumors due to somatic mutation are not heritable; only if the aberration is present constitutionally and in the patient's germline (egg or sperm cells) would there be a risk of inheritance for offspring, as in the case of constitutional reciprocal translocations leading to cancer predisposition syndromes.

☞PENETRANCE/GENOTYPE-PHENOTYPE CORRELATION:

- Phenotype associated with a chromosome disorder is correlated with the extent of DNA dosage, gene coding sequence, or gene regulatory region disruption.
- Chromosome aberrations that come to clinical significance in adulthood, usually display variable penetrance (evidence of any clinical abnormality) and expressivity (extent and nature of involvement of organ systems) among carriers.
- Monosomy and/or deletion is generally more severe phenotypically than trisomy and/or duplication.
- Mosaic aneuploidies display extremely variable penetrance and expressivity, and may go undetected.

## Management and Treatment

**Management:** Patients have a wide range of clinical symptoms from chromosomal abnormalities. They usually have more severe and multiple organ involvement and learning disabilities with larger deletions or duplications. Treatment is dependent on the unique features of each chromosome condition and may require a multidisciplinary approach.

☞PHARMACOGENETICS: Therapy selection and adjustment with imatinib (Gleevec) and dasatinib (Sprycel) is determined by the presence and proportion of the reciprocal translocation t(9;22)(q34;q11), known as the Philadelphia chromosome that creates a fusion of the *BCR* and *ABL* genes, present in chronic myeloid leukemia and acute lymphoblastic leukemia.

## Molecular Genetics and Molecular Mechanism

### Genetic Testing:

Clinical availability of testing

- Chromosome analysis, which will detect rearrangements of material greater than 5 Mb in size and all of the structural abnormalities detailed under the Summary section, is readily available through cytogenetic laboratories in any major medical institution or commercial laboratories.
- Further characterization of breakpoints and loss or gain of genetic material may be indicated and often accomplished with array CGH; array CGH analysis is available in more specialized molecular genetics and cytogenetic laboratories.

Clinical utility of testing

- Chromosome analysis by tradition cytogenetic of CGH analysis is a cost-effective test in couples with infertility or recurrent miscarriages, obviating the need for a protracted multidisciplinary workup and providing critical information for risk estimation of genetic abnormalities in offspring.

### *Future Directions:*

- Rapidly expanding whole genome sequencing data across multiple populations is detecting large numbers of interindividual structural aberrations notably CNVs that are now being studied and classified for their impact on complex phenotypes.
- Cancer genotyping continues to elucidate chromosome aberrations that contribute to neoplastic transformation, and with increasingly rapid and decreasingly costly whole genome analysis, large sets of tumor genotype data will aid in determining which chromosome abnormalities are related to pathogenesis and which incidentally accumulate in cancer progression.

### BIBLIOGRAPHY:

1. Gardner RJM, Sutherland GR. *Chromosome Abnormalities and Genetic Counseling*. 3rd ed. Oxford: 2004:59-360.
2. Rimoin DL, Connor JM, Pyeritz, et al., eds. *Emery and Rimoin's Principles and Practice of Medical Genetics*. 4th ed. 2002:1166.
3. Schinzel A. *Catalogue of Unbalanced Chromosome Aberrations in Man*. 2nd ed. New York, NY: Walter de Gruyter; 2001:23-24.
4. Eeles RA, Easton DF, Ponder BAJ, et al., eds. *Genetic Predisposition to Cancer*. 2nd ed. London, UK: Arnold; 2004:136-137.
5. Gersen SL, Keagle MB, eds. *The Principles of Clinical Cytogenetics*. 2nd ed. New Jersey, NY: Humana Press; 2005:327-328.
6. Pinto D, Marshall C, Feuk L, et al. Copy-number variation in control population cohorts. *Hum Mol Genet*. 2007;16 Spec No. 2: R168-R173.
7. Mardis ER, Ding L, Dooling DJ, et al. Recurring mutations found by sequencing an acute myeloid leukemia genome. *N Engl J Med*. 2009;361(11):1058-1066.

## Supplementary Information

### OMIM REFERENCES:

[1] 46,XX Gonadal Dysgenesis, Complete, SRY-Positive; SRY (#400045)

[2] Leukemia, Chronic Myeloid; CML, BCR (#608232)

### Alternative Names:

- Aneuploidy
- Chromosome Rearrangement
- Chromosome Translocation
- Genomic Structural Variation
- Genomic Dosage Aberration

***Key Words:*** Cytogenetics, aneuploidy, derivative chromosome, inversion, rearrangement, reciprocal translocation, robertsonian translocation, carrier, mosaicism

# 168 Hereditary Disorders of Connective Tissue

Maureen Murphy-Ryan and Noralane Lindor

## KEY POINTS

- *Disease summary:*
  - Hereditary disorders of connective tissue (HDCT) are a group of disorders in which genetic errors affect the proper formation of connective tissue, the intercellular material that holds human tissues together.
  - Connective tissue is a complex network of substances (including collagen, elastin, fibrillin, fibulin, and many others) produced by fibroblast cells. The specific combination and proportion of these elements differs from one tissue to another to create diverse mechanical properties and functions within the human body.
  - There is extensive overlap both clinically and genetically between the HDCT. A single gene can affect the connective tissue of multiple organ systems (pleiotropy). The clinical features often overlap with other connective disorders caused by mutations in different genes. Furthermore, a single gene may be linked to multiple distinct disorders based on the mutation type and genetic environment.
  - The ability to differentiate between the 40+ known HDCT has the capacity to significantly alter patient care.
- *Hereditary basis:*
  - The hereditary basis of HDCT varies by disorder, and can include autosomal recessive, autosomal dominant, X-linked, and de novo mutations. Refer to Table 168-1 for syndrome- and gene-specific details.
  - *Differential diagnosis:* Many different clinical findings may spur consideration of an underlying HDCT. Some of the most common findings are joint laxity, skin hyper- or inelasticity, vascular aneurysms, hernias, long bone overgrowth, and ophthalmologic pathology. The differential diagnosis for a suspected HDCT is not easily summarized. The major entities and causative genes and inheritance patterns are summarized in Table 168-1.

## Diagnostic Criteria and Clinical Characteristics

*Clinical Characteristics:* These are outlined in Table 168-1.

## Screening and Counseling

*Screening:*

**Tests to be considered once a patient is suspected to have HDCT**
- **Ophthalmologic evaluation** to assess for abnormalities of the lens, retina, vitreous, and refraction.
- **Radiographic imaging** including echocardiography to measure the aortic root to check for dilatation and examine the aortic arch for abnormalities such as tortuosity.
- **Computed tomography (CT) or magnetic resonance (MR) angiogram** of the cerebral, neck, thoracic, abdominal, and pelvic arteries.
  - If abnormal limited CT or MR angiogram, assess all other major arteries if any abnormality consistent with a HDCT is identified.
- **Skeletal evaluation** including skeletal survey, bone densitometry.
- **Brain imaging** to identify any structural abnormalities if neurologic signs are present.

- **Audiologic assessment** for patients with a differential diagnosis including disorders with hearing loss.
- **Genetic testing** if the narrowed differential includes disorders whose causative genes have available clinical or research genetic testing that will confirm the diagnosis and/or guide treatment.

*Counseling:* When counseling patients and families with a clinically or genetically diagnosed HDCT, it is important to explain the principles of inheritance, penetrance, availability of genetic testing, significance of all possible testing results, and any knowledge about correlations between specific genotypes and phenotypes. Specific counseling guidance for the more common HDCT are included in this text, and further information about these or other HDCT can be found by searching OMIM and genetests.org.

## Management and Treatment

Refer to individual disease chapters for disease-specific details.

*Genetic Testing:* Genetic testing is taking an increasingly important role in diagnosing hereditary disorders of connective tissue and guiding management as disease-specific treatments become available. Clinical testing is available for nearly all of the genes shown in Table 168-1 and it is anticipated that this list will continue to grow. Regularly updated information on the availability of genetic testing for specific disorders can be found at genetests.org.

*Table 168-1* **Genetic Differential Diagnosis**

| Syndrome | Gene Symbol | Associated Findings[a] |
|---|---|---|
| Familial abdominal aortic aneurysms | *COL3A1* (AD), loci 19q13, 4q31, 9p21 | Abdominal aortic aneurysm |
| Arterial tortuosity syndrome | *SLC2A10* (AR) | Generalized tortuosity of the arterial bed including aorta, arterial stenosis, abdominal aortic aneurysm, aneurysm of medium-sized arteries, ascending aortic dilatation, macrocephaly, characteristic facies, high-arched palate, micrognathia, keratoconus, inguinal and diaphragmatic hernias, intestinal elongation, joint laxity, joint contractures, muscular hypotonia, hyperelastic skin |
| Bicuspid aortic valve with thoracic aortic aneurysms | *NOTCH1, KCNJ2*, others (AD) | Ascending aortic dilatation, bicuspid aortic valve, aortic valve calcification |
| Congenital contractural arachnodactyly | *FBN2* (AD), unknown locus heterogeneity | Ascending aortic dilatation, mitral valve prolapse, cranial abnormality, ear dysmorphism "crumpled" with folded upper helix, high-arched palate, retro/micrognathia, keratoconus, myopia, arachnodactyly, joint contractions of knees and ankles that may improve with age, flexion contractures of small digital joints, hip contractures, thumb adduction, clubfoot, paradoxical patellar laxity, pyeloureteral junction stenosis, "marfanoid habitus," motor developmental delay, muscular hypoplasia, osteopenia/osteoporosis/fractures, pectus deformities, scoliosis, protrusio acetabuli, striae |
| Cutis laxa | *ELN* (AD), *FBLN5* (AD, AR-type 1), *FBLN4* (AR-type 1), *ATP6V0A2* (AR-type 2), *P5CS* (AR-type 2), *PYCR1* (AR-type 2), *ATP7A* (X-linked) | **Generally:** loose, redundant, inelastic skin, ascending aortic dilatation, medium vessel aneurysms, arterial tortuosity, enlarged anterior fontanel, hernias, diverticula, lung abnormalities, visceral prolapse, joint laxity or contractures, motor development delay, muscular hypotonia, osteopenia/osteoporosis/fractures (bone fragility), intellectual impairment/developmental delay<br>**AD:** TAA, inguinal hernia, emphysema<br>**AR1:** infantile emphysema, supravalvular aortic stenosis<br>**AR2:** characteristic facies, variable CNS involvement, microcephaly, skin features attenuate with age, neurologic symptoms emerge or worsen with age, late closure of large anterior fontanel<br>**X-linked:** occipital bony abnormalities (bilateral, symmetric wedge-shaped bony outgrowths beside the foramen magnum at the site of muscle attachment), failure to thrive due to chronic diarrhea, malabsorption, congenital hydronephrosis or urethral and bladder diverticula. |
| Familial ectopia lentis | *ADAMTSL4* (AR), *FBN1* (AD), *LTBP-2* (AR), *TGFBR2* (AD) | Lens dislocation, secondary glaucoma, myopia, mild skeletal symptoms, mitral valve prolapse, nonprogressive aortic root |
| Ehlers-Danlos, arthrochalasia type | *COL1A1* (AD), *COL1A2* (AD) | Early-onset congenital hip dislocation, hernias, extreme joint laxity, osteopenia/osteoporosis/fractures, pectus deformities, scoliosis, short stature, mildly hyperelastic skin, frequent fractures |
| Ehlers-Danlos, cardiac valvular type | *COL2A1* (AR) | Mitral valve prolapse, hernias, joint laxity, atrophic scars/delayed wound healing, easy bruising, hyperelastic skin |
| Ehlers-Danlos, classical type | *COL5A1* (AD), *COL5A2* (AD), *COL1A1* (AD) | Ascending aortic dilatation, mitral valve prolapse, joint laxity, pectus deformities/scoliosis, atrophic scars/delayed wound healing, easy bruising, hyperelastic skin, skin that is smooth, velvety, thin, fragile, translucent, and/or atrophic with cigarette paper scarring, characteristic facies (epicanthic folds, excess eyelid skin, prematurely aged appearance) |
| Ehlers-Danlos, dermatosparaxis type | *ADAMTS2* (AD) | Enlarged anterior fontanel, delayed phenotype onset, characteristic facies (eyelid fullness, epicanthal folds, downslanting palpebral fissures), retro/micrognathia, hernias, hollow organ rupture, joint laxity, short stature, extreme skin fragility, dental abnormalities, blue sclera, easy bruising, hyperelastic skin |

*(Continued)*

*Table 168-1 **Genetic Differential Diagnosis** (Continued)*

| Syndrome | Gene Symbol | Associated Findings[a] |
|---|---|---|
| Ehlers-Danlos, kyphoscoliotic type | *PLOD1* (AR) | Ascending aortic dilatation, joint laxity, gross motor development delay, muscular hypotonia, generalized muscle weakness, pectus deformities/scoliosis, hyperelastic skin, "marfanoid" habitus, normal neuromuscular testing, deficient lysyl hydroxylase activity |
| Ehlers Danlos, musculocontractural type | *CHST14* (AD) | Distinctive craniofacial dysmorphism, congenital contractures of fingers, clubfeet, severe kyphoscoliosis, muscular hypotonia, thin and hyperextensible skin, easy bruising, atrophic scarring, wrinkled palms, joint laxity, ocular involvement (anterior chamber abnormality, blue sclera), large anterior fontanel with delayed closure, normal lysyl hydroxylase activity |
| Ehlers-Danlos, progeroid type | *B4GALT7* (AR) | Characteristic progeroid facies, joint laxity, osteopenia/osteoporosis/fractures, pectus deformities/scoliosis, short stature, intellectual impairment/developmental delay, atrophic scars/delayed wound healing, easy bruising, loose yet hyperelastic skin |
| Ehlers-Danlos, spondylocheiro dysplastic type | *SLC39A13* (AR) | Characteristic facies, joint laxity, "marfanoid" habitus, muscular hypotonia, osteopenia/osteoporosis/fractures, short stature, atrophic scars/delayed wound healing, easy bruising, hyperelastic skin, skin that is smooth, velvety, thin, fragile, translucent, and/or atrophic with cigarette paper scarring, skin that may appear prematurely aged over the hands and feet, slender and tapering fingers, small joint contractures, substantial thenar and hypothenar atrophy with resultant limited fine motor skills, postnatal growth retardation, blue sclera, distinctive waddling gait with knee and hip pain |
| Ehlers-Danlos, vascular type | *COL3A1* (AD, AR) | Abdominal aortic aneurysm, medium-sized artery aneurysm, characteristic facies, lung manifestations (hemoptysis, spontaneous pneumothorax, bullae, blebs), hollow organ rupture (intestines, uterus), limited joint laxity, joint contractions, atrophic scars/delayed wound healing, extremely easy bruising, limited skin hyperelasticity |
| Ehlers-Danlos-like syndrome, tenascin-X type | *TNXB* (AR) | Mitral valve prolapse, severe diverticular intestinal disease (pancolonic) prone to rupture, GI bleeding, rectal prolapse, lung manifestations (COPD), joint laxity, easy bruising, hyperelastic skin, polyneuropathy |
| Familial thoracic aortic aneurysm and/or dissection | *ACTA2* (AD), FAA locus11q23-q24 (AD), *FBN1* (AD), *MYH11* (AD), *TAAD1* locus 5q13-q14 (AD), *TGFBR1* (AD), *TGFBR2* (AD), *MYLK* (AD) | Abdominal aortic aneurysm, medium-sized vessel aneurysm, ascending aortic dilatation, arterial tortuosity, hernias, pectus deformities/scoliosis, histologic medial necrosis (Erdheim cystic medial necrosis)<br>**ACTA2**: patent ductus arteriosus, bicuspid aortic valve, livedo reticularis, iris flocculi may be present<br>**TGFBR**: skeletal connective tissue disorder features more likely |
| Homocystinuria | *CBS* (AR) | Vascular thrombosis, stroke, lens dislocation (most often downward), myopia, arachnodactyly, joint laxity, "marfanoid" habitus, osteopenia/osteoporosis/fractures, pectus deformities/scoliosis, significant intellectual impairment/developmental delay, seizures, psychiatric disorders, striae, generalized hypopigmentation, pancreatitis, malar flush, livedo reticularis |
| Loeys-Dietz syndrome (LDS), types 1 and 2 | *TGFBR1* (AD), *TGFBR2* (AD) | **Craniofacial features** are more prominent in **LDS type 1** including cranial abnormality, hypertelorism, and oral clefting.<br>Both types: abdominal aortic aneurysm, medium-sized vessel aneurysm, ascending aortic dilatation, arterial tortuosity, myopia, retinal detachment, strabismus/blue sclera, recurrent hernias, lung manifestations (pneumothorax), hollow organ rupture (spleen, bowel, uterus), arachnodactyly, joint laxity, "marfanoid" habitus, pectus deformities/scoliosis, dural ectasia. Vascular risks are significant and similar to Ehlers-Danlos syndrome (EDS) vascular type.<br>**Cutaneous features** are more prominent in **LDS type 2** including atrophic scars/delayed wound healing, easy bruising, and translucent/velvety skin. |

*(Continued)*

*Table 168-1* **Genetic Differential Diagnosis (Continued)**

| Syndrome | Gene Symbol | Associated Findings[a] |
|---|---|---|
| Marfan syndrome/ MASS phenotype | *FBN1* (AD) | Abdominal aortic aneurysm, medium-sized artery aneurysm, ascending aortic dilatation, mitral valve prolapse, cranial abnormality, characteristic facies, high-arched palate, retro/micrognathia, lens dislocation (most often upwards), myopia, retinal detachment, hernias, lung manifestations, arachnodactyly, joint laxity, joint contractures, "marfanoid" habitus, muscular hypoplasia, pectus deformities/scoliosis, protrusio acetabuli, dural ectasia, easy bruising, striae<br>**MASS phenotype**: attenuated phenotype that does not meet criteria for Marfan syndrome, with many features but the **absence** of progressive abdominal aortic or medium-sized artery aneurysms, lens dislocation, lung manifestations, muscular hypoplasia, dural ectasia |
| Mitral valve prolapse syndrome | *FBN1* (AD), 16p12.1-p11.2 (AD), 11p15.4 (AD), 13q31.3-q32.1 (AD) | Mitral valve prolapse, mild joint laxity, long limbs, chest pain, dyspnea, thoracic cage deformity (narrow A-P diameter), dysrhythmia |
| Persistent patent ductus arteriosus with familial thoracic aortic aneurysm | *MYH11* (AD) | Ascending aortic dilatation, patent ductus arteriosus, sometimes PDA or AAA may be isolated |
| Stickler syndrome | *COL2A1* (AD), *COL9A1* (AR), *COL9A2* (AR), *COL11A1* (AD), *COL11A2* (AD) | Mitral valve prolapse, midfacial hypoplasia, oral clefting, retro/micrognathia, myopia, retinal detachment, vitreous abnormalities, cataracts, glaucoma, mild spondyloepiphyseal dysplasia, joint laxity, pectus deformities/scoliosis, precocious osteoarthritis, protrusio acetabuli, sensorineural and/or conductive hearing loss |
| Weill-Marchesani syndrome | *ADAMTS10* (AR), *FBN1* (AD) | Lens dislocation, myopia, retinal detachment, vitreous abnormalities, shallow orbits, microspherophakia, brachydactyly, joint contractures, short stature, congenital cardiac anomalies (MVP, prolonged QT interval, pulmonary and aortic valve stenosis) |

[a]Each associated finding has been noted in patients with clinically and/or genetically confirmed disorder, but may not be present in every patient with that disorder. Individual diagnostic criteria can be used to evaluate the significance of the presence or absence of a given clinical feature for diagnostic purposes.

AD, autosomal dominant; AR, autosomal recessive.

Gene names: In order of appearance

*COL3A1*, collagen type III alpha-1; *SLC2A10*, solute carrier family 2 member 10; *NOTCH1*, notch 1; *KCNJ2*, potassium inwardly rectifying channel subfamily J member 2; *FBN2*, fibrillin 2; *ELN*, elastin; *FBLN5*, fibulin 5; *FBLN4*, fibulin 4; *ATP6V0A2*, ATPase H+ transporting lysosomal V0 subunit a2; *P5CS*, pyrroline-5-carboxylate synthetase; *PYCR1*, pyrroline-5-carboxylate reductase 1; *ATP7A*, ATPase Cu++ transporting alpha polypeptide; *ADAMTSL4*, ADAMTS (a disintegrin-like and metallopeptidase with thrombospondin type 1 motif)-like protein 4; *FBN1*, fibrillin 1; *LTBP2*, latent transforming growth factor beta binding protein 2; *TGFBR2*, transforming growth factor beta receptor II; *COL1A1*, collagen type I alpha 1; *COL1A2*, collagen type I alpha 2; *COL2A1*, collagen type II alpha 1; *COL5A1*, collagen type V alpha 1; *COL5A2*, collagen type V alpha 2, a disintegrin-like and metallopeptidase (reprolysin type) with thrombospondin type 1 motif 2; *PLOD1*, procollagen-lysine 2-oxoglutarate 5-dioxygenase 1; *CHST14*, carbohydrate (*N*-acetylgalactosamine 4-0) sulfotransferase 14; *B4GALT7*, xylosylprotein beta 1,4-galactosyltransferase polypeptide 7; *SLC39A13*, solute carrier family 39 (zinc transporter) member 13; *COL3A1*, collagen type III alpha 1; *TNXB*, tenascin XB; *ACTA2*, actin alpha 2 smooth muscle aorta; *FAA* locus, familial aortic aneurysm locus; *MYH11*, myosin heavy chain 11 smooth muscle; *TAAD1* locus, thoracic aortic aneurysm and dissection 1 locus; *TGFBR1*, transforming growth factor beta receptor 1; *MYLK*, myosin light chain kinase; *CBS*, cystathionine-beta-synthase; *COL2A2*, collagen type II alpha 2; *COL9A1*, collagen type IX alpha 1; *COL11A1*, collagen type XI alpha 1; *COL11A2*, collagen type XI alpha 2; *ADAMTS10*, a disintegrin-like and metallopeptidase (reprolysin type) with thrombospondin type 1 motif 10.

**BIBLIOGRAPHY:**

1. Murphy-Ryan M, Psychogios A, Lindor NM. Hereditary disorders of connective tissue: a guide to the emerging differential diagnosis. *Genet Med.* 2010;12:344-354.

2. Summers KM, West JA, Peterson MM, Stark D, McGill JJ, West MJ. Challenges in the diagnosis of Marfan syndrome. *Med J Aust.* 2006;184:627-631.

3. Pearson GD, Devereux R, Loeys B, et al. Report of the National Heart, Lung and Blood Institute and National Marfan Foundation Working Group on research in Marfan syndrome and related disorders. *Circulation.* 2008;118:785-791.

4. Callewaert B, Malfait F, Loeys B, De Paepe A. Ehlers-Danlos syndromes and Marfan syndrome. *Best Pract Res Clin Rheumatol.* 2008;22:165-189.

5. Mizuguchi T, Matsumoto N. Recent progress in genetics of Marfan syndrome and Marfan-associated disorders. *J Hum Genet.* 2007;52:1-12.

6. Morava E, Lefeber D, Urban Z, et al. Defining the phenotype in an autosomal cutis laxa syndrome with a combined congenital defect of glycosylation. *Eur J Hum Genet.* 2008;16:28-35.

7. Beighton P, De Paepe A, Steinmann B, Tsipouras P, Wenstrup RJ. Ehlers-Danlos syndromes: revised nosology, Villefranche, 1997. Ehlers-Danlos National Foundation (USA) and Ehlers-Danlos Support Group (UK). *Am J Med Genet.* 1998;77:31-37.

8. Milewicz DM, Guo DC, Tran-Fadulu V, et al. Genetic basis of thoracic aortic aneurysms and dissections: focus on smooth muscle cell contractile dysfunction. *Annu Rev Genomics Hum Genet.* 2008;9:283-302.

9. De Paepe A, Devereux R, Dietz HC, Hennekam RC, Pyeritz RE. Revised diagnostic criteria for the Marfan syndrome. *Am J Med Genet.* 1996;62:417-426.

10. Donoso LA, Edwards AO, Frost AT, et al. Clinical variability of Stickler syndrome: role of exon 2 of the collagen COL2A1 gene. *Surv Opthalmol.* 2003;48:191-203.

11. Faivre L, Dollfus H, Lyonnet S, et al. Clinical homogeneity and genetic heterogeneity in Weill-Marchesani syndrome. *Am J Med Genet A.* 2003;123A:204-207.

12. Hinterseher I. Genes and abdominal aortic aneurysm. *Ann Vasc Surg.* 2011;25:388-412.

# Supplementary Information

## OMIM REFERENCES:

[1] Abdominal Aortic Aneurysms; COL3A1 (#100070)

[2] Arterial Tortuosity Syndrome; SLC2A10 (#208050)

[3] Bicuspid Aortic Valve With Thoracic Aortic Aneurysms; NOTCH1, KCNJ2 (#109730)

[4] Congenital Contractural Arachnodactyly; FBN2 (#121050)

[5] Cutis Laxa; AD: ELN, FBLN5 (#123700); AR1: EFEMP2/FBLN4, FBLN5 (#219100); AR2: ATP6V0A2, P5CS, PYCR1 (#219200)

[6] Familial Ectopia Lentis; ADAMTSL4, FBN1, LTBP2 (#129600)

[7] Ehlers-Danlos, Arthrochalasia Type; COL1A1, COL1A2 (#130060)

[8] Ehlers-Danlos, Cardiac Valvular Type; COL1A2 (#225320)

[9] Ehlers-Danlos, Classical Type; CL5A1, COL5A2, COL1A1 (#130000, mild #130010)

[10] Ehlers-Danlos, Dermatosparaxis Type; ADAMTS2 (#225410)

[11] Ehlers-Danlos, Kyphoscoliotic Type; PLOD1 (#225400)

[12] Ehlers-Danlos, Musculocontractural Type; CHST14 (#601776)

[13] Ehlers-Danlos, Progeroid Type; B4GALT7 (#130070)

[14] Ehlers-Danlos, Spondylocheiro Dysplastic Type; SLC39A13 (#612350)

[15] Ehlers-Danlos, Vascular Type; COL3A1 (#130050)

[16] Ehlers-Danlos-Like Syndrome; Tenascin-X Type; TNXB (#606408)

[17] Familial Thoracic Aortic Aneurysm and/or Dissection; AAD4: MYH11 (#132900), AAT6: ACTA2 (#611788), AAT1: 11q23.3-q24 (%607086); AAT2: 5q13-q14 (%607087); AAT7: MYLK (#613780)

[18] Homocystinuria; CBS (#236200)

[19] Loeys-Dietz Syndrome, Type 1; TGFBR1 (#609192), TGFBR2 (#610168)

[20] Loeys-Dietz Syndrome, Type 2; TGFBR1 (#608967), TGFBR2 (#610380)

[21] Marfan Syndrome; FBN1 (#154700)

[22] Mitral Valve Prolapse Syndrome; MMVP1: 16p12.1-p11.2 (%157700), MMVP2: 11p15.4 (%607829), MMVP3: 13q31.3-q32.1 (%610840)

[23] Persistent Patent Ductus Arteriosus With Familial Thoracic Aortic Aneurysm; MYH11 (#132900)

[24] Stickler Syndrome; STL1: COL2A1 (#108300), STL2: COL11A1 (#604841), STL3: COL11A2 (#184840), STL4: COL9A1 (#614134), STL5: COL9A2 (#614284)

[25] Weill-Marchesani Syndrome; WMS1: ADAMTS10 (#277600), WMS2: FBN1 (#608328)

## Alternative Names:

- For major alternative names of a clinical entity of interest, see Table 168-1 or refer to the OMIM entry (OMIM numbers above).

*Key Words:* Connective tissue disease, Ehlers-Danlos syndrome, Loeys-Dietz syndrome, Marfan syndrome, Cutis laxa, abdominal aortic aneurysms, arterial tortuosity syndrome, bicuspid aortic valve, thoracic aortic aneurysms, congenital contractural arachnodactyly, familial ectopia lentis, homocystinuria, MASS phenotype, mitral valve prolapse, patent ductus arteriosus, Stickler syndrome, Weill-Marchesani syndrome

# 169 Ehlers-Danlos Syndrome, Hypermobility and Classical Type

Howard Levy

## KEY POINTS

- *Disease summary:*
  - Ligamentous laxity predisposes to joint instability, subluxations, and dislocations.
  - Chronic pain and fatigue are common.
  - The classical type is distinguished from the hypermobility type by the presence of skin fragility, hyperelasticity, and atrophic scarring in the former.
  - Additional features may include easy bruising, prolonged bleeding, cardiovascular autonomic dysfunction, mild-to-moderate aortic root dilation, and functional bowel disorders.
- *Hereditary basis:*
  - Both types of EDS are inherited in an autosomal dominant pattern.
  - The genetic basis of most cases of hypermobility type EDS is unknown.
  - Mutations in one of the two genes for type V collagen account for half of cases of classical type EDS.
- *Differential diagnosis:*
  - Four other types of EDS are described in Table 169-1.
  - There are dozens of other genetic causes for ligamentous laxity, including (but not limited to) Marfan syndrome, Loeys-Dietz syndrome, Stickler syndrome, fragile X syndrome, and Turner syndrome.
  - Hypotonia, which itself is a feature of many genetic conditions, can also cause joint laxity, and may be difficult to distinguish from ligamentous laxity.

## Diagnostic Criteria and Clinical Characteristics

***Diagnostic Criteria (see Table 169-2):*** Joint laxity is semi objectively measured with the Beighton scale (1 point each for ability to place palms on the floor with knees straight; hyperextension of each elbow or knee >10 degrees; dorsiflexion of each fifth finger >90 degrees; passive apposition of each thumb to flexor surface of forearm). A score of 5 or more is considered positive, but males, older individuals, and those with arthritis and/or history of trauma typically have less laxity, so lower scores may be considered positive.

Skin elasticity is best measured in a location without excess or redundant skin (ie, not the elbow, back of hand, neck, or cheek). The volar wrist is a good option; normal is approximately 1 cm.

***Clinical Characteristics (see Table 169-1):*** Joint laxity, leading to instability, subluxations, and dislocations is common to all types of Ehlers-Danlos syndrome (EDS). Pain and fatigue, often out of proportion to physical examination and radiologic findings, are frequent and sometimes disabling. Both neuropathic pain and myofascial spasm are likely to occur. Migraines and temporomandibular dysfunction are also common.

Soft skin, prolonged bleeding, and easy bruising are also common to all types of EDS. The classical type is distinguished from the hypermobility type by the presence of skin hyperelasticity and fragility, as well as delayed wound healing, wound dehiscences, and atrophic ("cigarette paper") scars. Rupture or tearing of arteries, intestines, or uterus are not features of the hypermobility type, and only very rarely occur in the classical type.

Functional bowel disorders, including gastritis and irritable bowel syndrome, affect up to half of EDS patients.

Cardiac autonomic dysfunction, manifesting as neurally mediated hypotension and/or postural orthostatic tachycardia are also common. Mild-to-moderate aortic root dilation occurs in up to one-third of patients. Mitral valve prolapse, using modern diagnostic criteria, is not an associated feature of EDS.

## Screening and Counseling

***Screening/Diagnosis:*** In the current nomenclature, there are six distinct types of EDS. The hypermobility and classical types are the most common. Diagnostic evaluation is primarily based on clinical findings and family history. Molecular genetic testing can be helpful in the more rare types, but is not currently helpful in the hypermobility or classical types. Major features of each type are described in Table 169-3. See Fig. 169-1 for a clinical diagnostic algorithm that can help guide further testing/evaluation.

***Counseling:***

☞**INHERITANCE:** The hypermobility and classical types are inherited in an autosomal dominant pattern. Each first-degree relative (parent, sibling, and child) has a 50% chance of also being affected, regardless of sex. Among the other four types of EDS, the vascular and arthrochalasia types are also autosomal dominant; the kyphoscoliosis and dermatosparaxis types are autosomal recessive.

☞**PENETRANCE AND EXPRESSIVITY:** Clinical expression is highly variable, but at least some clinical manifestations can usually be found in obligately affected individuals, so penetrance is likely complete. Men tend to be less severely affected and thus less likely to come to medical attention, so most recognized cases are among women. At the milder end of the spectrum it can be hard to distinguish EDS from the looser end of the normal range

**Table 169-1 System Involvement**

| System | Manifestation |
|---|---|
| Musculoskeletal | Joint laxity/hypermobility, dislocations/subluxations, muscle spasm, pain, fatigue, osteoarthritis<br>Rarely tendon/muscle tears (classical type) |
| Skin & soft tissue | Soft, hyperelastic, and fragile with wound dehiscences, atrophic scars, and hernias (classical type) |
| GI | Irritable bowel syndrome, functional gastritis |
| Hematologic | Easy bruising, prolonged bleeding |
| Cardiac | Neurally mediated hypotension, postural orthostatic hypotension<br>Mild-to-moderate aortic root dilation (up to one-third of patients) |
| Obstetric | Increased laxity and pain in third trimester, rapid labor and delivery (all types)<br>Premature rupture of membranes (classical type) |

of joint mobility. What used to be called the benign joint hypermobility syndrome is now considered a mild manifestation of hypermobility type EDS.

☞**GENOTYPE-PHENOTYPE CORRELATION:** A small subset of hypermobility type EDS is due to haploinsufficiency of tenascin X. Clinical manifestations include joint laxity and soft skin, without easy bruising. No other genes have been associated with hypermobility type EDS, and no genotype-phenotype correlation has been identified in classical type EDS.

## Management and Treatment

Joint instability and trauma can be reduced (but not completely prevented) by minimizing resistance exercise and impact activity. Bracing is sometimes helpful for particularly unstable joints.

Treatments such as heat, cold, massage, ultrasound, electrical stimulation, acupuncture, and similar mechanical techniques can provide a few hours of pain relief. Pharmacologic management of pain may require a combination of several drug classes, including acetaminophen, nonsteroidal anti-inflammatory drugs (NSAIDs), skeletal muscle relaxers, and antineuropathic pain medications. Opioids should generally be reserved until all of the above have been maximized, and then added to the regimen, rather than replacing the other medications.

The long-term goal is to improve joint stability by increasing muscle tone. Exercises should be very low resistance, such as walking, bicycling, elliptical trainer, swimming, other water exercise, and other range of motion activities. Progress should be made slowly, by adding repetitions rather than resistance. It often takes months or even years of routine toning exercise (5 or more days per week) before patients notice improved stability and reduced pain.

Orthopedic surgeries designed to stabilize joints frequently fail outright or within 1 to 5 years. In addition, patients with the classical type are subject to intraoperative soft tissue fragility and postoperative wound healing problems, so elective or optional surgery is best avoided. When surgery is performed in patients with classical EDS, the surgeon should be prepared for complications. Sutures should not be pulled any tighter than necessary and should be left in approximately 1.5 to 2 times as long as usual.

An echocardiogram should be obtained at diagnosis and every 2 years until approximately age 25 to evaluate for aortic root dilation. If present, beta-blockers may be of value in preventing progression, although this has not been specifically studied in EDS.

Functional bowel disorders and cardiovascular autonomic dysfunction are treated the same way as in patients without EDS.

## Molecular Genetics and Molecular Mechanism

See Table 169-3 for genes associated with the various forms of EDS.

The majority of cases of hypermobility type EDS are of unknown etiology. Haploinsufficiency of tenascin X (TNXB) has been identified in a few individuals with joint laxity and soft skin, but without easy bruising. Tenascin X is an extracellular matrix glycoprotein that is thought be important in cell adhesion and spreading.

**Table 169-2 Major Supportive and Exclusionary Diagnostic Criteria for Hypermobility and Classical Type Ehlers Danlos Syndrome**

| Diagnostic Criteria | Hypermobility Type | Classical Type |
|---|---|---|
| Major (all are required): | • Joint laxity<br>• Soft skin | • Joint laxity<br>• Hyperelastic skin<br>• Fragile skin or atrophic scars |
| Supportive findings: | • Easy bruising<br>• High, narrow palate | • Soft skin<br>• Easy bruising<br>• High, narrow palate<br>• Hernias/soft tissue fragility |
| Exclusionary findings (suggestive of other diagnoses): | • Skin fragility<br>• Hyperelastic skin<br>• Poor wound healing<br>• Arterial, intestinal, and/or uterine rupture<br>• Other syndromic manifestations | • Other syndromic manifestations |

*Table 169-3 Types of Ehlers-Danlos Syndrome*

| Type | Former Name | Inheritance | Features | Associated Gene(s) |
|---|---|---|---|---|
| Hypermobility | Type III | AD | • Joint laxity<br>• Soft skin<br>• Easy bruising | Most unknown<br>Rarely *TNXB* (this form lacks easy bruising) |
| Classical | Types I & II | AD | • Joint laxity<br>• Soft skin<br>• Hyperelastic skin<br>• Fragile skin<br>• Atrophic scars<br>• Hernias/soft tissue fragility<br>• Easy bruising | *COL5A1, COL5A2* (50% of cases)<br>Others unknown |
| Vascular | Type IV | AD | • Joint laxity (primarily small joints)<br>• Soft skin<br>• Hyperelastic skin<br>• Fragile skin<br>• Atrophic scars<br>• Thin, translucent skin<br>• Arterial, intestinal and/or uterine rupture<br>• Extensive bruising | *COL3A1* |
| Kyphoscoliosis | Type VI | AR | • Joint laxity<br>• Soft skin<br>• Hyperelastic skin<br>• Fragile skin<br>• Atrophic scars<br>• Arterial rupture<br>• Severe, congenital hypotonia<br>• Marfanoid habitus<br>• Progressive scoliosis onset in first year of life<br>• Scleral fragility/ocular rupture (rare)<br>• Easy bruising | *PLOD1* |
| Arthrochalasia | Types VIIA & VIIB | AD | • Severe diffuse joint laxity<br>• Soft skin<br>• Hyperelastic skin<br>• Fragile skin<br>• Hypotonia<br>• Congenital bilateral hip dislocation<br>• Kyphoscoliosis<br>• Easy bruising | *COL1A1, COL1A2* (exon 6 only) |
| Dermatosparaxis | Type VIIC | AR | • Joint laxity<br>• Soft, doughy skin<br>• Severe skin fragility<br>• Sagging, redundant skin<br>• Easy bruising<br>• Premature rupture of fetal membranes<br>• Large hernias | *ADAMTS2* |

Modified from Beighton et al., 1998.

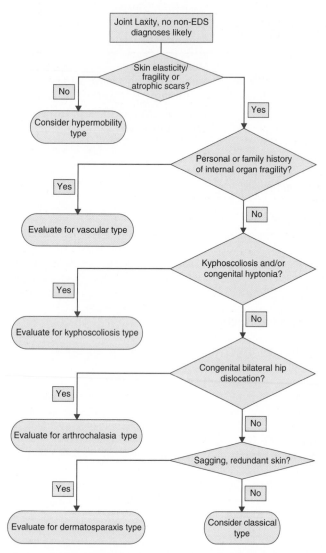

***Figure 169-1*** Ehlers-Danlos Syndrome Clinical Diagnostic Algorithm. Additional criteria are necessary to establish any one of these diagnoses.

In approximately half of patients with classical type EDS, a mutation in type V collagen (COL5A1 or COL5A2) can be identified. Type V collagen is a fibrillar collagen found primarily in skin, bones, and tendons. It interacts with and is thought to regulate the diameter of type I collagen fibrils.

***Genetic Testing:*** Clinical sequencing and deletion or duplication testing of TNXB is available on a limited basis, primarily in Europe. Since it appears to cause only a small minority of hypermobility type EDS-like syndromes, it is of very low clinical utility, and the hypermobility type is currently diagnosed based only on clinical evaluation.

Clinical sequencing with or without deletion or duplication testing of COL5A1 and COL5A2 is widely available. Identification of a mutation is useful for confirming the diagnosis. However, since

mutations cannot be found in half of classical type EDS cases, failure to identify a mutation in these genes carries no significant negative predictive value, and this test is also of low clinical utility.

## BIBLIOGRAPHY:

1. Sacheti A, Szemere J, Bernstein B, Tafas T, Schechter N, Tsipouras P. Chronic pain is a manifestation of the Ehlers-Danlos syndrome. *J Pain Symptom Manage.* 1997;14:88-93.

2. Voermans NC, Knoop H, van de Kamp N, Hamel BC, Bleijenberg G, van Engelen BG. Fatigue is a frequent and clinically relevant problem in Ehlers-Danlos syndrome. *Semin Arthritis Rheum.* 2010;40:267-274.

3. De Coster PJ, Martens LC, De Paepe A. Oral health in prevalent types of Ehlers-Danlos syndromes. *J Oral Pathol Med.* 2005;34:298-307.

4. Rowe PC, Barron DF, Calkins H, Maumenee IH, Tong PY, Geraghty MT. Orthostatic intolerance and chronic fatigue syndrome associated with Ehlers-Danlos syndrome. *J Pediatr.* 1999;135:494-499.

5. Wenstrup RJ, Meyer RA, Lyle JS, et al. Prevalence of aortic root dilation in the Ehlers-Danlos syndrome. *Genet Med.* 2002;4:112-117.

6. McDonnell NB, Gorman BL, Mandel KW, et al. Echocardiographic findings in classical and hypermobile Ehlers-Danlos syndromes. *Am J Med Genet A.* 2006;140:129-136.

7. Beighton P, De Paepe A, Steinmann B, Tsipouras P, Wenstrup RJ. Ehlers-Danlos syndromes: revised nosology, Villefranche, 1997. Ehlers-Danlos National Foundation (USA) and Ehlers-Danlos Support Group (UK). *Am J Med Genet.* 1998;77:31-37.

8. Tinkle BT, Bird H, Grahame R, Lavallee M, Levy HP, Sillence D. The lack of clinical distinction between the hypermobility type of Ehlers-Danlos syndrome and the joint hypermobility syndrome (a.k.a. hypermobility syndrome). *Am J Med Genet A.* 2009;149A:2368-2370.

9. Levy HP (Updated December 14, 2010). Ehlers-Danlos Syndrome, Hypermobility Type. In: GeneReviews at GeneTests: Medical Genetics Information Resource (database online). Copyright, University of Washington, Seattle. 1997-2011. http://www.genetests.org. Accessed August 16, 2011.

10. Wenstrup R, De Paepe A (Updated May 11, 2010). Ehlers-Danlos Syndrome, Hypermobility Type. In: GeneReviews at GeneTests: Medical Genetics Information Resource (database online). Copyright, University of Washington, Seattle. 1997-2011. http://www.genetests.org. Accessed August 16, 2011.

## Supplementary Information

### OMIM REFERENCES:

[1] Ehlers-Danlos Syndrome, Hypermobility Type (type III); (#130020)

[2] Ehlers-Danlos Syndrome, Classical Type (types I & II); COL5A1, COL5A2 (#130000, #130010)

### Alternative Names:

- Ehlers Danlos Syndrome, Hypermobility Type
  - Type III, Type 3, Benign Joint Hypermobility Syndrome
- Ehlers Danlos syndrome, Classical Type
  - Type I, Type 1, Gravis
  - Type II, Type 2, Mitis

## 170 Clinical Implications of Copy Number Variation in the Human Genome

Jung Sook Ha and Charles Lee

### Introduction

During the past 9 years, copy number variation (CNV) has emerged as a highly prevalent form of genomic variation. CNVs are smaller than the chromosomal aberrations observed microscopically by cytogeneticists, but larger than single-nucleotide polymorphisms (SNPs) and insertion or deletion (indel) mutations. Many CNVs are simply normal genetic variants that do not contribute to a clinically recognizable phenotype. Other CNVs predispose or are significantly associated to conditions of medical consequence.

In clinical genetics, the challenge has been to understand (and ultimately predict accurately) the relationship between genomic changes and clinical phenotypes and outcomes. This is compounded by the complexity of the data being generated by genome-wide genetic tests.

### Definition of Copy Number Variants

When the human genome was completed on April 14, 2003, 50 years after the discovery of the structure of the double helix, scientists concluded that they had deciphered the complete DNA sequence of essentially every human. This was based on the notion that the genomes of healthy individuals were 99.9% identical and that the major genetic differences between any two individual was in the form of scattered single base changes (SNPs). In 2004, two papers showed that the genomes of healthy individuals were actually a lot more different from one another than previously thought. Using genome-wide array comparative genomic hybridization (CGH) platforms, hundreds of genomic regions were found to vary between individuals—not significantly with respect to the actual DNA sequence—but rather with respect to the number of copies an individual had of each DNA segment. These CNVs are now operationally defined as a DNA segment, longer than 1 kb, with a variable copy number compared to a reference genome.

CNVs are scattered throughout the human genome and it has been estimated that as many as 1500 CNVs can be found in a single individual's genome. When one examines all CNVs in a given individual, there are clearly more smaller-sized CNVs compared to large-sized CNVs. While some CNVs in healthy individuals can be greater than 1 Mb in size, the median size of CNVs is approximately 2.9 kb. Taken together, when comparing the genomes of two individuals, approximately 0.8% of their genomes differ with respect to CNVs.

Simple CNVs can take the form of genomic losses (deletions) or copy number gains (duplications or amplifications). Duplications can occur in tandem or elsewhere on the same chromosome or even on different chromosomes (ie, insertional duplication). CNVs may involve whole genes, portion of genes, multiples of contiguous genes, regulatory elements, or none of the above. Clearly, the nature and extent of genomic material that is gained or lost is undoubtedly important for the phenotypic consequences.

The DNA sequences at the edges of CNVs are important as they often yield clues as to how the CNV was generated. For example, if a given CNV is flanked by nearly identical blocks of sequences (also known as segmental duplications or low copy repeats) or by Alu or LINE repetitive elements, misalignment of DNA strands during meiotic recombination can lead to a process called nonallelic homologous recombination (NAHR). This process was first suggested as the basis for genomic duplications that led to Charcot-Marie-Tooth disease type 1A (CMT1A). Such recurrent changes have now been associated with many other genomic disorders.

Other mechanisms have become appreciated for generating CNVs. With the advent of next-generation DNA sequencing, large-scale projects to sequence whole genomes (eg, the 1000 Genomes Project) has provided nucleotide-resolution breakpoint information for over 10,000 common CNVs. Based on this dataset, the majority of common deletions (~65%) are generated via nonhomologous end joining (NHEJ) mechanisms. For these CNVs, two base microhomologies were found at the CNV breakpoints. For more complex CNVs, microhomology-mediated break-induced replication is one mechanism that has been proposed.

### How Do CNVs Cause Disease

CNVs can cause quantitative (dosage) or disruptive effects. CNVs that are completely embedded within a gene (intragenic) or involve a single gene may have functional consequences that are similar to point mutations and exhibit classical Mendelian dominant or recessive traits. In some cases, CNVs can overlap parts of two different genes, leading to fusion genes that may have phenotypic consequences. For "genomic disorders," CNVs overlap multiple genes that are juxtaposed to one another.

Deletion of a genomic segment leads to hemizygosity for the deleted interval and may result in haploinsufficiency for a dosage-sensitive gene. Alternatively, deletion of a genomic segment may "unmask" a recessive mutation on the other allele leading to a clinical phenotype. Copy number gains (such as duplications) may create imbalances due to excess product of the duplicated gene(s) or, when intragenic, may alter the structure of a protein product. In cases of insertional duplications, it is possible that the extra copy of a gene becomes localized to (and thereby under the influence of) a regulatory element that substantially increases the expression level of that gene. A CNV can similarly disrupt (or disassociate) promoters, enhancers, repressors, or even disrupt local chromatin structure.

## Clinical Testing and CNVs

Microarray-based genomic copy number analysis is now a commonly ordered clinical genetic test. It is offered under various names such as "chromosomal microarray" (CMA), microarray karyotyping, or simply as array CGH (aCGH). aCGH is a term that refers specifically to the technology of hybridization of one person's DNA (eg, patient's DNA/test DNA) to another's (eg, DNA from healthy individual(s)/reference DNA). SNP arrays are also widely being used in such clinical tests, but since only the patient's DNA is hybridized to these arrays, they are technically not aCGH tests. Agilent, Inc., is currently the largest commercial vendor for aCGH platforms. Both Affymetrix, Inc., and Illumina, Inc., produce SNP arrays that are used for clinical testing.

When analyzing clinical microarray tests, clinical laboratory geneticists need to categorize each genomic gain or loss identified (ie, each CNV) as either likely benign, likely pathogenic, or of unknown clinical significance. CNVs that overlap critical regions of well-defined microdeletion or microduplication syndromes are likely to be pathogenic in nature. For all other CNVs, several factors need to be considered to assess whether the CNV is likely to be pathogenic or likely to be benign. First, is the CNV found in an affected or nonaffected parent or relative? Second, does the CNV overlap with a CNV found in past clinically recognized patients (eg, databases such as DECIPHER/ISCA) or is the CNV commonly found in healthy individuals (eg, Database of Genomic Variants). Finally, does the CNV overlap with an OMIM gene whose known function is related to one of the clinical phenotypes of the patient? Other risk factors for CNVs can be found in Lee et al. and Kearney et al.

In 2010, the International Standard Cytogenetic Array (ISCA) consortium put forth recommendations for standardizations for clinical microarray testing. A clinically effective microarray test has to balance sensitivity and specificity such that it maximizes the yield of pathogenic CNVs but minimizes the detection of benign CNVs found in the normal population. Clinical array tests are now usually designed to detect genomic imbalances of at least 50 kb in targeted genomic regions (eg, known Mendelian genes) and at least 250 kb for the rest of the genome; although genomic imbalances smaller than these can certainly be pathogenic, the application of higher-resolution microarray testing for clinical purposes is fraught with an exponentially increasing number of benign CNVs. Indeed, estimates are that more than 95% of all known benign CNVs are smaller than 500 kb.

The ISCA consortium subsequently recommended that clinical microarray testing be offered as a first-tier genetic test, in lieu of G-banded karyotyping. Clinical microarray testing costs are similar, or in some cases less than G-banded karyotyping but has an increased diagnostic yield rate, especially in cases of developmental delay or congenital anomalies (~19% in 36,325 microarray cases compared to ~3% for G-banded karyotyping). For prenatal genetic testing, microarray testing has also been shown to be very effective: identifying the pathogenic genomic imbalance in nearly 99% of cases with cytogenetically detected chromosomal aberrations and identifying clinically relevant genomic imbalances in 6% of fetuses with structural abnormalities. Since microarray testing does not require cell culturing or even live cells, turn around times are potentially shortened compared to karyotyping.

## CNVs, Disease Penetrance, and Variable Expressivity

Observing the phenotypic consequences of CNVs is the integral part of determining their clinical significance. However, for a given CNV, the phenotypic presentation is not always the same in every individual. Individuals carrying a presumed "pathogenic" CNV, but not exhibiting a clinical phenotype (ie, apparently unaffected) are said to exhibit "incomplete penetrance." Pathogenic CNVs that cause a range of clinical phenotypes, from mildly affected to severely affected, are said to exhibit "variable expressivity." The most common human microdeletion, del 22q11.21, is highly penetrant but has a wide range of phenotypic expression (ie, variable expressivity). On the other hand, a nearby microduplication has been found in a substantial number of individuals with essentially no clinical phenotype such that some question the clinical relevance of this particular genomic imbalance. This duplication CNV is said to be incompletely penetrant. Recent studies have further suggested that the existence of multiple large, rare CNVs can have a compound effect and result in more severe clinical presentation.

## Conclusions

In the past 9 years, we have appreciated a magnitude more of genetic variation in the human genome. Structural genomic variations (of which CNVs are the largest class) exist ubiquitously in everyone's genomes. Most CNVs do not appear to lead to clinically recognizable phenotypes but are thought to contribute collectively to one's ability to adapt to the environment, one's susceptibility to various diseases, and one's cognition and behavior. With an increased understanding and study of CNVs, geneticists have been able to make more associations with certain phenotypes and use the data from genetic patients and normal controls to more accurately interpret genome-wide genetic tests. With the advent of next-generation DNA sequencing in clinical diagnostics, our knowledge of CNVs will undoubtedly continue to increase, revealing the complexities of pathways and genetic interaction networks in disease presentation, and hopefully leading to more accurate genetic diagnoses and insights into new therapies.

### BIBLIOGRAPHY:

1. Iafrate AJ, Feuk L, Rivera MN, et al. Detection of large-scale variation in the human genome. *Nat Genet.* 2004;36:949-951.

2. Sebat J, Lakshmi B, Troge J, et al. Large-scale copy number polymorphism in the human genome. *Science.* 2004;305:525-528.

3. Freeman JL, Perry GH, Feuk L, et al. Copy number variation: new insights into genome diversity. *Genome Res.* 2006;16:949-961.

4. Conrad D, Pinto D, Redon R, et al. Common copy number variation in the human genome: mechanism, selection and disease association. *Nature.* 2010;464:704-12.

5. Lupski JR, de Oca-Luna RM, Slaugenhaupt S, et al. DNA duplication associated with Charcot-Marie-Tooth disease type 1A. *Cell*. 1991;66:219-232.

6. Hastings PJ, Ira G, Lupski JR. A microhomology-mediated break-induced replication model for the origin of human copy number variation. *PLoS Genet*. 2009;5:e1000327.

7. Lee C, Iafrate AJ, Brothman AR. Copy number variations and clinical cytogenetic diagnosis of constitutional disorders. *Nat Genet*. 2007;39:S48-S54.

8. Miller DT, Adam MP, Aradhya S, et al. Consensus statement: chromosomal microarray is a first-tier clinical diagnostic test for individuals with developmental disabilities or congenital anomalies. *Am J Hum Genet* 2010;86:749-764.

9. Wapner RJ, Martin CL, Levy B, et al. Chromosomal microarray versus karyotyping for prenatal diagnosis. *N Engl J Med*. 2012;367:2175-2184.

10. Girirajan S, Rosenfeld JA, Coe BP, et al. Phenotypic heterogeneity of genomic disorders and rare copy-number variants. *N Engl J Med*. 2012;367:1321-1331.

11. Mills RE, Walter K, Stewart C, et al. Mapping copy number variation by population-scale genome sequencing. Nature. 2011;59-65.

# 171 Genetic Privacy

Heather L. Harrell and Mark A. Rothstein

## KEY POINTS

- A variety of complex ethical and legal issues are included under the broad heading of "genetic privacy."
- Federal laws exist to protect individual genetic privacy and protect against discrimination.
- Emerging threats to genetic privacy include electronic health records, compelled disclosure, and direct-to-consumer genetic testing.

## Why Is Genetic Privacy Important

Numerous public opinion surveys in the last decade confirm that the public overwhelmingly supports the concept of genetic privacy. Genetic information is widely regarded as sensitive information that should not be readily accessible to any other individuals or entities without the explicit consent of the individual. Unauthorized access, use, or disclosure of genetic information may be considered to result in two types of harms. First is intangible harms, such as mental anguish, embarrassment, stigmatization, and undermining of personal and familial relationships, which can be lessened by limiting access to genetic information. In addition, there is also support for the principle that individuals should have a right "not to know" the predictive and sometimes unsettling information in their DNA. Second, the disclosure of genetic information may lead to tangible harms, such as adverse treatment by employers and various insurers, loss of government benefits, or disadvantage in educational or other opportunities. Collectively, these concerns are often referred to as "genetic discrimination." Many of the laws enacted to deal with genetic privacy focus on preventing genetic discrimination.

There is a close connection between genetic privacy (including discrimination) and research and clinical genetics. Individuals who believe they—or their children and other family members—might experience genetic discrimination are likely to forego genetic testing and other potentially beneficial medical interventions. Thus, legislative efforts to protect privacy and prohibit discrimination are less about redressing the relatively few cases of tangible harm than the widespread need to reassure individuals that they can avail themselves of genetic services without worrying about the social consequences.

## How Does the Law Define Genetic Information

The definition of genetic information selected by a legislature in a statute has important practical implications. A narrow definition, such as only the results of an individual's genetic test, would not extend protection to individuals who were subject to discrimination on the basis of a family history of a genetic disorder. On the other hand, a broad definition that included family history might be regarded as too far-reaching. The federal Genetic Information Nondiscrimination Act of 2008 (GINA), which prohibits discrimination in employment and health insurance on the basis of genetic information, defines genetic information as the results of the individual's genetic tests, the genetic tests of family members, and the health history of family members. Excluded from coverage is the individual's own health history. As a result, GINA only prohibits discrimination against asymptomatic individuals. Provisions of the Patient Protection and Affordable Care Act, effective in 2014, fill this gap by prohibiting exclusion from or termination of health insurance based on personal health status.

## Should Genetic Information Be Treated Separately

The difficulty of defining genetic information is only one of the reasons why it is problematic to enact genetic-specific legal protections. This approach, referred to as "genetic exceptionalism," has been the subject of much discussion in the literature. Critics point out that treating genetic information separately reinforces the stigma of genetic conditions. Supporters of genetic-specific laws note that much of the public regards genetic information as unique. Although most commentators recommend more general legislation to deal with health-based discrimination and privacy concerns, virtually all of the legislation enacted in the United States, at both the federal and state level, to deal with genetic privacy and discrimination, has been genetic specific. The most common explanation is simply that genetic privacy and nondiscrimination proposals have broad support, but more comprehensive legislation lacks such support and therefore is unlikely to be enacted.

## What Laws Protect Genetic Privacy

Several federal laws protect genetic privacy and prohibit genetic discrimination. Three of the most important of these laws are summarized in Table 171-2.

Numerous state laws also prohibit genetic discrimination. Virtually all of the states have enacted laws prohibiting genetic discrimination in health insurance and about two-thirds of the states have enacted laws prohibiting genetic discrimination in employment. Because this type of discrimination also is prohibited under federal law, the main value of the state laws is that they may have wider applicability. For example, GINA's prohibition on genetic discrimination in employment applies to employers with 15 or more employees, but several of the state laws also apply to smaller employers.

Twelve states (AL, AZ, FL, GA, MA, MI, NE, NM, NY, SC, SD, VT) have enacted laws purporting to protect genetic privacy. The laws vary considerably, but all are quite limited in protections and generally require informed consent before any genetic

*Table 171-1* **Definitions**

| | |
|---|---|
| Privacy | A condition of limited access to an individual or information about an individual |
| Right to privacy | Ethical and legal principles applicable to an individual's ability to control access to his or her person or information |
| Confidentiality | Duty of possessor of information disclosed in confidence not to redisclose the information without authorization |
| Security | Physical, electronic, and other means used to grant access to information to those authorized and deny access to those not authorized |

testing. There are exceptions for law enforcement, paternity determinations, and newborn screening. Some of the laws apply only in healthcare settings. See Table 171-1 for relevant definitions related to genetic privacy.

Although some of the statutes discussed earlier provide for individual remedies, another potentially viable legal action for an egregious privacy violation is to sue under the common law tort of invasion of privacy. Intrusion upon seclusion and public disclosure of private facts are the most appropriate types of invasion of privacy legal actions for invasion of genetic privacy. No successful cases have yet been brought under this theory involving genetic privacy.

## What Are Some Emerging Threats to Genetic Privacy

The largest threat to genetic privacy is the expected proliferation of genetic information in health records as the cost of genetic testing (including genome sequencing) declines and medical applications of genetic information increase. Three other threats to genetic privacy are the following:

*Electronic Health Records:* With the enactment of the federal Health Information Technology for Economic and Clinical Health (HITECH) Act in 2009, the United States has embraced the vision of an interoperable network of electronic health record (EHR) systems. EHRs hold great promise for improving efficiency and health outcomes, but they also present a challenge to privacy because they are comprehensive and longitudinal. Electronic health information does not disappear or become inaccessible when an individual moves or changes providers, and individuals and entities accessing health records can see a lifetime of information, including sensitive information with no current clinical utility. This includes family health histories, genetic test results, and medical histories of genetic disorders. One way of protecting privacy in EHRs would be to give individuals the ability to segment or sequester sensitive information in their health records. Besides a wealth of technological issues, there are numerous ethical and policy matters to resolve in limiting access to certain information in health records.

*Compelled Disclosures:* Although negligent or wrongful disclosures of health information through hacking hospital records or lost laptops often receive substantial publicity, an even greater threat to privacy is the compelled disclosure of health information. It is common for individuals to be required to sign an authorization to release their health records as a condition of applying for a job, health insurance, disability insurance, life insurance, long-term care insurance, workers' compensation, social security, or numerous other public and private commercial transactions and benefits. According to one estimate, each year in the United States there are at least 25 million compelled authorizations. Some of the authorizations are of unlimited scope; others have a more limited scope, but practical concerns make it easier for custodians of the records to release the entire file. Efforts to protect health privacy, including genetic privacy, must give serious consideration to the technological and policy challenges raised by compelled disclosures of health information.

*Direct-to-Consumer Genetic Testing:* In the last few years, several for-profit companies have begun to market genetic testing directly to consumers without a healthcare provider ordering the test. The tests may be performed for curiosity (eg, ancestry), predictive health, parentage, or other reasons. Full genome scans reporting the results of a few dozen alleles—and the risks they confer— have become common. Some consumers are not aware that the

*Table 171-2* **Federal Laws Protecting Genetic Privacy and Prohibiting Genetic Discrimination**

| Law | Key Provisions | Limitations |
|---|---|---|
| Genetic Information Nondiscrimination Act of 2008 | Prohibits genetic discrimination in employment and health insurance. | Does not apply to life insurance, long-term care insurance, disability insurance, or other potential uses of genetic information. Does not apply to individuals who are symptomatic. |
| Health Insurance Portability and Accountability Act of 1996 | Prohibits genetic discrimination in employer-sponsored group health plans. The HIPAA Privacy Rule limits uses and disclosures of protected health information. | Does not provide for individual remedies. |
| Americans with Disabilities Act | Prohibits discrimination on the basis of an expressed disability, that is, based on phenotype. | It is unlikely that a genetic predisposition will be considered as a disability. |

companies performing the tests usually are not subject to federal or state privacy laws because they are not considered healthcare providers or clinical laboratories. Moreover, genomic information is a valuable commodity and therefore there is a risk that the information will be sold or used for a secondary purpose.

## Conclusion

Although not all genetic information is sensitive, much of it is, and the amount of genetic information in health records and other files will continue to grow significantly. Genetic privacy is concerned with both intangible and tangible harms that could result from the nonconsensual access to, use, or disclosure of genetic information. Several laws attempt to protect genetic privacy and prohibit genetic discrimination, but these laws are inadequate in coverage, scope, procedures, and remedies. To provide their patients with information needed to weigh the social risks and benefits of genetic testing and other services, clinicians need to be aware of the issues surrounding genetic privacy.

**BIBLIOGRAPHY:**

1. Anderlik MR, Rothstein MA. Privacy and confidentiality of genetic information: what rules for the new science? *Ann Rev Genomics Hum Genet.* 2001;2:401-433.

2. National Conference of State Legislatures, State Genetic Privacy Laws. www.ncsl.org/programs/health/genetics/prt.htm.

3. Rothstein MA. Genetic exceptionalism and legislative pragmatism. *Hastings Cent Rep.* 2005;35(4):27-33.

4. Rothstein MA, ed. *Genetic Secrets: Protecting Privacy and Confidentiality in the Genetic Era.* Yale University Press; 1997.

5. Suter SM. Disentangling privacy from property: toward a deeper understanding of genetic privacy. *George Washington Law Rev.* 2004;72:734-814.

# 172 Race, Ancestry, and Genomics

Lynn B. Jorde

Race, ethnicity, and ancestry are often used in medicine and genetics, but their usefulness remains controversial. In this brief review, recent genetic findings relevant to these concepts are summarized. Individual ancestry is a more useful descriptor of one's genetic constitution than are race or ethnicity, and ancestry can now be estimated genetically. In some cases, direct assessment of genetic variation in individual patients can offer more accurate diagnosis and treatment than self-reported race, ethnicity, or ancestry.

## The Distribution of Human Genetic Diversity

On average, humans are heterozygous at about one in every 1000 DNA base pairs (bp). Thus, in terms of variation among single-nucleotide polymorphisms (SNPs), haploid human sequences are 99.9% identical but differ by about 3 million bp. In addition, each human is heterozygous for approximately 100 copy number variants (CNVs), which consist of contiguous segments of DNA sequence that are present in varying numbers of copies. Each CNV segment is at least 1000 bp in size, so CNVs account for an additional several million base-pair differences between haploid human sequences. Overall, the level of genetic diversity in humans is about half that of gorillas and central African chimpanzees, reflecting a relatively recent origin of our species, as well as the influence of bottlenecks in the size of human populations during our prehistory.

Because anatomically modern humans have a relatively recent origin not more than 200,000 years ago, and because our ancestors were located in a single continent, Africa, until 50,000 to 70,000 years ago, human populations are quite similar to one another. Most of our genetic variation, in fact, can be found within any major human population. About 85% to 90% of all human genetic variation would be observed, for example, in a sample of individuals from Great Britain or China. Only an additional 10% to 15% of variation is found if all human populations are assayed.

Population similarities can also be assessed by estimating the extent to which common SNPs (ie, those in which the frequency of the less common allele is >5%) are shared among major continental populations. These SNP alleles, which account for most human genetic variation, have attained high frequency because they originated a long time ago, before anatomically modern humans migrated out of Africa. Thus, the great majority of these SNPs are shared among individuals of African, Asian, or European origin and are not exclusive to a specific population. They differ only in frequency among populations. In contrast, most SNPs in which the less common allele is rarer (frequency <5%) have arisen since the major migration out of Africa, and insufficient time has elapsed for the allele to spread among all populations. These rarer alleles are much more likely to be specific to just one or a few human populations.

The African origin of humans predicts that more genetic variation should be found in Africa than anywhere else in the world. This is indeed the case, and genetic variation in human populations generally declines with greater distances from Africa (eg, Native Americans have less genetic diversity than do Asians or Europeans, who have less diversity than Africans). As expected, among SNPs that are not shared among major continental populations, more are found in African populations than in other continental populations. To better assess this diversity in genome-wide association studies (GWASs), SNP microarrays have been developed in which a larger number of African-specific SNPs have been included.

Genetic similarities among populations are generally correlated with their geographic location. Populations located close together are more likely to have common founders and are more likely to have shared migrants during their history. There are, however, numerous exceptions to this general correlation because of population movements, especially in the past several hundred years. In addition, because of our history of migration and genetic exchange, it is not usually possible to delineate precise boundaries between populations.

Because of these patterns, it is difficult to organize human genetic variation into discrete groups. For example, it has been common to use continental ancestry to group humans as Africans, Asians, Europeans, Native Americans, Australians, etc. These groups are often termed "races." The term "ethnicity" is sometimes used interchangeably with "race" but is also sometimes used for more specific ancestral designations (eg, Polish or Chinese). However, these labels can be inaccurate and misleading. Many North African populations are genetically more similar to Europeans than to sub-Saharan African populations, and some west Asian populations are more similar to Europeans than to East Asians. Furthermore, many human populations have undergone extensive migration and mixture during their recent history, causing highly variable ancestry. For example, while on average African Americans have about 20% European ancestry, some self-identified African Americans have considerably more than 50% European ancestry. Many human populations, such as Latinos, are not readily described by traditional racial or ethnic labels, since members of this population can have highly variable amounts of European, Native American, or African ancestry.

These patterns imply that individual ancestry is potentially a more accurate description than is designated membership in a broad category such as race or ethnicity. By analyzing thousands of SNPs (or several hundred selected SNPs that are known to vary greatly among populations), it is possible to estimate, at least approximately, the proportionate geographic ancestry of an individual. Such estimates can lead to a more accurate and appropriate assessment of an individual's genetic background when designing case-control disease studies.

## Genetic Variation and Phenotype

A relatively small number of SNPs vary substantially in frequency among human populations because of adaptation to specific environmental conditions. Examples include genes that affect hair, eye, and skin pigmentation; hereditary lactase persistence (which allows adults to digest dairy products); and adaptation to hypoxic conditions at high altitude. Many Mendelian diseases also vary in frequency among populations, typically as a result of founder effect, random genetic drift, or natural selection. Some notable examples are cystic fibrosis and hemochromatosis (higher prevalence rates in most European populations), Tay-Sachs and Gaucher diseases (higher prevalence in individuals of Ashkenazi Jewish descent), sickle cell disease (higher prevalence in Africans and circum-Mediterranean populations), and beta-thalassemia (higher prevalence in parts of Africa and southern Europe and South Asia). The latter two diseases are good examples in which natural selection, in this case for resistance to malaria, has significantly altered allele frequencies. Importantly, these diseases, like common SNPs, vary in frequency among populations but are not restricted to any specific human population.

A number of common diseases also vary in prevalence among human populations. Type 1 diabetes is especially common among individuals of European ancestry, for example, while type 2 diabetes is especially prevalent among some Native American and Hispanic populations. Prostate cancer, preterm birth, and hypertension are more common among African Americans. A substantial portion of this variation is due to nongenetic causes (eg, diet, exercise, access to health care), but there is also variation among populations in SNPs that are known to be associated with these diseases. At this time, these SNPs account for 10% to 50% of the variation in susceptibility to most common diseases, and the extent to which they vary in frequency among human populations is only partially known. As more information is gained about common and rare SNPs that are associated with common diseases, it may be possible to better estimate the genetic contribution to population variation in the prevalence of these diseases.

Physicians sometimes use their patient's self-reported ethnicity to help make decisions about diagnosis and treatment (eg, drug dosages, in which the optimal doses may differ, on average, among populations). There are now several examples in which direct testing of the genes that mediate drug response gives a more accurate assessment of optimum dosage in an individual patient than does ethnicity or race. As more such knowledge is gained, it can be anticipated that drug therapies will become more effective and less dependent on the use of sometimes misleading population categories.

**BIBLIOGRAPHY:**

1. Sachidanandam R, Weissman D, Schmidt SC, et al. A map of human genome sequence variation containing 1.42 million single nucleotide polymorphisms. *Nature*. 2001;409:928-933.

2. Lander ES. Initial impact of the sequencing of the human genome. *Nature*. 2011;470:187-197.

3. Li JZ, Absher DM, Tang H, et al. Worldwide human relationships inferred from genome-wide patterns of variation. *Science*. 2008;319:1100-1104.

4. Jorde LB, Watkins WS, Bamshad MJ, et al. The distribution of human genetic diversity: a comparison of mitochondrial, autosomal, and Y chromosome data. *Am J Hum Genet*. 2000;66:979-988.

5. Jakobsson M, Scholz SW, Scheet P, et al. Genotype, haplotype and copy-number variation in worldwide human populations. *Nature*. 2008;451:998-1003.

6. Gravel S, Henn BM, Gutenkunst RN, et al. Demographic history and rare allele sharing among human populations. *Proc Natl Acad Sci USA*. 2011;108(29):11983-11988.

7. Conrad DF, Jakobsson M, Coop G, et al. A worldwide survey of haplotype variation and linkage disequilibrium in the human genome. *Nat Genet*. 2006;38:1251-1260.

8. Durbin RM, Abecasis GR, Altshuler DL, et al. A map of human genome variation from population-scale sequencing. *Nature*. 2010;467:1061-1073.

9. Xing J, Watkins WS, Witherspoon DJ, et al. Fine-scaled human genetic structure revealed by SNP microarrays. *Genome Res*. 2009;19:815-825.

10. Sankar P, Cho MK. Genetics. Toward a new vocabulary of human genetic variation. *Science*. 2002;298:1337-1338.

11. Race, Ethnicity, and Genetics Working Group. The use of racial, ethnic, and ancestral categories in human genetics research. *Am J Hum Genet*. 2005;77:519-532.

12. Rotimi CN, Jorde LB. Ancestry and disease in the age of genomic medicine. *N Engl J Med*. 2010, 363:1551-1558.

13. Manolio TA, Collins FS, Cox NJ, et al. Finding the missing heritability of complex diseases. *Nature*. 2009;461:747-753.

14. The International Warfarin Pharmacogenetics Consortium. Estimation of the warfarin dose with clinical and pharmacogenetic data. *N Engl J Med*. 2009;360:753-764.

# 173 Population Genetics

Frederick R. Bieber

## KEY POINTS

- Application of population genetic principles is the key to the provision of traditional medical genetic services as it plays a role in
  - Determination of frequency of genetic diseases
  - Heterozygote carrier frequency estimation
  - Genetic disease risk prediction
  - Public health/epidemiology
  - Role of genes versus environment
  - Study of complex traits

## Number of Genotypes at a Single Locus

The number of genotypes at a locus in a population is defined by $n = k^2 + k/2$, where $k$ = # alleles at a specific locus

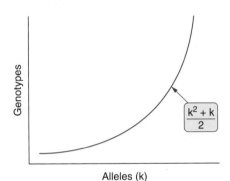

| Alleles at a Single Locus | Possible Genotypes in the Population |
|---|---|
| **Example:** 2 | 3 |
| 3 | 6 |
| 4 | 10 |
| 5 | 15 |
| 6 | 21 |
| 7 | 28 |
| 8 | 36 |

## Allele Frequencies

Actual allele frequencies in a population sample can be determined by the counting method. First, perform genotype studies on a randomly selected group of unrelated individuals, as shown in the example below using short tandem repeat (STR) genotype data:

**Example:**
- STR genotype data (N = 129 individuals)
  Allele designations "14-20" refer to # of STRs at a particular locus

### # Individuals with each genotype

| | 14 | 15 | 16 | 17 | 18 | 19 | 20 | Allele Frequency |
|---|---|---|---|---|---|---|---|---|
| 14 | 9 | | | | | | | 75 |
| 15 | 3 | 0 | | | | | | 6 |
| 16 | 19 | 1 | 1 | | | | | 46 |
| 17 | 23 | 1 | 14 | 9 | | | | 72 |
| 18 | 6 | 0 | 3 | 10 | 4 | | | 31 |
| 19 | 6 | 1 | 7 | 3 | 2 | 2 | | 23 |
| 20 | 0 | 0 | 0 | 3 | 2 | 0 | 0 | 5 |

From the data above, the frequency of the "14" allele in this sample = 75/258, and that of the "17" allele = 72/258.

**Standard Formula Notation Used in Population Genetics:**
- $f(A) = p$
- $f(a) = q$
- $f(A/a) = 2pq$
  The sum total of all alleles at a locus = 1
- $p + q = 1$
  Sum total of all genotypes in a population = 1
- $(p + q)^2 = 1$
- $(p + q)^2 = p^2 + 2pq + q^2 = 1$, where
- $p^2 = f(AA)$
- $2pq = f(Aa)$
- $q^2 = f(aa)$
- $p + q + r + \cdots + n = 1$ (sum of all allele frequencies adds to unity)
- $(p + q + r + \cdots + n)^2 = 1$ (sum of all genotype frequencies adds to unity)
- Genotype frequencies stabilize after one generation of random mating and remain constant with several assumptions (large population size, random mating, no mutation, selection, migration)
  - Change in allele or genotypic frequencies can occur if above assumptions deviate widely.

**Calculation of Allele Frequencies:** At a locus with only two alleles (A and a) calculation of allele frequencies can be performed knowing the number of individuals who are homozygous for the "A" and the "a" allele and how many are heterozygous. This relationship is shown below:

- Frequency of A, known as $p = f(AA) + \frac{1}{2} f(Aa)$
- Frequency of a, known as $q = f(aa) + \frac{1}{2} f(Aa)$

- $p + q = f(AA) + f(aa) + f(Aa) = 1$
- so $q = 1 - p$
- $p + q = 1$
- $p = 1 - q$, or $q = 1 - p$
- $(p + q)^2 = 1$
- $2pq \sim 2q$, for rare values of q

### Example:

Assume that the frequency of cystic fibrosis (CF) is 1/2500 liveborn infants in a large metropolitan area. We can calculate the expected frequency of heterozygote carriers in the population, first by solving for q, as follows:

The observed frequency of affected infants (aa) = $q^2$ = 1/2500 = 4/10,000 = 0.0004

If $q^2 = 0.0004$, then q = 0.02

Then the expected frequency of heterozygous carriers ($2pq \sim 2q$), or $(2 \times 0.02) = 0.04$ or 1/25

Thus, 1/25 individuals would be expected to be heterozygote carriers of a CF allele.

### Hardy-Weinberg Equilibrium:

- The Hardy-Weinberg equilibrium (HWE) predicts that the diploid genotype frequencies in diploid mating populations are found in predictable, based on individual allele frequencies.
- Demonstration that a population (or sample) is in HWE allows
  - Calculation of predicted genotype frequencies in a population
  - Certain probability calculations using the product rule
- Note that a population might not be in HWE if there are major deviations from important assumptions (eg, regarding population size, random mating, mutation, selection, migration)

### Tests to Determine If Allele Frequency Data Meets H/W Expectations:

- Exact test
- Likelihood ratio test
- Heterozygote or homozygote ratio
- Chi-square

### ☞Properties of a Population in Hardy Weinberg (Genetic) Equilibrium:

- Maximum heterozygosity is attained when p = q
  Take dH = 2 (1 − q) q, with regard to q
  $dH/dq = d(2q − 2q2)/dq = 2 − 4q$
  Set d = 0 (maximum likelihood function), to solve for q
  Then q = 0.50
- As p, q values move away from equality, the heterozygote class diminishes
  Where $2pq = p^2$, $2p(1 − p) = p^2$, then $p = 2/3$
  Beyond which $p^2 > 2pq > q^2$
- As rarer allele becomes less frequent, the heterozygote class carries greater proportion of that allele than does the homozygote class.
  $H/R = 2pq/q^2 = 2p/q$

### ☞Ratio of Heterozygotes to Homozygotes: The table below shows that in a population in HWE the expected ratio of heterozygotes to homozygotes for the recessive allele ($2pq/q2$) changes depending on the frequency of the recessive allele.

| q | $q^2$ | 2pq | $2pq/q^2$ |
|------|----------|------|------|
| .5 | .25 | .50 | 2 |
| .1 | .01 | .20 | 20 |
| .01 | .0001 | .02 | 200 |
| .001 | .000001 | .002 | 2000 |

**Deviations From Hardy-Weinberg Equilibrium:** While the HWE predicts stable genotype frequencies over many generations of mating, a number of factors can influence a change of allele frequencies and, by extension, the resulting genotype frequencies.

- **Nonrandom mating**
  - Population substructure
  - HWE predicts that a population will reach equilibrium genotypic frequencies after just one single generation of random mating. Nonrandom mating within a population would alter the genotype frequencies depending on the nature of the mating structure. Assortative mating structures include positive assortative mating, negative assortative mating, and inbreeding.
  - *Inbreeding* refers to the mating of individuals who share recent common ancestors. Inbreeding tends to result in an increase in *homozygosity* for all genes.
    - **The coefficient of relationship (R)** can be computed to determine the degree to which two individuals share parts of their genome due to common ancestry. It describes the *degree of kinship* in numerical terms. The value of R can be calculated based on the method of path analysis in which Mendelian expectations are used to compute the chance that a particular allele would be expected to be shared by individuals with knowledge of the pedigree information available, and then by extension to the whole nuclear genome.
    - **The inbreeding coefficient (F)** is computed for offspring of two individuals to estimate the *expected* percentage of *homozygosity* in the genome arising from a particular mating.
    - The value of F can be computed as F = ½ R. Values of R and F are shown below for common matings.

| Coefficient of Relationship of Two Persons (R) | Relationship of the Two Persons | Inbreeding Coefficient of Their Children (F = ½ R) |
|------|------|------|
| ½ | Parent-offspring | ¼ |
| ½ | Full siblings | ¼ |
| ¼ | Grandparent-grandchild | ⅛ |
| ¼ | Half siblings | ⅛ |
| ¼ | Aunt/uncle-nephew/ niece | ⅛ |
| ¼ | Double first cousins | ⅛ |
| ⅛ | Great grandparent-great grandchild | 1/16 |
| ⅛ | First cousins | 1/16 |

- **Mutation**
  - Responsible for introduction of new alleles
  - New alleles and their frequencies can be affected by selection and genetic drift
- *Mutation* by itself may have but a small effect on allele frequencies, as mutation rates at single nucleotides are often on the order $10^{-4}$ to $10^{-8}$ per locus per generation. Mutational changes serve to maintain rare alleles in a population even in the face of negative selective (eg, lethal mutations). Positive selective

advantage may favor some mutations if they increase genetic fitness (breeding or survival advantage).

- A general formula predicting the effects of mutation on allele frequency is shown below:

$$\Delta p = p_t - p_{t-1} = -u_{p_{t-1}}$$

- Note that allele A decreases and allele a increases in proportion to u
- $\Delta p$ gets smaller as p itself decreases
- After n generations, $p_n = p_0 e^{-nu}$ (where e = nlog)
- Thus, even after 10,000 generations with a low mutation rate (u = $10^{-5}$), the value of p decreases very slightly from fixation to about 90%.

$$p = p_0 e - (10^4) \times (10^{-5}) = p_0 e^{-0.1} = 0.904 p_0$$

- **Migration**
  - Genetic drift
  - Founder effects

Migration of individuals (leaving from or entering into a mating pool) can result in genotype frequency changes in one or more populations. Population substructure within a larger population can result in a reduction of *heterozygosity* in the overall *population*, even if the subpopulations are in HWE. This is known as the Wahlund effect, which can be the result of cultural or geographic barriers to random mating, followed by stochastic changes in allele frequencies in the smaller subgroups.

- **Small population size**
  - Random drift can be observed in small population groups due to stochastic effects or sampling errors. Allele frequencies can change rapidly in small contained groups, leading to **founder effects** when a small number of individuals with high genetic fitness (fertility) produce larger number of offspring.
- **Selection**
  - Can alter allele frequencies, often quickly
  - Can be directional, leading to loss of an allele, or balancing
- **Applications of population genetics to medical genetics**
  - Calculation of allele frequencies
  - Calculation of genotype frequencies
  - Carrier frequency estimates
    - Genetic disease risk prediction
    - Study of complex traits
  - Human evolution studies
    - Migration, admixture
  - Identity testing
  - Paternity testing
  - Kinship reconstruction
- **Parentage testing and kinship analysis**
  - Kinship analysis is performed routinely to assist in resolution of questions relating to parentage, immigration and probate disputes, and in human remains and missing persons' identification.
  - In the most straightforward of applications, paternity testing involves the analysis of numerous genetic markers (typically STRs) from a parentage trio (typically a known mother, her child[ren], and one or more possible biologic father).
  - After such DNA-based typing a parentage index (PI) is calculated as a likelihood ratio, that compares a *numerator* which computes that chance of observing the genotypes of the trio given that the tested male is the biologic father,

compared to the *denominator* which computes the chance of observing the genotypes if a randomly selected man is the biologic father. This likelihood ratio is commonly referred to as a paternity index. If the numerator greatly exceeds that the denominator then the result favors parentage, or other defined biologic relationship.

**Future Directions:**

- Moving into the era of genomic medicine (precision medicine)
  - Need to learn more about population specific allele and genotype frequencies
- Medical Anthropology
  - Study of human migration
- Identify loci valuable for genetic identity testing
  - Y-STR, Y-SNP, and mitochondrial DNA (mtDNA) population data
  - Define population structure
  - Medical forensics

**BIBLIOGRAPHY:**

1. AABB. *Guidance for Standards for Relationship Testing Laboratories*. 9th ed. Bethesda, Maryland: AABB; 2009.
2. Awadalla P, Gauthier J, Myers RA, et al. Direct measure of the de novo mutation rate in autism and schizophrenia cohorts. *Am J Hum Genet*. 2010;87:316-324.
3. Bieber FR, Brenner C, Lazer D. Finding criminals through DNA of their relatives. *Science*. 2006;312:1315.
4. Bailey-Wilson JE, Ballantyne J, Baum H. Bieber FR, et al. http://www.sciencemag.org/content/310/5751/1122.summary-coresp-1#corresp-1 LG.
5. Biesecker LG, Bailey-Wilson JE, Ballantyne J, et al. Epidemiology. DNA identifications after the 9/11 World Trade Center attack. *Science*. 2005;310(5751):1122.
6. Buckleton J, Triggs C, Walsh S. *Forensic DNA Evidence Interpretation*. Boca Raton, FL: CRC Press; 2005.
7. Yu C, Zhang S, Zhou C, Sile S. A likelihood ratio test of population Hardy-Weinberg equilibrium for case-control studies. *Genet Epidemiol*. 2009;33(3):275.
8. Consortium GP, Abecasis GR, Altshuler D, et al. A map of human genome variation from population-scale sequencing. *Nature*. 2010;467:1061-1073.
9. Evett I, Weir B. Interpreting DNA evidence. *Statistical Genetics for Forensic Scientists*. Sunderland, Massachusetts: Sinauer Associates; 1998.
10. Fisher RA. On the interpretation of $\chi^2$ from contingency tables, and the calculation of P. *J R Stat Soc*. 1922;85(1):87.
11. Fisher RA. *Statistical Methods for Research Workers*. London, UK: Oliver and Boyd; 1954.
12. Gjertson DW, Brenner CH, Baur MP, et al. ISFG: recommendations on biostatistics in paternity testing. *Forensic Sci Int Genet*. 2007;1(3-4):223.
13. Hardy GH. Mendelian proportions in a mixed population. *Science*. 1908;28(706):49.
14. Roach JC, Glusman G, Smit AF, et al. Analysis of genetic inheritance in a family quartet by whole-genome sequencing. *Science*. 2010;328:636-639.
15. Slooten K. Validation of DNA-based identification software by computation of pedigree likelihood ratios. *Forensic Sci Int Genet*. 2011;5(4):308.
16. Zhou JJ, Lange K, Papp JC, Sinsheimer JS. A heterozygote-homozygote test of Hardy-Weinberg equilibrium. *Eur J Hum Genet*. 2009;17(11):1495.

# 174 Transplantation Genetics and Genomics: Alloreactivity After Hematopoietic Stem Cell Transplantation

Jessica C. Shand and Terry Fry

## KEY POINTS

- *Disease summary:*
  - Hematopoietic stem cell transplantation (HSCT) is a curative therapy for a number of malignant and nonmalignant conditions including leukemia, bone marrow failure, severe immunodeficiencies, and other disorders involving the hematopoietic system such as thalassemia and sickle cell anemia.
  - The HSCT procedure involves multiple phases including a preparative regimen consisting of cytotoxic and immune-depleting agents followed by infusion of a hematopoietic graft. Recovery of neutrophils and platelets typically occurs within 2 to 4 weeks but full immunologic recovery can take months to more than a year.
  - Graft sources currently being used include bone marrow, peripheral blood stem cells collected via an apheresis procedure, and cryopreserved umbilical cord blood.
  - Graft-versus-host disease (GVHD) represents one of the major causes of morbidity and mortality after allogeneic HSCT. However, donor-versus-recipient alloreactivity can also contribute to the curative potential of HSCT via the graft-versus-leukemia (GVL) reaction.
  - Degree of donor and recipient matching at the human leukocyte antigens (HLA) system encoded on chromosome 6 has a significant impact on transplant outcomes including the risk of GVHD and relapse of malignancy.
  - GHVD can occur even when donor and recipient are fully HLA-matched as in the matched sibling donor setting illustrating the importance of other non-HLA minor histocompatibility antigens (miHAs) such as those encoded on the Y chromosome.
  - Donor killer immunoglobulin-like receptor genotype encoded on chromosome 19 can also influence the potency of the GVL effect and the risk of leukemia relapse.
  - Polymorphisms in other genes such as those encoding cytokines, cytokine receptors, and innate immune response genes among others can also influence transplant outcomes.

- *Genome-wide associations:*
  - The application of genome-wide association study (GWAS) to HSCT is relatively recent. Two studies have demonstrated that these approaches can be used to identify single-nucleotide polymorphisms (SNPs) that modulate outcomes following HSCT. Future studies will be needed to validate these findings in larger populations.

- *Pharmacogenomics:*
  - Patients are frequently on multiple medications during HSCT including agents with substantial toxicity. Metabolism and clearance of many of these agents can be affected by pharmacogenomic variants (Table 174-1). Many of the medications used in HSCT are dose adjusted to achieve a target range.

## Diagnostic Criteria and Clinical Characteristics

Primary factors affecting outcome after HSCT are GVHD, infection, organ toxicity, and relapse or recurrence of the underlying disease for which the HSCT is being performed. GVHD is a disorder arising from immunologic targeting of recipient tissues by donor cells. Due to better supportive care resulting in lower mortality from preparative regimen-related toxicity or infection, GVHD and relapse have become the primary causes of poor outcome. However, despite GVHD-associated morbidity and mortality, it is well established that donor immune reactivity against leukemia (the GVL effect) improves survival. Therefore, a major focus of HSCT research has sought to separate the harmful effects of GVHD from the beneficial effects of GVL at the molecular level. Genomics has played a role in this and other aspects of

HSCT for over two decades, since the initial observation that matching at the HLA system resulted in reduced GVHD and improved outcomes.

### Diagnostic Criteria for Graft-Versus-Host Disease:

**Diagnostic evaluation should include at least one of the following:**

- Scoring for GVHD is clinical, however, due to the large differential diagnosis and implications of delayed diagnosis for some of these conditions (eg, infection), prompt histologic confirmation of GVHD is often required to ensure appropriate therapy is initiated in a timely manner (Fig. 174-1).
- The diagnostic evaluation depends on the organ system involved.
- When there is cutaneous involvement, skin biopsies can be performed rapidly.
- Biopsies of the gastrointestinal tract or liver may also be necessary in the event that there are no skin manifestations or the skin biopsies are inconclusive.

**Table 174-1 Selected Pharmacogenetic Considerations in HSCT**

| Gene | Associated Medications | Variants | Effect |
|---|---|---|---|
| *MTHFR* (5,10-methylene tetrahydrofolate reductase) | Methotrexate | 677T 1298C | ↓GVHD ↑GVHD |
| *GST* (glutathione *S*-transferase) | Busulfan | GSTM1, GSTT1 GSTA1 | ↑VOD ↓Busulfan clearance |
| *CYP3A5* | Cyclosporine, tacrolimus | +6986AA rs4646450 C/C | ↑Cyclosporine levels ↑Tacrolimus levels |
| *ABCB1* ATP-binding cassette, subfamily B (MDR/TAP), member 1 | Cyclosporine, tacrolimus | C1236T lack of +1236CC | ↑Neurotoxicity ↓Treatment-related mortality |

- Chronic GVHD typically manifests with symptoms analogous to those seen in autoimmune diseases such as scleroderma and lupus. Biopsies of involved organs as well as evaluation of organ-targeted antibodies can aid in the diagnosis.

**And the absence of**

- Infections are the major entity in the differential diagnosis of GVHD as post-HSCT patients are highly immunocompromised and the symptomatology for both is nonspecific and overlapping.

- Sinusoidal obstructive syndrome (also known as veno-occlusive disease) must also be considered in the setting of hyperbilirubinemia.

**Clinical Characteristics:** GVHD can either be acute or chronic. Initially, acute and chronic GVHD were distinguished by the time in which they occurred following HSCT (acute <100 days). It is now recognized that these entities represent different clinical and pathologic conditions and should be distinguished on this basis

| Extend of organ involvement | | | |
|---|---|---|---|
| **Stage** | **Skin** | **Liver** | **Gut** |
| 1 | Rash on <25% of skin[a] | Bilirubin 2–3 mg/dL[b] | Diarrhea >500 mL/d[c] or persistent nausea[d] |
| 2 | Rash on 25%–50% of skin | Bilirubin 3–6 mg/dL | Diarrhea >1000 mL/d |
| 3 | Rash on >50% of skin | Bilirubin 6–15 mg/dL | Diarrhea >1500 mL/d |
| 4 | Generalized erythroderma with bullous formation | Bilirubin >15 mg/dL | Severe abdominal pain with or without ileus |
| **Grade**[e] | | | |
| I | Stage 1–2 | None | None |
| II | Stage 3 or | Stage 1 or | Stage 1 |
| III | - | Stages 2–3 or | Stages 2–4 |
| IV[f] | Stage 4 | Stage 4 | - |

a. Use "rule of nines" or burn chart to determine extent of rash.

b. Range given as total bilirubin. Downgrade one stage if an additional cause of elevated bilirubin has been documented.

c. Volume of diarrhea applies to adults. For pediatric patients, the volume of diarrhea should be based on body surface area. Downgrade on stage if an additional cause of diarrhea has been documented.

d. Persistent nausea with histologic evidence of GVHD in the stomach or duodenum.

e. Criteria for grading given as minimum degree of organ involvement required to confer that grade.

f. Grade IV may also include lesser organ involvement with an extreme decrease in performance status.

**Figure 174-1** Center for International Blood and Marrow Transplantation Research. 'Acute GVHD Scoring System

rather than time post-HSCT. Acute GVHD is graded according to a number of scoring systems with the modified Glucksberg criteria most commonly used (Fig. 174-1). The target organs utilized are skin, liver (hyperbilirubinemia), and gastrointestinal tract. Chronic GNHD was originally characterized as limited (skin only) or extensive (other organs systems besides skin involved) but the recently developed National Institute of Health (NIH) Consensus Criteria is more predictive of outcome.

## Management and Treatment

**Management:** Prevention of GVHD is one of the most important considerations in HSCT. Donor lymphocytes (mainly T cells) contained in the graft and reactive against the recipient are the primary cells contributing to acute GVHD with inflammation of the target organs from the preparative regimen initiating the cascade of events leading to GVHD. Removal of T cells is effective at preventing GVHD but results in prolonged lymphocyte deficiency and increased risk of graft failure, infection, and relapse of malignancy. The most common type of transplant utilizes a T cell-containing unmanipulated graft with immunosuppression given to the recipient for GVHD prophylaxis. Typical prophylactic regimens include, but are not limited to, a calcineurin inhibitor (cyclosporine A or tacrolimus) plus another agent such as methotrexate, mycophenolate mofetil or sirolimus. T-cell–targeted antibodies such as antithymocyte globulin or alemtuzumab (anti-CD52) are also used, most commonly with unrelated donors where there is likely to be greater genetic disparity and potential alloreactivity (see section later for a discussion of donor-recipient matching). Although the molecular risk factors for chronic GVHD have not been well characterized, acute GVHD represents the greatest clinical risk factor. It should be noted that the development of acute or chronic GVHD is associated with a reduced risk of relapse in patients with malignancy. Thus, the intensity of GVHD prophylaxis is often tailored based on the underlying condition for which the HSCT is being performed.

**Therapeutics:** Corticosteroids are the mainstay of therapy for GVHD. Topical steroids can be used when GVHD is limited to the skin but other organ involvement generally requires systemic therapy. Methylprednisolone at 1 to 4 mg/kg/d is a typical regimen, often combined with a calcineurin inhibitor. There is limited data indicating that doses of corticosteroids higher than 2 mg/kg/d are more effective. Response typically occurs in 2 to 5 days but approximately 50% of patients will be steroid refractory. In this situation second-line therapy depends on the clinical setting and what agents are already being used in a given patient. Mycophenolate mofetil and sirolimus are often considered as part of the second-line therapy. Monoclonal antibodies targeting T cells, interferon gamma, tumor necrosis factor (TNF), and the interleukin-2 receptor have also been used. While responses to these agents occur, results in larger series have largely been disappointing. Thus, numerous experimental approaches are being explored for steroid-refractory acute GVHD.

☞**PHARMACOGENETICS:** Many of the medications used in HSCT are dose adjusted based on levels. Busulfan pharmacokinetics are often measured with the first dose and adjustments made to achieve a target exposure. In addition, calcineurin inhibitors and sirolimus are dosed to target trough levels. There is more recent data that trough levels of mycophenolate and its metabolites can predict toxicity. Nonetheless, there is extensive literature on the impact of both donor and recipient genetic polymorphisms on outcomes (Table 174-1).

## Molecular Genetics and Molecular Mechanism

***Genetic Testing:***

☞**MAJOR HISTOCOMPATIBILITY ANTIGENS (HUMAN LEUKOCYTE ANTIGENS):** HSCT was one of the first conditions in which genetic testing was utilized clinically following the identification of the highly polymorphic major histocompatibility locus in mice and the recognition that donor-recipient disparity at this locus resulted in "wasting syndrome" following bone marrow transplantation. The human counterpart is known as the HLA complex (located at chromosome 6p21.3) and is among the most polymorphic loci in the genome. The first successful HSCT in humans was performed in 1968 using a presumed full haplotype-matched sibling donor. With the advent of unrelated donor transplantation, it was recognized that the incidence of acute GVHD was directly linked to the degree of mismatch at the class I HLA loci A and B and the class II locus, DRB1 with the lowest risk in "6 out of 6" ("6/6") matched transplants. Initially, typing was performed using panels of HLA-reactive antibodies, known as serologic typing. Polymerase chain reaction (PCR)-based typing has identified increasing numbers of HLA allotypes. It was subsequently recognized that mismatch at additional HLA loci (the class I HLA-C and class II HLA-DQB1) resulted in the ability to identify 10/10 matched unrelated donors. Currently, "high-resolution" typing can distinguish over 1700 HLA-A alleles, 2300 HLA-B alleles, 1200 HLA-C alleles, and 150 HLA-DRB1 alleles (http://hla.alleles.org/). Optimal selection of an unrelated donor involves high-resolution typing at HLA-A, -B, -C, -DRB1, and -DQB1. Some studies have indicated that transplants using donors matched at all of these loci carry an approximately equivalent risk of GVHD to transplants using haplotype-matched related donors. Recently, match at the class II locus, DPB1 (resulting in a 12/12 match), has also been shown to be associated with a reduced risk of GVHD although the likelihood of identifying such donors from the unrelated registry is extremely low except for selected populations such as Japan where certain haplotypes are highly prevalent.

☞**MINOR HISTOCOMPATIBILITY ANTIGENS:** The fact that GHVD still occurs in up to 25% of sibling donors fully matched at the major HLA loci presumes that other so-called miHAs can serve as target antigens for GVHD. A number of miHAs have been identified in humans and have been shown to contribute to the development of acute and chronic GVHD. They have also demonstrated therapeutic potential in the GVL effect. The genes encoding a complex of male-specific antigens on the Y chromosome are among the best-studied miHAs. It has been observed that male recipients of female bone marrow transplant have both higher risks of GVHD and lower risks of relapse. Another prototypic miHA is HA-1, a nonapeptide with a polymorphic allele (HA-1$^H$) that binds the HLA-*0201 locus with greater affinity than other variants, creating the potential for GVHD in HA-1$^H$ recipients with mismatched donors. Donor-recipient mismatch at loci with homozygous gene deletions, such as in the *UGT2B17* locus (which is deleted in ~30% of Caucasians with European ancestry), have also shown a potential for increased risk of GVHD depending on the manner in which the associated peptides are processed and presented to donor antigen-presenting cells. Small, heterogeneous studies have shown variable associations of HA-1 and *UGT2B17* mismatch with GVHD, suggesting a need for larger studies that account for immunogenetic

**Table 174-2  Selected Gene Polymorphisms That May Affect HSCT Outcomes**

| Candidate Gene (location) | Associated Variant | Functional Significance | Associated Disease Phenotype | Selected Study |
|---|---|---|---|---|
| **Immunoregulatory genes** | | | | |
| IL10 (1q31-32); IL10Ra (11q23); IL10Rb (21q22.11) | Promoter microsatellite polymorphisms | Increased level of Th2-type immunosuppressive cytokine | Decreased aGVHD | Goussetis et al. *Bone Marrow Transplant.* May 2008;41(9):821-826. |
| TNF (6p21.3) | Microsatellite SNPs (position -308) | Increased secretion of proinflammatory cytokine targeting CTLs to gut and skin | Increased aGVHD (grade II-IV) | Goyal et al. *Biol Blood Marrow Transplant.* Jul 2010;16(7):927-936. |
| IL23R (1p31.2) | SNP (1142G>A) Arg381Gln | Decreased level of Th17-type proinflammatory cytokine from donor T cells | Decreased aGVHD (grade II-IV) Decreased risk of infection | Elmaagcli AH et al. *Bone Marrow Transplant.* May 2008;41(9):821-826. |
| MBL2 (10q11.2); MASP2 (1p36.3-p36.2) | Multiple variants | Recognition of fungal surface proteins | Increased risk of invasive fungal infection post-HSCT | Grannell M et al. *Exp Hematol.* Oct 2006;34(10):1435-1441. |
| **Minor histocompatibility antigens** | | | | |
| HY complex (Yq11.1-11.3) | Polymorphism with X chromosome | Recognized by female CTLs as alloantigen in skin graft rejection and GVHD | aGVHD, cGVHD, enhanced GVT/GVL, decreased risk relapse | Markiewics et al. *Bone Marrow Transplant.* Feb 2009;43(4):293-300. |
| HMHA1 (19p13.3) | Nonhomologous coding SNP | Recognized as alloantigen by donor CTLs | aGVHD | Tait et al. *Transplant Proc.* 2001;33:1760-1761. |
| UGT2B17 (14q13) | Homozygous deletion | Processed as alloantigen by donor APCs | aGVHD, cGHVD | McCarrol et al. *Nat Genet.* Dec 2009;41(12):1341-1344. |
| TYMP (22q13) | Nonsynonymous coding SNP (Arg → His) | Alternatively translated peptide recognized by allo-CTL | aGVHD, enhanced GVL | Slager EH et al. *Blood.* Jun 15 2006;107(12):4954-4960. |

SNP, single-nucleotide polymorphism; cSNP, coding single-nucleotide polymorphism; aGVHD, acute graft-versus-host disease; cGVHD, chronic graft-versus-host disease; APC, antigen-presenting cells; CTL, cytotoxic T lymphocytes.

and other factors when determining risk. Examples of miHAs are presented in Table 174-2. Recent GWASs will likely identify additional miHAs of clinical significance and these are discussed later.

☞**POLYMORPHISMS IN IMMUNE-RESPONSE GENES:** The post-transplant environment represents a unique milieu in which inflammation from the conditioning regimen, alloreactivity, and products from bacteria such as lipopolysaccharide result in GVHD. Donor and host factors that determine the immune response are central to this process. Recent studies suggest that polymorphisms in genes involved in cytokine or chemokine expression, regulation of innate immunity and susceptibility to opportunistic infection may produce differential GVHD and relapse outcomes. Representative examples are provided in Table 174-2, though continued large external validation series are needed to confirm their biologic and prognostic significance. There is consistent evidence that polymorphisms in the *IL10* promoter increase secretion of this immunoregulatory cytokine and can decrease the risk of acute GVHD. There is also strong evidence that variants in TNF, a key proinflammatory mediator of alloreactivity-directed tissue pathology,

significantly increase the risk of developing acute GVHD after adjusting for comorbid clinical factors. Mutations in innate pattern recognition receptors for bacterial and fungal proteins, such as mannose-binding lectin 2 (*MBL2*) and nucleotide oligomerization domain-like receptors (*NOD2*) may also have significant effects on transplant-associated mortality. Certain polymorphisms appear to have different effects in particular populations, as evidenced by a recent Japanese study demonstrating that polymorphisms in *NOD2*, a gene involved in pattern recognition of bacterial proteins, may increase the susceptibility to severe acute GVHD in Caucasian but not Japanese populations.

☞**KILLER IMMUNOGLOBULIN-LIKE RECEPTORS:** Like T cells, natural killer (NK) cells can also contribute to the GVL effect following HSCT. However, unlike T cells, which recognize antigen using a highly specific, genetically rearranged receptor, NK cells mediate cytotoxicity based on lack of self-recognition. The inhibitory receptors on NK cells that recognize self-antigens (often HLA-C molecules) thus reducing NK reactivity are encoded by a polymorphic set of receptors known as killer immunoglobulin-like receptors (KIRs) on chromosome 19p13. The number of inhibitory receptors available is dependent on the KIR haplotypes that have been shown to contribute to risk of autoimmunity and viral clearance. In HSCT, donor KIR reactivity based on donor KIR haplotype and the presence or absence of ligands for donor KIR on recipient tissues (including malignant cells) influences the risk of relapse. Increasing complexity in this system such as the importance of activating receptors some of which are also encoded on chormosome 19p13 is recognized. Ongoing multi-institutional trials are prospectively evaluating whether KIR haplotype can be used as additional criteria in donor selection to reduce relapse risk.

### Future Directions:

☞**GWAS:** Refinements in HLA typing and, in particular, identification of additional important loci, have improved the ability to select optimal donors. Furthermore, additional polymorphic loci encoding immune response genes in both donors and recipients that contribute to transplant outcomes have also been identified and these genes may be used as additional donor selection criteria in the future. These candidate gene approaches have improved outcomes following HSCT such that results using extremely well-matched unrelated donors (when available) are similar to matched sibling donors. Two recent GWAS have identified additional factors that may contribute to transplant outcomes. It remains to be seen whether validation studies in larger populations will confirm the results of these studies.

### BIBLIOGRAPHY:

1. Miller JS, Warren EH, Ritz J, et al. NCI First International Workshop on the Biology, Prevention and Treatment of Relapse after Allogeneic Hematopoietic Stem Cell Transplantation: report from the Committee on the Biology Underlying Recurrence of Malignant Disease Following Allogeneic HSCT: graft-versus-tumor/leukemia reaction. *Biol Blood Marrow Transplant*. 2010;16:565-586.

2. Cahn JY, Klein JP, Lee CJ, et al. Prospective evaluation of 2 acute graft-versus-host (GVHD) grading systems: a joint SociétéFrançaise de Greffe de Moëlle et ThérapieCellulaire (SFGM-TC), Dana Farber Cancer Institute (DFCI), and International Bone Marrow Transplant Registry (IBMTR) prospective study. *Blood*. 2005;106:1495-1500.

3. Hansen J. Genomic and proteomic analysis of allogeneic hematopoietic cell transplant outcome. Seeking greater understanding of the pathogenesis of GVHD mortality. *Biol Blood Marrow Transplant*. 2009;15:1-7.

4. Ogawa S, Matsubara A, Onizuka M, et al. Exploration of the genetic basis of GVHD by Genetic Association Studies. *Biol Blood Marrow Transplant*. 2009;15;39-41.

5. Mullally A and Ritz J. Beyond HLA: the significance of genomic variation for allogeneic hematopoietic stem cell transplantation. *Blood*. 2007;109:1355.

6. Hansen JA, Chien JW, Warren EH, et al. Defining genetic risk for graft-versus-host disease and mortality following allogeneic hematopoietic stem cell transplantation. *Curr Opin Hematol*. 2010;17:483-492.

7. Morishima S, Ogawa S, Matsubara A, et al. Impact of highly conserved haplotype on acute graft-versus-host disease. *Blood*. 2010;115:4664-4672.

8. Mullighan CG, Bardy PG. New directions in the genomics of allogeneic hematopoietic stem cell transplantation. *Biol Blood Marrow Transplant*. 2007;13:127-144.

## Supplementary Information

### Alternative Names:
- Bone Marrow Transplantation
- Umbilical Cord Blood Transplantation
- Peripheral Blood Transplantation

*Key Words:* Graft-versus-host disease, bone marrow, alloreactivity, human leukocyte antigen, minor histocompatibility antigens, natural killer cells

# 175 Personalized Medicine in Clinical Practice

Omri Gottesman and Erwin Bottinger

## KEY POINTS

- *Progress in research:* The past decade has yielded unprecedented new insights into the role of genetics in disease risk and treatment response. Some of these insights are ready to be utilized in clinical care.
- *Focus for initial translation:* Pharmacogenomics, common disease risk stratification, and rare diseases are the three main conceptual areas being addressed for initial implementation strategies of personalized medicine.
- *Barriers and solutions:* Barriers to translation include a lack of provider education and resources to implement this new knowledge. Solutions involve incorporating personalized medicine into undergraduate and postgraduate curricula and the development of computational resources to simultaneously analyze data and evidence to provide useable clinical decision support at the point of care.

## Background

Following a decade of extraordinary advances in genomics and healthcare information technology, a series of fundamental changes in medical practice are coming, promising to transform the way in which health care is delivered, transitioning to the era of Personalized Medicine.

Our knowledge and understanding of the genetic influences on common disease risk and therapeutic efficacy of pharmacologic agents has increased dramatically in the past decade. Since the completion of the Human Genome Project in 2003, genomics research has exploded, yielding an evergrowing number of genomic variants that are associated with an individual's risk for a disease or their response to a medication. This began in earnest with the development of high-throughput genotyping technology and the subsequent success of genome-wide association studies (GWASs) in identifying large numbers of genomic variants with potential clinical utility. The most common genetic variations among people are single-nucleotide polymorphisms (SNPs) ("snips"). Each SNP denotes a difference in a single nucleotide. For example, in a stretch of DNA, a SNP may replace the nucleotide adenine (A) with guanine (G). A phenotype is an observable or measurable characteristic of an individual, such as height, weight, blood pressure, lipid levels, a disease including its manifestations, or response to medication. Comparison of the frequencies of SNPs between cases and controls for a given phenotype has yielded a large number of variants that are associated with risk for a wide range of phenotypes including cardiovascular disease, diabetes, kidney disease, hyperlipidemia, and hypertension, many of which have been replicated successfully in multiple populations. This phenomenon is likely to continue for some time as the $1000 genome nears reality and comprehensive individual genotype and molecular ("omics") data becomes the norm in clinical care. Today we stand on the brink of a paradigm shift in health care, transitioning from the era of population-based medicine to the era of Personalized Medicine.

Personalized medicine aims to optimize the health care provided to an individual by basing decisions about their care on all available patient data, including genomic, molecular, clinical, and environmental data. This represents a sea change from the utilitarian approaches of evidence-based medicine to date. On the whole, current clinical guidelines tend to summarize evidence that is applicable on a population level. As an example, the UK National Institute for Health and Clinical Excellence (NICE) recommends that the first-line treatment for elevated blood pressure (>140/90 mm Hg) in a Caucasian male under the age of 55 is an angiotensin-converter enzyme (ACE) inhibitor. Whilst this recommendation is based on the best available evidence, the evidence considers what the best treatment option is for a group, rather than an individual. Because variations in individuals' genetic profiles may correlate with differences in how individuals develop diseases and respond to treatment, personalized medicine has the potential to facilitate the tailoring of health care to the individual. In the example above, rather than recommending treatment for any Caucasian male under the age of 55 with high blood pressure, personalized medicine would aim to recommend a specific drug at a specific dose with a specific blood pressure threshold for starting treatment in a specific individual.

## From Base Pairs to Bedside—the Road to Implementation

The transition of both genomics and personalized medicine from the realms of research into mainstream clinical care has begun. As the concept of integrated personalized medicine becomes a reality, genomic and molecular tests that could potentially guide providers in making clinical decisions are being validated and approved for use by professional bodies and federal agencies. There are three major conceptual areas of personalized medicine translation characterized by different opportunities, challenges, and current progress: pharmacogenomics, common disease risk prediction, and rare diseases defined by a prevalence of less than 0.05%.

***Pharmacogenomics:*** The first wave of clinically useful genomic variants that have started to gain acceptance are those associated with response to medication. Pharmacogenomics is the field of genomics that deals with how individual genetic variation may play a role in that individual's response to a medication. This variability in response can range from complete lack of effect to reduced efficacy to serious adverse drug reactions. To date, there are more than 30 commonly prescribed drugs that have had their FDA-label modified to include information about pharmacogenomics, with new amendments to existing drugs being considered.

Pharmacogenomic-guided prescribing has significant potential for reducing adverse drug reactions (ADRs) and increasing therapeutic efficacy. For example, it has been shown that loss-of-function polymorphisms in the hepatic cytochrome CYP2C19 enzyme, which metabolizes clopidogrel (Plavix) from its inactive prodrug to its active metabolite, are responsible for variations in rates of stent thrombosis following percutaneous interventions for obstructive coronary artery disease. Loss of function was associated with a greater than threefold increase in the risk of stent thrombosis and death at 1 year. In addition it has been demonstrated that genome-guided prescribing can reduce adverse events and save costs simultaneously. Abacavir, a commonly used HIV medication is known to cause severe hypersensitivity in 4% to 8% of patients. HLA B*5701 is a known genetic risk factor for abacavir hypersensitivity in Caucasians and in a cost-saving analysis, genotype-guided prescribing reduced the incidence of hypersensitivity reactions, offering cost savings of approximately $29,000 per patient.

### Common Disease Risk Prediction and Personalized Preventive Medicine:

Though pharmacogenomics represents the first-wave of genomic medicine that can be integrated into routine clinical care, reports evaluating the clinical utility of genomic risk prediction models for common diseases are just beginning to emerge. For example, a recent study that used a risk-weighted, multilocus genetic risk score based on a 13-SNP panel was able to identify individuals who were at an approximately 70% increased risk of a first coronary heart disease event. Perhaps most encouraging is the finding that the genetic risk score was able to improve risk reclassification in individuals who were at intermediate risk based on traditional risk assessed by Framingham risk score. The 13-SNP panel-based reclassification shifted 15% to 20% of individuals above or below treatment thresholds for lipid-lowering drugs recommended in current practice guidelines and thus potentially altered their treatment. Similar scores have been tested in type 2 diabetes. The major challenge for efforts to develop improved diagnostic and prognostic tools for common diseases lies in the modest effect sizes of the common variants so far discovered and therefore the limited proportion of heritable variance, which they explain. Thus, at the time of this writing, clinical application of genomic risk scores to predict incident diseases is still investigational. It is hoped and anticipated that with advances in genotyping technology and the discovery of rarer variants of larger effect, tests will emerge to estimate an individual's risk for developing a disease, such as type 2 diabetes or heart disease. It is hoped that addition of validated genomic variant information will improve the ability of established risk prediction models to accurately assess the likelihood of onset of a common disease in an individual in the future. Anticipated personal and public health benefits will be more precise and effective allocation of primary prevention strategies and discovery and efficient evaluation of new preventive interventions. This will usher in the promise of true preventive medicine.

### Rare Diseases:

The application of genomics in rare diseases, defined by a population prevalence of <0.05%, will be driven by the increasingly affordable ability to interrogate the sequence of all coding regions (exons) or the entire genome of individuals for mutations that can plausibly underlie manifestations of a rare disease. Thus, with the anticipated rapid spread of whole exome and whole genome sequence information, genomics will likely dramatically redefine the identification and management of thousands of rare diseases.

## Barriers and Solutions to Implementation

**Provider Education:** Despite a clear role having been established for pharmacogenomics in the efficacy and toxicity of numerous drugs, the implementation of pharmacogenomic tests in clinical practice lags far behind the increasing knowledge base. There are a number of factors that may account for this lag. Though genetics has long played a part in undergraduate and postgraduate medical education, this has on the whole been limited to education about long-understood genetic defects that cause overt disease, such as cystic fibrosis or chromosomal abnormalities, such as Down syndrome. Genomics is a new field and its rapid ascent from research to clinical practice has left the current provider workforce "genomically illiterate." As a result, studies surveying the knowledge, skills, and confidence of the clinical workforce in implementing genomic medicine have revealed a deficit that must be addressed. A recent study that surveyed primary care physician's awareness and opinions of direct-to-consumer (DTC) genetic testing was extremely illuminating about the current state of affairs. DTC genetic testing refers to genetic tests that are marketed directly to consumers, without necessarily involving a medical professional in the ordering process. In the survey, 20% of physicians had patients ask questions about DTC testing or bring in test results and only 15% felt prepared to answer questions about DTC testing. The growing market for DTC genetic testing promotes awareness of genetic diseases and allow consumers to take a more proactive role in their health care, however these tests have significant risks with potentially uninformed or vulnerable patients being misled by the results of unproven or invalid tests. Thus, reliable up-to-date education and practical guidance in genomics and its clinical applications are essential to prepare trainees and physicians to apply personalized medicine competently in clinical care. The current textbook is poised to become a valuable practice-oriented reference resource in clinical genomics for healthcare providers.

**Practical Guidance:** While genomic education is a cornerstone for personalized medicine, the current mismatch of emerging clinical validity, established patient enthusiasm, and lagging physician knowledge require effective clinical support tools that consolidate and translate genomic knowledge and integrate this knowledge into existing clinical workflows that will allow clinicians to make informed decisions at the point of care. The increasing prevalence of electronic health records (EHRs) and related technologies offers an appealing solution. One of the highly anticipated quality improvement advantages offered by EHRs is the potential for point-of-care clinical decision support (CDS). CDS provides clinicians with person-specific knowledge that is presented at appropriate times, such as when a provider is about to prescribe a new medication. To date, much of this has centered on drug-drug or drug-allergy interactions. However, with the coming wave of disease-risk and drug-response associated genomic variants, CDS has the potential to provide the necessary level of genome-informed, patient-personalized guidance to providers at the point of care that will be necessary in the era of personalized medicine.

## Summary

There is a growing consensus that a fundamental change in medical practice is coming, away from broad disease concepts and treatments and toward evidence-based personalized medicine. The prospect of genome-guided medicine is fast becoming a reality as the science advances and the technology cost plummets. This approach will require infrastructure for large-scale data mining and integration, data analysis and associated clinical decision support, as well as provider and patient education. Genomics education will be complemented and supported at the point of care by customized electronic medical record (EMR)-enabled clinical decision support tools to guide the provider with individual-level, evidence-based healthcare decisions.

## BIBLIOGRAPHY:

1. Hindorff LA, Sethupathy P, Junkins HA, et al. Potential etiologic and functional implications of genome-wide association loci for human diseases and traits. *Proc Natl Acad Sci U S A*. 2009;106:9362-9367.

2. http://www.nice.org.uk/nicemedia/live/13561/56015/56015.pdf

3. Kawamoto K, Lobach DF, Willard HF, Ginsburg GS. A national clinical decision support infrastructure to enable the widespread and consistent practice of genomic and personalized medicine. *BMC Med Inform Decis Mak*. 2009;9:17.

4. Green ED, Guyer MS. Charting a course for genomic medicine from base pairs to bedside. *Nature*. 2011;470:204-213.

5. Flockhart DA, Skaar T, Berlin DS, Klein TE, Nguyen AT. Clinically available pharmacogenomics tests. *Clin Pharmacol Ther*. 2009;86:109-113.

6. http://www.fda.gov/drugs/scienceresearch/researchareas/pharmacogenetics/ucm083378.htm

7. Simon T, Verstuyft C, Mary-Krause M, et al. Genetic determinants of response to clopidogrel and cardiovascular events. *N Engl J Med*. 2009;360:363-375.

8. Hughes DA, Vilar FJ, Ward CC, Alfirevic A, Park BK, Pirmohamed M. Cost-effectiveness analysis of HLA B*5701 genotyping in preventing abacavir hypersensitivity. *Pharmacogenetics*. 2004;14:335-342.

9. Ripatti S, Tikkanen E, Orho-Melander M, et al. A multilocus genetic risk score for coronary heart disease: case-control and prospective cohort analyses. *Lancet*. 2010;376:1393-1400.

10. Meigs JB, Shrader P, Sullivan LM, et al. Genotype score in addition to common risk factors for prediction of type 2 diabetes. *N Engl J Med*. 2008;359:2208-2219.

11. Mrazek DA, Lerman C. Facilitating clinical implementation of pharmacogenomics. *JAMA*. 2011;306:304-305.

12. http://ghr.nlm.nih.gov/handbook/testing/directtoconsumer.

13. Powell KP, Cogswell WA, Christianson CA, et al. Primary care physicians' awareness, experience and opinions of direct-to-consumer genetic testing. *J Genet Couns*. 2012;21:113-126.

14. Osheroff JA, Teich JM, Middleton B, Steen EB, Wright A, Detmer DE. A roadmap for national action on clinical decision support. *J Am Med Inform Assoc*. 2007;14:141-145.

## Supplementary Information

***Key Words:*** Personalized medicine, genomic medicine, preventive medicine, electronic medical records, clinical decision support

# 176 Genomics and Evidence-Based Medicine

W. Gregory Feero

## KEY POINTS

- *The intersection between genomics and personalized medicine is in an early stage.* Challenges to applying the principles of evidence-based medicine (EBM) to the assessment of genomics include the rapid pace of technology advancement, the rarity of most monogenic conditions, and the complexity of human genetic variation underlying common conditions.
- *Analytic validity, clinical validity, and clinical utility are important concepts related to the performance of molecular diagnostic testing.* Analytic validity describes the ability of a test to reliably detect the presence of a given genomic variation or biomarker, whereas clinical validity describes the relationship of the variant or maker with a trait or disease. Clinical utility is a term describing the ability of a genomic technology to improve health outcomes.
- *The United States Preventive Services Task Force (USPSTF) and Evaluation of Genomic Applications in Practice and Prevention (EGAPP) are developers of rigorous evidence-based guidelines for genomic tests and interventions.* Insurer technology assessment groups, professional societies, and disease advocacy organizations are also valuable sources of evidence-based recommendations; however, the rigor of the methodology employed in guideline development and the evidence base supporting these recommendations can be variable.

The intersection of genomic technologies with mainstream health care is growing exponentially. This is occurring at a time where there is a tremendous amount of scrutiny regarding healthcare costs. This is particularly true from public funders (particularly state Medicaid programs) where budget shortfalls are prompting elimination of some traditional services. It is not surprising that health professionals, insurers, and the public are viewing all new technologies through a lens of value—that is, the extent to which resources invested yield measurable improvements in health outcomes. The paradigm of EBM offers approaches for evaluating the benefits and harms of any new technology entering health care, and increasingly these precepts are being applied to evaluate genomic technologies.

## Evidence-Based Medicine Versus Genomic Medicine

*"EBM is...the conscientious, explicit, and judicious use of current best evidence in making decisions about the care of the individual patient. It means integrating individual clinical expertise with the best available external clinical evidence from systematic research."* (David Sackett et al., 1996)

This definition of EBM, penned by a founding father of the movement, provides a brief grounding in the major tenets of the field. As a discipline, EBM affords a rigorous approach for ordering, digesting, assessing, and succinctly disseminating the vast amount of knowledge available regarding healthcare technologies. Functionally, EBM is often employed to dissect a disparate knowledge base to yield a dichotomous yes or no answer regarding the value of using a particular technology for a well-defined purpose in health care. EBM is a relatively new field; many of the concepts and tools of EBM were pioneered by individuals at McMaster University in the late 1980s. In the United States, perhaps the pre-eminent organization basing its work on EBM is the United States Preventive Services Task Force (USPSTF). The approaches pioneered by groups like the USPSTF and the Cochrane Collaboration have been adopted by a wide range of professional societies, insurer technology assessment groups, and governmental bodies worldwide. The output of rigorous EBM evaluations of new technologies has served as the substrate for planning for biomedical research, clinical guideline development, regulatory determinations and reimbursement decisions. In the 21st century, it seems unlikely that any major health professional organization in the United States would not state that it adheres to the tenets of EBM to the greatest extent possible. Since the advent of EBM there have been growing pains between EBM and emerging biomedical technologies. Genomics and personalized medicine offers no exception to this. However, it cannot be overemphasized that in no way is Dr. Sackett's definition of EBM contrary to the precepts of genomics and personalized medicine.

Those that ascribe to the Western medical tradition will agree that healthcare providers should strive to combine the most up-to-date scientific information for a given condition with an understanding of the characteristics of the patient before them to make logically defensible decisions to optimize health outcomes. Likewise, most would agree that, when ethically and economically feasible, all new technologies should be subject to rigorous clinical trials designed to measure health outcomes such as morbidity and mortality (so-called "patient-oriented evidence"). EBM holds that all clinical trials are not created equal, and that the gold standard for evidence is the double-blind, placebo-controlled randomized trial. According to the precepts of EBM, the ideal evidence base supporting clinical decisions rests on meta-analysis of multiple well-designed trials conducted on a sufficient number of individuals of diverse biologic and socioeconomic backgrounds to be assured that the results are applicable to the patient in question. Such high standards have been met for a wide variety of types of health interventions (Table 176-1). To date there are only a few genomic interventions that have met such a high evidentiary bar.

Adapting the paradigms of EBM to genomic or personalized medicine is challenging. The most obvious reason for this is the rapid pace of discovery. It takes considerable time and resources to conduct clinical trials with endpoints of morbidity and mortality, and the rush to bring technologies to clinical care is substantial.

*Table 176-1  Selected Evidence-Based Recommendations for Conditions Related to Cardiovascular Disease*

| Condition | Intervention | Intended Use | Recommendation | Source |
|---|---|---|---|---|
| Hyperlipidemia | Laboratory testing | Screening | "The US Preventive Services Task Force (USPSTF) strongly recommends screening men aged 35 and older for lipid disorders." | United States Preventive Services Task Force |
| Nicotine dependence | Counseling | Primary prevention | "The USPSTF strongly recommends that clinicians screen all adults for tobacco use and provide tobacco cessation interventions for those who use tobacco products." | United States Preventive Services Task Force |
| Hypertension | Drug therapy | Treatment | "Thiazide-type diuretics should be used as initial therapy for most patients with hypertension, either alone or in combination with one of the other classes (ACEIs, ARBs, BBs, CCBs) demonstrated to be beneficial in randomized controlled outcome trials." | Joint National Committee on Prevention, Detection, Evaluation, and Treatment of High Blood Pressure |
| Myocardial infarction | Drug therapy | Secondary prevention | "Prescribe aspirin in patients with stable coronary artery disease if there are no medical contraindications." | The Institute for Clinical Systems Improvement (ICSI) |

Many genomic technologies are too new for such trials to have been completed. New genomic technologies often come to clinical care with an evidence base consisting of biologic plausibility, epidemiologic associations, and a few small trials with surrogate markers as proxy endpoints for health outcomes. Such trials can be subject to bias and occasionally surrogate markers fail to accurately predict actual health outcomes. The story of the use of CYP2C19 genotyping to guide clopidogrel dosing to prevent stent thrombosis provides an example of this. Early studies suggested a possible correlation between genotype and meaningful health outcomes. Subsequent studies showed an association between genotype, dosing, and a surrogate endpoint (such as platelet aggregation) and several small clinical trials suggested a mixed picture of clinical benefit from dosage adjustment. A subsequent meta-analysis of existing studies suggest there may be no benefit to adding the expense of genotyping to current clinical practice, though very likely the story will continue to evolve as the evidence base expands.

A less obvious but critical issue separates the current practice of EBM from genomics and personalized medicine. Fundamentally, EBM is predicated on applying the mean results from clinical trials to an individual that may or may not represent that mean. Current traditional clinical trials seek information from larger and larger population groups to determine the efficacy and effectiveness of a proposed intervention, and only very crudely examine trial data for subgroups, and may disregard outliers. When results from such trials are used to create care guidelines, and such guidelines are applied to large numbers of individual patients, population health outcomes are improved. However, all healthcare providers have had the experience where a front-line therapy for a condition fails in an individual or an example where an individual benefits unexpectedly from an intervention with low likelihood of effectiveness. Personalized medicine predicated on knowledge of the individual patients' genetic makeup seeks to achieve a more precise match between the individual and the evidence of benefit. There is ample reason to believe that, on occasion, outliers and small subgroups in

trials that derive benefit may share genomic variations. That same variation may, in fact, reside the individual patient sitting before the healthcare provider, and account for an unexpected benefit or harm.

Clear examples of the consequences of individual genomic variation on therapeutic efficacy have arisen in cancer care, examples include epidermal growth factor receptor (EGFR) mutation testing in non–small cell lung cancer and *KRAS* mutation testing in colorectal cancer. Without the ability to peer into the genomic underpinnings of these cancers to select for individuals that might derive benefit, erlotinib, and cetuximab, respectively, may have been rejected as therapeutic options. Current clinical research studies are generally not designed to identify benefits that accrue to genetically distinct subpopulations in large studies, but this is beginning to change. EBM and genomic medicine will need to develop new approaches for developing clinical trials as well as care guidelines to ensure that individuals as well as populations derive maximal benefit from genomic advances.

## Mapping Genomic Technologies to the Language of EBM

A high-quality diagnostic test of any kind must be accurate, predict a clinically meaningful outcome, and add value to the management of an individual. For various historical and technical reasons, there are semantic differences between the terms used to describe molecular diagnostics and other types of testing. The term analytic validity is used to refer to the performance characteristics of a given test, such as accuracy and reproducibility (Table 176-2). That is to say, does the test measure what it claims to measure, and on repeated measurement of the same sample is the outcome similar? An example of analytic validity would be a metric for the error rate in accurately reading the nucleotide present in a particular position in the genome using a particular

**Table 176-2** *Terminology Related to the Performance of Genomic Tests and Biomarkers*

| Test Attribute | Definition | Related Concept |
| --- | --- | --- |
| Analytic validity | Accuracy in measuring a given genomic variation or biomarker | Accuracy, reproducibility, precision |
| Clinical validity | Relationship between the presence of a genomic variation or biomarker and a trait or condition | Sensitivity, specificity, positive predictive value, negative predictive value |
| Clinical utility | Ability of a genomic intervention to improve health outcomes | Efficacy, effectiveness, cost-effectiveness, number needed to treat, number needed to screen |

sequencing technology—conceptually this is not much different than the error bars on a serum sodium or cholesterol measurement.

Clinical validity is often used to describe the strength of the association between a given result from a molecular diagnostic test and a clinical attribute (phenotype). For example, there is substantial evidence supporting an association between the presence of the Δ *F508* mutation in its homozygous state and cystic fibrosis. In contradistinction, there is considerably less evidence supporting the link between some uncommon variations in the *BRCA1* gene and development of breast cancer. The attribute of clinical validity is somewhat analogous to the concepts of sensitivity and specificity—and the related concepts of positive predictive value (PPV) and negative predictive value (NPV) commonly used to describe how well a laboratory test performs in detecting the presence of absence of disease. For example, it could be said that testing for the Δ *F508* mutation in homozygous state has a high sensitivity, specificity, PPV, and NPV for classic cystic fibrosis, whereas a variant of unknown significance in the *BRCA1* gene may have very poor predictive value for development of breast cancer.

The term clinical utility is broadly used to describe whether or not a given genomic technology (diagnostic or otherwise) changes health outcomes. It is perhaps the most intuitive and important concept to the practicing healthcare provider, and is the focus of the application of EBM in genomic and personalized medicine. Without demonstrated utility of some sort, genomic technologies have the potential cause to harm directly or by adding cost and complexity to an already immensely complex healthcare system. Not surprisingly, this term is the most controversial, as not all can agree on what constitutes an adequate outcome change to declare utility is present. Arguments have been made that a determination of favorable utility should be predicated only hard measures such as reductions in morbidity, mortality, and healthcare cost savings. Others have argued that utility might encompass softer outcomes such as patient satisfaction, achieving a diagnostic label, or facilitating nonmedical decision making on the part of a patient. This has led to the development of another term—"personal utility." Clinical utility might be thought to encompass traditional EBM measures and concepts such as the number needed to treat or screen and cost-effectiveness among others. It is generally regarded that a high analytic and clinical validity are necessary but not sufficient for a molecular diagnostic to be accepted as having high clinical utility. For example, a given single-nucleotide polymorphism (SNP) associated with type 2 diabetes risk might be very accurately measured by a diagnostic platform, and might have been shown in many genome-wide association studies (GWASs) to be highly significantly associated with increased risk of diabetes yet have essentially no utility due to a very low effect size (eg, an odds ratio of 1:1). This point is often lost in less responsible marketing materials associated with molecular diagnostic tests. Additionally, healthcare providers should be aware that there is no US federal governmental body that assures commercially available laboratory developed tests have utility.

## Evaluation of Genomic Applications in Practice and Prevention (EGAPP) Pilot

In recognition of the need for publically accessible evidence-based recommendations regarding emerging genomic technologies, the Office of Public Health Genomics of the US Centers for Disease Control and Prevention (CDC) established EGAPP pilot project. The organization is modeled after the USPSTF and is formulated around an independent multidisciplinary working group that makes use of rigorous and transparent methods for evaluating and making recommendations regarding the evidence supporting the use of genomic technologies for a defined clinical purpose. EGAPP works in conjunction with two other related bodies, the EGAPP stakeholder group, and a federal steering committee. These groups help select topics and interact with various communities at all points during the deliberative process, but have no say in the final recommendation. Comprehensive structured evidence reviews have been conducted to date through contracts with the Evidence-Based Practice Centers established by the Agency for Healthcare Research and Quality (AHRQ). To date numerous evidence reports with recommendations have been generated. Some, including the first report regarding the use of pharmacogenomic testing to guide depression therapy, have generated controversy by exposing gaps in the evidence supporting use of commercially available genomic tests.

Several lessons can be learned from the EGAPP project. First, a single body, employing traditional EBM approaches for evaluating evidence, is likely not agile enough to keep pace with the rapidly expanding spectrum of genomic applications. Next, the spectrum of expertise required to evaluate new technologies is remarkable, and often metrics that define quality are just now evolving. Finally, coming to consensus regarding what constitutes adequate clinical utility is a challenging process requiring input from a diversity of stakeholder organizations. Managing potential conflict of interest in such deliberations becomes a major challenge.

*Evidence-Based Guidelines for Care:* There are a wide variety of clinical guideline development methods, ranging from expert opinion-based approaches to consensus development to evidence-linked approaches. By the standards of the EBM community, the best guidelines are those that are transparently linked to the evidence from which they were derived. Such guidelines have a number of characteristics. First, the guidelines are usually developed around a well-defined question about a given intervention in a specific population. This is a double-edged sword in that it allows for a rigorous evidence evaluation and synthesis; on the other hand, it can limit the extent to which the guideline may be generalized to diverse populations or even slight variations in the technology being examined. Second, a predefined analytic framework is used for gathering, synthesizing, and rigorously evaluating the evidence base. The framework and methods are specified to an extent that permits a third party to duplicate the process, and generally the group that completes the review is distinct from the body that sits in judgment of the evidence. Third, there is a transparent process for drawing conclusions from the evidence base with an active process for managing conflicts of interest in the group that develops the final guideline. Fourth, guidelines are given ratings regarding their strength using a standardized scale, most often this reflects the strength of the evidence on which the guideline is based. There are a variety of such scales or criteria for rating guidelines and evidence—one of the more commonly used and recognized in primary care is the Strength of Recommendation Taxonomy (SORT) rating system. Finally, high-quality guidelines have an explicit link between the evidence base and the actual recommendation. For some technologies there are studies that directly link the intervention with improved health outcomes, in other cases a chain of evidence is constructed. The final product is subject to peer review and publication, often in a high-profile journal.

There are comparatively few guidelines for genomic technologies that meet the highest standards of EBM, examples include recommendations from USPSTF and EGAPP (Table 176-3). A diversity of guidelines relying on various less robust evidentiary requirements exists for many genomic technologies. Such guidelines may be based on technology assessments generated by commercial insurer technology assessment groups to guidelines based on expert opinion generated by disease advocacy organizations or evidence reviews conducted by members of medical specialty societies. It should be recognized that groups noted for generating the most rigorous EBM recommendations will often not address a subject until there is a sufficient evidence base of clinical trials. Therefore, for technologies relevant to rare conditions, or for new technologies, only expert opinion or consensus level guidelines may be available. Often clinical decisions will need to be made using suboptimal evidence; this is true for any rapidly advancing area of biomedical science. Healthcare professionals should always use sound clinical judgment when applying guidelines to patients; this is particularly the case with those based on consensus or expert opinion.

**Table 176-3** *Selected USPSTF and EGAPP Guidelines for Genomic Interventions*

| Condition | Intervention | Recommendation | Source |
|---|---|---|---|
| Breast cancer | Referral | "The USPSTF recommends that women whose family history is associated with an increased risk for deleterious mutations in *BRCA1* or *BRCA2* genes be referred for genetic counseling and evaluation for *BRCA* testing." | USPSTF |
| Hemochromatosis | Genetic testing | "The USPSTF recommends against routine genetic screening for hereditary hemochromatosis in the asymptomatic general population." | USPSTF |
| Hyperlipidemia | Biomarker testing | "The USPSTF recommends screening men aged 20 to 35 for lipid disorders if they are at increased risk for coronary heart disease." . . . "A family history of cardiovascular disease before age 50 in male relatives or age 60 in female relatives." | USPSTF |
| Colorectal cancer | Genetic/biomarker testing | "The EGAPP Working Group found sufficient evidence to recommend offering genetic testing for Lynch syndrome to individuals with newly diagnosed colorectal cancer to reduce morbidity and mortality in relatives." | EGAPP |
| Venous thromboembolism | Genetic testing | "The EGAPP Working Group found adequate evidence to recommend against routine testing for factor V Leiden (FVL) and/or prothrombin 20210G>A (PT) in the following circumstances: (1) adults with idiopathic venous thromboembolism (VTE). In such cases, longer-term secondary prophylaxis to avoid recurrence offers similar benefits to patients with and without one or more of these mutations. (2) Asymptomatic adult family members of patients with VTE and an FVL or PT mutation, for the purpose of considering primary prophylactic anticoagulation." | EGAPP |

## Conclusions

The clinical applications of genomics and personalized medicine have arisen largely in the context of medical genetics and medical subspecialty environments. Until recently, these disciplines have focused on the study and care of individuals suffering from rare, or at least uncommon, single gene disorders. Small case series and data on biologic plausibility have occasionally been the only available sources of information to guide critical clinical decision making. As such, there has not been a tradition of adherence to the formal approaches of EBM. The expansion of genomic technologies into the realm of common disease is radically altering the landscape of medical genetics to include the domains where EBM approaches to care are the gold standard. Over time medical genetics, genomics, personalized medicine, and EBM will be strengthened by the intersection to the benefit of patients, the healthcare system, and society.

BIBLIOGRAPHY:

1. ACCE Model Process for Evaluating Genetic Tests. www.cdc.gov/genomics/gtesting/ACCE/. Accessed June 5, 2012.

2. Armstrong K. Can genomics bend the cost curve? *JAMA.* Mar 14 2012;307:1031-1032.

3. Cochrane Collaboration. www.cochrane.org/. Accessed June 5, 2012.

4. Ebell MH, Siwek J, Weiss BD, et al. Strength of recommendation taxonomy (SORT): a patient-centered approach to grading evidence in the medical literature. *Am Fam Physician.* 2004;69:548-556.

5. Evaluation of Genomic Applications in Practice and Prevention. www.egappreviews.org/. Accessed June 5, 2012.

6. Institute for Clinical Systems Improvement. www.icsi.org/index.aspx. Accessed June 5, 2012.

7. Nissen SE. Pharmacogenomics and clopidogrel: irrational exuberance? *JAMA.* 2011;306:2727-2728.

8. Sackett DL, Rosenberg WM, Gray JA, Haynes RB, Richardson WS. Evidence based medicine: what it is and what it isn't. *BMJ.* 1996;312:71-72.

9. SACGHS Documents, Reports and Correspondence. http://oba.od.nih.gov/sacghs/sacghs_documents.html. Accessed June 5, 2012.

10. The Seventh Report of the Joint National Committee on Prevention, Detection, Evaluation, and Treatment of High Blood Pressure (JNC 7). www.nhlbi.nih.gov/guidelines/hypertension/. Accessed June 5, 2012.

11. United States Preventive Services Task Force. www.uspreventiveservicestaskforce.org/. Accessed June 5, 2012.

12. White B. Making evidence-based medicine doable in everyday practice: finding the evidence you need is getting easier than you ever thought possible. *Fam Pract Manag.* 2004;11:51-58.

# 177 MicroRNA in Cancer

Serge P. Nana-Sinkam and Carlo M. Croce

## KEY POINTS

- *Summary:*
  - (miRNAs or miRs) are 18 to 25 noncoding RNAs that have the capacity to regulate mRNA through degradation or inhibition of translation. miRNAs represent only one member of a larger family of noncoding RNAs many of whose function has yet to be elucidated.
  - Given the potential redundancy between a miRNA sequence ("seed" sequence) and multiple target mRNA sequences, miRNA can simultaneously target tens to hundreds of genes. As a result, it is estimated that more than 30% of the human genome is targeted by miRNA.
  - miRNAs have been implicated in the regulation of fundamental cellular processes including differentiation, growth, survival, and angiogenesis.
  - While, patterns of miRNA expression are being used for both diagnostic and therapeutic purposes, several challenges remain in the translation or miRNA biology to targeted therapies.
- *MicroRNA as diagnostic and prognostic biomarkers:*
  - The global deregulation of miRNAs across malignancies supports their role in tumor development. These patterns of expression are being leveraged for both diagnostic and prognostic purposes.
- *Therapeutic applications for microRNA:*
  - Given their capacity to simultaneously regulate multiple genes and thus essential biologic functions, miRNAs are reasonable candidates as targeted therapies. However, both minimizing off-target effects as well as achieving target organ or disease specificity are important challenges to effective miRNA therapy.
- *Delivery systems:*
  - The majority of miRNA-based approaches to therapy have been conducted in vitro and in animal models of disease are still far from reaching human application. However, in one case, systemic delivery of miRNA-based agents has now reached clinical trial. Currently, a pharmaceutical-led clinical trial targeting the liver-specific *miR-122* (SPC3649) is being tested as a therapy for Hepatitis C.
- *miRNAs and chemotherapeutics:*
  - miRNAs may also have a role as either predictors or modifiers of response to traditional therapeutic agents.

## Molecular Genetics and Molecular Mechanism

miRNAs or miRs are 18 to 25 noncoding RNAs that have the capacity to regulate mRNA through degradation or inhibition of translation. miRNAs represent only one member of a larger family of noncoding RNAs many of whose function has yet to be elucidated. The critical role for miRNAs in the development and progression of both solid and hematologic malignancies is increasingly apparent based on patterns of global deregulation, see Table 177-1. In addition, by targeting critical hallmarks to tumor development and progression, miRNAs may function as either tumor suppressors or oncogenes. miRNA biology is also being applied to nonmalignant disease involving the cardiac, endocrine, neurologic, and respiratory systems to name a few. There are several mechanisms for miRNA deregulation including chromosomal deletions, amplifications, and translocations, epigenetic modification, impaired processing, miRNA polymorphisms, and environmental factors. Some of the first expression studies in miRNA were conducted in hematologic malignancies. Investigators first observed that *miR-15a* and *16-1* were located in a chromosomal region that was either deleted or downregulated in 68% of patients with chronic lymphocytic leukemia (CLL). This pattern of expression was associated with a more indolent form of disease. Since that initial observation, several other prognostic miRNAs including *miR-29c* and *miR-223* have been identified in CLL. These patterns of miRNA expression

are being leveraged for both diagnostic and prognostic purposes. For example, Yanaihara et al. determined that increased *miR-155* and low *let7a-2* expression correlated with poor survival in adenocarcinoma of the lung. A separate independent study identified five miRNAs (*miR-25, miR-34c-5p, miR-191, let-7e,* and *miR-34a*) that predicted survival in lung cancer. Deregulated miRNAs also correlate with survival in colorectal carcinoma with *miR-21* being validated as prognostic biomarker in two independent cohorts. An important caveat, however, to these expression studies is the continued requirement for larger studies demonstrating reproducibility in miRNA signatures.

*Noninvasive Detection of miRNA:* Noninvasive testing for solid malignancies remains highly sought after. Technology for the noninvasive detection of miRNA has rapidly evolved in the last few years. As a result, investigators are now routinely examining blood, sputum, and urine for miRNA expression patterns. It is hypothesized that such patterns may provide some scientific insight into pathogenesis of disease or serve as either diagnostic or prognostic biomarkers. Based on their relative stability in circulation, miRNAs may be reasonable as biomarkers. To date, deregulated circulating miRNAs have been described in lymphoma, lung cancer, breast cancer, and prostate cancer. A few studies have also suggested that circulating miRNA may be critical to cell-cell communication. While the studies to date are encouraging, investigators must still address key limitations including determining the ideal assay for detection, compartment for detection (cells vs serum vs plasma), and their physiologic relevance.

*Table 177-1* **MicroRNAs in Select Solid and Hematologic Malignancies**

| Disease | Upregulated | Downregulated |
|---------|-------------|---------------|
| CLL | *miR-155* | *miR-15a/16-1, miR-29b, miR-181b, miR-34* |
| AML | *miR-10a/b, miR-29, miR-155* | *miR-181, miR-204* |
| Breast cancer | *miR-9, miR-21, miR-182, miR-17-92, miR-155* | *Let-7, miR-9, miR-10b, miR-125b, miR-126, miR143/145* |
| Colorectal cancer | *miR-21, miR-155, miR-183, miR-17-92* | *Let-7, miR-34, miR-143* |
| Pancreatic cancer | *miR-21, miR-155, miR-196a/b* | *Let-7, miR-15a/16-1, miR-34* |
| Lung cancer | *miR-155, miR-21, miR-17-92, miR-221, miR-222* | *Let-7, miR-1, miR-29, miR-126* |
| Ovarian cancer | *miR-200* | *Let-7, miR-125b, miR-145* |
| Hepatocellular cancer | *miR-21, miR-221/222* | *miR-1, miR-26a, miR-122, miR-125a* |

***miRNA as Targeted Therapeutics:*** The majority of miRNA-based approaches to therapy have been conducted in both in vitro and murine models of disease. As a result, we are still in the early phases of potential human application. miRNA-based targeting in cancer is based on the premise of either repletion of a miRNA with tumor suppressive properties of suppression of oncogenic miRNA. Delivery systems may take the form of systemic, targeted, or local therapy each of which carry distinct advantages and disadvantages. Systemic delivery of miRNA-based agents has now reached clinical trial. A DNA-LNA *miR-122* anti-miRNA (SPC3649) in the only nonhuman primate model of chronic hepatitis C virus (HCV) infection resulted in a potent reduction (300-fold) in HCV burden. These promising results have subsequently led to a pharmaceutical-led clinical trial targeting the liver-specific *miR-122* (SPC3649) as a therapy for hepatitis C. As opposed to direct targeting, another feasible approach is the use of miRNAs as either predictors or modifiers of response to traditional therapeutic agents. During the course of therapy, tumors may acquire resistance thus rendering chemotherapy ineffective. In vitro data would suggest that miRNA may be used to overcome resistance or provide synergistic benefit to traditional treatment. Several examples exist to support this approach. For example, in vitro, *miR-155* and *miR-21* manipulation have been used to alter drug response in breast and pancreatic cancer, respectively. More globally, patterns of miRNA expression may also distinguish between drug responsive and nonresponsive individuals. In one study, a panel of 37 miRNAs distinguished patients with CLL who either responded or did not respond to fludarabine.

***Genetic Testing:*** No role yet exists for genetic testing for miRNA.

***Future Directions:*** miRNAs are novel noncoding RNAs that regulate gene expression and are involved in the pathogenesis of both malignant and nonmalignant disease. It is important to recognize that miRNAs represent only one of a family of noncoding RNAs many of whose function remain unknown. Recently, investigators have identified two other noncoding RNA family members termed ultraconserved regions (UCRs) and long-intervening noncoding RNAs (lincRNAs). These longer noncoding RNAs are being implicated in cancer progression and gene regulation. Studies are ongoing to further our understanding of their function but it is likely that they will have an important role in disease development. Given their ability to regulate tens to hundreds of genes and thus biologic pathways, miRNAs are being integrated into ongoing clinic trials to assist in further defining disease molecular heterogeneity and as predictors of response to therapy. While the majority of miRNA-based therapeutic studies have been conducted in the laboratory, miRNAs have now reached clinical application in phase 1 human studies. A continued refinement of our understanding of how miRNAs target select genes, and where miRNAs may fit within the human genome as modifiers of disease as well as improving current modalities for tissue-specific delivery are all essential to translating this interesting biology to human application.

**BIBLIOGRAPHY:**

1. Bartel DP. MicroRNAs: genomics, biogenesis, mechanism, and function. *Cell.* 2004;116:281-297.

2. Lee RC, Feinbaum RL, Ambros V. The C. elegans heterochronic gene lin-4 encodes small RNAs with antisense complementarity to lin-14. *Cell.* 1993;75:843-854.

3. Croce CM. Causes and consequences of microRNA dysregulation in cancer. *Nat Rev Genet.* 2009;10:704-714.

4. Calin GA, Cimmino A, Fabbri M, et al. MiR-15a and miR-16-1 cluster functions in human leukemia. *Proc Natl Acad Sci U S A.* 2008;105:5166-5171.

5. Stamatopoulos B, Meuleman N, Haibe-Kains B, et al. microRNA-29c and microRNA-223 down-regulation has in vivo significance in chronic lymphocytic leukemia and improves disease risk stratification. *Blood.* 2009;113:5237-5245.

6. Yanaihara N, Caplen N, Bowman E, et al. Unique microRNA molecular profiles in lung cancer diagnosis and prognosis. *Cancer Cell.* 2006;9:189-198.

7. Yu SL, Chen HY, Chang GC, et al. MicroRNA signature predicts survival and relapse in lung cancer. *Cancer Cell.* 2008;13:48-57.

8. Schetter AJ, Leung SY, Sohn JJ, et al. MicroRNA expression profiles associated with prognosis and therapeutic outcome in colon adenocarcinoma. *JAMA.* 2008;299:425-436.

9. Yu L, Todd NW, Xing L, et al. Early detection of lung adenocarcinoma in sputum by a panel of microRNA markers. *Int J Cancer.* 2010;127:2870-2878.

10. Mitchell PS, Parkin RK, Kroh EM, et al. Circulating microRNAs as stable blood-based markers for cancer detection. *Proc Natl Acad Sci U S A.* 2008;105:10513-10518.

11. Boeri M, Verri C, Conte D, et al. MicroRNA signatures in tissues and plasma predict development and prognosis of computed

tomography detected lung cancer. *Proc Natl Acad Sci U S A.* 2011;108:3713-3718.

12. Sieuwerts AM, Mostert B, Bolt-de Vries J, et al. mRNA and microRNA expression profiles in circulating tumor cells and primary tumors of metastatic breast cancer patients. *Clin Cancer Res.* 2011;17:3600-3618.

13. Rak J. Microparticles in cancer. *Semin Thromb Hemost.* 2010;36:888-906.

14. Trang P, Wiggins JF, Daige CL, et al. Systemic delivery of tumor suppressor microRNA mimics using a neutral lipid emulsion inhibits lung tumors in mice. *Mol Ther.* 2011;19:1116-1122.

15. Obad S, dos Santos CO, Petri A, et al. Silencing of microRNA families by seed-targeting tiny LNAs. *Nat Genet.* 2011;43:371-378.

## Supplementary Information

**Alternative Names:**
- miRNA
- miR
- Noncoding RNA

# 178 Genetic Syndromes of Childhood in Adults

Peter J. Mc Guire and Kurt Hirschhorn

## KEY POINTS

- With improvements in medical care, children with genetic diseases now live longer.
- Transition of care of pediatric patients with chronic diseases to adult providers presents challenges, especially in the care of pediatric genetic diseases.
- Adult patients with monogenic diseases diagnosed in childhood require an interdisciplinary approach to medical care.
- Medical management of other adult-onset conditions not related to the primary diagnosis must be addressed.
- The astute physician must sometimes differentiate between medical issues related to the primary genetic diagnosis and other nonrelated pathologic conditions.

## Introduction

Although the majority of conditions seen in adult medicine are multifactorial in nature, many monogenic disorders are becoming more frequent in adults due to improvements in health care, leading to longer survival of affected children.

There are two general scenarios where an adult physician may see a patient with a childhood genetic disorder:

1. When the patient is diagnosed in childhood and requires continuing care into adulthood (eg, Down syndrome).
2. When a new patient presents whose syndrome was not diagnosed in childhood.

Table 178-1 is a survey of genetic conditions that present in childhood and may continue into adulthood. This table is in no way intended to be exhaustive, but rather, gives an overview of the various monogenic and chromosomal disorders that may present to the adult physician. Further details of these conditions can be found in Online Mendelian Inheritance in Man (OMIM; http://www.ncbi.nlm.nih.gov/omim/).

## Summary

In recent years, a great deal of progress has been made in the identification of genetic syndromes in children. Many of these syndromes are lifelong chronic conditions that require a medical home for the coordination of care. This often involves a multidisciplinary team of healthcare professionals. As patients with genetic syndromes become older, the focus often changes from the management of medical issues to the development of coping skills, educational planning, independent living, respite care, and even reproductive options. The transition to the care of an adult physician can be difficult, but not insurmountable.

Table 178-1 highlights many common genetic syndromes that present in childhood and can continue into adulthood. This table is not inclusive, but rather is intended to give the reader an appreciation of the spectrum of disorders which may continue into adulthood. At times, the adult physician is faced with an unknown diagnosis, and must decide whether to pursue the diagnosis due to syndrome-related medical issues. It must also be emphasized that patients with genetic syndromes also suffer from many common multifactorial disorders (eg, diabetes or hypertension) which are discussed in other chapters of this book. This emphasizes the fact that not all medical findings should be attributed to the syndrome, and should be investigated and managed appropriately.

**Table 178-1  Genetic Syndromes of Childhood in Adults**

| | OMIM # (Reference) | Heredity | Genes Involved | Disease Mechanism | Clinical Details | Management | Genetic Testing (Detection) |
|---|---|---|---|---|---|---|---|
| **Neurologic** | | | | | | | |
| *Ataxia telangiectasia* | 208900 | AR | *ATM* | Lack of protein product leads to increased dsDNA breaks and lack of coordination of cell cycle | Progressive cerebellar ataxia, conjunctival telangiectasias, immunodeficiency, increased risk of leukemia, and lymphoma. Death by 3rd decade. | IVIG for immunodeficiency, avoid radiation, supportive therapy | Mutation analysis (>95%) |
| *Duchenne (**DMD**) and Becker (**BMD**) muscular dystrophy* | **DMD** 310200 **BMD** 300376 | XLR | *DMD* | Dystrophin binds muscle membrane proteins. **DMD:** lack of dystrophin **BMD:** abnormal quality or quantity of dystrophin | **DMD:** onset <5 y with proximal muscle weakness, calf hypertrophy, DCM, wheelchair 2nd decade, vent dependent/death 3rd decade **BMD:** later-onset myopathy, DCM may occur in isolation, + wheelchair 2nd decade, death 5th-6th decade | Supportive therapy, steroids may prolong walking 2-3 y | Gene deletion: DMD (65%), BMD (85%) Gene duplication: DMD (6%) Mutations: DMD (30%) |
| *Fragile X* | 300624 | X-linked triplet repeat | *FMR-1* | **Full mutation:** >200 CGG repeats silences gene by methylation **Premutation:** 59-200 CGG repeats | **Full mutation:** Males—DD, MR, PDD spectrum, characteristic facies, macroorchidism at puberty Females—milder phenotype **Premutation:** Males—tremor ataxia syndrome >50 y Females—premature ovarian failure | Supportive therapy, no treatment for tremor ataxia syndrome and premature ovarian failure | Targeted mutation analysis (>99%) |
| *Friedreich ataxia* | 229300 | AR triplet repeat | *FRDA* | **Disease causing:** 66-1700 GAA triplet repeats form stable DNA structure that inhibits transcription | Progressive degeneration of dorsal root ganglia and corticospinal and spinocerebellar tracts, optic nerve atrophy, hypertrophic cardiomyopathy, diabetes. Wheelchair bound in 15-20 years after first symptoms, death in early adulthood usually due to hypertrophic cardiomyopathy. | Supportive therapy | Targeted mutation analysis (98%) |

*(Continued)*

Table 178-1 Genetic Syndromes of Childhood in Adults (Continued)

| | OMIM # (Reference) | Heredity | Genes Involved | Disease Mechanism | Clinical Details | Management | Genetic Testing (Detection) |
|---|---|---|---|---|---|---|---|
| Neurofibromatosis | 162200 | AD | NF1 | Loss of function mutations (>500) disables ras GTPase control of cellular proliferation | Café-au-lait spots, neurofibromas (including plexiform), optic gliomas, Lisch nodules, bone malformations. Clinical diagnostic criteria | Surgery for bone malformations and neurofibromas. Risk of malignant transformation of neurofibromas. | Mutation analysis of gDNA and mRNA (90%) |
| Spinal cerebellar ataxias | ~30 distinct clinical entities in OMIM | AD | >25 loci identified | Multiple mechanisms including CAG repeat expansions, mutations, and deletions | Progressive gait ataxia, poor coordination of hands, speech, and eye movements, cerebellar atrophy | Supportive therapy | Ataxia panels available |
| Tuberous sclerosis | 191100 | AD | TSC1, TSC2 | Altered tumor suppressor function | Hypomelanotic macules, facial angiofibroma, Shagreen patch, ungual fibroma, subependymal nodules, cortical tubers, giant cell astrocytomas, seizures, cardiac rhabdomyomas, renal angiomyolipomas, polycystic kidney disease (contiguous gene deletion). May be mild course, seizures: infantile spasms, onset <2 y, or poor control has an increased risk of LD. | Renal US q1-3 y, + renal CT/MRI | Mutation analysis: TSC1–familial (30%), sporadic (15%) TSC2–familial (50%), sporadic (60%-70%) |
| **Renal** | | | | | | | |
| Collagen IV-related nephropathies (Alport syndrome and thin basement membrane nephropathy) | XL: 301050 AR: 203780 AD: 104200 | XL AD AR | **XL:** COL4A5 **AR/AD:** COL4A3, COL4A4 | Abnormal type IV collagen in the basement membrane of glomeruli | Ranges from isolated hematuria (thin basement) to progressive renal failure, cataracts, and deafness (Alport). ESRD: 90% by 40 y Deafness: 90% SN deafness by 40 y | Nephrology follow-up, renal transplantation, management of deafness | Mutation analysis: COL4A5 (>80%) COL4A3/ COL4A4 (100%) |

| Disease | OMIM | Inheritance | Gene | Mechanism | Clinical features | Management | Testing |
|---|---|---|---|---|---|---|---|
| *Polycystic kidney disease* | ADPKD: 173900 ARPKD: 263200 | AD AR | *PKD1, PKD2, PKHD 1* | **ADPKD**: abnormal polycystin complex resulting in altered calcium homeostasis **ARPKD**: unclear | **ADPKD**: bilateral renal cysts, cysts in the liver, seminal vesicles, pancreas, intracranial aneurysms, 50% renal replacement therapy by 60 y. **ARPKD**: fetal/neonatal death, pulmonary hypoplasia from oligohydramnios, renal failure, hepatic fibrosis, 30%–50% mortality in peri/neonatal period. | Nephrology follow-up, renal transplantation | Mutation analysis: PKD1 and PKD2 (>88%) |
| *Congenital nephrosis* | 256300 | AR | *NPHS1, NPHS2, WT1, LAMB2* | Disruption of podocyte foot processes or slit membrane | Congenital nephrotic syndrome with renal failure. High mortality in first year of life. Infection risk high. | Periodic albumin infusions; diuretics; dialysis; transplant by 3 y; monitor for infection and treat aggressively | Detection rates not available. |
| **Hematologic** | | | | | | | |
| *Factor V Leiden* | 188055 | AD | *F5* | Slowed inactivation of factor 5 due to mutation at APC cleavage site -> increased thrombin. Homozygosity increases risk. | Venous thromboembolism. Risk increased by concurrent thrombophilic disorders. Pregnancy loss, DVT. | Warfarin or LMW heparin for recurrent venous thromboembolism. | Targeted mutation analysis (100%) |
| *Hemophilia A* | 306700 | XLR | *F8* | Reduced or absent factor VIII | Hemarthroses, intracranial bleeding, deep tissue hematomas; prolonged PTT | IV factor VIII prophylactically for severe disease and in trauma | Targeted mutation analysis—intron 22-A inversion (48%) Mutation analysis (43%) |
| *Hemophilia B* | 306900 | XLR | *F9* | Reduced or absent factor IX | Hemarthroses, intracranial bleeding, deep tissue hematomas; prolonged PTT | IV factor IX prophylactically for severe disease and in trauma | Mutation analysis (97%) |

*(Continued)*

Table 178-1 **Genetic Syndromes of Childhood in Adults (Continued)**

| | OMIM # (Reference) | Heredity | Genes Involved | Disease Mechanism | Clinical Details | Management | Genetic Testing (Detection) |
|---|---|---|---|---|---|---|---|
| *Sickle cell anemia* | 603903 | AR | *HBB* | Glu6Val point mutation leads to distorted deoxygenated Hgb leading to a characteristic sickle shape of RBCs | Vaso-occlusive crises leading to pain crises, long bone pain, dactylitis, acute chest syndrome, priapism, stroke, MI. Long term: anemia, jaundice, cholelithiasis. NB: variable presentation with thalassemias | Acute episodes: hydration, pain control, antibiotics for acute chest syndrome. Long term: penicillin prophylaxis, hydroxyurea, transfusions | Targeted mutation analysis for Glu6Val. Frequency of mutation will differ based on ethnicity. |
| *von Willebrand disease* | 193400 | AD (most) | *VWF* | Deficiency of von Willebrand factor: normally aids in platelet adherence for nl blood clotting | 7 subtypes with bleeding, easy bruising, prolonged bleeding time, especially after surgery or tooth extraction; nl platelet count | Plasma-derived clotting factor concentrates, +desmopressin, fibrinolytic inhibitors, OCPs for menorrhagia. | Type 1 (most frequent): sequencing (60%–65%) |
| *Alpha thalassemia* | 141800 | AR | *HBA1, HBA2* | Decreased or absent alpha chains for Hgb formation **Hb Bart:** loss of all 4 alpha chains **HbH:** loss/dysfunction of 3 alpha chains **Alpha trait:** loss/dysfunction of 2 alpha chains **Silent carrier:** loss/dysfunction of 1 alpha chain | **Hb Bart:** hydrops fetalis, neonatal death **HbH:** hemolytic anemia **Alpha trait:** low MCV, low MCH **Silent carrier:** none or mild anemia Trait protective against malaria (aa/– or a-/a-) mild anemia, microcytosis) aa/– more common in SE Asians than Africans (a-/a-) | **Hb Bart:** no Rx, recommend termination **HbH:** transfusion during hemolytic crises, + splenectomy, antibiotics | Targeted mutation analysis for common deletions, detection varies by population |

| Beta thalassemia | 141900 | AR | *HBB* | Decreased or absent beta chains for Hgb formation $\beta^0$–when no HbA present $\beta^+$–if some HbA present | **Thalassemia major:** severe microcytic anemia and hepatosplenomegaly in first 2 years of life, crew cut skull on x-ray **Thalassemia minor:** milder anemia that only rarely requires treatment with blood transfusion | Thalassemia major: transfusions with chelation | Targeted mutation analysis detection varies by population. Sequencing (99%) |
|---|---|---|---|---|---|---|---|
| **Dermatologic** | | | | | | | |
| *Ichthyosis* | 242300 308100 146800 604777 | AR, XL | *TGM1, ALOXE3, ALOX12B, ICHTHYIN, ABCA12,* and *CYP4F22* | Multiple mechanisms involved in maintenance of cornified layer of the epidermis | A continuum of thick scaly skin that may range from severe with restriction of movement to milder forms. Harlequin ichthyosis (severe and often fatal form), lamellar ichthyosis (LI), and nonbullous congenital ichthyosiform erythroderma (NCIE). | Treatment of infections, petrolatum-based creams/ointments, + alpha-hydroxy acid or urea preparations to promote peeling and thinning of the stratum corneum | Mutation analysis: TGM1 (90% LI) ALOX12B (6%) ALOXE3 (4%) ABCA12 (1-2% LI, >93% HI) ICHTHYIN (1%-2% negative for TGM1) |
| *Incontinentia pigmenti* | 308300 | XLD | *NEMO* | Lack of NF-κB leads to apoptosis in cells | **Major:** skin changes: erythema > blister > hyperpigmented streaks > atrophic skin patches **Minor:** hypo/andontia, alopecia, wooly hair, nail pitting, retinal neovascularization. Male fetuses miscarry | Retinal exams first 1-2 years, cosmetic dentistry | Deletion/duplication analysis (80%) |

*(Continued)*

Table 178-1 Genetic Syndromes of Childhood in Adults (Continued)

| | OMIM # (Reference) | Heredity | Genes Involved | Disease Mechanism | Clinical Details | Management | Genetic Testing (Detection) |
|---|---|---|---|---|---|---|---|
| Oculocutaneous albinism | **OCA1A:** 203100 **OCA1B:** 606952 **OCA2:** 203200 | AR | *TYR, OCA2* | **OCA1A:** no melanin synthesis **OCA1B:** some melanin synthesis **OCA2:** some melanin synthesis | **OCA1A:** white hair and skin, decreased iris pigment, foveal hypoplasia, decreased visual acuity, nystagmus, strabismus. **OCA1B:** milder than OCA1A **OCA2:** eye problems similar to OCA1A, better vision, skin/eye pigmentation normal | Yearly eye exams, sun screen, skin cancer monitoring | Mutation analysis: TYR (OCA1A 2 mutations 83%, 1 mutation 17%; OCA1B 2 mutations 37%, 1 mutation 63%) |
| **Chromosomal/ Microdeletion** | | | | | | | |
| Angelman syndrome | 105830 | Imprinted | *UBE3A* | Loss of maternally imprinted contribution to PWS/AS region by common deletion, UBE3A mutation or imprinting defect. Abnormal ubiquitin protein degradation. | Microcephaly, MR, speech impairment, ataxia, seizures, inappropriate happy behavior | Management of medical issues, PT, OT, ST, antiepileptic medications | FISH/CGH (68%) UPD studies (7%) UBE3A sequencing (11%) |
| Klinefelter syndrome | Bojesen, Gravholt, 2007 | Chromosomal, 46 XXY | | Meiotic nondisjunction, maternal > paternal origin, AMA effect | Tall stature, gynecomastia, decreased facial hair, learning problems, delayed motor and language skills, small fibrosed testes resulting in azoospermia and infertility, osteopenia | Testosterone: bone density, secondary sex characteristics, libido, energy level, muscle mass, increased cholesterol. ICSI: can used to retrieve sperm from testicular biopsy | Karyotype |

| Disorder | OMIM | Inheritance | Gene | Mechanism | Clinical features | Management/Screening | Testing |
|---|---|---|---|---|---|---|---|
| *Prader-Willi syndrome* | 176270 | Imprinted | *SNURF-SNRPN, MKRN3 MAGEL2, NDN* | Loss of paternally imprinted contribution to PWS/AS region by common deletion, UPD or imprinting defect. | Hypotonia at birth with feeding problems, hyperphagia and obesity during childhood, MR, OCD, hypogonadism, hypothalamic insufficiency | Management of medical issues (OCD, OSA, DM, osteopenia) | 3-5 Mb deletion (70%) matUPD (15%) PWS imprinting center (1%-2%) |
| *Trisomy 21* | 190685 | Chromosomal: de novo trisomy (95%), robertsonian translocation (5%) | *Multiple genes in the Down syndrome critical region (DSCR)* | | Dysmorphic features, varying degrees of MR, hypotonia, growth delay, congenital heart defect, duodenal atresia, Hirschsprung disease, early-onset Alzheimer, transient myeloproliferative disorder, ALL | Thyroid monitoring: birth, 6 months, yearly. Celiac: screen 24 months. Atlantoaxial instability: assess at 3 and 5 years. Audiologic and ophthalmic monitoring. | Karyotype |
| *Turner syndrome* | Bondy, 2007 | Chromosomal, 45,XO | | X chromosome genes escape X-inactivation | Dysmorphic features, short stature, congenital lymphedema of hands and feet, webbed neck, coarctation of aorta, gonadal dysgenesis, renal anomalies, hypothyroidism | Short stature: GH Cardiovascular: initial ECHO in newborn period. Management of medical issues. | Karyotype |
| **Pulmonary** | | | | | | | |
| *CFTR-related disorders* | **CF:** 219700 **CBAVD:** 277180 | AR | *CFTR* | Dysfunction membrane chloride channel leads to thick secretions. Mutation classes: I–reduced or absent synthesis II–block in protein processing III–block in CFTR regulation IV–altered conductance | Cystic fibrosis: elevated sweat chloride test, chronic airway infection including sinusitis, end-stage lung disease, meconium ileus, pancreatic insufficiency, male infertility. CBAVD: congenital bilateral absence of the vas deferens. | Antibiotics, bronchodilators, steroids, mucolytics, lung transplant, pancreatic enzymes and fat-soluble vits | Targeted mutation analysis (25 mutation panel): Ashkenazi Jewish (97%) Caucasian (88%) African American (69%) Hispanic American (57%) Asian American (NA) |

*(Continued)*

Table 178-1 *Genetic Syndromes of Childhood in Adults (Continued)*

| | OMIM # (Reference) | Heredity | Genes Involved | Disease Mechanism | Clinical Details | Management | Genetic Testing (Detection) |
|---|---|---|---|---|---|---|---|
| *Alpha-1 antitrypsin deficiency* | 107400 | AR | *SERPINA1* | Loss of protease inhibition by AAT protein. PI alleles:<br>**PI\*M:** normal allele<br>**PI\*Z:** (p.E342K) deficiency allele | Obstructive jaundice and transaminitis in childhood, COPD and cirrhosis in adulthood. Isoelectric focusing of PI types:<br>**PI MM:** normal individuals<br>**PI MZ:** slight increased risk for decreased lung function among heterozygotes<br>**PI SZ:** increased risk of COPD among smokers<br>**PI ZZ:** clinical disease, plasma AAT ~18% | Liver transplantation, COPD management with bronchodilators and steroids | Targeted mutation analysis: PI\*Z, PI\*S (95%) |
| **Cardiac** | | | | | | | |
| *Brugada syndrome* | 601144 | AD | *SCN5A* | Lack of expression or increased inactivation of cardiac sodium channels | Nocturnal agonal breathing, syncope, ST-segment abnormalities in V1-V3, sudden cardiac death 40 y, SIDS | Implantable defibrillator, antiarrhythmics | Mutation analysis: SCN5A (20%-25%) |
| *Dilated cardiomyopathy* | 115200 601154 600884, others | AD, AR, XL | *ACTC1, DES, LMNA, MYH7, TNNT2, others* | Mutations in sarcomeric proteins involved in cardiac contractile mechanism | Heart failure, arrhythmias, thromboembolic disease | Pharmacologic therapy, pacemaker, implantable cardiac defibrillator, cardiac transplantation | Mutation analysis: multiple genes involved |
| *Familial hypertrophic cardiomyopathy* | 192600 | AD | *MYH7, MYBPC3, TNNT2 TNNI3, TPM1, others* | Mutations in sarcomeric proteins involved in cardiac contractile mechanism | Adolescents/adults: chest pain, palpitations, orthostasis, syncope, progressive heart failure, sudden cardiac death | Pharmacologic therapy, pacemaker, implantable cardiac defibrillator, cardiac transplantation | Mutation analysis: multiple genes involved |

| Disorder | OMIM | Inheritance | Gene(s) | Molecular pathogenesis | Clinical features | Management | Testing |
|---|---|---|---|---|---|---|---|
| Long QT | **LQT1:** 192500 **LQT2:** 152427 **LQT3:** 603830 | AD: Romano-Ward AR: Jervell/Lange-Nielsen | *KCNQ1, KCNH2, SCN5A, KCNE1, KCNE2* | **RWS:** LQT1: mutations in KCNQ1 or KCNE1, abnormal IKs potassium channel function LQT2: mutations in KCNH2 or KCNE2, IKr potassium channel dysfunction LQT3: mutations in SCN5A, abnormal INa channel function **JLN:** mutations in KCNQ1 or KCNE1, abnormal IKs potassium channel function | **RWS:** QT prolongation and T-wave abnormalities on the ECG and the ventricular tachycardia torsade de pointes (TdP). **JLN:** severe bilateral SNHL, prolonged QT interval, arrhythmia, syncope, sudden death | **RWS:** Pharmacologic therapy, pacemaker, implantable cardiac defibrillator **JLN:** cochlear implants, pharmacologic therapy, pacemaker, implantable cardiac defibrillator. | Mutation analysis: RWS (~70%) JLN (94%) |
| Noonan syndrome | 163950 | AD | *PTPN11, SOS1, KRAS, RAF1* | Constitutive activation of the RAS MAP kinase pathway due to gain-of-function mutations | Dysmorphic features, short stature, pulmonic valve stenosis, hypertrophic cardiomyopathy, renal malformations, bleeding diathesis, myeloproliferative disorder, cryptorchidism | Cardiac care, orchiopexy, GH treatment | Mutation analysis: PTPN11 (60%) KRAS (5%) SOS1 (10%-15%) RAF1 (3%-8%) |
| DiGeorge/velo-cardiofacial | 188400 | AD | *Multiple genes in 22q11 region, TBX1* | Common 3 Mb deletion leading to abnormal development of pharyngeal arches due to TBX1 dosage | Congenital heart defects: TOF, IAA B, conotruncal defects; immune dysfunction, hypocalcemia, renal anomalies, DD, psychiatric disorders, feeding problems, cleft palate | Cardiac care for CHD, palate repair, calcium supplements, caution with live vaccines | FISH/MLPA (>95%) |

*(Continued)*

Table 178-1 Genetic Syndromes of Childhood in Adults (Continued)

| | OMIM # (Reference) | Heredity | Genes Involved | Disease Mechanism | Clinical Details | Management | Genetic Testing (Detection) |
|---|---|---|---|---|---|---|---|
| **Metabolic/ Endocrine** | | | | | | | |
| *Acute intermittent porphyria* | 176000 | AD | HMBS | Defect in heme synthesis. Neurotoxicity of PBG metabolites? | Adolescent onset with acute attacks of abdominal pain, muscle weakness, neuropathy, psychiatric disturbance. Risk of hepatocellular carcinoma. | Stop precipitant of attack. IV dextrose and hemin. | Mutation analysis: HMBS (>98%) |
| *Androgen insensitivity syndrome* | **CAIS:** 300068 **PAIS:** 312300 | XLR | AR | Point mutations impair androgen binding to androgen receptor | May range from complete to partial androgen insensitivity. **CAIS:** undermasculinization of the external genitalia at birth, abnormal secondary sexual development in puberty, cryptorchidism, infertility in individuals with a 46,XY karyotype. **PAIS:** underviralized or ambiguous genitalia in 46, XY. | Prepubertal gonadectomy for cryptorchidism. HRT to maintain feminine characteristics (estrogen), or promote virilization (testosterone) and prevent bone loss (estrogen or testosterone). Discussion of sex assignment surgery in **Partial.** | Mutation analysis: AR (>95%) |
| *Congenital adrenal hyperplasia* | 201910 | AR | CYP21A2 | Production of cortisol is blocked with buildup of 17-OH progesterone which is converted to androgens. | **Classic:** Virilization and precocious puberty in females. Salt wasting crises at birth. Childhood virilization in males. **Nonclassic:** variable postnatal virilization | Hydrocortisone with stress doses. Discuss sex assignment surgery in virilized females. | Mutation analysis: CYP21A2 (>80%-98%) |

| Disease | OMIM | Inheritance | Gene(s) | Pathophysiology | Clinical features | Treatment | Mutation analysis |
|---|---|---|---|---|---|---|---|
| *Congenital hypothyroidism* | 275200 218700 | Sporadic AR | *DUOX2, PAX8, SLC5A5, TG, TPO, TSHB, TSHR* | Thyroid dyshormonogenesis | Untreated patients have profound MR, severe impairment of linear growth and bone maturation, spasticity, gait abnormalities, dysarthria or mutism, and autistic behavior. | Thyroid hormone replacement | Mutation analysis: DUOX2 (NA) PAX8 (NA) SLC5A5 (NA) TG (NA) TPO (NA) TSHB (NA) TSHR (NA) |
| *Fabry disease* | 301500 | XLR | *GLA* | Deficiency of alpha-galactosidase with progressive lysosomal deposition of globotriaosylceramide in cells throughout the body | Acroparesthesias, angiokeratomas, hypohidrosis, corneal and lenticular opacities, and proteinuria. ESRD usually occurs in men in the 3rd-5th decade. | Carbamazepine or gabapentin for acroparesthesias, ACEi for proteinuria. ERT using recombinant or gene-activated human alpha-Gal A enzyme. | Mutation analysis: GLA (100% males, unknown females) |
| *Gaucher disease* | **Type 1:** 230800 **Type 2:** 230900 **Type 3:** 231000 | AR | *GBA* | Deficiency of glucocerebrosidase with progressive lysosomal deposition of glucosylceramide in cells throughout the body | **Type 1:** osteopenia, focal lytic or sclerotic lesions, osteonecrosis, hepatosplenomegaly, anemia and thrombocytopenia, lung disease, and the absence of primary central nervous system disease. **Types 2 and 3:** + neurologic disease with onset before age 2 years, type 2 death 2-4 y, type 3 death 3rd-4th decade. Carrier rate is 1:18 in Ashkenazi Jews. | ERT using recombinant glucosylceramidase enzyme. Miglustat for individuals who are not candidates for ERT. Transfusions/splenectomy for pancytopenia, analgesics for bone pain, joint replacement therapy. Bone marrow transplantation. | Targeted mutation analysis: GBA (>98%) Mutation analysis: GBA (99%) |

*(Continued)*

Table 178-1  Genetic Syndromes of Childhood in Adults (Continued)

| | OMIM # (Reference) | Heredity | Genes Involved | Disease Mechanism | Clinical Details | Management | Genetic Testing (Detection) |
|---|---|---|---|---|---|---|---|
| Kallmann syndrome | 308700 147950 | XLR, AD | KAL, FGFR1 | Anosmin (KAL) and FGFR1 are critical in development of olfactory bulb. | Low FSH/LH, testosterone (males), estradiol (females). MRI: hypoplasia of olfactory bulbs/tracts **Type 1:** hypogonadotropic hypogonadism with anosmia, mirror hand movements, ataxia, GU abnormality **Type 2:** hypogonadotropic hypogonadism with anosmia, MR, cleft lip/palate, cryptorchidism, choanal atresia, congenital heart disease, hearing loss | Endocrine evaluation for gonadal steroid levels. Multidisciplinary management of associated medical/surgical issues. | Mutation analysis: KAL (5%-10%) FGFR1 (~10%) |
| Maple syrup urine disease | 248600 | AR | BCKDHA, BCKDHB, DBT | Deficiency of branched-chain ketoacid dehydrogenase leads to ketoacidosis and buildup of toxic leucine metabolites | Acute episodes of ketonuria, encephalopathy, lethargy, coma with increased protein load due to dietary nonadherence, infection, overrestriction. The phenotype is classified as classic or intermediate. Alloisoleucine on plasma amino acid analysis. | Synthetic amino acid formula devoid of branched-chain amino acids — valine, isoleucine, and leucine. Restriction of natural protein. Thiamine-responsive variants. Sick day regimens. Monitor plasma amino acids. | Mutation analysis: BCKDHA (~95%) BCKDHB (~95%) DBT (~95%) |

| | | | | | | | |
|---|---|---|---|---|---|---|---|
| *Phenylketonuria* | 261600 | AR | *PAH* | Deficiency of phenylalanine hydroxylase results in elevated phenylalanine and neurotoxic phenyllactate and phenylpyruvate. | Suboptimal/untreated individuals have learning deficits and mental retardation. Poorly controlled adults experience problems with concentration. | | |
| *Urea cycle disorders* | **NAGS:** 237310 **CPS1:** 2237300 **OTC:** 311250 **ASS1:** 215700 **ASL:** 207900 **ARG1:** 207800 | AR XLR | *NAGS, CPS1, OTC, ASS1, ASL, ARG1* | Deficiency in 1 of 6 urea cycle enzymes leads to hyperammonemia. | Acute episodes of hyperammonemic encephalopathy, coma, and death following increased protein load due to dietary nonadherence, infection, over-restriction. | Synthetic essential amino acid formula combined with dietary protein restriction. Detoxification medications. Sick day regimens. Monitor plasma amino acids, ammonia and LFTs. | Mutation analysis: NAGS (NA) CPS1 (NA) OTC (NA) ASS (96%) ASL (NA) ARG1 (NA) |
| *Wilson disease* | 277900 | AR | *ATP7B* | Loss of ATP7B impairs copper excretion with deposition of copper in tissues and oxidative damage | Kayser-Fleisher rings, low serum copper and ceruloplasmin, high urinary copper. Liver disease ranging from hepatitis to failure. Basal ganglia disease due to copper deposition. | Copper chelation, liver transplant | Mutation analysis: ATP7B (98%) |
| **Musculoskeletal** | | | | | | | |
| *Achondroplasia* | 100800 | AD | *FGFR3* | Constitutive activation of FGFR3 leads to growth suppression | Short stature, frontal bossing, macrocephaly, rhizomelic shortening, trident-shaped hand, midface hypoplasia, sleep apnea, spinal cord compression, narrowing of interpediculate distance. | Management of orthopedic issues: leg lengthening, hip replacement, spinal fusion, suboccipital decompression. | Mutation analysis: FGFR3 (98%) |

*(Continued)*

**Table 178-1 Genetic Syndromes of Childhood in Adults (Continued)**

| | OMIM # (Reference) | Heredity | Genes Involved | Disease Mechanism | Clinical Details | Management | Genetic Testing (Detection) |
|---|---|---|---|---|---|---|---|
| Ehlers-Danlos | **Type I:** 130000<br>**Type II:** 130010<br>**Type III:** 130020<br>**Type IV:** 130050<br>**Type VI:** 225400 | AD | **Type I:** COL5A1<br>**Type II:** COL5A2<br>**Type III:** TNXB<br>**Type IV:** COL3A1<br>**Type VI:** PLOD1 | **Types I and II:** dominant negative effect with abnormal collagen interfering with normal collagen.<br>**Type III:** abnormal dermal elastic fibers.<br>**Type IV:** abnormal type III procollagen<br>**Type VI:** deficient cross-linking of collagen | Abnormal collagen on dermal fibroblasts.<br>**Types I and II:** joint hypermobility leading to sprains/subluxation/dislocations, easy bruising, atrophic scars, aortic root dilatation.<br>**Type III:** joint hypermobility, velvety skin, easy bruising, narrow palate, aortic root dilatation and MVP.<br>**Type IV:** (vascular type) arterial rupture, intestinal rupture, uterine rupture<br>**Type VI:** kyphoscoliosis, hyperextensible skin, scarring, rupture of globe. | Physical therapy, joint bracing, avoid extreme movements, cardiac assessment (types I, II, III), eye exam (type VI). | Mutation analysis:<br>COL5A1 (30%)<br>COL5A2 (50%)<br>COL3A1 (98%-99%) |
| Loeys-Dietz syndrome | 609192 | AD | TGFBR1, TGFBR2 | Abnormal TGFβR signaling | Aortic dissection occurs at smaller aortic diameters than observed in Marfan syndrome. Cerebral, thoracic, and abdominal arterial aneurysms and/or dissections. Pectus deformity, scoliosis, joint laxity, arachnodactyly, talipes equinovarus, bifid uvula. | Beta-blockers to reduce hemodynamic stress. Frequent ECHO, MRA to monitor vessel disease. | Mutation analysis:<br>TGFBR1 (95%)<br>TGFBR2 (95%) |
| Marfan syndrome | 154700 | AD | FBN1 | Dominant negative forms of fibrillin and activation of TGFβ leads to abnormal tissue formation | Diagnosed by the Ghent criteria.<br>Tall stature, arachnodactyly, pectus deformity, lens dislocation, lumbosacral dural ectasia (MRI), aortic root dilatation (ECHO). | Beta-blockers for aortic root dilatation, ophthalmologic evaluation | Mutation analysis:<br>FBN1 (70%-90%)[a] |

| Disease | OMIM | Inheritance | Gene | Mechanism | Clinical features | Treatment | Mutation analysis |
|---|---|---|---|---|---|---|---|
| *Nemaline myopathy* | 609284 256030 161800 609285 | AD, AR | *ACTA1, CFL2, NEB, TNNT1, TPM2, TPM3* | Dysfunctional anchoring proteins in muscle lead to myopathy | Congenital/childhood/adulthood onset of head/neck and proximal weakness, hypotonia, decreased DTRs. Nemaline bodies in the sarcoplasm on muscle biopsy. | | Mutation analysis: ACTA1 (>90%) NEB (NA) TNNT1 (NA) TPM2 (NA) TPM3 (NA) |
| *Osteogenesis imperfecta* | **Type I:** 166200 **Type II:** 166210 **Type III:** 259420 **Type IV:** 166220 | AD, rare AR | *COL1A1, COL1A2* | Premature stop codons (type I) and missense mutations (types II, III, IV) alter collagen structure | 7 types distinguishable by clinical features. Bone fractures with minimal trauma, short stature, blue sclera, dentinogenesis imperfecta, hearing loss. | Bisphosphonates to decrease bone loss, GH. Orthopedic management of fractures. | Mutation analysis: Type I: (~ 100%) Type II: (98%) Type III: (60%–70%) Type IV: (70%–80%) |
| **Immunologic** | | | | | | | |
| *Common variable immunodeficiency* | 240500 | | *TNFRSF13B (TACI), ICOS, CD19, TNFRSF13C (BAFFR)* | Deficiency of regulatory molecules specific for immune development and function | Onset after 24 months with humoral immune deficiency resulting in increased susceptibility to infections. Sinopulmonary infections, meningitis, systemic bacterial infections, recurrent eye or skin infections, or gastrointestinal symptoms. Abnormal T-cell function and immune dysregulation. Autoimmune phenomena, lymphomas. | IVIG infusion | Mutation analysis: TNFRSF13B (100%) ICOS (100%) CD19 (100%) |
| *Familial Mediterranean fever* | 249100 | AR | *MEFV* | Mutations result in increased IL-1 responsiveness | Recurrent febrile attacks with inflammation of serosal surfaces: peritonitis, synovitis, pleuritis. Amyloidosis. At-risk groups include Armenians, Turkish, Arabs, North African Jews, Iraqi Jews, Ashkenazi Jews. | Colchicine maintenance | Mutation analysis: MEFV (90%) |

(Continued)

Table 178-1 Genetic Syndromes of Childhood in Adults (Continued)

| | OMIM # (Reference) | Heredity | Genes Involved | Disease Mechanism | Clinical Details | Management | Genetic Testing (Detection) |
|---|---|---|---|---|---|---|---|
| X-linked agammaglobulinemia | 300755 | XLR | BTK | BTK protein is expressed in multiple hematopoietic cell lineages and plays a role in development | Recurrent respiratory tract infections including sinusitis, pneumonia and otitis media. Cellulitis, sepsis, and meningitis. | IVIG infusion | Mutation analysis: BTK (92%) |
| **Hearing/Vision** | | | | | | | |
| Congenital hearing loss | 220290 | AR | GJB2 (Cx26), GJB6 (Cx30) | Gap junction loss results in buildup of toxic metabolites and hair cell death | Mild-profound SNHL | Hearing aids, cochlear implants, sign language | Mutation analysis: GJB2 (100%) GJB6 (100%) |
| Leber hereditary optic neuropathy | 535000 | Mitochondrial | MTND1, MTND4, MTND5, MTND6 | Degeneration of the ganglion cell layer of the retina and optic nerve due to mitochondrial dysfunction | Blurred or clouded vision progressing to retinal dystrophy and optic atrophy | No treatment available, faster progression with alcohol and smoking | Targeted mutation analysis: MTND (~95%) |
| Usher syndrome | **Type I:** 276900 **Type II:** 276901 **Type III:** 276902 | AR | Majority: MYO7A, USH2A | Degeneration of rod and cone functions of the retina | **Type I:** congenital profound SNHL, balance problems, retinitis pigmentosa (RP) onset first decade **Type II:** congenital mild-severe SNHL, RP onset late 2nd-3rd decade **Type III:** progressive later-onset SNHL, balance problems, variable-onset RP | Vitamin A may slow progression of blindness. Cochlear implants, hearing aids for SNHL. | Mutation analysis: MYO7A (~90%) USH2A (~35%-75%) |

| | | Inheritance | Gene(s) | Pathophysiology | Clinical features | Management | Molecular testing |
|---|---|---|---|---|---|---|---|
| **Gastrointestinal** | | | | | | | |
| Inflammatory bowel disease (see relevant chapter for further details) | Ishihara, 2009 | Multifactorial | **Crohn Disease:** *CARD15, TNFSF15, IL23R, ATG16L1, IRGM, OCT-NPTPN2, HLA (DR7, DRB3\*0301, DQ4, DRB1\*0103)* **Ulcerative colitis:** *IL23R* | Genes involved in immunity and maintenance of gastrointestinal mucosal barrier | **Crohn disease:** discontinuous transmural mucosal inflammation from mouth to anus with cobblestoning, fissure formation, and granuloma formation. **Ulcerative colitis:** continuous colonic mucosal ulceration with gland destruction and crypt abscesses. | Salicylates, antibiotics, steroids, immunomodulators. Nutritional management. Surgery for fistula formation. | NA |
| Familial adenomatous polyposis | 175100 | AD | *APC* | Abnormal APC protein allows high levels of cytosolic beta catenin to migrate to the nucleus and activate c-Myc and cyclin D1 | 100-1000 adenomatous polyps in childhood-adolescence. Malignant transformation inevitable. Colon cancer by 4th decade in untreated. **Attenuated FAP:** fewer, more proximal polyps. **Gardner syndrome:** polyposis with osteomas and soft tissue tumors. **Turcot syndrome:** colon cancer and CNS tumors | Colectomy by late adolescence. | Mutation analysis: APC (>90%) |

a Although molecular testing is done on occasion, Marfan syndrome is a clinical diagnosis

875

## BIBLIOGRAPHY:

1. Bojesen A, Gravholt CH. Klinefelter syndrome in clinical practice. *Nat Clin Pract Urol*. 2007;4:192.

2. Bondy CA. Care of girls and women with Turner syndrome: a guideline of the Turner Syndrome Study Group. *J Clin Endocrinol Metab*. 2007;92:10.

3. Ishihara S, Aziz MM, Yuki T, Kazumori H, Kinoshita Y. Inflammatory bowel disease: review from the aspect of genetics. *J Gastroenterol*. 2009;44:1097.

# 179 Clinical Interpretation of Genomic Data

Joseph V. Thakuria and Michael F. Murray

## KEY POINTS

- *Genomic technology:*
  - Advances in DNA sequencing technology have led to improved accuracy as well as decreased costs and have resulted in the recent introduction of individual whole genome, whole exome, and large gene panel sequencing from certified reference laboratories for clinical molecular diagnosis.

- *Data filtering:*
  - Bioinformatic filtering of the over 3 billion nucleotide base pairs found in any genome is required to identify causal mutations. Currently, most analysis focuses on the estimated 4000 genes (out of a total of ~20,000 genes) in the human genome implicated in human disease.

- *Informed consent:*
  - Prior to testing patients should be informed of (a) potential disclosure of nonpaternity, consanguinity, and/or unrelatedness to one or more family members, (b) the possibility of finding either a diagnosis or predisposition to a disease unrelated to the reason that sequencing was ordered, (c) limitations of current sequencing approaches (even when genetic etiology is strongly suspected), and (d) potential risk of genetic discrimination affecting either insurability and employment. They should also be informed of the US Federal law (GINA) which seeks to protect against the existing genetic discrimination.

- *Incidental findings:*
  - Diagnostic use of this technology is made more complex by the uncovering of numerous incidental findings (some with unknown significance and others with an established pathogenic effect) present in any individual genome.
  - Recent ACMG recommendations on release of incidental findings advises the return of "known pathogenic" and "expected pathogenic" variants identified across 56 well curated genes.

- *Genetic counseling:*
  - Appropriate genetic counseling to address incidental findings and informed consent issues is necessary both prior to as well as following medical genomic testing in a patient.

- *Periodic reanalysis:*
  - The rapidly evolving knowledge base allows providers to discuss with patients the expectation that future reanalysis of the same genomic dataset will yield additional valuable insights into the health implications of the data for the patient. Many predict that annual reanalysis will become the norm.

- *Results disclosure:*
  - Allowing patients to "opt out" for disclosure of abnormal results (even when findings are incidental or secondary) is generally not the norm in medicine. While controversial, there may be special instances in medical genomics where providing an "opt out" option for abnormal results is appropriate - such as when incidental findings for an adult-onset disease in a pediatric patient is discovered. Even in these cases, however, disclosure to the parents/guardians is generally favored over suppression of these results.

- *Sanger sequencing:*
  - The use of traditional DNA sequencing approaches to genetic diagnosis (ie, Sanger sequencing) continues to have a clinical role in the diagnosis of many well-studied conditions. Currently, pathogenic mutations generated from next-generation sequencing (NGS) are usually confirmed with an alternative method of clinical sequencing before being medically acted upon and Sanger sequencing is often considered the "gold standard" for confirmation.

- *Limitations of NGS:*
  - Current technology does not perfectly represent the complete genome or exome due to technical limitations. At this time, clinical exome sequencing on average covers 92-99% or more of targeted coding areas of genes and provides a diagnostic yield in around one-quarter of cases when applied to highly selected scenarios of "diagnostic unknowns." Some causative mutations, such as trinucleotide repeat expansions in disorders like Huntington Disease, may be better identified by other methodologies like Southern blots.

## Genome Types and Sources

*Nuclear and Mitochondrial Genomes:* Genomes can be nuclear or mitochondrial. Nuclear genomes are sequenced from DNA in a cell's nucleus. Mitochondrial genomes are sequenced from circular DNA found in mitochondria organelles in the cytoplasm and are maternally inherited. At 37 kb, mitochondrial genomes are much smaller than the approximately 3 Gb haploid nuclear genome. Mitochondrial genomes can also have large sequence variation (a) between individuals, (b) within the same individual in different tissues, and/or (c) within the same tissue (a phenomena termed heteroplasmy). In this chapter we refer to nuclear genomes unless otherwise specified.

***Germline and Somatic Mutations:*** Comparison of germline mutations (those that are transmitted to offspring) against somatic mutations (those accumulated over one's lifetime) has been shown to have clinical impact specifically in oncology. Studying these changes to the normal germline genome is expected to refine molecular characterization of cancers and lead to more targeted and individualized treatments. An important challenge is distinguishing "driver" mutations (those mutations causing tumors and enabling disease progression) from "passenger" mutations (mutations arising from tumor progression with neutral effect that are not present in the germline genome). Identifying somatic mutations that are pharmacogenetically informative may also lead to safer and better targeted cancer treatment regimens.

***DNA Source:*** DNA can be extracted from any tissue in the body. Traditionally, DNA extracted from leukocytes in whole blood is the sterile source of DNA for most clinical testing. When DNA is derived from nonsterile sources, clinicians should be aware that DNA sequence from normal flora may mistakenly be confused for host sequence from either sequencing or bioinformatics error. Obtaining DNA from a nonsterile site, such as with buccal swab or saliva sample, however, has the advantage over blood draw of being less invasive and has been used for large-scale genomic research studies.

## Basic Individual Genome Statistics

- Average basic genomic statistics have been shown to be generally uniform across individuals and diverse ethnic populations. The difference between any two unrelated individuals on the single nucleotide level is less than 0.1%. Diversity between individuals is greatly increased, however, when factoring in structural chromosomal rearrangements or insertions and deletions, and RNA transcript variation. Because of this similarity, analysis detecting pathogenic variants can be prioritized on the proportionately smaller number of variants that are either novel (ie, not seen in standard reference genomic databases) and/or have low minor allele frequencies.
- A human haploid genome has roughly 3.2 billion bases. The number of single-nucleotide variants against the reference genome is 3.5 to 4 million changes per genome. The number of single-nucleotide variants causing nonsynonymous changes (ie, those causing a change in amino acid and potentially deleterious) averages greater than 9500/genome.
- Clinical interpretation of genomes always requires some degree of bioinformatic filtering to identify those changes most likely to cause disease or influence disease severity. Often described as trying to "find a needle in a haystack," distinguishing causal variants from a potentially large number of false-positive variants is a major challenge in clinical genome analyses.

## Genomic Disease Architecture

***Coding Regions:*** Focusing genomic sequencing and/or data filtering on coding regions, representing approximately 1.5% to 2% of the genome that codes for protein is a reasonable first pass for most clinical situations as over 85% of known disease-causing mutations are found here. Sequencing exomes (ie, the 180,000 exons in the human genome) instead of whole genomes reduces cost and storage requirements. At the time of this writing, exome sequencing is more common in clinical use than whole genome sequencing.

The trade-off for this approach, however, is potentially missing a pathogenic variant(s) in noncoding regions and losing potentially important gene-regulatory information.

With the increase of competitive pricing, it is likely that clinical WGS will become preferable to exome sequencing. In selected cases, WGS may be a good follow-up test when exome sequencing is not diagnostic. Further, the disease contribution of noncoding regions is likely to be generally underestimated because of the difficulty traditional Sanger sequencing historically has had comprehensively capturing these large noncoding sequence segments. Prioritizing which regions of a genome are clinically analyzed (ie, on the basis of coding region, known causal genes, and/or mutation type) should be guided by disease-specific information when available.

Determining which genetic changes in noncoding regions are pathogenic is also more challenging as the presence and/or type of protein change produced may be less obvious. In addition, presumably lower selection pressure in these noncoding areas can potentially make analysis of evolutionary conservation less informative.

Currently, clinical molecular genetics laboratories offering exome sequencing are generally reporting 92% to 97% coverage of targeted exome regions at a sequencing depth sufficient enough to allow confident zygosity calls. The sequence accuracy within these regions is typically reported at 99.9%. False-positive rates are relatively high at 5% to 10%. Diagnostic yield from exome sequencing across cases appears to be around 25% at the present time (and as high as 50% in carefully selected cases).

***Functional Effects:*** A gene is a contiguous portion of DNA that codes for protein and is considered a functional part of the genome. While the existence of pathogenic sequence variations outside of genes are well documented, the majority of known disease mutations are either within genes or within close enough proximity (eg, within 50 kb) of a nearby gene to affect function. Recently published data from ENCODE highlights the progress being made at better categorization of noncoding regions affecting gene function and expression. The data suggest functional elements in noncoding sequence throughout the genome may have been underestimated (ie, reside >50 kb from the gene it regulates). With respect to clinical analyses of genomic data however, the majority of known genetic disease is still overwhelmingly in coding regions at the present time and therefore is still typically prioritized in most clinically focused analyses. More clinical outcomes data are needed to study the clinical impact of these regulatory regions.

***Gene Prioritization:*** From roughly 20,000 genes in the human genome, only around 3000 to 4000 genes are robustly associated with highly penetrant inherited diseases at present. Prioritizing analyses in genes specifically known to cause the patient's pathogenic phenotype before looking genome—wide to discover a gene without previous disease association is reasonable—especially when the number of cases analyzed is low and/or familial genomic references are not available.

***Variant Classes and Mutation Classes:*** To date, most well-recognized monogenic disorders are caused by single-nucleotide changes in coding regions as well as pathogenic chromosomal deletions, and, to a lesser extent, insertions.

## Variant Filtering Algorithms

- Variant filtering algorithms aim to reduce the large number of genomic variants found in any individual's genome down to a small and manageable number likely to contain the causal pathogenic variant(s). A variety of these have proven successful in molecular diagnosis and medical discovery. Several basic variant filtering strategies have proven successful across a wide range of genetic disease when used in combination and are described later.

**Case or Control Data:** Whether the aim is to (a) comprehensively screen an individual genome for any serious, medically important mutation, or (b) to identify a disease-specific causative mutation(s), case or control data is typically the strongest line of evidence in determining causality. Unfortunately, utilizing case-control data from the literature is labor intensive and typically requires some degree of manual review. In critical review of the literature emphasis should be placed on (a) sample sizes, (b) availability of general population screening data, (c) how well controls were phenotyped and if they were of advanced age, (d) the allele frequency of the variant of interest, (e) prevalence of the disease studied, and (f) quality of the sequence data.

**Locus-Specific Databases (LSDBs):** In addition to case or control (ie, clinical outcomes) data from the literature, currently much (and for some diseases, the majority) of variant evidence for pathogenicity reside in the unpublished databases of private academic and commercial laboratories doing the clinical sequencing. Obviously, just as it is for single gene sequencing, this is valuable data in clinically interpreting genomic data—especially when combined. Several efforts are underway to incentivize clinical laboratories to make more of this data available. At present, no single variant database is inclusive of all known pathogenic human mutations. Efforts to create more comprehensive disease-specific as well as general disease pathogenic variant databases are underway but challenging to create for a variety of reasons. Ideally, a single comprehensive database of known pathogenic variants would simplify genomic analyses by enabling genomes to be parsed against one database for all variants known to have clinical evidence of pathogenicity.

**Familial Analyses:** Familial data supporting pathogenic variants through disease segregation with the mutation within a family (or across families) can be part of the reported case or control data in the literature. When published case-control data does not exist, the next best clinical outcomes evidence for causality can come from familial analyses comparing the patient's (or study subject's) genome against that of affected and unaffected family members. This is typically helpful when the disease of interest either shows a simple Mendelian pattern of inheritance or is believed to be the result of a de novo mutation (ie, a mutation arising new in the family during conception of the proband). Familial analyses can be challenging if the disease phenotype is common and may not truly be tracking with the shared familial mutation.

To save on sequencing costs, some groups have successfully elected to perform linkage analysis with genotyping chip technology on family members to narrow down the size of the candidate pathogenic region and then perform targeted NGS of the area.

**Common Risk Variants Versus Mendelian Mutations:** When critically evaluating the case-control literature, it is helpful to make the broad distinction between the two groups of variants. Mendelian mutations reported in the literature are generally (a) monogenic, (b) highly penetrant, (c) rare (allele frequency <1%-5% for autosomal dominant disease), and (d) causative of a disease with rare or unusual phenotype. They are typically medically actionable and have reproductive importance.

Common risk variants typically (a) have high allele frequency, (b) are low penetrant, (c) occur in noncoding regions, and (d) are poorly predictive (relative risk [RR] <2) for a common disease.

These variants are linked to disease through genome-wide association study (GWAS), and are felt to contribute too many risk factors for common diseases.

Not making the important distinction between these two types of variants in a clinical setting is a common pitfall in analyses leading to numerous false positives.

**Variant Frequency:** In general, the frequency of a genomic variant in the general population is inversely proportional to pathogenicity and can therefore aid in estimating pathogenicity in clinical cases. Common variants are likely to be benign and pathogenic variants are likely to be rare. There are exceptions however, common variants are not always benign (especially with respect to carriers of recessive disorders and reproductive counseling) and, of course, rare variants are not always pathogenic.

Setting frequency thresholds should be guided by suspected Mendelian inheritance pattern when appropriate. For example, in suspected autosomal dominant disease, allele frequency cutoffs should be more stringent (eg, <1%-5% minor allele frequency [MAF]) than when autosomal recessive inheritance is suspected (ie, where allele frequency in unaffected carriers can be as high as 10%-20%).

Additionally, due to sampling bias, reported allele frequencies will vary between studies especially if the sample size is not statistically large enough. Complicating matters, reported allele frequencies vary between ethnic groups across different studies and are not always similar even within ethnic groups across different studies (especially when an ethnicity is under-represented).

Obviously, when using too strict a frequency threshold to determine pathogenicity, causative variants may erroneously get excluded. Despite these limitations, successful genomic parsing of disease genomes using stringent allele frequency filtering has already led to successful clinical molecular diagnosis and genomic discovery for rare Mendelian disorders in several studies.

**Protein Prediction:** Another important filtering mechanism routinely used to narrow down the list of causative variants is the utilization of software that helps predict how pathogenic the gene's protein product will be based on a variety of factors related to the mutation that are scored and weighed differently across different bioinformatic tools.

Factors that these tools consider include (a) the degree to which the sequence is evolutionarily conserved across species, (b) whether the nucleotide change is from a purine to a pyrimidine or vice versa (ie, transitions vs tranversions), and (c) if a resulting amino acid change results in a change in either electrical charge or hydrophobicity for the molecule.

**Clinical Ascertainment Bias:** Because of historical clinical ascertainment bias, some variants reported as pathogenic in both the literature and databases may be found to be benign in patients who have had NGS for other reasons when adequate outcomes data from screening of the general population are not yet available.

## Biologic Confounders

**Genetic Heterogeneity:** Genetic disease caused by mutations in one of several different genes present challenges in clinical interpretation when one or more candidate hits are identified in a patient's genome or exome.

**Genetic Pleiotropy:** When single genes cause a wide range of disease phenotypes, interpreting the clinical significance of mutations in these genes in the context of personal and family history becomes more complex.

*Reduced Disease Penetrance:* Pathogenic variants may be difficult to identify when disease has reduced penetrance (where a subset of individuals with the pathogenic mutation will not manifest disease).

*Variable Disease Expressivity:* When a genetic disease has a wide spectrum of disease severity and manifestations between different individuals, this also poses challenges in clinical interpretation of genomic data. For example, high disease expressivity can be problematic when studying disease segregation in a family if there is variable age of onset.

## Platform or Technology Confounders

Platform and technology confounders described later summarize general concepts important for clinicians who are engaged early in a clinical genomic interpretation pipeline. Typically, they are either performing the NGS in a clinical laboratory setting and/or are the first to receive the "raw" or minimally processed NGS data. Clinicians who primarily (a) interpret summarized NGS reports with candidate variants already annotated, (b) review summarized results in the context of patient's medical and family history, (c) counsel and report genomic results to patients, and (d) medically manage and treat the patient and extended family members should also be familiar with these confounders. In many cases, though, these confounding factors will have already been considered by the clinical laboratory performing the NGS and generating the summarized clinical report.

*Coverage:* To a large degree, greater confidence in nucleotide base determination or "base calling" at a specific single-nucleotide position is a direct function of the number of times the nucleotide is redundantly called at that position. When this redundancy is 10-fold (10×) or more, accurately determining zygosity at that position becomes more probable. Coverage of at least greater than 30 to 35× is what is typically expected in NGS for clinical use. Several laboratories offering clinical exome sequencing provide an average of 70× coverage or greater. Confirmation of the suspected pathogenic variant(s) with Sanger sequencing is typically included in pricing as is a limited clinical interpretation focused on the medical indication leading to NGS.

*Chromosomal Phasing:* Accurate phasing of potentially pathogenic variants is still not reliable with NGS at the time of this writing. Efforts to increase sequence read length may eventual lead to routine and accurate phase determination—particularly important for autosomal recessive disorders. For now, as in traditional single gene sequencing, the most accurate way to determine the phase of a variant in clinical situation is parental testing whenever possible.

*Pseudogenes:* Pseudogenes represent evolutionarily nonfunctional gene copies with high sequence homology to their functional gene counterparts. Such homology can cause both chemical sequencing (especially in the annealing phase) and bioinformatic (particularly with alignment) confounding errors. Several studies analyzing representative areas of the genome extrapolate that 10,000 to 20,000 pseudogenes exist in the human genome. Because a relatively small subset of functional genes are believed to be responsible for a large fraction of the total number of pseudogenes (perhaps through sharing a common retrotransposon origin), the confounding impact of pseudogenes is lower than what might otherwise be expected.

*Bias Toward Single-Nucleotide Variants:* As noted earlier, indels, chromosomal rearrangements, and repetitive regions have higher NGS error rate due to both sequence chemistry and bioinformatics. For this reason, NGS diagnostic yield is higher when the molecular etiology is a single-nucleotide variant. In fact, many clinical NGS providers currently limit analyses to single-nucleotide variants.

## Computational or Bioinformatic Confounders

*Data Formats:* A variety of genomic data formats are available. Comparisons across individual genomes should ideally be made on datasets sharing the same format. Conversion of genomic datasets into a shared format prior to analyses may introduce error. When data formats lack nucleotide-specific coverage information and other alignment data, confidence in base calls is decreased. To varying degree, different formats include nucleotide-specific coverage and other information relevant to alignment accuracy.

*Data Compression:* Excluding data with high storage requirements and low likelihood of clinical importance from genomic data files help decrease cost as well as processing needs. Data often considered for exclusion in order to compress genomic files include (a) raw sequencing images, (b) noncoding data, (c) reference alleles, and (d) indels (which are usually still provided as separate files when bioinformatically excluded). Lack of these data can present problems in base call confidence or when causative mutations are found in these excluded regions.

*Alignment:* Alignment, or the bioinformatic process of accurately placing short-sequenced reads (typically 35-250 bp vs 650-800 bp with conventional Sanger sequencing) against its corresponding position in genomic reference sequence, can introduce additional error when reads are inaccurately placed. When base calls differ between different datasets due to alignment error or because different alignment tools (with different base-calling thresholds) are used, molecular diagnosis may be challenging—even in cases strongly suspected to have an identifiable molecular cause.

*Variant Annotation and Manual Curation:* Variants can be automatically annotated to genetic disease databases as noted earlier. While many are extremely helpful and routinely used in clinical practice, at present, all of these have limitations, are incomplete, and prone to error. In most cases, some degree of manual curation is required. Research into ways to leverages crowdsourcing more efficiently to curate a wide range of pathogenic and benign mutations found is underway in the Personal Genome Project study and other projects. These curations can be found in GET-Evidence, a publicly available Wiki-like resource for genomic variant interpretation.

*Reference Genomes:* The UCSC hg19 genomic reference is likely the most commonly used reference in clinical genomic analyses currently. Not surprisingly, clinical interpretation relies heavily on comparison with a reference sequence. When affected and unaffected family members are available to serve as patient-specific familial genomic references, potential diagnostic yield is increased.

Most current genomic references are based on Caucasian ethnicity. The first human sequence draft generated from the Human Genome Project, a 13-year effort that began in 1990 and cost over $3 billion, was composite of WBC-derived DNA where roughly 70% of sequence came from RP11, an anonymous male donor from Buffalo, NY, with the remaining sequence library being represented by two males and two females; with each gender randomly selected from a pool of 20 individuals each.

The use of ethnically matched reference genomes in clinical analyses may lower the number of false positives generated in any medical genome analyses. Efforts to create (a) major allele reference genomes, (b) patient-specific familial references, and (c) "healthy" reference genomes (in which pathogenic and risk alleles are removed) are underway by our group and others which hopefully further decreases false positives in clinical genomic analyses.

## Current Clinical NGS Offerings

- *Laboratories:* There are a growing number of clinical laboratories offering whole genome and whole exome testing for clinical use. There are research laboratories that other this testing too, outside of a CLIA environment, however such testing is not for use in clinical care.
- *Cost, TAT, and common platform:* The cost of clinical whole genome sequencing is approximately $7500. Exome sequencing providers generally deliver exome sequencing at a cost of less than $5000 per case. Turn-around time is generally 4 to 12 weeks.
- *Other genomes:* Some laboratories offer sequencing and comparative genomic analyses between tumor and germline genomes in the same individual. Mitochondrial genome sequencing is sometimes included in exome sequencing depending on the sequencing provider.

## Future Directions

Expanding clinical indications and incorporating genomic data into routine clinical care will present unique challenges to existing healthcare delivery systems.

**Expanding Clinical Indications:** As the full genetic disease contribution for any individual should be increasingly decipherable from clinical analysis of genomic and other datasets (eg, proteomics), it seems inevitable that in the coming years (especially as prices continue to drop, sequence accuracy improves, and more cases of clinical utility are documented), indications for NGS will expand and ultimately it is likely to be offered as a health screening option for most adults.

Currently, depending on variant filtering stringencies, an average of 5 to 25 variants indicating carrier status for established autosomal recessive disorders can be expected to be found in any whole genome or exome that are currently medically actionable in terms of reproductive planning and offering expanded testing to family members.

Recent ACMG recommendations on release of incidental findings advise the return of "known pathogenic" and, for some genes, "expected pathogenic" variants identified across 56 genes found in patients, and even healthy family members (presumably sequenced for comparison against an affected proband), with exome or whole genome data ordered for a different primary clinical indication. The number of genes in which return of secondary findings is recommended can be expected to grow over time and should lead to genomic screening options in healthy individuals. Disorders caused by mutations in these genes include inherited cancers, connective tissue disorders (specifically those associated with cardiovascular events), cardiomyopathies, cardiac arrhythmia, familial hypercholesterolemia, and malignant hyperthermia.

Further, screening for highly penetrant and well-established pathogenic mutations is likely to have some clinical benefit at relatively small sample sizes. Estimates are that as many as 10% of analyzed human genomes will have this type of significant finding.

More prospective clinical data is needed to determine whether the risks and costs associated with follow-up of genomic incidental findings is enough to offset potential benefits. Furthermore, as prospective clinical data from genomic screening of the general population accumulates over time, accurate determination of variant pathogenicity will increase and risk from follow-up of incidental findings should proportionately decrease.

**BIBLIOGRAPHY:**

1. ENCODE Project Consortium, Dunham I, Kundaje A, et al. An integrated encyclopedia of DNA elements in the human genome. *Nature.* 2012;489:57-74.
2. ACMG Board of Directors. Points to consider in the clinical application of genomic sequencing. *Genet Med.* 2012;14:759-761.
3. Ball MP, Thakuria JV, Zaranek AW, et al. A public resource facilitating clinical use of genomes. *Proc Natl Acad Sci U S A.* 2012;109:11920-11927.
4. Dewey FE, Chen R, Cordero SP, et al. Phased whole-genome genetic risk in a family quartet using a major allele reference sequence. *PLoS Genet.* 2011;7:e1002280.
5. Ashley EA, Butte AJ, Wheeler MT, et al. Clinical assessment incorporating a personal genome. *Lancet.* 2010;375:1525-1535.
6. Green RC, Berg JS, Grody WW, et al. ACMG recommendations for reporting of incidental findings in clinical exome and genome sequencing. *Genet Med.* 2013;15:565-574.

# 180 Genetic Risk Profiling in the Genomics Era

Anthony A. Philippakis

## KEY POINTS

- *Overview:*
  - The past 5 years have been a time of tremendous progress in our understanding of the genetic basis of polygenic traits, with over 1100 genomic loci having been associated with over 165 complex (ie, polygenic) traits. While this has led to huge advances in our understanding of the mechanisms of disease, the clinical application of this information to risk prediction has been more limited. The reasons for this are outlined here. Since a detailed discussion of genetic risk for every disease is beyond the scope of this chapter, we focus on a few illustrative examples.
- Genome-wide association studies (GWAS) have dramatically increased our understanding of the mechanisms of common human diseases.
- Applying these results to clinical medicine is difficult due to both incomplete heritability and an incomplete understanding of the genetic basis of human disease.
- Further studies are needed to better understand how genetically based risk prediction can be effectively applied to the management of human diseases. Studies are also needed that address the ethics of genetic disclosure and its psychologic effects on patients.

## Basic Definitions and Principles

***Modes of Inheritance: Monogenic Versus Polygenic:*** Monogenic traits are those which are determined by a single gene. Examples include diseases such as cystic fibrosis and Duchenne muscular dystrophy, as well as benign traits such as having attached earlobes. Polygenic traits, in contrast, are the result of many genes. Examples again include both diseases such as type 2 diabetes mellitus, as well as nondisease traits such as stature. Note that polygenic traits, although frequently quantitative (eg, blood pressure or low-density lipoprotein [LDL] cholesterol), can also be binary (eg, coronary artery disease or schizophrenia). For nonquantitative polygenic traits, a threshold model is frequently used to explain modes of inheritance.

***Heritability:*** In its most simplistic formulation, the variation of any trait can be partitioned into a genetic component ($G$) and an environmental component ($E$). Heritability refers to the proportion of trait variation that can be attributed to genetic variation (ie, $G/(G + E)$), and its value ranges from 0 (ie, no genetic contribution) to 1 (completely genetic). Although the variation of a trait can be directly measured, the heritability must be indirectly inferred. There are many methods for this, but one of the most common is through the comparison of monozygotic and dizygotic twins; if the correlation for the trait among monozygotic twins is higher than that among dizygotic twins, then the trait is more heritable (the interested reader is encouraged to refer to *Genetics and Analysis of Quantitative Traits* for a further discussion of this method, which is known as *Falconer's formula*).

***Genome-Wide Association Study:*** A new method developed in recent years to identify genetic variants that increase or decrease the likelihood of a polygenic trait. In a typical GWAS, one begins with a collection of individuals with a given trait (such as coronary artery disease), as well as a collection of controls. In each individual from the case and control populations, a large number of genetic variants (typically on the order of 1 million) throughout the genome are assayed, and those variants that are most over- or under-represented among cases are determined. Thus, a GWAS is a type of case-control study that seeks to discover genetic variants associated with disease.

***Odds Ratio:*** The fundamental unit for reporting the effect size of a genetic variant on a trait. It expresses the proportion of individuals in the case group who carry a given allele relative to the proportion in the control group. When the odds ratio (OR) is greater than 1, a given allele is more frequent in the case group; conversely, when the OR is less than 1, it is more common in the control group.

☞**SUCCESSES AND LIMITATIONS OF GWAS:** Prior to 2005, fewer than a dozen genetic loci outside of the human leukocyte antigen (HLA) had been reproducibly associated with polygenic traits; since then, over 1100 genetic loci have been associated with over 165 traits. The key to this progress was the advent of the GWAS, which allowed polygenic traits to be mapped at a rate that was previously unimaginable. However, while GWASs have led to breathtaking progress in our understanding of the mechanisms of disease, their clinical applicability has been disappointing to many. The central issue is that the ORs of the vast majority of discovered loci are small, generally less than 1.5. Moreover, even in aggregate, the loci that have been associated with most diseases seem to explain only a small fraction of the observed heritability. This does not by any means imply that the discovered loci are biologically unimportant; for example, the *HMGCR* locus whose gene product is the target of statins has a common variant that only affects LDL by a modest 2.8 mg/dL, yet it is clearly an important locus in the biology of lipid metabolism. Instead, it suggests that many of the variants discovered through GWASs are weakly penetrant, and that it is their biologic relevance, rather than their clinical utility, that is of greatest importance.

Thus, even though a large number of loci have been discovered, and even though the studies have been performed in very large sample sizes (often in over 100,000 individuals), only a small amount of genetic risk is currently explained. For example, in type 2 diabetes mellitus (T2DM), 39 loci have been associated with the disease as of early 2011. Together, these loci explain at most approximately

25% of the heritability of the disease. Given that the disease is itself only about 60% heritable (although this can vary depending on the characteristics of the sampled population), this implies that at most approximately 15% of variance in disease incidence can be explained by these 39 loci, a fraction that is too small to be clinically useful in predicting who is most at risk for T2DM.

It is currently unclear where the "missing heritability" lies for polygenic traits. GWASs performed to date have focused on common variants, and it is possible that there are other, rarer variants of larger effect that explain the missing heritability. For example, an intriguing recent study by Alkuraya and colleagues discovered that rare but highly penetrant homozygous mutations in the gene *DNASE1L3* cause a disease that phenocopies systemic lupus erythematosus. Similarly, it is possible that interactions among genes or between genes and the environment will explain the bulk of the missing heritability. Finally, many postulate that modifications to DNA ("epigenetics"), rather than DNA variation itself, will be more important than previously realized.

Thus, despite the success of GWASs as a tool for discovering the mechanisms of disease, translating these discoveries into risk profiling has proven more difficult. The following examples demonstrate cases where people have attempted risk profiling for polygenic traits, highlighting both successful and unsuccessful attempts.

### Example 1: Type 2 diabetes and limitations to the use of genetics in risk prediction

The works of Meigs et al. and Lyssenko et al. represent early, but carefully done, studies evaluating the utility of genetic variables in predicting who is mostly at risk for the development of T2DM. Both groups began with the premise that the heritability of T2DM is substantial, suggesting that genetic variables might be an effective tool to predict who is mostly at risk for T2DM. However, there are many clinical variables that are also predictive of T2DM, such as body mass index (BMI), age, gender, a family history of T2DM, and fasting blood glucose level. This begs the question of the degree to which genetic variables add to clinical variables in risk prediction.

Meigs et al. examined patients in the Framingham population, using the "area under the curve" (AUC) as a measure of predictive accuracy. This is a commonly used statistical measure for evaluating classification methods, with a value of 1 implying perfect classification and a value of 0.5 being no better than random (an AUC of 0 implies perfectly inaccurate classification). The authors evaluated a genetic risk score based on 18 loci known to influence the risk of T2DM (the total number of validated loci at the time of the study) and found that this score in addition to information on patient gender (a genetic variable) had an AUC of only 0.595. A score based on clinical variables alone, however, had an AUC of 0.9, and was not significantly improved by adding genetic variables. Thus, T2DM appears to be "predictable" but clinical variables are much more useful than genetic variables.

The study of Lyssenko et al. took a similar approach, but focused on Scandinavian populations. They also looked at a genetic score based on 11 loci associated with T2DM, as well as clinical variables. Similar to Meigs et al., they also noted that the addition of clinical factors resulted in only a slight improvement in the AUC, increasing its value in this population from 0.74 to 0.75.

There are some limitations to these studies. First, they were done at a time when very few loci for T2DM had been discovered; one could imagine that such genetic risk scores will continue to improve as more loci are discovered. Second, these studies were performed in adults, and many of the clinical variables utilized in

risk prediction for T2DM (such as fasting glucose levels or BMI) become manifest only slightly before the development of the disease. Thus, one would expect a genetic risk score to have greater utility relative to clinical variables in, say, a newborn. Nevertheless, these studies highlight the limited utility of genetic variables in risk prediction for T2DM because of (1) incomplete heritability, (2) incomplete knowledge of the genetic basis of T2DM, and (3) the fact that much of the information that could be gained from genotyping can also be obtained from clinical variables such as BMI and a positive family history.

### Example 2: Age-related macular degeneration as a candidate for risk prediction

One of the most successful applications of GWAS methodology has been age-related macular degeneration (AMD). In 2005, a series of seminal papers demonstrated an association between complement factor H (CFH) and AMD, with unusually large ORs of approximately 3.5. Prior to these studies, there had been no appreciation for the possible role of the complement cascade in the progression of AMD. Moreover, additional loci in other genes involved in the complement cascade were subsequently found to be associated with AMD in better-powered follow-up GWASs, strengthening the original result.

A study by Seddon and colleagues in 2007 sought to rigorously evaluate the degree to which *CFH*, as well as another loci *LOC387715* that had previously been linked to AMD, could be used to predict who was mostly at risk for the disease. Moreover, they sought to examine whether there was any interaction between these loci and two traditional risk factors for AMD, obesity and smoking. Using a cohort of 1466 individuals that were followed prospectively for 6 years for the development of AMD, the authors began by genotyping potential risk alleles at each of these two loci. For the *CFH* locus, rates of progression to AMD were 10% for those individuals homozygous for the nonrisk allele (study participants were aged 55-80 years), 18% for heterozygotes, and 30% for individuals homozygous for the risk allele. Similarly, for the *LOC387715* locus, rates of progression were 9.5% for individuals homozygous for the nonrisk allele, 24% for heterozygotes, and 44% for individuals homozygous for the risk allele. Individuals homozygous for risk alleles at both genes had a nearly 50% progression rate. There was no evidence for genetic interaction (epistasis) between the loci; although somewhat surprising from a view of model organism genetics, where epistasis is commonplace, it is consistent with a prior study examining these loci. The authors further demonstrated that 71.8% of the risk was attributable to these loci, and that these loci alone could be used to classify which individuals would progress to AMD with an AUC of 0.758.

The authors next looked at the impact of the clinical variables BMI and smoking. They found that both smoking (OR 1.2) and BMI greater than 25 (OR 1.5) increased risk of progression to AMD, irrespective of genotype. When information about genetic background was included, they found that risks largely operated in an additive fashion, without statistical evidence for interaction. Here, being a carrier of all four risk factors, including BMI greater than 25, smoking, and being homozygous for the risk alleles at both loci, carried an OR of 19 for risk of progression to AMD. Adding BMI and smoking covariates to a genetic model modestly increased the attributable risk to 81.2% from 71.8%, but increased the AUC for classification to only 0.768 from 0.758.

Unlike the case of T2DM, the preceding results suggest that genetic variables appear to be more informative than clinical variables in risk prediction for AMD. Thus, AMD represents a disease where there may eventually be a role for genetic risk profiling. This will require two advances, however: (1) Although the risk prediction model described earlier was promising, it is unclear whether it is sufficiently accurate for clinical use. Already, the same authors of that study have published a follow-up study using both more genetic loci and more clinical variables, and they have demonstrated that it has greater accuracy. The clinical utility of this model, or a similar model, will need to be prospectively tested and independently validated. (2) Even more important will be understanding how the prediction of disease risk informs clinical management. Perhaps patients will be more successful at quitting smoking or losing weight if they learn that they are at increased risk for blindness. Alternatively, there is the possibility that intervening on the disease at a preclinical stage might improve outcomes. Further studies are also required to demonstrate these possibilities empirically.

***Example 3: Alzheimer disease and the psychologic effects of risk prediction*** Apolipoprotein E (ApoE) is a protein that, when combined with fat, becomes a lipoprotein. There are three common variants of ApoE, known as ApoE2, ApoE3, and ApoE4. The ApoE4 allele has been associated with an increased risk of Alzheimer disease (AD), with an OR of approximately 3 in the heterozygous state, and approximately 15 in the homozygous state. Within the world of polygenic diseases, the ApoE4 allele is unusual for both being common (frequency of 15% among Caucasians) and having a large effect size. Moreover, the association of this allele with AD was one of the earliest loci to have been associated with a polygenic disease.

Given that the risk allele is common and has a large effect it is, in many respects, an ideal locus to use for risk prediction. The difficulty lies in the fact that knowledge of one's genotype is not currently clinically actionable, and it is thus rare that ApoE is genotyped in a clinical setting. Even in a research setting, many individuals have expressed their desire not to know their genotype at this locus. For example, when the genome of James Watson (codiscoverer of the structure of DNA) was sequenced, he asked that his allele at this locus not be revealed. Similarly, the well-known linguist Stephen Pinker volunteered to have his genome sequenced, but also asked that this locus be blinded.

The REVEAL study sought to evaluate the effect of genotype disclosure at the *ApoE* locus in an empirical way. The authors assembled a cohort of 162 asymptomatic patients (mean age 54) who all had a parent with AD. All subjects went through genetic counseling and genetic education prior to enrollment. The group was randomized in a 2:1 ratio to a group who was and was not disclosed their genotype at the *ApoE* locus, respectively. Among the 111 subjects that were disclosed their ApoE genotype, three individuals were homozygous for the ApoE4 genotype and 50 were heterozygous. The primary endpoints of the study were changes in the subjects' anxiety and depression symptoms measured at 6 weeks, 6 months, and 1 year. Contrary to what might have been expected, there were no significant differences in anxiety and depression, both between the disclosure and nondisclosure groups, as well as between the nondisclosure group and the disclosure subgroup carrying the ApoE4 allele.

There are at least two limitations to this study: (1) It was small and possibly underpowered to discern differences in the primary endpoint, and (2) there is the potential for sample bias, given that those who agreed to the study might be least disturbed by learning the results. At the same time, this study was remarkable for the care it took in educating study participants about genetics and genetic testing prior to enrollment; as such it can be considered a prototype

for future studies. Perhaps more importantly, the data support the psychologic safety of disclosing data about genetic risk to patients, even if the result is not clinically actionable. Given the current lack of guidelines for deciding which loci have sufficient clinical utility to justify disclosure to patients, this study provides valuable empirical data to suggest that disclosure of genetic information in a clinically monitored way can be done without harm.

## Summary Points

Predicting risk of disease has been a long-standing goal of clinical medicine, and recent breakthroughs in human genetics have opened up the possibility that genetic variables could be used for risk prediction. The preceding examples provide reasons for being cautious, however. Specifically,

1. There are currently a few diseases where a sufficient fraction of heritability has been explained in order for this information to be clinically useful. Moreover, it is possible that much of the information that could be learned from genetics might also be encapsulated by clinical variables.
2. Even in cases where genetic variables augment risk prediction, it is not yet clear how this information could be made clinically actionable.
3. More studies are required to understand the psychologic effects on patients of disclosing genetic information, which cannot be changed (unlike BMI or smoking), and may not be clinically actionable. The REVEAL study provides an important prototype for this.

Thus, it is crucial that medical professionals approach the oncoming flood of genomic information in an evidence-based manner. As with other new diagnostic modalities, it is important that controlled studies be performed to discover where and how this information can be best applied. The preceding examples suggest that we should focus on diseases where (1) genetic information greatly augments clinical variables, (2) there is the possibility of clinical intervention on presymptomatic disease, and (3) there is an understanding of what the psychologic effects of the disclosure of genetic information might be. A promising candidate is coronary artery disease, as many loci have been discovered that increase or decrease risk for the disease, there are many available interventions, and family history has already been extensively utilized as risk factor.

Moreover, as it becomes possible to affordably sequence whole genomes in a clinical setting, the preceding issues will become ever more important. A typical individual contains over 6 million variants (out of 3 billion letters), and we are only at the beginning of understanding which of these affect our risk for disease, and which are benign. Already, computational tools such as PolyPhen are being applied in a clinical setting to predict rare and highly penetrant coding mutations causing monogenic diseases, but there is still a great deal of work to be done before such computational approaches can be applied to polygenic traits.

Developing reliable methods for genomically based risk prediction is likely to be one of the most challenging, yet important, goals of medicine for the coming decade. While the rate of scientific and technologic progress provide many reasons for being optimistic, empirically guided clinical studies are needed to make this goal a reality.

**BIBLIOGRAPHY:**

1. Lander ES. Initial impact of the sequencing of the human genome. *Nature*. 2011;470:187-197.

2. Falconer DS. *Introduction to Quantitative Genetics*. 2nd ed., London, UK: Longman;1981.

3. Lynch M, Walsh B. *Genetics and Analysis of Quantitative Traits*. Sunderland, MA: Sinauer;1998.

4. Manolio TA. Genomewide association studies and the assessment of the risk of disease. *N Eng J Med*. 2010;363:166-176.

5. Almgren P, Lehtovirta M, Isomaa B, et al. Heritability and familiality of type 2 diabetes and related quantitative traits in the Botnia Study. *Diabetologia*. 2011;54:2811-2819.

6. Al-Mayouf SM, Sunker A, Abdwani R, et al. Loss-of-function variant in DNASE1L3 causes a familial form of systemic lupus erythematosus. *Nat Genet*. 2011;43:1186-1188.

7. Manolio TA, Collins FS, Cox NJ, et al. Finding the missing heritability of complex diseases. *Nature*. 2009;461:747-753.

8. Meigs JB, Shrader P, Sullivan LM, et al. Genotype risk score in addition to common risk factors for prediction of type 2 diabetes. *N Eng J Med*. 2008;359:2208-2219.

9. Lyssenko V, Jonsson A, Almgren P, et al. Clinical risk factors, DNA variants, and the development of type 2 diabetes. *N Eng J Med*. 2008;359:2220-2232.

10. Edwards AO, Ritter R 3rd, Abel KJ, Manning A, Panhuysen C, Farrer LA. Complement factor H polymorphism and age-related macular degeneration. *Science*. 2005;308:421-424.

11. Klein RJ, Zeiss C, Chew EY, et al. Complement factor H polymorphism in age-related macular degeneration. *Science*. 2005;308:385-389.

12. Haines JL, Hauser MA, Schmidt S, et al. Complement factor H variant increases the risk of age-related macular degeneration. *Science*. 2005;308:419-421.

13. Hageman GS, Anderson DH, Johnson LV, et al. A common haplotype in the complement regulatory gene factor H (HF1/CFH) predisposes individuals to age-related macular degeneration. *Proc Natl Acad Sci USA*. 2005;102:7227-7232.

14. Gold B, Merriam JE, Zernant J, et al. Variation in factor B (BF) and complement component 2 (C2) genes is associated with age-related macular degeneration. *Nat Genet*. 2006;38:458-462.

15. Seddon JM, Francis PJ, George S, Schultz DW, Rosner B, Klein ML. Association of *CFH Y402H* and *LOC387715 A69S* with progression of age-related macular degeneration. *JAMA*. 2007;297:1793-1800.

16. Maler J, George S, Purcell S, et al. Common variation in three genes, including a noncoding variant in CFH, strongly influences risk of age-related macular degeneration. *Nat Gen*. 2006;38:1055-1059.

17. Seddon JM, Reynolds R, Yu Y, Daly MJ, Rosner B. Risk models for progression to advanced age-related macular degeneration using demographic, environmental, genetic, and ocular factors. *Ophthalmology*. 2011;118:2203-2211.

18. Farrer LA, Cupples LA, Haines JL, et al. Effects of age, sex, and ethnicity on the association between apolipoprotein E genotype and Alzheimer disease. *JAMA*. 1997;278:1349-1356.

19. Green RC, Roberts JS, Cupples LA, et al. Disclosure of APOE genotype for risk of Alzheimer's disease. *N Eng J Med*. 2009;361:245-254.

20. Ramensky V, Bork P, Sunyaev S. Human non-synonymous SNPs: server and survey. *Nucleic Acids Res*. 2002;30:3894-3900.

# 181 Epigenetics and Clinical Medicine

Fowzan S. Alkuraya

## KEY POINTS

- Epigenetics refers to heritable mechanisms that influence the activity of DNA but do not include the DNA sequence itself.
- Despite being a relatively young field, epigenetics has provided critical insights into gene regulation and addressed important gaps in our understanding of how static DNA sequence is normally interpreted in a dynamic fashion, both temporally and spatially.
- Imprinting disorders and cancer are examples of germline and somatic epigenetic disorders, respectively. In addition, there is a growing appreciation of epigenetic consequences of a number of "single" gene disorders such as fragile-X syndrome, Immunodeficiency, centromeric instability and facial anomalies (ICF), and Rett syndrome.
- The demonstration that the epigenetic signature of a given cell can be completely reversed to the level of pluripotency is the ultimate proof of the plasticity of the epigenome and its candidacy for therapeutic intervention to treat epigenetic disorders and make inroads in regenerative medicine.

## Introduction

The phenomenon of marked phenotypic and functional differences between the different cell types of the human body presents a major challenge in the field of biology. If DNA truly functions as the "operation manual," how do cells that share the same copy of the manual act so differently? Indeed, the initial enthusiasm in decoding this manual through the Human Genome Project has inadvertently fueled the perception, especially among nongeneticists, that deciphering the DNA sequence is the ultimate answer to biologic diversity. However, the remarkable progress made in this regard left many questions unanswered and only emphasized that DNA sequence represents only the most basic level of analysis of the human genome and that higher-order organization is key to its proper function, much like how the amino acid sequence of a protein is only meaningful in the context of its tertiary structure. The term "epigenetics" describes mechanisms that influence the activity of DNA that do not include the DNA sequence itself. While the original use of the term was more vague and inclusive of environmental factors, the term is nowadays limited to heritable molecular mechanisms although environmental factors are increasingly recognized as major modulators of these molecular mechanisms. More specifically, the "epigenome" refers to the constellation of covalent modifications of DNA and the histone proteins that help pack DNA on the chromosome as well as the newly discovered noncoding transcripts that function to modulate the transcriptional activity of DNA. So while the first-order organization of DNA (ie, DNA sequence) is essentially the same in all cells of the human body, the context in which the sequence occurs varies greatly, conferring tissue-specific "epigenomes" that in turn determine the transcriptional signature of a cell (transcriptome) as well as the profile of proteins it produces (proteome).

Despite its relatively young age, the field of epigenome has provided invaluable insight into the transcriptional regulation of DNA and the pathogenesis of several rare and common disorders. This chapter will summarize our current understanding of the epigenetic mechanisms, how they operate in disease and health and how relevant they are to the practice of medicine in the 21st century.

## Epigenetic Mechanisms

*Methylation:* This is perhaps the best-understood and the longest studied epigenetic mechanism. Methylation refers to the addition of a methyl group to the cytosine residues in DNA. Interestingly, this is usually restricted to cytosine that exists in the context of CpG dinucleotides which are widely spread in the human genome. Methylating these dinucleotides is thought to represent an important defense mechanism that protects the genome from the harmful expression of sequences that have parasitized the human genome in ancient times such as retroviral DNA-derived sequences. Importantly, CpG dinucleotides also exist in so-called "CpG islands," stretches of DNA characterized by high CG content. A high percentage of CpG dinucleotides are present in 70% of all known human gene promoters. In contrast to CpG found in repetitive DNA elements which are methylated, CpG islands are usually unmethylated except under special circumstances. This lack of methylation confers a permissive environment of transcription and represents an important transcriptional regulatory mechanism.

Methylation also refers to the addition of methyl group to lysine residues in the histone proteins around which DNA is wrapped. This particular form of methylation can be associated with a more "open" or "closed" configuration of the chromatin depending on various factors including the specific lysine residues being methylated. It is important to mention here that there is a correlation between histone methylation and DNA methylation, where the latter can induce the former to effect a closed chromatin configuration to silence expression.

*Acetylation:* In this covalent modification, an acetyl group is added to lysine residues on histone proteins that results in a relaxed chromatin configuration that is characteristic of transcriptionally active DNA. Acetylation tends to be more dynamic than methylation, which tends to be more stable, although this has been challenged in recent years.

*Others:* Histone proteins can also be covalently modified by sumoylation and phosphorylation although these are much less studied epigenetic mechanisms. In addition, there is increasing interest in the effect of noncoding RNA in transcriptional regulation of DNA, another mechanism that adds to the complexity of the epigenome.

# Epigenetics in Health

The epigenome represents the missing link between the genome and the remarkably diverse transcriptome and proteome by regulating how genes and DNA sequences in general are transcribed in the different body tissues. A similarly important function served by the epigenome is evident during development where the temporal dimension of transcriptional regulation is highly critical. Thus, both embryonically and later in life, epigenetics can be thought of as the cellular memory that determines the fate of the cell and its descendants as well as their function. It is appropriate to mention here that early reproductive cloning experiments in mammals have challenged the long held view that such "memory" is irreversible. Indeed, the capacity of the chromatin of a mature adult mammary cell nucleus to be reprogrammed and regain its potential to drive the normal process of development and differentiation of an entire mammalian organism (eg, the sheep Dolly), is the ultimate proof of the reversibility of the epigenetic marks. It is exciting to think of health-related applications of this reversibility, including the exploding field of induced pluripotent stem cells (iPS) and their use in regenerative medicine. As mentioned earlier, epigenetics plays a critical role in safeguarding against the harmful transcription of certain elements of DNA such as DNA repeats and transposons, thus preserving the integrity of the genome stability. Lastly, epigenetics is the means by which the female body keeps only one of the two X chromosomes active to achieve balance with the male counterpart who naturally possesses only one X chromosome. A combination of extensive methylation as well as use of transcripts that "coat" the X chromosome that is destined to inactivation ensures full silencing of that chromosome with the exception of loci that are known to have biallelic expression in females.

# Epigenetics in Diseases

In this section, we will enumerate a few clinically relevant examples of diseases that have at their core impaired epigenetic regulation and how our improved understanding of epigenetics has helped facilitate their diagnosis and perhaps prediction and treatment.

***Imprinting Disorders:*** Until relatively recently, the classical teaching of genetics involved the one gene-two alleles-one protein (50% contribution by each allele) paradigm. While several aspects of this paradigm are being challenged by new revelations, we will focus our discussion on the two alleles-one protein part. For the overwhelming majority of genes, it remains true that the two alleles of each gene act together to generate the normal 100% level of the transcript and, if the gene is protein-coding, the protein. However, a small subset of genes (<100 identified in humans so far) seem to depart from this rule and are characterized by mono-, rather than biallelic expression, a process called imprinting. In its simple form, the allele inherited from only one parent is expressed in a nonrandom gender-specific fashion that is true to all cells of the individual. Further investigation of this intriguing phenomenon documented that it can be further fine-tuned where the monoallelic expression is limited to a subset of tissues. Little is known about

the rationale of this phenomenon and interested readers are referred to a number of interesting papers that discuss several hypotheses put forth to explain it. However, we do know that this phenomenon is epigenetic rather than genetic in nature. In other words, the DNA sequence of the two alleles can be identical but it is the epigenetic context that marks one allele for transcription and the other for silencing. DNA methylation appears to be the universal epigenetic mechanism involved in imprinting. Usually, imprinted genes exist in clusters part of which is paternally expressed and part is maternally expressed as determined by the methylation pattern of nearby differentially methylated region (DMR). On its surface, this phenomenon presents a dilemma. Take the *IGF2/H19* locus on 11p15 as an example. Normally, only the paternal *IGF2* allele is active (*H19* has the exact opposite pattern of imprinting). One of the mechanisms that underlie Beckwith-Wiedemann syndrome (BWS, characterized by the triad of omphalocele, large tongue and somatic overgrowth, among others) is biallelic expression of *IGF2*. Theoretically, each child has a 25% risk of inheriting the active *IGF2* allele of his maternal grandfather through his mother and the active *IGF2* allele of his paternal grandfather through his father, which translates to a 25% risk of BWS. Obviously this is not true, so there has to be a mechanism to protect against this otherwise very high risk of imprinting defects. We have mentioned in the beginning of this chapter the important features of reversibility of the epigenetic mark. Indeed, a very interesting phenomenon of "erasure" and "resetting" occurs in the gametes to ensure that gametes of each parent carry the correct gender-specific mark on both alleles regardless of which grandparent they were inherited from. In other words, all sperms have a male-specific mark on the *IGF2* locus and all eggs have a female-specific mark to ensure the propagation of the normal imprint from one generation to another. Failure of this mechanism is called imprinting center defect. For example, the critical interval for Angelman and Prader-Willi syndrome (PWS) (two phenotypically distinct syndromes that share similar pathogenesis) on 15q11 is an imprinted locus. An imprinting center defect in the father can impair the resetting of male-specific imprint in sperm, resulting in 50% of sperms carrying a paternal grandmother's chromosome 15 with its female-specific imprint. Fertilization by this sperm of an egg with the normal female-specific imprint on chromosome 15 will result in a fetus with two chromosome 15 copies that both carry a female-specific imprint. The resulting phenotype is PWS. When a similar defect impairs the switch to maternal imprint in eggs, the risk will be for a fetus with both copies of chromosome 15 carrying a paternal imprint resulting in Angelman syndrome (AS). Nevertheless, imprinting center defects are rare causes of PWS and AS. A much more common cause (75% of the cases) is deletion of the critical interval on the paternal chromosome 15 in PWS or the maternal chromosome 15 in AS. The end result is the same, that is, loss of paternal contribution in PWS and loss of maternal contribution in AS. A third mechanism is when one parent literally contributes both copies of chromosome 15, a phenomenon called uniparental disomy (UPD). As one would expect, UPD should have no consequences unless there are imprinted genes on the involved chromosome (there is of course the possibility of homozygosity for autosomal recessive mutations in the case of isodisomy but this is beyond the scope of this chapter). Indeed, UPD has been observed for every single chromosome and it is only with the very few chromosomes that carry an imprinted locus that a phenotypic abnormality was observed as a result. Thus, epigenetics has provided an explanation for imprinting disorders that defy analysis when only DNA sequence was considered. Additionally, there is active research in the reversal of the abnormal imprint as a way to treat patients who are born with these disorders, at least those with functional rather than structural loss of critical interval, that is, those with imprinting center defects and UPD.

**Single Gene Methylation Disorders:** Similar to imprinting disorders, there are human diseases that are known to be the result of abnormal methylation-induced silencing of certain genes. Cancer will be discussed separately as this section will only list examples of where the abnormality only affects one gene as the primary event.

☞**FRAGILE-X SYNDROME:** In this X-linked intellectual disability disorder, the number of CGG repeats in the 5'UTR of *FREM1*, usually variable within the population, exceeds a threshold beyond which extensive methylation of the promoter of the gene (which is CpG island-containing) occurs, causing a shutdown of its transcription. This repeat expansion also mediates fragility of the corresponding X-chromosome band under special culture conditions, hence the name of the disease. Interestingly, there are rare cases where the repeat expansion fails to induce methylation and intellectual disability does not occur. This has facilitated the development of diagnostic assays that are specifically based on the methylation signature of this disorder rather than the repeat length and 100% sensitivity and specificity has been reported. In addition, knowing that methylation is the mechanism through which the repeat expansion operates has encouraged research in potential therapeutics that can remove this abnormal epigenetic modification and restore normal *FREM1* expression.

**Single Gene Disorders that Affect Epigenetics:**

☞**RETT SYNDROME:** This is an X-linked dominant neurodevelopmental disorder characterized by profound regression after a short period of normal development during infancy in females. The disease is caused by mutations in *MECP2* which encodes a member of the methyl CpG-binding protein (MBP) family that functions to induce higher-order compaction of chromatin surrounding genomic regions with methylated CpG. The resulting gene silencing is believed to be critical for the proper function of postnatal neurons and several studies have demonstrated the perturbed transcriptional signature of these neurons in patients with *MECP2* mutations. These new revelations have renewed interest in drug development for patients with Rett syndrome since their neurons are intact but dysfunctional.

☞**ICF SYNDROME:** Immunodeficiency centrosomal instability facial dysmorphism syndrome is a rare autosomal recessive secondary to DNMT3B deficiency (mutations in ZBTB24 have also been reported more recently). This protein is involved in the de novo methylation of DNA. Consistent with its pivotal role, mice that completely lack this protein die in early embryonic stages and all reported human mutations are predicted to retain some residual function. Intriguingly, the resulting hypomethylation is not widespread but rather limited to the pericentromeric repeat DNA on just three chromosomes. How this results in the various phenotypic features of the disorder remains to be explained.

**Epigenetics and Common Disorders:**

☞**CANCER:** The longest studied epigenetic perturbation in any human disease is methylation in cancer where it was noticed more than 25 years ago that cancers are characterized by abnormal methylation patterns. Both hypomethylation and hypermethylation are observed and it is now widely believed that each abnormality serves a different role in cancer pathogenesis. Hypomethylation affects the widely distributed CpG dinucleotides and is thought to remove the normal defense mechanism against the expression of

harmful DNA elements resulting in genomic instability, a characteristic finding in cancerous cells. Hypermethylation, on the other hand, is directed toward CpG island-containing promoters and several tumor suppressor genes were found to be silenced in cancer by this mechanism. There is mounting evidence that the methylation abnormalities are at the basis of cancer rather than a mere secondary phenomenon. The introduction to the clinical practice of cancer therapy that specifically targets these methylation aberrations further highlights the medical relevance of research in the area of cancer epigenetics.

☞**METABOLIC SYNDROME:** Perhaps the most intriguing link between epigenetics and common diseases is the increasingly recognized role of epigenetics in serving as the intermediary between environmental risk factors in early life and the occurrence of the metabolic syndrome. The first link was published 20 years ago when overwhelming epidemiologic evidence was found to support low birth weight as a risk factor for the development of diabetes mellitus and coronary artery disease later in life. Despite the compelling epidemiology of this phenomenon, a molecular explanation was lacking. However, in recent years it was found that early-life stressors (maternal malnutrition most notably) modulate the epigenetic profile of fetal cells, primarily though histone modification rather than DNA methylation. The downstream gene targets of this modification are still being elucidated but are likely to involve a number of genes that play key role in the pathogenesis of metabolic syndrome including those involved in beta-cell development in pancreas. Surprisingly, and despite the dynamic nature of histone modification, these changes appear to be transmitted across generations although whether this transmission is direct or indirect is hotly debated. However, this represents an exciting opportunity to mechanistically explain the effect of exposure to adverse environmental factors very early in life on the development of the metabolic syndrome. More interestingly, this has fueled interest in blocking this vicious cycle by adjusting early-life environment, most notably through dietary means.

## Summary

Epigenetics represents a fertile area of clinical medicine that has only recently been explored. No doubt the coming years will transform our understanding of the role of epigenetics in the pathogenesis of an increasing number of common diseases. In addition, new treatment modalities that are based on epigenome modification are likely to be developed as a result.

**BIBLIOGRAPHY:**

1. Ong CT, Corces VG. Enhancer function: new insights into the regulation of tissue-specific gene expression. *Nat Rev Genet.* 2011;12:283-293.
2. Suzuki MM, Bird A. DNA methylation landscapes: provocative insights from epigenomics. *Nat Rev Genet.* 2008;9:465-476.
3. Feil R, Fraga MF. Epigenetics and the environment: emerging patterns and implications. *Nat Rev Genet.* 2012;13:97-109.
4. Baylin SB, Jones PA. A decade of exploring the cancer epigenome—biological and translational implications. *Nat Rev Cancer.* 2011;11:726-734.
5. Ferguson-Smith AC. Genomic imprinting: the emergence of an epigenetic paradigm. *Nat Rev Genet.* 2011;12:565-575.
6. López Castel A, Cleary JD, Pearson CE. Repeat instability as the basis for human diseases and as a potential target for therapy. *Nat Rev Mol Cell Biol.* 2010;11:165-170.

7. Zhu H, Lensch MW, Cahan P, Daley GQ. Investigating monogenic and complex diseases with pluripotent stem cells. *Nat Rev Genet.* 2011;12:266-275.

8. Gluckman PD, Hanson MA, Cooper C, Thornburg KL. Effect of in utero and early-life conditions on adult health and disease. *N Engl J Med.* 2008;359:61-73.

9. De Sario A. Clinical and molecular overview of inherited disorders resulting from epigenomic dysregulation. *Eur J Med Genet.* 2009;52:363-372.

10. Ballestar E. An introduction to epigenetics. *Adv Exp Med Biol.* 2011;711:1-11.

11. Augui S, Nora EP, Heard E. Regulation of X-chromosome inactivation by the X-inactivation centre. *Nat Rev Genet.* 2011;12:429-442.

12. Plath K, Lowry WE. Progress in understanding reprogramming to the induced pluripotent state. *Nat Rev Genet.* 2011;12:253-265.

## Supplementary Information

**OMIM REFERENCES:**

[1] Beckwith-Wiedemann Syndrome; (#130650)

[2] Rett Syndrome; (#312750)

[3] ICF Syndrome; (#242860)

[4] Angelman Syndrome; (#105830)

[5] Prader-Willi Syndromes; (#176270)

[6] Fragile X Syndrome; (#300624)

**Key Words:** Gene regulation, epigenome, induced pluripotent stem cells (iPS), methylation, acetylation

# 182 The Clinical Potential of Stem Cells in Reproductive Medicine

Raymond M. Anchan and Behzad Gerami-Naini

## KEY POINTS

- Embryonic and patient-specific induced pluripotent stem cells (iPSCs) hold great potential for cell-based therapies due to their ability to generate the tissues and cell types of developing organs.
- In addition to embryonic stem cells (ESCs), some adult tissue-specific stem cells can also be potentially utilized for organ repair and therapeutic applications.

## Introduction

The continued advance of stem cell therapy in clinical medicine will require robust and renewable sources of stem cells. The origin of this source could be from ESCs, tissue-specific stem cells, or iPSCs. Since the only current source for the derivation of human embryonic stem cells (hESCs) remains discarded human tissue from in vitro fertilization (IVF) clinics, there is a close relationship between reproductive medicine and the field of stem cell biology. A continual supply of normal hESCs lines and iPSCs are essential to developing cell-based therapies to address general health concerns as well as those in reproductive medicine. Some of the potential target therapeutic applications in reproductive medicine include advancing treatments for oocyte development atresia diminishing gonadal function and urinary tract disorders associated with aging or premature ovarian failure.

In addition, there are less well-defined sources of stem cells from reproductive tissue such as ovarian stem cells and fetal stem cells that persist in maternal blood during fetal microchimerism, that might prove useful for cell-based therapies in health and reproductive function. In this chapter we briefly discuss some of the available types of stem cells and the clinical potential of this field.

## Types of Stem Cells

***Embryonic Stem Cells:*** ESCs were originally isolated from mouse, and hESCs are now derived from discarded human embryos from assisted reproductive technology (ART) clinics. The hallmark of hESCs is their ability to self-renew, proliferate on mitotically inactivated mouse embryonic fibroblast (MEF) feeders, and differentiate under permissive culture conditions into virtually any cell type of the human body. In the mouse model, the transfer of ESCs into a gestational carrier has demonstrated the ability of these cells to contribute to several tissue types as reflected by the birth of resultant chimeric mice, which can then go on to reproduce demonstrating germline contribution of these ESCs.

ESCs give rise to variety of cell types of the adult organism (ectoderm, mesoderm, and endoderm). Thus the potential applications of hESCs has captured the imagination of scientists and the medical community with the hope of developing cell-based therapies for diseases involving degenerative cellular mechanisms.

The challenges to be met before achieving these hopes include (1) ethical issues, (2) evidence of chromosomal instability in culture, (3) concerns about antigen matching of donor cells, (4) concerns about possible teratoma formation post-transplant, and (5) concern for zoonoses given culturing techniques.

***Adult Tissue-Specific Stem Cells:*** While the current literature has significantly concentrated on the potential of ESCs, there is a large population of stem cells or progenitor cells that are tissue specific and continue generating the progenitor cells even during adulthood which are called adult stem cells. In contrast to ESCs which are pluripotent, which can self-renew and potentially generate a broad range of tissue types from all three germ layers, ectoderm, mesoderm, and endoderm, the emerging data indicates that tissue-specific stem cells can be reprogrammed for development of various tissue types outside of the homotypic tissue by a process called transdifferentiation. Classic regenerative studies in amphibian development have demonstrated that tissue-specific progenitors are involved in repair of damaged organs by the transdifferentiation process.

***Endometrial Stem Cells:*** The fact that the endometrial lining replenishes itself suggests the presence of a population of endometrial stem cells within the epithelium and stroma involved in the regenerative process of the endometrium. The identity and existence of such cells was initially confirmed by a functional assay transplanting such cells into host animals and growing endometrium. This population of cells is now suspected to have the capacity to not only form endometrium, but also potentially treat other disorders such as Parkinson disease. The injection of endometrial stem cells in the brains of mice with Parkinson symptoms suggests that these cells differentiate into dopaminergic cells to ameliorate such symptoms in the mice. Additionally, stromal stem cells have been isolated from the endometrium that are Stro-1 positive and have the ability to differentiate into various connective tissue such as bone and skin as well as participating in angiogenesis. Such results raise exciting possibilities for the therapeutic applications of these cells.

***Placental Tissue and Umbilical Cord Stem Cells:*** Placenta, which is a potent endocrine organ during pregnancy, also harbors large populations of placental tissue stem cells as well as hematopoietic stem cells. The advantage of these stem cells is that one could use discarded tissue postpartum to harvest such progenitors and expand the cells for storage and therapeutic applications. For several years the presence and utility of umbilical cord stem cells have been established. These cells are typically harvested at the time of infant delivery and stored for expansion. Such cells have successfully been employed to treat various diseases, including neurologic and cardiovascular disorders, by transplant therapy. A primary advantage of placental tissue, umbilical cord, and amniotic fluid stem cells (AFSCs) is that these are autologous to the infant and semiallogeneic to siblings or parents. This allows easier tissue matching for transplant therapy. Moreover, given the primitive antigenic identity of these cells they potentially are less immunogenic relative to adult tissue and might prove advantageous for transplant therapy with a lower likelihood for rejection.

***Amniotic Fluid Stem Cells:*** The amniotic fluid has long been discarded at the time of delivery. In recent years various groups of researchers have identified significant regenerative medicine applications for amniocytes. It has been demonstrated that with appropriate culture conditions the amniotic fluid cells may be directed toward generating mesenchymal stem cells. Such enriched populations of mesenchymal stem cells have been used with the help of biodegradable scaffolds to bioengineer structures such as bladder flaps, tracheal implants, and muscular diaphragmatic flaps for transplant therapy. A detailed analysis of human amniotic fluid indicates the presence of distinct subpopulations of stem cells with unique antigenic identity suggestive of hematopoietic stem cells, myogenic progenitors, neural stem cells, and a small percentage (0.9%), but confirmed presence of AFSCs that are both c-Kit and Oct4 immunoreactive. While these AFSCs share antigenic properties with ESCs, functionally they have been shown to behave differently by being able to generate cell types and organs representative of all three germ layers (endoderm, mesoderm, and ectoderm). However, teratoma formation has remained a primary concern in employing ESC derivatives in regenerative medicine. Collectively, placental tissue, umbilical cord, and AFSCs have the advantage of host or recipient antigenic matching and inability to generate teratomas, both of which have proven to be barriers in the translational application of ESCs. Despite these limitations, ESCs remain the gold standard of differentiation and serve to address basic developmental questions regarding gene regulatory networks for directed differentiation and organ development.

***Induced Pluripotent Stem Cells:*** In 2007, Yamanaka revolutionized the field of stem cell biology by demonstrating that retroviral introduction of four pluripotency genes (*Oct3/4*, *Sox2*, *Klf4*, and *cMyc*) into adult fibroblasts reprogrammed these somatic cells into pluripotent cells. These inducing genes were termed pluripotency inducing factors (PIF) and the derivative stem cells were termed iPSCs. Since these initial reports the relative ease of reprogramming somatic cells with these PIFs has triggered a scientific race to identify different somatic cell types that may be reprogrammed into iPSCs.

A key observation relating to efficiency of reprogramming is that more primitive cell types such as adipose tissue stem cells (ADSCs), neural stem cells (NSCs), or AFSCs reprogram at a more efficient and rapid rate than relatively older somatic cells. Furthermore some of these cell types may be reprogrammed with less than the full cohort of four PIF genes. While the originally reported efficiency of MEF reprogramming or human keratinocyte reprogramming was 0.001% and 0.01%, respectively, taking as long as 3 weeks for colony emergence, we and other groups show that both mouse and human amniocytes may be reprogrammed in to amniocyte-derived iPSCs (AdiPSCs) with a severalfold improved efficiency of 0.5% in as short as 5 days postinfection. Moreover,

preliminary studies suggest that this reprogramming of AdiPSCs may be achieved with as few as two genes similar to that observed for neural stem cells in the mouse system.

An obvious advantage to iPSCs is that they are patient specific and may be generated for patients in a rapid manner at the time of medical necessity. Such iPSCs may then be used for autologous stem cell therapy (Fig. 182-1). For example, amniocyte-derived iPSCs may be used to generate tissue for use not only in the developing fetus, but also for the parents as semiallogeneic transplants.

Another advantage of iPSC lines is that there is no need to obtain discarded human embryos to generate iPSC lines. Additionally iPSC lines from diseased tissue such as derived from a patient with Parkinson disease, amyotrophic lateral sclerosis or diabetes may allow us to better understand the pathophysiology of the disease at a cellular level and facilitate drug testing in a laboratory before extending this to clinical trials. Recognizing the clinical limitations of employing virally reprogrammed cells in translational medicine, much of the recent focus has been trying to develop efficient protocols for reprogramming somatic cells using either viral-free systems or chemical inducers of pluripotency.

## Summary and Reflections

While conventional medical therapies have continued to advance at a rapid rate, many of the limitations we encounter in degenerative disease processes appear to require replacement of lost cells. Whether it is dopaminergic neurons in Parkinson patients or gametes in patients with gonadal failure, we are limited in our treatment protocols without the ability to replenish these cells. Decades of research have investigated regenerative mechanisms with the hope of unlocking genetic pathways that would allow us to differentiate desired cell types and tissue from developmentally primitive populations of stem cells. With the isolation of ESCs and development of protocols to reprogram terminally differentiated stem cells in to iPSCs we have entered a new and exciting realm of regenerative biology. The close relationship between reproductive medicine to the field of stem cell biology results from the need for discarded human embryos being the only source for generating new and normal hESC lines. Furthermore, health concerns in reproductive medicine such as oocyte atresia, diminishing gonadal function, and urinary tract disorders with aging in women may be addressed with cell-based therapy using stem cells. Additionally various reproductive tissue provide a rich source for generating different types of stem cells that could be employed in developing therapies for reproductive health. Less understood populations of reproductive stem cells include ovarian stem cells and fetal stem cells that persist in the mother as fetal microchimerism. Both these groups of stem cells are areas of ongoing investigation. Isolation and characterization of these stem cell populations will not only provide us with other robust sources of stem cells but will enhance our understanding of antigenic identity, modifications of immune surveillance that allow persistence of fetal cells in maternal circulation, and mechanisms that underlie targeting of stem cells to areas of tissue injury to initiate regenerative processes for cell replenishment as is believed to be the case with ovarian and bone marrow stem cells.

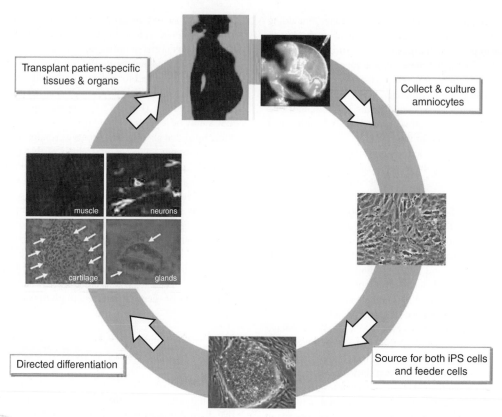

*Figure 182-1* Patient-Specific Stem Cell Therapy Using Human Amniocytes in an Autologous System. An ideal approach for an autologous cell-based therapy is illustrated in this diagram. In this model discarded amniocytes are obtained as a byproduct of routine antenatal screening. They are cultured and then reprogrammed in vitro to become patient-specific iPSCs. These patient-specific AdiPSCs may then be maintained and expanded on amniocyte feeder cells from the same patient and subsequently banked for use in cell-based therapies to generate new tissues and organs as needed.

### BIBLIOGRAPHY:

1. Thomson JA, Itskovitz-Eldor J, Shapiro SS, et al. Embryonic stem cell lines derived from human blastocysts. *Science.* 1998;282:1145-1147.

2. Yamanaka S. Strategies and new developments in the generation of patient-specific pluripotent stem cells. *Cell Stem Cell.* 2007;1:39-49.

3. Anchan RM, Quaas P, Gerami-Naini B, et al. Amniocytes can serve a dual function as a source of iPS cells and feeder layers. *Hum Mol Genet.* 2011;20:962-974.

4. Pincus G, Enzmann EV. The comparative behavior of mammalian eggs in vivo and in vitro: I. The activation of ovarian eggs. *J Exp Med.* 1935;62:665-675.

5. van den Hurk R, Zhao J. Formation of mammalian oocytes and their growth, differentiation and maturation within ovarian follicles. *Theriogenology.* 2005;63:1717-1751.

6. Jensen F, Willis MA, Albamonte MS, Espinosa MB, Vitullo AD. Naturally suppressed apoptosis prevents follicular atresia and oocyte reserve decline in the adult ovary of Lagostomus maximus (Rodentia, Caviomorpha). *Reproduction.* 2006;132:301-308.

7. Tilly JL, Johnson J. Recent arguments against germ cell renewal in the adult human ovary: is an absence of marker gene expression really acceptable evidence of an absence of oogenesis? *Cell Cycle.* 2007;6:879-883.

8. Gargett CE, Chan RW, Schwab KE. Endometrial stem cells. *Curr Opin Obstet Gynecol.* 2007;19:377-383.

9. Wolff EF, Gao XB, Yao KV, et al. Endometrial stem cell transplantation restores dopamine production in a parkinson's disease model. *J Cell Mol Med.* 2011;15:747-755.

10. Meng X, Ichim TE, Zhong J, et al. Endometrial regenerative cells: a novel stem cell population. *J Transl Med.* 2007;5:57.

11. Cairo MS, Wagner JE. Placental and/or umbilical cord blood: an alternative source of hematopoietic stem cells for transplantation. *Blood.* 1997;90:4665-4678.

12. Sodian R, Weber S, Markert M et al., Pediatric cardiac transplantation: three-dimensional printing of anatomic models for surgical planning of heart transplantation in patients with univentricular heart. *J Thorac Cardiovasc Surg.* 2008;136(4):1098-1099.

13. Chua SJ, Bielecki R, Yamanaka N, Fehlings MG, Rogers IM, Casper RF. The effect of umbilical cord blood cells on outcomes after experimental traumatic spinal cord injury. *Spine (Phila Pa 1976).* 2010;35:1520-1526.

14. Kunisaki SM, Jennings RW, Fauza DO. Fetal cartilage engineering from amniotic mesenchymal progenitor cells. *Stem Cells Dev.* 2006;15:245-253.

15. De Coppi P, Bartsch G Jr., Siddiqui MM, et al. Isolation of amniotic stem cell lines with potential for therapy. *Nat Biotechnol.* 2007;25:100-106.

16. Kim JB, Zaehres H, Wu G, et al. Pluripotent stem cells induced from adult neural stem cells by reprogramming with two factors. *Nature.* 2008;454:646-650.

# 183 Effectively Integrating Genomic Clinical Decision Support into the EHR

Joseph Kannry, Andre Kushniruk, Joshua C. Denny, Mark Hoffman, Howard Levy, and Marc S. Williams

## Introduction

This chapter will look at the present state and challenges of integrating genomic test results and genomic decision support (GDS) into an electronic health record (EHR). The fundamental premise of this chapter is that EHRs are becoming increasingly prevalent and that any intervention that seeks to change clinical outcomes will have to do so through the EHR. Where possible in this chapter, the present state and challenges will be compared and contrasted in commercial and internally developed EHRs. Commercial EHRs while significantly more prevalent may have initially less flexibility to accept genomic test results and to provide GDS especially in the age of regulated meaningful use. The meaningful use of EHRs is defined by the CMS EHR incentive program funded through the HITECH acts as part of the American Recovery and Reinvestment Act of 2009. For purposes of this chapter, we define GDS as a form of computerized clinical decision support or clinical decision support system (CDSS). This chapter will also examine the present state of and challenges with usability in regards to genomic test results and genomic CDS.

## Opportunities and Need for Genomic Decision Support

Until recently, the use of genetic and genomic information was largely restricted to diagnostic guidance or esoteric treatment guidance, in which the only consumer of the information is an expert in that field (eg, oncology, genetic medicine for rare diseases). One of the earliest examples of implementation of genetic medicine is with azathioprine and thiopurine methyltransferase (TPMT) activity, which can be tested through genetics as well as enzyme activity. However, a recent growing body of evidence points to common medications as targets for genomic guidance, including clopidogrel, warfarin, and simvastatin. Each of these has been a top grossing medication worldwide within the last decade, and can be commonly prescribed by a diverse group of practitioners, including specialists and primary care physicians. Indeed, the body of genetic evidence is growing, and, as of first-quarter 2012, the US Food and Drug Administration lists pharmacogenetic information in the structured product labels of 99 medications. The future of personalized medicine envisions a time in which many medications have potential pharmacogenetic influences. Given a growing list of medications with pharmacogenetic influences and more individuals exposed to potential prescribing conditions, there is a need to develop and maintain genomic CDS that will enable easy access to the current evidence-based practices for safe and effective prescribing. Indeed, one can argue that the diversity and complexity of genomic testing and results is an ideal candidate for CDS for several reasons: (1) the complexity is difficult for a broad community to maintain, (2) proper interpretation of genetic test results requires knowledge of specific allele changes and combinations that currently are not expressed in self-evident nomenclature (eg, *CYP2C19*\*2 represents a poor metabolizing variants while *CYP2C19*\*17 is a hypermetabolizing variant), (3) the ability to incorporate, within CDS, drug-genome, drug-drug, and drug-drug-genome interactions to a level of complexity not easily synthesized by a human, and (4) the field changes rapidly.

## Genomics and Clinical Decision Support

Portions of the section on genomic and CDS were adapted from Hoffman and Williams, 2011.

CDS refers broadly to providing clinicians and/or patients with clinical knowledge and patient-related information, intelligently filtered, or presented at appropriate times, to enhance patient care. CDS does not require a computer or EHR and is simply anything that supports a clinical decision. A CDSS refers to computerization of CDS, where the CDS can be viewed as the content paired with a computerized delivery system. A CDSS incorporates patient-specific data, a rules engine, and a medical knowledge base to produce a patient-specific assessment or recommendation for clinicians. CDS can be grouped in three general categories: passive, asynchronous, and active.

***Passive Decision Support:*** Passive decision support consists of nonmandatory resources available at the time of care in the EHR. Two examples of passive decision support are electronic resources (E-resources) and context specific.

E-resources are electronic content collections within the patient record. These E-resources can contain external collections, links to the system's medical libraries, and patient education resources, internally developed care guidelines, protocols, laboratory, and formulary information. Links to these resources take the user to the resource home page where a search query can begin. Resources are queried until an answer is found adding to the time needed to find an answer. This is a significant issue as Levy and colleagues (2008) found that busy clinicians want a resource that provides an answer within 2 to 3 minutes of search initiation. These authors also found issues with accuracy and completeness of genomics content in the commonly used online resources.

To decrease the time needed to find answers to clinical questions, informaticists realized that where the clinician is navigating in the patient EHR could provide context for the question being asked allowing "presearch" of content libraries. This presents the clinician with a filtered set of resources that minimize search time. This approach can be called context-specific passive decision support (eg, InfoButtons). InfoButtons or equivalent capabilities appear in locations relevant to the most commonly asked questions—the problem list, laboratory results and medication list (including medication ordering). The preferred content resource can be changed based on a determination by the knowledge managers about which resource is most likely to provide the best answer for a given question. In the case of an InfoButton in the problem list associated with the problem "Diabetes" the preferred content could be internally developed best practice guidelines of the specific healthcare system, or a professional society. For genetic conditions such as Marfan syndrome, the preferred content could be Genetics Home Reference (a concise, simplified resource) or GeneReviews (more complete and detailed information but tailored more for genetics professionals). Genomic content experts could create content specific to best care practices for the system.

Passive decision support can facilitate the clinician's access to information needed to answer a clinical question, but requires the clinician to recognize that a clinical question exists. The remaining types of CDS are the most amenable to computerization. For the purposes of this chapter CDSS and asynchronous and active decision support will be used interchangeably. Active and asynchronous CDS are designed to provide the clinician with information he/she needs to know but was never requested.

***Active CDS:*** Active (or synchronous) CDS describes a workflow in which a clinician process, such as prescribing a medication, is monitored in real time by rules of logic and clinician behavior is influenced based on the logic embedded in a rule. The most widely recognized approach is pop-up alert windows warning the user of a potentially risky decision, such as an allergy or drug-drug interaction (DDI). Other modalities are gaining favor (to avoid "alert fatigue"), including workflow logic in which warnings and alerts are embedded into the user navigation through the EHR application. For example the contents of an application window may vary based on genomic risks or additional screening procedures may be added to order lists.

Pharmacogenomic testing for the drug carbamazepine (Tegretol) demonstrates how active CDS can work. It is known that patients who carry a specific human leukocyte antigen (HLA) type (B*1502) are at increased risk for an adverse drug reaction. If a clinician uses a computerized medication order system and chooses carbamazepine an algorithm is run represented by the logic model in Fig. 183-1. The information in the left hand box is automatically collected by the program from various parts of the electronic data warehouse (EDW) (Table 183-1).

In this case the indication is psychomotor epilepsy. If the patient is female over a predetermined age and the drug presents a risk to a fetus the clinician would be prompted to order a pregnancy test. Ethnicity is requested because HLA-B*1502 has a significantly higher prevalence in many Asian populations. If testing has been done previously and the patient carries the *HLA-B*1502* allele, the

**Table 183-1  *Data Elements for Tegretol Dosing***

| *Information Needed* | *Reason Needed* |
|---|---|
| Age | Dosing algorithm |
| Weight | Dosing algorithm |
| Sex | Risk for pregnant women |
| Pregnant? (if female) | Risk for pregnant women |
| Clinical indication | Generate list of appropriate alternative medications |
| Ethnicity | Population risk |
| Drug allergies | Prior history of reaction |
| Interacting medications | Dosing and safety |

clinician sees the alert represented in the right hand box of Fig. 183-1. If the InfoButton is clicked (this is the blue circle with the white "i") the clinician is taken to the FDA alert's abstract. There is also a link to alternative medications. If this is clicked, the system will look at the indication for treatment and other factors and would propose clonazepam as the recommended alternative, given its equivalence to carbamazepine in the treatment of psychomotor seizures. Alternatively, if the HLA-B*1502 test had not been done previously the clinician would be alerted to order this test before prescribing carbamazepine. If the patient was not of Asian ethnicity, the query about the HLA-B*1502 would not have triggered and the prescribing would have proceeded with consideration of the other factors.

A unique aspect of germline genetic or genomic testing is that the test only needs to be done once in a patient's lifetime. An article by Riegert-Johnson et al. identified a significant issue with genetic tests being repeated, resulting in wasted resources. An examination at Intermountain Healthcare looking at two thrombophilia tests showed that roughly 5% of these tests represented duplicates (Williams et al., unpublished data). When additional data were examined a small number of clinicians were identified that were responsible for a disproportionate number of these duplicate tests. CDSS could be used to alert and educate the clinicians that such testing is needlessly duplicative. Changes in behavior can be monitored prospectively to ensure that test ordering behavior has changed.

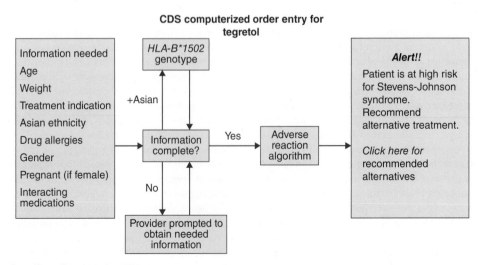

**CDS computerized order entry for tegretol**

***Figure 183-1*** Flowchart for Carbamazepine CDS.

**Asynchronous CDS:** Asynchronous CDS involves the system monitoring behaviors, perhaps assembling data that was not completely available at the time of clinician or patient interaction and comparing this to rules or algorithms crafted to identify opportunities to improve clinical care, recognize patient safety issues, or close targeted care gaps. The output of asynchronous CDS can be messages to the clinician generally within the EHR at a time the clinician is not expecting the message nor seeing the patient. Several pregenomics and pre-HIPAA studies have successfully sent results via alphanumeric paging. When celecoxib (Celebrex) was removed from the market it was important to identify and contact patients taking the medication, a nearly impossible task for a clinician using paper records. With EHRs, CDSS could message each physician with target population patients and potentially contact patients directly through a personal health record (PHR). Asynchronous CDS can deliver monthly dashboards about a clinician's patient population with a given disease, such as diabetes presenting information such as hemoglobin $A_{1c}$, eye examinations, medications, etc. This allows clinicians to take actions such as recalling the patient, placing orders etc. Care gaps can be tracked over time guide for further action.

Genomic data may purport to multiple opportunities for asynchronous CDS. Current and future programs in genomic testing may test multiple variants simultaneously. Examples will be described below.

## Challenges to the Implementation of Genomic Decision Support

**Systems Issues for genomic CDS:** Previously we defined GDS as a form of computerized clinical decision support or CDSS. In order to move toward GDS, EHR systems will require a number of enhancements. The legacy of commercial EHRs traces back to early needs to better support administrative transactions. These transaction-oriented systems were not designed to enhance the care of individual patients. Some internally developed EHR suppliers began to take a person-centric approach to their system architecture in the 1980s to 1990s. This shift enabled users to more readily assemble an accurate picture of diagnostic and therapeutic events associated with a specific patient allowing contributions from EHRs to the individualization of care.

EHR developers are actively assessing innovations needed to ensure that EHR systems can fully support the integration of genetic information into patient care. There are distinct categories of EHR developers. (1) The academic or large private institution model with an EHR highly tailored to the unique needs of the institution, sometimes through a ground-up design of a unique system. EHRs developed in this model have the benefit of agility and build as needed, although resources needed for support are significant. Successful strategies developed in these contexts often prove difficult to deploy more widely because of the site-specific customization. (2) EHRs developed through a commercial model for installation in a wide variety of settings. These systems must be flexible enough to meet the needs of a wide variety of organizations, must ensure that they meet the legal and regulatory requirements of a system that is distributed commercially and must enable information exchange of a subset of their data elements across platforms at the sacrifice of customization for institutional workflows. Regardless of the development model, EHR developers have realized that improvements in

foundational capabilities will enhance the ability to better support personalized medicine.

**Discretely Stored Genetic Test Results:** One foundational capability that is necessary to enable both asynchronous and synchronous decision support is the discrete storage of consistently codified genetic and genomic test results. Meaningful Use Stage 1 regulations includes the requirement that systems highlight the discrete storage of laboratory results. The proposed Meaningful Use Stage 2 regulations strengthen the requirement significantly. While there are many interpretations of discrete data, this requirement will encourage all EHR developers to review their ability to store genomic data discretely. Many laboratory information systems (LIS) and EHR implementations have operated under the assumption that it was adequate to store genetic and genomic test reports as purely textual documents. While this is useful in the context of a physician invoking the medical record of a patient, even in the most advance EHRs routine processing of text documents by natural language processing (NLP) for CDSS is not available. Discrete storage of genomic test results in a machine-readable format is an important prerequisite for (1) widespread availability of GDS, (2) as a means of exchanging data between clinical organizations and laboratories, (3) facilitating continuity of care across patient venues. Another challenge that remains is these tests may be subject to varying and revised interpretation as new knowledge about variants is generated. These types of results may need additional security to ensure privacy and confidentiality to comply with human subjects' protections, local, state, and federal regulations.

**Codification of Genetic Test Results:** To enable the exchange of genetic test results across systems, genetic information must utilize appropriate standardized terminology. The systematized nomenclature of medicine—clinical terms (SNOMED-CT) has a strong representation of clinical conditions, The logical observation identifiers' names and codes (LOINC), with some exceptions, provides reasonable coverage of possible genetic test procedures and the clinical bioinformatics ontology (CBO) provides a semantically structured vocabulary representing the physical observations of the diagnostic laboratory. For example, a clinician might order a cystic fibrosis screening panel that is associated with a LOINC code. The laboratory performing the testing can associate the presence or absence of the 87 mutations in the testing panel that they utilize with CBO concept codes. The final report confirming carrier status for cystic fibrosis or risk of congenital absence of the vas deferens might be associated with one or more SNOMED-CT codes. For continuous traits, such as cytochrome P450 or TPMT enzyme activity, variants may be represented in terms of human-readable interpretations of the expected phenotype for the individual (eg, rapid, extensive [normal], intermediate, or poor metabolizer). Currently, different nomenclatures may be used for different CYP450 enzymes. Mapping such as phenotypic information while retaining raw genetic information could allow decoupling of GDS to specific variants, thus allowing GDS to be more robust to new variants for which there is guidance.

**Interfacing Clinical Systems: The Exchange of Genetic Data Across Clinical Systems:** Structured genetic test orders and results enable better care when integrated with existing standards for exchange of clinical data. Health Level 7 (HL7) is a widely accepted standard messaging protocol used to exchange information between clinical information systems. HL7 has a proposed model for communication of genomic results that can use the coding systems outlined earlier. It is beyond the scope of this chapter to examine and/or speculate how data exchange would occur across transitions of care, in Regional Health Information Organizations (RHIOs), or the nascent National Health Information Network (NHIN), but standards will clearly be central to this effort.

**Family History:** Genetic and genomic data have direct and lasting relevance to family members of the patient. While a variety of stand-alone pedigree generation and analysis applications are available integration of structured and machine-readable family history into EHR has been limited. The recent release of a web-enabled family history application by the US Surgeon General has generated renewed interest in integrating family history capability with both EHR and PHR. The proposed regulations for Meaningful Use Stage 2, list structured entry of data for family history as a menu item. Menu items (ie, elective) in Meaningful Use, usually become objectives (required) in the next stage, so the US government is stating that within 5 years structured entry of family history will be required.

## Example of Currently Available Genomic CDS

In 2010, Vanderbilt implemented the Pharmacogenomic Resource for Enhanced Decisions in Care and Treatment (PREDICT) program, which has as its goal prospective, multiplexed genetic testing of individuals at high risk to receive medication for which there is known pharmacogenetic guidance. An important aspect of the PREDICT program is that patients are tested with a multiplexed platform that contains 184 variants in 34 pharmacogenes to allow for multiple opportunities to provide genomic guidance now and in the future. Providers order genomic testing on patients as they are about to undergo cardiac catheterization (about 40% of which end up receiving clopidogrel), or based on a risk score calculation suggesting that the patient is at increased risk to receive one of three medications with pharmacogenetic guidance (clopidogrel, warfarin, or simvastatin). This prospective algorithm calculates, based on past medical history and demographics, an individual's risk of receiving warfarin, simvastatin, or clopidogrel within the next 3 years. Genetic testing is performed within a Clinical Laboratory Improvement Amendment (CLIA) certified laboratory, and only results with high concordance and sufficient evidence are implemented. Genomic CDS guidance exists in the form of decision support prompts (see Fig. 183-2 for an example of clopidogrel CDS) that execute when a provider attempts to prescribe a medication for which genomic guidance exists and the patient has genetic information available. In addition, patients who have had genetic testing have these variants displayed in their patient summary, between the "Allergy and Adverse Reactions" and "Current medications" section. Genetic variants are displayed with the genetic test result (eg, *CYP2C19*\*2 homozygote), the phenotypic interpretation (eg, "poor metabolizer, at increased risk of clopidogrel failure"). Since the internal representation of these results are based on the genotype results, the phenotypic descriptions can be updated when new knowledge is available (eg, if a new drug was to be found relevant to an existing variant in the EHR) or additional drug-genotype interaction pairs are added. When updates are done, it is considered a new laboratory result and contains the date of the revised interpretation. In the 1.5 years since implementation, the PREDICT program has tested nearly 5000 patients.

Other efforts at genomic CDS are underway across several other institutions including St. Jude's Children's hospital (which provides GDS around *TPMT* and *CYP2D6* poor metabolizers), and other sites in the eMERGE network. Mount Sinai Medical Center is seeking to integrate genomic test results and decision support within the commercial EHR. This project using mostly off the shelf functionality with data from an external system, ensures integration at the point of care without requiring the user to access external systems. Geisinger Health System is in the process of implementing genotyping of *IL28B* coupled with hepatitis C viral genotyping to guide therapeutic intensity in patients with chronic hepatitis C without cirrhosis (Williams, personal communication). The Mayo clinic has studied the use of genotyping to assist in the use of antidepressant medications.

## General Issues With the Usability of CDS

Alert fatigue was referenced earlier, and is one of the most common challenges facing effective CDS. This occurs when an active CDS system provides alerts with information that is not deemed important by the clinician for decision making. Perhaps the most familiar example of irrelevant alerts includes many DDI alerts. When DDI alerts were first deployed in EHRs, virtually every prescription order generated information about a potential interaction. The alerts generated additional work by the clinician to deal with DDI alerts even though the vast majority of the interactions were not clinically important. This could result in important DDIs being overlooked in the course of dealing with other trivial alerts, or, more commonly, requests to have the CDS disabled. Alert fatigue is a symptom of a larger problem which is disruption of clinical workflow. As Bates stated in his Ten Commandments article, CDS should not force the user to change direction (meaning to stop what they are doing and addressing an unrelated alert or reminder). The best CDSS presents the right information to the right clinician at precisely the right time in the course of clinical care in a useable fashion so that the CDSS is transparent to the user. While this problem is not unique to genomics, it is important to note that the rapid increase and sheer volume of knowledge related to genomic information will challenge existing paradigms of local development and deployment of CDS and may require externally developed CDS modules that integrate with commercial EHRs. Finally, usability, something not often assessed is an important factor in CDS utilization and acceptance.

**Introducing Usability:** The usability of health information technologies is a critical factor in the acceptance of and adoption by clinicians of technologies such as EHRs and CDS. Lack of usability has been cited as being a major factor in the acceptance or rejection of systems such as EHRs by healthcare providers. Health information systems having poor usability have been cited for adversely affecting patient safety, interrupting clinician workflow, and resistance to adoption by end users.

**Defining Usability:** Usability can be defined as being a measure of ease of use of a system in terms of a system's effectiveness, efficiency, enjoyability, safety, and learnability. In order to improve the usability of health information systems, a range of methods have been applied in health informatics. These two main approaches to usability engineering are: (1) usability testing, and (2) usability inspection. Usability testing involves observing representative users of an information systems (eg, physicians) while they interact

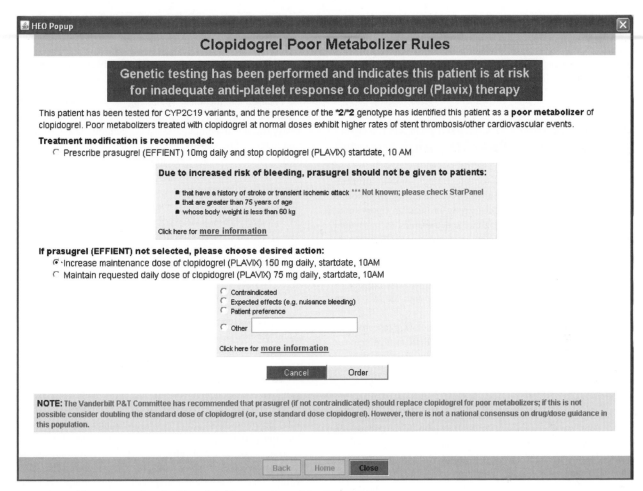

***Figure 183-2*** Decision Support for Clopidogrel Guidance as Part of the PREDICT Program.

with an information system or resource being tested (eg, an EHR or clinical guidelines) to carry out representative tasks (eg, deciding on treatment for a patient while using an EHR). A range of studies employing usability testing have been conducted to assess the usability of a wide range of healthcare information systems, such as electronic patient records, educational software, web-based clinical guidelines, and various forms of clinical information systems. New low-cost and easy-to-deploy methods for conducting usability testing rapidly have opened up the possibility of testing healthcare systems with representative users prior to widespread system deployment. This testing may be done in real settings (eg, hospital rooms, clinics, emergency rooms etc) and may involve realistic patient cases, prior to their widespread deployment in order to ensure the usability and safety. Usability inspection refers to another complementary set of methods (eg, heuristic evaluation and cognitive walkthrough) that involve an analyst methodically "stepping" or "walking through" a user interface or system while identifying and noting potential usability issues and problems (eg, problems with navigation or understanding of how to use a system). Both usability testing and usability inspection methods are ideally applied in an iterative manner and as early in system design as possible, that is, with results of cycles if usability testing and inspection feeding back in to redesign and improvement of healthcare

systems and user interfaces before their ultimate release to clinician users. For example, recent work in conducting usability analyses of a CDS tool embedded within an institutional EHR indicate that successive round of usability testing are needed in order to streamline and improve the effectiveness of the clinical decision support, and improve the "fit" of the system within clinician's workflow before releasing CDS tool on a widespread basis.

In the context of studying CDSS that may provide support to physicians about genomic information (eg, alerts or reminders produced by an EHR about a patient's genomic data), methods from usability engineering (eg, usability testing) can be used to help in determining user needs when working with systems under design or development. For example, physicians can be observed while they interact with mock-ups of early designs for EHRs or CDSs, with the results of these observations (eg, analysis of user interactions indicating specific usability problems) can be fed back into system design and refinement.

Usability testing methods have also been used as a method to detect and prevent a new class of errors, known as technology-induced errors prior to deploying systems in order to ensure system safety and prevent inadvertent medical error. Technology-induced errors are errors that are typically not detected by traditional computer testing but rather appear when health information technology is deployed in complex healthcare settings. Such errors have been shown to be associated with poor system usability and poorly designed user interfaces. Approaches based on usability testing have lead to early detection of technology-induced error that information systems might inadvertently cause.

# Useable Genomics: Usability of Genomic Test Results and Clinical Decision Support

There is considerable potential for integrating genomic information with EHRs. Such integration would enable the use of genomic information at point of care and thereby provide an opportunity for health professionals to tailor medical therapies to individual patients. For example, currently a range of software has been developed for use by genetic specialists and counselors for incorporating results from genomic analysis. The possibility for this type of information to be made accessible at point of care by physicians on a widespread basis has been increased through the increasing prevalence of EHR systems.

Research is beginning to be targeted at integrating research and technological advances in genomics with the EHR as a vehicle for presenting and displaying relevant genomic information at point of care. For example, approaches to the detection of adverse drug reactions (ADRs) can be coupled the use of EHR systems designed to serve as repositories of information about an individual's health status and health care. ADRs refer to expected or unexpected untoward outcomes that occur as a result of drug therapy. Research has accumulated regarding predicting ADR using genomic information. Experts from the fields of genomic research, health informatics, and human-computer interaction will be needed to jointly work on developing new approaches for such integration and design of effective user interfaces for presenting genomic information at point of care in order for information to be effectively presented and that do not lead to "cognitive overload."

In addition to its potential for providing safer healthcare the potential for cost-savings from improved decision making in the clinic offers considerable impetus for conducting work in integrating genomic data with EHRs. Such research could have important impact and potential for the translation of genomic results into improved health and more effective health services.

**Known Challenges in Producing Usable Genomic Test Results and Clinical Decision Support:** Specific issues related to usability that will need to be addressed in order to realize the potential for integration of genomic data with the EHR include the following:

- Selection and presentation of genomic data in a way understood by clinicians at point of care and that is most pertinent to the patient case at hand (this will require studies of clinician information needs for genomic data)
- Triggering of alerts and reminding about genomic aspects of patient cases in a way that is useful for physicians and that does not interfere with their clinical workflow
- Avoidance of cognitive overload through intelligent filtering, presentation, and summarization of only genomic information most relevant to patient cases
- Integration of genomic data with conventional patient data in a seamless manner
- Ability of the CDS to adapt its presentation of information to varied classes of users (eg, primary care physicians, specialists etc)

- Appropriate training and support for new users of CDS that incorporate genomic data, including alerting and remaindering forms of CDS
- Ability for end users to provide feedback into refinement of GDS and reporting of potential error

Focused on the most promising front in personalization of health delivery, new approaches will be needed to develop and assess design of computer-assisted, genome-based clinical decision making. Specifically, there will be a need to develop new user interfaces and software tools to bring genomic information to bear at the point of care by clinicians, in particular physicians. To do this will require innovative methods to assess healthcare professionals' information needs and information seeking. Furthermore, there will be a need to develop and evaluate the usability of prototype systems to explore the most effective possibilities for directly interfacing genomic data with electronic health records. A focus of this work will need to be on the development of models of user interaction that will allow for integration of genomic information into clinical decision making in a way that fits with health professional cognitive processes (eg, information seeking and decision making) and clinic workflow. This is currently an unmet need, as no electronic health record products have been deployed that embody an integrated system or interface for bringing genomic data into routine use by health professionals at point of care.

To address issues around providing personalized medicine using electronic health records, the information needs of clinicians will have to be assessed in order to understand which (and how) genomic information is best presented to promote effective decision making within the context of the clinical encounter (ie, at point of care). Specifically, this will involve the need to develop and test novel user interactions with novel prototype interfaces, using a range of modifiable and customizable EHRs. For example, work has been conducted in developing links to genetic information resources within an electronic health record systems using "InfoButtons" links to genetic resources for clinician users of the EHR. Plans for development of other systems are underway to create decision support in the form of EHR alerts for medications based on analysis of genomic data. Such prototype systems will need to be tested with a set of representative, virtual patient scenarios in a simulated, real-world environment (ie, a clinic), in which genomic and clinical information relevant to specific patient cases will be presented to subjects (ie, physicians) using different representations (eg, automated alerts and reminders, flagged potential ADR information, statistical information). During these clinical simulations subjects could be observed and recorded as they interact with the patient scenarios and information presented (including genomic information). Following this, subjects could be asked to specify prescriptions and/or tests for the virtual patients in the scenarios. The results could be analyzed to provide input into the design and refinement of usable data management models, user interfaces, and interaction modes that are representative of real-world clinical scenarios and situations.

A focus of this research will need to be on development of useful and understandable formats for presenting information and assessing the impact of information presented on decision making and assessing the physicians' decisions to understand, apply, or ignore information presented. Early work along these lines has been reported by Scheuner et al., who have interviewed clinicians about their information needs and how integration of genomic data has considerable potential to improve delivery of personalized health care. However, despite the importance of this work, there has been very few reported studies to date of genomic information needs of clinicians that could inform the integration of genomic data with the EHR. The study of the human factors and usability factors that could enable this integration within the EHR and support effective user interactions is currently in its infancy. Such research will be needed in order to lead to design and implementation of effective genomic-enabled EHRs.

## Summary and Conclusions

Genomics through the vehicle of personalized medicine has the ability to transform health care. However, until recently the only clinical user of such information was an expert in that field (eg, oncology, genetic medicine for rare diseases). Ensuring that the widely growing volume of genomics information is in the hands of clinicians at the point of care will require successful integration of the genomic test results and decision support (GDS) into the EHR. Yet many challenges remain for successful EHR integration. Some of these challenges arise from the early state of the field in knowledge, workflow, structuring of data, interface development (ie, the transmission of information from one clinical system to another) and development of standards. An example of these challenges is workflow. It is unclear how we want to use tests that are run once in the lifetime of the patient but potentially interpreted many times. Significant work remains to be done on structuring family history. Just as we have seen the transformation of disease management from the level of the patient to that of the population, we can expect the same with findings from genomic test results and decision support.

This chapter assumes that we will want genomic results at the point of care with the knowledge and support that GDS provides. In this chapter, we defined GDS as a form of computerized clinical decision support or CDSS. Ideally CDSS should deliver the right information to the right clinician at the right time. For GDS, the right time and right clinician has yet to be defined. For example, some germline genetic or genomic testing needs to be done once in a patient's lifetime. Once it is done, when and where is the right time to use it for decisions support: If a patient has an increased risk of heart disease, which visit (eg, every visit) is the clinician reminded by GDS of the increased risk of heart disease? Which clinicians need to be reminded? Primary care providers or cardiologists? Or all clinicians touching the patient? At what point do genomic test results migrate from test results triggering GDS to items on the problem list? If the test demonstrates cystic fibrosis, is it enough to add cystic fibrosis to the problem list and stop reminding the provider about the genomic findings?

Whatever form genomic tests result and GDS take in the EHR, they must be provided in both a form that is usable and useful. The best way to ensure this is to conduct rigorous and frequent usability testing. However, integrating usability testing in commercial systems in operational environments has been challenging. The peer reviewed literature to date clearly indicates that not nearly enough usability testing for CDSS interventions occur. Most importantly, usability correlates with user errors.

Ultimately the user needs to understand and wants to use genomic data whether it is presented in the form of genomic test results or decision support. This need will come from education of the user which is in a sense what this book is about. This chapter provides a window on the current state of and use of future tools that will enable educated clinicians to use genomic data at the point of care in the EHR.

## Bibliography:

1. Medicare and Medicaid programs; electronic health record incentive program. Final rule. *Fed Regist.* 2010;75:44313-44588.

2. Anon. Genomics. Table of Pharmacogenomic Biomarkers in Drug Labels. http://www.fda.gov/Drugs/ScienceResearch/ResearchAreas/Pharmacogenetics/ucm083378.htm. Accessed March 9, 2011.

3. Hoffman MA, Williams MS. Electronic medical records and personalized medicine. *Hum Genet.* 2011;130:33-39.

4. Osheroff JA, Teich JM, Middleton B, Steen EB, Wright A, Detmer DE. A roadmap for national action on clinical decision support. *J Am Med Inform Assoc.* 2007;14:141-145.

5. Kannry J. Medical informatics : an executive primer. In: Ong KR, ed. *Computerized Physician Order Entry and Patient Safety: Panacea or Pandora's Box?* Chicago, IL: HIMSS; 2007:316.

6. Hunt DL, Haynes RB, Hanna SE, Smith K. Effects of computer-based clinical decision support systems on physician performance and patient outcomes: a systematic review [see comments]. *JAMA.* 1998;280:1339-1346.

7. Randolph AG, Haynes RB, Wyatt JC, Cook DJ, Guyatt GH. Users' Guides to the Medical Literature: XVIII. How to use an article evaluating the clinical impact of a computer-based clinical decision support system. *JAMA.* 1999;282:67-74.

8. Cimino JJ. Infobuttons: anticipatory passive decision support. *AMIA Annu Symp Proc.* 2008;1203-1204.

9. Del Fiol G, Williams MS, Maram N, Rocha RA, Wood GM, Mitchell JA. Integrating genetic information resources with an EHR. *AMIA Annu Symp Proc.* 2006;904.

10. Locharernkul C, Loplumlert J, Limotai C, et al. Carbamazepine and phenytoin induced Stevens-Johnson syndrome is associated with HLA-B*1502 allele in Thai population. *Epilepsia.* 2008;49:2087-2091.

11. Riegert-Johnson DL, Macaya D, Hefferon TW, Boardman LA. The incidence of duplicate genetic testing. *Genet Med.* 2008;10:114-116.

12. Kuperman GJ, Hiltz FL, Teich JM. Advanced alerting features: displaying new relevant data and retracting alerts. *Proc AMIA Annu Fall Symp.* 1997;243-247.

13. Kuperman GJ, Teich JM, Bates DW, et al. Detecting alerts, notifying the physician, and offering action items: a comprehensive alerting system. *Proc AMIA Annu Fall Symp.* 1996;704-708.

14. Kuperman GJ, Teich JM, Tanasijevic MJ, et al. Improving response to critical laboratory results with automation: results of a randomized controlled trial. *J Am Med Inform Assoc.* 1999;6:512-522.

15. Shabot MM, LoBue M. Real-time wireless decision support alerts on a Palmtop PDA. *Proc Annu Symp Comput Appl Med Care.* 1995;174-177.

16. Shabot MM, LoBue M, Chen J. Wireless clinical alerts for physiologic, laboratory and medication data. *Proc AMIA Symp.* 2000;789-793.

17. Hoffman MA. The genome-enabled electronic medical record. *J Biomed Inform.* 2007;40:44-46.

18. Gardner RM, Pryor TA, Warner HR. The HELP hospital information system: update 1998. *Int J Med Inform.* 1999;54:169-182.

19. McDonald CJ, Overhage JM, Tierney WM, et al. The Regenstrief Medical Record System: a quarter century experience. *Int J Med Inform.* 1999;54:225-253.

20. Safran C, Sands DZ, Rind DM. Online medical records: a decade of experience. *Methods Inf Med.* 1999;38:308-312.

21. Slack WV, Bleich HL. The CCC system in two teaching hospitals: a progress report. *Int J Med Inform.* 1999;54:183-196.

22. Teich JM, Glaser JP, Beckley RF, et al. The Brigham integrated computing system (BICS): advanced clinical systems in an academic hospital environment. *Int J Med Inform.* 1999;54:197-208.

23. Morgan MW. The VA advantage: the gold standard in clinical informatics. *Healthc Pap.* 2005;5:26-29.

24. Miller RA, Waitman LR, Chen S, Rosenbloom ST. The anatomy of decision support during inpatient care provider order entry (CPOE): empirical observations from a decade of CPOE experience at Vanderbilt. *J Biomed Inform.* 2005;38:469-485.

25. Medicare and Medicaid Programs; Electronic Health Record Incentive Program—stage 2. Proposed rule. *Fed Regist.* 2012;77:13698-13827.

26. Mitchell DR, Mitchell JA. Status of clinical gene sequencing data reporting and associated risks for information loss. *J Biomed Inform.* 2007;40:47-54.

27. Hoffman M, Arnoldi C, Chuang I. The clinical bioinformatics ontology: a curated semantic network utilizing RefSeq information. *Pac Symp Biocomput.* 2005:139-150.

28. Shabo A. The implications of electronic health record for personalized medicine. *Biomed Pap Med Fac Univ Palacky Olomouc Czech Repub.* 2005;149:S251-S258.

29. Giovanni MA, Murray MF. The application of computer-based tools in obtaining the genetic family history. *Curr Protoc Hum Genet.* 2010;Chapter 9:Unit 9.21.

30. Pulley JM, Denny JC, Peterson JF, et al. Operational implementation of prospective genotyping for personalized medicine: the design of the Vanderbilt PREDICT Project. *Clin Pharmacol Ther.* 2012;92:87-95.

31. Rundell JR, Staab JP, Shinozaki G, et al. Pharmacogenomic testing in a tertiary care outpatient psychosomatic medicine practice. *Psychosomatics.* 2011;52:141-146.

32. Kannry J. Effect of e-prescribing systems on patient safety. *Mt Sinai J Med.* 2011;78:827-833.

33. Saleem JJ, Patterson ES, Militello L, Render ML, Orshansky G, Asch SM. Exploring barriers and facilitators to the use of computerized clinical reminders. *J Am Med Inform Assoc.* 2005;12:438-447.

34. Patterson ES, Doebbeling BN, Fung CH, Militello L, Anders S, Asch SM. Identifying barriers to the effective use of clinical reminders: Bootstrapping multiple methods. *J Biomed Inform.* 2005;38:189-199.

35. Kushniruk AW, Patel VL. Cognitive and usability engineering methods for the evaluation of clinical information systems. *J Biomed Inform.* 2004;37:56-76.

36. Preece J. Human-computer interaction. Wokingham, England; Reading, Mass: Addison-Wesley Pub. Co.; 1995.

37. Kushniruk A. Evaluation in the design of health information systems: application of approaches emerging from usability engineering. *Comput Biol Med.* 2002;32(3):141-149.

38. Kushniruk AW, Borycki EM. Low-cost rapid usability engineering: designing and customizing usable healthcare information systems. *Healthc Q.* 2006;9:98-100, 102.

39. Borycki E, Kushniruk A. Identifying and preventing technology-induced error using simulations: application of usability engineering techniques. *Healthc Q.* 2005;8 Spec No:99-105.

40. Nielsen J. *Usability Engineering.* Boston, MA: Academic Press; 1993.

41. Mann DM, Kannry JL, Edonyabo D, et al. Rationale, design, and implementation protocol of an electronic health record integrated clinical prediction rule (iCPR) randomized trial in primary care. *Implementation Sci.* 2011;6:109.

42. Kushniruk AW, Triola MM, Borycki EM, Stein B, Kannry JL. Technology induced error and usability: the relationship between usability problems and prescription errors when using a handheld application. *Int J Med Inform.* 2005;74(7-8):519-526.

43. Glaser J, Henley DE, Downing G, Brinner KM, Community PHCWotAHI. Advancing personalized health care through health information technology: an update from the American Health Information Community's Personalized Health Care Workgroup. *J Am Med Inform Assoc.* 2008;15:391-396.

44. Belmont J, McGuire AL. The futility of genomic counseling: essential role of electronic health records. *Genome Med.* 2009;1:48.

45. Rothstein MA. *Pharmacogenomics: Social, Ethical, and Clinical Dimensions.* Hoboken, NJ: Wiley-Liss; 2003.

46. Impicciatore M. Pharmacogenomic can give children safer medicines. *Arch Dis Child.* 2003;88:366.

47. Scheuner MT, de Vries H, Kim B, Meili RC, Olmstead SH, Teleki S. Are electronic health records ready for genomic medicine? *Genet Med.* 2009;11:510-517.

48. Kannry J, Kushniruk A, Koppel R. Meaningful usability: health care information technology for the rest of Us. In: Ong K, ed. *Medical Informatics: An Executive Primer.* 2nd ed. Chicago, IL: HIMSS; 2011.

49. Kushniruk A, Triola M, Stein B, Borycki E, Kannry J. The relationship of usability to medical error: an evaluation of errors associated with usability problems in the use of a handheld application for prescribing medications. *Medinfo.* 2004;11(pt 2):1073-1076.

# 184 Genetic Assessment at the End of Life

John M. Quillin, Joann Bodurtha, and Thomas J. Smith

## KEY POINTS

- *Prevalence of genetic disease at the end of life:*
  - Inherited factors contribute about 20% to mortality in the population. About 5% to 10% of common causes of mortality, such as cancer, are associated with strong individual genetic risks with implications for surviving family members.
- *Rationale for genetics assessment:*
  - Current genetic tests are not fully clinically sensitive but can be very informative for breast, ovary, and colorectal cancers. It is typically most useful to begin testing with an affected family member. Once affected family members have died, opportunities for genetics assessment, or obtaining genetic material for future testing, may be lost, so DNA banking may be a viable option.
- *Options for genetics assessment:*
  - *Record* patient and family history that may be relevant for genetic history. For example, "S-I-D-E": *S*imilar conditions in other family members, *I*nherited diagnoses described in the family, *D*eaths at an early age, and *E*xtreme laboratory values. Collect these information for three generations of relatives on both the maternal and paternal sides of the family. *Bank DNA* for patients suspected to have a genetic condition and consider genetics consultation for the patient and/or family. This will allow future testing for the benefit of surviving family members.

## Introduction

Recognition of the genetic component of disease is increasing in clinical practice. Completion of the Human Genome Project has led to an acceleration of clinically available genetic tests with varying validity and utility. Despite increasing recognition of a genetic component for many diseases, current genetic testing still will not detect a familial mutation for many families, even among patients meeting clinical criteria for genetic disorders. Current genetic testing is often most informative if it begins with a family member most suspected to have a genetic disorder. This may include a patient dying from a condition suspected to have a genetic link. Genetic testing may not currently be available, and/or time may not be sufficient to facilitate genetic testing at the end of life. Recording available family history and banking DNA can be critical for the health of surviving family members.

## Screening and Counseling

This section addresses two aspects of genetic screening at the end of life: (1) identifying patients who might benefit from DNA testing and/or DNA banking, and (2) talking with patients and family members about genetic screening at the end of life.

***Identifying Genetic Conditions at the End of Life:*** For every patient, collect past medical history information and family medical history including at minimum all first-degree (full siblings, children, parents) and second-degree (aunts/uncles, nieces/nephews, grandparents, grandchildren, half-siblings) relatives. Encourage patients to collect, store, and update their family health histories. A useful tool for family history collection is "My Family Health Portrait" (https://www.familyhistory.hhs.gov/fhh-web/home.action). A helpful mnemonic for family history screening is S-I-D-E:

**S:** Any family members with health conditions that are *S*imilar to the patient's condition?

**I:** Any family members with diagnoses of *I*nherited conditions?

**D:** Any family members who *D*ied at an early age or were diagnosed with a disease at an earlier-than-typical age?

**E:** Does the patient or any family members have *E*xtreme laboratory values that could suggest, for example, an inherited metabolic disease?

The S-I-D-E mnemonic is also a reminder to ask about *both* the maternal and paternal sides of the family, even for conditions that are more common or exclusive to one sex or the other, such as breast cancer or prostate cancer. Table 184-1 presents a list of specific conditions in patients and/or family members that suggest a hereditary component.

Consider DNA banking (see later) if the family history presents a known inherited condition affecting the patient, the patient has a condition that is present in two other close relatives, or the patient has one other relative with the same condition if it is rare or diagnosed at an earlier-than-typical age. DNA banking may be helpful if

- The patient is affected with a condition that appears to be hereditary
- The family has not already tested positive for a genetic mutation, and
- The patient has identifiable family members who could benefit from knowing their genetic susceptibility.

***Talking with Patients and Families About Genetic Screening at the End of Life:*** Discussing a possible genetic component may be difficult for some patients and families for many reasons. The possibility of a hereditary component to disease may be unexpected, either because the diagnosis may be new or the doctors may not have discussed it. Patients and family members may feel guilty or angry at the idea that disease may be passed in the family. Others may be more concerned about the actual process of obtaining a DNA sample (usually a blood draw). On the other hand, patients may find genetics assessment an opportunity to provide helpful information for future generations, a gift of their legacy.

Although there is no consensus on the best way to approach patients and families about genetics assessment at the end of life,

*Table 184-1 Indications for Hereditary Disease Among End-of-Life Patients*

| Patient or Family Characteristic | Indication for Hereditary Risk | Example of Indication or Genetic Diagnosis |
| --- | --- | --- |
| Age at diagnosis | Earlier-than-expected age for the disease | Breast cancer or colorectal cancer <50 years old |
| Other relatives with the same condition | For common diseases, 3 close relatives, including the patient, or 2 close relatives with at least one diagnosed at a young age | Female patient with heart attack before 50 and sister who died from heart attack<br>Kidney or adrenal gland cancer |
| Number of primary cancers (not metastases) | More than one primary cancer in the patient | Patient with breast cancer and ovarian cancer |
| Birth defects | One major or multiple minor birth defects | Spina bifida |
| Hearing or vision | Congenital hearing loss or vision loss without an environmental explanation | Patient fails newborn screen for hearing loss |
| Cognition | Intellectual disability (IQ <70) or autism | Suspected fragile X syndrome |
| Stature | Unusually tall or short compared to relatives | Suspected achondroplasia |
| Skin pigmentation | Unusual neurocutaneous markings or more pigmentary changes than expected | ≥6 café-au-lait spots that could represent neurofibromatosis type 1 |
| Musculature | Congenital myopathy or muscular dystrophy | Suspected Duchenne muscular dystrophy |
| Heart | Cardiomyopathy or arrhythmia without clear-cut cause, or at an earlier-than-expected age<br>Sudden death that is unexplained | Hypertrophic cardiomyopathy |
| Connective tissue | Hyperflexibility or multiple fractures or dislocations with minimal trauma | Osteogenesis imperfecta |
| Bleeding | Excessive bleeding or clotting not associated with medication or comorbidity | Factor V Leiden–associated hypercoagulability |
| Neurologic abnormalities | Seizures without a known etiology | Tuberous sclerosis |

most likely a straightforward discussion will be appreciated and appropriate: "I'd like to talk with you about your family health history. Some health conditions tend to run in families and knowing your health history and seeing if it is connected to your illness could help others in your family to stay healthy. Most diseases are not strongly genetic, but sometimes it is helpful to have a genetic test or store a blood sample for testing later."

## DNA Banking

DNA banking involves obtaining a tissue sample, usually blood, and storing the extracted DNA. This sample can be used in the future for genetic testing or research. **DNA banking at the end of life can be useful because many genetic tests are not fully clinically sensitive. Therefore, testing the affected relative first tells other family members whether genetic testing will help them.** DNA banking can help to ensure that tissue is available for testing after the affected person has died.

Usually DNA banking involves drawing a couple of tubes of blood and sending the sample to a DNA banking facility. Often there is an informed consent form explaining important information such as length of storage, privacy assurances, and who can access the sample in the future. It is important for family members

to agree on who will have access to the sample and any related test results in the future. DNA banking typically costs about one hundred or a couple hundred dollars, and it is not usually covered by insurance. Some storage facilities charge an additional annual fee for storage. Helpful information about DNA banking can be found at the National Society of Genetic Counselors website (http://www.nsgc.org) and the GeneTests website (http://www.genetests.org). The GeneTests website also includes a listing of facilities offering DNA banking.

## Genetic Counseling and Testing

When a patient is suspected to have a genetic condition, if there is time and availability consider a medical genetics consult and related genetic counseling for the patient and/or family. Genetic consultation and counseling may be an option for the family after the patient has died, too. Medical geneticists are physicians with specialty training in genetics who can facilitate diagnoses through family history interview, physical examination, and review of related medical tests. They are certified through the American Board of Medical Genetics. Genetic counselors are typically masters trained and certified through the American Board of Genetic Counseling. Genetic counselors specialize in assessing genetic risks and communicating with patients and family members about their risks and the natural history of relevant genetic diseases. Genetic nurses have specialty training in genetics assessment and communication, too.

Because clinical genetic tests, in contrast to DNA banking, are highly specific, often not fully sensitive, and typically more expensive, an accurate clinical diagnosis or suspicion is critical before selecting a genetic test. Genetic specialists such as those listed here can facilitate this assessment and test selection, in addition to working with patients and families for informed consent. The American College of Medical Genetics website (http://www.acmg.net) can be searched to find a nearby medical geneticist, and the National Society of Genetic Counselors website (http://www.nsgc.org) can be searched to find a nearby genetic counselor. Testing will continue to evolve. The GeneTests website (http://www.genetests.org) also contains a directory of laboratories offering genetic tests and updated reviews of many genetic conditions.

### BIBLIOGRAPHY:

1. GeneTests: Medical Genetics Information Resource (database online). Educational Materials: About Genetic Services. Copyright, University of Washington, Seattle. 1993-2009. http://www.genetests.org. Accessed October, 2009.

2. My Family Health Portrait: A Tool from the Surgeon General (online). Educational Materials: About Genetic Services. https://www.familyhistory.hhs.gov/fhh-web/home.action. Accessed October, 2009.

3. National Society of Genetic Counselors: The Leading Voice, Authority and Advocate for the Genetic Counseling Profession (database online). DNA Banking. Copyright, National Society of Genetic Counselors, Inc. 1995-2009. http://www.nsgc.org. Accessed October, 2009.

4. Lillie AK. Exploring cancer genetics and care of the family: an evolving challenge for palliative care. *Int J Palliat Nurs*. 2006; 12:70-74.

5. McGinnis JM, Williams-Russo P, Knickman JR. The case for more active policy attention to health promotion. *Health Aff (Millwood)*. 2002;21:78-93.

6. Quillin JM, Bodurtha JN, Smith TJ. Genetics assessment at the end of life: suggestions for implementation in clinic and future research. *J Pall Med*. 2008;11:451-458.

7. Quillin JM, Bodurtha JN, Smith TJ. Genetic screening and DNA banking at the end of life. *Fast Facts and Concepts* [serial online]. August 2008; 206. http://www.eperc.mcw.edu/fastfact/ff_206.htm. Accessed August, 2011.

8. Quillin JM, Bodurtha JN, Siminoff LA, Smith TJ. Exploring hereditary cancer among dying cancer patients—a cross-sectional study of hereditary risk and perceived awareness of DNA testing and banking. *J Genet Couns*. 2010;19:497-525.

9. Skirton H, Frazier LQ, Calvin AO, Cohen MZ. A legacy for the children—attitudes of older adults in the United Kingdom to genetic testing. *J Clin Nurs*. 2006;15:565-573.

## Supplementary Information

***Key Words:*** Genetic screening, genetic testing, DNA banking, end of life, palliative care

# INDEX

Page numbers in **bold** indicate the start of the main discussion of the topic; those followed by *f* or *t* indicate figures or tables, respectively.